CLINICAL METHODS AND INTERPRETATION IN MEDICINE

CLINICAL METHODS AND INTERPRETATION IN MEDICINE

Ashis Kumar Saha MD (Cal) DTM & H (Cal) FICP
Associate Professor
General Medicine
KPC Medical College
Kolkata, West Bengal, India

Foreword

Subhas Chandra Hazra

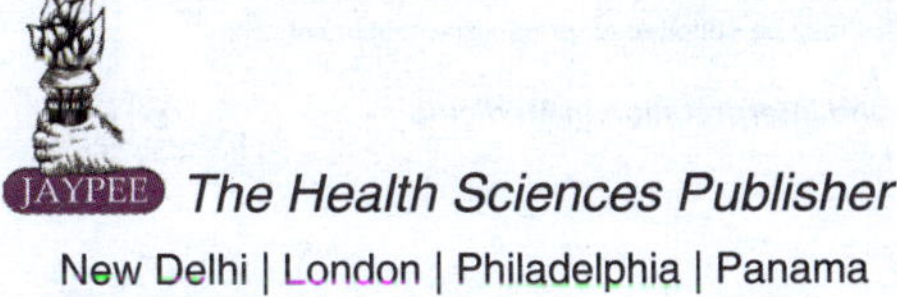

JAYPEE *The Health Sciences Publisher*

New Delhi | London | Philadelphia | Panama

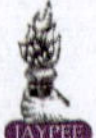 **Jaypee Brothers Medical Publishers (P) Ltd.**

Headquarters

Jaypee Brothers Medical Publishers (P) Ltd.
4838/24, Ansari Road, Daryaganj
New Delhi 110 002, India
Phone: +91-11-43574357
Fax: +91-11-43574314
E-mail: jaypee@jaypeebrothers.com

Overseas Offices

J.P. Medical Ltd.
83, Victoria Street, London
SW1H 0HW (UK)
Phone: +44-20 3170 8910
Fax: +44(0) 20 3008 6180
E-mail: info@jpmedpub.com

Jaypee-Highlights Medical Publishers Inc.
City of Knowledge, Bld. 237, Clayton
Panama City, Panama
Phone: +1 507-301-0496
Fax: +1 507-301-0499
E-mail: cservice@jphmedical.com

Jaypee Medical Inc.
The Bourse
111, South Independence Mall East
Suite 835, Philadelphia
PA 19106, USA
Phone: +1 267-519-9789
E-mail: jpmed.us@gmail.com

Jaypee Brothers Medical Publishers (P) Ltd.
17/1-B, Babar Road, Block-B
Shaymali, Mohammadpur
Dhaka-1207, Bangladesh
Mobile: +08801912003485
E-mail: jaypeedhaka@gmail.com

Jaypee Brothers Medical Publishers (P) Ltd.
Bhotahity
Kathmandu, Nepal
Phone: +977-9741283608
E-mail: kathmandu@jaypeebrothers.com

Website: www.jaypeebrothers.com
Website: www.jaypeedigital.com

Clinical Methods and Interpretation in Medicine

First Edition: **2015**

ISBN: 978-93-5152-628-5

Printed at : Samrat Offset Pvt. Ltd.

Foreword

It is my great pleasure and honor to write a few words about *Clinical Methods and Interpretation in Medicine*, which is an excellent made-easy book, written by Dr Ashis Kumar Saha.

I am sure that reading the lucid description in the book, undergraduates and postgraduates will be able to prepare themselves in a systematic way for the final examination as well as for real life.

I think after reading the book thoroughly, the student will be able to take the history from any type of patient along with proper and systematic examination to come to a diagnosis, so that proper management will be possible.

In this respect, I strongly appreciate and feel that the book will really be a good guide, written in a concise and comprehensive manner, and this will help all the students to make a strong and basic foundation on which future pillar of knowledge can be made to stand erect.

I appreciate and praise the whole-hearted effort and honest work, sincerity, endeavor, enthusiasm and patience in bringing out the book for the learners of Medicine.

Subhas Chandra Hazra MD (Cal)
Head
Department of General Medicine
KPC Medical College
Kolkata, West Bengal, India

Preface

At last, by the grace of Almighty God, I have succeeded in bringing out the first edition of *Clinical Methods and Interpretation in Medicine*.

The idea behind the preparation of the book is to give proper, concise, comprehensive and complete picture of all the systems of the body. At the same time, the book aims at helping the students learn proper history-taking from all types of patients including physically handicapped and emotionally fragile patients. To treat a patient, a sound knowledge of medical science, optimum clinical skills and good interpersonal skills are required. The book will help the students become good clinicians in future.

According to my clinical experience, many candidates including the brilliant ones, often fail to succeed in the examination due to lack of adequate technique of taking history from a patient, analysis of symptoms, detection of signs as well as answering the questions of the examiners. In spite of theoretical knowledge, the students are occasionally unable to communicate properly with the patients. So, it is necessary to develop the clinical and practical knowledge vis-à-vis the theory. Keeping this in mind, I have decided to write the book with enormous number of pictures to memorize the various methods and symptoms.

The book has been written with a view to entertain the wide variety of readers from the medical students to postgraduates. It includes a detailed method of proper history-taking and physical examinations, and tips of interpretation of various clinical features to come to a diagnosis.

I do not claim that the book is enough for the whole clinical medicine. So, the students need to consult the standard textbook for consultation. But, for examination purpose, the book is surely helpful for optimum preparation.

I would like to invite constructive criticism from valuable readers, so that any error or omission in the book may be corrected.

Ashis Kumar Saha

Acknowledgments

I am extremely grateful to my mother, who inspired me to perform such a job, so that I shall be within the mindframe of teacher- and student-community forever. This was aided by encouragement and inspiration of my father as well as teacher, Professor Tushar Kanti Saha, teacher-cum-philosopher and guide, Professor Sukumar Mukherjee for writing this book.

Professor Alakendu Ghosh, Professor Subhas Chandra Hazra, Professor Malay Maitra, Professor Avijit Banerjee, Professor Sagar Bose, Professor Pushpa Maitra and Dr Nirmalya Roy have given me immense inspiration during my writing the book. I am thankful to Professors Malay Maitra and Avijit Banerjee, who have helped in editing the chapters on *Respiratory System* and *Cardiovascular System* respectively.

Dr Anirban Mazumdar helped me in providing the pictures for my book.

My patients have helped me enormously during taking pictures of their physical examinations.

My father-in-law, Dr SK Saha constantly inspired me to write such a book which would be helpful for the students across the country.

My sons Subhrakanti Saha and Abhrakanti Saha provided constant and proper moral support to me for my project work.

My special thanks to M/s Jaypee Brothers Medical Publishers (P) Ltd, New Delhi, India, for their constant encouragement and keen interest shown in completing this clinical treatise.

Last but not least, without whose constant support and sacrifice it was not possible to write and bring the book in the light of the day, and for which no amount of appreciation is sufficient, it is none else but my wife Kalyani Saha.

Contents

12. Thyroid Gland 1281

CHAPTER 1

Art of Interviewing to a Patient

Good communication of the interviewer is of paramount importance in spite of latest diagnostic technology. The importance of skill of interview is developed recently because:

- This interview takes the doctor very nearer to patient's mind, so that the patient can trust, can say everything of his own life
- Patient can discuss everything of his personal details of illness
- This can reduce the patient's psychological illness and anxiety, resolves symptoms.

Communication Means Good and Successful Interview

By interview, the interviewer:

- Should get all informations regarding patient's illness
- Should know how he or she gradually develops this illness
- After allowing the patient to narrate the illness from its commencement, the interviewer starts leading questions pointing towards the specific illness
- Should be aware of the patient's social, economic and cultural factors, because anything hidden in these factors may be responsible for the patient's illness
- Should know about the patient's educational status—because, some question may not be understandable to the patient, in that case, interviewer has to narrate the question, so that the patient can understand what the interviewer wants
- Should know about the patient's language, because asking the patient in his own words, he will be gradually nearer to the interviewer and the patient can express everything to him
- Can use some slang words according to the patient's background education and social status
- Can use some phrases or words to gain confidence of the patient.
- Avoid 'if', 'would', 'could', because, these are nonsense language
- Should know, whether the patient is deaf and dumb
- Should know the impact of this illness in his personal, social and marital life

- Should be cheerful, friendly to the patient
- Should allow the patient, at the beginning, to narrate the illness in his own words. Interviewer should not interfere in this, rather he could nod, smile and in few cases, relevant questioning may gain confidence of the patient during narrating the story. From the story, the interviewer may get clue regarding the patient's illness, so interviewer must be keen to the patient's problem—related story
- Should respect the patient's age, sex, educational status, legal status, belief, culture and economic status
- If the patient's story is vague, start some leading questions, like, 'where', 'when', 'how', these are more effective rather than questioning like 'why'.

When the interviewer does not know the patient's language, he can use interpreter. He:
- Should know the medical terminology
- Should be of same sex and comparable age
- Should share same understanding and belief regarding patient's problem
- Is a bridge between the interviewer and the patient regarding spanning of ideas, emotions and problems
- Must be of patient's choice—because in few cases—family member may be of patient's choice. Because he is most closure to the patient, so that, important problems regarding social, sexual and personal history can be collected by family members of patient's choice—this may be very confidential.

Rule of Five Vowels

Rule of five vowels are important for the interviewer.
- *Audition:* This corresponds to the careful listening patient's story.
- *Evaluation:* This corresponds to sorting of important, relevant and useful data, which is corroborating with patient's chief complaint.
- *Inquiry:* This corresponds to the interviewer's leading questions to the patient to probe the areas of history, which requires more clarification.
- *Observation:* This corresponds to the patient's behavior during conversation with the interviewer. He also watches the patient's attitude and behavior to answering the leading questions.
- *Understanding:* This is most important, because, the interviewer must be sympathetic to the patient, he should accept the patient's presenting complaint and situation responsible for the complaint.

The interviewer should be sympathetic to the patient's description regarding antisocial behavior, which may include:

Drug Addiction, Unlawful Action and Aberrant Sexual Behavior

The interviewer should not question such as, 'why'—it may stop the patient, because he comes to know that the interviewer is unsuitable listener. On the other hand, 'I understand'—phrase from interviewer may be a good signal to the patient, so that the patient will be keener to describe this nature more vividly.

Patient's body language is also very important during interview, because:
- Patient may frown, when he becomes annoyed to some leading questions produced by the interviewer
- Patient may keep his right palm on the left chest—when he tries to speak something—which is really true
- While asking about his addiction, patient may show his tongue, as if he is ashamed of or frown
- Patient may fist on a table—while he is saying something, which should be emphasized
- Patient may sometimes rub his eyes—when he tries to avoid or refuse the questions, which may harm the patient
- If the patient wants to avoid the particular question during the interview, he may start removing dust from the bed or from his or her clothes
- Patient of Middle East may speak with drooping eyelids; it shows the lack of attentiveness.

Like patient's body language, interviewer's body language is also important, because:
- From interviewer's posture, gesture, eye contact, tone of voice, patient can understand the interest, attention, and understanding of the interviewer
- Interviewer should not be in hurry
- Interviewer's approach, dress, cleanliness, facial appearances are also important to the patient
- The interviewer's room is also very important, because—the patient may not give proper history in a room having several patients, or in waiting room or in busy emergency department.

In that case, interviewer has to take the patient a lonely room or has to draw a curtain around them to maintain the privacy.

During history taking, touching the patient is very useful, because it can grow confidence, attention and understanding between the patient and the interviewer. But touch is varied according to the age and sex.

In all ages and all sexes, placing the hand on the shoulder of the patient can do no harm. As the patient grows older, touching is more important.

In the age of biomedical advancement, the clinician usually writes costly investigations (both laboratory and radiological) without taking proper history from the patient or without doing proper physical examination—this may help the patient to feel of being neglected, rejected and properly unattended.

Sometimes the patient is advised to be admitted in any hospital wearing hospital dress, keeping his or her dentures, hearing aids and other personal belongings away from him—this may loose the belief of the patient and looses the morale of the patient much more.

Sometimes the clinician may be overworked, tired after days work. In that case, he or she may give less attention to the patient; in that case, he has to depend on investigations.

In other words, history taking is the cognitive skill of the interviewer; it is a powerful diagnostic skill.

Before seeing the patient, interviewer should collect the data from the patient's medical records, like, age, sex, occupational status, address, medication list, details of allergies, any past diagnoses and treatment schedule, if any.

The above collected data may be incomplete or may not match with the data, which you will collect from the patient—but this will help the interviewer to give proper care to the patient.

Symptoms refer to:
- *Definite symptoms:* What the patient feels, it should be described in detail by the patient
- *Constitutional symptoms:* This commonly occurs in body systems—such as fever, chill, weight gain or loss, sweating, etc.

Approach to a Patient for History Taking and Examination

- Interviewer should wear white coat with named badge. He should address the patient with Mr/Mrs/Dr/Ms, handshake with him and say his aim
- Bed around the patient and surroundings are properly lighted. The patient's privacy should be assured
- The interviewer must be sure that the patient is not deaf or dumb. Patient should lie in comfortable position or sitting in the chair.
- Interviewer should sit in front of the patient in a chair, 3 to 4 feet from the patient in relaxed position
- In case of bed-ridden patient, elevate the head end of the bed and try to lower the bedside rail, so that it cannot interrupt the interview

- After introduction, interviewer should ask the patient—"For which problem, he has been admitted here?" If the patient tells the interviewer to see his hospital records, he should ask the patient about his previous health, followed by remodeling of first question "he want to hear from the patient's own voice?"
- After interviewer asks the patient to narrate the chief complaint in a specific format, followed by past history, social, personal, drug, dietary history and so on.

Two types of questioning usually should be done:

1. *Open type questioning:* This type of question is required to gather general information. This question is required for opening the interview. Questions are:
   - What about your headache?
   - What about your stomach pain?
   - What about your sensation during headache or stomach pain?
2. *Direct questioning:* This type of question points towards the chief complaint. To elaborate it:
   - Where the pain has been started primarily and where it has been radiated?
   - Whether the chest pain aggravates with respiration?
   - Whether the stomach pain aggravates with intake of food?

Format of the History

There are two types of format:

1. *Disease-orientated approach:* This emphasizes disease process that promotes the patient to seek for medical advice.
2. *Patient-orientated approach:* This is more complete and comprehensive approach, where complete history is needed to know the cause of impact on the chief complaint, e.g. if patient complains of shortness of breath—history of onset, duration, type, frequency, aggravating and relieving factors of that pain has to be gathered to get the vivid picture of the chest pain.

So the format of the patient related history is:

- Patient's details
- Chief complaints/presenting problems
- History of present illness
- History of past illness
- Family history
- Personal history
- Psychological and spiritual history
- Occupational and environmental history
- Sexual, gynecological and reproductive history
- Drug history
- Immunization history

Patient's Details

It includes:

- Name
- Age
- Sex
- Religion
- Address
- Occupation
- Date of admission
- Date of examination

Chief Complaints

- It is brief statement with duration for which he or she has been admitted for in specified institution.
- If the chief complaint is more than one, then they should be arranged in chronological order with respect to duration. For example,
  - ❖ Pain in upper abdomen for 4 days
  - ❖ Nausea and vomiting for 2 days
  - ❖ Loose motion for 1 day.

History of Present Illness

It is important to know that the patient was well before the onset of illness. Patient often does not remember the exact date of onset and duration of illness. In that case, it is necessary for the interviewer to correlate the symptom with any known or memorable event. For example, whether the pain starts during, before or after *pooja* vacation.

Each principal symptom has to be described in relation to:

OLD CARTS: It means:

O = Onset

L = Location

D = Duration

C = Character

A = Aggravating/relieving factors

R = Radiation

T = Timing

S = Associated factors.

If the patient has more than one complaint, then according to the chronology, they should be described in separate paragraph.

During the present illness, if any medication is taken, it should be described in generic name with specific dosage, route and frequency. If any remedy or aggravation occurred with these medications, this should also be described.

Any allergy due to intake of recent medication such as, skin rash, nausea, if present or not, it should also be described.

History of Past Illness

It should be divided into two parts:

1. *Childhood history:*
   - ❖ *Communicable diseases:* Chickenpox, measles, rubella, mumps, whooping cough, if occurred, the time of occurrence, course and treatment.
   - ❖ Any severe bacterial illness involving lung, gastrointestinal tract, nervous system—should be thoroughly interviewed.
2. *Adult illness:* It should be divided into:
   - ❖ *Medical history:*
     - Acute or chronic infection
     - Asthma
     - Any disease requiring hospitalization.
   - ❖ *Surgical history:* Any type of operation—open, laparoscopic or endoscopic.
   - ❖ *Gynecological history:* Any type of major or minor operation.

Past medical illness composed of three components:

1. *Diagnosis:* Lobar pneumonia
2. *Evidence:* Fever, cough, rusty sputum, breathlessness
3. *Management:* Antibiotics

History of admission in any hospital for medical, surgical, obstretical, gynecological or psychological reasons—the interviewer may ask directly regarding emotional or nervous problem and any counseling therapy was performed or not.

The importance of taking past medical history is to link this with present history of illness, if any.

Any surgical procedure, date, hospital name, if possible, should be obtained.

Family History

It includes the history of:

- Parents
- Grandparents
- Siblings
- Children
- Grandchildren.

The diseases to be enquired are:

- Cardiac—coronary artery disease, hypertension
- Renal—chronic renal disease
- Endocrinological—thyroid disease, diabetes
- Lung—tuberculosis

- Skin—atopic dermatitis
- CNS—convulsion, strokes
- Metabolic—hyperlipidemia.

Personal History

- *Educational status:* Age of onset of schooling, upto which level the patient is educated
- Occupational status.
- *Marital status:*
  - Whether the patient is married or not?
  - If married, for how many years he is married?
  - How many issues are present with this patient?
  - Whether the siblings are suffering from any illness?
  - Whether the illness is correlated with the patient's present complaint?
- *Dietary history:* The following questions are to be asked to the patient:
  - Whether the patient is vegetarian or nonvegetarian?
  - What is his routine diet?
  - Does he take diet with high fiber content, e.g. whole grain, bread, cereal, fresh fruit, vegetables, bran?
  - Does he take extra salt in his diet?
  - How much saturated fat present in his diet?
  - How much and type of fish or meat (chicken, mutton) present in his daily diet?
  - Does he take boiled food or fried food? If so, when?
  - Does he take caffeine containing food daily, if yes, what is the frequency of intake?

    For example, coffee, tea, cola, chocolate. Caffeine containing foods are responsible for fatigue, palpitation, lightheadedness, headache, irritability.
  - Whether the patient has special or restricted diet?
  - What sort of oils is used during cooking of food?
  - How often the patient uses to take outside food?
  - Occasionally, disease-related questions are to be asked:
    - Patient with coronary artery disease should avoid saturated fat, dietary oils, egg yolk, fried food.
    - Patient with diabetes mellitus, the following interrogations should be required:
      - Insulin or oral antidiabetic drugs
      - Dietary restriction
      - Any past history of hypoglycemia
      - What type of food exchanges the patient uses to follow?

    Dietary allergy history: It is necessary to ask the patient about allergy to food. Common foods those are associated with allergy are peanuts, shellfish, eggs, brinjal, soy, milk.

The allergic reactions are:

- *Involving respiratory tract:* Rhinorrhea, sneezing, wheezing, respiratory distress due to laryngeal edema.
- *Gastrointestinal symptoms:* Diarrhea, vomiting, pain abdomen, nausea.
- *Skin:* Angioedema, urticaria, erythematous skin eruptions.
- Food allergy should be differentiated from abdominal bloating. This may be upper abdominal or lower abdominal bloating.
- *Upper abdominal bloating:* It is usually acute. Ingestion of gas during swallowing of food or liquid (aerophagia) due to:
  i.   Rapid intake of food
  ii. Smoking
  iii. Talking during intake of food
  iv. Intake of carbonated beverage.
- *Lower abdominal bloating:* It is usually chronic.

Loose motion or flatulence, postprandial cramping abdominal pain are usually due ingestion of sugar (xylose, sorbitol), high fibers and lactase deficiency (may be due to intake of yogurt, ice cream, cheese).

The following percent of foods is usual guide for a person:

• Carbohydrate	45–65% of total calories
• Fat	20–35% of total calories
• Protein	10–35% of total calories
• Sodium	= 3.8 gram of salt per day
• Cholesterol	<300 mg per day

- *Addiction history:*
  - *Smoking:* The question should be:
    - For how many years, the patient is taking cigarette?
    - How many cigarettes per day he is taking?
    - What type of tobacco he is taking, cigarette, cigar, *bidi*, chewing tobacco?
    - Does he change the type of cigarette in recent years?
    - Did he try to stop the smoking? If so, what was his feeling?
    - Does the smoking relate with bowel movement or cheerfulness?
  - *Alcohol history:* The question should be:
    - What type of alcohol?
    - How much alcohol taken by the patient per day?

From the history of alcohol intake, the interviewer can correlate the present illness with the alcohol intake, e.g. if the patient is suffering from jaundice, or severe pain in upper abdomen, it may be due to alcohol related hepatitis, or acute pancreatitis or alcohol related gastritis. It may relate with the patient's emotional reaction.

So heavy alcohol intake may be associated with the following medical problems:
- Coronary artery disease
- Alcohol-related liver disease
- Cardiac arrhythmias
- Hemorrhagic or ischemic strokes
- Hypertension
- Pancreatitis.

CAGE questioning, this is the screening questions for alcohol abuse:

C = Has he ever felt the need to cut down of alcohol drinking?

A = Has the patient ever been annoyed by criticism of his drinking?

G = Has he felt guilty conscious for drinking?

E = Has he ever taken alcohol after rising from the bed (eye opening) in the morning to become steady and get rid of the hang over?

Two or more positive answers to CAGE questionnaire suggest alcohol misuse—sensitivity is 43 to 94 percent, specificity is 70 to 96 percent.

Detection of alcohol misuse can be done by getting history of:
- Syncope
- Convulsion
- Accidents
- Conflict in job
- Relationship with others.

Alcohol intake can be measured in two methods:
1. *First method:* It is inaccurate and underestimate intake.
2. *Second method:* It is the direct calculation of the alcohol content of the drinks.

Method I: One glass of = 1 unit of alcohol.

Method II: 1 unit of alcohol = 10 mL of pure alcohol.

x percent proof = x units of alcohol per liter = 10x mL of pure alcohol.

30 percent proof spirit = 30 units of alcohol per liter = 300 mL of pure alcohol.

1 liter or 1000 mL of spirit contains 40 units of pure alcohol.

1 mL of spirit contains 40/1000 units of pure alcohol.

750 mL of spirit contains 40 × 750/1000 units of pure alcohol = 30 units of pure alcohol.

In case of wine:
If alcohol content of wine is 12 percent, i.e. 1000 mL contains 12 units of pure alcohol.

So, 750 mL contains 12 × 750/1000 mL = 9 units of pure alcohol.

Recommended safe drinking:
21 units per week for men.
14 units per week for women.

Average weekly intake of above 50 units in men and 40 units in women—hazardous drinking.

❖ *History of drug abuse:* In contrast to alcohol abuser, drug abusers are more likely to magnify their use. The following questions should be asked regarding drug abuse:
- What types of drug used?
- How long he has started?
- For how many days, he is taking drug heavily?
- Approximately when he has started drug abuse?
- Why he has started to take the drug heavily?
- At which time, he uses to take the drug?
- What is his feeling after taking the drug?
- Whether he has tried to get rid of the drug?
- What is his feeling after leaving the drug abuse temporarily?
- Is there any convulsion after withdrawal of the drug?
- Does he take the drug in single dose or in divided doses?
- Is he taking only single drug for addiction?

Interviewer must be well conversant about the drugs, used for addiction. When cocaine is being used for addiction—orally or intravenously, interviewer should know about the toxicity of the above drugs—whether given orally or intravenously.

Normally used drug can be used as a drug of addiction, e.g. propranlol or metoprolol are usually used as antihypertensive, but they can be used to relieve stage fright.

- Sleep history.

Psychosocial and Spiritual History

- *Psychosocial history* includes:
  - ❖ Education
  - ❖ Life experience
  - ❖ Relationship with other individual
  - ❖ Schooling
  - ❖ Religious belief
- *Spiritual history:* Spirituality helps the patient to cope up with chronic disease, debilitation and dying. The spirituality may be in the form of meditation and prayer.
  - ❖ This reduces the stress

* Early recovery from the surgical pain
* Faster recovery from illness.

Occupational and Environmental History

Occupational history is responsible for 3,50,000 new cases per year in United States. But one may incorrectly describes the illness due to some other cause, because of long latency between exposure and onset of illness. Many occupational diseases have been discovered up till now. Some of these are:

* Bladder carcinoma—in aniline dye worker
* Malignant mesothelioma—person exposed to asbestos
* Malignant neoplasm in nasal cavities—woodworkers
* Hepatic angiosarcoma—person exposed to vinyl chloride
* Pneumoconiosis—coal workers
* Silicosis—sandblasters
* Bassinosis—cotton industry workers
* Ornithosis—bird breeders
* Bronchial asthma—person exposed to dust, pollen
* Khangri cancer—in the inner lip, exposed to tobacco chewers
* Toxic hepatitis—workers of plastic industries
* Friedlander's pneumonia—exposed to pigeon and parrot danders.

Environmental pollution is also responsible for mortality and morbidity of human being world wide, e.g.

* Chernobyl—due to high radiation
* Minamata bay, Japan—due to mercury poisoning
* Hopewell, Virginia—due to poisoning with pesticides chlordecone
* Bhopal, India—due to gas leak methylisocyanate

To recognize the disease as environmental or occupational hazards, the following interrogations are necessary:

* What is his job?
* How long he is in his job?
* In his job, with what material he is working?
* Does he work with proper precaution during his work?
* Description of surroundings around his working place.
* Where is his house? Whether his house is nearer to the coal mine, shipyard, any factories?
* How long he is living in that place?
* What is his hobby? Whether he likes bird or animal?
* If bird, which bird, and if animal, which animal?
* Whether he is working with lead, asbestos, fumes, dust, flower?

Sexual, Gynecological and Reproductive History

This history is most important for complete evaluation of the patient.

Sexual history taking is important for following reasons:
- Sexual drive is sensitive indicator of well-being.
- Sexual dysfunction is responsible for anger, anxiety and depression
- Child's sexual abuse should be identified as early as possible
- Older adult is not sexually inactive, he may enjoy sexual contact.

The following questions may discover the patient's sexual activity:
- Is the patient sexually active?
- If yes, ask about his sexual partner.
- Is he satisfied with his sexual partner? If not, what is the problem? Is it from his side or from her partner's side?
- Has the patient more than one sexual partner?
- If yes, are they of same sex or either male or female sex?
- Whether the patient uses the condom during intercourse?
- In last 6 months, how many sexual partners he had?
- In his life time, how many sexual partners he had?
- Has he ever sexually transmitted disease?
- Whether he has treated or tested for sexually transmitted disease. If so, why?

Menstrual history:
- Age of menarche
- Menstrual flow
- Duration of flow
- Any pain preceding or during menstruation
- If yes, when it subsides?

Obstetric history:
- Number of pregnancies
- Number of abortion
- Number of deliveries
- Age of 1st pregnancy
- Frequency of pregnancies
- Abortion—whether spontaneous or, induced
- Complication of pregnancy
- Postpartum condition of the patient.

Drug History

Any history of intake of drug with dosage, duration, frequency, any history of associated drug allergy should be taken. From drug history, interviewer can think of:

- Any past medical history
- Any relation of past history with present illness
- If there is drug allergy, avoid the drug throughout the life
- If any flare up of previous disease, which may indicate inadequately treated disease, may be in the form of dosage or duration of treatment
- In case of chronic disease, like, hypertension, diabetes, hyperlipidemia, whether the drugs are continued or not
- If not, the present illness may be the consequences of above chronic disease.

Drug may produce drug and nutrient interactions. This should be interrogated to the patient during interview. So the following questions should be asked to the patient:

- Whether the patient is taking minerals, herbs or dietary supplements for any ailment, if so, why?
- What is the dose of the above drugs?
- Whether the patient experience any side effect during this drug intake?
- Who is the person responsible for the above prescription of the drug?

Drug may influence the nutrients in the following ways:
- Avoiding intake of the food—due to nausea, vomiting or feeling of bad smell of the food.
- Abnormal absorption of the food is due to:
  - Increased intestinal motility
  - Competitive inhibition of the food by the drugs
  - Alteration of the intestinal pH
  - Alteration in excretion.

Drugs	Nutrients affected
• Aluminum hydroxide	Phosphate
• Sulfasalazine, methotrexate	Folate
• Neomycin, mineral oil, cholestyramine	Fat soluble vitamins
• Neomycin	Vitamin B_{12}
• Mineral	Water, electrolytes, fat and fat soluble vitamins
• Isoniazid	Vitamin B_6 deficiency
• Frusemide, thiazides	Potassium, magnesium, calcium
• Phenobarbital, phenytoin	Calcium, folate, vitamin D

Immunization History

- From birth to childhood age, whether all immunizations were done or not. If done, the interviewer should see the immunization card
- In adult, yearly influenza vaccination should be done in patient with cardiovascular, pulmonary, renal, hematological disorders.
- Patient with chronic renal disease and older (65 years), should receive pneumococal vaccine once only
- Patient with alcoholism, myeloma, lymphoma, cirrhosis, functional asplenia should receive pneumococcal vaccine
- Only in case of functional asplenia or anatomical asplenia pneumococcal vaccine should be taken in every 6 years.

Hepatitis B vaccination should be given to:
- Intravenous drug users
- Dialysis staff
- Staff of endoscopy unit
- Sexual partner of hepatitis B virus carrier
- Multiple sexual partners
- Hemophiliac patients
  Haemophilus influenzae type B vaccine to be given to children.

Live vaccine MMR not to be given:
- To immunocompromised patients
- To patient receiving steroid therapy
- To generalized malignancy
- To pregnant mothers.

History Taking from Different Type of Patients

History Taking from Silent Patient

Patient may be silent due to following causes:
- *Due to problem from interviewer's side:*
  - ❖ When the questions are short and are thrown in rapid succession.
  - ❖ When the question makes the patient annoyed.
  - ❖ When the question is not understandable to the patient.
- *From the patient's side:*
  - ❖ To remember past events.
  - ❖ To recollect past thought serially.
  - ❖ Patient thinks whether the interviewer can be trusted to give the details of himself.
  - ❖ In case of depressed patient, the interviewer has to question regarding the cause of his depression.

In this case, the interviewer has to gain confidence of the patient, so that patient will give proper informative history.

During interviewing with this type of silent patients, it is often necessary to watch the facial expression of the patients.

Sometimes, the interviewer should be silent for sometime when the patient starts emotional reactions like, crying, annoying during answering the questions. This allows the patient to release the tension and gives proper history when questioning will be started. So interviewer must be cooperative, attentive and very kind to the patient.

History Taking from the Confused Patient

Sometimes the patient may confuse the interviewer in the following processes:

- When the patient gives affirmative answer to all the direct questions from the interviewer, he has to say the meaning of the questions, so that the patient will answer to the point.
- In some cases, patient's answer is vague, loss of ideas, loss of thought, difficult to understand the meaning of the answer or difficult to understand the language, e.g. patient may give history like:
  - ❖ Something crawling over the body
  - ❖ Tingling sensation in different parts of the body in different times.

In case of mentally ill patient (depression, anxiety, neurosis, manic depressive psychosis): The history may be inconsistent and may give different types of history of illness having no sequential chronological order.

In this type of patient, the interviewer should not spend time to gather detailed history, rather than giving much time for mental status examination.

History Talking from Talkative Patient

- First, the interviewer should allow the patient to narrate the whole history. Only thing the interviewer has to nod at regular interval and to hear very cautiously the speech and take out the necessary points from the very elaborative history
- The interviewer should listen and think—whether there is any flight of ideas, disorganized thought
- He has to watch, whether the patient is anxious, impatient while talking
- After listening to the elaborative history, the interviewer has to make a structure containing points in the history, and then he has to ask the direct questions to clarify them, e.g. the patient has told regarding the chest pain which is aggravated with exertions. Again he has told that he has retrosternal chest pain exacerbated

by intake of food. So the interviewer has to know that which pain is earlier
- If possible, the interviewer has to call the patient next day to listen the extra points regarding the history.

History Taking from the Patient Who is Crying

- Crying is the burst of emotion, frustration. Crying is therapeutic. Allowing the patient to cry, the interviewer has to wait, and to provide a tissue paper to rub his or her eyes
- After recovering from the crying episode, most patient starts telling story
- Only the interviewer has to boost at regular intervals during conversation.

History Taking from Angry Patient

- Anger is the outburst of patient who is ill, lack of control in his personal life, feeling of loneliness. But he expresses his anger to the interviewer, if he is late in his chamber or hospital
- In that case, interviewer should not stop him rebuking, rather accepts the angry feelings and accept bad talk without being angry in return in clinic or hospital
- Better the interviewer should avoid the angry patient to join with the other persons in chamber
- After the patient become calm and quiet, the interviewer should tell and confess his guilt and he promises not to do like this in future
- Some angry patients become disruptive. He or she can disturb the atmosphere of the hospital and the clinic.

In this case, the interviewer (clinician) has to call security guard to control the situation by taking the patient in the other room and makes him or her to understand the cause.

When the rapport will be established between the patient and the interviewer, the patient will be calm and quiet and starts giving history.

History Taking from the Patient with Low Literacy

Firstly, the interviewer has to know whether the patient has:
- Language barrier
- Diminished vision
- Learning disorder
- Lack of education.

If the patient is not blind, there is no language barrier, lack of education or low literacy is the prime cause. This can be tested by the following methods:

- Can the patient read the question given by the interviewer?
- Can he fill in the blanks in a form given?
- The interviewer gives any book or text in up side down to the patient and asks him to read.

History Taking from the Patient with Impaired Hearing

Firstly, the interviewer has to know about:
- Language of communication
- Level of education
- Level of schooling
- If the patient is blind unilaterally, the interviewer has to sit on the side in which ear he is not blind
- The room must be calm and quiet, the sound of television, radio or any if present, should be stopped
- If deaf person can read the lips of the interviewer, he can understand what the interviewer wants to say.

History Taking from Psychotic Patient

This patient usually suffers from hallucination, delusion, flight of ideas, feeling of persecution. So the interviewer has to calm, quiet, understand the patient as much as possible. Some patient is not floridly psychotic. So there are several clues, which are very helpful for the interviewer to diagnose the patient as psychotic:
- Speech pattern
- Speech organization
- Flight of ideas
- Distraction from the questions
- Patient cannot complete answer, the question, rather he unnecessarily asks questions.

History Taking from the Demented and Delirious Patient

- Demented patient has lost his intellectual memory, becomes confused from their surroundings
- Delirious patient has altered level of consciousness—as a result of which he behaves incorrectly with his surroundings

   Both types of patients suffer from fear. Hence, during questionnaire to these patients, the interviewer must be calm, quiet and beware of that type of questions, which may be harmful to the patients
- Patient with organic mental syndrome is lucid, occasionally becomes disorientated, has defect in attention, memory and thought.

   In this type of patient, record the questions and answers. After few minutes, the interviewer asks similar questions and he should check whether the patient gives similar answer or not. This proves that the patient is suffering from inattention.

History Taking from Acutely Ill Patient

It is better to take relevant questions during rapid physical examination, because there is no time to ask the patient the detailed history and perform detailed examination as it may defer the urgent management.

As the patient becomes stabilized, the interviewer can take detailed history and will do accordingly.

History Taking from Patient Suffering from Cancer

Patient with cancer has five major concerns:
1. Loss of control makes the patient helpless.
2. Alienation—this feelings arising from reaction of the people around him.
3. Perception of pain—patient has intense fear of having pain.
4. Fear of mutilation—women with mastectomy may suffer from a fear of rejection by the community as no longer being a complete woman.
5. Patient always thinks of his inevitable mortality very soon, because the pathologic process always progresses very fast.

Physician is always afraid of the patient, because he may ask the progress of the disease. But physician must be sympathetic to his emotional reaction.

History Taking from Aphasic Patient

- If the patient is aphasic, it may be motor or sensory
- If it is sensory, then it is not possible for the interviewer to get the history from the patients, so in that case, he has to depend upon the patient's party
- If the patient's aphasia is of motor type, it must be confirmed by giving a pen and a paper and ask him to write 'yes' or 'no' to the simple questions like, 'are you male', or 'have you married?' If the patient comprehend the question, then the interviewer ask the patient a series of questions and allow him to give answer in the form of nodding of head, or 'yes' or 'no' in writing.

History Taking from Alcoholic Patient

Alcoholic patient is physically handicapped, because:
- He may suffer from various diseases related to gastroenterological system and liver, cardiovascular system and respiratory system
- He is sexually inadequate

Alcoholic patient is psychologically handicapped, because:
- He feels alone
- He is abandoned by his family members and friends.
  Alcohol is his day and night friend.

In this case, interviewer should be particular in asking history, because, it may make the patient annoyed, explosive.

◼ Approach to a Patient for Physical Examination

Make-up of the Patient's Mind

- Give your identification as a medical student
- Give proper security to the patient
- You must be calm and quiet in spite of occasional irritable behavior of the patient
- Give assurance to the patient that you will examine the whole body keeping privacy. Because he has to examine the whole body in spite of no abnormality in any system other than the involved system for which he has been admitted in this hospital
- Draping of the patient is very essential for keeping the privacy of the patient. You should examine the areas one after another, e.g. when you want to examine abdomen, cover the other parts of the body. Again you want to examine the left breast, cover the rest of the body. This helps in the following ways:
  - ❖ This helps to concentrate the examination area
  - ❖ This draws confidence of the patient
  - ❖ This draws respect from the patient.
- You should be gentle, systematic and professional while doing physical examination
- After examination is over, you should not interpret the findings with the friends or with the teacher in front of the patient, because the patient may wrongly interpret your discussion
- Again, you should not react badly by seeing any foul smelling lesion
- Take permission from the patient before examining the private parts of the patient, e.g. pubic area, femoral pulse
- During physical examination, you must watch the facial expression of the patient—whether he is angry, sensitive or cooperative.

Proper Lighting in the Examination Area

- Proper lighting should be in your examination room, so that both of you are comfortable
- Room should be calm and quiet, so that heart sounds and lung sounds can be heard easily

- Two types of lighting are useful during physical examination:
  1. Tangential light is required for seeing:
     - Jugular venous pulsation
     - Thyroid gland
     - Apical impulse.

     Because, it can shadow on the surface—so that contour, elevation, depression, pulsations may be noticed.
  2. Direct lighting.

Details of Instruments used in Examination

- Blood pressure instrument
- Torch light
- Thermometer
- Watch
- Stethoscope, having earpiece, fits strongly without pain, and bell and diaphragm should be good and interchangeable
- Tape
- Tuning fork
- Cotton
- Pin
- Hammer
- Two glasses containing cold and warm water respectively
- Pencil and paper
- Gloves for rectal examination
- Ophthalmoscope
- If required, otoscope.

Postexamination

- Patient should be comfortable in his previous position
- If the patient is bedridden, bed should be down. Side rails should be raised, so that the patient will not fell down.

Primary position of the patient and the examiner:
- Patient should be examined from his right side. This position is important for having following advantages:
  - ❖ It is reliable to see jugular venous pulse from right
  - ❖ Placement of hand for palpation of apical impulse is comfortable
  - ❖ Palpation of abdominal organs, such as liver, spleen, and kidney is easier and comfortable
  - ❖ The examiner can move for examination of the extremities to the foot end or left hand side.
- Patient should be examined from head to toe—sequentially, because if you jump from one part to another part, leaving area in between, there is every chance of missing some important finding in that area.

- *In case of bedridden patient:*
  - ❖ The examiner should examine head, neck and anterior chest in supine position
  - ❖ The examiner should examine posterior chest, back of the head in right or left lateral position
  - ❖ Roll the patient to supine or patient's comfortable position.
- *In case of mobile patient:*
  - ❖ *Sitting position:*
    - General survey
    - Examination of head
    - Examination of neck
    - Thyroid gland
    - Cervical lymph node
    - Anterior and posterior part of chest
    - Breast
    - Few parts of nervous system examination—mental status, orientation, cranial nerves, cerebellar function, upper extremities
    - Palpation of aortic and pulmonary area.
  - ❖ Lying supine with head end of the body raised to 45 degree position—Jugular venous wave, carotid artery, tricuspid area
  - ❖ Supine position with 30° elevation of the head end and rotation slightly towards left—mitral area for murmur and other abnormal sound
  - ❖ In sitting position with leaning forward—tricuspid and aortic area.
  - ❖ *Lying in supine position in flat bed:*
    - Face
    - Anterior neck
    - Anterior thorax
    - Breast
    - Abdomen
    - Axillae
    - Pubic area
    - Genital area
    - Upper and lower extremities
    - Plantar response.
  - ❖ *Supine with flexed, abducted and externally rotated hip and knee flexed position:*
    - Pelvic examination
    - Rectal examination.
  - ❖ *Lying on left lateral position:*
    - Rectal examination
    - Prostate examination.

The following techniques of examination are usually done:

- *Inspection:* It means close observation of:
  - ❖ Skin
  - ❖ Facial expression
  - ❖ Body habitus
  - ❖ Eye movements
  - ❖ Any thoracic asymmetry, deformity, fullness, abnormal movement
  - ❖ Abdomen—size, shape, lesion, venous prominence
  - ❖ Cardiovascular system—jugular venous pulsation, abnormal precordial pulsation, aortic and pulmonary area
  - ❖ Height
  - ❖ Weight
  - ❖ Body mass index.
- *Palpation:* Pressure by the palm of the hands assess:
  - ❖ Skin elevation
  - ❖ Temperature
  - ❖ Pulse
  - ❖ Lymph nodes
  - ❖ Size of the organs and tenderness
  - ❖ Any mass any where in the body
  - ❖ Abnormal palpable cardiac sounds, thrill
  - ❖ Palpable pleural rub, rhonchi.
- *Percussion:*
  - ❖ Chest percussion for evaluation of different notes
  - ❖ Abdominal percussion for any fluid in the abdomen.
- *Auscultation:*
  - ❖ Lung sounds
  - ❖ Heart sounds
  - ❖ Peristaltic sound
  - ❖ Any bruit in the abdomen
  - ❖ Venous hum.
- *Auscultopercussion:*
  - ❖ To delineate stomach size
  - ❖ To diagnose hydropneumothorax.

Analysis of Data

- Data collected from history—subjective data
- Data collected from physical examination—objective data

Now compilation of subjective and objective data can be done in the following ways. If patient complains of chest pain, it may arise from:

- Heart and associated great vessels
- Lung and pleura

- Esophagus
- *Musculoskeletal structure:*
  - ❖ If pain is associated with exertion—think of cardiovascular disease
  - ❖ If pain alters with respiration—think of respiratory (pleural), and musculoskeletal structure
  - ❖ If pain arises during carrying heavy bag—think of musculoskeletal structure
  - ❖ If pain arises during swallowing and in retrosternal area—think of esophagus
  - ❖ If there is fever, weight loss, anorexia, then there is no definite history of structure or area involvement.

Detection of Processes or Causes from History of Present Illness

- *The following processes or causes are:*
  - ❖ Congenital
  - ❖ Inflammatory
  - ❖ Vascular
  - ❖ Trauma
  - ❖ Infection
  - ❖ Nutritional
  - ❖ Metabolic
  - ❖ Neoplastic
  - ❖ Degenerative
  - ❖ Toxic.

  If a patient complains of headache, then it may signify:
  - ❖ Infection
  - ❖ Vascular
  - ❖ Trauma
  - ❖ Metabolic
  - ❖ Neoplastic
  - ❖ Nutritional.

  If there is associated vomiting and neck rigidity, then it may suggest:
  - ❖ Infection
  - ❖ Vascular—subarachnoid hemorrhage
  - ❖ Degenerative process—cervical spondylosis.

  If associated loss of consciousness it may suggest:
  - ❖ Vascular
  - ❖ Traumatic
  - ❖ Associated cerebral involvement in case of meningitis.
- *Pathophysiological process:*
  - ❖ Congestive cardiac failure
  - ❖ Migraine.

- *Psychological:*
  - ❖ Anxiety
  - ❖ Depression.

Working Out to Establish the Diagnosis

- After getting history of present illness, relevant other history and findings of physical examination, it is necessary to perform necessary hematological, biochemical, serological (both routine and special), invasive and noninvasive radiological investigations for clinching the proper diagnosis or narrowing the differential diagnoses.
- *These depend upon the nature of symptom:*
  - ❖ If it is vague, a large number of investigations are necessary to come to a diagnosis.
  - ❖ If the complaints are projected towards:
    - Specific structure or structures
    - A specific process
    - A specific cause.

    Then a limited number of investigations may be necessary to come to a diagnosis.
- So a plan of future events like, investigations for confirmation of structural diagnosis and management are necessary having a specific cause and process. This should be discussed with patient or patient's party for:
  - ❖ Seeking his or her opinion
  - ❖ Willingness to perform future investigations, whichever and whenever these are necessary.

    If the patient, his or her party are knowledgeable or understand the problem, then he or she will proceed.

Clustering of Data and its Challenges

- *Problem:* After clustering of data, it may fit into one or several problems.
  - ❖ *Age of the patient:*
    - If the patient is young, the patient probably is suffering from one disease.
    - If the patient is older, he or she may suffer from multiple diseases.
  - ❖ *Timing of illness:*
    - If the patient suffers from pharyngitis 1 month ago, recent history of fever, cough, chest pain may not be related to previous pharyngitis.
    - If the patient now presents with discharge from penis followed by penile ulcer after 3 weeks—think of primary syphilis or gonorrhea.

- If similar patient develops lymphadenopathy and skin rash after 2 months—think of secondary syphilis.
- *Involvement of different systems due to complaints, which relate to different systems:*
  - ❖ Symptoms related to one body system.
  - ❖ Symptoms related to more than one body systems, e.g. patient may complains of chest pain, palpitation—which may relate to cardiovascular system, but if this patient also develops loose motions—it may relate to gastrointestinal system.
- *Occasionally, single disease may explain involvement of different systems:* An alcoholic patient present with jaundice, ascites, previously diagnosed as cirrhosis of liver, present with decreased micturition and unconsciousness. In this case, it may be due to:
  - ❖ Involvement of brain due to increase blood ammonia level
  - ❖ Decreased micturition due to hepatorenal syndrome unless proved otherwise.

After collection of data—both subjective and objective, the interviewer should compose the data with proper interpretation.

By asking several relevant questions, he should exclude some of the differential diagnoses before doing investigations.

A clear well-organized clinical data is very necessary for patient's future care.

Physical Examinations

GENERAL SURVEY

■ Temperature

Normal Temperature

According to more recent study, Mackowlak et al.—normal temperature ranges from 96.5°F to 98.6°F (36°C to 37°C). Deviation of temperature by more than 4°C above or below the normal is warning cellular dysfunctions.

Site of Measuring Temperature

- Rectum, mouth, ear, axilla and groin
- Rectal temperature is about 0.6°F higher than that of the oral or groin reading. It is much higher in mouth breather or tachypneic patient, because oral temperature is low in this patient
- Axillary temperature is about 1.0°F less than that of oral value. Normal axillary temperature ranges between 97.8°F to 98.4°F
- Fever is said to be present when oral temperature is above 98.6°F or rectal temperature is above 100.5°F.

Diurnal Variation of Body Temperature

- *For daytime workers:* Minimum temperature at 3:00 to 4:00 am rises slowly to maximum between 8:00 to 10:00 pm
- *For night-time workers:* This pattern is reversed. This transition from one pattern to another requires several days.

Causes of Decrease or Increase in Oral Temperature

- Tachypneic patient (tachypnea decrease oral temperature by 0.5°C for every 10 breaths per minute)
- Recent ingestion of hot or cold substances.

Tympanic Membrane Temperature (Measured by Infrared Tympanic Thermometer)

- It is lower than the oral temperature
- It can be best suited for core temperature
- It can be lowered by cerumens and varied according to the time of recordings.

Axillary Temperature

- It should be avoided because it is very inaccurate
- In hemiparesis patient, affected site always exhibits lower temperature.

Time of Recording of Oral Temperature

- Three minutes for old thermometer model
- One minute for new thermometer model.

Temperature Physiology

- Hypothalamus maintains a set-point for temperature
- Autonomic nervous system regulates the blood flow from the internal organs to skin and the sweat glands.

Temperature loss may be conductive or evaporative.
- Conductive heat loss can be done by:
  - ❖ Dilatation of capillaries
  - ❖ Increasing blood flow towards cutaneous capillaries.
- Evaporative loss can be done by production of sweat.
  At that time the patient requires shade, cooler environment and to be less active.
  When the body temperature is low, the patient tries to increase the core temperature by:
- Shivering—generates heat in muscles
- Behavioral adaptations—like putting on clothes or entering warm environment.

Pathophysiology of Elevated Temperature

Release of endogenous pyrogen (Interleukin-I) triggered by tissue necrosis, infection, inflammation and tumors increase the temperature set-point. Onset of fever is marked by: chill, shivering and rigor due to vasoconstriction.

When set-point is reached, skin becomes warm, moist and flushed; in some cases skin temperature is normal or subnormal, but core temperature is markedly elevated. Temperature elevation is usually accompanied by tachycardia, he becomes comfortable in warm environment.

New set-point and the fever curve dynamics depend upon particular pathophysiologic process that varies according to the disease process.

As the disease resolves gradually, the set-point of temperature resolves temporarily or permanently, marked by sweat and flushing of the body.

Night sweats is the exacerbation of normal diurnal variation in temperature. It is marked by decline of fever at night.

Night sweat occurs in:
- Chronic infectious disease
- Chronic inflammatory disease
- Malignancies.

Febrile response unable to occur in:
- Older patients
- Chronic renal failure
- Immunosuppressive patients
- NSAIDs user.

Patterns of Fever

- *Continuous fever:* A fever with diurnal variation of 1°F to 1.5°F (0.5°C to 1.0°C) and *never touches the baseline.*
  Example: Lobar pneumonia (Fig. 2.1).

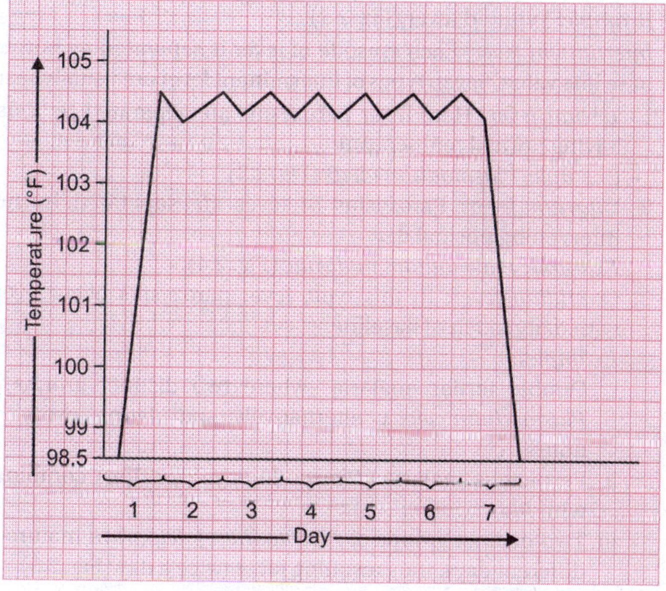

FIG. 2.1 Continuous temperature

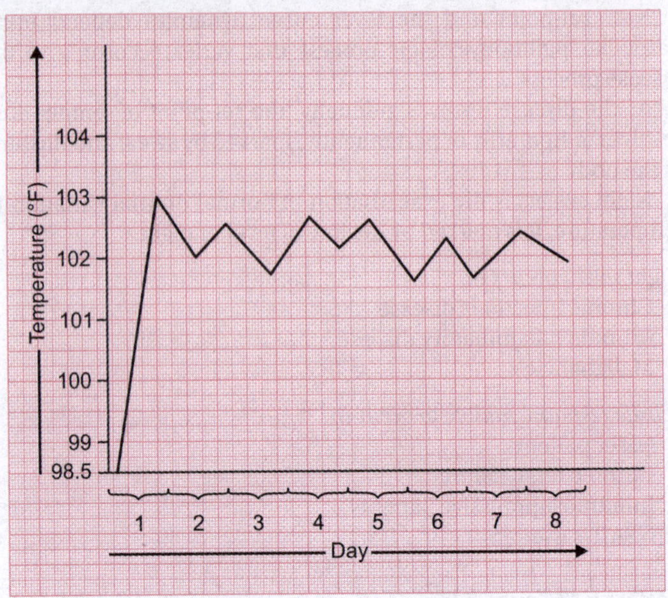

FIG. 2.2 Remittent temperature

- *Remittent fever:* A fever with diurnal variation of 2.5°F (1.1°C) and never touches the base line
  Example: Typhoid fever (Fig. 2.2)
- *Intermittent fever:* Each episode of fever is separated by normal base line value. Seven types of intermittent fever are usually seen:
  1. *Tertian fever:* Here fever paroxysms are separated by a day having normal temperature
     Example: Plasmodium vivax (Fig. 2.3)
  2. *Quartan fever:* Paroxysms of fever are separated by two intervening normal day
     Example: Plasmodium malariae (Fig. 2.4)
  3. *Quotidian fever:* In this type, fever paroxysms occur every with daily touch of baseline.
     Examples:
     i. Double tertian malaria—where two distinct groups of *Plasmodium vivax* alternatively sporulating every 48 hours
     ii. Pernicious malaria (*Plasmodium falciparum*) combined with *Plasmodium vivax*
     iii. Two distinct groups of *Plasmodium falciparum* mature in different days, thus resulting fever twice a day (Fig. 2.5).

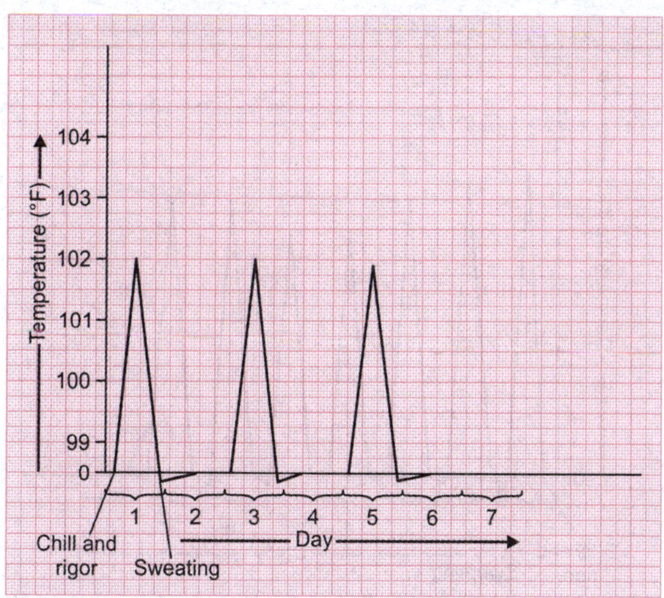

FIG. 2.3   Tertian temperature

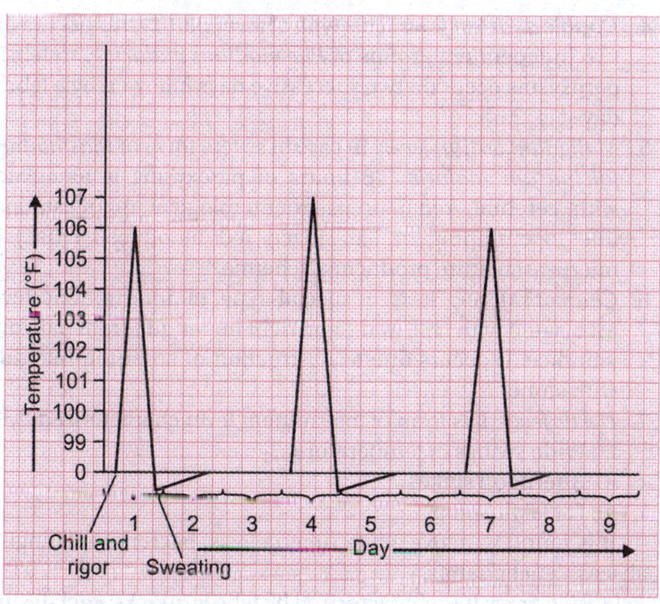

FIG. 2.4   Quartan temperature

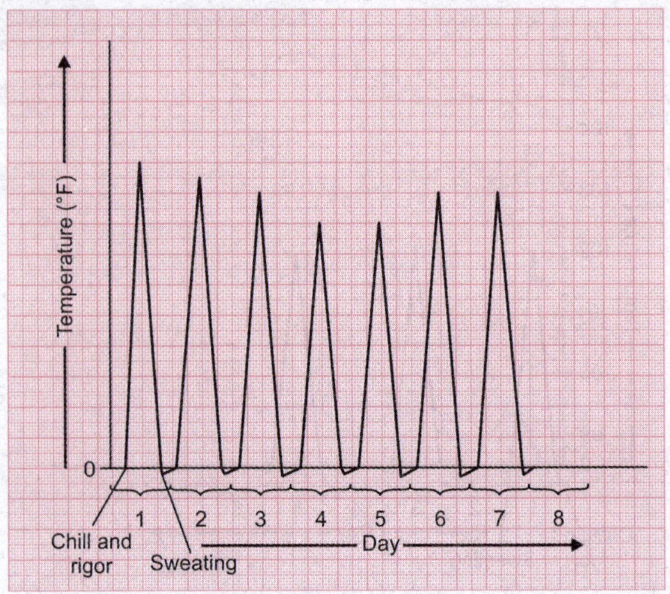

FIG. 2.5 Quotidian fever

4. *Double quartan fever:* This type of fever paroxysms occur with two independent groups of *Plasmodium malariae,* so febrile paroxysms occur on two successive days followed by a febrile day (Fig. 2.6)

5. *Malignant tertian fever:* In case of severe form of *Plasmodium falciparum malaria,* 48 hours of paroxysms is associated with cerebral, renal or gastroenterological manifestations due to clumping of parasitized red blood cell (RBC) in microvasculature producing ischemia

6. *Charcot's fever:* It is a special type of intermittent fever associated with chill and rigor, right upper quadrant pain and jaundice. It occurs due to obstruction of common bile duct with stone

7. *Hectic fever:* It is form of intermittent fever characterized by:
   i. Wide swings of temperature
   ii. Afternoon spikes
   iii. Facial flushing.
   It is found in active acute tuberculosis, bacterial meningitis, abscess, encephalitis.

- *Relapsing fever:* It is characterized by febrile attacks, each lasting for several days separated by afebrile intervals of some duration.

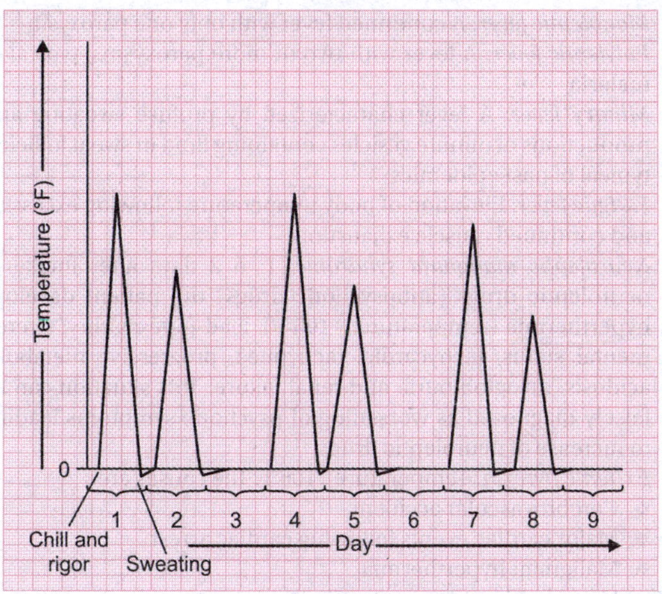

FIG. 2.6   Double quartan fever

Example:
❖ Infections: Brucellosis, Borreliosis, relapsing typhoid, tuber-
culosis
❖ Hodgkin fever
❖ Mediterranean fever.
- *Pel-Ebstein fever:* In this case episodes of fever last for several
hours to several days followed by afebrile period of days or
weeks. It is also called relapsing fever. It occurs in 17 percent of
Hodgkin's disease
- *Factitious fever:* It occurs in hospitalized patients attempting to
malinger, although the cause is obscure. This can be suspected:
❖ When a series of high temperatures are recorded in an atypical
pattern
❖ When the temperature is not associated with other signs
of fever. The patient usually dips the thermometer in warm
water, or place it in contact with heat source, heated the bulb
by friction, bed clothes or with mucous membrane of the
mouth.
- *Undulant fever:* Long and wavy temperature due to Brucellosis

- *Monoleptic fever:* A continued fever with only one paroxysm
- *Polyleptic fever:* A fever with two or more paroxysms, typical of malaria
- *Miliary fever:* A fever characterized by profuse sweating and productions of minute vesicles containing fluid in sweat follicles, typical of past epidemics
- *Fatigue fever:* Elevation of body temperature following excessive and continued muscle exhaustion
- *Neuroleptic malignant syndrome:* 1 to 2 days after intake of neuroleptic drugs (antipsychotic drugs) the patient develops hyperthermia (temperature > 106°F), lead-pipe rigidity, altered mental status, tachycardia, tachypnea, progressive metabolic acidosis, myoglobinuria and renal failure. This situation can be falsely diagnosed as worsening of psychotic symptoms leading to increase of neuroleptic drugs
- *Extreme pyrexia:* Temperature >106°F. The causes are:
  - ❖ Cerebrovascular accident
  - ❖ Major cardiac events following cardiac arrest
  - ❖ Malignant hyperthermia
  - ❖ Neuroleptic malignant syndrome.
- *Malignant hyperthermia:* This inherited disorder of muscle sarcoplasmic reticulum cause rapid increase in intracellular calcium. Following exposure to inhaled succinylcholine anesthetics patient precipitates sustained muscle contraction. As a result the patient develops rigidity, hyperthermia, rhabdomyolsis, metabolic acidosis and hemodynamic instability. It may also occur in Gram negative sepsis
- *Heat exhaustion:* When the patient undergoes exertion in hot and humid environment, there is loss of fluid and electrolytes and decreased ability to dissipate body heat. The patient is usually younger; he develops palpitation, faintness, headache, nausea, vomiting and cramps, low blood pressure, diaphoresis, ashen, cool moist skin and dilated pupils. Core body temperature is elevated but less than 104°F
- *Heat stroke:* There is failure of thermoregulatory system to produce sweating, as a result the core body temperature rises rapidly. The provocating factors are:
  - ❖ Cardiovascular disease
  - ❖ Anticholenergic drugs
  - ❖ Diuretics.

The patient is usually elderly, deleterious or comatose, skin is hot and dry.

Clinical Occurrence of Fever

• Congenital	Familial mediterranean fever, familial periodic fever, prophyrias
• Endocrine	Hyperthyroidism, pheochromocytoma
• Infections	Bacteria, fungal, viral, rickettsial, parasitic (localized or systemic)
• Inflammatory	SLE, Still's disease, acute rheumatic fever, vasculitis, serum sickness, sarcoidosis
• Mechanical/traumatic tissue necrosis	Myocardial infarction, pulmonary infarction, stroke, exercise
• Metabolic reaction	Gout
• Neoplastic	Leukemia, lymphoma, solid tumors
• Neurologic seizures	
• Psychological	Factitious fever

Fever of Unknown Origin

The following criteria must be met to diagnose it as fever of unknown origin:

- The illness must be more than three weeks duration
- Temperature must be repeatedly >38.3°C (100.9°F)
- No diagnosis has been reached after 3 out patient visits or at least 7 days stay in hospital.

Causes of Pyrexia of Unknown Origin

• Noninfectious infectious inflammatory disease	SLE, Still's disease, sarcoidosis, Crohn's disease, polymyalgia rheumatica, vasculitis (Giant cell arteritis, Wegener's disease, polyarteritis nodosa)
• Infections	Tuberculosis, urinary tract infection, HIV, subphrenic abscess, cytomegalovirus, cholangitis
• Neoplasm	Leukemia, lymphoma, Hodgkin's disease, adenocarcinoma
• Miscellaneous	Habitual hyperthermia, subacute thyroiditis, Addison's disease, drug fever

Temperature Pulse Dissociation

This occurs when a rise in temperature is not matched with equivalent rise in heart rate. Normally for each degree of temperature rise there is 10 beats/minute rise in heart rate. When this does not occur, it is called fever with relative bradycardia. *The causes are:*

- *Infectious diseases:* Salmonellosis, brucellosis, legionellosis, *Mycoplasma pneumoniae,* meningitis with increased intracranial pressure
- *Iatrogenic:* Digitalis, beta-blockers.

Hypothermia

The factors responsible are:
- Decreased hypothalamic set point
- Excessive heat loss
- Insufficient heat generation
- Environmental condition
- Behavioral factors.

Effects

- Failure of cellular metabolism
- Impairs brain function particularly judgment.
  As a result, there is failure to take proper measures to cold exposure, this can lead to fatal hypothermia.
- Protection from ischemic tissue injury. This is used in surgical procedure. True hypothermia occurs when body temperature is below 95°F (35°C).

At this low level of temperature body is unable to generate heat, thus the core temperature continues to fall.

Types of Hypothermia

- *Mild hypothermia:* Temperature 89.6°F to 95°F
- *Moderate hypothermia:* Temperature 82.4°F to 89.5°F
- *Severe hypothermia:* Temperature <82°F.

Temperature of this degrees are missed by routine thermometers, thus require thermistors.

Causes of Hypothermia

• Endocrine	Hypothyroidism hypoglycemia
• Idiopathic	Advanced age
• Infectious cases	Sepsis
• Mechanical/traumatic exposure and immersion	
• Hypothalamic injury	Trauma, hemorrhage
• Burn	
• Metabolic/toxic	Drug overdoses, antipyretics
• Neoplastic	Brain tumors
• Neurologic	Stroke
• Psychosocial	Homelessness, poverty
• Vascular	Strokes

Signs and Symptoms of Hypothermia

Mild	Moderate	Severe
• Confusion	Consciousness diminished	Unresponsive
• Tachypnea	Dilirium	Loss of reflexes
• Tachycardia	Bradycardia	Appeared–dead
• Vasoconstriction	Shivering–stopped	Hypotension
• Lethargy	Cold diuresis	Very cold skin
• Shivering	Tachypnea	Pulmonary edema
• Ataxia		Respiratory failure
• Dysarthria		Ventricular fibrillation
• Fine motor incoordination		

■ Anthropometry

Height

Human being grows by linear growth in:
- Infancy
- Childhood
- Adolescence, and ends with closure of the epiphyses of the long bones of the extremities.

Linear growth requires the presence of:
- Growth hormone
- Nutrition (protein, calories, calcium, vitamin D, phosphorus).

Mature height is determined by:
- Genetic factors
- Environmental factors, mainly nutrition.

With advancement of age, there is gradual loss of height due to:
- Hormone—independent loss of bony mineral density
- Loss of muscle tone
- Strength affecting posture
- *Pathological stress:*
  - ❖ Osteoporosis
  - ❖ Spinal compression.

Height should be measured from infancy through childhood. It should be plotted in the form graph, from which one can determine the nature of growth at a point of time. After stability of growth will be reached, height should be measured once a year till the age of 60 years.

Methods of Measuring the Height (Figs 2.7 and 2.8)

- Patient should be erect so that his or her heel, buttock and scapulae will touch the wall

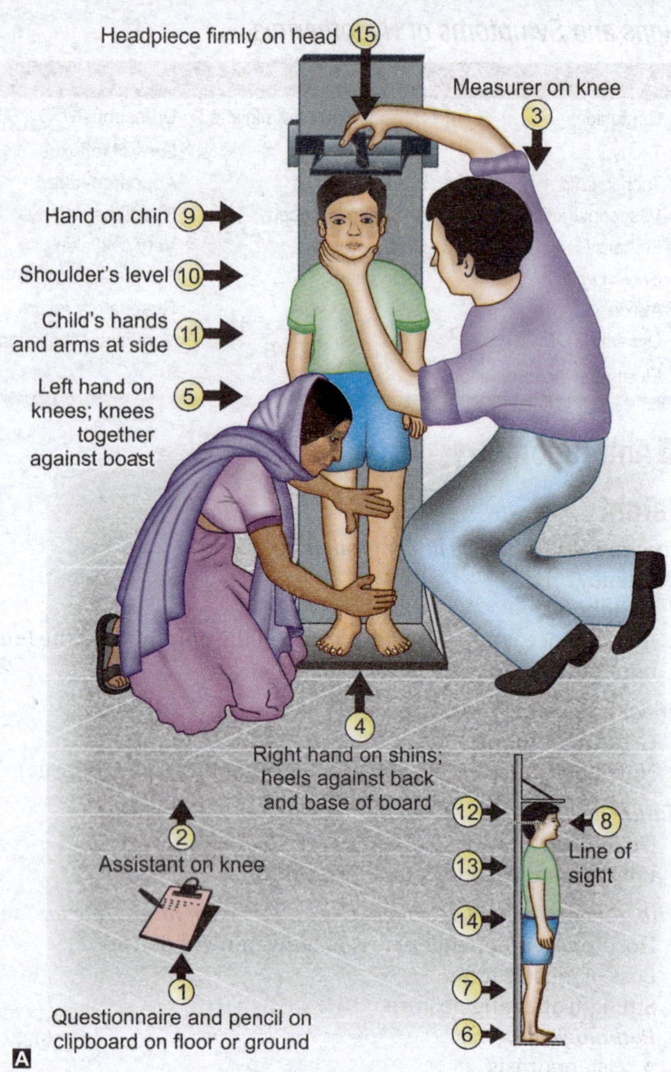

- Head should be in neutral position so that occiput will never touches the wall
- Height is the distance between the floor and the point horizontal with the highest point of the scalp
- Compress the hair to eliminate the overestimating height
- Height should be recorded in centimeter or inches.

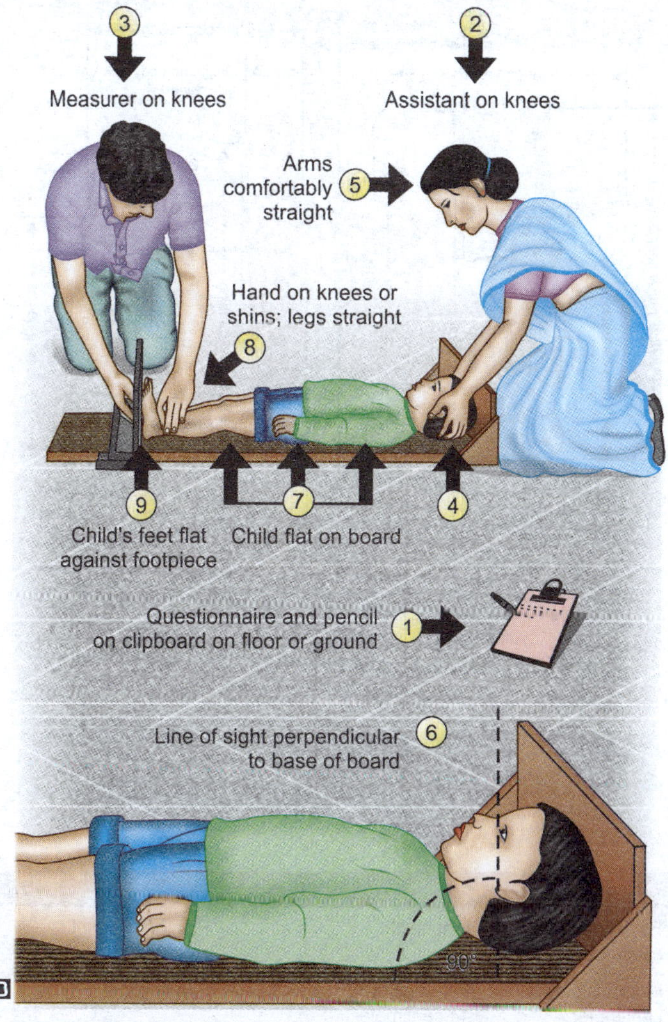

FIGS 2.7A AND B   Height measurement

Pathological States of Height

- *Short stature:* It may be due to:
  - Decrease in growth hormone production
  - Decreased tissue responsiveness to hormone
  - Impaired nutrition.

  Expected stature can be measured in scales or adding 6.5 cm for boys, and subtracting 6.5 cm for girls from the mid-parental height.

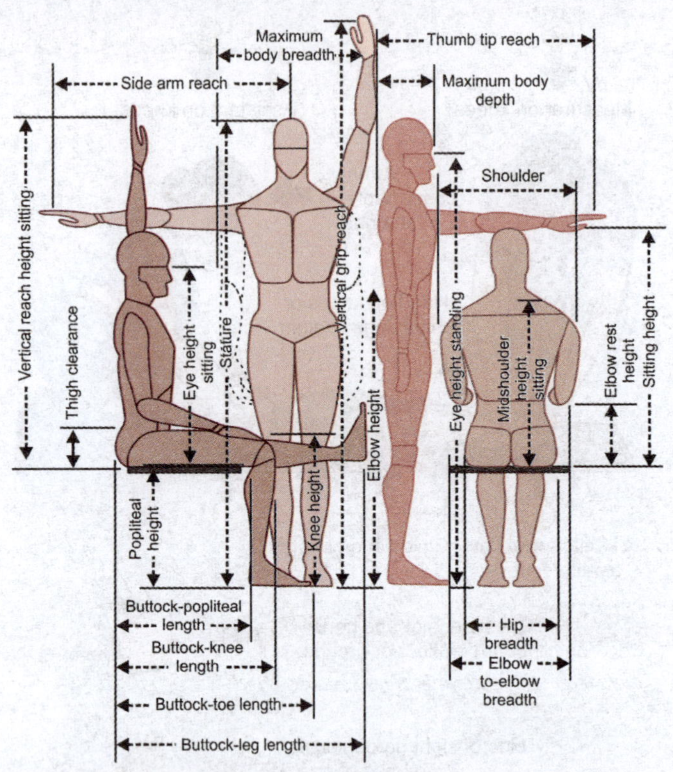

FIG. 2.8 L4-body measurements

	For a boy	For a girl
• Father's height in centimeter	Plot height	Plot (height – 14 centimeter)
• Mother's height in centimeter	Plot (height + 14 centimeter)	Plot height
• Mid-parental height in centimeter	(Father's height + mother's height)/2 + 14	(Mother's height + Father's height)/2 – 14
• Adult target range in centimeter	MPH+/–10 cm	MPH+ /–8.5 cm

- *Accelerated linear growth:* Linear growth accelerates during early and late phase, this can be seen from the routine use of growth chart of that child plotted during childhood. Significant deviation of this growth rate results from increased growth hormone production as a result from pituitary adenoma.

- *Excessive height:*
  - ❖ *Gigantism:* This growth occurs as a result of excess linear growth at the open epiphyses (linear growth excess of the predicted by parental height) due to excess production of growth hormone from pituitary tumor
  - ❖ *Acromegaly:* When the epiphyses closes, the growth occur in hands, skull, mandible and soft tissue thickening without increasing the height.

Loss of Height

Decreased height after skeletal maturity may occur from:

- Loss of long bone growth
- Loss of cartilage in lower extremity joints (hips and knees)
- Loss of vertebral height
- Loss of intervertebral spaces
- Excessive spinal curvatures.

• Long bones	Trauma, surgery, osteomalacia
• Cartilage	Rheumatoid arthritis, osteoarthritis
• Intervertebral discs	Herniated discs, desiccated disc, disc infection
• Vertebrae	Osteoporosis, osteomalacia, Paget's disease, traumatic fractures, compression, multiple myeloma
• Spinal curvature	Scoliosis, pregnancy, abdominal muscle weakness, myositis, poliomyelitis

Weight

Total body weight is thought as a series of compartments:

- Total body water is 60 percent of body weight in male, 50 percent of body weight in female and 80 percent of body weight in newborn
- Since fat contains less body water, obese person has less body water as compared to lean person.

• Intracellular fluid—40% of body weight (or 60%)	Extracellular fluid—20% of body weight (or 00%)
• 2/3rd of body water	1/3rd of body water

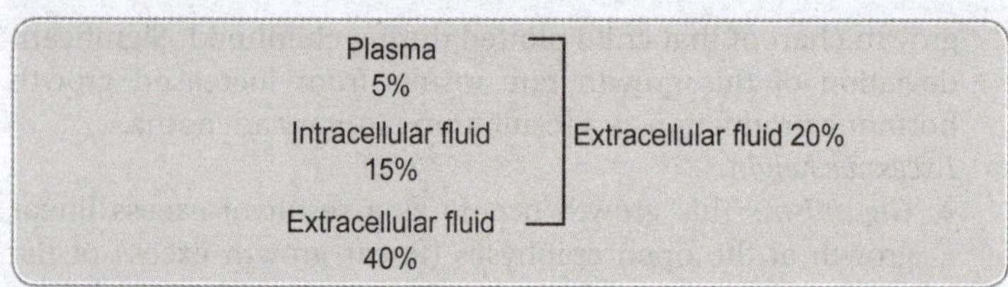

Distribution of Fluid Volume

Fluid type	Total	ICF	ECF	Interstitial	Plasma
Percent of body weight	60%	40%	20%	15%	5%
Vol for 70 kg weight	42 L	28 L	14 L	10.5 L	3.5 L

Weight loss should be measured at each visit to establish a baseline range and to detect any significant changes.

Weight may be acute usually due to acute loss of body tissue, rapid diuresis or acute dehydration.

Percent of weight loss = [(usual weight – current weight)/(usual weight)] × 100

Significant involuntary weight loss can be defined as more than 5 percent of body weight 1000 preceding 6 months or more than 10 percent of body weight in last 1 year.

Weight loss may be due to:
- Decreased intake
- Maldigestion
- Malabsorption
- Increased metabolic utilization
- Increased loss of calories.

Several questions to be asked:
- Ask the patient whether weight loss occur within very short period
- If so, within how many months
- Whether the patient record his last weight
- Ask whether the patient losses his appetite also at the time of weight loss
- Ask whether patient notices the change the size of clothes
- Review the patient's daily intake of food and drinks and any change of activities
- Look for the striae or loose skin over the abdomen or arms.

Causes of Weight Loss

• Endocrine	Hyperthyroidism, adrenal insufficiency, diabetes
• Idiopathic	Advanced age (normal adult lose his weight after the age of 60 years), debilitating disease
• Inflammatory	SLE, rheumatoid arthritis, vasculitis
• Infections	Tuberculosis, AIDS, CAH, intestinal parasites
• Metabolic/Toxic	Uremia, CCF, emphysema, advanced liver disease
• Increased physical activity	
• Malabsorption	
• Dieting	Decreased intake, starvation
• Mechanical/traumatic bowel obstruction	Dysphagia, odynophagia, dental and chewing problems
• Neoplastic	Decreased appetite and increased utilization
• Neurologic	Hypothalamic disorders, multi-infarct dementia
• Psychological dieting	Dementia, anorexia nervosa, bulimia, depression, poverty

- Weight gain is a part of normal growth in childhood and adolescence, and failure to weight gain is normal at that age
- As skeletal maturity is reached, weight gain continues till the skeletal muscle mass increases to adult size, especially in men
- After reaching the adult mass, further weight gain indicates pathological condition.
- Energy content of:
  - ❖ Fat—9 kcal/g
  - ❖ Alcohol—7.5 kcal/g
  - ❖ Carbohydrate—4.5 kcal/g
  - ❖ Protein—4.5 kcal/g.

Causes of Weight Gain

• Increased intake	Overeating, insulinoma, hyperthyroidism, treatment of diabetes, hypothalamic injury, anabolic steroids
• Decreased metabolic demand	Hypothyroidism, hypogonadism, inactivity, confinement
• Salt and water retention	CCF, renal failure, nephritic syndrome, portal hypertension with ascites, idiopathic edema, diuretic rebound, venus insufficiency with dependent edema

Body Mass Index (BMI)

Proportion of height to weight.
- *Normal range:* 18 to 24.9
- *Overweight:* 25.0 to 29.9
- *Obese:* >30.

In younger subject >25, BMI is associated with cardiovascular risk.

Importance of BMI

High BMI is associated with following serious problem:
- Hypertension
- Dyslipidemia
- Type II diabetes
- Female infertility
- Sleep apnea
- Cardiovascular disease
- Osteoarthritis.
- *Various organ cancers:* Endometrial, breast, prostate and colon.
- Lower extremity venus stasis
- Idiopathic intracranial hypertension
- Gastroesophageal reflux
- Urinary stress incontinence
- Gallbladder disease.

Cut-off of BMI

According to New England Journal Study:
- Lowest death rate if BMI < 19
- Risk of death > 20 percent, if BMI 19 to 24.9
- Risk of death > 30 percent, if BMI 25 to 26.9
- Risk of death > 60 percent, if BMI 27 to 28.9
- Risk of death > 100 percent, if BMI >29.0.

Measurement of BMI

It can be measured by dividing weight in kg by height in meters square (BMI = weight in kg/height in meter square).

Following formula is:

$$BMI = \frac{Weight\ (Ibs)}{\{Height\ (inches)\}^2}$$

or,

$$\frac{Weight\ (kg)}{Height\ (m^2)}$$

Conversion formula: 2.2 lbs = 1 kg; 1.0 inch = 2.54 cm; 100 cm = 1 meter.

Distribution of fat in the body
Fat disposition may be (Fig. 2.9):

Central distribution:
- Bihumeral diameter is greater than bitrochanteric diameter.
- Subcutaneous fat has descending distribution—mostly concentrated in the upper half of the body (neck, cheek, shoulder, chest, and upper abdomen).

Peripheral distribution:
- Bitrochanteric diameter is greater than bihumeral diameter.
- Subcutaneous fat has ascending distribution, mostly concentrated in the lower half of the body (lower abdomen, pelvic girdle, buttock and thigh).

Importance of fat distribution in the body
Normal women have more subcutaneous fat than men, and have peripheral distribution.

With weight gain, fat tends to distribute diffusely subcutaneously in women, but in men it will be distributed in the internal organs and omentum (visceral obesity), so they have central obesity.

This visceral adipose tissue is grossly different from the subcutaneous fat to play pathophysiological role in the body in the form of:
- Hyperlipidemia
- Insulin resistance
- Cardiovascular disease
- Other metabolic diseases
- Arm circumference (Fig. 2.10) method as described.

Waist circumference
Measure tape between the last rib and the iliac crest at minimal inspiration.

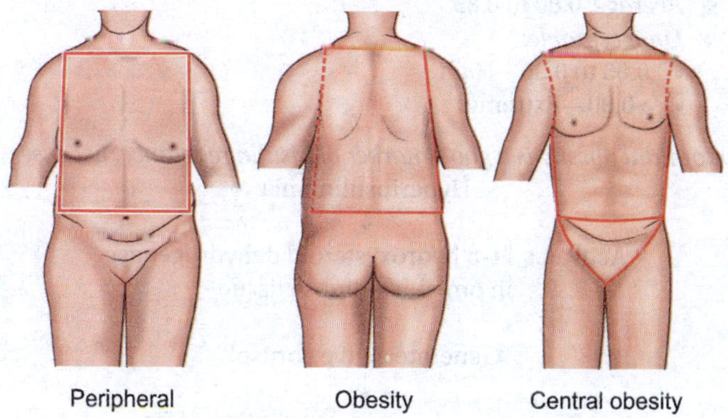

FIG. 2.9 Body mass index

According to above measurement, narrowest waist level just above the umbilicus.

Hip circumference
Tape measure at the widest part of the buttocks.

Importance of waist and hip circumference
- *Waist/hip ratio >1.0—risk for men and women:* Apple shape (extra weight around stomach) is more dangerous than pear shape (extra weight around hip and thigh)
- Waist circumference is much more risk for future cardiovascular diseases than BMI alone
- *According to British study,* Waist/hip ratio >0.99 in nonsmoker men and >0.90 in nonsmoker women is associated with 40 percent risk for cardiovascular diseases/death than lower waist/hip ratio <0.8
- Cut-off value of waist/hip ratio <0.83 for women and <0.9 for men
- Comparing with BMI, there is three-fold increase in population risk factor for myocardial infarction.
- *Cardiovascular risk factor on waist/hip ratio:*
  Male:
  - ❖ *Acceptable:*
    - <0.85—Excellent
    - 0.85 to 0.90—Good.
  - ❖ *Average:* 0.90 to 0.95.
  - ❖ *Unacceptable:*
    - 0.95 to 1.0—High.
    - >1.0—Extreme.
  Female:
  - ❖ *Acceptable:*
    - <0.75—Excellent
    - 0.75 to 0.80—Good.
  - ❖ *Average:* 0.80 to 0.85
  - ❖ *Unacceptable:*
    - 0.85 to 0.90—High
    - >0.90—Extreme.

Abdominal obesity is a good marker of insulin resistance, because:

Hyperinsulinemia

↓

Activates 11-β hydroxysteroid dehydrogenase
in omental adipose tissue

↓

Generate active cortisol

↓

Promote cushingoid distribution of fat

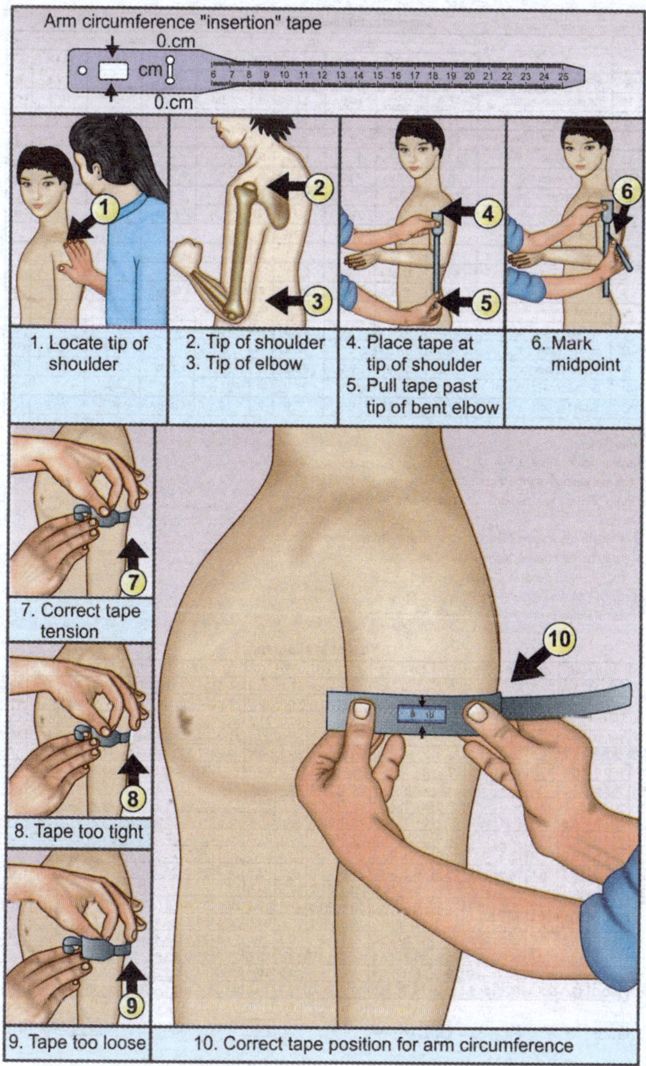

FIG. 2.10   Arm circumference

No correlation of BMI with waist/hip ratio
Within three BMI categories (normal, overweight, obese) (Fig. 2.11):
High waist circumference values (>102 cm for men and >88 cm for women) are associated with hypertension, diabetes, dyslipidemia than normal values of waist circumference (<102 cm for men and <88 cm for women).

Selected anthropometric dimensions

ID	Description	Male					Female				
		Med	SD	MIN	MAX	GP	MED	SD	MIN	MAX	GP
A	Height	69.1	2.44	59.5	77.6	a	63.2	2.48	55	73	d
B	Shoulder breadth	17.9	0.91	14.6	22.8	a	13.4	1.22	8.7	19.3	d
C	Hip breadth (seat)	15.3	1.11	12	21.3	b	14.6	1.04	12.1	20.6	c
C	Hip breadth (stand)	13.2	0.73	8.3	15.8	a	15	1.03	11.8	18.9	e
C	Hip breadth (seat	13.9	0.87	11.4	18.1	a					
D	Foot breadth	3.8	0.19	3.2	4.7	a					
E	Arm span	70.8	2.94	58.3	82.3	a					
F	Arm reach	34.6	1.65	27.6	39.8	d	31.8	1.29	28.3	35.4	e
G	Chest depth	9	0.75	6.7	13	a					
H	Hand breadth	3.5	0.16	3	4.1	a					
I	Forearm–hand	18.9	0.81	15.4	22.1						
J	Buttock–knee	23.6	1.06	18.5	27.6	a	22.6	0.96	19.7	26.7	e
K	Seat length	18.9	0.96	15.4	23.1	b	18.2	1.04	15.2	22.2	c
L	Sitting knee Height	21.7	0.99	17.3	24.8	a	17.2	1.07			d
M	Foot length	10.5	0.45	8.9	12.2	a	9.6	0.4	8.9	10.9	e
N	Erect sit height	36	1.29	29.9	40.2	a	34.1	1.02	30.7	34.4	e
P	Shoulder Hgt (seat)	13.3	1.14	18.9	27.2	a	24.6	3.02			d
Q	Seat height	19	0.89	15.6	22	b	18.1	0.89	15.4	20.6	c

Notes:

Source: Mc cormick, 1964

" Normal sitting height is about 2" less than erect height

Group "c" data are medians. Groups "d" and "e" data are means

Groups:

a. 4000 Air force flying personnel, Herzbeng, Daniels and Churchill

b. 1959 Civilian males, Hooten and staff

c. 1908 Civilian females, Hooten and staff

d. 10,042 Civilian females, O' Brien and Shelton

e. 447 Female pilots, Randall, Damon, Benton and Pratt

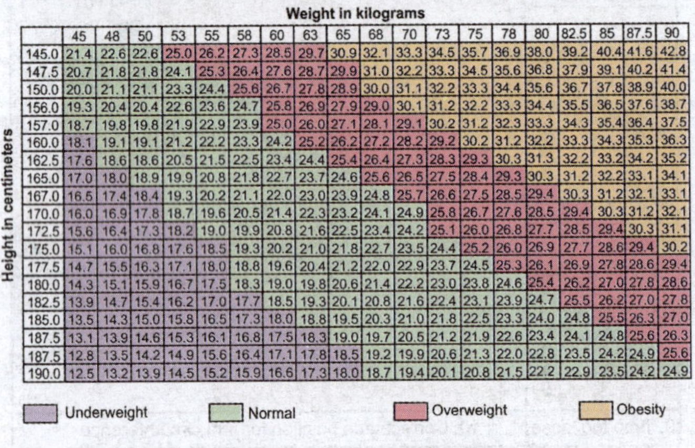

Weight in kilograms

Height in centimeters	45	48	50	53	55	58	60	63	65	68	70	73	75	78	80	82.5	85	87.5	90
145.0	21.4	22.6	22.6	25.0	26.2	27.3	28.5	29.7	30.9	32.1	33.3	34.5	35.7	36.9	38.0	39.2	40.4	41.6	42.8
147.5	20.7	21.8	21.8	24.1	25.3	26.4	27.6	28.7	29.9	31.0	32.2	33.3	34.5	35.6	36.8	37.9	39.1	40.2	41.4
150.0	20.0	21.1	21.1	23.3	24.4	25.6	26.7	27.8	28.9	30.0	31.1	32.2	33.3	34.4	35.6	36.7	37.8	38.9	40.0
156.0	19.3	20.4	20.4	22.6	23.6	24.7	25.8	26.9	27.9	29.0	30.1	31.2	32.2	33.3	34.4	35.5	36.5	37.6	38.7
157.0	18.7	19.8	19.8	21.9	22.9	23.9	25.0	26.0	27.1	28.1	29.1	30.2	31.2	32.3	33.3	34.3	35.4	36.4	37.5
160.0	18.1	19.1	19.1	21.2	22.2	23.3	24.2	25.2	26.2	27.2	28.2	29.2	30.2	31.2	32.2	33.3	34.3	35.3	36.3
162.5	17.6	18.6	18.6	20.5	21.5	22.5	23.4	24.4	25.4	26.4	27.3	28.3	29.3	30.3	31.3	32.2	33.2	34.2	35.2
165.0	17.0	18.0	18.9	19.9	20.8	21.8	22.7	23.7	24.6	25.6	26.5	27.5	28.4	29.3	30.3	31.2	32.2	33.1	34.1
167.0	16.5	17.4	18.4	19.3	20.2	21.1	22.0	23.0	23.9	24.8	25.7	26.6	27.5	28.5	29.4	30.3	31.2	32.1	33.1
170.0	16.0	16.9	17.8	18.7	19.6	20.5	21.4	22.3	23.2	24.1	24.9	25.8	26.7	27.6	28.5	29.4	30.3	31.2	32.1
172.5	15.6	16.4	17.3	18.2	19.0	19.9	20.8	21.6	22.5	23.4	24.2	25.1	26.0	26.8	27.7	28.5	29.4	30.3	31.1
175.0	15.1	16.0	16.8	17.6	18.5	19.3	20.2	21.0	21.8	22.7	23.5	24.4	25.2	26.0	26.9	27.7	28.6	29.4	30.2
177.5	14.7	15.5	16.3	17.1	18.0	18.8	19.6	20.4	21.2	22.0	22.9	23.7	24.5	25.3	26.1	26.9	27.8	28.6	29.4
180.0	14.3	15.1	15.9	16.7	17.5	18.3	19.0	19.8	20.6	21.4	22.2	23.0	23.8	24.6	25.4	26.2	27.0	27.8	28.6
182.5	13.9	14.7	15.4	16.2	17.0	17.7	18.5	19.3	20.1	20.8	21.6	22.4	23.1	23.9	24.7	25.5	26.2	27.0	27.8
185.0	13.5	14.3	15.0	15.8	16.5	17.3	18.0	18.8	19.5	20.3	21.0	21.8	22.5	23.3	24.0	24.8	25.5	26.3	27.0
187.5	13.1	13.9	14.6	15.3	16.1	16.8	17.5	18.3	19.0	19.7	20.5	21.2	21.9	22.6	23.4	24.1	24.8	25.6	26.3
187.5	12.8	13.5	14.2	14.9	15.6	16.4	17.1	17.8	18.5	19.2	19.9	20.6	21.3	22.0	22.8	23.5	24.2	24.9	25.6
190.0	12.5	13.2	13.9	14.5	15.2	15.9	16.6	17.3	18.0	18.7	19.4	20.1	20.8	21.5	22.2	22.9	23.5	24.2	24.9

Underweight   Normal   Overweight   Obesity

FIG. 2.11   Weight and height

So other factors come into play are:

- Age
- Race
- Poverty
- Income status
- Smoking
- Alcohol intake.

Malnutrition on the basis of BMI:
- *Marginal malnutrition:* BMI 17 to 18.4
- *Moderate malnutrition:* BMI 16.0 to 16.9
- *Severe malnutrition:* BMI <16.0.

Subjective global assessment (SGA) of nutritional status detects:
- Loss of subcutaneous fat
- Loss of muscle mass
- Shifting of intravenous fluid.

Subcutaneous fat can be measured in:
- Triceps region in the arm
- Mid-axillary line at the costal margin
- Interosseous and palmar areas of the hand
- Deltoid of the shoulder.

Loss of subcutaneous fat can be diagnosed by:
- Lake of fullness
- Skin loosely fit over the deep tissue.

Loss of muscle mass can be detected by palpation of muscles:
- Quadriceps femoris
- Deltoids
- It can detect muscle wasting.

Loss of fluid from the intravascular spaces can be detected by:
- Ankle for edema
- Sacral region for edema
- Abdominal wall for parietal edema
- Ascites.

Above three SGA are recorded and graded as:
- Normal (0)
- Mild (1+)
- Moderate (2+)
- Severe (3+).

In some cases, the distribution of adipose tissue can serve as a clue to the diagnosis:
- Truncal obesity, round facies, prominent hump of fat over the upper back:
  - ❖ Cushing's disease
  - ❖ Iatrogenic steroids
  - ❖ Use of protease inhibitors in the treatment of HIV.
- Localized accumulation of fat at the sites of repetitive insulin injection (lipodystrophy).

Metabolic Syndrome

The presence of three or more of these five abnormalities defines metabolic syndrome:
- Obesity
- Hypertension

- Low LDL
- Elevated cholesterol
- Elevated triglycerides
- Elevated fasting glucose.

Posture

- *Patient with pancreatitis:* Patient lies in fetal position on one side with knees and legs bend over
- *Patient with peritonitis:* Patient becomes still and avoid movement that worsens pain
- *Patient with intestinal obstruction:* Patient becomes restless
- *Patient with renal and peritoneal abscess:* Patient bends towards the side of the lesion
- *Patient with inflamed appendix, diverticulum, terminal ileum, from Crohn's disease, i.e. abnormality around the ileopsoas muscle:* Patient uses to lie supine with knee flexed and hip externally rotated—Psoas sign. It may occur due to tubercular abscess originating in the spine and spreading along the muscle—this is called cold abscess
- *Patient with meningitis:* Patient lies on one side with neck extended, thigh flexed at the hips and leg bent at the knees
- *Patient with large pleural effusion:* Patient uses to lie on the affected side to maximize excursion of the unaffected lung. This however worsens hypoxemia
- *Patient with small pleural effusion:* Patient uses to on the unaffected side, because direct pressure may worsen the plural pain
- *Patient with large pericardial effusion:* (Especially cardiac tamponade) sit up on the bed and lean forward, a posture referred as "The praying Muslim position"
- *Patient with tetralogy of Fallot:* Patient often assumes squatting position, trying to avoid cyanotic spells, e.g. after exercise.

Apparent Age

Conditions those Make Older than Apparent Age

- Cigarette smoking
- Chronic exposure to sunlight
- *Progeria (Hutchinson-Gilford syndrome):*
  - ❖ Affect 1 in 8 million children, accelerating the aging process by 6 to 8 times.

- ❖ Symptoms begin around 18 to 24 months. *Features are:*
  - Stunted growth
  - Alopecia
  - Receding chin
  - Small face
  - Pinched up nose.
- Atherosclerotic heart disease
- Cardiovascular disease
- *Werner's syndrome:*
  - ❖ Autosomal recessive disease of DNA replication
  - ❖ Premature aging and death at 40 or 50 years
  - ❖ Growth is normal until puberty
  - ❖ Then they start aging rapidly, having:
    - Wrinkling of the skin
    - Loss of hair
    - Early cataract
    - Thin extremity
    - Thick trunk
    - Face is like bird.

Conditions those Make Younger than Apparent Age

- Hypogonadism and other endocrine disorders—producing arrest of development
- Panhypopituitarism
- Anorexia nervosa
- Immune suppressive agents.

Toxic Looking Patients

- Anxious, flushed, sweaty, febrile, having tachycardia, rapid and shallow respiration
- Poisoning (salicylate intoxication)
- Thyroid storm
- Psychotic crisis
- Heat stroke.

Facies

It is Latin word—indicates peculiar often pathognomonic facial feature of a particular disease.

The different types of facies are:

Congenital

• *Facial borvina*	1. Large cranial vault, 2. Large forehead, 3. High bregma, 4. Occasional hypertelorism (due to enlarged sphenoid). *Greig syndrome:* Associated congenital malformations: Osteogenesis imperfecta, syndactyly, polydactyly, scapular elevation, mental retardation.
• *Elfin facies* (Fig. 2.12)	1. Flat face, 2. Broad forehead, 3. Hypertelorism, 4. Short and upturned nose, 5. Low set ears, 6. Puffy cheek, 7. Wide mouth, 8. Patulous lips, 9. Hypoplastic teeth, 10. Deep husky voice. *William's syndrome:* Patient is mentally retarded, short stature, congenital supravalvular aortic stenosis, and hypercalcemia.
• Cherubic facies	Child-like face due to familial fibrous dysplasia of the jaws—enlargement in childhood and regression in adulthood.
• *Hound dog facies*	A degenerative disease of elastic fibers, as a result skin becomes progressively loose and hanging like folds—like hound dog. *Facial appearance:* 1. Antimongoloid facies, 2. Everted nostrils, 3. Prominent ears, 4. Prominent epicanthic folds, 5. No joint laxity. *Congenital disease: Cutis laxa:* Premature aging.

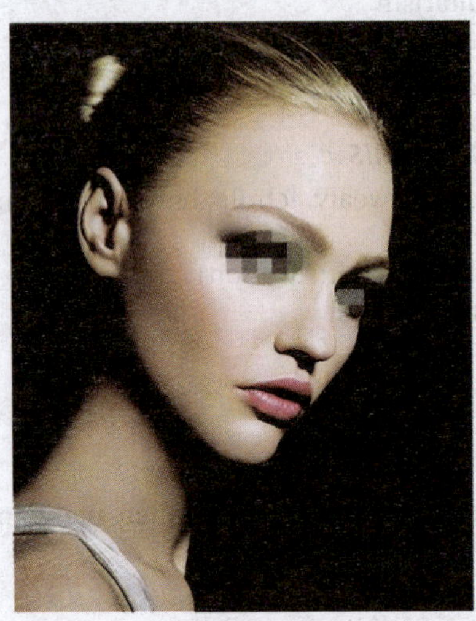

FIG. 2.12   Elfin facies

• *Hurloid facies*	Gargoyle like facies—Type! mucopolysaccharidosis: because of lack of L-iduronidase—these patients accumulate intracellular deposits. *Hurler's syndrome:* Dwarfism, kyphosis, limited joint motion, spade like-hands, corneal clouding, hepatosplenomegaly, mental retardation.
• *Morquio's facies* (Fig. 2.13)	Mucopolysaccharidosis—Type IV; 1. Face is coarse, 2. Large mouth, 3. Antiverted nose, 4. Short neck. *Morquio's syndrome:* Chest and limb deformities (short stature, kyphosis, pectus carinatum, protruded abdomen, genu valgum), hepatosplenomegaly, increased urinary excretion of mucopolysaccharidosis, neutrophils containing Intracytoplasmic metachromatic granules.
• *Potter's face*	Hypertelorism, prominent epicanthic folds, low set ears, receding chins, flattened nose. *Potter's syndrome:* Bilateral renal agenesis, pulmonary hypoplasia, cardiac malformations (VSD, endocardial cushion defect, Fallot's tetralogy, PDA).
• *Down's syndrome* (Fig. 2.14)	1. Oblique orbital fissure, 2. Prominent epicanthic folds, 3. Small ears, 4. Flat nasal bridge, 5. Protruding tongue, 6. Brushfield spot in iris. Other features are: Short stature, single palmer crease, curved little finger, endocardial cushion defect, increased gap between 1st and 2nd toes.

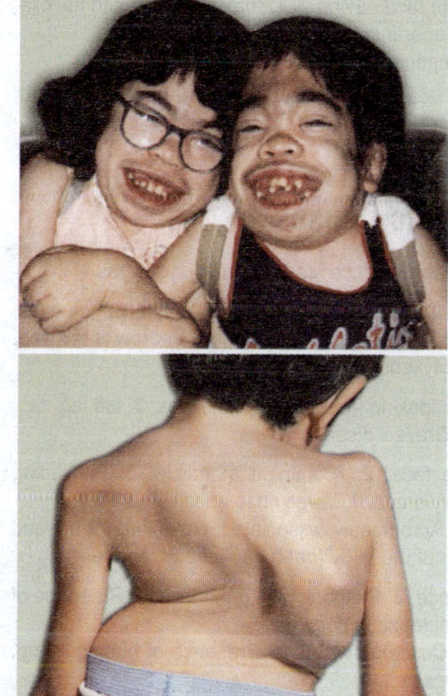

FIG. 2.13 Morquio's facies

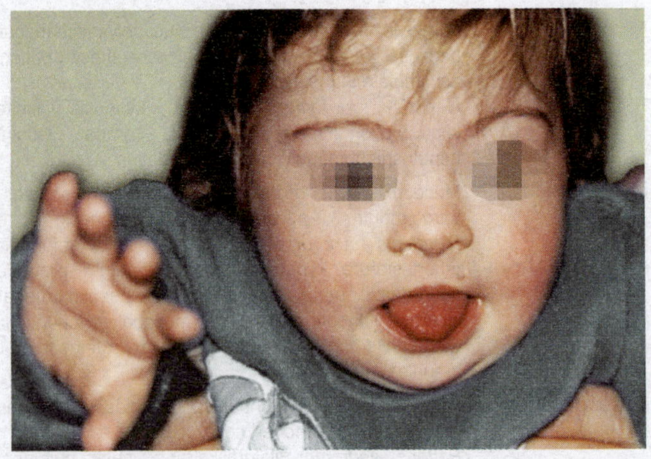

FIG. 2.14 Down's syndrome

Infectious Facies

• *Facies leonina* (Fig. 2.15)	• Lion like face, prominent ridges, furrows on the forehead and cheeks • Advanced lepromatous leprosy
• *Facies antonina*	• Alteration in the eyelids and anterior eye • Lepromatous leprosy
• *Scaphoid face*	• Disc like face having: 1. Depressed nose and maxilla, 2. Protuberant forehead, 3. Prominent chin • Advanced lepromatous leprosy
• *Tetanus face*	This is called risus sardonicus—opened mouth, transversely tightened lips

Endocrine and Metabolic Causes

Renal face	Puffy and swollen face, coarse hair, boggy eyes
Myxedematous face (Fig. 2.16)	1. Puffy and swollen face, 2. Coarse hair, 3. Boggy eyes, 4. Dry and rough skin, 5. Lateral third eyebrow is missing. *Disease:* Myxedema
Graves' disease	1. Anxious looking face, 2. Exophthalmos, 3. Lid lag *Disease:* Graves' disease
Acromegalic face (Fig. 2.17)	1. Coarse face, 2. Prominent mandible, 3. Protruding supraciliary areas, 4. Large nose and lips *Disease:* Acromegaly associated conditions: Enlarged acral parts of the body (head, face, hand, and feet)
Cushing's face	1. Moon face, 2. Plethoric oily round face, 3. Presence of acne, 4. Increase in body hair *Disease: Cushing syndrome:* Presence of buffalo hump, central obesity

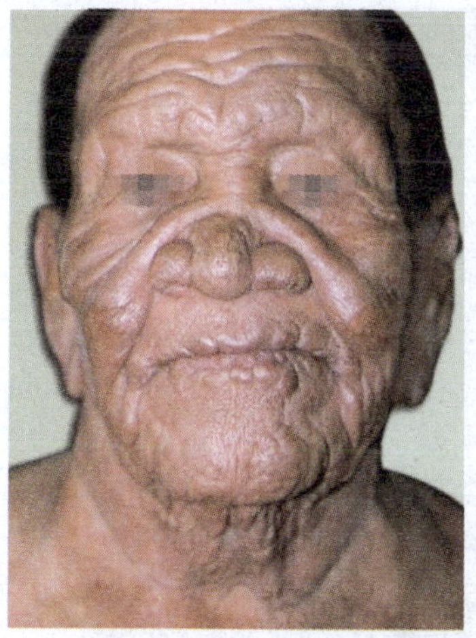

FIG. 2.15   Facies leonina

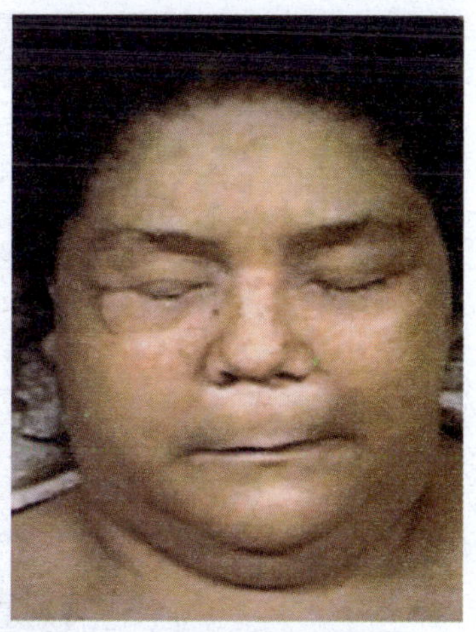

FIG. 2.16   Myxedematous face

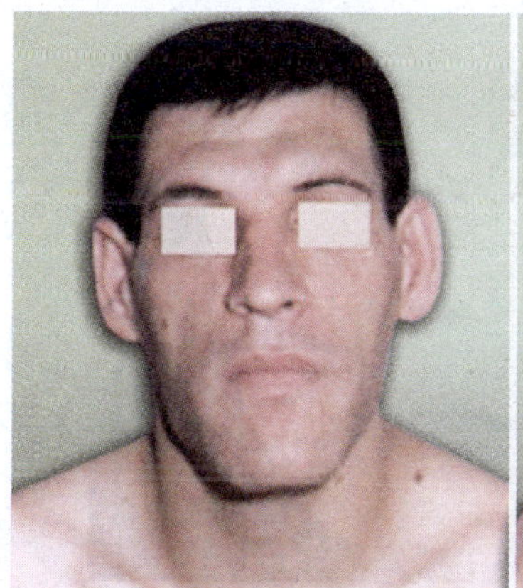

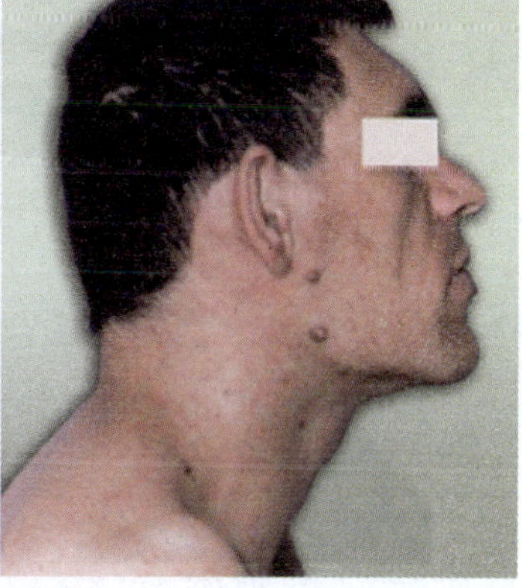

FIG. 2.17   Acromegalic face

Rheumatologic Faces

Scleroderma face *(Fig. 2.10)*	1. Skin is tightly drawn so that wrinkle disappears 2. Sharp nose, 3. Areas of hyperpigmentation, 4. Patchy areas of hypopigmentation, 5. Opening of mouth is narrow, 6. Areas of telangiectasia *Disease:* Scleroderma
Facies of SLE *(Fig. 2.19)*	Butterfly such as rash over the bridge of the nose including malar areas *Disease:* Systemic lupus erythematosus

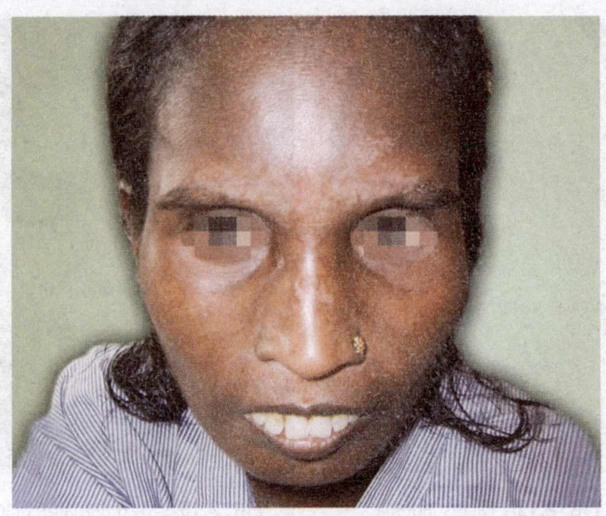

FIG. 2.18 Scleroderma face

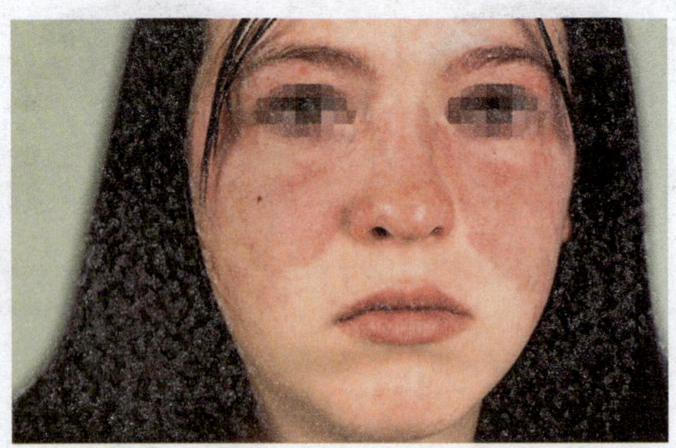

FIG. 2.19 Facies of SLE

Cardiovascular Facies

Aortic face	Pale and shallow face of aortic regurgitation.
Corvisart's face	Puffy, cyanotic, swollen eyelids, shiny eyes.
De Musset's face	Bobbing motion of head with each heart beat *Disease:* Aortic regurgitation, may be in tricuspid regurgitation.
Mitral facies (Fig. 2.20)	Acrocyanotic face, due to peripheral desaturation as a result of low cardiac output. In this process, the parts involved are: Nose, lip, cheeks, hands and feet. When mitral stenosis involves right side of the heart producing right-sided heart failure and tricuspid regurgitation, face becomes shallow, overtly icteric.

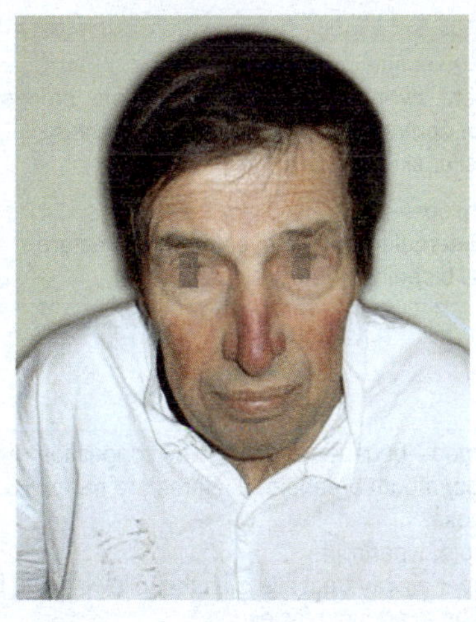

FIG. 2.20 Mitral facies

Neurologic Facies

Parkinson's face	Apathic, mask like.
Myasthenic face (Fig. 2.21)	1. Saggling of the corner of the mouth, 2. Drooping of the eyelids, 3. Weakness of the facial muscles producing apathic look. *Disease:* Myasthenia gravis.
Myopathic face	1. Protruding lips, 2. Drooping eyelids, 3. Ophthalmoplagia, 4. Relaxation of facial muscles (Hutchinson's face).
Steinert's face	1. Frontal balding, 2. Cataract, 3. Bilateral muscle wasting, 4. Thin and beak like nose, 5. Tenting upper lip, 6. Tendency of the mouth to hang over. *Disease:* Myotonic dystrophy.

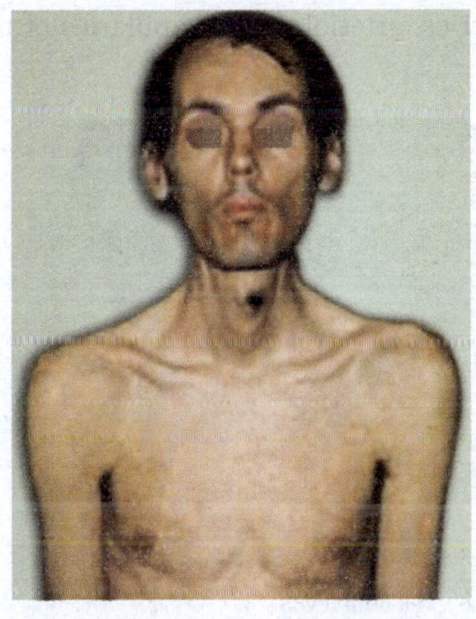

FIG. 2.21 Myasthenic face

Traumatic Face

Battle sign	Bruise present over or behind the mastoid process—ipsilaterally or contralaterally of basilar skull fracture. *Disease:* Basilar skull fracture.
Raccoon eyes (Fig. 2.22)	Periorbital bruises—due to capillary fragility. *Causes:* 1. External trauma to eyes, 2. Skull fracture, 3. Intracranial bleeding, 4. Amyloidosis.

Miscellaneous

Facial adenoid (Fig. 2.23)	1. Mouth is open—because upper airway congestion make them obligatory mouth breahers, 2. Nares are narrow, 3. Pinched up nose. *Cause:* Adenoid hypertrophy. In case of upper airway tract allergies the following can be seen in addition to adenoid facies: i. *Dennie's line:* Horizontal creases under both eyelids. ii. *Nasal pleat:* Horizontal creases just above the tip of the nose. iii. *Allergic shiner:* Bilateral infraorbital shadow due to chronic venous congestion.
Saddle nose (Fig. 2.24)	Congenital or acquired erosions and destruction of nasal bones and cartilage producing depression of nasal bridge. *Causes:* 1. Congenital syphilis, 2. Wegner's granulomatosis, 3. Relapsing polychondritis.

■ Lymph Node

Anatomy of Lymphatic System

Lymphatic channels and lymph nodes are a discontinuous circulation. It has:

- Efferent loops are the arteries, arterioles and capillaries of the vascular system

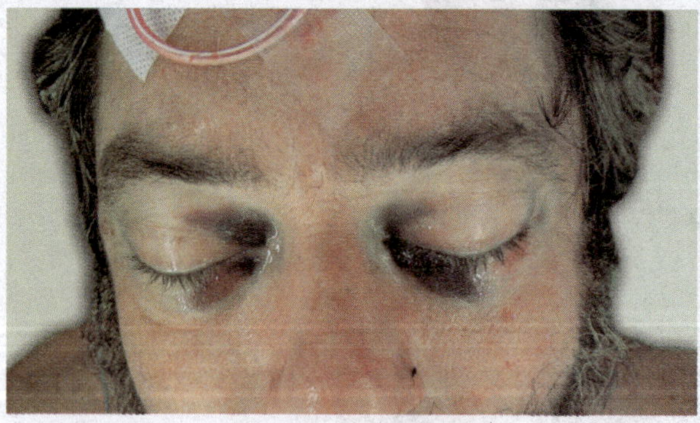

FIG. 2.22 Raccoon eyes

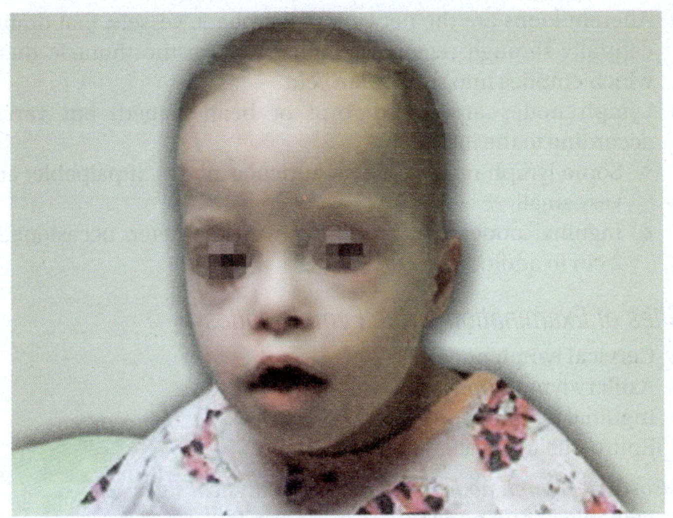

FIG. 2.23 Facial adenoid

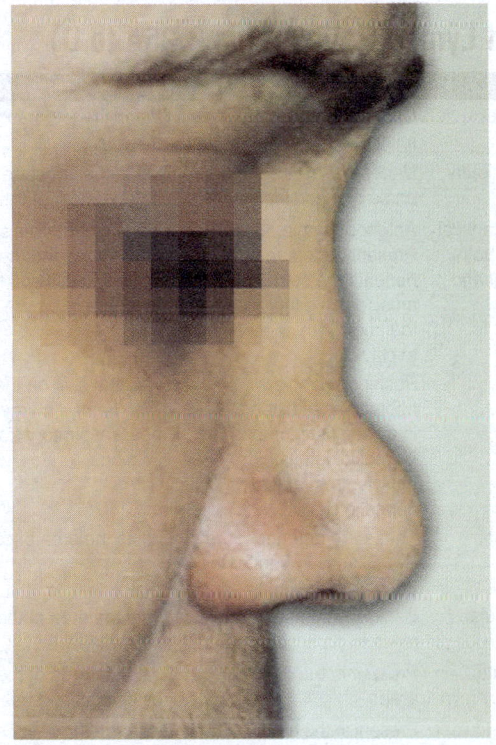

FIG. 2.24 Saddle nose

- Afferent loops are the network of lymphatic vessels, that drains centrally through regional lymph nodes to the thoracic duct, which empties into subclavian vein
- Lymph nodes are round, oval or bean-shaped, but varies according to the location
  - ❖ Some lymph nodes, like preauricular nodes, if palpable, are very small
  - ❖ Inguinal nodes are larger—1 cm in diameter, occasionally 2 cm in adult.

Sites of Examination of the Lymph Nodes

- Cervical lymph nodes
- Axillary lymph nodes
- Inguinal lymph nodes
- Epitrochlear lymph nodes.

Disorder of lymph nodes produces three physical signs:
1. Palpable lymph nodes
2. Red streak in the skin from superficial lymphangitis
3. Lymph edema.

Cervical Lymph Nodes (Figs 2.25A to D)

Sites	Anatomic location	Drainage area
• Submental	Under the chin in the midline on either side.	Drains the teeth and intraoral cavity.
• Submandibular	Under the jaw near the angle of mandible.	Drains the structure on the posterior floor of the mouth.
• Anterior cervical (Jugular) both superficial and deep	Anterior triangle nodes. Present on top and beneath the sternomastoid muscles on either side of the neck from angle of jaw to clavicle.	Drains the internal structures of the throat and the posterior pharynx, tonsil and thyroid gland.
• Posterior cervical	Posterior triangle nodes. These extend in a line posterior to sternocleidomastoid muscle, from mastoid bones to clavicle.	Drain the skin on the back of the head, enlarged during upper respiratory tract infections.
• Preauricular	These are anterior to the ear. Slightly in front of the tragus of the pinna.	Drains the area of conjunctiva.
• Postauricular	Behind the pinna on the mastoid process.	Drain the area of the eye and external ear.
• Suboccipital	Present in the occipital area.	Drain the area of the scalp of posterior part of head.
• Supraclavicular	Present in the hollow of the clavicle, just lateral to where it joins the sternum.	Drain the thoracic cavity and abdomen.

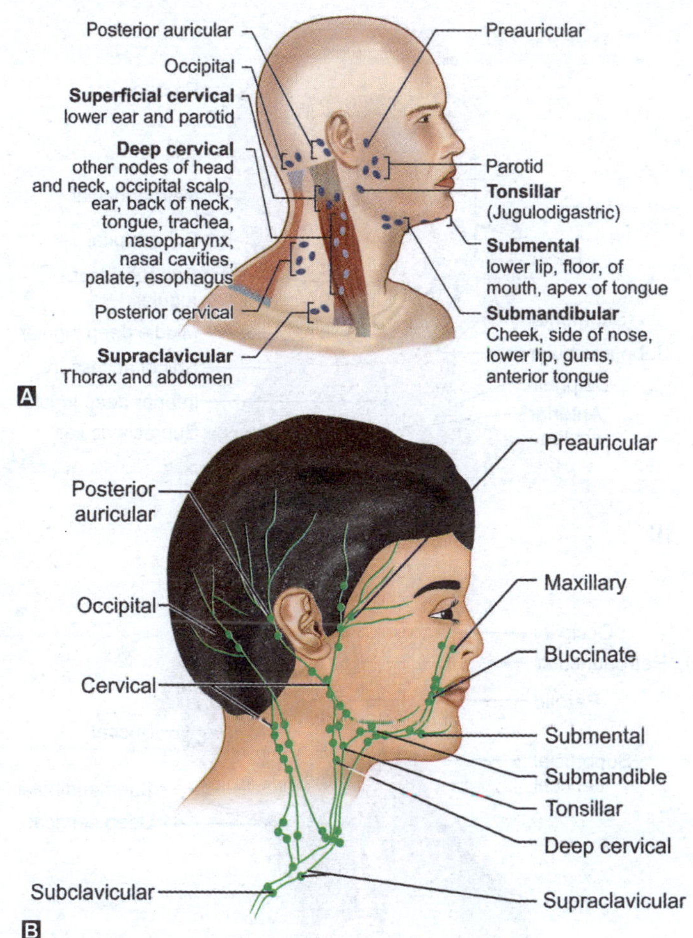

FIGS 2.25A AND B Cervical lymph nodes

Methods of Palpation of Cervical Lymph Nodes (Figs 2.26A to I)

- By using the pulp of the fingers examine both sides of the head and neck simultaneously by sliding the fingers over the area of attention
- Apply steady and gentle pressure
- Examine all cervical sites by following anterior and posterior aspects of the underside of jaws and neck

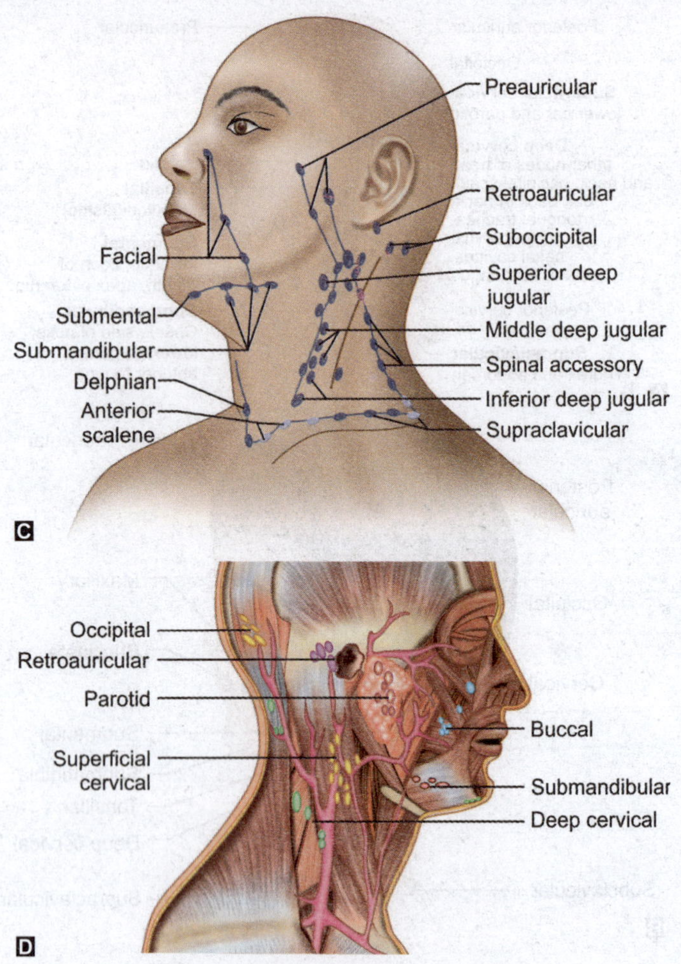

FIGS 2.25C AND D Cervical lymph nodes

- Using the pad of 2nd and third fingers palpate the preauricular nodes with gentle rotatory motion
- Then examine the posterior auricular nodes and occipital nodes.
- Palpate anterior superficial and deep cervical chains, located anterior and superficial to sternocleidomastoid
- Then palpate posterior cervical chain along the anterior edge of trapezius and posterior edge of sternocleidomastoid
- During cervical region palpation flex the head end turn towards the side of examination.

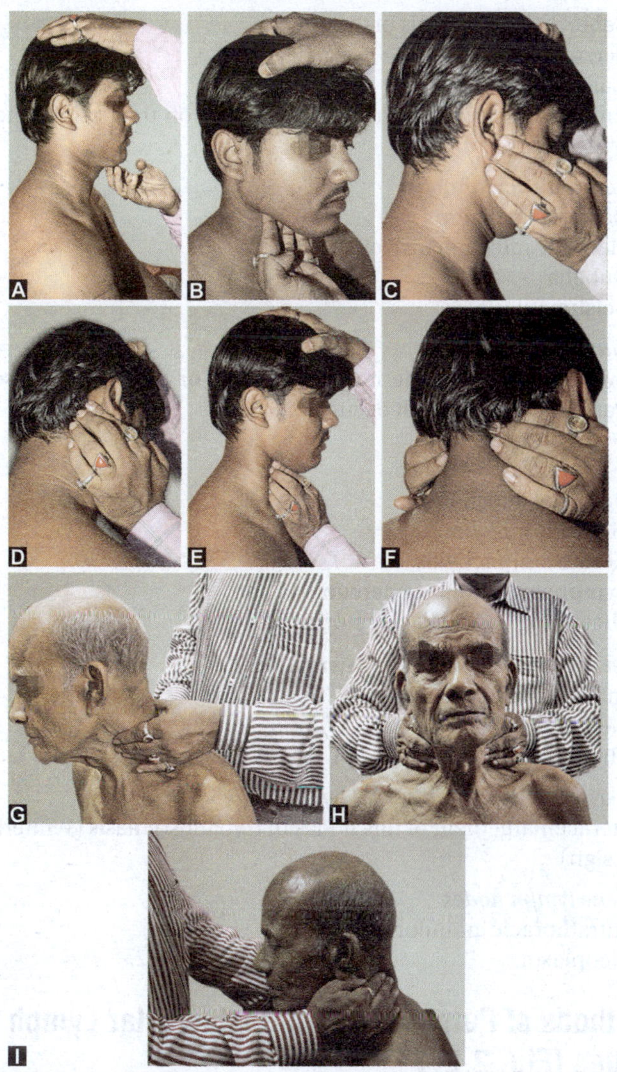

FIGS 2.26A TO I Methods of palpation of cervical lymph nodes. (A) Submental node; (B) Submandibular nodes; (C) Preauricular nodes; (D) Postauricular nodes; (E) Anterior cervical nodes; (F) Suboccipital nodes; (G) Anterior triangle nodes from behind I; (H) Anterior triangle nodes from behind II; (I) Posterior triangle nodes from front

Significance of Cervical Group of Lymph Nodes

Suboccipital nodes

- Ringworm of scalp
- Bites in pediculosis capitis

- Seborrheic dermatitis of the scalp
- Secondary syphilis
- Cancer

Enlarged lymph node may give pressure on the occipital nerve may produce headache.

Posterior auricular nodes
- Bacterial infection
- Herpetic infection of acoustic meatus
- Rubella
- Leishmaniasis.

Preauricular nodes
- Swelling on this node in conjunctivitis or pink eye represents Parinaud syndrome. It occurs in:
  - ❖ Tularemia
  - ❖ Cat-scratch disease
- Bacterial infections
- Herpetic infections
- Keratoconjunctivitis
- Lymphogranuloma venereum.
- Ulcerating basal cell carcinoma.

Anterior sternocleidomastoid lymph node
- Infection of oral cavity
- Neoplasm of oral cavity
- Thyroid cancer.

Posterior sternocleidomastoid lymph node
Bilateral enlargement of this nodes in trypanosomiasis (Winterbottom sign).

Scalene lymph nodes
- Intrathoracic granuloma
- Neoplasm.

Methods of Palpation of Supraclavicular Lymph Nodes (Fig. 2.27)

Two methods of palpation are:

1. The patient is allowed to sit up, head straight up and arms down. Palpate from behind—allow optimal adaptation of your hand to the patient's anatomy.
2. *Palpation from front:* In supine patient, where absence of gravity mobilizes the node and makes it more accessible. If the node is not palpable, patient is asked to cough or to perform Valsalva maneuver. This may pop a deeply seated node; make it palpable by your hand.

Drainage area: Head, arm, chest wall and breast.

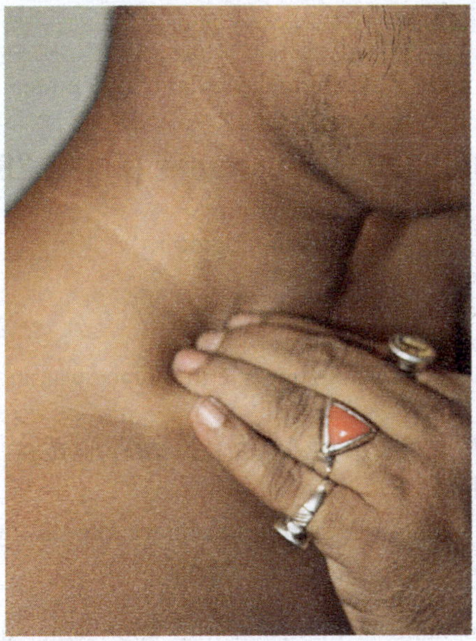

FIG. 2.27 Supraclavicular nodes 3

Significance of Supraclavicular Lymph Nodes

- *Right supraclavicular lymph nodes enlarge due to tumor of:*
  - ❖ Ipsilateral breast
  - ❖ Ipsilateral lung
  - ❖ Mediastinum
  - ❖ Esophagus

Because of bilateral crossed drainage, right node enlargement is due to lung cancer involving left lobe.

- *Left supraclavicular lymph node enlargement is due to tumor of:*
  - ❖ *Thorax:*
    - Esophagus
    - Ipsilateral lung involvement
    - Ipsilateral breast.
  - ❖ *Abdomen:*
    - Stomach
    - Liver
    - Gallbladder
    - Pancreas
    - Kidney
    - Intestine
  - ❖ *Pelvis:*
    - Ovaries
    - Testes

- Endometrium
- Prostate.

Troisier's node is left supraclavicular lymph node.

Axillary Group of Lymph Nodes (Fig. 2.28)

- Anterior group or pectoral group
- Posterior group or subscapular group
- Lateral group
- Medial group
- Apical group or central group.

Drainage area: Afferent from upper limb, thoracic wall and the breast.

Methods of Palpation of Axillary Lymph Nodes (Figs 2.29A and B)

- Relax the patient's left arm and axillary muscles by holding his left wrist with your left hand
- Elevate the patient's arm away from the chest wall
- Place your hand in the axilla with approximated fingers and palm towards his chest wall
- Push your approximated fingers towards the apex of the axilla to palpate central group
- Then his left hand is allowed to rest on your examining hand and your released left hand is used to support him from behind the shoulders

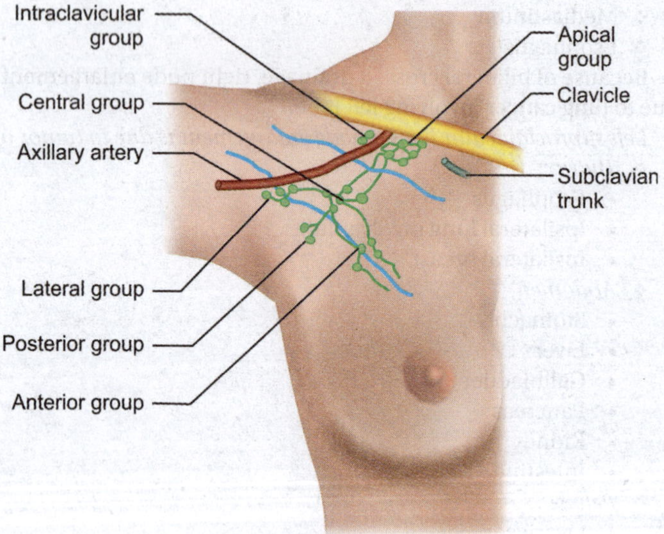

FIG. 2.28 Axillary nodes 4

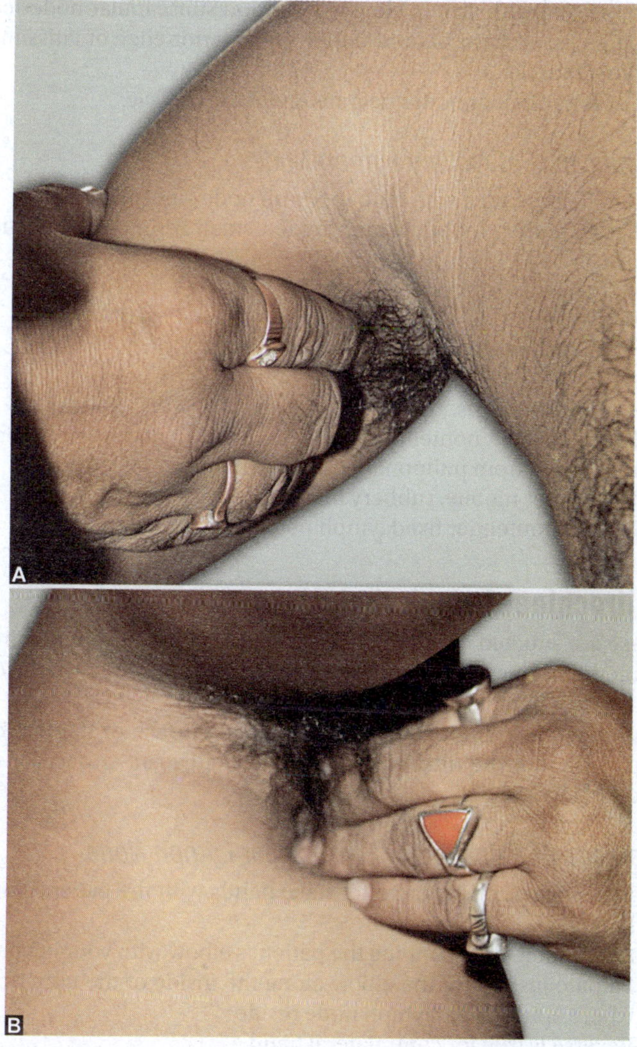

FIGS 2.29A AND B   Method of palpation of axillary nodes 8

- Then your pulp of the fingers are allowed to follow along the thoracic cage to feel for the enlarge lymph nodes
- Lateral group can be palpated along the axillary vein by elevating the patient's arm
- In patient's arm in elevated position, pectoral group can be palpated along the lateral edge of pectoralis major muscle

- In patient with arm in elevated position subscapular nodes can be palpated from behind under the anterior edge of latissimus dorsi muscle
- For infraclavicur nodes palpate under the clavicle.

Significance of Axillary Lymph Nodes

- Small nontender, soft, mobile lymph node—normal people
- Large, tender, mobile lymph node—small wounds or infection of arm:
  - ❖ Cat-scratch fever
  - ❖ Tularemia
  - ❖ Staphylococcal infection
  - ❖ Streptococcal infection
  - ❖ Sporotrichosis.
- Hard, fixed, nontender matted lymph nodes—secondary metastasis from pulmonary or breast tissue
- Nontender mobile, rubbery in consistency—lymphoma
- Matted nontender fixed lymph node—tuberculosis.

Epitrochlear Lymph Nodes

These are situated on the medial surface of the arm 3 cm proximal to medial humeral epicondyle, in the groove between the biceps and triceps brachii.

Draining areas: Lymphatic from the ulnar surface of the forearm and the hand, the little and ring fingers, adjacent surface of the middle finger.

Methods of Palpation of Epitrochlear Lymph Node

- By using your right hand to shake hands with the patient's right hand
- At the same time cupping the patient's elbow with your left hand
- Palpate just above the elbow along the inside of the upper arm where epitrochlear lymph node reside
- Reverse is true for contralateral hand.

Alternate Methods

- Support the patient's right wrist with the left hand
- Grasp the partially flexed elbow with right hand
- Use the thumb to feel the epitrochlear node
- Examine the left epitrochlear node with left thumb.

Significance of Enlarged Epitrochlear Node

It depends upon whether it is isolated or generalized. But this node enlargement is not benign.

The most common causes are:
- Infectious mononucleosis
- Non-Hodgkin lymphoma.

The other causes are:
- Sarcoidosis
- HIV
- Connective tissue diseases.

Historically, the conditions associated are:
- Secondary syphilis (father-in-law sign)
- Lepromatous leprosy
- Rubella
- Leishmaniasis.

Lower Extremity Lymph Nodes

Inguinal Lymph Nodes

- Lymphatic of the lower limb follows the venous supply
- It consists of both superficial and deep systems. Deep nodes cannot be palpable
- Superficial nodes are divided into two groups (Figs 2.30A and B):
  1. Horizontal group lies below the inguinal ligament on the anterior aspect. It drains superficial portions of the lower abdomen and buttock, the external genitalia excluding the testes, the anal canal, perianal area and the lower vagina.
  2. Vertical groups are situated near upper part of saphenous vein. Afferents come from lower limb, along the great saphenous vein, penis, scrotum and perineal region.

Significance of Enlarged Inguinal Lymph Nodes
Adult, who uses to walk in the outdoor.

Infections:
- Cellulitis
- *Venereal disease:*
  - Syphilis
  - Chancroid
  - Genital herpes
  - Lymphogranuloma venereum.
- *Cancers:*
  - Lymphoma
  - Melanoma
  - Carcinoma of penis or valva.
  In above cases, biopsy of the node is informative.

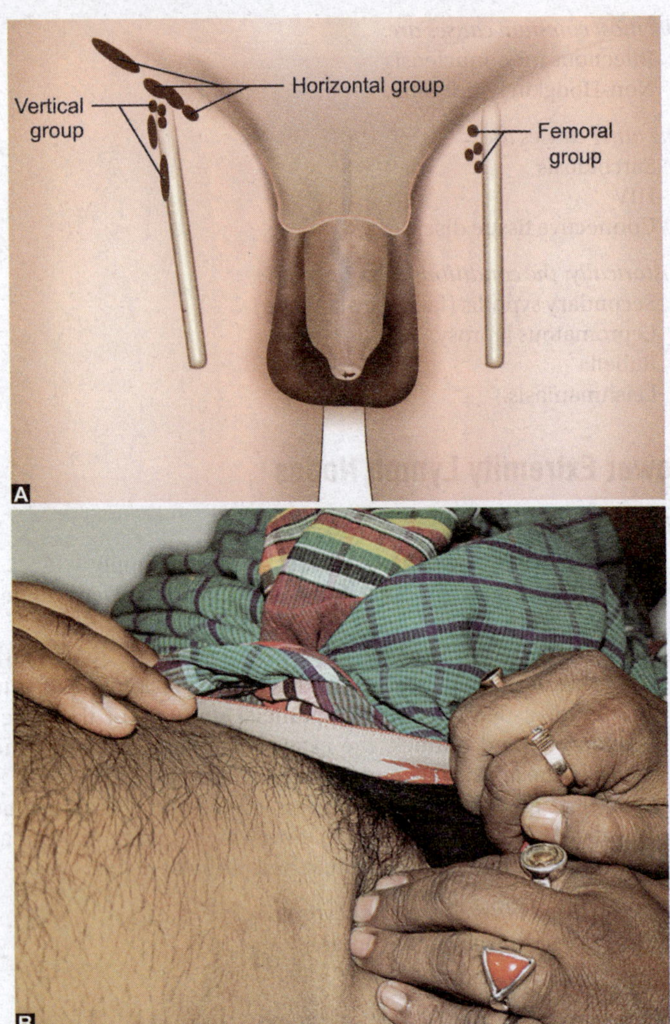

FIGS 2.30A AND B (A) Inguinal and femoral group of lymph nodes, (B) Method of palpation of inguinal lymph nodes

Node of Rosenmüller-Cloquet
A deep inguinal lymph node near to femoral canal, when enlarged pathologically, may be mistaken as inguinal hernia.

Femoral Lymph Nodes

- Femoral nodes are medial to inguinal lymph nodes and closer to genital area
- They are much less significant
- Their enlargement is associated with dermatophytosis of the foot.

Popliteal Lymph Nodes (Fig. 2.31)

- Popliteal nodes are very difficult to palpate
- Use both hands to palpate the node in inguinal fossa, when knee flexed to less than 45°
- They are of little significance.

Sister Mary Joseph's nodule

- It is periumbilical node or hard mass—it represents direct or lymphoid metastasis from intrapelvic or intra-abdominal tumor
- This is first reported by William J Mayo, based on the observation by his scrub nurse, sister Mary Joseph
- Umbilicus has multiple anatomic, vascular and embryologic connections. The causes are:
  - ❖ Adenocarcinoma of stomach
  - ❖ Ovarian cancer
  - ❖ Large bowel cancer
  - ❖ Pancreatic cancer.

In 14 to 33 percent of cases, umbilical metastasis is the first and diagnostic manifestation of occult neoplasm.

Dolphin Nodes (Fig. 2.32)

- There are cluster of pharyngeal nodes
- *Site:* Located on thyroid membrane, anterior to cricothyroid ligament, just above the thymus
- They are easily palpable if enlarged
- They at times may be confused with pyramidal lobe of the gland

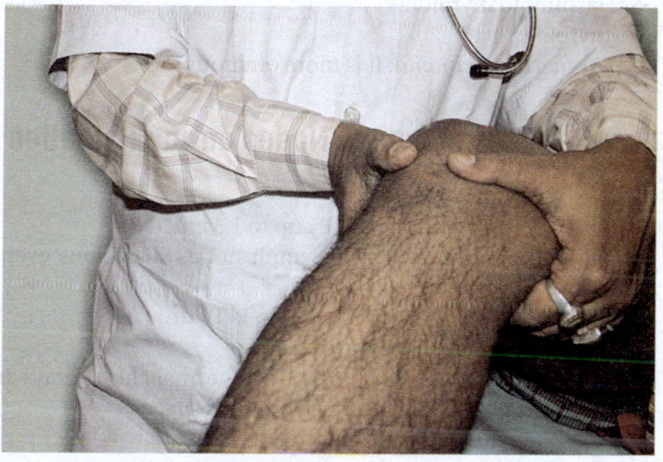

FIG. 2.31   Popliteal lymph nodes

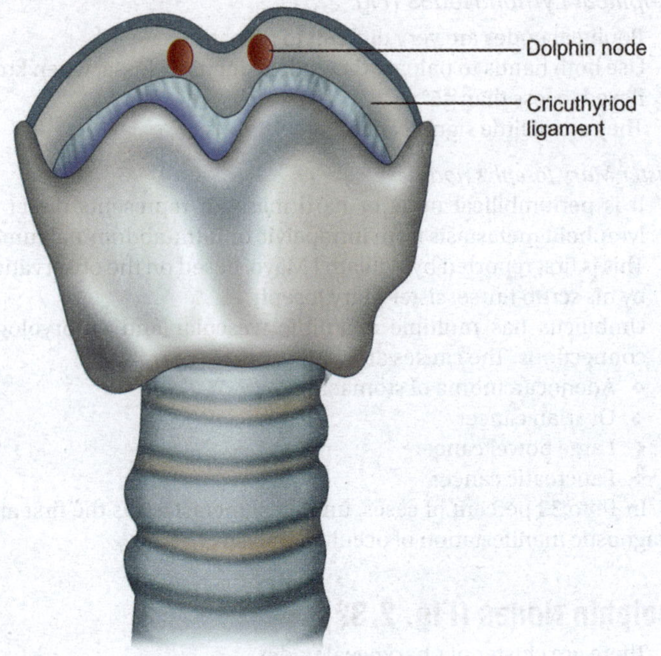

FIG. 2.32 Dolphin nodes 8

- They drain thyroid and larynx
- Palpable Dolphin nodes represent:
  - ❖ Subacute thyroiditis
  - ❖ Hashimoto thyroiditis
  - ❖ Thyroid cancer
  - ❖ *Laryngeal carcinoma:* It is more ominous sign.

Characteristics of Lymph Nodes during Palpation

Size

- Inguinal lymph node—normally up to 1.5 cm
- Preauricular and epitrochlear lymph nodes suspicious even if they are 0.5 to 1.0 cm
- Large and benign nodes are common in IV drug users
- Nodes <1 cm is never neoplastic
- In children, nodes >2 cm along with abnormal chest X-rays and absence of ear, nose and throat symptoms suggest:
  - ❖ Granulomatous disease (cat-scratch disease, sarcoidosis)
  - ❖ Cancers (mostly lymphoma)

Duration

Longer the duration, it is present, less likely it is in risk of neoplasm or granulomatous disease. In few cases, lymphoma regresses temporarily.

Consistency

- Soft—infectious or inflammatory disease
- Rock like—primary or metastatic malignancy
- Firm and rubbery—Hodgkin's disease
- Fluctuant/tense ballon-like tender—lymphadenitis
- Fluctuant nodes fistulize through skin—sinuses
- Buboes—Gonorrhea, syphilis, plague.

Matting

Fusion into scalloped mass transforms individual node into conglomerates.
- Neoplastic (metastatic or lymphoma)
- Inflammatory (sarcoid)
- Chronic infection (tuberculosis, lymphogranuloma venereum).

Relationship with Surrounding Tissue

Adherence to surrounding subcutaneous tissue and skin show—neoplastic lesion.

Pain/tenderness

It is due to rapid growth and painful capsular stretching. Occurs in:
- Suppurative inflammation
- Hemorrhage into necrotic center.

So, tenderness cannot differentiate benign from neoplastic lesion.

In other words:
- *Benign nodes:* Small, discrete, nontender, mobile, soft
- *Neoplastic nodes:* Large, nontender, rock-hard, matted fixed, rubbery
- *Inflammatory:* Tender, firm, occasionally fluctuant, matted and fixed.

Normally, palpable lymph nodes are:
- Submandibular nodes
- Inguinal nodes
- Axillary nodes occasionally.

Lymph node enlargement occurs due to:
- Stimulation by regional or systemic immune response
- Direct infection of the node lead to suppuration

- Deposition of intracellular or extracellular material
- Infiltration with neoplastic cells.

Lymphadenopathy

Presence of abnormal lymph nodes in terms of:
- Size
- Consistency
- Number.

Lymphadenopathy may be:
- *Localized:* When enlargement of the lymph node occur in a single region or one group in a single region. This is most common.
  - ❖ *Ulceroglandular syndromes:* It is due to cutaneous inoculation of infectious agents followed by spread through subcutaneous lymphatics producing inflammation and indurations of the nodes
  - ❖ *Acute cervical lymphadenopathy:* Localized infections of scalp, face, mouth, teeth, pharynx associated with inflamed draining nodes
  - ❖ *Genital lesion with satellite nodes:* Syphilis, chancroid, herpes simplex, lymphogranuloma venereum, tuberculosis associated with enlarged draining nodes
  - ❖ Suppurative lymphadenopathy.
- *Generalized lymphadenopathy:* When enlargement occur in two or more contagious sites: Due to systemic process—infectious, inflammatory or neoplastic.

• Hematological malignancy	Lymphoma Leukemia Angioimmunoblastic lymphadenopathy
• Collagen vascular disease	Rheumatoid arthritis Sarcoidosis Systemic lupus erythematosus
• Infections	Syphilis HIV Tuberculosis Infectious mononucleosis Cytomegalovirus infection Toxoplasmosis Brucellosis Histoplasmosis Coccidioidomycosis
• Drugs	Phenytoin Cephalosporin Penicillin Sulphonamide

General characteristics that can help to interpret an abnormal nodes:
- A—Age of the patients
- L—Location of abnormal lymph nodes
- L—Length of time the nodes have been present
- A—Associated symptoms—whether local or extranodal
- G—Presence or absence of generalized lymphadenopathy
- E—Extranodal sites
- S—Presence or absence of splenomegaly and or, fever.

Few lymph nodes remain enlarged after infection. They are:
- Tonsillar lymph nodes
- Submandibular lymph nodes
- Submental lymph nodes.

They are small, <1 cm, nontender, rubbery in consistency.

They are sequelae of past infection, like pharyngitis or dental infection.

Shotty Lymph Nodes

They are small, like tiny peas, nontender, nonstony or hard, equal, mobile, round, well demarcated, found in cervical region in children with viral illness. They may outlast the illness by several weeks. It is of no clinical importance.

Differential Diagnosis of Unexplained Lymphadenopathy

CHICAGO
- *(C) Cancer:*
    - *Hematological malignancy:*
        - Hodgkin's lymphoma
        - Non-Hodgkin's lymphoma
        - Acute and chronic lymphatic leukemia
        - Multiple myeloma
        - Waldenstorm macroglobulinemia
        - Systemic mastocytosis.
    - *Metastatic solid tumor:*
        - Breast
        - Lung
        - Prostate
        - Renal cell.
- *(H) Hypersensitivity syndrome.*
    - Scrum sickness
    - Drug sensitivity (diphenylhydantoin, carbamazepine, gold, allopurinol, indomethacin, sulphonamide)
    - Silicon reaction
    - Graft-versus-host disease
    - Vaccination related.

- *(I) Infections:*
  - ❖ *Viral:*
    - Infectious mononucleosis
    - CMV
    - Infective hepatitis
    - Adenovirus
    - Herpes zoster
    - HIV
    - Postvaccinal lymphadenitis.
  - ❖ *Bacterial:*
    - Cutaneous infections—*Staphylococcus, Streptococcus*
    - Cat-scratch fever
    - Chancroid
    - Tuberculosis
    - Atypical mycobacteria
    - Primary syphilis
    - Secondary syphilis.
  - ❖ Chlamydial infection—Lymphogranuloma Venereum
  - ❖ Protozoal—Toxoplasmosis
  - ❖ Mycotic—Histoplasmosis
  - ❖ Rickettsial—Scrub typhus
  - ❖ Helminthic—Filariasis.
- *(C) Connective tissue diseases:*
  - ❖ Rheumatoid arthritis
  - ❖ SLE
  - ❖ Mixed connective tissue disease
  - ❖ Dermatomyositis
  - ❖ Sjögren syndrome.
- *(A) Atypical lymphoproliferative disorder:*
  - ❖ Angiofollicular lymph node dysplasia
  - ❖ Angioimmunoblastic lymphadenopathy
  - ❖ Angiocentric immunoproliferative disorders
  - ❖ Wegener granulomatosis.
- *(G) Granulomatosis:*
  - ❖ Tuberculosis
  - ❖ Histoplasmosis
  - ❖ Cryptococcosis
  - ❖ Cat-scratch fever
  - ❖ Silicosis.
- *(O) Other unusual cases:*
  - ❖ Idiopathic pseudotumor of lymph node
  - ❖ Histiocytic necrotizing lymphadenopathy
  - ❖ Sinus histiocytosis with massive lymphadenopathy.

■ Clubbing

Definition

It is a bulbous swelling of connective tissue of the terminal phalanges with loss of normal angle of the nail bed and nail (acute angle becomes obtuse). The angle is called Lovibond angle.

Involvement

- It may involve fingers or toes or both
- It may be bilateral symmetrical or unilateral
- It may involve single digit.

Causes of Clubbing

- *Cardiovascular causes:*
  - ❖ Congenital cyanotic heart disease
  - ❖ Causes of right to left heart shunt
  - ❖ Subacute bacterial endocarditis
  - ❖ Infected aortic bypass graft.
- *Lung causes:*
  - ❖ *Intrathoracic causes:*
    - Bronchiectasis
    - Lung abscess
    - Bronchogenic carcinoma
    - Pneumoconiosis
    - Interstitial fibrosis
    - Chronic bronchitis
    - Metastatic lung disease
    - Cystic fibrosis
    - Sarcoidosis.
  - ❖ *Extrathoracic causes:*
    - Empyema
    - Hodgkin's disease
    - Mesothelioma.
- *Gastrointestinal causes:*
  - ❖ *Luminal:*
    - Inflammatory disease
    - Carcinoma of esophagus
    - Achalasia.
  - ❖ *Hepatic causes:*
    - Cirrhosis
    - Primary biliary cirrhosis.
- *Malignancies:*
  - ❖ Thyroid malignancy
  - ❖ Hodgkin's disease
  - ❖ Chronic myeloid leukemia.

- *Miscellaneous:*
  - ❖ Pregnancy
  - ❖ Acromegaly.
- Idiopathic
- Normal
- Genetic.

Causes of Painful Clubbing

Bronchogenic carcinoma

Causes of differential clubbing: In congenital cyanotic type heart disease—due to pumping of desaturated blood to either upper or lower limb—only affected hands or feet will show clubbing.

The disorders are:
- *Patent ductus arteriosus with pulmonary hypertension:* In this case, desaturated blood produces cyanosis and/or clubbing of affected feet and spares the hands
- *Origin of great vessels from right ventricle:* In this case reverse shunt affects upper limb and spares feet
- If right ventricular origin of great vessels are associated with patent ductus arteriosus and ventricular septal defect and pulmonary hypertension.
  - ❖ Oxygenated blood from left ventricle enters the pulmonary trunk through the ventricular septal defect

    ↓

    This blood shunts through patent ductus arteriosus into descending aorta

    ↓

    To the lower extremities

    ↓

    No cyanosis or clubbing in the lower extremities

    ↓

  - ❖ Deoxygenated blood from right ventricle

    ↓

    Enters ascending aorta and brachiocephalic vessels

    ↓

    Hands become cyanotic and clubbed

So this is reverse differential cyanosis.

Causes of Unilateral Clubbing

- Aneurysm of aorta or subclavian arteries
- Pancoast tumor
- Lymphangitis
- Surgical arteriovenous fistula (less common).

Diagnostic Features of Clubbing

- *Angle between the base of the nail and surrounding skin*—called Lovibond's angle (unguophalangeal angle)—Normally, this angle is <180° (Fig. 2.33).

  In clubbing, this angle is obliterated or obscured.

  This can be visualized by keeping a paper or pencil over the angle.

  Normally, there is a window between nail and pencil or paper. This angle cannot be visualized in clubbing.
- *Ballotability of nail bed:* Increased sponginess of the base of the nail bed. This can be detected by (Fig. 2.34):

  When the skin proximal to nail bed is compressed, nail sinks deep towards the bone.

  Upon release, it springs upward and backward, it is just like pushing and releasing ice cube down a pot of water.
- *Abnormal phalangeal depth ratio (Fig. 2.35):* This is the ratio of distal phalangeal depth measured at the cuticle (DPD).

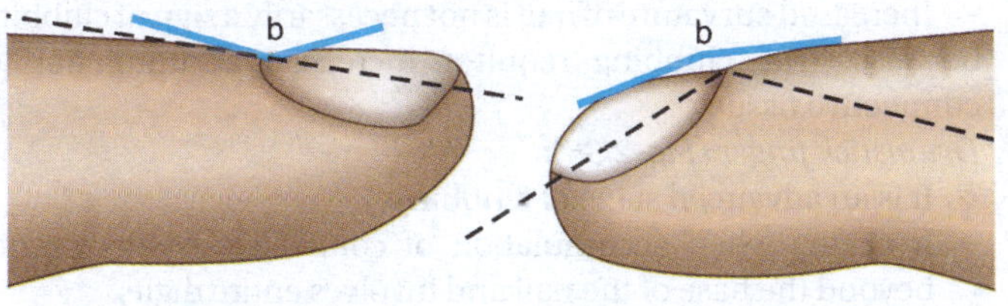

FIG. 2.33   Lovibond angle

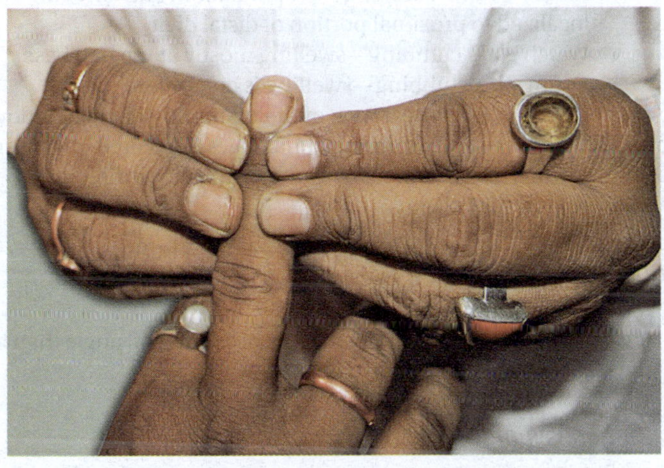

FIG. 2.34   Method of ballotability

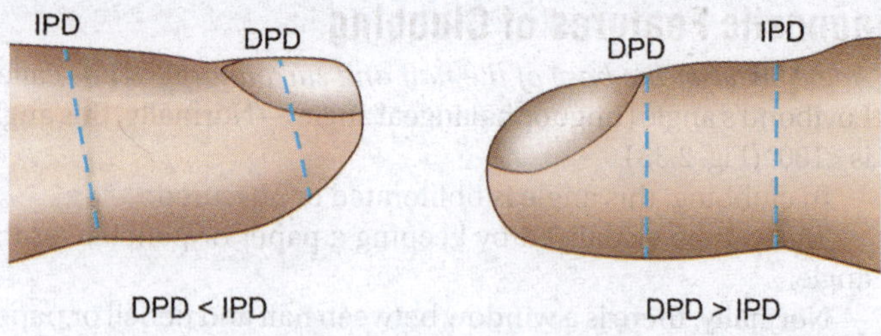

FIG. 2.35 Phalangeal depth ratio

Interphalangeal depth is measured at interphalangeal joint (IPD).

- ❖ Normally DPD/IPD is 0.895—it means gradual tapering of finger tip from distal interphalangeal joint
- ❖ In clubbing, DPD/IPD is >1.0, it is found in children with cystic fibrosis (85%).

  Ballotability is not exclusive indication because it can be found in elderly patient with no clubbing.

  Increased curvature of nail is not necessarily a sign of clubbing because, true clubbing requires increased accumulation of connective tissue.

- *Drumstick finger (Fig. 2.36):*
  - ❖ It is an advanced stage of clubbing
  - ❖ It occurs when accumulation of connective tissue extends beyond the base of the nail and involves entire digits
  - ❖ Depending on the sites of accumulation, few terms have been created:
    - • Parrot beak's clubbing—accumulation and swelling are localized to proximal portion of distal digit
    - • Watch glass clubbing—swelling mostly at the nail base
    - • Drum stick clubbing—swelling is circumferential.

Schamroth's sign: Disappearance of the diamond-shaped window, normally present when terminal phalanges of paired digits are juxtaposed, this is described by South African cardiologist, Leo Schamroth (Fig. 2.37).

Congenital Clubbing

- It is relatively common
- It is characterized by more by the loss of subungual angle than by the ballotment.

Pathogenesis of Clubbing

Normally, large platelets are filtered by pulmonary vasculature. But in any situation of pulmonary damage, vascular shunt, these large

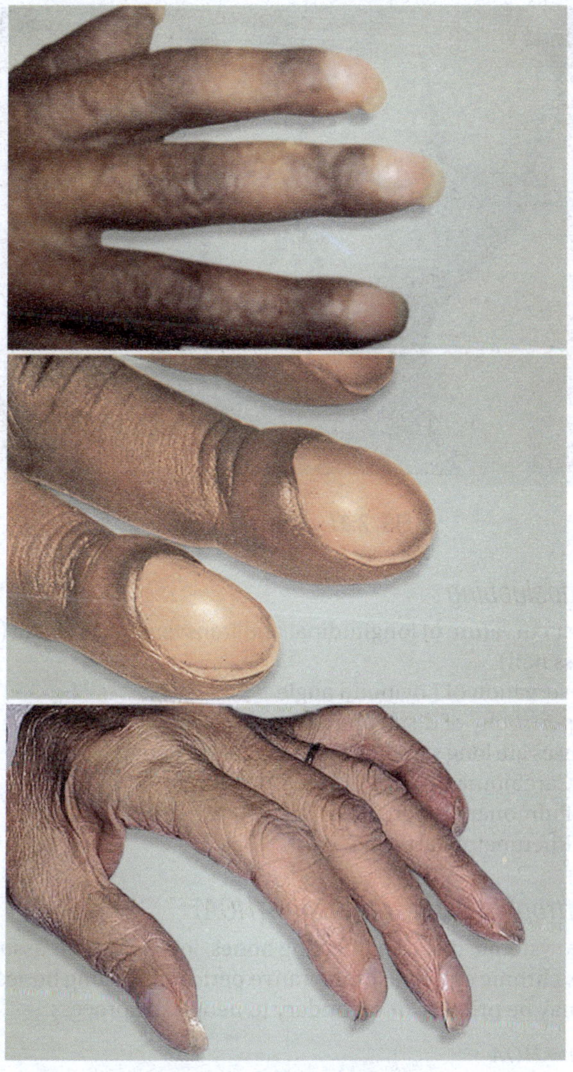

FIG. 2.36 Clubbing

platelets escape filtration and reach the distal digits, they clump, release mediators and produce fibrovascular response, proliferation of fibrovascular tissue at the base of nail bed.

In case of infected dialysis shunt or infective endocarditis, platelet clumps originate directly on the damaged vascular surface, escape and lodge in the digital vessels and trigger fibrovascular response.

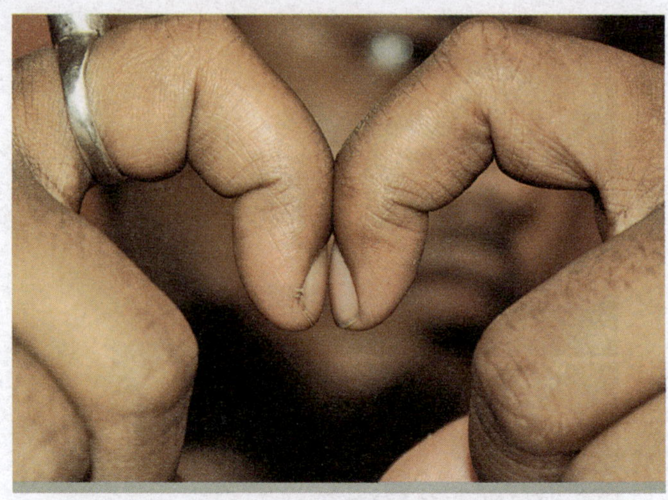

FIG. 2.37 Schamroth's sign

Pseudoclubbing

- Over curvature of longitudinal and transverse axes of nail (watch glass nail)
- Preservation of Lovibond angle
- Hypertrophy of distal phalanx
- Causes are long standing and debilitated condition, such as:
  - ❖ Carcinoma of lung
  - ❖ Pulmonary tuberculosis
  - ❖ Rheumatoid arthritis.

Hypertrophic Osteoarthropathy (HOA)

- It is systemic disorder affecting bones, joints and soft tissues
- It is chronic systemic proliferative periostitis of long bones
- It may be primary or secondary to neoplastic process.

Primary HOA

It is congenital autosomal dominant disorder called pachy-dermoperiostosis.

Pachydermoperiostosis: It is subperiosteal new bone formation, especially distal end of long bones.

Associated skin changes are:

- Thickening and furrowing oiliness of facial forehead and skin
- Seborrheic hyperplasia.

Secondary HOA

- Bronchogenic carcinoma
- Lymphoma

- Mesothelioma.
- Metastatic cancer.

Bones predominantly affected in HOA

Diaphysis of long bones is affected. The bone involved in descending disorder are:

- Radius
- Ulna
- Tibia
- Fibula
- Humerus
- Femur
- Metacarpals
- Metatarsals
- Proximal and middle phalanges.

Other diagnostic features include:

- Symmetrical arthritis like changes in ankle, wrist, knee, elbows.
- Coarsening of subcutaneous tissues in distal portions of arms and legs.
- Neurovascular changes in hands feet (chronic erythema, paresthesias, increased sweating).

Association between clubbing and HOA

Some diseases are associated with clubbing and HOA, e.g.

- Bronchogenic carcinoma
- Lung abscess
- Cystic fibrosis
- Bronchiectasis
- Diseases not associated with HOA—pulmonary interstitial fibrosis.

Hypertrophic osteoarthropathy is occasionally symptomatic:

- In few cases, frank bony pain and tenderness
- Pretibial skin is shiny, thickened and warm to touch
- Autonomic manifestations may be present.

Thyroid acropachy: Acroperipheral, Pachy—thick:

- It is thickening of peripheral tissues.
- It occurs in 1 percent of Graves' disease—associated with other infiltrative manifestations, such as myxedema of feet and hands and exophthalmos.
- It may be associated with clubbing and periosteal new bone formation.

It can be differentiated from HOA

- It usually involves hands and feet, rather than long bones
- It is usually painless
- Joints are not involved.

Cyanosis (Fig. 2.38)

Normal Hb percent 100 cc blood = 15 g

   1 g of hemoglobin combines with 1.33 cc of O_2

   15 g of hemoglobin combines with $1.33 \times 15 = 19.95 = 20$ cc of O_2.

Normally Arterial Blood is 95 percent saturated

  100 percent saturation = 15 g of oxyhemoglobin.

$$1 \text{ percent saturation} = \frac{15}{100} \text{ of oxyhemoglobin}$$

$$95 \text{ percent saturation} = \frac{15 \times 95}{100} \text{ of oxyhemoglobin}$$

$$= 14.25 \text{ of oxyhemoglobin}$$

So 0.75 g of hemoglobin is reduced hemoglobin.

Venous blood is 70 percent saturated.

  100 percent saturation = 15 g of oxyhemoglobin.

$$1 \text{ percent saturation} = \frac{15}{100} \text{ of oxyhemoglobin}$$

$$70 \text{ percent saturation} = \frac{15 \times 95}{100} \text{ of oxyhemoglobin}$$

$$= 10.5 \text{ of oxyhemoglobin}$$

So reduced Hb percent in venous blood

$$= (15 - 10.5) = 4.5 \text{ g}$$

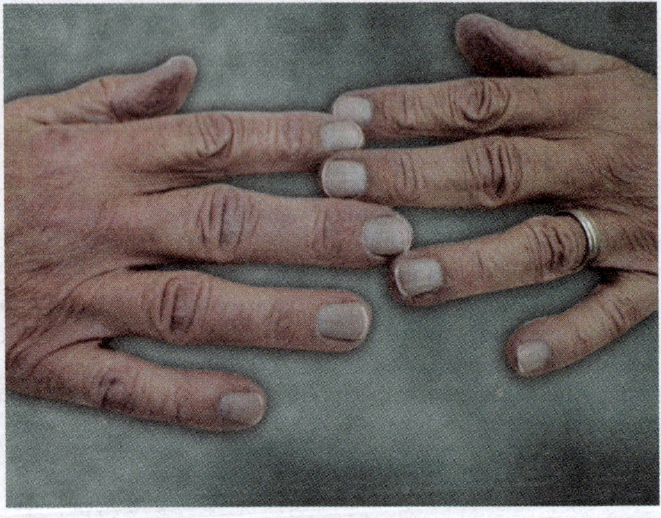

FIG. 2.38 Cyanosis

So reduced Hb% in capillary blood

$$= \frac{\text{Arterial reduced Hb\% + Venous reduced Hb\%}}{2}\ g$$

$$= \frac{0.75 + 4.5}{2}\ g = 2.6\ g$$

Cyanosis is the bluish discoloration of skin and mucous membrane when—reduced hemoglobin in capillary blood is >14 g %. There are other two types of abnormal hemoglobin in the blood.
These are:
- Methemoglobin
- Sulfhemoglobin.

So cyanosis, occurs also when:
- Methemoglobin > 1.5 gm%
- Sulfhemoglobin > 0.5 gm%.

Total amount of reduced hemoglobin depends upon the red cell mass:
- In polycythemia rubra, due to very high red cell mass, reduced hemoglobin content is also increased—producing central cyanosis at higher level of O_2 saturation
- In extreme anemia, when hemoglobin is ≤5 gm%, central cyanosis will never appear, because
Total red cell is decreased enormously
↓

Hemoglobin content is very low
In this case, in spite of very low arterial PO_2, total amount of reduced hemoglobin will never reach less than 5 gm%.

Three types of cyanosis are usually seen:
1. *Peripheral cyanosis:*
   - ❖ *Areas to be examined:*
     - Tip of nose
     - Ear lobule
     - Outer surface of lips
     - Cheeks
     - Peripheral part of body—extremities.
   - ❖ *Intensity of cyanosis depends upon:*
     - Thickness of the skin
     - Status of capillaries and venules of skin
     - Subpapillary venous plexus.
       This color in cyanosis—a mixture of red color of oxyhemoglobin and blue color of reduced hemoglobin—producing purplish color.
   - ❖ *Pathophysiology:*
     - Cutaneous vasoconstriction is due to:
       - Low cardiac output—in congestive cardiac failure, shock

- Vasospastic disorder—in extreme cold and Raynaud's phenomenon.

    Here arterial oxygen saturation is normal but venous oxygen saturation is very low due to low flow.

- *Vascular obstruction:*
    - Venous obstruction

        ↓

        Stagnation of blood in vein

        ↓

        Venus blood is of low O_2 content

        ↓

        Peripheral cyanosis
    - Arterial obstruction

        ↓

        Sudden fall in arterial pressure so that pulse is absent distal to obstruction. Very low amount of blood goes to periphery

        (Common causes are: Atrial fibrillation, vascular heart disease myocardial infarction)

        ↓

        Less amount of O_2 is supplied to peripheral tissue

        ↓

        Peripheral cyanosis
    - Embolism
    - *Thrombosis:* Atherosclerosis collagen disease
    - Arterial wall injury, myeloproliferative disorder.

    But in chronic obstruction, or obstruction is slowly progressing, surrounding collapsed collaterals open and reduce the intensity of cyanosis.
- ❖ Temperature of extremities is cold and calm.

2. *Central cyanosis:*
   - ❖ *Areas to be examined:*
       - Skin—tip of nose, earlobes, outer surface of lips, cheeks and extremities
       - Mucous membrane:
           - Inner surface lips
           - Tip of tongue
           - Bulbar conjunctiva.
   - ❖ *Temperature:* Peripheral extremities are cold.

       Central cyanosis appears when arterial oxygen saturation is below 85 percent.
   - ❖ *Mechanism of central cyanosis:* Central cyanosis appears due to three causes:
       i. *Anoxic cyanosis:* Inadequate oxygen supply to blood from lung due to following pathologic mechanism:

- *Ventilation/perfusion mismatch:*
  - Poor ventilation—COPD
  - Poor perfusion—pulmonary embolism.
- *Abnormalities in diffusion:*
  - Decrease in total surface area of lung due to rupture of alveoli
  - Thickening of interstitial area—pulmonary edema, pulmonary fibrosis.

ii. *Shunt or admixture cyanosis:* Free admixture of venous and arterial blood due to right to left heart shunt:
  - Pulmonary venous blood is fully saturated—due to 100 percent saturation in lung
  - Inhalation of 100 percent oxygen—cannot reduce cyanosis.

iii. Replacement cyanosis:
  - Concentration of methemoglobin and sulfhemoglobin are high >0.5 gm%
  - Arterial oxygen saturation is normal
  - Central cyanosis may be associated with:
    - Polycythemia
    - Clubbing.

3. *Mixed cyanosis*

Here both central and peripheral cyanosis coexist. The diseases producing mixed cyanosis:

- Left ventricular failure

↓

Increased left atrial pressure

↓

Increased pulmonary venous pressure

↓

Increased pulmonary capillary pressure

↓

Pulmonary edema

↓

Decrease O_2 content due to diminished transport of O_2 from alveoli to blood

↓

Central cyanosis.

Low cardiac output

↓

Peripheral vasoconstriction

↓

Decreased tissue perfusion of oxygen

↓

Peripheral cyanosis

- Chronic bronchitis and emphysema

  $\downarrow$

  Diminished transport of oxygen from lung to capillary blood

  $\downarrow$

  Central cyanosis

In long-standing cases, it produces pulmonary hypertension

$\downarrow$

$\uparrow$ Right ventricular diastolic pressure

$\downarrow$

$\uparrow$ Right atrial pressure

$\downarrow$

Peripheral cyanosis

Acrocyanosis

- The cyanosis occurs in acral parts of limbs due to exposure to cold
- It may be associated with excessive sweating
- Pain may be present.

Erythrocyanosis

It is a vasomotor (autonomic) disorder characterized by:
- It occurs in female in cold weather
- Bluish discoloration of legs, along with coldness
- The affected area will have burning pain and itching.

Intensity of Central Cyanosis

It depends upon:
- *Temperature* $\uparrow$ temperature $\rightarrow$ $\uparrow$ vasodilatation $\rightarrow$ $\downarrow$ cyanosis
  $\downarrow$ Temperature $\rightarrow$ vasoconstriction $\rightarrow$ cyanosis
- *Exercise:* Exercise

  $\downarrow$

  Decreases peripheral vascular resistance

  $\downarrow$

  Increase shunting of blood from right to left across the defect

  $\downarrow$

  Decrease O_2 content of arterial blood
- *Fetal hemoglobin:*
  If increase concentration of fetal hemoglobin

  $\downarrow$

  Increased affinity for O_2

  $\downarrow$

  Decreased release of O_2 into tissues

  $\downarrow$

  Cyanosis

- *Volume of right to left heart shunt:*
  If volume of right to left heart shunt is >25 percent of left ventricular output
  ↓
  Central cyanosis
- *pH of blood:* If blood pH is acidic
  ↓
  Shifting of oxygen hemoglobin dissociation curve to left
  ↓
  Cyanosis
- *Blood 2,3-diphosphoglycerate increases*
  ↓
  Shifting of oxygen—hemoglobin dissociation curve to left
  ↓
  Oxygen release to tissue will be low
  ↓
  Cyanosis.

Cyanosis Tardive

It occurs in:
- Congenital heart disease
- Eisenmenger syndrome.
  Cyanosis occurs first in the second decade of life.

Differential Cyanosis

This can be defined by:
Cyanosis in some parts of the body, no cyanosis of other parts. This differential cyanosis can be subdivided into following types:
- *Cyanosis of lower limbs with little or no cyanosis of upper arms and face:*
  ❖ *Patient having congenital patent ductus arteriosus—develops pulmonary hypertension:* PDA is funnel shaped communication between pulmonary artery—connected at narrow end and aorta proximal to left subclavian artery at its wide end (Fig. 2.39).
    Normal PDA closes within 15 to 18 hours of birth of baby due to:
    - High oxygen tension of lung as a result of spontaneous respiration producing high O_2 content of blood.
    - Decreased prostaglandin levels due to placental ligation.
    - Increased metabolism of prostaglandin.
      Normally, the PDA in adult circulates blood from aorta to pulmonary artery producing left to right shut.

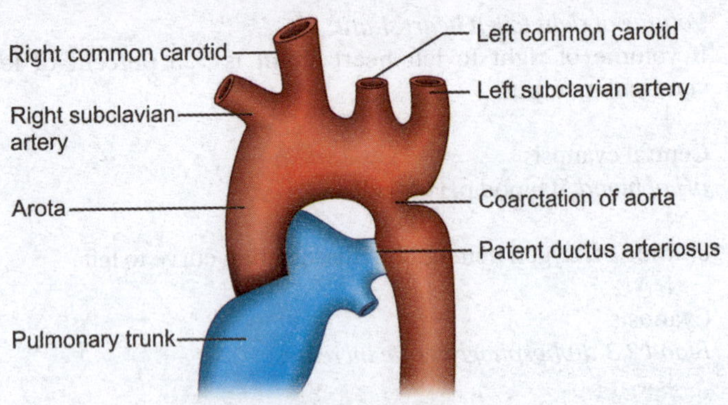

FIG. 2.39 Patent ductus arteriosus

But if patient develops pulmonary hypertension, blood flows from pulmonary artery to aorta—producing differential cyanosis, i.e.

- Face and right upper limb in normal in color
- Left arm and lower limbs are cyanosed.

❖ *Coarctation of aorta:* It is the narrowing in the region of the ligamentum arteriosus, remnant of ducts arteriosus, distal to the origin of left subclavian artery.

As a result pressure is descending aorta is low femoral pulse is of low volume and delayed in appearance in comparison to radial artery.

If patent ductus arteriosus is present—blood flows from high pressure site, pulmonary artery to low pressure zone, descending aorta, producing right to left heart shunt and differential cyanosis, i.e.

- Both upper limbs are normal in color
- Both lower limbs are cyanosed.

● *Reversed differential cyanosis:*

❖ Cyanosis of both upper limbs are higher than both lower limbs:

The causes are:

- Transposition of great arteries with preductal narrowing of aorta (coarctation or interrupted aortic arch) and reverse flow through patent ductus arteriosus (from pulmonary artery to aorta).

In TGA, there is ventriculoarterial discordance—as a result:

- *Deoxygenated blood flows* → right atrium → across tricuspid valve → right ventricle → aorta → systemic arteries.
- *Oxygenated blood flows* → left atrium → across mitral valve → left ventricle → pulmonary artery → to lung.

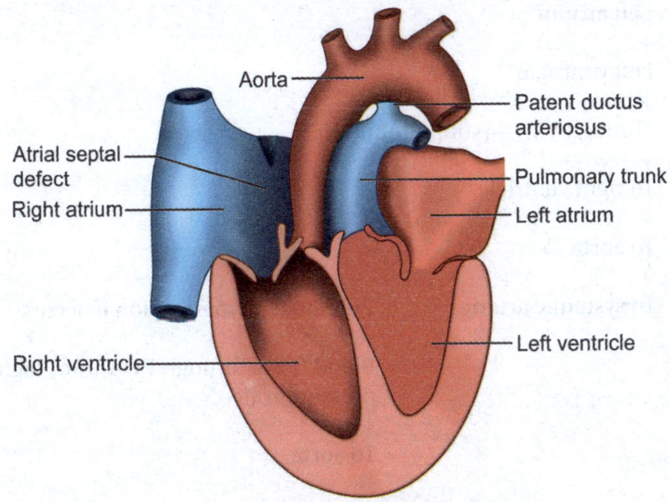

FIG. 2.40 Transposition of great vessels: PDA and ASO

In absence of ASD, VSD and PDA, there is no shunting of blood. Therefore, life is incompatible.

If bidirection is present, patient can survive (Fig. 2.40). In case of pulmonary artery hypertension if there is PDA → blood flows from pulmonary artery to aorta—producing reverse differential cyanosis, i.e.
  - Upper limbs are cyanotic
  - Lower limbs are normal in color.
- In transposition of great arteries.
  Pulmonary hypertension patent ducts arteriosus.
- *Double outlet right ventricle (DORV):* Here both pulmonary artery and aorta arise from right ventricle.

Here deoxygenated blood flow through pulmonary artery and aorta, if there is no VSD present.

If there is VSD, in DORV:
(Subpulmonic)
Blood
↓
Right atrium
↓
Right ventricle
↓
Pulmonary artery and aorta
↓
Blood flows through lungs
↓

Left atrium
↓
Left ventricle
↓
Through VSD—(subpulmonic)
↓
To right ventricle
↓
To aorta →
↓
To systemic arteries   Pulmonary hypertension if occurs
↓
Blood flows through PDA from high-pressure zone
↓
To aorta

Evaluation of Cyanosis

Skin or mucous membrane mimicking cyanosis:

- *Smokers lips:* There is bluish discoloration in chronic smoker.
- *Bluish skin:* Due to deposition of silver salt can be differentiated by pressure:
  - ❖ Cyanotic skin blanches
  - ❖ Silver deposited skin cannot blanch.
- *Pigmented tongue:* It is patchy in distribution rather than generalized.

Age of Cyanosis

- *At birth:* CHD, TOA
- *2 to 5 months of age:* TOF.
- *Bimodal distribution:*
  - ❖ 2 to 5 months of age—Eisenmenger syndrome with VSD
  - ❖ >10 years age—Eisenmenger syndrome with VSD
  - ❖ >20 years age—Eisenmenger syndrome with ASD.
- *Old age:* Cor pulmonale.
- *>30 to 50 years:* VSD with PH, ASD with PH.

Distribution of Cyanosis

- *Generalized cyanosis:*
  - ❖ Peripheral
  - ❖ Central
  - ❖ Mixed
  - ❖ Replacement cyanosis.

- *Cyanosis in lower limb:*
  - ❖ PDA pulmonary hypertension
  - ❖ Coarctation of aorta with PDA.
- *More in UL:* TGA with narrowing of aorta PDA and reverse flow.

Presence of any factor responsible for cyanosis:
- Exercise
- Heavy eating
- Straining at defecation
- Exposure to cold—Raynaud's phenomenon
- Diurnal variation:
  - ❖ In the morning—chronic bronchitis, TOF
  - ❖ Midnight—pulmonary edema.
- Position—in supine position—bronchial asthma.

Onset

Sudden
- Foreign body obstruction
- Laryngo—tracheobronchitis
- Postnasal drip at night
- Pulmonary edema.

Causes of Cyanosis

Patho-physiology	M	I	N	T
	Malformation	Inflammation	Neoplasm	Traumatic toxication
1. Decreased intake of oxygen	Foreign body	1. Acute laryngo-tracheo-bronchitis 2. Chronic bronchitis and emphysema 3. Asthma 4. Whooping cough		1. Pneumoconiosis 2. Lipoid pneumonia 3. Pneumothorax 4. Suffocation
2. Decreased absorption of oxygen		1. Sarcoidosis 2. Fibrosis of lung 3. Alveolar proteinosis 4. Emphysema	1. Oat cell carcinoma 2. Metastatic carcinoma	
3. Decreased perfusion in lung	1. Congenital heart disease, ToF		1. Hemangioma	
4. Decreased combining power of blood				1. Copoisoning 2. Methemoglobinemia 3. Sulfhemoglobinemia

Pseudocyanosis

Bluish tinge of skin and mucous membrane not associated with hypoxemia or peripheral vasoconstriction. The causes are:

Metals

- Silver nitrate
- Silver iodide
- Silver lead.

Drugs

- Phenothiazine
- Chloroquine hydrochloride
- Amiodarone
- Colloidal silver for urinary tract infection.

Sulfhemoglobin

- Intense blue color of skin
- Caused by binding of sulfur with hemoglobin, so that oxygen cannot be bound
- Unlike methemoglobin, reduced hemoglobin is in Fe^{++} state.

Raynaud's phenomenon: It is due to tonic muscular contraction of digital arteries, mainly of fingers (may occur in toes) due to vasospasm in exposure to extreme cold.

Causes

- Primary Raynaud's phenomenon
- Secondary Raynaud's phenomenon due to:
  - ❖ Occlusive vascular disease
  - ❖ Collagen vascular disease
  - ❖ Thoracic outlet syndrome
  - ❖ Occupational hazards—exposed to high frequency vibrations
  - ❖ Cryoglobulinemia
  - ❖ Drugs—propranolol, ergot.

Primary Raynaud's phenomenon

- Mainly young female—in teenage and menopause
- Extremely sensitive to cold
- Bilateral symmetrical
- Mainly present in fingers
- Color change to white—during early phase of loss of vascularity.

  Blue → In early recovery phase due to circulated deoxygenated blood

  Red → In late phase—due to vasodilatation after spasm.

Secondary Raynaud's phenomenon
- Abrupt onset
- Unilateral
- It occurs in men.

If ischemic change is progressively increased:
- Gangrene and ulceration from prolonged tissue hypoxia.

Methemoglobinemia

- Normal methemoglobin content is <1 percent
- Methemoglobin level (3-15%)—discoloration—pale, gray, blue
- At 15 to 20 percent—methemoglobin level—slaty gray cyanosis
- At 25 to 50 percent—CNS manifestations like—headache, dyspnea, syncope, weakness, and confusion
- At 50 to 70 percent—cardiovascular—abnormal rhythm CNS—seizures, coma metabolic acidosis.

Physiology

Each hemoglobin composed of 4 polypeptides and 4 heme groups. Iron is present in two forms in heme group:
1. Ferrous form or reduced form
2. Ferric form or oxidized form.

In ferrous state iron combines with oxygen by taking one electron to form oxyhemoglobin—in tissue—oxygen is released from iron and revert it to ferrous form.

In ferric state—iron looses electrons, to become oxidized and form methemoglobin. It lacks electron to bind with oxygen, so no oxygen is being transported.

In spite of constant oxidant stress, low level of methemoglobin is maintained by two important mechanisms:
1. Hexose monophosphate shunt pathway within the RBC—through this pathway oxidizing agents is reduced by glutathione—prior to formation of methemoglobin.
2. *Two enzyme systems:* Diaphorase I and diaphorase II.

Diaphorase I and diaphorase II require NANH and NADPH respectively to reduce iron from ferric state and ferrous state:

Diaphorase II activation is activated by cofactor methelene blue.

Pathophysiology

- Oxidized form reduces the oxygen carrying capacity of Hb
- Ferric heme group impairs the release of oxygen from nearby ferrous heme group
- Methemoglobin impairs the release of oxygen to tissues and shift the oxygen dissociation curve to the left.

When methemoglobin increases progressively to 70 percent
↓
There is evidence of cellular hypoxia
↓
Death.

Causes

Congenital:

Lack of cellular protective abilities

- NADH methemolgobin reductase deficiency.
- Hemoglobin M disease → hemoglobin is not able to be reduced
- Pyruvate kinase deficiency → impairment of glycolytic pathway
- It G-6PD deficiency → may have impaired production of NADPH in hexose monophosphate shunt.

Acquired

- Children <4 years of age have underdeveloped NADH methemoglobin reductase system
  ↓
  In GI infection—overgrowth of bacteria
  ↓
  Produces oxidant stress.
- *Adult:*
  - ❖ *Pharmacologic agent:*
    - Anesthetic agents (Benzocaine, Lidocaine)
    - Chloroquine
    - Dapsone
    - Nitrites
    - Nitrates
    - Nitroglycerin
    - Phenacetin.
  - ❖ *Environmental agent:*
    - Aniline dyes
    - Aromatic amines
    - Chlorate
    - Chlorobenzene.

Diagnosis can be done by:

- Decreased O_2 saturation in presence of normal PO_2
- Spectroscopic analysis of methemoglobin—band appears at 630 mm—decreased after addition of reducing agent
- When venous blood is starred for 15 minutes, a chocolate brown color is formed.

Sulfhemoglobinemia

Slaty gray cyanosis occurs when sulfhemoglobin content is > 0.5 g/dL in blood.

Kansas hemoglobin: Central cyanosis occurs when mutant hemoglobin (Kansas hemoglobin) is present in high concentration. This hemoglobin has low affinity for oxygen. So less oxygen is delivered to tissue producing cyanosis.

◼ Anemia

Anemia can be defined as a feeling of weakness, fatigue, malaise dyspnea associated with constellation of signs evidenced by pallor of mucous membrane of conjunctive, skin, nail bed, koilonychias, jaundice (due to breakdown of red blood cells), pica (consumption of nonbased items shut as dirt, paper, wax, grass, ice and hair) due to low hemoglobin context in blood.

Pallor can be seen in the following areas (Figs 2.41A to C):
- Lower palpebral conjunctiva
- Dorsum of the tongue and buccal mucous membrane
- Palmar crease
- General surface of the skin.

WIIOs hemoglobin threshold used to define anemia:
1 g/dL = 0.6206 mmol/L

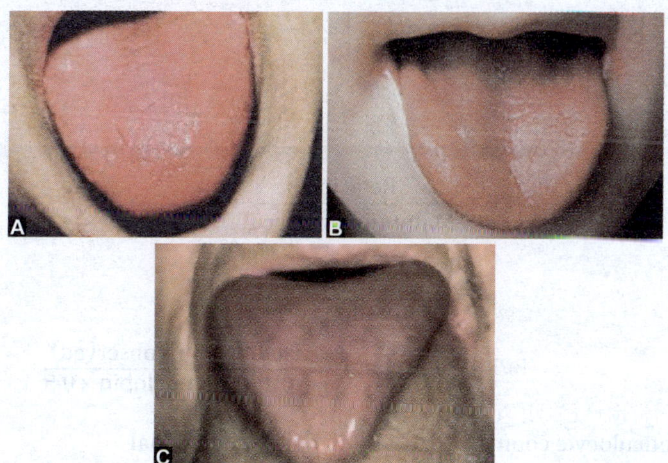

FIGS 2.41A TO C (A) Nutritional anemia, (B) Vitamin B_{12} deficiency anemia, (C) Iron deficiency anemia

Age or gender group	Hb% g/dL	Hb-threshold (mmol/L)
• Children (0.5–5 years)	11.0	6.8
• Children (5–12 years)	11.5	7.1
• Teens (12–15 years)	12.0	7.4
• Women, nonpregnant (>15 years)	12.0	7.4
• Women pregnant	11.0	6.8
• Men (>15 years)	13.0	8.1

Following laboratory tests should be used to quantity and type of anemia:

- *Reticulocyte count:* Normal level—0.5 to 1.5 percent
- *Reticulocyte index (also called corrected reticulocyte index):* Calculated value to diagnose anemia, because raw reticulocyte want is misleading in anemia patient.

Calculation:

$$\text{Retic index} = \text{Retic count} \times \frac{\text{Hct}}{\text{Normal Hct}}$$

$$45 = \text{Normal hematocrit}$$

Next step is to correct longer lifespan of prematurely released reticulocytes in the blood—a phenomenon of increased red blood cell production. This relies on a table:

Hct	Retic survival (days) – Maturation correction
• 36–45	1.0
• 26–35	1.5
• 16– 25	2.0
• ≤15	2.5

$$\text{RPI} = \frac{\text{Retic index}}{\text{Maturation correction}}$$

$$= \frac{\text{Retic count} \times \dfrac{\text{Hct}}{\text{Normal Hct}}}{\text{Maturation correction}}$$

$$\text{RPI} = \text{Retic count} \times \frac{\text{Hemoglobin (observed)}}{\text{Normal hemoglobin} \times 0.5}$$

Reticulocyte count = 1.0 to 2.5—in normal individual

Reticulocyte count = <1—decreased reticulocyte production

Reticulocyte count >2.5—increased RBC destruction leading to increased production of RBC.

Erythrocyte Sedimentation Rate (ESR)

$$\text{ESR (mm/hr)} = \frac{\text{Age (years)} + 10 \text{ (if female)}}{2}$$

Age	20	55	90
Men	12	14	19
Women	18	21	23

Normal range
Newborn—0 to 2 mm/hour
Neonatal to puberty—3 to 13 mm/hour

Serum Folate Level

- Normal—5 to 20 ng/mL.
- Negative balance/Deplete stores/Tissue deficiencies/Anemia is <3 ng/mL.

RBC folic acid level (ng/mL)
- Normal >200
- Negative balance <200
- Deplete stores/Tissue deficiency/Anemia = <200.

Vitamin B$_{12}$ Deficiency (pg/mL):

- Serum cobalamin—200 to 900
- Negative balance—150 to 500
- Deplete stores—100 to 300
- Tissue deficiency—50 to 250
- Anemia—50 to 250.

Nail

Anatomic Details of Nails (Figs 2.42A to C)

Lunula: While half-moon at the proximal edge of nail bed
Cuticle: Thin skin adherent to nail at the proximal portion
Nail grows: 0.1 to 0.15 mm/day.

Methods of Examination of Nail Bed

Although finger nails are more informative than toenails, but examine both carefully.
- Examine with out pressure thoroughly.
- Blanch fingertips to see any pigmented lesion, changes color (which would argue for discoloration of vascular bed rather than nail plate).

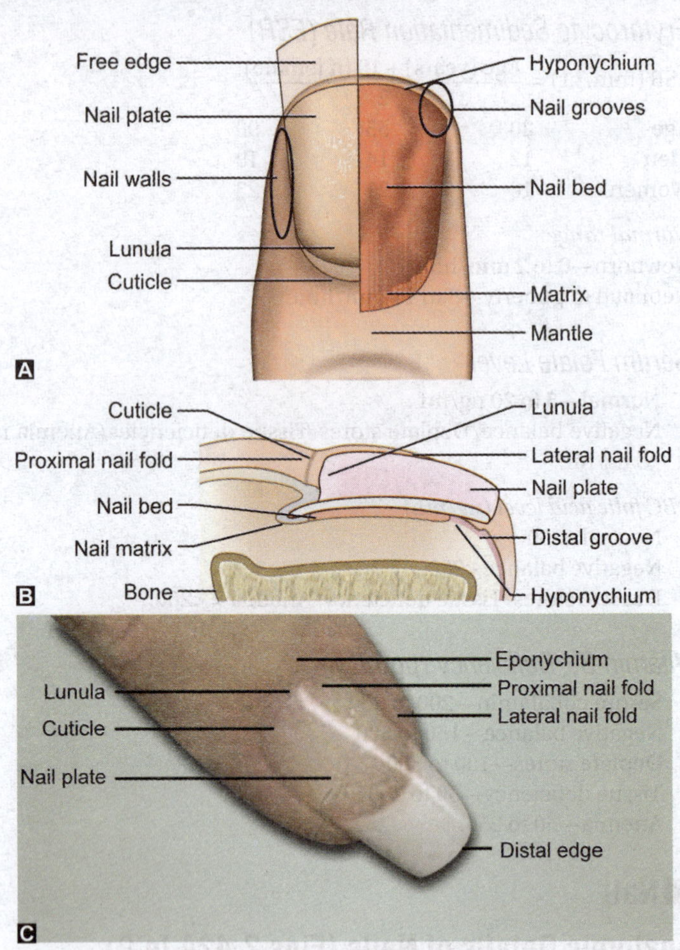

FIGS 2.42A TO C Nail structure

- Place a pencil right against finger pulp and shine it through nail. If upon illumination, discoloration disappears, it is more likely to be in vascular bed than in soft tissue or matrix.
- Scrap the nail plate surface and do KOH preparation to exclude fungal infection.
- See any surface changes.

Systemic causes of changes in shape or growth of nails:
- *Clubbing*—described in detail before.

Koilonychia (spoon nails) (Fig. 2.43)

- Iron deficiency anemia
- Hemochromatosis
- Raynaud's disease
- SLE
- Trauma
- Nail-patella syndrome
- Normally in infant.

Onycholysis (Fig. 2.44)

Separation of nail plate from nail bed. It begins at the free edge, progresses proximally, causing a traumatic uplifting of the distal plate. It results white discoloration of the affected area, causing secondary infection.

Causes:

- Psoriasis
- Hyperthyroidism
- Sarcoidosis
- Amyloidosis
- Connective tissue disorders
- Trauma
- Reaction to acrylic nails or nail hardness.

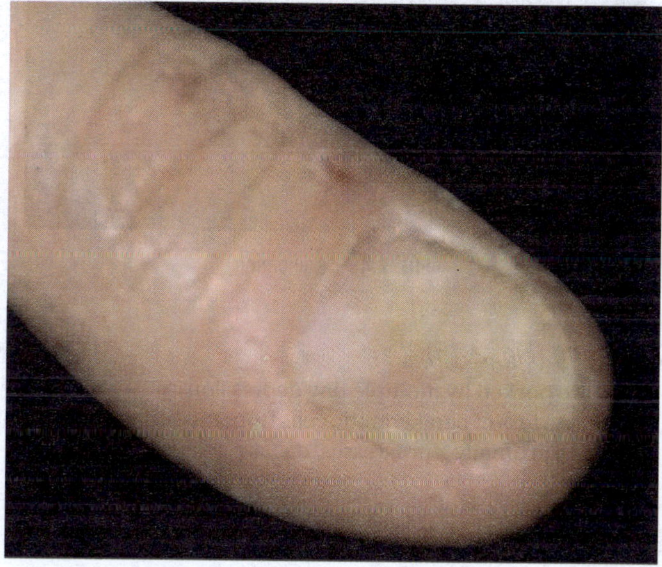

FIG. 2.43   Koilonychia (spoon nails)

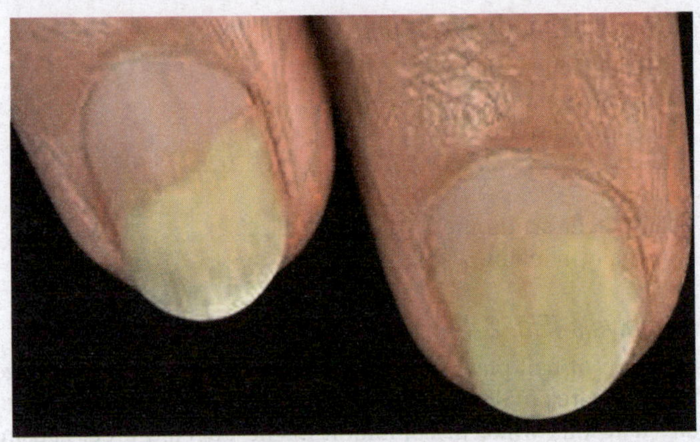

FIG. 2.44 Onycholysis

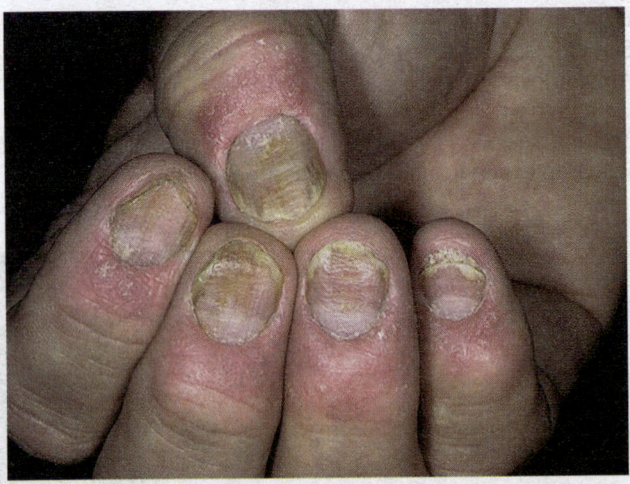

FIG. 2.45 Nail pitting

Nail Pitting (Fig. 2.45)

- Nails are pocked by multiple tiny depression
- It is due to loss of parakeratotic cells from the surface of nail plate
- It starts proximally—progresses, distally
- *Causes:*
  - ❖ Psoriasis
  - ❖ Alopecia areata
  - ❖ Incontinentia pigmenti
  - ❖ Reiter syndrome.

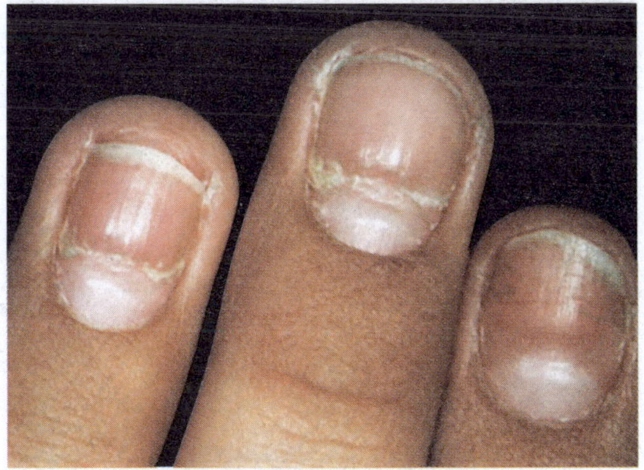

FIG. 2.46 Beau's lines

Beau's Lines (Fig. 2.46)

- It is transverse grooves on the finger nails of patients recovering from serious fillness.
- It is causes or produced by transient intermittent inflammation of matrix resulting in arrested growth.
- Grooves progresses distally, finally moving out as the nail elongates.
- *Causes:*
  - ❖ Severe systemic illness
  - ❖ Raynaud's disease
  - ❖ Pemphigus
  - ❖ Trauma.

Yellow nails (Figs 2.47A and B)

- Heaped up thickened appearance
- Excessive transverse curvature
- Loss of lunula
- Yellowish/greenish discoloration
- Eventually nail thickens and detaches.

Causes:
- Infection *Pseudomonas*
- Lymph edema of extremities
- Respiratory involvement—sinusitis chronic bronchiectasis
- Pleural effusions
- Internal malignancies

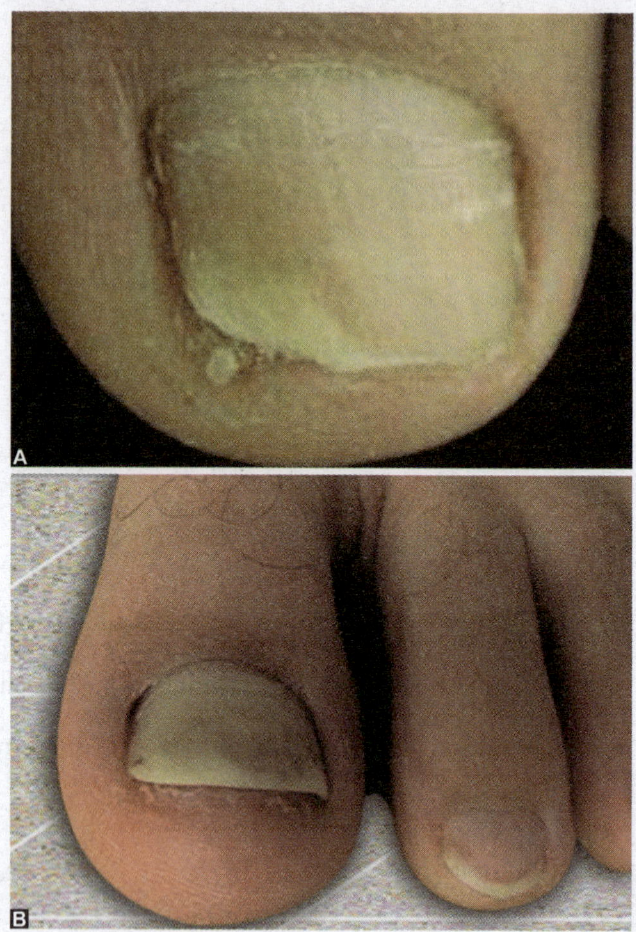

FIGS 2.47A AND B Yellow nails

- Rheumatoid arthritis (due to drugs like penicillamine and gold salts)
- Nephrotic syndrome.
  Microvascular permeability with protein leakage link the yellow nail syndrome with infection, pleural effusion, hypoalbuminemia, lymph edema.

Brittle Nails (onychorrhexis) (Fig. 2.48)
It is distal plate split into layers with irregular, frayed and firm borders resembling dry skin.

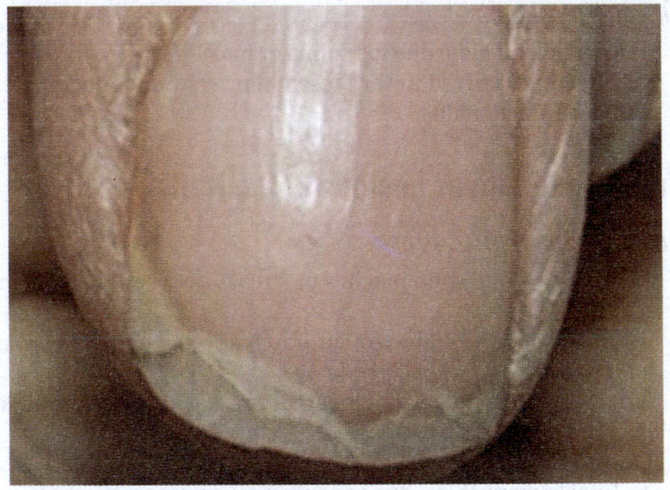

FIG. 2.48 Brittle nails (onychorrhexis)

Causes:
- Twenty percent adult in old ages
- It may be congenital
- Strong solvents
- Repeated immersion in water (dishwashers)
- Dysmetabolic states:
  - ❖ Hyperthyroidism
  - ❖ Malnutrition
  - ❖ Iron deficiency
  - ❖ Calcium deficiency.

Longitudinal Ridging of Nails
- Ridges typically extend from proximal nail fold to distal plates
- They are usually multiple, on may be single
- *Causes:*
  - ❖ Normal variant—older than 50
  - ❖ Also in younger subject
  - ❖ Lichen planus—single ridge.

Nail Beading
- It is due to rapid matrix turn over
- It is rare in early rheumatoid arthritis, but common in late RA
- Drugs—itraconazole.

Onychogryphosis

- Thickened nail plate due to trauma or infection
- Nail becomes curved inward resembling claw and pinching the nail bed (pincer nails).

Transverse Linear Lesions of the Nails

Leukonychia (Fig. 2.49):

- It is due to white spot, patches or streaks between the nail and nail bed
- It is produced by bubbles of air trapped in the nail plate layers after trauma
- It may involve whole nail (global) or present as lines (striate) or dots (punctate)
- *Causes:*
  - ❖ Total leukonychia—due to congenital dominant disorder
  - ❖ Striate or punctate—due to trauma.

Beau's Lines (Fig. 2.46)

Previously described.

Bitten Nail (Fig. 2.50)

- They present as transverse indentation
- They present as absence of free nail edge

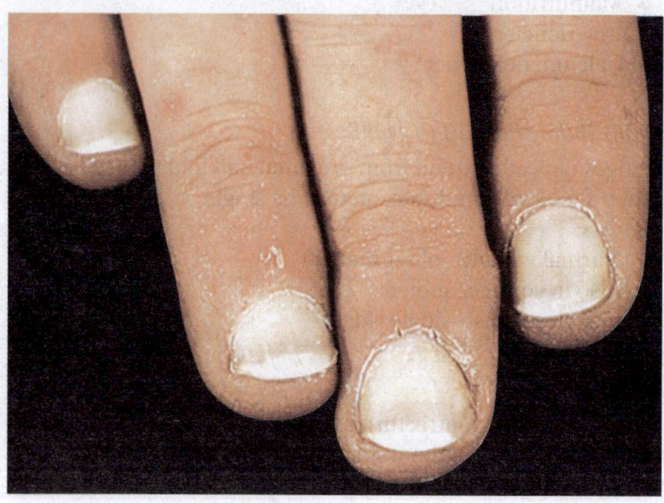

FIG. 2.49 Leukonychia

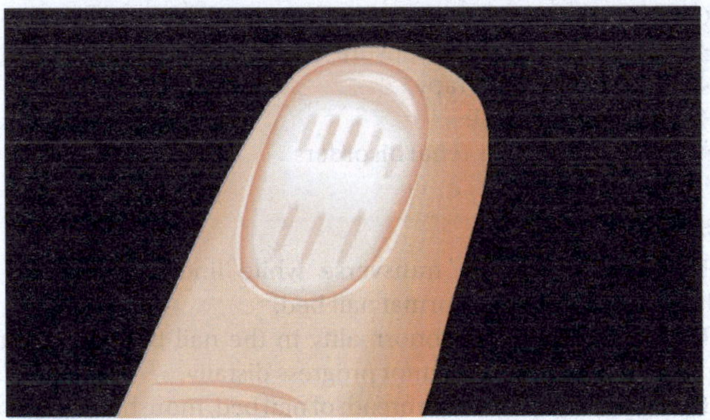

FIG. 2.50 Bitten nail

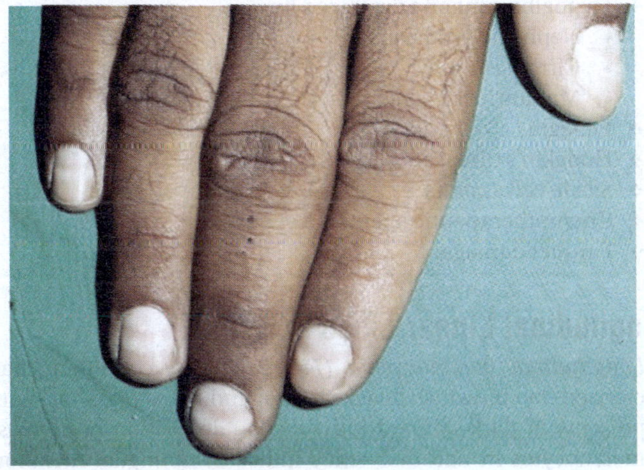

FIG. 2.51 Mees lines

- *Causes:*
  - ❖ Nervous biting
  - ❖ Chewing.

Mees Lines (Fig. 2.51)

- Transverse white line distal to the cuticle
- This is also called Raynaud's line or Aldrich's lines
- These lines are present in nail plate
- These lines progress distally.

- *Causes:*
    - ❖ Arsenic or thallium exposure
    - ❖ Cancer chemotherapy
    - ❖ Hodgkin's disease
    - ❖ Severe cardiac or renal disorders.

Merck's Lines

- Two arcuate narrow transverse white lines—parallel to the lunula, separated by normal nail bed.
- They reflect vascular abnormality in the nail bed, not the nail plate, hence this line cannot progress distally.
- They typically span entire breath of nail bed, more homogeneous, contour similar to that of distal lunula.
- They resolute after resolution of hypoalbuminemia.
- *Causes:*
    - ❖ Hypoalbuminemia produced by:
        - • Nephritic syndrome
        - • Cirrhosis
        - • Malnutrition.
    - ❖ Pellagra
    - ❖ Hodgkin's disease
    - ❖ Sickle cell anemia
    - ❖ Chemotherapeutic agents
    - ❖ Parquet damage.

Longitudinal Linear Lines in Nails

- *Longitudinal melanonychia (Fig. 2.52A):* A condition characterized by brownish/blackish longitudinal streaks or bands presents in dark-skinned individuals—deposition of increased melanocytes in nail bed—may indicate subungual melanoma when it is in doubt, biopsy of nail matrix and bed to be taken.

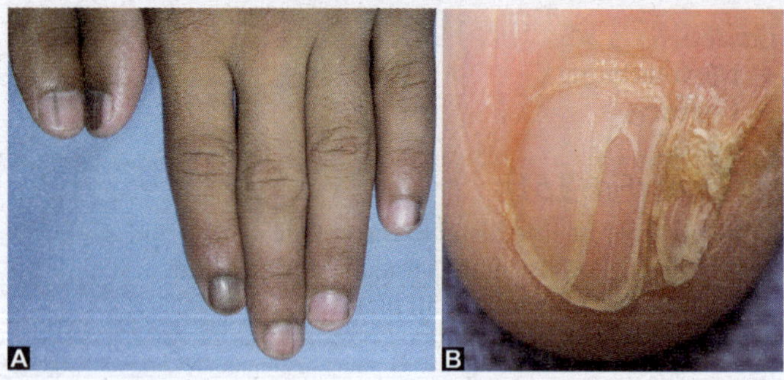

FIGS 2.52A AND B   (A) Longitudinal melanonychia, (B) Lichen planus of nail bed

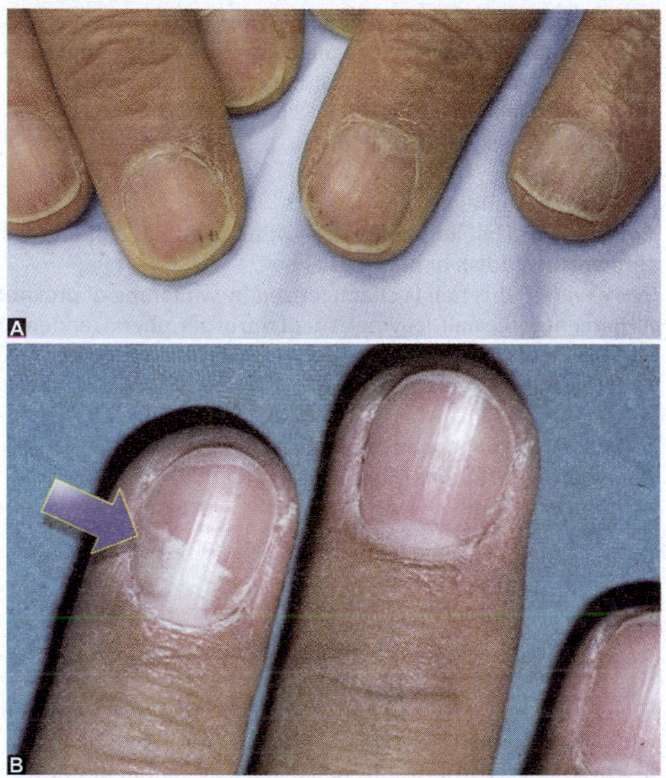

FIGS 2.53A AND B   (A) Splinter hemorrhage in nail, (B) Azure half-moon
in nail bed

- *Lichen planus of nail bed (Fig. 2.52B):* Thinning of nail plate, leading to longitudinal grooving and ridging.

Vascular and Nail Bed Changes

- *Splinter hemorrhage (Fig. 2.53A):* Linear red hemorrhagic streak extending from free margin of nail bed towards the proximal end. It can be found:
  - ❖ Subacute bacterial endocarditis
  - ❖ Trichinosis
  - ❖ Trauma
  - ❖ SLE
  - ❖ Rheumatoid arthritis
  - ❖ Antiphospholipid syndrome
  - ❖ OCP use
  - ❖ Psoriasis
  - ❖ Pregnancy

Difference between traumatic splinters and embolic splinter is:
  ❖ Traumatic splinters extend all the way into edge of the nail
  ❖ Embolic splinters are fully contained within the nail bed.
- *Azure half-moon in nail bed (Fig. 2.53B):*
  ❖ Wilson's disease—bluish lunula
  ❖ Quinacrine
  ❖ Silver poisoning.
- *Lindsay line:* Half and half nails—white proximal half and dark (brownish, reddish or pink) distal half.
- *Terry's nails:* This nail is characterized by whitening of proximal 80 percent of the nail, leaving a small rim of peripheral reddening, sharply demarcated as Lindsay lines. This nail is found in:
  ❖ Heart failure
  ❖ Cirrhosis
  ❖ Noninsulin dependent diabetes.
- *Longitudinal striations (Fig. 2.54):* It is found in:
  ❖ Alopecia areata
  ❖ Vitiligo
  ❖ Atopic dermatitis
  ❖ Psoriasis.

Nail Infections

- *Tinea unguium (Figs 2.55 and 2.56):* A dermatophytic infection of nail bed characterized by:
  ❖ Onychauxis (hypertrophy of nail plate by keratin pile-up)
  ❖ Onycholysis (separation of nail plate from nail bed)

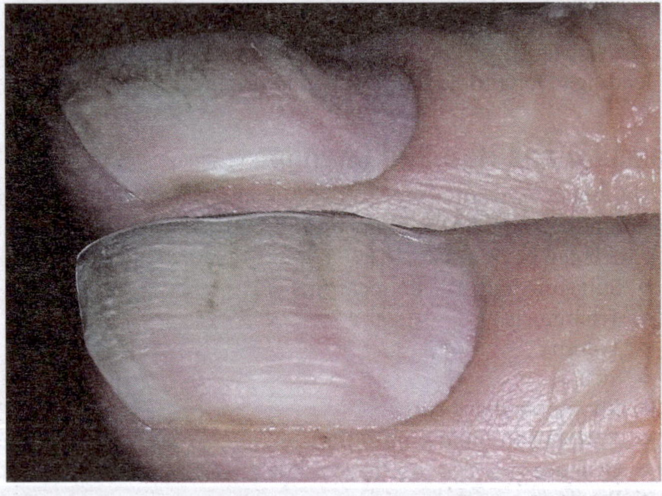

FIG. 2.54 Longitudinal striations

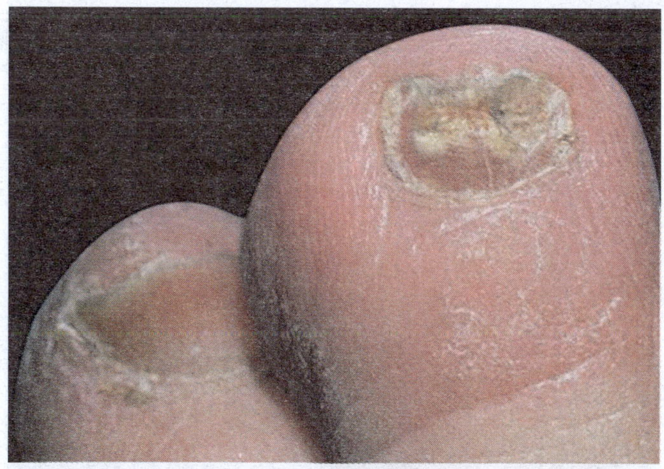

FIG. 2.55 Dermatophytosis of nail

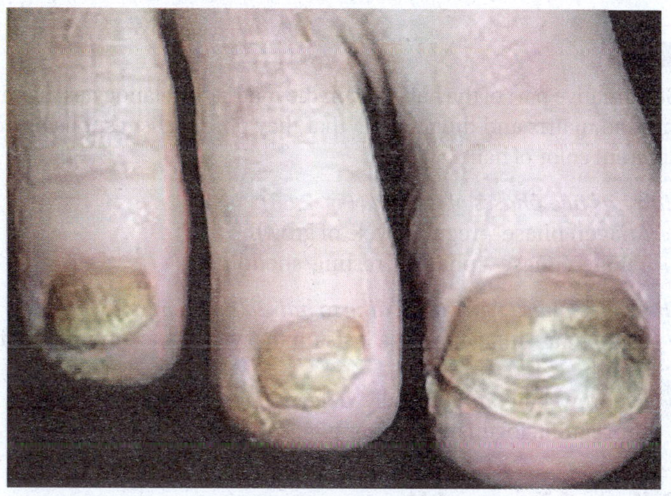

FIG. 2.56 Onychauxis

* ❖ Dysmorphic, thickened, broken and discolored nails (white, yellow, brown or blue)
* ❖ Browning of the plate
* ❖ Ridging and white spots.

Diagnosis can be done by: Scraping and KOH preparations.

* *Paronychia (Fig. 2.57):* Chronic infection with redness, swelling and tenderness.
* *Blue lines:* It is caused by—minocycline therapy.

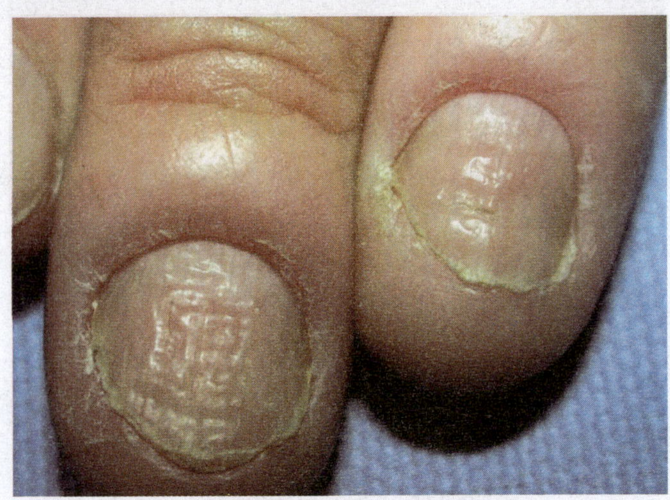

FIG. 2.57 Nail paronychia

■ Hair

Germinative part of the hair shaft in the matrix—melanocytes migrate into the matrix and the melanin that they produce is responsible for different color of hair.

Hair has two phases of growth (Fig. 2.58):
1. Anagen phase—regular cycle of growth.
2. Telogen phase—phase of resting/shedding.

The above phases vary according to hair in different body parts:
- Scalp hair—anagen phase lasts up to 5 years—accounting for its length
- Eyebrow hair and sexually determined hair—anagen phase is short and telogen phase is long.

Different Types of Hair

- *Lanugo hair (Fig. 2.59):* It covers the fetus, shed about 1 month before full term.
- *Vellus hair (Fig. 2.60):* Lanugo hairs are replaced by vellus hair, which covers much of body surface.
- *Terminal hair:* They replace the vellus hair in the scalp.
- *Curlier hair (Fig. 2.61):* At puberty, vellus hair of pubic region are replaced by coarser, darken curlier hairs. They begin:
  - ❖ In girls—earlier (11.5 years average)
  - ❖ In boys—later (13.5 years average)

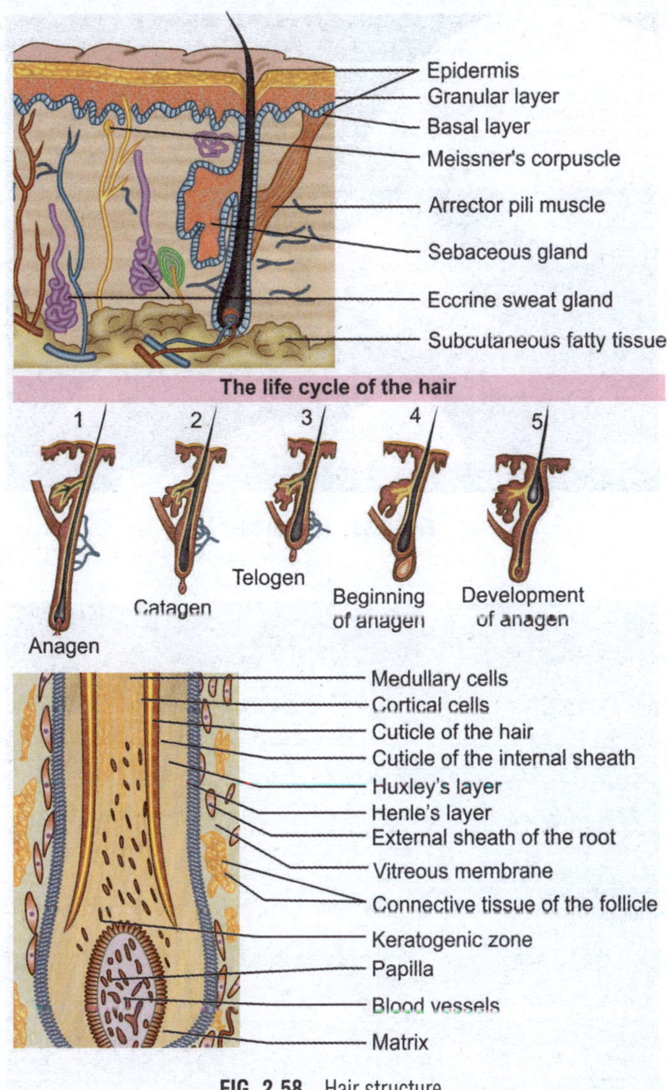

FIG. 2.58   Hair structure

This curlier hair growth depends upon adrenal androgen production (adrenarche). This occurs in absence of gonadotropin production.

- *Axillary hair*: It appears 2 years after the start of pubic hair growth and in boys coincide with the development of facial hair.
- *Body hairs:* It develops and get maturity throughout the years of sexual maturity.

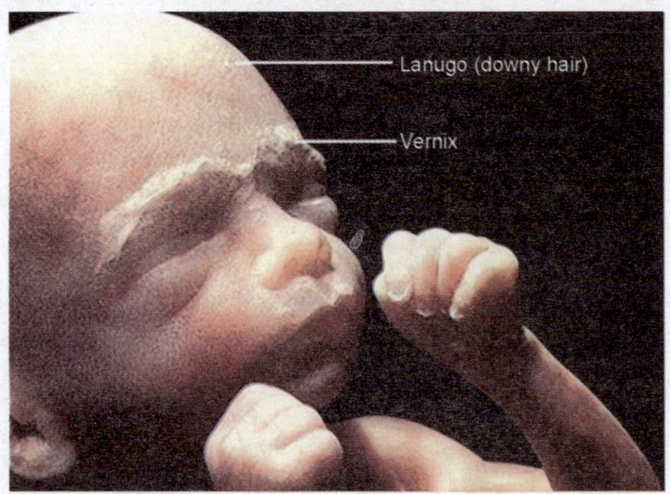

FIG. 2.59   Lanugo hair

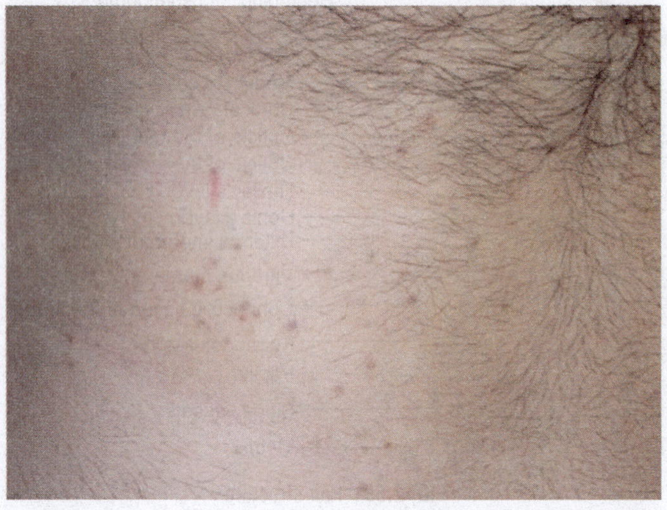

FIG. 2.60   Vellus hair

Types of Hair Varies According to Races

- Asian—straight hairs
- Negroids—curly hairs
- European—wavy hairs
- Mongoloid—spare facial and body hairs.

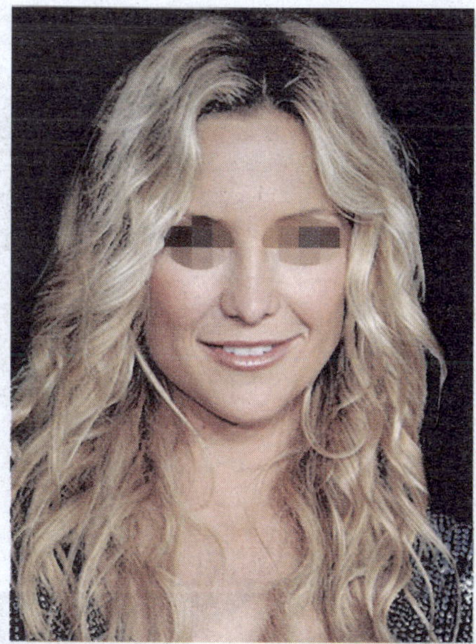

FIG. 2.61   Curlier hair

Common Abnormalities

Scalp Hair

- *Temporal recession (Figs 2.62A and B):*
  - ❖ Common in males
  - ❖ Progressing to thinning of hair over the crown
  - ❖ It is androgen dependent
  - ❖ Not reversed by castration in maturity.
- *Frontal recession (Fig. 2.63):*
  - ❖ Loss on thinning of hair at puberty
  - ❖ It occurs in myotonic dystrophy.
- *Alopecia:*
  - ❖ Alopecia areata (Figs 2.64A and B):
    - • It is local disease of scalp
    - • Hair fall out in patches
    - • In active disease—hairs shaped like exclamation marks, found periphery of bold area, which is clean and smooth
    - • It may cause total scalp baldness (Alopecia totalis) (Fig. 2.65)
    - • It may be associated with total loss of body hair (Alopecia universalis).
  - ❖ Alopecia associated with fungal infection. In this condition hair broken off close to skin

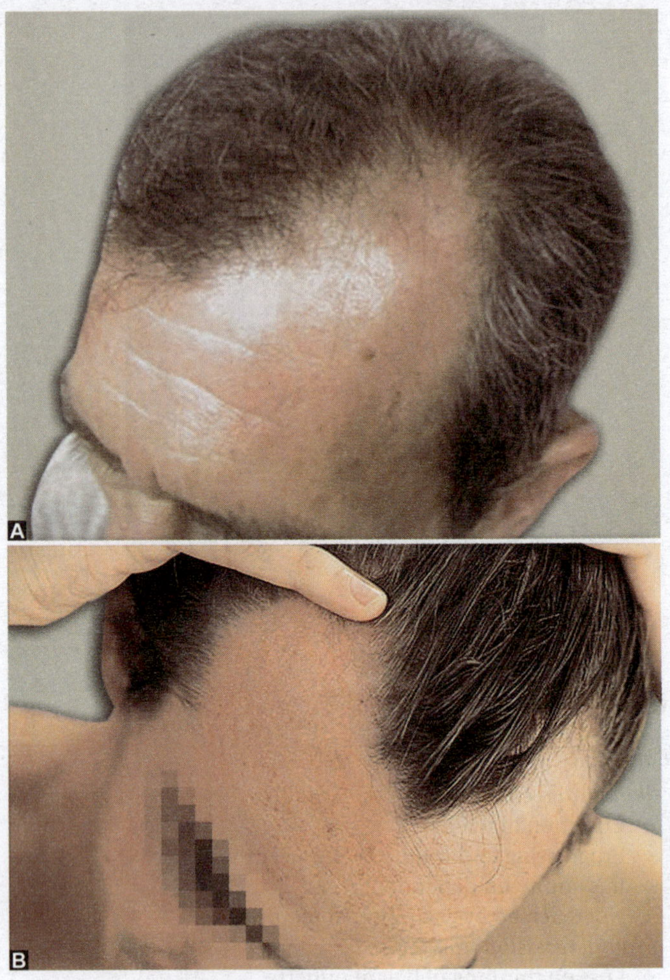

FIGS 2.62A AND B   (A) Temporal recession, (B) Male hair loss

- ❖ Alopecia may be associated with scarring (Figs 2.66A to D)—DLE
  Traction alopecia—due to traction and tear of hair—cause: Psychological
- ❖ Alopecia may be associated with lice infestation—in this condition scalp is itchy and posterior cervical lymphadenopathy. In lice infestation nits are adherent to hair, where dandruff is easily shed.

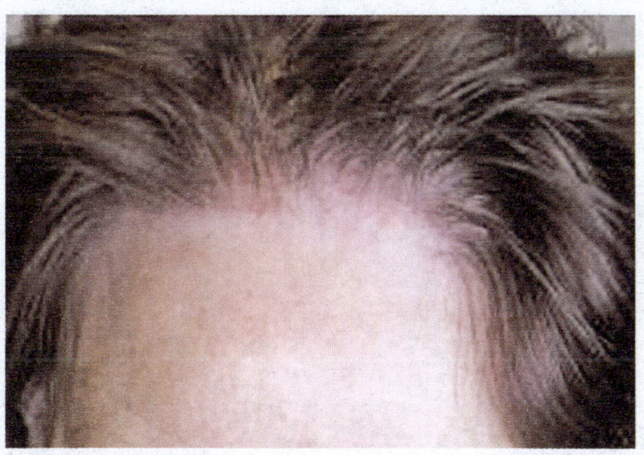

FIG. 2.63 Frontal recession

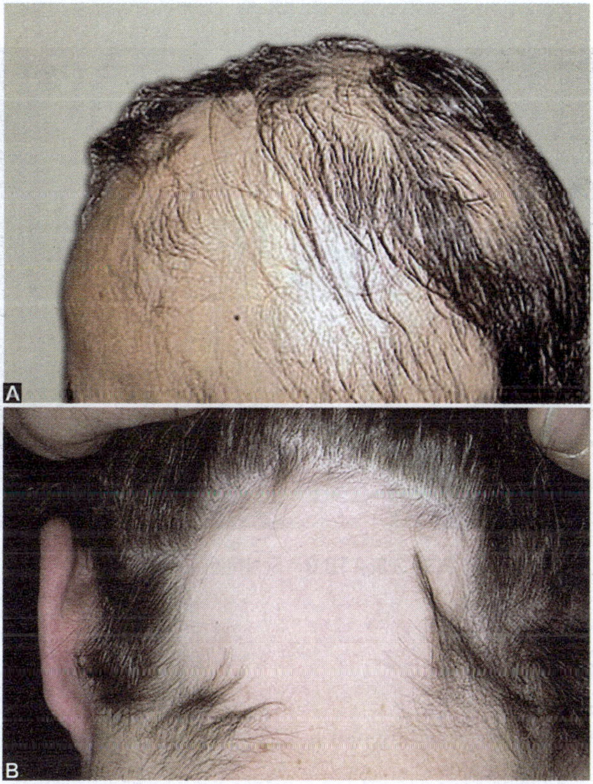

FIGS 2.64A AND B (A) Alopecia areata, (B) Dermnet NZ figure of
alopecia areata

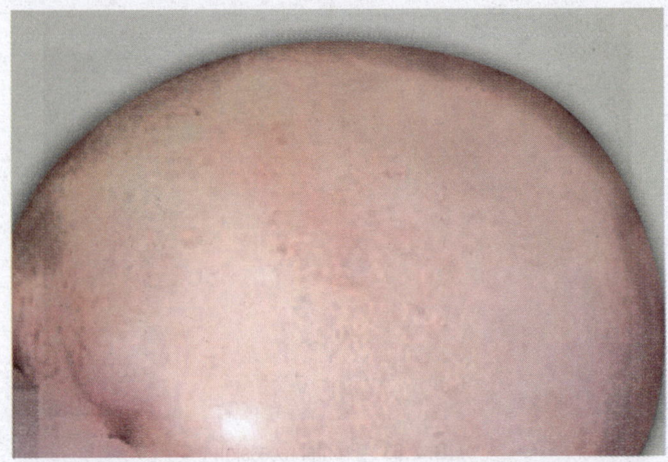

FIG. 2.65 Alopecia totalis

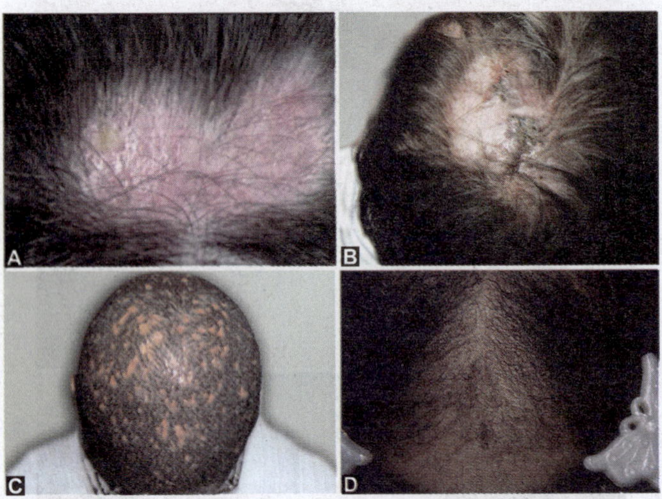

FIGS 2.66A TO D Scarring alopecia

Facial and Body Hair

- *Hirsutism (Fig. 2.67):*
  - ❖ Excessive growth of hair in face, trunk and limbs, the pattern seen in males.
  - ❖ Pubic hair spreads from its flat topped distribution upwards towards umbilicus described as male escutcheon.

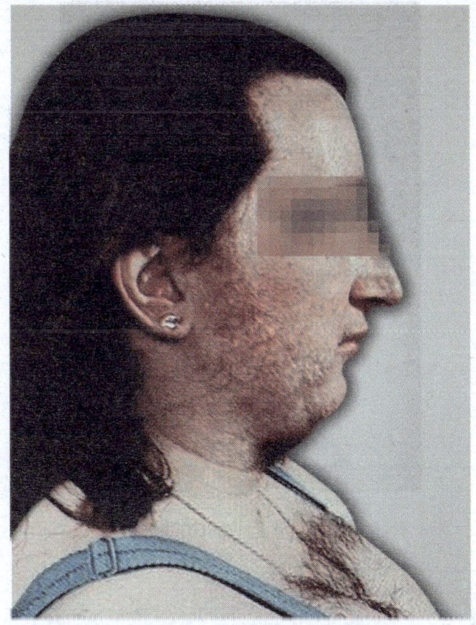

FIG. 2.67 Hirsutism hair

- ❖ This is caused by:
  - Higher than average level of testosterone
  - Psychological.
- ❖ Coarsening of facial hair—during menopause.
- *Hirsutism with virilization* (Development of masculine physical features): Seen in female:
  - ❖ Enlargement of clitoris
  - ❖ Menstrual irregularity or cessation
  - ❖ Sign of androgen secreting or pituitary tumor.
- *Hypertrichosis (Fig. 2.68):*
  - ❖ Excessive growth of coarse hair.
  - ❖ It may be due to:
    - Drugs (Minoxidil, cyclosporine)
    - Trauma
    - Cutaneous porphyria.
- *Secondary sexual hair:*
  - ❖ Face in male, axilla and pubis of both sexes
  - ❖ Diminished in:
    - Old age
    - Hypopituitarism
    - Hypogonadism
    - Cirrhosis.
- *Eyebrows:* Thinning of outer third of eyebrows—hypogonadism.

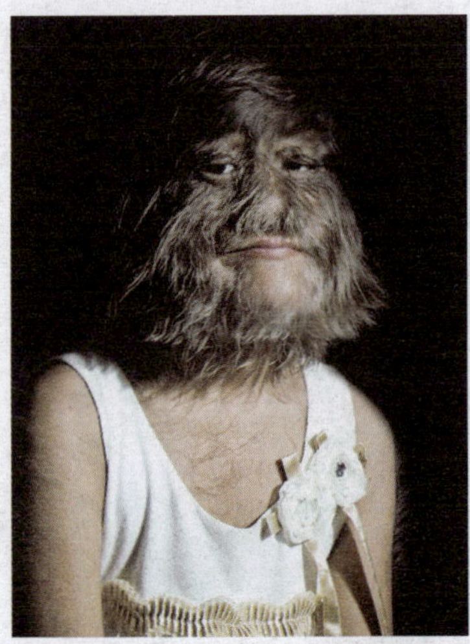

FIG. 2.68 Hypertrichosis

Edema

Fluid movement between intravascular space and extravascular spaces occurs through the capillaries.

The efflux of fluid across the capillary wall is governed by:
- Hydrostatic pressure transmitted by arterial blood pressure through the precapillary arteriole
- Capillary permeability
- Oncotic pressure of interstitial fluid.

The influx of fluid across the capillary wall is governed by:
- Oncotic pressure of the flowing blood—contains protein
- Hydrostatic pressure of interstitial fluid—tissue pressure.

In heart failure:

Increased central venous pressure

↓

Increased capillary pressure

↓

Accumulation of fluid interstitial fluid

↓

Renal hypoperfusion

↓

Activation of renal angiotensin—system

↓

Accumulation of sodium and water

In nephrotic syndrome, liver failure, malabsorption, protein losing enteropathy, severe burns, malnutrition:

Hypoalbuminemia
↓

Exudation of fluid into interstitial spaces
↓

Edema
↓

Renal hypoperfusion
↓

Activation of renal angiotensin—system
↓

Accumulation of Na^+ and water in blood vessels
↓

Transudation of fluid in extravascular spaces
↓

Edema

In liver failure:

Portal hypertension
↓

Splanchnic pooling
↓

Decreased effective circulating blood volume
↓

Renal hypoperfusion
↓

Activation of renal-angiotensin system
↓

Increased Na^+ and water retention
↓

Increased plasma volume
↓

Increased transudation of fluid
↓

Edema
Hypoalbuminemia
↓

Exudation of fluid in interstitial space
↓

Edema

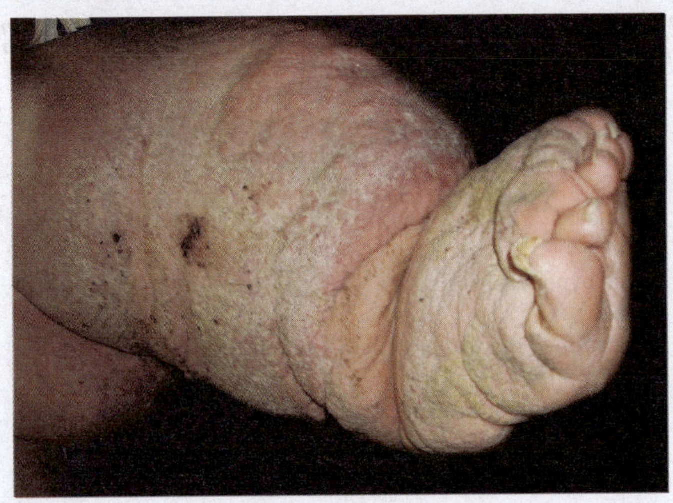

FIG. 2.69 Lymphatic edema leg

In inflammation:
 Increased capillary permeability
 ↓

 Increased movement of albumin and other colloid protein as well as fluid into interstitial spaces
 ↓

 Increased shifting of fluid and electrolytes out of capillaries into the interstitium

Lymphatic obstruction (Fig. 2.69):
 Accumulation of lymph rich in protein into the interstitial spaces
 ↓

 Increased in interstitial oncotic pressure
 ↓

 Drawing of fluid into interstitial spaces
 ↓

 Edema

Distribution of fluid in the interstitial fluid depends upon:
- Underlying cause
- Shifting effect of gravity
- Capacity of the tissue in which it accumulates.
 In congestive heart failure, edema appears as ankle swelling.

In the upright posture:

Increased capillary pressure transmitted to lower limbs
↓
Favors the regional accumulation of excess fluid in loose connective tissue around the ankles.

In the night:

Patient is in recumbent position
↓
Redistribution of transcapillary and gravitational forces towards sacral region and resolve of edema round the ankles
↓
Producing sacral edema.

If left ventricle fails:

Transudation of fluid into interstitial spaces in the lung
↓
From there fluid passes in to alveolar spaces
↓
Producing pulmonary edema
↓
Fluid accumulates in the dependent (basal) portion of lung
↓
Collapse of basal alveoli during expiration

During inspiration opening of collapsed alveoli produces basal crepitations.

In superior venacaval obstruction (Fig. 2.70):
Facial puffiness in common, especially, during waking in the morning.

In hypoproteinemic states—gross generalized edema—Anasarca.

Symptoms of Edema

- *If edema is generalized:*
  ❖ Tight-fitting shoes
  ❖ Frank swelling of the legs
  ❖ Unexplained weight gain
  ❖ It may be associated with symptoms linked to underlying causes like heart failure, liver, kidney, bowel, nutritional disease.
- *If edema in localized:* In case of venous thrombosis, regional lymphatic obstruction, inflamed area of swelling.

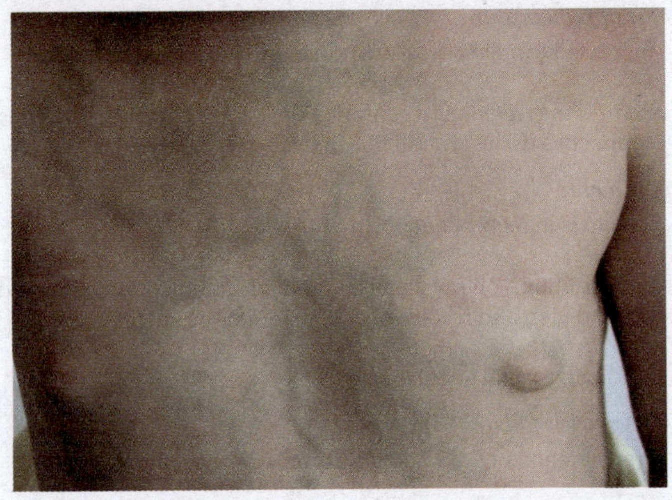

FIG. 2.70 Superior venacaval obstruction edema

- Fluid accumulation in pleural spaces:
  ❖ Breathlessness.
- Ascites may be noticed as:
  ❖ Increase abdominal girth
  ❖ Weight gain
  ❖ Eversion of umbilicus.

Signs of Edema

In ambulant patient having generalized edema:

Free fluid accumulates behind the medial malleolus. The area between medial malleolus and tendo-Achilles is usually concave.

As the fluid starts accumulating, this area becomes flattened, followed by convex.

Mild pedal edema can be diagnosed by palpation—press with the ball of your thumb in the area 5 cm above the medial malleolus for 10 seconds. After releasing, the pressure, the pit should persist for >5 seconds (Figs 2.71A and B).

Other areas of palpation are:
- Over the dorsum of foot.
- Behind the medial malleolus.

  In suspicion of edema, measure the legs to identify the edema and to follow its course.

  With flexible tape, measure:
- Forefoot
- The smallest possible circumference above the ankle

- Largest circumference at the calf
- Mid thigh—measured distance above the patella with the knee extended.

Compare the sides with each other.

A difference of more than 1 cm just above the ankle.

A difference of more than 2 cm at the calf is unusual—in normal people and suggest edema.

Veins of the lower legs have valves that protect the vessels from pressure effect of the column of blood from right ventricles.

Damaged valves or incompetent valves in the deep and perforating veins in the lower limb → produces marked increase

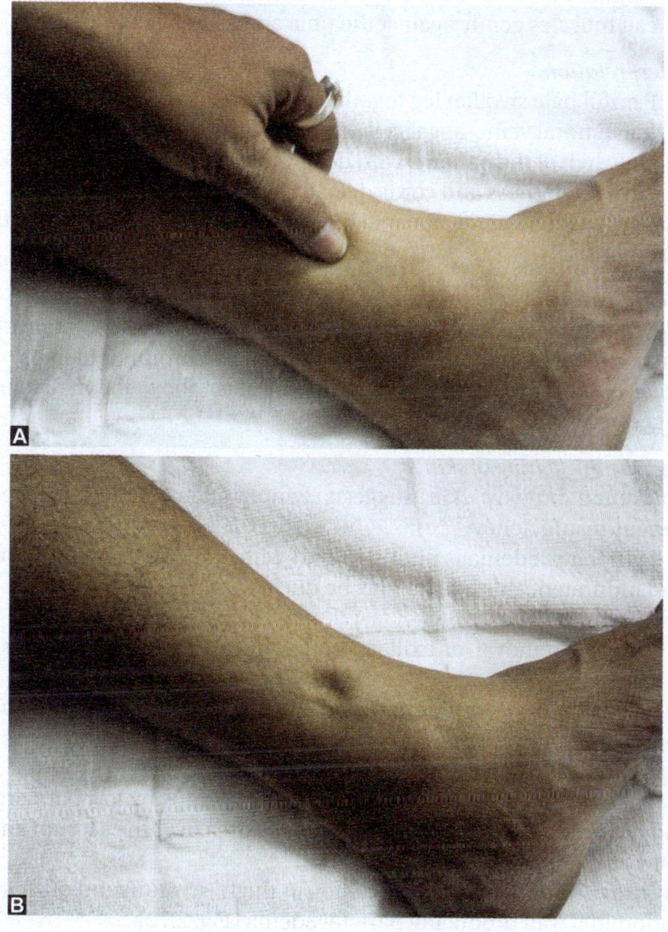

FIGS 2.71A AND B   Pedal edema

in hydrostatic pressure → produces pedal edema with dilated vein (varicose veins).

In deep venous thrombosis:

Localized edema: Here the extent of edema suggests location of occlusion:

- If lower leg or ankle is swollen—occlusion at popliteal veins
- If entire leg is swollen—iliofemoral veins are occluded.

Identify any venous tenderness that may accompany deep venous thrombosis.

- Palpate the groin medial to femoral pulse for tenderness of the fermoral vein.
- Palpate the calf in flexed leg and relaxed knee position. Press the calf muscles gently against the tibia and search for tenderness.

Interpretation:

- Painful pale swollen leg together with tenderness in groin—over the femoral vein—suggest iliofemoral thrombosis.
- Only half of the patients with deep venous thrombosis in the calf have tenderness and cords deep in the calf.

Calf tenderness is nonspecific, and may be present without thrombosis.

Identification of color of skin:

Identify the local area of tenderness: Local swelling, redness, warmth and a subcutaneous cord—suggest superficial thrombophlebitis.

Color of skin: Brownish discoloration or ulcer above the malleolus suggests chronic venous insufficiency.

Feel the thickening of skin:

Thickened browny skin suggests lymph edema and advanced venous insufficiency.

Lymphatic edema is pitting to start with, later on it is nonpitting and indurated. This edema may be due to:

- Filariasis
- Surgical removal of axillary nodes in the treatment of breast cancer.

In recumbent posture: Edema is less obvious around the ankles and most prominent over the sacrum and low back.

This can be diagnosed by following methods:

Patient should sit well forward in the bed exposing low back and sacral area. Press with the thumb into the area over the sacrum and low back.

In case of anasarca: Edema extends to thigh, scrotum and anterior abdominal wall producing parietal edema (Fig. 2.72).

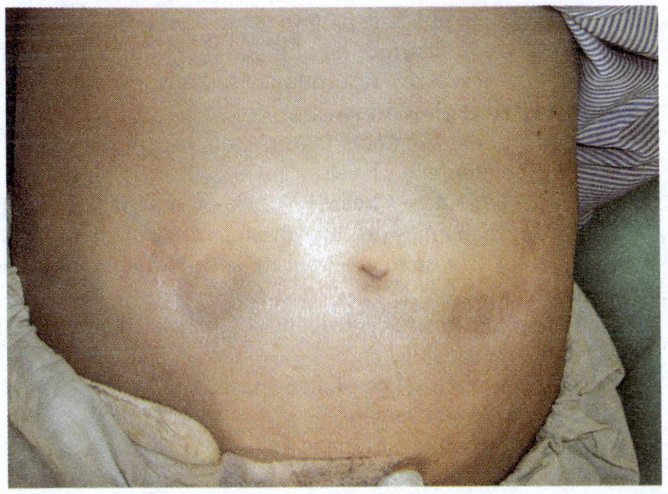

FIG. 2.72   Parietal edema

Causes of Edema

Generalized Edema

- Hypoproteinemia—fall in concentration of albumin in blood predisposes to edema.
  - ❖ Kwashiorkor—inadequate protein intake
  - ❖ Dietary restriction of protein
  - ❖ Pyloric obstruction with vomiting
  - ❖ Failure of digestion of dietary protein results from—impairment of exocrine secretion of pancreas as in chronic pancreatitis.
  - ❖ Failure of absorption of product of protein digestion, e.g.
    - Crohn's disease
    - Gluten enteropathy
    - Extensive small bowel resection.
  - ❖ Reduced synthesis of albumin in hepatocellular disease including cirrhosis.
  - ❖ Excessive loss of protein in urine:
    - Nephrotic syndrome
    - Removal of body fluids especially ascites.
  - ❖ Excessive loss of protein from gut:
    - Protein loosing enteropathy.
- *Fluid overload:*
  - ❖ Cardiac causes:
    - Impairment of renal blood flow
    - Reduction in renal blood flow

- Alteration in pulsatile pattern of renal perfusion
  Alteration in distribution of blood flow within the kidney promotes excessive resorption of sodium and water.
- Increased venous pressure:
  - In right-sided heart failure—this can be detected by inspection of neck vein
  - In left-sided heart failure—pulmonary venous congestion may produce dyspnea and cough
- *Effect of aldosterone:* Due to secondary hyper-aldosteronism
- *Antidiuretic hormone:* Evidence of increase in antidiuretic hormone
- *Lymphatic factor:* Lymphangiectasia
  - Incompetent valves.
  - Poor lymphatic drainage.
- Osmotic pressure
- Chronic passive congestion in liver
- Reduction in albumin synthesis
- Poor appetite
- Loos of protein in the edema fluid and in the urine.
  The protein content of interstitial fluid may rise to as much as 1 g/dL compared with 0.02 g/dL in normal interstitial fluid.
- ❖ *Renal causes:*
  - Expansion of circulating fluid volume and extracellular space
  - Increased tubular reabsorption of sodium.
- *Iatrogenic:* Excessive fluid replacement, if given intravenously. The danger is greatest in infants and young children.
- *Localized edema:*
  - ❖ *Venous causes:*
    - External pressure upon a vein
    - Venous thrombosis
    - Incompetence of the valves due to previous thrombosis.
  - ❖ *Lymphatic causes:* In presence of lymphatic obstruction. Water and solutes are reabsorbed into capillaries, but the protein remains, until its concentration approaches that in the blood.

↓

Fibrous tissue proliferate in the interstitial spaces

↓

Whole part becomes hard and no longer pits on pressure (Lymphatic edema)—due to obstruction by filarial worms.
Usually, one or both legs, female breast, external genitila are involved.
Skin becomes rough and thick—producing elephantiasis.

❖ *Inflammatory causes:*
Damage of tissues by injury, infection, ischemia, chemical, such uric acid
↓
Liberation of histamine, bradykinin
↓
Increases vasodilatation
↓
Increased capillary permeability
↓
Exudation of fluid into interstitial spaces with high protein content.

This edema is associated with classical signs of inflammation, redness, heat and pain.

❖ *Allergic causes:* Increased capillary permeability
↓
Exudation of fluid containing protein and eosinophils into the extracellular spaces.

Example: Angioedema—produce edema of face and lips.

This condition may be life threatening, if tongue and glottis are involved.

The differences between hypoproteinemic edema and fluid overload edema is:

In hypoproteinemic edema, JVP is normal.

In fluid overload edema, JVP is raised.

Neck Vein

Neck veins should be assessed:
- To estimate central venous pressure
- To evaluate venous pulse.

Central Venous Pressure Measures

- Right atrial pressure
- Right ventricular filling pressure
- Right ventricular end-diastolic pressure (in absence of tricuspid valvular stenosis).

Internal jugular vein should be evaluated for assessing pulse and central venous pressure, because this vein is indirect contact with right atrium.

Value to internal jugular venous (IJV) distension are:
- Noninvasive assessment of internal jugular vein to estimate:
  - ❖ Central venous pressure
  - ❖ Intravascular volume.

- Evaluation of wave form of pulse to estimate:
    ❖ Right ventricular function
    ❖ Right atrial function
    ❖ Tricuspid valves
    ❖ Pulmonary valves.
    ❖ Pericardial constriction.

Situations when IJV evaluation are very difficult:
- Short neck
- Fatty neck
- During mechanical ventilation
- Widespread respiratory swings—during status asthmaticus or any other type of respiratory distress.

Right internal jugular in the vein of choice because (Fig. 2.73):
It is direct continuation of right atrium and act:
- As manometer of central venous pressure
- As conduit of right atrial pulsation.

Left internal jugular vein is not of choice because:
- It may be partially compressed between the sternum and aortic arch.

External jugular vein is not used for evaluation of central venous pressure because (Fig. 2.74):
- It may be compressed because it passes through various facial planes.
- In patient with increased sympathetic vascular tone, vein may be constricted so that it may not be visible.
- It is far away from right atrium, so it is not in the straight line with right atrium.

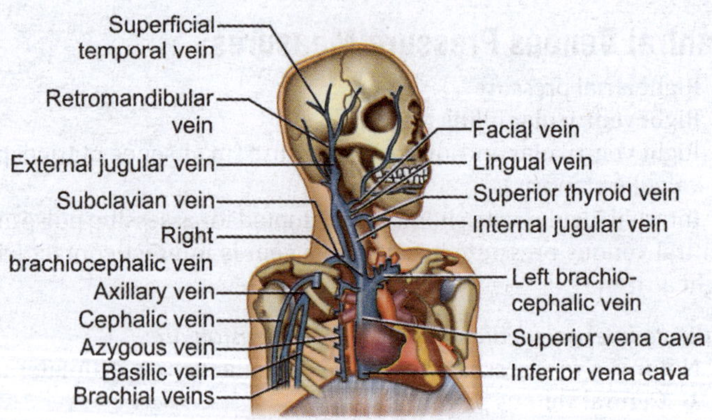

FIG. 2.73   Neck vein anatomy

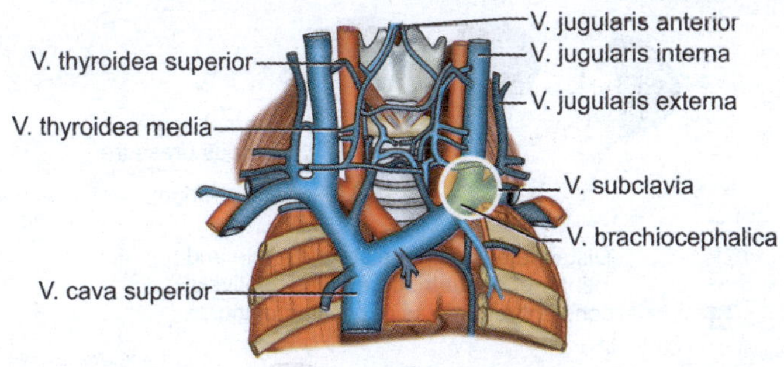

FIG. 2.74   Neck vein anatomy

- External jugular vein has valves so it does not interfere with the normal flow of blood towards heart, but it interferes with the flow of blood in reverse direction, hence evaluation of venous pulse.

Anatomy of Internal and External Jugular Veins

- External jugular vein lies above the sternocleidomastoid muscle, courses obliquely from behind and laterally towards the angle of jaw.
- Internal jugular vein lies below the sternocleidomastoid muscle, crossing it vertically in the straight line.

At the junction of internal jugular vein with subclavian vein, between the two heads of sternocleidomastoid there is a dilatation.

Method of position and measurement of internal jugular vein (Figs 2.75A and B):
- Head should be supported, so that neck muscles will be completely relaxed.
- Trunk should be inclined and raised at an angle at which top of the column of blood in internal jugular vein is visible just above the clavicle, but below the jaw level. So inclination will be varied according to CVP:
  - ❖ In patient with normal CVP—the angle will be 30° to 45° above the horizontal.
  - ❖ In patient with elevated CVP—the required angle will be >45°.
    - In patient with severe venous congestion, he has to sit upright and has to take deep inspiration to lower the meniscus down, to give full view.
    - In few patient, even in sitting position, upper level of venous pulsation is still behind the angel of jaw, where it will flicker the ear lobe.
  - ❖ In patient with low CVP—the inclination angle is between 0° to 30°.

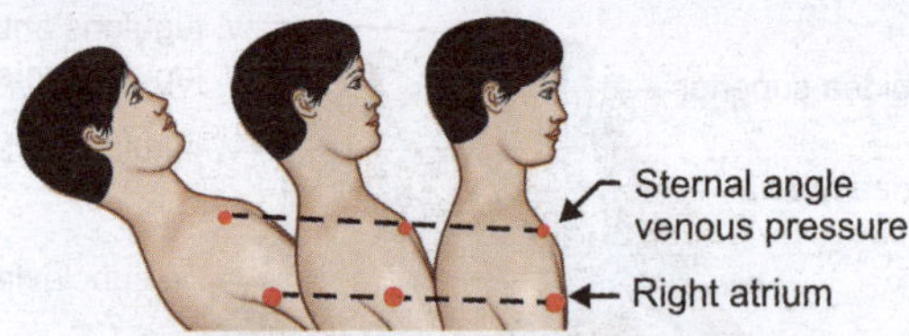

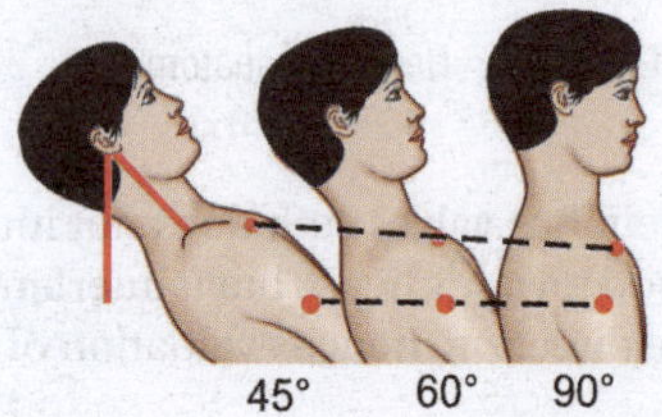

FIGS 2.75A AND B   Positions during measurement of internal jugular vein

- ❖ In patient with very low CVP—vein is empty, and pulsation will not be visible at all.

Differentiation between carotid pulse and internal jugular venous pulse:
- *Waveform is different:*
  - ❖ Venous pulse is diffuse, bifid, having trough, moving upwards and inwards
  - ❖ Carotid pulse—localized, single, upward and outward lift.
- *Relation with patient's position:*
  - ❖ Venous blood level moves down while the patient is gradually sit up and blood level moves up while the patient is gradually lie down
  - ❖ Carotid pulse never varies with position.
- *Response to respiration:*
  - ❖ If the patient is not suffering from any intrathoracic disease, top of venous waveform descends down during deep inspiration
  - ❖ Carotid pulse has no relation with respiration, except pulsus paradoxus, in this case also this variation is rarely visible.
- *Response to palpation:*
  - ❖ Venous pulsation is best seen, but not felt
  - ❖ Carotid pulse—best felt than seen.

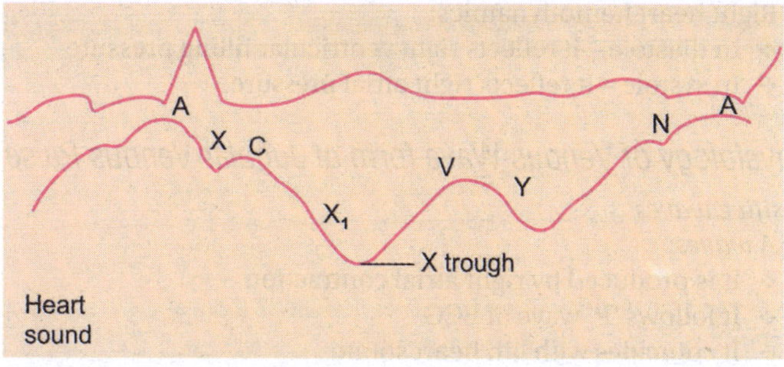

FIG. 2.76 Normal jugular venous wave pattern

- *Response to abdominal pressure:*
  - ❖ Carotid pulse will not be changed
  - ❖ Jugular venous pulse will be changed.

Evaluation of Venous Pulse

Inspection and venous pulse wave form:
- Level of venous column
- Timing of venous pulse
- Amplitude of venous pulse
- Respiratory variation of venous pulse
- Palpation and relation with carotid (left) and right radial artery
- Auscultation and relation with heart sounds.

It is easier to record venous wave form because:
The fluctuation in venous pressure is so mild (3–7 mm Hg) that peaks and troughs of venous pulse can be easily recorded.

The wave form of venous pulse:
Normal jugular venous wave (Fig. 2.76).
- *On venous tracing:*
  - ❖ Three positive waves—(A, C and V waves)
  - ❖ Three negative waves—(X, X_1 and Y waves)
  - ❖ A wave is followed by X decent
  - ❖ C wave is followed by X_1 decent
  - ❖ V wave is followed by Y decent.
- *At bedside:*
  - ❖ Two positive waves (A and V waves, A is taller than V)
  - ❖ Two negative waves (X_1 and Y waves, X_1 is steeper than Y).

Physiology of Venous Pulse

It is the relationship between:
- Volume of blood in venous system
- Vascular tone

- Right heart hemodynamics:
  - ❖ In diastole—it reflects right ventricular filling pressure
  - ❖ In systole—it reflects right atrial pressure.

Physiology of Venous Wave form of Jugular Venous Pulse

Positive waves
- *A waves:*
  - ❖ It is produced by right atrial contraction
  - ❖ It follows 'P' wave of ECG
  - ❖ It coincides with 4th heart sound
  - ❖ It precedes 1st heart sound and carotid upstroke.
- *C waves:*
  - ❖ It is produced by:
    - Budging of tricuspid cusp into right atrium—due to isometric contraction of right ventricle
    - Small part is produced by transmitted carotid pulsation.
  - ❖ The interval between 'A' and 'C' coincides with P-R internal.
- *V waves:*
  - ❖ Tricuspid valve is closed; blood begins to fill right atrium, increasing the pressure in right atrium.
  - ❖ It peaks immediately after S_2 (second heart sound).

Negative Waves
- *X descent:* It occurs between 'A' and 'C' positive waves.
- *X_1 descent:*
  - ❖ It is due to right atrial relaxation. It is produced by pulling of valve cusps and atrial floor into right ventricle during right ventricular isometric contraction
  - ❖ It takes place between 1st and 2nd heart sound
  - ❖ It takes place during ventricular systole.
- *Y descent:*
  - ❖ If occurs due to opening of tricuspid valve and flowing of blood from right atrium to right ventricle
  - ❖ It coincides with third heart sound.

Influence of respiration on jugular venous pressure:
Inspiration increases venous reform
↓
This in turn distends the right side of the heart
↓
Right atrial and right ventricular contraction becomes stronger
↓
As a result venous pulse becomes more visible
↓
Positive waves (A and V) become prominent and negative waves (X and Y) become brisk.

Diseases diagnosed by venous pulse.

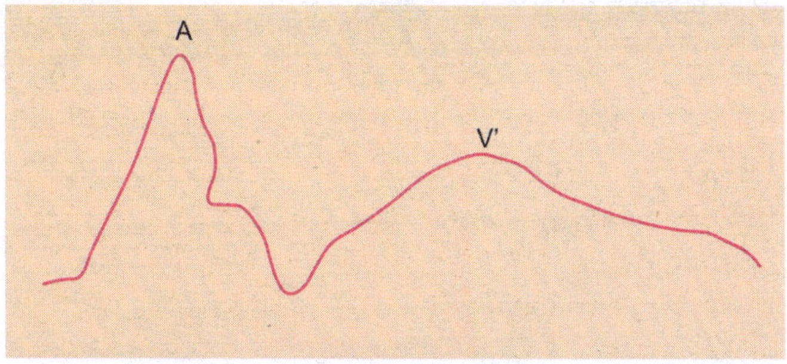

FIG. 2.77 Tricuspid stenosis prominent A wave

■ A Wave

- *Giant 'A' wave (Fig. 2.77)*
  - ❖ Tricuspid stenosis
  - ❖ Increased right ventricular end diastolic pressure—due to strong atrial contraction against stiff right ventricle:
    - Pulmonary stenosis
    - Primary pulmonary hypertension
    - Chronic pulmonary disease
    - Pulmonary embolism.
  - ❖ Marked left ventricular hypertrophy producing bulging of interventricular septum into right ventricle producing right ventricular filling more difficult:
    - Aortic stenosis
    - Systemic hypertension
    - Hypertrophic obstructive cardiomyopathy (Bernheim effect).
- *Cannon wave (Fig. 2.78)*
  - ❖ *Regular cannon wave:*
    - It occurs when right atrium contracts against closed tricuspid valve
    - Junctional rhythm
    - VY with 1:1 retrograde conduction.
  - ❖ *Intermittent cannon wave:* It occurs due to right atrial:
    - Complete AV block
    - Classic AV dissociation
    - VT
    - VPB.
- *Absent 'A' wave*
  - ❖ Atrial fibrillation—due to flickering of atrial muscles.
- *'V' waves:*
  - ❖ It occurs in tricuspid regurgitation—'V' wave becomes very dominant with brisk Y descent—In serve regurgitation

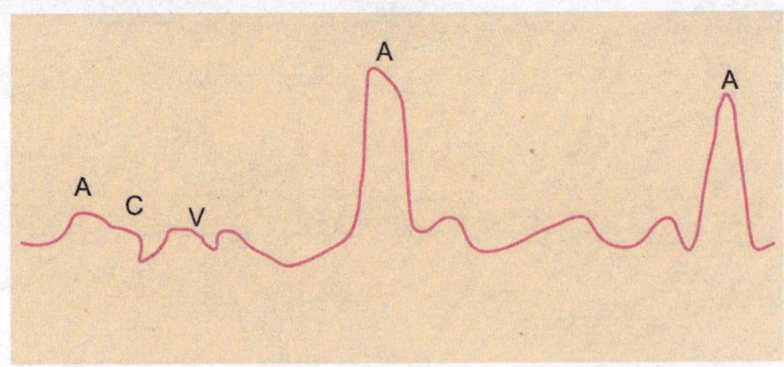

FIG. 2.78 Irregular Cannon waves in complete AV block

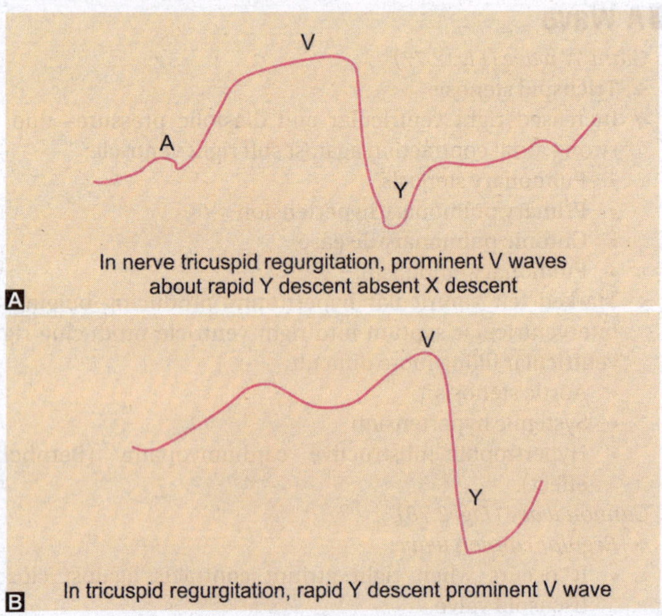

FIGS 2.79A AND B Tricuspid regurgitation

C wave becomes merged with 'V' wave with absent X descent and produce 'CV' wave—it is called "venous corrigan". It may produce bobbing of earlobes—"Lancisi sign" (Figs 2.79A and B).

Equally prominent A and V waves

- *Atrial septal defect:* In this disease 'V' wave in high pressure left atrium is transmitted through perforated interatrial septum to right atrium—from there to Jugular veins
- Right ventricular failure.

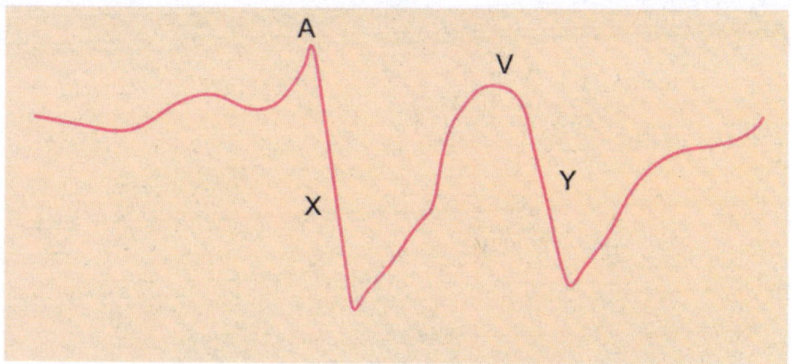

FIG. 2.80   Constrictive pericarditis rapid X and Y descent

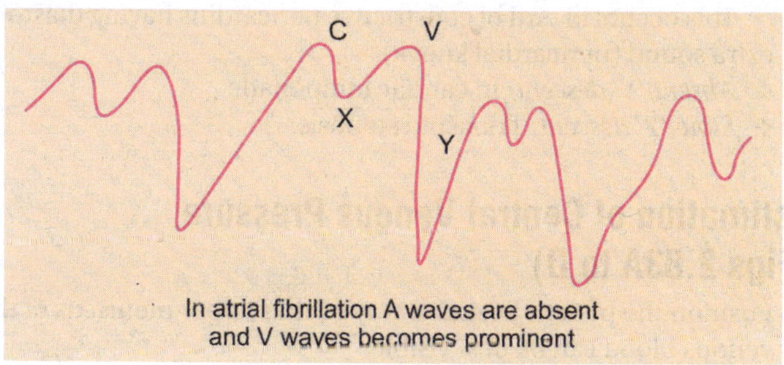

FIG. 2.81   Atrial fibrillation

- *X descent:*
  - ❖ *Prominent X descent:*
    - Constrictive pericarditis (Fig. 2.80)
    - Cardiac tamponade.
      It occurs due to prominent right ventricular contraction in closed and fixed space.
  - ❖ *Absent 'X' descent:*
    - Tricuspid regurgitation
    - Cardiomyopathy
    - Atrial fibrillation (Fig. 2.81)

In cardiomyopathy, right ventricular contraction is not forceful enough to pull down atrial floor.

- *Y descent:*
  - ❖ *Prominent 'Y' descent:*
    - *Constrictive pericarditis:* A brisk 'Y' descent—called Friedreich's sign (Fig. 2.82).

In combination with prominent 'X' descent it will produce 'W' sign—two steep trough.

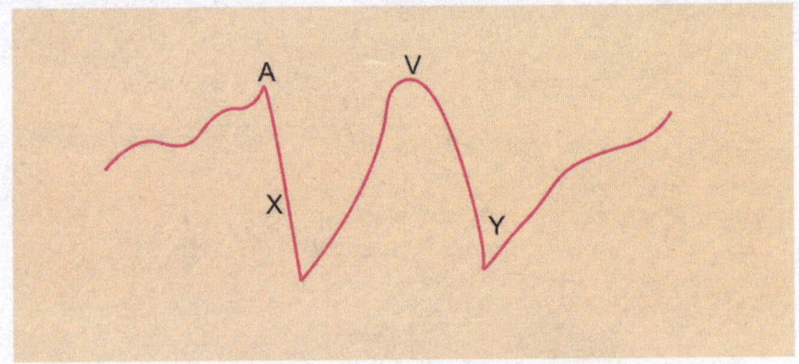

FIG. 2.82 Constrictive pericarditis

This occurs in ⅓rd of constrictive pericarditis having diastolic extra sound (pericardial knock)

- *Absent 'Y' descent:* In cardiac tamponade
- *Slow 'Y' descent:* Tricuspid stenosis.

Estimation of Central Venous Pressure (Figs 2.83A to D)

- Position the patient in such a way so that upper meniscus of the venous blood can be best visible.

  Normally 45° angle is taken as reference angle, because at this angle upper level of venous column is best seen.
- Finding sternal angle—as reference point—junction of the manubrium with the body of sternum. This point help to provide zero standard for jugular venous pressure.

  Zero standard for central venous pressure lies in center of right atrium.
- Measure the vertical distance between top of venous column and level of sternal angle—place one ruler—horizontally parallel to venous meniscus and other ruler vertically touching the sternal angle.
  - This height is generally normally <3 cm
  - Distance between sternal angle and center of right atrium is 5 cm
  - So normal CVP is 5 + 3 = 8 cm blood or water (by multiplying it by 0.8 to convert to mm of Hg).

Faster way to asses central venous pressure (Fig. 2.84)
While patient is in setting position, visible neck veins indicate CVP >7 cm water. It is pathologic. Because, clavicle lies 2 cm above sternal angle, hence if it is not visible, CVP is normal. If it is visible— it is abnormal.

Relation of CVP with respiration
During inspiration, intrathoracic pressure decreases

↓

It lowers jugular venous pressure

Alternative method of measuring CVP
- *Von Recklinghausen's maneuver:* Ask the patient to lie in supine position with palm of one hand laid down over the thigh and

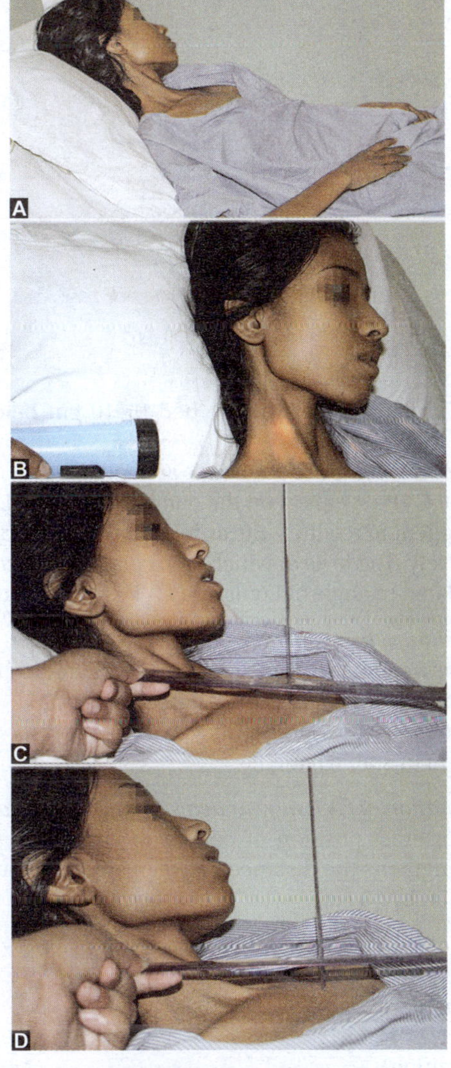

FIGS 2.83A TO D Neck vein

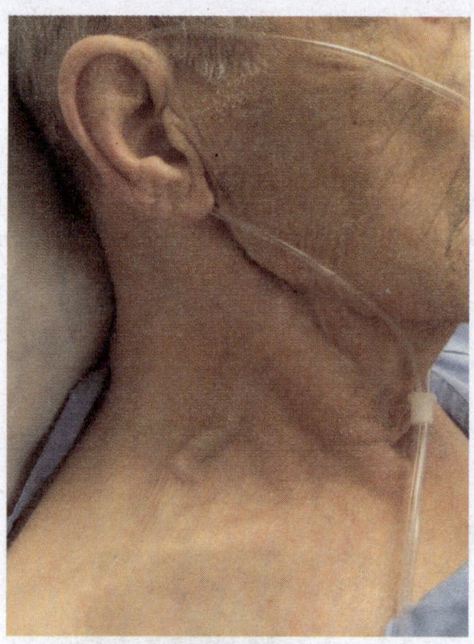

FIG. 2.84   Elevated JVP

other hand laid down over the bed (5–10 cm below the first hand):

- ❖ High CVP, if veins of both hands are engorged
- ❖ Normal CVP, if veins of on the hand are engorged.
- Ask the patient to recline—the arm is allowed to be raised slowly and passively. The level at which veins of the hand collapsed—it can be related to angle of Louis and CVP is measured.

Precision of clinical assessment of CVP

Difference between bedside estimation of CVP and catheter based estimation of CVP is 4 cm H_2O in 90 percent cases.

But interobserver variability may be as high as 7 cm. This is problematic in unstable patient.

Bedside estimation of CVP may underestimate CVP, because:

Semi-erect or erect position of patient to visualizes meniscus of neck vein, lengthens the distance between angle of Louis and zero reference point by >3 cm.

Significance of low central venous pressure

Causes of low central venous pressure:

- *Intravascular volume depletion:*
  - ❖ *GI tract:*
    - Vomiting
    - Diarrhea.

❖ *Urinary:*
  - Diuretics
  - Diabetes insipidus
  - Uncontrolled diabetes mellitus.

Significance of high central venous pressure
- *Superior venacaval obstruction:* No jugular venous pulse and abdominal hepatojugular reflux is negative.
- *Obstruction to right ventricular inflow:*
  - ❖ Tricuspid stenosis
  - ❖ Right atrial myxoma
  - ❖ Cardiac tamponade
  - ❖ Constrictive pericarditis.
- *Tricuspid regurgitation.*
- *Decreased right ventricular compliance:*
  - ❖ Factors those cause elevation right ventricular and diastolic pressure:
    - Pulmonary stenosis
    - Pulmonary hypertension
    - Right ventricular infarction/failure.
- *Left ventricular failure:* Patient presenting with dyspnea, angina, high central venous pressure indicates left ventricular failure.

Prognostic significance of abnormal jugular venous pressure
Together with third heart sound, abnormal jugular venous pressure is an ominous prognostic sign of adverse outcome.

Neck veins in cardiac tamponade
Distended neck vein together with dyspnea/tachypnea, tachycardia and clear lungs—have 5 differential diagnoses:
1. Right ventricular infarction
2. Massive pulmonary embolism
3. Constrictive pericarditis
4. Tension pneumothorax
5. Cardiac tamponade.

All above except cardiac tamponade present with:
- Kussmaul's sign positive in ½ of cases
- Pulsus paradoxus <21 mm Hg.

But cardiac tamponde presents with:
- Negative Kussmaul's sign
- Pulsus paradoxus >21 mm Hg.

Significance of pedal edema without increased CVP
- It reflects—renal or hepatic origin of edema, because cardiac edema presents with pedal edema and raised CVP
- Hepatic and renal originated edema many present with ascites also.

Significance of raised CVP in postoperative patient
Raised CVP in postoperative patient signifies:
- Right ventricular infarction
- Pulmonary edema.

Jugular findings in right ventricular infarction
- Right ventricular filling pressure is increased due to ischemic necrosis of muscle, RV is unable to handle incoming venous flow, so jugular venous flow is increased. This is highly specific; but low sensitivity.
- Jugular venous wave form shows prominent 'A' wave, it also shown prominent 'X' and 'Y' descents—so steep—almost mimic constrictive pericarditis. It is highly specific. Rapid 'Y' descent has low sensitivity for right ventricular infarction.
- Positive Kussmaul's sign with raised JVP.
- Abdominojugular test may be positive.
- If associated tricuspid regurgitation:
  - Giant 'V' wave
  - Pulsatile liver
  - Earlobe bobbing.

Hepatojugular reflux
Physiology: Steady pressure on the abdomen

↓

Shift the blood from splanchnic bed to thorax

↓

To jugular vein

↓

To right atrium

↓

To right ventricle

In case of slightly elevated jugular venous pressure, the raised pressure becomes overt.

Uses of hepatojugular reflux:
- Subclinical right ventricular failure
- Silent tricuspid regurgitation
- Symptomatic left ventricular failure.

Compression on liver during abdominojugular reflux is detrimental in patient with passive hepatic congestion; because:

Compression on the stretched glisson's capsule may elicit pain and valsalva response.

Hence anywhere, over the periumbelical area, compression may be given to elicit.

Method of performing abdominojugular reflux:
- Position the supine patient in inclined position at a degree, so that the venous column can be best monitored.

- Patient is asked to relax, breath normally through mouth. This will avoid false positive increase in jugular venous pressure caused by valsalva maneuver.
- Apply pressure over the abdomen in periumbelical area with palm of the hand having fingers widely apart—gradual and progressively increasing pressure for at least 15 seconds. Direction of pressure is firm, inward, cephalad, soon reaching pressure 30 to 35 mm of Hg.
- Throughout the maneuver (before, during and after compression) observe the column of blood in internal and external jugular vein.
- Also look for softening of 1st heart sound during application of pressure.

Value of abdominojugular reflux:
- *This reflux is positive when:*
  - ❖ There is increase in JVP >3 cm in height and it is sustained throughout 15 seconds of pressure.
  - ❖ During release of abdominal pressure, there is abrupt fall of jugular venous pressure and the drop must be > 4 cm.
- *This reflux is negative when:*
  - ❖ No change in JVP
  - ❖ Sustained change in JVP but it is not more than 3 cm
  - ❖ Pressure >3 cm of height—but it is sustained during 1st phase of abdominojugular pressure, but returns to normal during rest of the compression.

Significance of positive abdominojugular reflux:
In patients presenting with dyspnea/angina:
- Positive abdominojugular reflux favors biventricular failure with pulmonary capillary wedge pressure >15 mm Hg.
  In these patients:
  - ❖ Low ejection fraction
  - ❖ Low stroke volume
  - ❖ Increased left atrial pressure
  - ❖ Increased pulmonary capillary wedge pressure
  - ❖ Right atrial pressure.

Negative abdominojugular reflux—favors against increased left atrial pressure.
- In absence of left ventricular failure, positive test signifies inability of right atrium and right ventricle to handle the increased venous return—diagnoses may be:
  - ❖ Increased right ventricular preload (increased intravascular volume).
  - ❖ Decreased right ventricular compliance (right ventricular hypertrophy).

- ❖ Decreased/impaired right ventricular systolic function (right ventricular infarction).
- ❖ Increased right ventricular after load (pulmonary hypertension).

Positive test signifies:
- Right atrial pressure > 9 mm Hg
- Right ventricular and diastolic pressure >12 mm Hg.
  It occurs in:
  - ❖ Tricuspid regurgitation
  - ❖ Tricuspid stenosis
  - ❖ Restrictive cardiomyopathy
  - ❖ Constrictive pericarditis.

Abdominojugular pressure should be given for 15 seconds because:
CVP will be stabilized with in 15 seconds. So it is unnecessary to maintain pressure for 1 minute.

Kussmaul's respiration:
Normally during inspiration, the intrathoracic pressure becomes negative, so it produces a sucking effect on venous return.

But in few conditions, there is paradoxical increase in intrathoracic pressure and raised JVP during inspiration because right ventricle cannot handle the influx of venous blood. The causes are:
- Corpulmonale (acute or chronic)
- Restrictive cardiomyopathy
- Constrictive pericarditis
- Tricuspid stenosis
- Right ventricular infarction.

Association of pulsus paradoxus and Kussmaul's sign
Kussmaul's sign:
- It never occurs in pure tamponade (if it is associated with epipericardial fibrosis)
- It occurs in constrictive pericarditis (pure case).

Pulsus paradoxus does not occur in:
- Pure totally dry constructive pericarditis
- Right ventricular infarction.
  So cut off value of pulsus paradoxus >21 mm Hg.

Association between Kussmaul's sign and abdominojugular reflux
In above both cases, pathophysiology are same. They occur in peripheral venous constriction with increase in central venous pressures secondarily such as:
- Serve heart failure producing pump failure
- Various mechanical impediments—constrictive pericarditis, tricuspid stenosis, and corpulmonale (acute and chronic).

Venous hum:
- Functional murmur produced by turbulent flow of blood in the internal jugular vein
- It is continuous
- Sometimes it is so harsh that it is associated with a palpable thrill
- It is best heard on the right side of neck just above the clavicle
- It can be audible over the parasternal and sternal areas both right and left.

To elicit venous hum:
- Patient is to sit up with head turned away from the side of auscultation
- Hum vanishes upon inclination, maneuvers those reduces venous return, e.g.
  - Pressing over the jugular vein distal to hum
  - Performing valsalva.

Mechanism of venous hum:
- It is produced by compression of internal jugular vein by transverse process of atlas
- It occurs in patient with high cardiac output and increased venous flow
- It occurs in young adult (25%). 31 to 60 percent of normal children.

Jaundice—to be described in Chapter 5 Gastrointestinal System.
Pulse—to be described in Chapter 4 Cardiovascular System.

Respiratory System

◼ Thorax (Fig. 3.1)

It is superior part of the trunk between neck and abdomen.

Thoracic cavity contains heart and great vessels, lungs, thymus, distal part of trachea and most of the esophagus.

Thoracic cavity is bounded:
- Anteriorly by sternum and ribs
- Laterally by ribs
- Posteriorly by ribs and vertebrae
- Inferiorly by diaphragm and ribs margins
- Superiorly by clavicles and soft tissues of the neck.

Thoracic wall consists of:
- Skin
- Fascia
- Muscles
- Nerves
- Vessels
- Bones.

Functions of Thoracic Wall

- Protections of thoracic and abdominal organs
- Resists intrathoracic pressure generated by elastic recoil of lungs and respiratory movements
- Provides attachment for supporting the weight of the upper limbs
- Provides attachment for many of the muscles of upper limbs, neck, abdomen, back and muscles of the respiration.

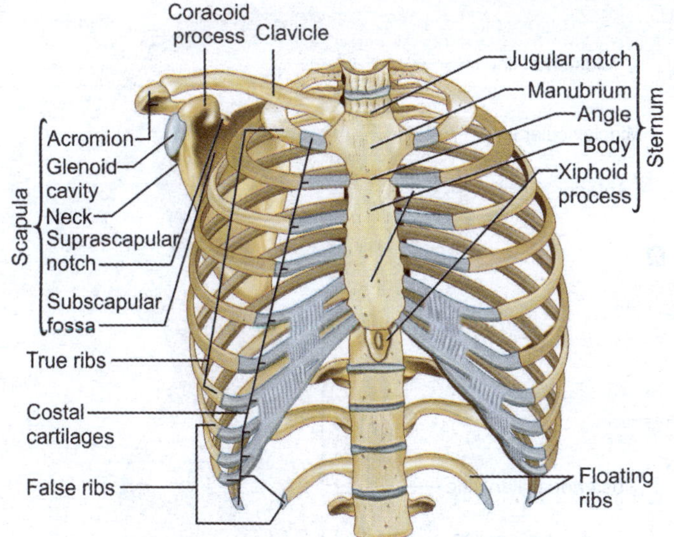

FIG. 3.1   Thoracic cavity

Thoracic Aperture

Thoracic cavity communicates with neck and upper limb through superior thoracic aperture called thoracic inlet.

- Structures entering and leaving the inlet are trachea, esophagus, nerves, and vessels
- Its anteroposterior diameter is 6.5 cm and transverse diameter is 11 cm
- It slopes anteriorly downwards.

Thoracic cavity communicates with abdomen through inferior thoracic aperture called thoracic outlet.

- Thoracic outlet is being separated from abdomen completely by the diaphragm
- The structures pass out and enter into thoracic cavity through the thoracic outlet by perforating the diaphragm.

Surface Anatomy of the Thoracic Wall (Figs 3.2A to C)

Several imaginary lines on the thoracic wall:

- *Anterior midsternal line:* It indicates the intersection of the medial plane with anterior chest wall
- *Midclavicular line:* This line passes through the midpoints of clavicle parallel to anterior midsternal line
- *Anterior axillary line:* This line passes along the anterior axillary fold, formed by border of the pectoralis major muscle.

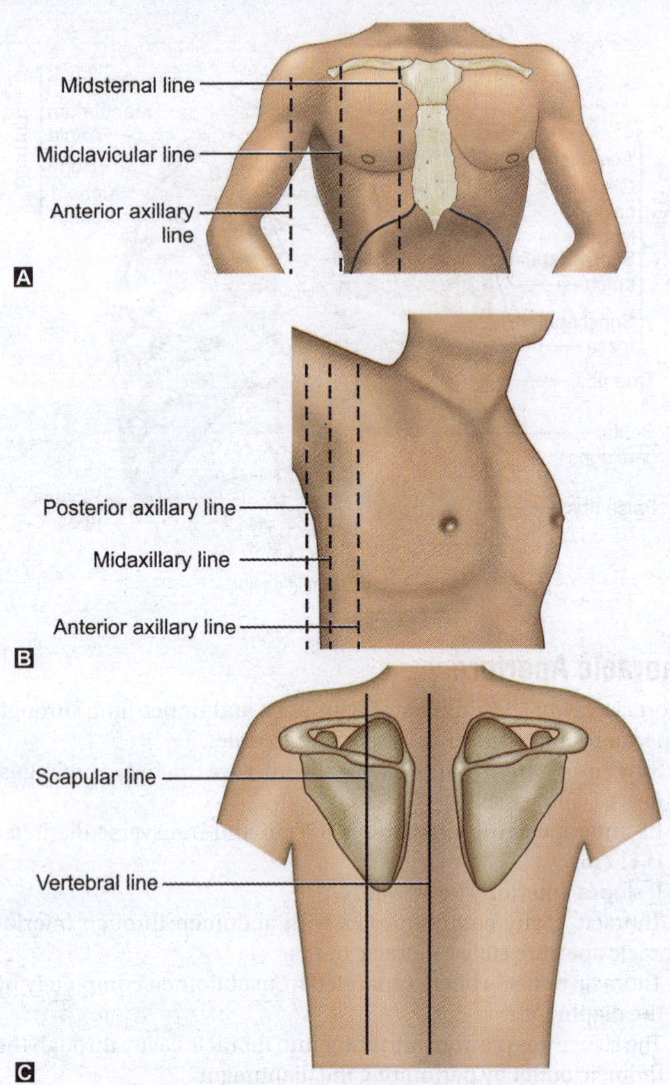

FIGS 3.2A TO C   Surface anatomy of thoracic wall

- *Midaxillary line:* This line passes along the posterior axillary fold, formed by latissimus dorsi and teres major muscles, as they span back to humerus
- *Posterior median line:* It is a vertical line at the intersection of median plane with vertebral column
- *Scapular line:* It is parallel to posterior median line and cross the inferior angle of the scapula.

Bones of the Thorax: Sternum (Fig. 3.3)

- *Three parts are:*
  - i. Manubrium
  - ii. Gladiolus
  - iii. Xiphoid.

  Manubrium is joined with gladiolus by fibrocartilage, mobility of this joint is slight.

  Gladiolus is joined with xiphoid cartilage may be calcified at later life.
- *Shape:* Looking like ancient Greek sword—manubrium is the handle, gladiolus is the blade, xiphoid cartilage is the tip
- *Shape of the xiphoid cartilage:* Lance-shaped or bifid, angulates forward.

Ribs (Fig. 3.4)

- It is flattened bone
- Its vertebral end has head, neck and double tubercle
- Its sternal end has costal cartilage
- Its head produces bipartite arthrodial (gliding) joint with two adjacent vertebral bodies and adjacent intervertebral disc
- Its neck tubercle produces arthrodial joint with transverse process of upper vertebra

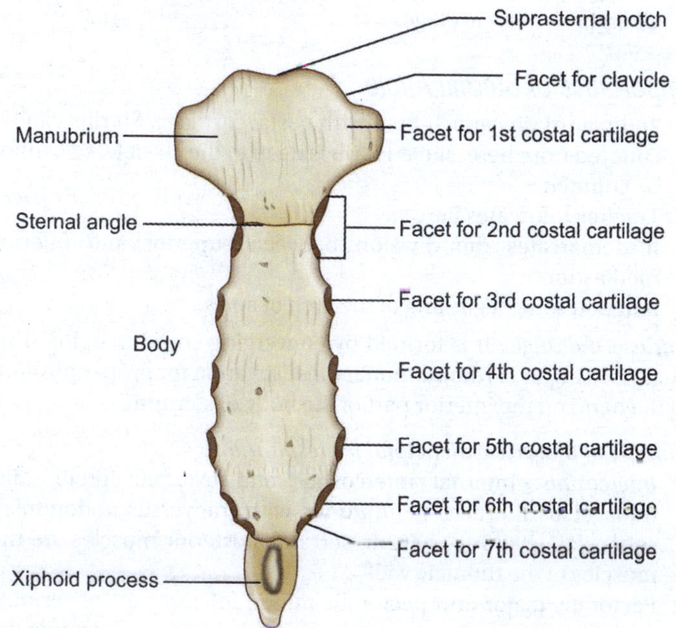

FIG. 3.3 Sternum

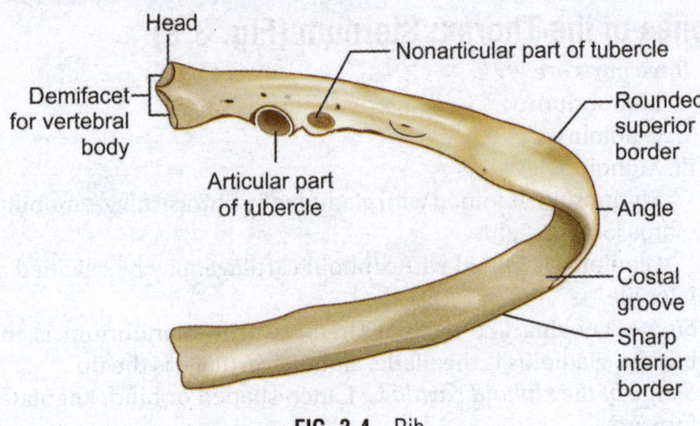

FIG. 3.4 Rib

- Sternal edges of first to seventh ribs join with sternum—they are true vertebrosternal joints
- 8th to 10th ribs are vertebrochondral; their sternal ends join with costal cartilage of the above adjacent ribs
- 11th and 12th ribs, because their anterior edge is free
- Joint of sternal edge of 1st rib with sternum is synarthrodial, because it is fixed. Other joints (2nd to 7th ribs) are arthrodial, these are mobile
- 2nd rib at its sternal edge joins with interface of manubrium and gladiolus—fibrocartilage.

Importance of Sternal Angle

- 2nd pair of ribs attach here with costal cartilage. So ribs can be counted from here, since 1st rib is deep to the clavicle, so cannot be counted
- Trachea bifurcates here
- It demarcates the division between superior and inferior mediastinum
- It denotes the beginning of the arch of aorta.

Infrasternal angle: It is formed by converging costal margins. This angle is used for cardiopulmonary resuscitation for proper position of the hand on the inferior part of the body of sternum.

Muscles of thoracic wall helpful for respiration
- *Intercostals:* Internal intercostals and external intercostals, transversus thoraces (continuous with tranversus abdominis), subcostal, levator costarum, serratus posterior muscles are the muscles of the thoracic wall
- Pectoralis major and pectoralis minor, inferior part of serratus anterior—act as accessory muscles of respiration—expands the thoracic cavity during forceful respiration

- The scalene muscles of respiration—fix these ribs and help the muscles connected below to be more effective in elevating lower ribs during forceful inspiration.

Respiratory passage: It consists of:
- Nose
- Nasopharynx
- Mouth
- Oropharynx
- Larynx
- Trachea
- Bronchial tree supplying the alveoli.

Description of Bronchial Tree (Fig. 3.5)

- Trachea bifurcates at the level of manubrium sterni by a dividing septum called carina
- Right bronchus is more vertical than left bronchus—hence more vulnerable to lodge the foreign body
- Right bronchus divides into three lobar bronchi, supplying three lobes of the lung:
  1. Upper lobe
  2. Middle lobe
  3. Lower lobe.
- Left bronchus divides into two lobar bronchi, upper lobe and lower lobe

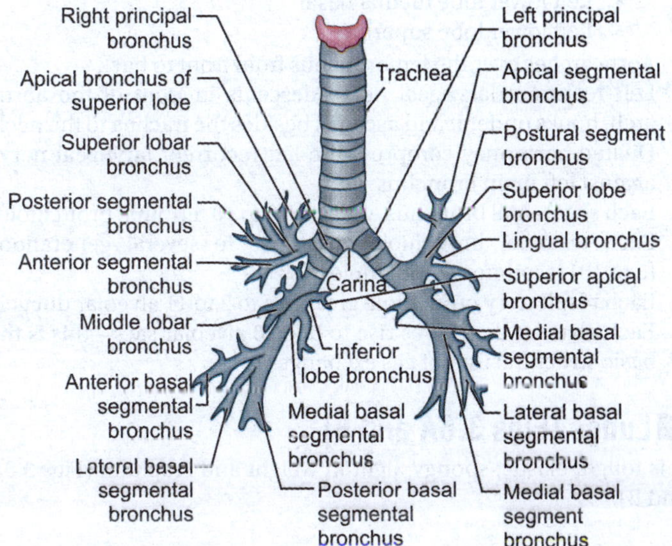

FIG. 3.5   Bronchopulmonary segment

- Each main bronchus is divided into segmental bronchi supplying the respectable bronchopulmonary segments
- The segment is pyramidal in shape with its apex towards the root and base towards the pleura. These segments are:
  - *Right upper lobe bronchus:*
    - Right upper lobe apical
    - Right upper lobe anterior
    - Right upper lobe posterior.
  - *Right middle lobe bronchus:*
    - Right middle lobe medial
    - Right middle lobe lateral.
  - *Right lower lobe bronchus:*
    - Right lower lobe anterior basal
    - Right lower lobe posterior basal
    - Right lower lobe lateral basal
    - Right lower lobe superior.
  - *Left upper lobe bronchus:*
    - Left upper lobe apical
    - Left upper lobe anterior
    - Left upper lobe posterior
    - Left upper lobe superior
    - Left upper lobe inferior.
  - *Left lower lobe bronchus:*
    - Left lower lobe anterior basal
    - Left lower lobe posterior basal
    - Left lower lobe lateral basal
    - Left lower lobe medial basal
    - Left lower lobe superior.
- Aorta arches over the left bronchus from front to back
- Left recurrent laryngeal nerve descents in front of the aortic arch, hooks under it and ascends besides the trachea to the neck. Dilated aorta may compress the left recurrent laryngeal nerve against left main bronchus
- Each segmental bronchus ends into 6 to 10 terminal bronchioles
- Each terminal bronchiole gives rise to several generations (5 to 10) respiratory bronchioles
- Each respiratory bronchiole gives rise to 2 to 11 alveolar ducts
- Each alveolar duct gives rise to 8 to 10 alveolar sacs—this is the basic structural unit of gas exchange.

■ Lungs (Figs 3.6A and B)

It is tough, elastic, spongy, light in weight and crepitant (Figs 3.6A and B).

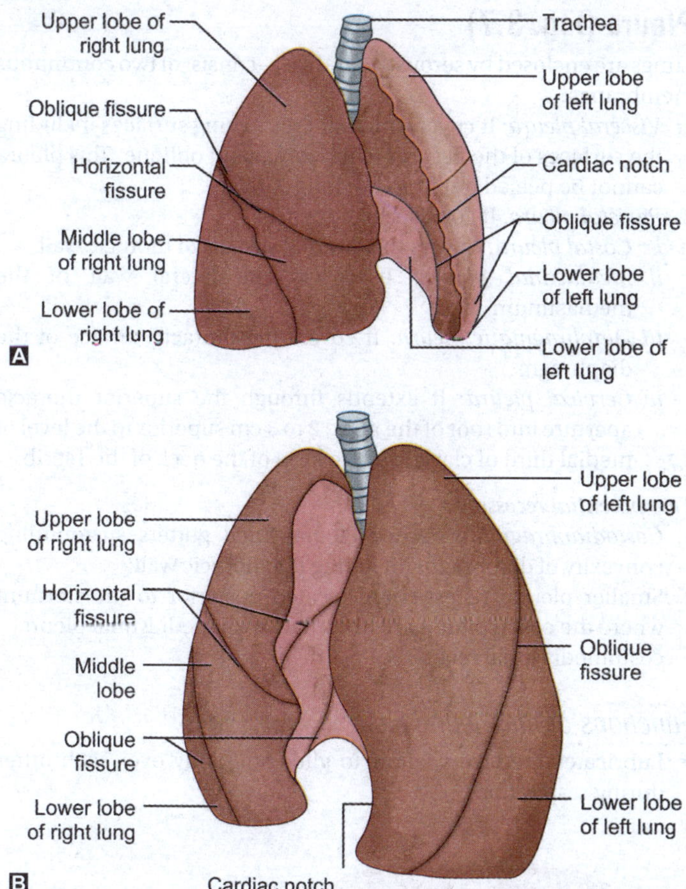

FIGS 3.6A AND B   (A) Lungs viewed from right; (B) Lungs viewed from left

Right lung is divided into three lobes:
1. Upper lobe
2. Middle lobe
3. Lower lobe.

Left lung is divided into two lobes:
1. Upper lobe
2. Lower lobe.

Each lobe is separated from the other of the same lung by lobar fissure—Infolding of the visceral pleura.

Shape of both the lungs are similar, but medial edge of left lung has an inferior indentation—cardiac notch.

Pleura (Fig. 3.7)

Lungs are enclosed by serous pleural sac—consist of two continuous membranes:

1. *Visceral pleura:* It covers and adheres to lung surfaces including the surfaces of the fissures—horizontal and oblique. This pleura cannot be peeled out from the lung surface.
2. *Parietal pleura:* It consists of four parts:
   i. *Costal pleura:* Covers the internal surface of thoracic wall
   ii. *Mediastinal pleura:* It covers the lateral wall of the mediastinum
   iii. *Diaphragmatic pleura:* It covers the thoracic surface of the diaphragm
   iv. *Cervical pleura:* It extends through the superior thoracic aperture into root of the neck, 2 to 3 cm superior to the level of medial third of clavicle at the level of the neck of the 1st rib.

Two potential recesses:
1. *Costodiaphragmatic recess:* Pleural-lined gutters surrounding convexity of diaphragm including the thoracic wall
2. Smaller pleural recesses are located posterior to the sternum where the costal pleura are in contact with mediastinal pleura—costomediastinal recess.

Functions of the Pleural Fluid

- Lubricates the layers, allow to glide smoothly over each other during respiration

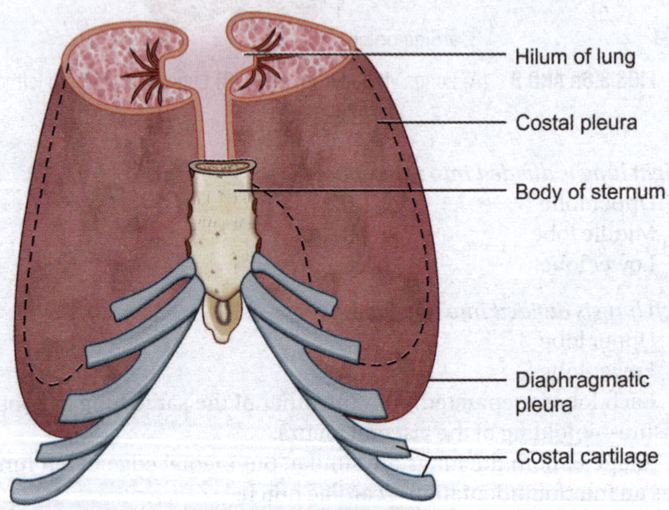

FIG. 3.7   Pleura

- Its surface tension so that the lungs fill with air, when thorax expands.

Root of the lung
The root of the lung is formed by the structures entering into and emerging from the lung, consists of:
- Pulmonary artery
- Superior and inferior pulmonary vein
- Bronchus.

Mediastinum

It occupies center of thorax, bounded laterally by mediastinal pleura and contains all thoracic viscera and structures except the lungs.

It extends from superior thoracic inlet to the diaphragm below, anteriorly sternum and costal cartilage to posteriorly thoracic vertebrae.

It is arbitrarily divided by an imaginary plane extending anteriorly from the sternal angle to 4th intervertebral disc posteriorly into:
- *Superior mediastinum:* It contains:
  - Superior vena cava
  - Brachiocephalic vein
  - Arch of aorta
  - Thoracic duct
  - Trachea
  - Esophagus
  - Thymus
  - Vagus nerve
  - Left recurrent laryngeal nerve
  - Phrenic nerve.
- *Inferior mediastinum* is subdivided by pericardium into:
  - *Anterior mediastinum:*
    - Remnant of thymus
    - Lymph nodes
    - Fat
    - Connective tissue.
  - *Middle mediastinum:*
    - Pericardium
    - Heart
    - Root of great vessels
    - Arch of azygos vein
    - Main bronchi.
  - *Posterior mediastinum:*
    - Azygos and hemiazygos veins
    - Esophagus
    - Thoracic aorta

- Vagus nerve
- Sympathetic trunk
- Splenic nerves.

Ventilation and Lung Mechanics

- Ventilation is defined as exchange of air between atmosphere and alveoli
- Flow of air is directly proportional to difference between atmospheric pressure and alveolar pressure, and inversely proportional to resistance to airflow, i.e.
- *Flow of air (F)*/$(P_{atmos} - P_{alv})$/Resistance (R)
- Atmospheric pressure is 760 mm Hg at sea level
- Alveolar pressure is less than atmospheric pressure during inspiration
- Alveolar pressure is higher than atmospheric pressure during expiration.
  Pleural pressure is also important.
1. Alveolar pressure—intrapleural fluid pressure (transpulmonary pressure) is the determinant of lung size.
2. Atmospheric pressure—alveolar pressure is the determinant of airflow.

During Inspiration

Diaphragm and inspiratory intercostals muscles contract
↓
Thorax expands
↓
Intrapleural pressure more subatmospheric
↓
Increased transpulmonary pressure
↓
Lung expands
↓
Alveolar pressure becomes subatmospheric
↓
Airflow into alveoli.

During Expiration

Diaphragm and intercostals muscles stop contracting
↓
Chest wall recoil inward
↓
Intrapleural pressure back towards the preinspiration value
↓

Transpulmonary pressure back towards preinspiration value

↓

Lung will recoil to preinspiration size

↓

Alveolar pressure becomes more than the atmospheric pressure

↓

Airflow out of the lungs.

Lung Volumes (Figs 3.8A and B)

- *Tidal volume:* During quiet breathing, the volume entering the lungs during inspiration is approximately equal to the volume of air leaving during expiration (450 mL)
- *Inspiratory reserve volume:* The maximal amount of air that can be inhaled above tidal volume during deep inspiration (amount – 3000 mL)
- *Expiratory reserve volume:* Maximal amount of air that can be exhaled during forced expiration after normal inspiration (amount – 1500 mL)
- *Residual volume:* Amount of air that is present after forceful expiration (amount – 1000 mL)
- *Functional residual capacity:* Expiratory reserve volume + Residual volume
- *Inspiratory capacity:* Tidal volume + Inspiratory reserve volume
- *Vital capacity:* Tidal volume + Inspiratory reserve volume + Expiratory reserve volume
- *Total lung capacity:* Tidal volume + Inspiratory reserve volume + Expiratory reserve volume + Residual volume.
  or
  Vital capacity + Residual volume.
  or
  Inspiratory capacity + Functional residual capacity.
- *Dead space air:* The amount of air present in the airways after full expiration (amount – 150 mL).
  So, fresh air entering the alveoli in one inspiration:
  450 – 150 mL = 300 mL.

Mechanism of Breathing

- *Muscles of respiration:*
  - ❖ Inspiration
  - ❖ Expiration.
- Elastic properties of the lung
- Elastic properties of the chest wall
- Airway resistance
- Tissue resistance.

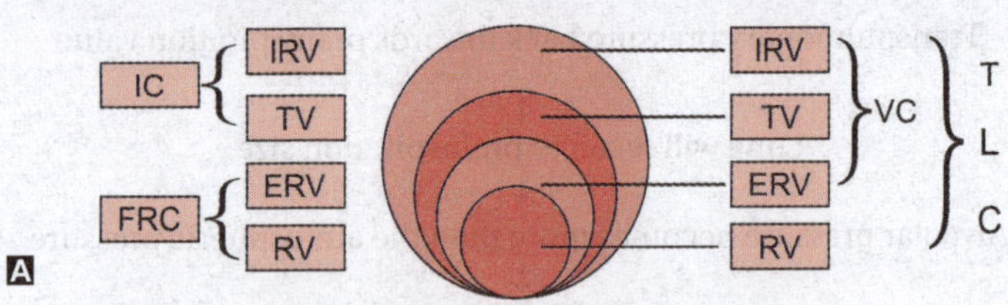

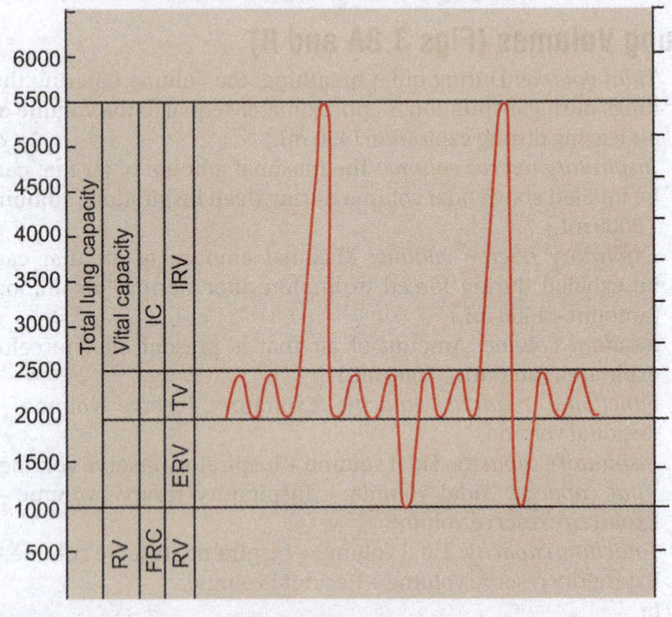

FIGS 3.8A AND B Lung volume

- *Work of breathing:*
  - ❖ Work of breathing of lung
  - ❖ Total work of breathing.

Respiratory Expansion of Thorax

Anteroposterior Expansion of Thorax

- 1st rib and sternum are fixed by scalene muscles
- Contraction of external and internal intercostals muscles narrows the intercostals spaces at the costovertebral joints about an axis passing through neck of the ribs
- Ribs are pulled upwards and forward like pump handle

- Since ribs slope inferiorly, their elevation results in anteroposterior movement of sternum with slight movement at manubriosternal joints in young people.

Lateral Expansion of Thorax

- During inspiration, 1st rib and sternum are fixed, each pair of ribs acts as semicircular plane rotating on anteroposterior axis
- Narrowing of the interspaces by intercostals muscles produce rotation of ribs in both anteroposterior and transverse axes rotating the middle part of the ribs, this is called bucket handle movement
- Lower ribs are more oblique and interspaces are wider, hence it is more evident in lower ribs.

Vertical Expansion of Thoracic Cavity

- Edge of the diaphragm is fixed to lower ribs center, forms a dome in the thoracic cavity
- During inspiration, thoracic wall diverge and flattening of the dome increases the vertical diameter of thorax. During normal inspiration, diaphragm descends about 1 cm. During forceful inspiration diaphragm descends about 10 cm downwards
- During expiration, central dome is high and thoracic wall converge—producing decrease in diameter of thoracic cavity
- During coughing, laughing, vomiting and defecation muscles of expiration—rectus abdominis, internal and external oblique muscles, transversus abdominis muscles contract, as a result intra-abdominal pressure is increased. Diaphragm is pushed upwards.

Lung Compliance

Magnitude of change in lung volume (VL) produced by a given change in transpulmonary pressure,

i.e. $CL = \Delta VL / \Delta (P_{alv} - P_{ip})$

The greater the lung compliance, the easier is to expand the lungs at any transpulmonary pressure.

Normal compliance of human lung is 200 mL/cm of water.

Compliance of the lung depends upon:

- *Stretchability of lung tissue:* So loss of lung tissue or stiffening of the lung produces decrease compliance
- *Surfactant:*
  - ❖ It is a dipalmitoylphosphatidylcholine
  - ❖ It is produced by Type II alveolar cells
  - ❖ It lowers the surface tension of the alveolar lining layer

❖ Deep breathing increases its secretion by stretching the Type II alveolar cells. Its secretion is small in case of shallow breathing
❖ *Loss of surfactant produces:*
  • Areas of atelectasis—producing stiff lung
  • Alveoli are filled up with exudates.

Regional Difference in Ventilation

Intrapleural pressure is less negative at lung base than apical area due to weight of the lung. So during inspiration, pressures near the bases are high and it is required to expand the lung bases than the apices. So basal region of the lung ventilates more than the apices.

Airway resistance: Frictional resistance to airflow is a major factor while flowing through the airways. Pressure required to produce laminar flow through the tube is governed by the following formula:

$$\text{Pressure required:} \quad \frac{\text{Length} \times \text{Viscosity} \times \text{Flow}}{\text{Radius} \times \text{Radius} \times \text{Radius} \times \text{Radius}}$$

• It is evident from the above equation that, radius in the most dominant variable for determining the resistance. Because just halving the radius there is 16 fold increase in the pressure
• Whereas, doubling the length of the tube produce doubling of pressure required
• Flow rate is linearly related to pressure. Because doubling of pressure is required for doubling the flow.

But in turbulent flow states:
• Greater increase in pressure is required to increase the flow
• Gas density also has a role. Because in case of gas of low density, resistance will be decreased (helium and oxygen mixture)
  Linear flow will occur in case quiet breathing through the mouth.

Nonlinear flow occurs in:
• Breathing through the nose
• Breathing through the narrowed airways
• In case of increase flow rate during exercise.

Chief site of airway resistance: Major site of resistance occurs at the medium size bronchi. Very small bronchioles contribute little resistance because of their large cross-sectional areas. However in case of asthma and chronic obstructive lung disease, major resistance occurs at smaller airways.

Factors Determining the Airway Resistance

• *Lung volume:* As the lung volume is reduced, airway resistance in smaller airways rises rapidly. At low lung volume, smaller airways at the bottom of the lung close completely where the lung is less expanded

- Contraction of the bronchial smooth muscles occurs through stimulation of receptors in the trachea and large bronchi
- Parasympathetic over activation
- Fall in P_{O_2} in the alveolar gas
- Increased density of the gas.

Control of ventilation (Fig. 3.9):
- *Sensors:*
  - Central chemoreceptors
  - Peripheral chemoreceptors
  - Lung receptors
  - Other receptors.
- *Central controllers:*
  - Brainstem
  - Cortex
  - Other parts of the brain.
- *Effector:* Respiratory muscles.
- *Responses in special conditions:*
  - Response to carbon dioxide
  - Response to oxygen
  - Response to pH
  - Response to exercise.

Central controller:
- *Brainstem:*
  - *Medullary respiratory center:* Situated beneath the floor of 4th ventricle it has two groups of cells:
    1. Dorsal respiratory group in the nucleus of tractus solitarius—it generates basic inspiratory pattern.
    2. Ventral respiratory group in the nucleus ambiguous and nucleus retroambiguous—responsible for active respiration at increased breathing rates. These cells are quiescent during normal breathing. But during forceful respiration, these cells are active.

       After abolishment of all afferent impulses, the above inspiratory cells send repetitive burst of active potentials, which is responsible for contraction of respiratory muscles.
  - *Pontine centers:* These are for fine tuning of the dorsal respiratory group. There are two centers:
    1. *Apneustic center:* Promotes inspiration. In case of brain injury, it is responsible for apneustic breathing.
    2. *Pneumotaxic center:* It inhibits inspiration. It controls respiratory rate and volume.
- *Cortex:* Both sensory and motor cortex override the function of brain stem within limits
- *Other parts of brain:* Limbic system and hypothalamus—change the pattern of breathing during emotion, fear, cry, and rage.

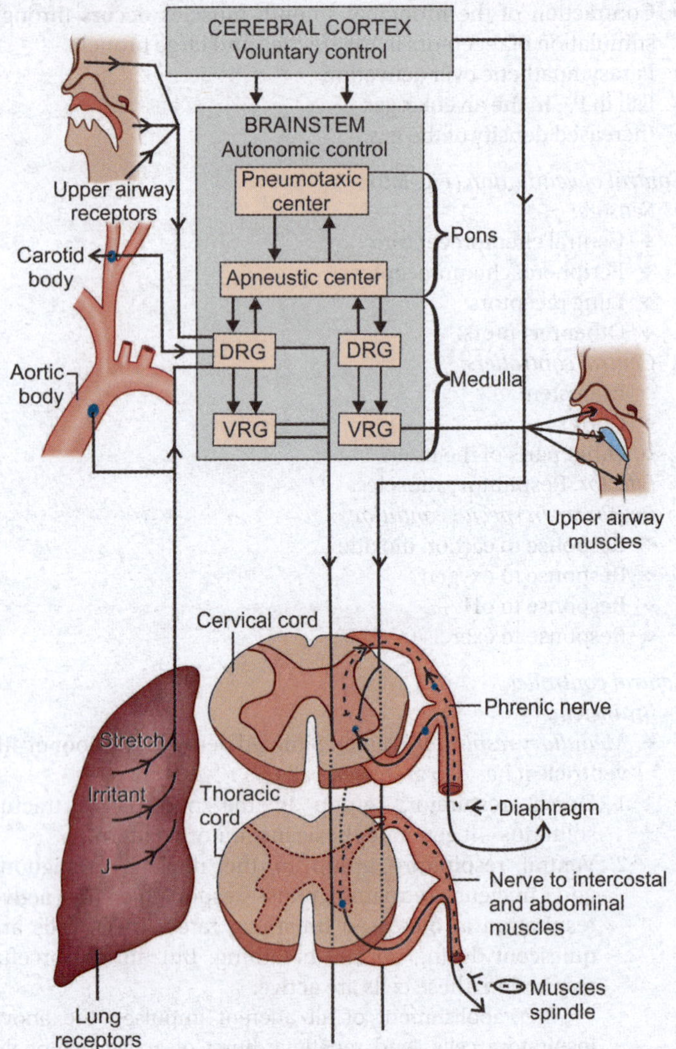

FIG. 3.9 Respiratory control system

Abbrevations: DRG, dorsal respiratory group of nucleus; VRG, ventral respiratory group of nucleus

Sensors

- *Chemoreceptor:* There are two types of chemoreceptor.
  1. *Central chemoreceptor:*
     - Located near ventral surface of medulla
     - Sensitive to the P_{CO_2} in the tissue but not P_{CO_2} of the blood
     - Responds to change in pH of extracellular fluid/cerebrospinal fluid (CSF) when CO_2 diffuses out of the capillaries.
       - Normal pH of CSF is 7.32

- CSF has less buffering capacity, because it contains less protein. So change in pH of CSF is greater than that of blood at any change in P_{CO_2}
- Again the change in pH of CSF occurs more promptly than change in arterial pH by renal compensation. Hence in chronic lung disease with long standing CO_2 retention—patient has low ventilation for his or her arterial P_{CO_2}.

2. *Peripheral chemoreceptor:*
   - Carotid bodies at the bifurcation of the common carotid arteries. It contains two types of glomus cells:
     i. Type one cells contain dopamine and are close apposition to endings of the afferent carotid sinus nerves.
     ii. Type two cells are rich in capillaries.
   - Aortic bodies below the aortic arch—responsible for fall in arterial pH.

- *Lung receptors:*
  - *Pulmonary stretch receptor (slow adapting receptor):*
    - Present in airway smooth muscle
    - They are activated in response to distension of lung
    - The impulse travels via vagus nerve (large myelinated fibers)
    - Main response is slowing of respiratory frequency—due to increase in expiratory time—known as Hering-Breuer inflation
    - Recent work suggests that these reflexes are largely inactive in adult human unless tidal volume exceeds 1 liter, as in exercise.
  - *Irritant receptor (rapidly adopting pulmonary stretch receptor):*
    - These lie in between airway epithelial cells
    - Stimulated by noxious gases, cigarette smokes, inhaled dust, and cold air
    - Impulses travel by myelinated vagal nerve fibers
    - Effector response is bronchoconstriction.
  - *J receptor:*
    - These are situated in the alveolar walls close to the capillaries
    - These are nonmyelinated C fibers
    - These are stimulated by chemicals in pulmonary circulation
    - Effector response is rapid shallow breathing and dyspnea.
  - *Bronchial C fibers:*
    - These are present in the bronchial wall close to bronchial circulation
    - Stimulated by chemicals in bronchial circulation
    - Effector response is rapid shallow breathing, broncho-constriction and mucus secretion.

- *Other receptors:*
  - ❖ *Nose and upper airway receptor:*
    - These are present in nose, nasopharynx, and larynx
    - Stimulated by chemical and mechanical stimuli
    - Effector responses are sneezing, coughing, and broncho-constriction.
  - ❖ *Joint and muscle receptor:*
    - Impulses from moving limb
    - Stimulates ventilation during exercise.
  - ❖ *Gamma system:*
    - Muscle spindles in the intercostals and diaphragm stimulated in response to elongation of muscle fibers
    - It controls strength of contraction, may produce dyspnea.
  - ❖ *Arterial baroreceptor:*
    - Increase in the arterial blood pressure, can cause reflex hypoventilation and apnea, when aortic carotid sinus baroceptors are being stimulated
    - Decrease of blood pressure produces hyperventilation.
  - ❖ *Pain, temperature receptors:*
    - Pain receptor stimulation produces period of apnea followed by hyperventilation
    - Heating or warming the skin produce hyperventilation.

Blood Gas Exchange (Fig. 3.10)

Responses in special conditions

- *Responses to CO_2:*

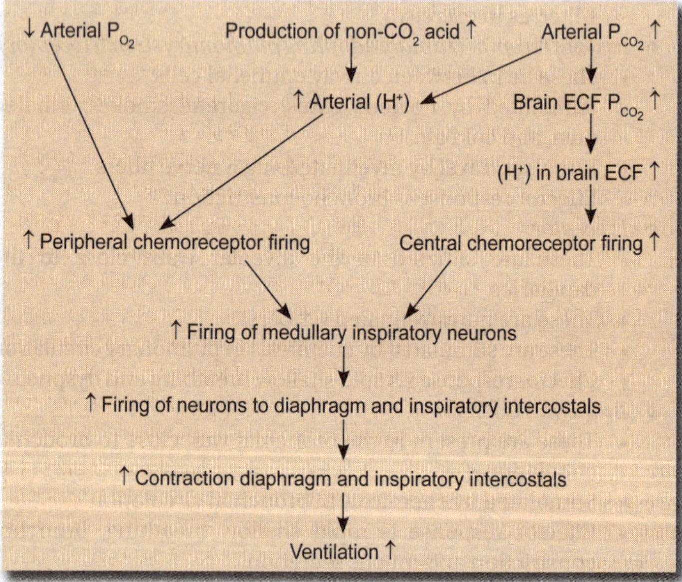

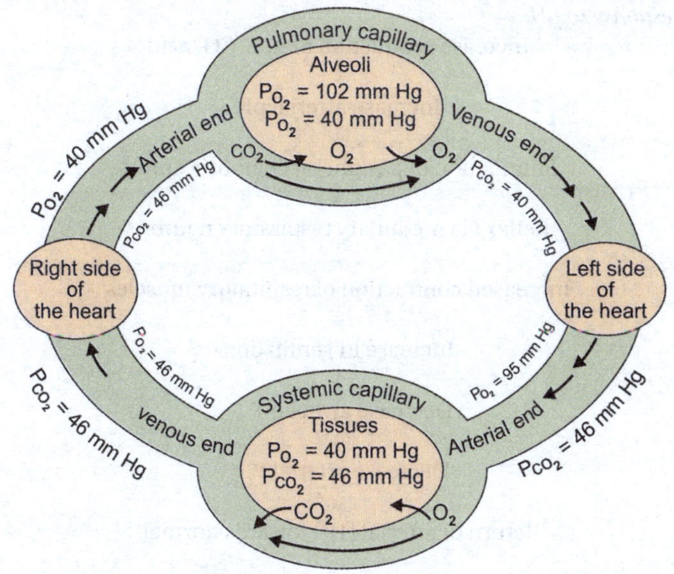

FIG. 3.10   Blood gas exchange

Ventilatory response to CO_2 is reduced by sleep, increasing age, genetic, racial and personality factors.
Trained athlete and drivers have low CO_2 sensitivity.

- *Response to oxygen:*

Decreased O_2 in the inspired air
↓
Decrease in alveolar P_{O_2}
↓
Decreased arterial P_{O_2}
↓
Stimulation of peripheral chemoreceptor
↓
Medullary respiratory neurons are stimulated
↓
Increased firing of neurons to diaphragm and inspiratory intercostals
↓
Increased contraction of respiratory muscles and diaphragm
↓
Increased ventilation
↓
Return of arterial and alveolar P_{O_2} towards normal

Reduction of arterial P_{O_2} may be accompanied by rise in P_{CO_2}— stimulates ventilation.

Response to pH:

$$\text{Increase production of non-}CO_2 \text{ acid}$$
$$\downarrow$$
$$\text{Increase arterial pH}$$
$$\downarrow$$
$$\text{Stimulation of peripheral chemoreceptors}$$
$$\downarrow$$
$$\text{Reflex via medullary respiratory neurons}$$
$$\downarrow$$
$$\text{Increased contraction of respiratory muscles}$$
$$\downarrow$$
$$\text{Increase in ventilation}$$
$$\downarrow$$
$$\text{Decrease alveolar } P_{CO_2}$$
$$\downarrow$$
$$\text{Decrease arterial } P_{CO_2}$$
$$\downarrow$$
$$\text{Return of arterial } (H^+) \text{ towards normal.}$$

■ Physiology of Pleural Fluid Absorption and Reabsorption

Amount of fluid in normal human being pleural cavity is 1 to 20 mL. The amount of fluid to be present in pleural space depends upon:

- Hydrostatic pressure
- Osmotic pressure
- Tissue pressure that is not known.

In case of parietal pleura:

- Capillaries around the parietal pleura = 30 cm of water
- Pleural pressure = – 5 cm of water in between the pleural layer
- So net pressures = 30 – (–5) = 30 + 5 = 35 cm of water. It is responsible for driving the fluid into the pleural cavity
- Colloid pressure in capillaries = 34 cm of water
- Colloid osmotic pressure of the pleura = 8 cm of water
- So net pressure = (34–8) cm of water = 26 cm of water, which is responsible for driving the fluid from the pleural space into pulmonary capillaries
- So, balance force is 35 – 26 = 9 cm of water, which directs the fluid from the parietal pleura into pleural cavity.

In case of visceral pleura:

- Capillaries (bronchial and pulmonary vessels) around the visceral pleura = 11 cm of water
- Pleural pressure = –5 cm of water
- So, net hydrostatic pressure from visceral pleura towards the pleural cavity is 11– (–5) = 11 + 5 = 16 cm of water

- Colloid osmotic pressure in capillaries = 34 cm of water
- Colloid osmotic pressure in pleural cavity = 8 cm of water
- So, net pressure is 34 – 8 = 26 cm of water, which is responsible for driving the fluid from pleural into pulmonary capillaries
- So, balance force is 26 – 16 = 10 cm of water, which is responsible for driving the fluid from pleural cavity to pleural capillaries.

Normal Values

Respiratory pressure is always expressed in relation to atmospheric pressure (760 mm Hg).

Intrapleural Pressure

- *At the end of normal inspiration:* –6 mm Hg = (760 – 6) mm Hg = 754 mm Hg
- *At the end of normal expiration:* –2 mm Hg = (760 – 2) mm Hg = 758 mm Hg
- *At the end of forced inspiration:* –30 mm Hg = (760 – 30) mm Hg = 730 mm Hg
- *At the end of forced expiration:* +50 mm Hg = (760 + 50) mm Hg = 810 mm Hg
- *At the end of forced inspiration with closed glottis:* –70 mm Hg = (760   70) mm Hg = 690 mm Hg.

Intra-alveolar Pressure

Intra-alveolar pressure is equal to atmospheric pressure so:
- *In normal respiration:* –1 mm Hg = (760 – 1) mm Hg = 759 mm Hg
- *In normal expiration:* +1 mm Hg = (760 + 1) mm Hg = 761 mm Hg
- *During forced inspiration with closed glottis (Müller's maneuver):* –80 mm Hg
- *During forced expiration with closed glottis:* +100 mm Hg
- At the end of inspiration and expiration, pressure is equal to atmospheric pressure = 760 mm Hg.

■ Vascular System (Fig. 3.11)

Precapillary pulmonary vessels are divided into three subtypes:
1. *Elastic arteries:* These include:
   Main pulmonary artery and its following branches extending approximately to the junction of bronchi and bronchioles:
   ❖ Lobar branches
   ❖ Segmental branches
   ❖ Subsegmental branches.
   As it enters the lung parenchyma, its medial wall is lost.

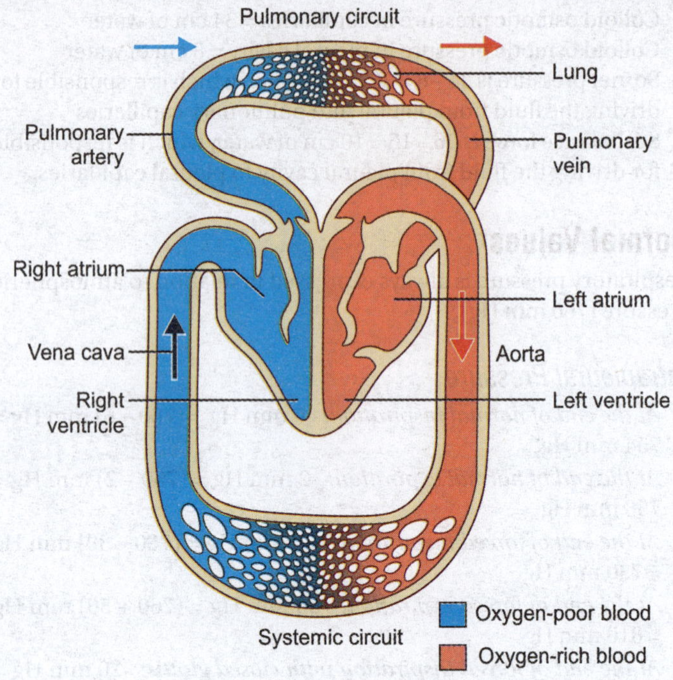

FIG. 3.11 Pulmonary vasculature

2. *Muscular arteries:* They have external diameter of 70 to 500 μm and have well developed layer of circular smooth muscle cells between elastic lamina. Below 70 μm diameter, these vessels gradually loose smooth muscles, becomes arterioles, having intima and elastic lamina.
3. *Arterioles:* Within the acinus, it divides along with accompanying branches of acini and give some accessory branches. These branches are terminated around alveolar sac; break up into capillaries around alveoli.

Other Accessory Vessels

These are supplementary branches of pulmonary artery directly penetrate into lung parenchyma. These branches arise from the entire length of arterial tree and increase towards periphery. So the branching ratio (average number of daughter branches originating from one parent branch) increases as the vessel size decreases. Proximally ratio is 3:1 distally the ratio is 3.6.

Pulmonary Veins

Pulmonary vein arises from capillaries of the arteriolar network. Supplementary vessels also join the vein in their course through the lung.

Two large superior pulmonary veins drain the blood from:
1. Middle and upper lobe of right lung
2. Upper lobe of left lung.

Two large inferior pulmonary veins drain the blood from: lower lobes of both the lungs.

Bronchial Arteries

Two to four bronchial arteries directly arise from:
- Aorta
- Intercostals vessels.

Near the hila, these branches to form intercommunicating network of circular arc around the main bronchi from these arterial network, intrapulmonary arteries radiate—these branches present within peribronchial connective tissue and divide along the branches of airways up to terminal bronchioles.

Thoracic Lymph Nodes (Fig. 3.12)

- *Parietal lymph nodes:* These nodes are subdivided into three groups:
  - i. *Anterior parietal (internal mammary lymph nodes):*
    - *Situation:* Upper portion of thorax behind anterior inter-costal spaces bilaterally
    - *Drainage area:* Anterior chest wall, medial portion of breast, certain portion of diaphragm, upper anterior abdominal wall.
  - ii. *Posterior parietal lymph nodes:*
    - Present adjacent to rib heads in posterior intercostal spaces (intercostal nodes) or adjacent to vertebrae (juxta-vertebral)
    - *Drainage area:* Intercostal spaces, parietal pleura, vertebral column.
  - iii. *Diaphragmatic nodes:* Diaphragm and upper part of abdomen.

Visceral Lymph Nodes

These are divided into three groups:
1. *Anterosuperior mediastinal nodes.* These groups drain the structures of anterior pericardium, thymus, diaphragmatic and mediastinal part of the heart and anterior portion of hila.
2. *Posterior mediastinal (periesophageal) lymph nodes and periaortic nodes: Drainage areas:* Posterior portion of diaphragm, pericardium, esophagus and lower lobes of lungs.

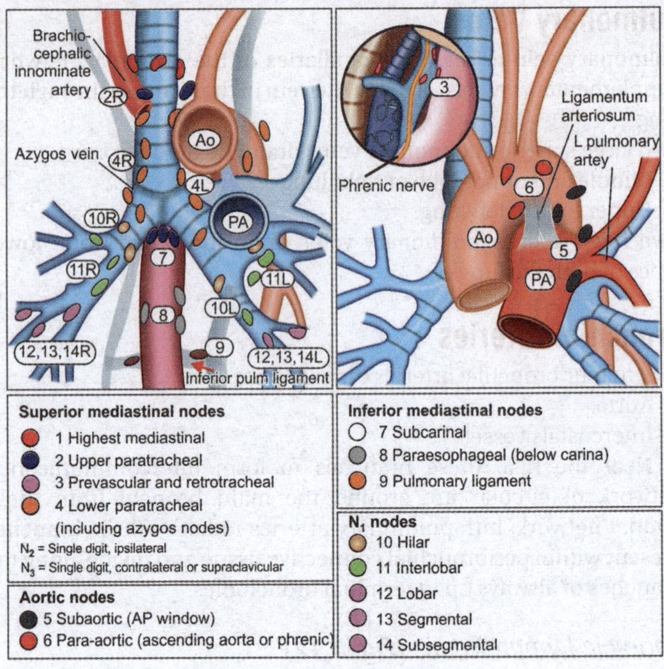

FIG. 3.12 Thoracic lymph nodes

3. *Tracheobronchial lymph nodes:* These are subdivided into following subgroups:

❖ *Paratracheal:* Afferent from bronchopulmonary nodes, tracheal bifurcation nodes, trachea, esophagus, right and left lung directly

❖ *Tracheal bifurcation (carinal) nodes:* Situated in precranial, and subcranial fat and around the circumference of right and left main bronchi

❖ *Aortopulmonary window nodes:* Divided into medial, lateral and superior groups. Afferent from bronchopulmonary nodes, mediastenal nodes, heart, pericardium, esophagus and lungs

❖ *Hilar nodes:* Located around the main bronchi. Afferent from all lobes of lungs.

Size of the nodes:

- Upper paratracheal and left paraesophageal nodes should be declared enlarged when the diameter is >7 mm
- Anterior mediastinal nodes are >8 mm
- Lower paratracheal and right paratracheal nodes are >10 mm
- Subcarinal nodes are >11 mm.

SYMPTOMS OF RESPIRATORY DISEASES

Seven principal symptoms are:
1. Cough
2. Sputum production or not
3. Hemoptysis
4. Chest pain
5. Breathlessness
6. Wheeze
7. Hoarseness.

Cough

It is an explosive expiration to protect the lung from aspiration and to promote secretion and other constituent upwards toward the mouth. The necessary stimulation usually arises from larynx to second order of bronchi.

Cough is a type of protective as well as cleansing mechanism:
- *Cause:* It arises from irritation of cough receptors in the trachea, pharynx, larynx, and bronchi by:
  ❖ Infection
  ❖ Inflammatory exudates in the airways or parenchyma
  ❖ Tumor
  ❖ Foreign body, inhaled particles
  ❖ Parietal pleura—on rare occasion during aspiration of pleural effusion
  ❖ Cerumen in the external ear
  ❖ Pressure on the external wall of bronchus.
- *Frequency and severity of cough depend upon several factors:*
  ❖ Situation and nature of the lesion
  ❖ Presence or absence of sputum production
  ❖ Presence of coexisting abnormalities, e.g.
    • Vocal cord paralysis
    • Impairment of ventilatory function
    • Pleural pain.

Cough may be voluntary, involuntary or combination of two.

Involuntary mechanism usually involves:
- *Mechanical and chemical.* Inhalation of irritants like, smoke, dust, distortions of airways by pulmonary fibrosis or atelectasis. Smokers are more vulnerable, because they have underlying pharyngitis, laryngitis, or tracheobronchitis
- *Tracheobronchial inflammation:* It is due to infection, inhalation of irritant
- *Psychogenic:* Anxiety.

Questions to be asked regarding cough:
- Whether cough is sudden in onset or gradually increasing?
- Whether cough is productive or nonproductive?
- How long it is persisting, if persists, duration?
- How long the cough is used to persist?
- Associated symptoms if present, what it is?
- Whether cough is associated with hemoptysis?
- Associated comorbid conditions, like diabetes, hypertension, coronary heart disease, etc.
- Whether the patient smokes? If so, what does he smoke? How much he smokes per day and how long?
- Does the cough start after eating?
- Is the cough worse in any position?
- What factor relieves cough?
- Are there any associated symptom with cough, like fever, headache, night sweat, rhinorrhea, weight loss, hoarseness of voice?

Causes and Characteristics of Cough

Causes	Characteristics
Epiglottal disease	Barking cough
Pharynx	Pharyngitis—upper respiratory tract symptoms like, sneezing, nasal allergy, sore throat
Larynx	Laryngitis, whooping cough, croup, Laryngeal tumor. Harsh, barking, painful, persistent, associated with stridor Left-sided vocal cord paralysis—Bovine cough, inefficient, low pitched accompanied by hoarseness of voice
Trachea	Tracheitis producing dry painful cough, sore throat, running nose (stridor)
Bronchus and alveoli	Bronchitis—dry or productive on most of the days for >3 consecutive months and for >2 years, worse in morning, sputum is mucoid
	Asthma—dry with scanty and sticky sputum, worse at night
	Bronchogenic carcinoma—cough with productive or nonproductive for month or years, with occasional hemoptysis
	Brochiectasis—long-standing cough with large amount of mucoid or foul smelling purulent sputum, amount changes with posture
	Lobar pneumonia—proceeded by upper respiratory tract symptoms, cough painful and dry at first, followed by productive later
	Bronchopneumonia—cough is dry or productive
	Exacerbation of chronic bronchitis—cough, first dry then mucoid followed by purulent

Contd...

Contd...

Causes	Characteristics
	Alveolar cell carcinoma—cough productive or nonproductive for weeks to years, occasionally large quantity watery sputum is produced
	Tuberculosis or fungal infection—cough with productive sputum, occasionally blood tinged
Benign tumor	Inefficient, nonproductive, occasionally hemoptysis
Interstitial tissue	Interstitial disease (infiltration, fibrosis)—cough, nonproductive, persistent, distressing
Mediastinum	Mediastinal tumor—breathlessness and cough due to compression on trachea or bronchi
	Aortic aneurysm—Brassy cough
Gastrointestinal cause	Gastroesophageal reflux—nonproductive cough following intake of heavy meals or recumbency. It is usually accompanied by heart burn, belching
	Associated with eating and drinking—neuromuscular disease of upper esophagus
Foreign body	When in upper airway—cough associated with stridor and asphyxia. Later in lower airways—nonproductive and localized wheeze
Cardiovascular	Left ventricular failure—cough aggravated in supine position, reduced in recumbent position
	Pulmonary infarction—cough associated with hemoptysis may be pleural effusion
Drug	Angiotensin converting enzyme inhibitor—nonproductive cough, usually in women, may start with commencement of drug on years after use
Debility and weakness	Inadequate coughing
Time of cough	Morning: Smoking Nocturnal: Postnasal drip, congestive cardiac failure

Type of Cough

Dry hacking cough	Allergy, viral infection, anxiety neurosis, tumor, interstitial lung disease
Chronic productive	Bronchiectasis, lung abscess, chronic bronchitis, bacterial pneumonia, tuberculosis
Barking	Epiglottic disease
Morning cough	Smoking
Nocturnal cough	Congestive cardiac failure
Stridor	Tracheal obstruction
Associated with eating or drinking	Upper esophageal muscular disease
Inadequate coughing	Debility, weakness
Wheezing	Asthma, allergy, chronic obstructive lung disease

Mechanism of Cough

Rapid inspiration followed by following processes in rapid sequences:

- Closure of glottis
- Contraction of thoracic and abdominal expiratory muscles
- Abrupt increase of intrathoracic pressure (100–200 mm Hg)
- Sudden opening of glottis
- Explosion of burst of air through mouth.

Production of sound during cough by:

- Vibration of intra-airway secretions
- Vibrations of tracheobronchial walls
- Vibration of parenchyma.

Neural Pathways in the Development of Cough

Afferent pathways

- 5th nerve carrying impulses from nose and sinuses
- 9th nerve carrying impulses from posterior pharynx
- 10th nerve carrying impulses from larynx, trachea, bronchi, pleura, and pericardium
- Phrenic nerve carrying impulses from trachea, bronchi, esophagus, stomach, and pleura.

Most of the receptors are concentrated in the larynx with gradual decrease in concentration of receptors down the tracheobronchial tree.

Efferent pathways

- 10th nerve carrying impulses to larynx, trachea, and bronchi
- Phrenic nerve carrying impulses to diaphragm
- Spinal motor nerve to expiratory muscles of the rib cage.

Controlling center: Medullary center (voluntary control).

Effectiveness of cough is determined by lung volume at which it occurs.

Damage of reflex pathways

- Bronchiectasis damage the irritant receptors on the bronchial wall
- Narcotics and anesthetics decrease the sensitivity of the receptors
- Tracheostomy eliminates the glottis closure
- Neuromuscular disease weakens the respiratory muscles
- Age weakens the respiratory muscles.

■ Sputum

Sometimes there is difficulty in distinguishing sputum production from:
- Gastroesophageal reflux
- Postnasal drip
- Saliva.

Regarding sputum one has to ask the patient:
- Show me what you have to do to get phlegm up
- If patient denies sputum—a cough producing rattle (loose cough)—suggests its presence.

Following informations have to be asked regarding sputum:
- *Amount:*
  - ❖ It may be very large (a teacupful per day)
    Causes:
    - Bronchiectasis
    - Lung abscess
    - Bronchoalveolar cell carcinoma.
  - ❖ Very small amount (one to two spits per day)
    - Early phase of pneumonia
    - Bronchial asthma.
  - ❖ Child usually swallows sputum.
- *Character:*
  - ❖ *Clear, watery, frothy sputum (serous):*
    - Acute pulmonary edema
    - Bronchoalveolar cell carcinoma (profuse).
  - ❖ *Clear, gray/white, frothy (mucoid):*
    - Chronic bronchitis—chronic obstructive pulmonary disease (COPD)
    - Chronic asthma
    - Tumors
    - Tuberculosis.
  - ❖ *Yellow, green, brown sputum:* Lung infections—all types—bronchopulmonary infection in bronchiectasis and chronic bronchitis
  - ❖ *Rusty sputum:* Pneumococcal pneumonia
  - ❖ *Pink frothy sputum, frothy sputum with streak of blood:* Pulmonary edema
  - ❖ *Black colored sputum:* Town dweller
  - ❖ *Red current jelly: Klebsiella pneumoniae* infection
  - ❖ *Pink blood tinged sputum:* Streptococcal or staphylococcal pneumonia
  - ❖ *Bloody sputum:* Pulmonary emboli, tuberculosis, bronchiectasis, bleeding disorders.

- *Viscosity:*
  - ❖ *Highly viscous:*
    - Early stage of lobar pneumonia
    - Bronchial asthma
    - Chronic bronchitis.
  - ❖ *Small bronchial cast like twigs:* Bronchopulmonary aspergillosis associated with asthma.
- *Taste or odor:* Foul smelling sputum:
  - ❖ Lung abscess
  - ❖ Infected bronchiectasis
  - ❖ Infection with anaerobic organism.

Questions to be asked regarding sputum:
- What is the color of the sputum?
- How often do you bring it up?
- How much do you bring it up?
- Do you have trouble getting it up?
- Is it foul smelling?
- Does it contain blood?

■ Hemoptysis

Coughing of blood is called hemoptysis.

Differences Between Hemoptysis and Hematemesis

Hemoptysis	Hematemesis
Coughing of blood	Vomiting of blood
Bright red and frothy	Blackish and not frothy
No food particle present	Food particles are present
Alkaline pH	Acidic pH
Prodromal symptom, like coughing	Associated with nausea or vomiting
Associated with dyspnea	Associated with nausea

Difference Between Hemoptysis of Nasal Bleeding

Hemoptysis	Epistaxis
Coughing of blood	Trickle of blood through mouth when it comes to pharynx
No associated nasal bleeding	Associated with bleeding from anterior nares

Sometime nasal bleeding is swallowed and then coughed up and diagnosed as hemoptysis.
- *Questions to be asked in hemoptysis:*
  - ❖ Whether if is coughed out or vomited out?
  - ❖ What is the amount of blood coughed out per day?

- ❖ How often it is coughed out per day?
- ❖ Whether it is increasing in amount per day?
- ❖ Whether coughing of blood is sudden?
- ❖ Whether this episode is recurrent? If so, how often it occurs?
- ❖ Whether the blood is in the form of clot or blood-tinged?
- ❖ Are there any associated symptoms like, nausea, vomiting, or coughing?
- ❖ Is there any family history of tuberculosis?
- ❖ Any history of travel by airplane?
- ❖ Any history of bleeding disorder?
- ❖ Any history of systemic disease like, liver disorders, collagen vascular disease?
- ❖ Any history of pain in the legs, prolonged bed riding?
- ❖ In case of female, any history of use of oral contraceptives?

Pointers to the Significance of an Episode of Hemoptysis

Probably serious	Probably not serious
• Middle aged or elderly	• Young adult
• Chronic smoker	• Nonsmoker
• Spontaneous	• Not spontaneous
• Recurrent episodes	• Single episode
• Large amount	• Small amount
• No recent infection	• Recent infection

Causes of Hemoptysis

Infective inflammatory cause in bronchus	Bronchitis, bronchiectasis
Infections in lung parenchyma	Tuberculosis, pneumonia, lung abscess
Fungal disorders	Aspergillosis, Fungal ball in healed tuberculous cavity, bronchiectatic area, and cystic residue of sarcoidosis
Noninfective inflammatory	Wegener's granulomatosis, good pasture syndrome
Tumor	Tracheal tumor, laryngeal tumor, bronchial adenoma, bronchogenic carcinoma
Vascular disorder	Pulmonary infarction, arteriovenous malformations, aortic aneurysm penetrating into tracheobronchial tree
Cardiac cause	Mitral stenosis left ventricular failure
Hematological	Blood dyscrasia
Trauma	Foreign body
Drugs	Anticoagulant
Liver	Amebic liver abscess perforating into right-sided pleural cavity producing sputum which is anchovy sauce like

- *Associated conditions:*
  - ❖ *Pulmonary embolism:*
    - Sudden onset of pleuritic chest pain
    - Dyspnea.
  - ❖ *Pulmonary tuberculosis:*
    - Fever
    - Weight loss
    - Cough
    - Sputum.
  - ❖ *Bronchiectasis:*
    - Long history of sputum production
    - Hemoptysis associated with recurrent purulent sputum.
  - ❖ *In acute pulmonary congestion,* sputum is pink and frothy.
    In chronic pulmonary congestion, sputum contains alveolar macrophages containing hemosiderin granules.

■Chest Pain

Pain fiber is not present in lung and visceral pleura.

- *Pain fiber arises from:*
  - ❖ Parietal pleura
  - ❖ Mediastenal structures
  - ❖ Chest wall.
- *Causes of chest pain:*
  - ❖ Central
  - ❖ Noncentral
  - ❖ *Central/retrosternal:*
    - Tracheitis
    - Mediastinitis
    - Mediastinal tumors
    - Medistinal emphysema
    - Esophageal disorders
    - Diseases of great vessels.
  - ❖ *Noncentral:*
    - *Pleural:*
      - Tuberculosis
      - Pneumonia
      - Pulmonary infarction
      - Malignant tumors.
    - *Chest wall:*
      - Rib fractures
      - Costochondritis
      - Direct invasion of chest wall or rib by metastatic tumors
      - Spinal nerve root involvement by:
        - Vertebral collapse
        - Herpes zoster.
      - Coxsackie B virus infection (Bornholm disease).

Description Pain According to Sites

Pleural Pain

- It occurs due to stretching of the inflamed pleura rubbing against each other
- Stabbing or sharp in nature
- It is aggravated by coughing, laughing, and straining
- It sometimes spreads along the intercostal nerves supplying the affected area
- In case of inflammation of diaphragmatic pleura due to inflammation above or below the pleura, pain usually radiates to the respective shoulder
- If central part of outer diaphragmatic pleura is involved, pain radiates to the abdomen
- Associated signs are fever, malaise, pulmonary signs.

Chest Wall Pain

It may arise from:
- *Intrathoracic:*
  - Pleura
  - Lungs
  - Pericardium
  - Heart
  - Chest wall.
- *Extrathoracic:* Below the diaphragm.
  Pleural pain: Described above.

Musculoskeletal pain:
- Pricking or stabbing in nature
- Worse on twisting, turning or rolling over the bed, may be aggravated by breathing
- Affected muscle is tender on gentle pressure
- History of fall with evidence of rib fracture, point tenderness and crepitus on the affected area.

Bornholm disease
- Viral infection of intercostal muscles
- Severe pain.

Tietze's disease
Pain and swelling of upper costal cartilage.

Severe constant pain, not relating to breathing but interferes sleep:
Malignant disease involving chest wall.

Severe pain according to root distribution:
Herpes zoster.

It may be associated with vesicles formation.

Central chest pain—due to involvement of mediastenal structures—probably due to pressure on these structures.

Pain Arising from Large Airways

- Retrosternal
- Burning in nature, occasionally incapacitating
- Aggravated by coughing, cold air.

Pain Arises from Pulmonary Sulcus Tumor

- Pain along the distribution of 8th cervical, 1st and 2nd thoracic nerves
- Horner's syndrome
- Bone destruction
- Small muscle of hand atrophy.

Questions to be asked on chest pain:
- Site of pain
- Type of pain
- Referred pain
- Intensity
- Aggravating factors
- Relieving factors.

Difference between pleural pain and chest wall pain:

Pleural pain	Chest wall pain
• Pleural pain is associated with pleural rub	• Chest wall pain is not associated with pleural rub
• Pleural pain is associated with coughing	• Chest wall pain is not associated with coughing
• Pleural pain is not associated with local chest wall tenderness	• Chest wall pain associated with local chest wall tenderness

Cardiac Pain

- *Myocardial ischemia:*
  - ❖ Compressive, oppressive type pain
  - ❖ Radiating to the left arm, shoulder, or neck
  - ❖ No relation to breathing
  - ❖ Severe in nature.
- *Pericardial pain:*
  - ❖ Retrosternal or left-sided pain
  - ❖ It is aggravated by deep breathing

- ❖ It is relieved by leaning forward
- ❖ Associated with rub which is synchronous with each heart beat.
- *Postpericardiotomy pain:*
  - ❖ Occurs within few days to few weeks after surgery
  - ❖ It is retrosternal in nature
  - ❖ It is radiated towards left side
  - ❖ It is aggravated by deep breathing
  - ❖ Associated features—fever, high sedimentation rate.
- *Miscellaneous pain:*
  - ❖ *Gastroesophageal reflux:*
    - Retrosternal pain
    - Burning in nature
    - Aggravated after eating and in recumbent position.
  - ❖ *Aortic dissection:*
    - Acute sharp, tearing pain
    - Radiation to shoulder
    - Associated with cardiovascular collapse.
  - ❖ *Arthritis of cervical spine:*
    Pain radiating to shoulder and arm.
  - ❖ *Pain in the thoracic spine:*
    - *Due to metastatic tumor:*
      - Bilateral in distribution
      - Tenderness in palpation.
    - *Due to herpes zoster:*
      - Severe pain distributed along the affected nerve
      - Unilateral in distribution.

Breathlessness

Difficulty in breathing or shortness of breath.

- Some patients complain about 'tightness'—it may mean pain in chest or breathlessness. In that case doctor has to ask directly whether 'tightness' means chest pain or breathlessness
- Patient with pleuritic chest pain complains of breathlessness, in that case it is necessary to know that whether breathlessness is due to chest pain or not
- There is little correlations between tachypnea and dyspnea. But there is close correlation between hypoxia and dyspnea. For example, tachypneic person may not be breathless if there is no hypoxia. Again patient with normal respiratory rate may be breathless, if there is hypoxia
- There is often little correlation between dyspnea and severity of hypercapnea. Normally rise in arterial Pa_{CO_2} induces hyperventilation in normal person, but in patient with Type

II respiratory failure if fails to do so because brainstems is less responsive or unresponsive to changes in arterial P_{CO_2}

- Stimulation of pulmonary stretch receptors in the alveolar capillary wall (J receptors) may mediate breathlessness, e.g. in pneumonia, pulmonary edema, thromboembolism.

Factors Causing Production of Breathlessness

Increased Work of Breathing

- *Airflow obstruction:*
  - ❖ *Large airway obstruction:*
    - Tracheal obstruction.
  - ❖ *Small airway obstruction:*
    - Bronchial asthma
    - Chronic bronchitis
    - Emphysema.
- *Decreased pulmonary compliance:*
  - ❖ Pulmonary edema
  - ❖ Pulmonary fibrosis
  - ❖ Extrinsic allergic alveolitis.
- *Restricted chest expansion:*
  - ❖ *Bony disease:*
    - Kyphoscoliosis
    - Ankylosing spondylosis.
  - ❖ *Muscular disease:*
    Respiratory muscle paralysis.

Increased Ventilatory Drive

- *Ventilation/perfusion mismatch:*
  ↓

  Causing increase in rate and depth of respiration.
  - ❖ Consolidation
  - ❖ Lung collapse
  - ❖ Pulmonary edema
  - ❖ Pulmonary thromboembolism.
- *Hyperventillation resulting from stimulation of respiratory center by chemical or rural stimuli:*
  - ❖ *Increased hydrogen ion concentration in arterial blood:*
    - Metabolic acidosis.
  - ❖ *Increased arterial P_{CO_2} concentration:*
    - Respiratory acidosis.
  - ❖ *Decreased arterial Pa_{O_2}*
    - Due to decreased Pa_{O_2} delivery—to tissues:
      - Anemia

- Shock
- Stroke.

❖ *Decreased arterial Pa_{O_2} via aortic, carotid and brainstem chemoreceptor:*
  - Pneumonia.
❖ *Increased central nervous system arousal:*
  - Exertion
  - Thyrotoxicosis
  - Emotion.
❖ *Pulmonary J receptor stimulations:*
  - Pulmonary edema
  - Pneumonia
  - Pulmonary thromboembolism.
- *Breathlessness associated with impaired respiratory muscle function and diaphragm:*
  ❖ Poliomyelitis
  ❖ GB syndrome
  ❖ Cervical transaction
  ❖ Muscular dystrophies
  ❖ Myasthenia gravis.

Questions to be asked regarding dyspnea:
- Is breathlessness recent or present for some time?
- How long the patient has shortness of breath?
- Whether the shortness of breath is sudden in onset?
- Whether the shortness of breath is constant?
- In what position the shortness of breath is exacerbated?
- How many stairs the patient can ascend without shortness of breath?
- Is there associated symptoms, like, cough, chest pain, wheeze, palpitation, or hoarseness?
- Whether breathlessness is constant or waxing and waning?
- Which specific work, like asbestos work, sandblasting, woody work, work in dusty atmosphere—patient cannot do without breathlessness?
- Any history of smoking?
- Any history of contact with tuberculosis?
- What makes the breathlessness worse?
- Which factor or factors relieve the patient from breathlessness?

Duration of Breathlessness in Differential Diagnosis

- *Immediate:* Within minutes:
  ❖ Pulmonary embolism
  ❖ Pulmonary edema
  ❖ Pneumothorax—tension pneumothorax.

- *Within minutes to hours:*
  - ❖ *In children:*
    - Epiglotitis
    - Trachitis
    - Laryngitis
    - Laryngotracheobronchitis.
  - ❖ *In adults and children:*
    - Asthma
    - Pulmonary edema due to left ventricular failure
    - Pulmonary infarction due to massive embolism
    - Pneumonia
    - Acute exacerbation of chronic bronchitis
    - *Cardiac cause:* Myocardial infarction, arrhythmia, non-compensated valvular heart disease
    - Hyperventilation syndrome.
- *Within days to weeks:*
  - ❖ All above acute causes may produce subacute obstruction
  - ❖ Superior caval syndrome
  - ❖ Pulmonary vascular disease—hypersensitivity pneumonias.
- *Chronic (months to years):*
  - ❖ *Pulmonary vascular diseases:*
    - Hypersensitivity pneumonitis
    - Pulmonary vasculitis.
  - ❖ Chronic obstructive pulmonary disease (COPD)
  - ❖ *Cardiac cause:* Valvular heart disease.
  - ❖ *Diffuse parechymal diseases:*
    - Idiopathic pulmonary fibrosis
    - Sarcoidosis
    - Pulmonary tuberculosis
    - Bronchiectasis
    - Idiopathic pulmonary hypertension
    - Veno-occlusive disease.
- *Systemic disease:*
  - ❖ Anemia
  - ❖ Beriberi
  - ❖ Thyrotoxicosis.

Variability of Dyspnea

Dyspnea may be variable—throughout the day or in a particular time of the day, from night to day. Variability of dyspnea is highly characteristic of bronchial asthma. It can be aggravated by smoke, house dust, exercise (it is a potential trigger factor in children), fumes, emotions.

Questions to be asked to patient with bronchial asthma:
- Does anything make any difference in asthma?
- What happens when you are worried or upset?
- Does patient's chest wake him at night?
- Does cigarette smoke make any difference?
- Does household spray affect the patient?
- What happens when sweeping or dusting the house?
- Does exposure to cats and dogs make any difference?

Severity of Dyspnea

Questions to be asked:
In what way breathlessness restricts the patient's activities:
- Can they go upstairs—troubled—after how many steps?
- Whether dyspnea occurs in the same floor? If so, after how many steps?
- Can go shopping?
- Can wash their car?
- Can do gardening? It is useful mainly in summer, as it is possible to grade activity from pulling out few weeds to digging potato patch.

Orthopnea

Dyspnea occurs at supine position, which will be relieved by erect position. It can be measured by following methods:
- The number of pillows required by the patient to relieve from breathlessness
- The degree of head elevation at which the breathlessness is relieved using goniometer.

Patient with chronic bronchitis—becomes orthopneic and admits to not having slept flat for years.

In normal people—while lying in flat position, breathe more with diaphragm and less with chest wall.

In patient with severe airways obstruction, diaphragm is already flat and inefficient and may draw the inwards and downwards.

So when this patient lies down, chest wall cannot expand upwards adequately against gravity, patient may become breathless. So orthopnea is associated with:
- Obesity
- Asthma
- Pulmonary hypertension
- Left-sided heart failure
- COPD
- Diaphragmatic paralysis.

Hyperventilation Syndrome

Features suggestive of hyperventilation syndrome:
- Breathlessness at rest
- Breathlessness is severe with mild exertion as with greater exertion
- More difficulty in breathing in than breathing out
- Light headedness
- Tinnitus
- Peripheral and circumpolar parenthesia
- Cold and moist hands and feet
- Constant tiredness and generalized weakness
- Chest tightness, heaviness, and palpitation
- Abdominal cramping and bloating
- Urgency and frequency in defecation and maturation.

Factors responsible for breathlessness in pneumonia:
- Pyrexia—stimulating respiratory center
- Pleuritic pain—limiting chest wall expansion
- Increased work of breathing—stiff lung
- Ventilation/perfusion mismatch
- Stimulation of pulmonary J receptors
- Hypoxemia—low Pa_{O_2}
- Septic shock.

Factors responsible for breathlessness in pulmonary edema:
- Ventilation/perfusion mismatch
- Increased work of breathing—stiff lung
- Stimulation of pulmonary J receptors
- Hypoxemia—low Pa_{O_2}
- Carcinogenic shock
- Hypoventilation.

Causes of breathlessness
- *Physiological:*
  - Exercise
  - High altitude.
- *Pathological:*
  - Anemia
  - Obesity
  - Respiratory disorder
  - Cardiac disorders.
- *Psychological:* Hyperventilation syndrome

- *Pharmacological:*
  - ❖ Drug-induced respiratory distress
  - ❖ Drug-induced cardiac disorders.

Aggravating and relieving factors of breathlessness:
- *Breathlessness which improves at the weekend or holiday:*
  - ❖ Occupational asthma
  - ❖ Extrinsic allergic alveolitis.
- *Breathlessness increased after coughing, laughing or exertion or following exposure to smoke, dust, pollen or danders:*
  - ❖ Bronchial asthma
  - ❖ Chronic bronchitis.
- *Breathlessness awakens the patient from sleep (PND):*
  - ❖ Bronchial asthma
  - ❖ Pulmonary edema
  - ❖ Severe COPD.

Acute breathlessness, diagnostic value of associated symptoms:
- *With chest pain lateralized and pleuritic:*
  - ❖ Pneumonia
  - ❖ Pulmonary infarction
  - ❖ Pneumothorax
  - ❖ Rib fracture
  - ❖ Pleural effusion.
- *With chest pain, central and nonpleuritic:*
  - ❖ Myocardial infarction
  - ❖ Massive pulmonary embolism.
- *Without chest pain, cough and wheeze:*
  - ❖ Pulmonary embolism
  - ❖ Tension pneumothorax
  - ❖ Metabolic acidosis.
- *Without chest pain, but with cough and wheeze:*
  - ❖ Bronchial asthma
  - ❖ Chronic bronchitis
  - ❖ Pulmonary edema.

Questions to be asked for assessing severity of breathlessness:
- Whether sleep disturbed by breathlessness?
- Whether breathlessness occurs at rest?
- Whether breathlessness hampers normal conversation?
- Whether dressing or washing produce breathlessness?
- Whether patient can walk on flat area without stopping?
- Whether patient can climb upstairs without stopping?
- Which activity is hampered by breathlessness?

Grading of Dyspnea (American Thoracic Society Scale):

Description	Grade	Degree
• Not troubled by shortness of breath when hurrying on the level or walking up a slight hill	0	None
• Troubled by shortness of breath when hurrying on the level or walking up a slight hill	1	Mild
• Walks more slowly than the people of same age on the level because of breathlessness or has to stop for breath when walking at his own space	2	Moderate
• Stops for breath after walking about 100 yards or after few minutes on the same level	3	Severe
• Too much breathless to leave the house, breathless on dressing or undressing	4	Very severe

Wheeze

It is a musical sound produced by passage of air through narrowed bronchi—when it is heard from a distance, it is called wheeze.

It occurs in expiratory phase of respiration, when slight bronchoconstriction occurs physiologically after strenuous exercise.

It occurs in:
- *Asthma:* Due to bronchospasm and mucosa edema and loss of elastic support. Asthma is associated with wheezing, but not all wheezing is asthma
- Obstruction by intraluminar material, like foreign body or secretions.

Well-localized wheeze, unchanged by coughing—obstruction by intraluminal foreign body or tumor.

The following questions to be asked for wheezing:
- At what age it has been started?
- Whether it has started suddenly or not?
- How frequently it occurs?
- Is there any precipitating factors like, food, emotions, odors?
- How it can be terminated?
- Is there any history of heart disease?
- Any smoking history?
- Any history of nasal polyp?

Decrease in wheezing is usually due to:
- Either opening of the airway, or
- Progressive closing of the partially obstructing airways producing 'silent chest', which is a bad sign.

◼ Hoarseness

It is harsh aspiratory and expiratory sounds produced by passage of air through partially obstructed major bronchi and can be heard from distance easily. The causes are:

- Laryngeal edema
- Laryngeal carcinoma suggested by progressive hoarseness of voice over weeks to months. Patient is usually smoker, taking cannabis. Patient complains of dysphagia, hemoptysis or ear pain
- Foreign body in larynx
- *Chronic laryngitis:* Hoarseness over months to years. History of recurrent laryngitis
- *Singer's node:* Patient is usually singer or gives voice strain during singing, use alcohol, fumes. It occurs over months to years
- *Functional:* Sign of stress
- *Vocal cord paresis:* History of surgery occurs after weeks to months, complains of bovine cough
- *Myxedema:* Over months to years, associated with other signs of myxedema
- *Acromegaly:* Due to swollen vocal cords, associated other signs of acromegaly
- *Sicca syndrome:* Due to dry mouth and eyes.

Symptoms Related to Upper Respiratory Tract

Nose and Nasopharynx

- *Whether there is intermittent nasal obstruction:*
  - ❖ Mucosal edema
  - ❖ Excessive mucus secretion.
- *Whether the nasal obstruction is persistent:*
  - ❖ Adenoid enlargement
  - ❖ Nasal polyp.
- *Whether the nasal obstruction changes with posture:* Posterior nasal polyp
- *Whether the patient takes breathe through mouth:*
  - ❖ Posterior nasal polyp
  - ❖ Large adenoid.
- *Whether the patient complains of excessive sneezing:* Allergic rhinitis
- *Whether sneezing is associated with headache:* Infection of nasal sinuses.

Larynx

- *Hoarseness:* It may be from slight hoarseness to complete loss (aphonic) of voice

Questions to be asked:
- ❖ Duration of hoarseness
- ❖ Factors or events which precede the onset—voice abuse, heat, cold, chronic cough, operations in neck or throat
- ❖ Whether hoarseness is improving, worsening or static.
- *Cough:*
  - ❖ *Barking cough*—tumor in larynx
  - ❖ *Bovine cough*—recurrent laryngeal nerve paralysis.
- *Laryngeal stridor:* It is high pitched crowing sound heard during inspiratory phase
  Causes are:
  - ❖ Foreign body lodged between the vocal cords
  - ❖ Laryngeal spasm—this can be judged from patient while he is giving history
  - ❖ Laryngeal edema
  - ❖ Laryngitis.
- *Laryngeal pain:*
  - ❖ *Mild pain:* Acute laryngitis
  - ❖ *Constant severe pain:*
    - • Laryngeal tuberculosis
    - • Laryngeal carcinoma.

Trachea

- Pain referred to behind sternal manubrium—intense after coughing and subsides soon after cough becomes productive—Tracheitis
- Tracheal stridor—differs from laryngeal stridor:
  - ❖ Low-pitched sound heard best during inspirations accentuated by coughing—obstructing lesion in trachea.

Best Way of Hearing Tracheal Stridor
- Patient should be asked to cough, and then breathe deeply in and out
- By very careful listening near patient's mouth during 1st few seconds after coughing—presence of stridor at an early stage.

■ Other Important Points in History

- *Fever:*
  - ❖ Character of rise of temperature
  - ❖ Whether associated with chill and rigor, or night sweat
  - ❖ Any defervescence or not. If so, how it remits?
    It may occur in:
    - • Infection—acute or chronic (pulmonary tuberculosis, pneumonia, etc.)
    - • Malignancy

- Connective tissue disease.
  ❖ Associated pain and swelling in legs—DVT.
- *Weight loss:* It may occur in:
  ❖ Carcinoma
  ❖ Infection—tuberculosis
  ❖ Chronic airflow abstraction—presumably from increased respiratory effort. It may occur in this disease due to:
    - Impaired appetite
    - Divert calories to respiratory muscles.
- *Weight gain:*
  ❖ Cushing's syndrome
  ❖ Hypothyroidism.
- *Edema:* Whether peripheral or central. It starts as dependant edema in early phase, later on as the disease progresses, it involves whole body. The causes may be cardiac, renal, hepatic.

Symptoms Suggestive of Sleep Apnea Syndrome

- Excessive day time somnolence.
  Caused by sleep disturbance:
  ❖ Chest pain
  ❖ Breathlessness
  ❖ Cough.
- Intellectual deterioration
- Early morning headache
- Snoring
- Social deterioration.
  Cause:
  ❖ Obesity
  ❖ Hypertrophied tonsils.

History Suggestive of Having Sleep Apnea Syndrome

- Is the patient snores?
- How frequent the patient snores?
- Whether this snoring disturbs the other nearby people?
- Is there evidence of breath holding during snoring?
- Is the patient tired during daytime or tired after sleeping?
- Is any history of falling asleep during driving?
- Whether the patient is suffering from high blood pressure?

Tiredness, snoring and sleepiness suggest diagnosis of sleep apnea syndrome.

Early morning headache is due to poor quality of sleep leads to day time somnolence and carbon dioxide retention.

Past History

- *Tuberculosis:*
  - ❖ Current symptoms may be due to relapse
  - ❖ History of operation—thoracoplasty and phrenic crush—producing lifelong thoracic deformity
  - ❖ Bronchial damage producing bronchiectasis
  - ❖ Fungal ball (aspergillosis) in tubercular cavity.
- *Pneumonia and pleurisy:* Caused by:
  - ❖ Bronchiectasis
  - ❖ Bronchial tumor
  - ❖ Aspiration of esophageal content (achalasia cardia)
  - ❖ Aspiration of pharyngeal content or vomit (bulbar palsy)
  - ❖ Alcoholism
  - ❖ Hypogammaglobulinemia
  - ❖ Multiple myeloma.
- *Measles or whopping cough:*
  - ❖ It can produce pneumonia in early childhood
  - ❖ It can cause wheeze bronchitis or bronchiectasis.
- *Wheezy bronchitis or recurrent bronchitis in childhood:* Recurrence of bronchial asthma in adult who have history of childhood asthma or wheezy bronchitis in common.
- *Chest injuries:* Traumatic hemithorax—leads to pleural thickening and splints of chest (frozen chest).
- *Recent history of general anesthetics or loss of consciousness:* Inhalation or aspiration of oropharyngeal secretion or foreign body leads to:
  - ❖ Aspiration pneumonia
  - ❖ Lung abscess.
- *Pregnancy, surgery:* Pulmonary embolism
- Comparison of recent chest radiograph with previous radiograph.

Social History

Smoking

- It is important cause of COPD and bronchogenic carcinoma.
  Questions to be asked:
  - ❖ Age at which it has been started?
  - ❖ Age at which it was given up, it patient stops smoking?
  - ❖ Number of cigarettes or cigar per day?
  - ❖ Amount of tobacco per week?
  Regarding passive smoking the questions are:
  - ❖ How much time spared in home with smokers?
  - ❖ For how many days, the persons are exposed?
  - ❖ Whether the person exposed is child or adult?

It may produce bronchial asthma in childhood and intercurrent infections.

Pets and Hobbies

- ❖ Exposure to pigeons, parrots and other caged birds can cause:
  - Extrinsic allergic alveolitis
  - Bronchial asthma
  - Allergic rhinitis
  - Pneumonia (psittacosis).
    Cause may be exposure to protein material derived from feathers and droppings.
- ❖ *Acute symptoms* usually seen in pigeon fanciers who, few hours after cleaning out the birds, develop cough, breathlessness, flu like symptoms
- ❖ *Chronic symptoms* seen in budgerigar owners—because they exposed continuously to low dose of antigen—they complain of progressive breathlessness. You may extend your enquiries beyond home because patient may be exposed to birds belonging to friends and relations.

Occupational History

The leading question is 'what work do you do?' This question is important in two ways:

1. Respiratory disease may affect patient's ability to work but may also be the result of the occupation.
2. Any job involving exposure to noxious agents of respirable size potentially damages the respiratory tract. Most obvious example is pneumoconiosis in coal miners.
   Next question is 'How long you work in that job?'
   For example, in case of asbestosis—the interval between exposure to asbestos and development of asbestosis and mesothelioma is 30 years.

Occupational Cause of Lung Diseases

Occupation	Agent	Disease
• Mining	Coal dust	Pneumoconiosis
• Quarrying	Silica dust	Silicosis
• Foundary work	Silica dust	Silicosis
• Asbestos (mining, healing building, demolition ship building)	Asbestos fibers	Asbestosis, mesothelioma, lung cancer

Contd...

Contd...

Occupation	Agent	Disease
• Farming	Actinomycetes	Alveolitis
• Paint spraying	Isocyanates	Asthma
• Plastic manufacture	Isocyanates	Asthma
• Soldering	Aluminum	Restrictive lung disease

- History of shortness of breath, cough and chills a few hours after forking out fodder for cattle in the winter called farmer's lung—caused by agent—microaerophilic actinomycetes contaminated stored damp hay
- Bagassosis—mouldy sugar cane
- Other occupational risk factors—mushroom workers, malt workers and wood workers—antigen varies in each case.

Family History

- Family history of asthma, hay fever and eczema
- Family history of cystic fibrosis or alfa 1 antitrypsin deficiency—rare cause of emphysema
- Tuberculosis is common in Asian and African migrants, particularly in their first 10 years in the country
- Tuberculosis is more common in conditions of poverty
- Heterosexuals having symptoms of AIDS
- Family history of pulmonary hypertension
- History of cancer, sickle cell anemia
- History of diabetes, which may lead to cardiac or respiratory problem
- History of recent viral illness, like, influenza.

Drug History

- Use of bronchodilators and steroids in airways obstruction
- Use of aspirin, nonsteroidal anti-inflammatory drugs (NSAIDs) in patient with bronchial asthma
- ACE inhibitors in chronic cough—maker worse
- Beta-adrenergic blocking drugs in bronchial asthma—makes the condition worse
- Use of steroid therapy in tuberculosis and infection
- History of pneumococcal vaccination.

Personal History

- Intravenous drug user or sexual malpractices may be responsible for unusual pulmonary disorder
- Toxicities of immunosuppressive drugs.

CHEST INSPECTION

■ Abnormalities in Respiration

Rate of Respiration (Fig. 3.13)

- Normal respiratory rate—20 ± 5 breaths/minute.
- Tachypnea—more than 25 breathes/minute with shallow breathing. It is commonly seen in:
  - ❖ Lung disease
  - ❖ Pain
  - ❖ Sepsis
  - ❖ Obesity
  - ❖ Anxiety
  - ❖ *Fever:* Respiratory rate increases 4 breath/minute for every 1 degree rise in body temperature.
- Bradypnea—less than 10 breaths/minute—occurs in:
  - ❖ Hypothyroidism
  - ❖ Narcotic use
  - ❖ Sedation
  - ❖ Diabetic coma.
- *Apnea:* Absence of respiration for at least 20 seconds while awake.

  Absence of respiration for at least 30 seconds while asleep.
  - ❖ *Central apnea:* Neuromuscular dysfunction
  - ❖ *Obstructive sleep apnea:* Airway obstruction induced by rapid eye movement sleep.

Abnormalities in Depth of Respiration

- *Hyperpnea:* A rapid and deep inspiration.
  - ❖ *Acidotic breathing:*
    - Increased anion gap metabolic acidosis
    - Methanol poisoning
    - Aspirin intoxication
    - Ethlene glycol toxicity
    - Diabetic ketoacidosis
    - Uremic ketoacidosis
    - Lactic acidosis.

Difference between hyperpnea and hyperventilation:

- *Hyperventilation:* Where vital capacity compromised, thus breath is shallow and increase in rate
- *Hyperpnea:* Due to increase in tidal volume, rate and death are increased
- *Hypopnea:* Respirations is shallow.

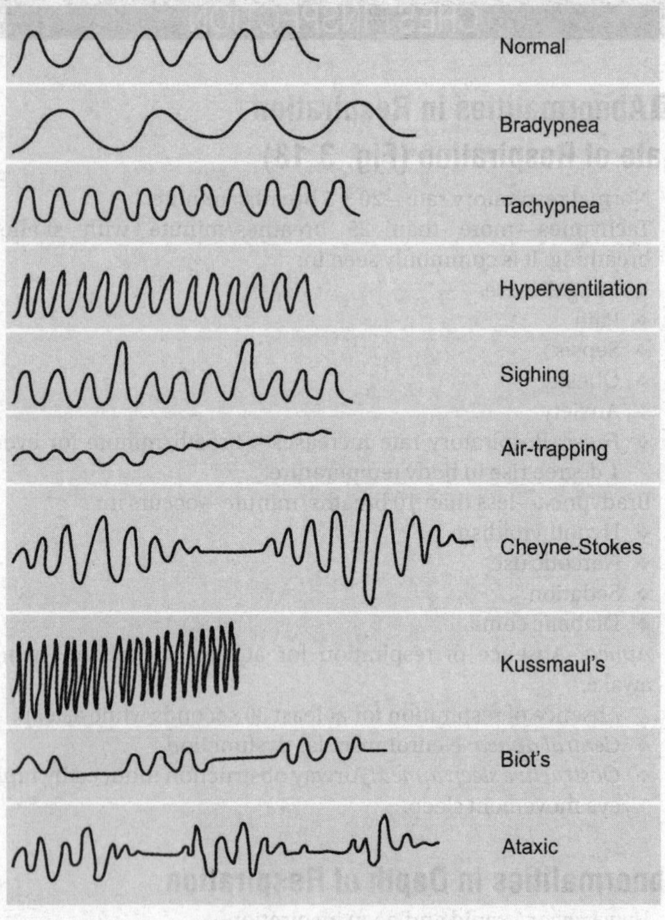

FIG. 3.13 Types of breathing

Causes:
* ❖ Impending respiratory failure
* ❖ Obesity.

Abnormalities in Rhythm and Pattern of Respiration (Fig. 3.13)

Moving downward in rostrocaudal fashion, from uppermost to lowermost neurological center the most common abnormalities are:

* *Cheyne-Stokes respiration:* Progressive increase in rate and depth of respiration eventually culminating in peak followed by progressive decrease in rate and depth of respiration followed by apnea.

Crescendo decresendo pattern last for 30 sec, apneic period last for shorter periods.

Causes:

❖ Aging
❖ Simple sleep
❖ High altitude
❖ *Neurological disorders:* Meningitis, bilateral or unilateral cerebral infarction, hemorrhage, traumatic brainstem lesion. *Cause:* Heightened sensitivity of respiratory center to CO_2 stimulation.

- *Biot's respiration:* Hyperventilation or hyperpnea followed by apnea—without cresendo-decresendo pattern.

Causes:

❖ Meningitis
❖ Medullary compression.

Worse prognosis—resulting complete apnea and cardiac arrest.

- *Apneustic breathing:* Deep inspiratory phase followed by breath holding period and rapid exhalation.

Cause: Brainstem lesion.

- *Central hyperventilation:* Pattern of hyperpnea and tachypnea (deep and rapid respiration)—but it is not as fast as Kussmaul's breathing.

Causes: Midbrain and upper pontine lesion.

- *Ataxic breathing:* Totally anarchic respiration—fibrillation of respiratory center, sudden shift from hyper- to hypoventilation and from hyperpnea to hypoapnea (agonal respiration)

Causes: Medullary damage.

- *Grunting respiration:* Preterminal grunting or gurgling sound produced by the patient to clear secretions

❖ It is a death rattle—sign of severe pneumonia with impending respiratory failure, muscle fatigue and death
❖ More frequent in children—short and low pitched noise produced by forced expiration against closed glottis. Grunt is due to sudden opening of glottis and loud rush of air from larynx.

- *Pursed-lip respiration:* Patient is at risk of expiratory airway closure and air trapping, so they resort to pursed-lip exhalation, as it they are inflating a balloon. This increases intra-airway pressure—induces positive end expiratory pressure.

Physiologic Impact of Pursed-lip Respiration

- It increases arterial O_2, decreases CO_2—it behaves like E-PAP or Bi-PAP-machine
- It reduces respiratory rate
- It increases tidal volume—decreases dyspnea.

Nasal flaring: It is outward motion of nostrils—associated motion of accessory respiratory muscles.

It is a sign of respiratory distress.

■ Abnormalities in Posture

Orthopnea

Orthop (upright), pnea (breathing)

Dyspnea aggravated in lying down position, relived by upright position.

Causes

- *Congestive cardiac failure:* Pooling of blood to the dependent areas of the body—reduces venous return and ventricular load. But when LVF degenerates into biventricular failure, producing right ventricular failure, thus producing relief from orthopnea and pulmonary edema
- *Pulmonary causes:*
  - ❖ Pneumonia
  - ❖ Bilateral diaphragmatic paralysis
  - ❖ Pleural effusion
  - ❖ Bilateral apical lung disease

  Sitting positions improves vital capacity and pulmonary compliance

  ↓

  Since these areas are best ventilated, sittings positions improves ventilation/perfusion (V/Q) matching and gas exchange.
  - ❖ *In COPD patient sitting position* improves:
    - Gas-exchange and lung mechanics by increasing use of accessory respiratory muscles
    - These patients do so by grasping the sides of the bed or by pushing with the elbows over the thighs.
  - ❖ *In acute asthma:* It is the good predictor of poor outcome. Because these patients have worse pulmonary function.
- *Nonpulmonary or noncardiac:*
  - ❖ Obesity
  - ❖ Massive ascites
  - ❖ Bilateral phrenic nerve paralysis.

Paroxysmal Nocturnal Dyspnea

Characterized by nocturnal spell (paroxysm) of acute dyspnea (air hunger). After 1 to 2 hours of sleep patient awakens, sit upright, lowers the legs by the side of the bed, opens the window to catch the fresh air, after few minutes, he expectorates small amount of frothy sputum, occasionally pink frothy sputum, he feels better enough to go back to sleep.

Mechanism

In upright posture, peripheral pooling of blood, reduces the venus return, reduces pulmonary congestion.

Causes
- Acute left ventricular failure
- Bilateral apical and bullous lung diseases—both basilar perfusion and lung mechanics are improved.

Platypnea

Plat (flat) pnea (respiration). Difficulty in breathing while sitting up and relieved by recumbent position.

Significant of Platypnea

- *Right to left intrapulmonary shunts:* In these cases upright posture increases perfusion to lower lobes and worsens the ventilation/ perfusion (V/Q); as a result oxygen desaturation occurs leading to dyspnea; conversely platypnea improves V/Q matching and relieves dyspnea. It occurs in:
  - ❖ Multiple recurrent pulmonary emboli
  - ❖ Pleural effusion
  - ❖ Cirrhosis
  - ❖ Arteriovenous malformation.
- *Intracardiac right to left heart shunt:* In case of atrial septal defect associated with increased pulmonary resistance—as in case of pleuropericardial or pericardial effusion or postlobectomy or postpneumonectomy.
  Upright posture reduces the shunt by:
  - ❖ Redirecting the blood through atrial septum
  - ❖ Decreasing the pressure over right atrium.
  Supine posture has opposite effect.

Trepopnea

Trepo (twisted) and *pnea* (breathing)—twisted respiration. Patient's inability to lie in supine or prone position and preference to lie in lateral decubitus position.

Physiology Behind Trepopnea

Increased perfusion in dependent lung—producing better V/Q matching, better oxygenation and relieves dyspnea.

Causes
Unilateral lung collapse from: In these situations patient feels better when the good lung is dependent.

- Endobronchial obstructing lesion
- Massive pleural effusion
- In congestive cardiac failure from dilated cardiomyopathy (patient is in right lateral decubitus position—feels better because this position relieves pressure on the left lung by enlarged heart)
- *When mediastinal or endobronchial tumors* compress the airways in particular position, patient prefers lateral decubitus position in particular position.

Contraindication to good lung down: In unilateral lung disease due to spilable material, e.g. pneumonia (pus), hemorrhage (intra-alveolar blood), and position with good lung down—produces intrabronchial spread of pus or blood to good lung making the condition worse.

So in these cases, patient should lie I diseased lung down to prevent spillage of material to good lung.

Abnormalities in Respiratory Musculature

Abnormal muscles in use are:
- Muscles of diaphragm
- Intercostal muscles.

They produce:
- Abdominal paradox
- Respiratory alternans.

Abdominal Paradox

In normal respiration—abdominal and thoracic walls expand during inspiration and contract during expiration—chest expansion is greater in upright position and abdominal expansion greater in supine position.

But in bilateral diaphragmatic paralysis

During inspiration: Chest wall expands and abdomen is pulled in because diaphragm is pulled in or sucked in as passive membrane.

During expiration: Chest wall contract and diaphragm is pulled out. This is called rocking motion.

Detection of Rocking Motions

- It can be detected by placing one hand on patient's chest and one hand on patient's abdomen
- It can be detected by simple inspection.

The patient with abdominal paradox becomes orthopneic to compensate respiratory discomfort.

In impending respiratory failure abdominal paradox has 95 percent sensitivity and 91 percent specificity.

- *In case of chronic obstructive lung disease:* During early phase of expiration there is inward movement of abdominal wall followed by outward movement of the same in late phase of expiration.

This rocking movement—reflect worse pulmonary function and requires mechanical ventilation and the patient may die.

Respiratory Alternans

Patient exhibits alternate use of either diaphragm or intercostals—producing chest and abdomen rocking in one way or the other way.

This motion occurs with or without abdominal paradox. This motion occurs in respiratory muscle weakness with impending respiratory failures.

Asymmetry in Thoracic Expansions

This can be detected during deep inspiration, because this abnormality cannot be detected during normal respiration.

This can be:

- Total hemithorax
- Local lagging in chest expansion.

Causes

- Atelectasis
- Pneumonia
- Pleural effusion
- Large pneumothorax.

Abnormalities in Chest Cage

Chest cage is composed of:

- Spine
- Sternum
- Ribs.

Abnormalities of Spinal Column

This occurs in:

- Sagittal plane
- Frontal plane
- Both.

Abnormalities Occur in Frontal Plane (Figs 3.14A to E)

Lateral spinal curvature called scoliosis, scoliosis may have:

- Single curvature
- Two curvatures—primary and secondary, i.e. compensatory curvature.

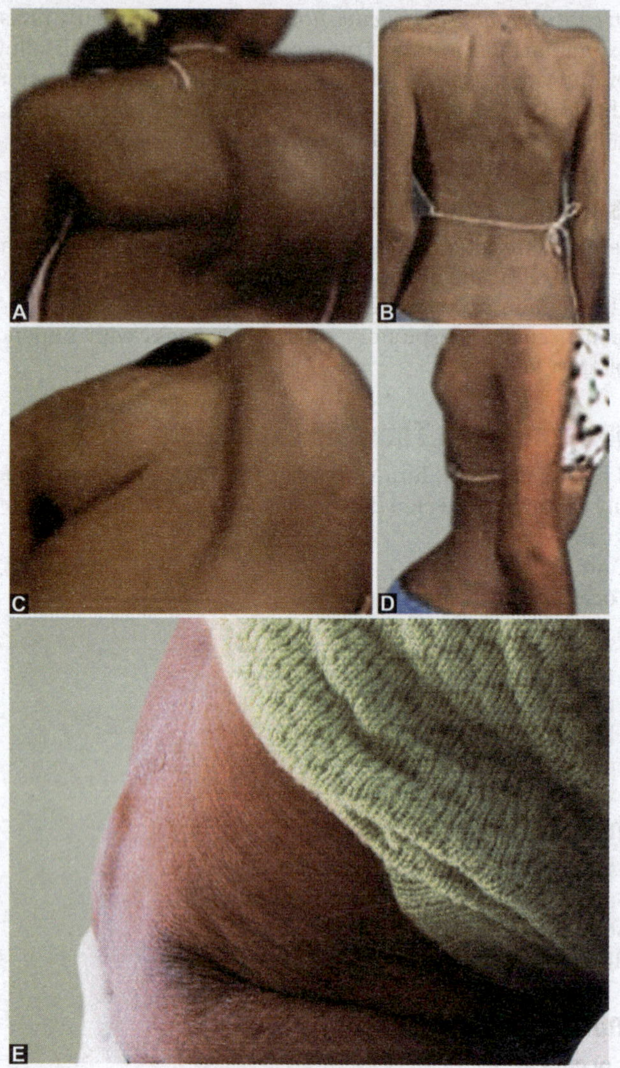

FIGS 3.14A TO E Scoliosis

Scoliosis may be fixed because of bony and/or muscle deformity.

Scoliosis may be mobile because of unusual muscle contraction.

Chest radiograph is the best way to measure kyphoscoliosis. Cobb's angle of scoliosis is important to measure the degree of scoliosis.

Measurement of Cobb's Angle (Fig. 3.15):
Two lines drawn parallel to:
- Upper border of highest
- Lower border of lowest vertebral bodies of primary curvature.

Another two lines are drawn perpendicular to the original lines.

The angle between the two above lines is called Cobb's angle.

Cobb's angle of 10° is the minimum angulations for a definition of scoliosis.

Cobb's angle of >100° represents severe deformity.

Causes of Kyphoscoliosis

- *Neuromuscular:*
  - Muscular dystrophy
  - Cerebral palsy
  - Poliomyelitis
  - Friedreich ataxia.
- *Vertebral:*
  - Osteoporosis
  - Osteomalacia
  - Vitamin D resistant rickets
  - Neurofibromatosis.

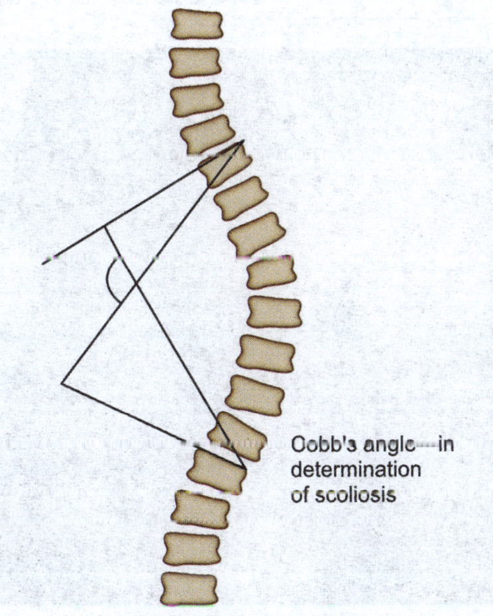

FIG. 3.15 Cobb's angle

- *Connective tissue diseases:*
  - ❖ Marfan syndrome
  - ❖ Ehlers-Danlos syndrome
  - ❖ Morquio syndrome.

Consequences of Spinal Abnormalities

Any of spinal abnormalities
↓
Compromisation of respiratory mechanics
↓
Localized hypoventilation
↓
V/Q mismatch
↓
Localized hypoxemia
↓
Pulmonary hypertension
↓
Right-sided heart failure.

■ Abnormalities of the Sternum

- *Funnel chest (Fig. 3.16):* It is also called pectus excavatum. This is characterized by depression or inward displacement of lower half of sternum, often visible during deep inspiration.

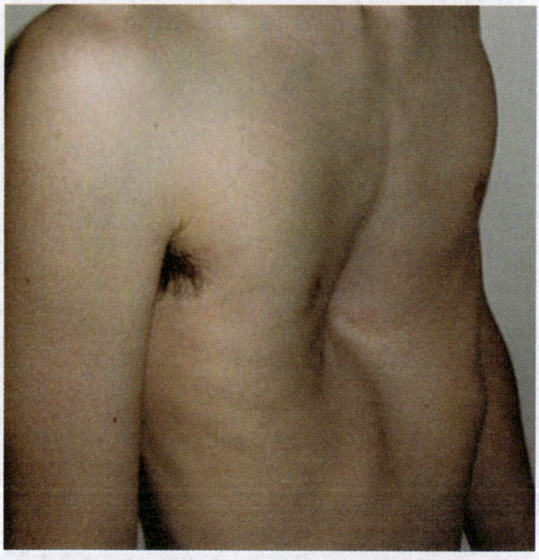

FIG. 3.16   Funnel chest

This may be associated with depression of upper part of abdomen producing pot belly appearances.

Consequences:

❖ It compress lungs producing distortion of lung mechanics
❖ It compress right ventricle and displace right ventricle towards left.

Causes:

❖ Congenital
❖ Rickets
❖ Marfan syndrome
❖ Acromegaly
❖ Scoliosis.

Symptoms produced as a result of above consequences:

❖ Cosmetic problem
❖ Psychological problem
❖ Severe defect produces tachyarrhythmia caused by compression of right ventricle and pulmonary artery
❖ Right ventricular strain pattern is ECG
❖ Pulmonary flow murmur
❖ Compensatory increase in respiratory rate and shift towards diaphragmatic respiration

↓

Increase work of breathing

↓

Fatigability.

● *Pigeon chest (pectus carinatum) (Fig. 3.17):* This is characterized by sternal protrusion from cartilage overgrowth with forward sternal projection and secondary flattening of either side of chest.

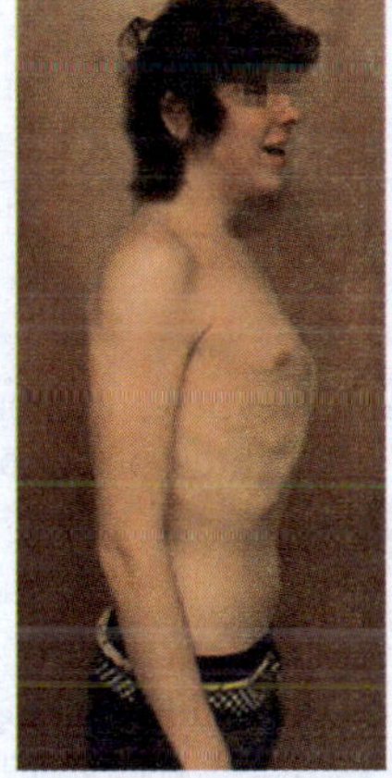

FIG. 3.17   Pectus carinatum

Causes:
- ❖ Rickets
- ❖ Osteomalacia
- ❖ Noonan syndrome
- ❖ Marfan syndrome.

Clinical Consequences

- Pain due to forward buckling of sternum and ribs
- Rigid chest—which is fixed in full inspiration

$$\downarrow$$

Pockets of hypoventilation

$$\downarrow$$

Chance of asthma

$$\downarrow$$

Increased respiratory infection

- Greater use of diaphragmatic and intercostal muscles of respiration during strenuous exercises

$$\downarrow$$

Easy fatigability.

■ Abnormality of the Ribs

Two types of abnormalities:
1. Slope related
2. Rib related.

Slope: Normal slope is:
- Oblique, at 45° angle
- Ratio of AP and transverse diameter 0.7 to 0.85.

Modification of Slope

Barrel chest: Rib cage is almost round, AP diameters ≈ TD diameter.

Causes:
- Emphysema
- Chronic bronchitis
- Status asthmaticus.

Mechanism

Excessive pull on rib and sternum by accessory muscles of respiration (scalene and sternocleidomastoid) increase the anteroposterior diameter, so that their ratio becomes close to 0.90.

Clinical Significance

Horizontal rib slope may compromise lung function, making ventilation less efficient.

Ribs

Rachitic Rosary

This is characterized by thickening of costochondral junctions forming two rosary like lines of beads across the anterior chest (Fig. 3.18A).

Harrison's Groove

First described by English Physician Edward Harrison in 1820.

This is horizontally orientated depression at the site of diaphragmatic costal insertion caused by phrenic pull on ribs weakened by rickets. Resulting indentations extends bilaterally from xiphoid process to the axillae—making the chest like body of violin (Fig. 3.18B).

Causes:
- Rickets
- Laryngeal stenosis in pediatric age group due to excessive diaphragmatic pull.

Hoover's Groove

This is characterized by bilateral depression on thoracic cage of by inward pulling by flattened diaphragm.

Causes
- *In rachitic children*—groove is produced by normal pulling by diaphragm on soft bones.
- *In patient with COPD*—it is associated with severe dyspnea in exercise and in rest.

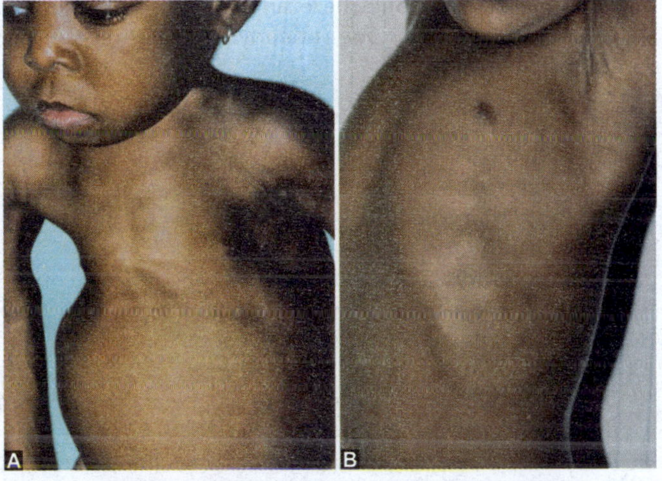

FIGS 3.18A AND B   (A) Ricket; (B) Harrison's groove

Normal movement of lower rib cage during inspiration:
- In quiet inspiration, costal margin moves very little
- In deep inspiration, lower ribs move outward and upward
- In few healthy subjects, they may move little inward at the end of peak inspiration. This movement is grossly exacerbated in COPD patient.

Hoover's Sign

This is paradoxical inward movement of lateral rib cage in patient with COPD during inspiration due to traction by flattened diaphragm on the lateral rib margins. As a result subcostal angle (the angel between xiphoid process and costal margins) becomes acute.

Diseases producing the Hoover's signs
- COPD
- Emphysema   } Produce bilateral Hoover's sign
- Large pneumothorax
- Large pleural effusion. } Produce unilateral Hoover's sign.

■ Abnormalities of Chest Surfaces

- *Abnormalities in color:*
  - *Pallor:* Due to anemia—in effective oxygenation
  - *Cyanosis:* Hallmark of insufficient ventilation resulting hypercapnia and reduced hemoglobin >5.5 g/100 mL
  - *Diaphoresis:* Ineffective oxygenation.
- *Abnormalities in pigmentation:* Hyperpigmented skin tightly drawn and covered with telangiectasia or vitiligo—in these patients hand skin should be examined—the most common cause is scleroderma. The underlying lung diseases are consequences of:
  - Vasculitis
  - Pulmonary hypertension
  - Cor pulmonale.
- *Bulging or sinking:*
  - *Focal expiratory building*—pneumothorax
  - *Diffuse expiratory building*—COPD
  - *Focal inspiratory sinking*—focal airway obstruciton
  - *Diffuse sinking*—upper airway obstruction
  - *Paradoxical motion of thorax*—flail chest.
- *Collateral circulation:*
  - *In superior vena cava obstruction*—collateral flow occurs on the chest wall in caudal direction (Fig. 3.19).
  - *In IVC obstruction*—collateral flow occurs in cephalic direction.

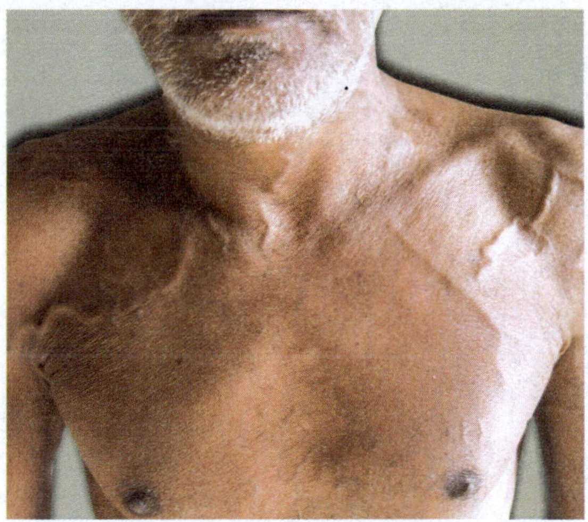

FIG. 3.19 Superior vena cava obstruction

- *Chest wall fistula:* In empyema necessitates in this case, pus burrows outside producing a subcutaneous abscess that finally ruptures.

Inspection of neck
Two things to be noted:
1. Accessory muscle of respiration
2. Neck veins.
Accessory muscles of respiration are:
- Scalene and sternocleidomastoid for inspiration
- Abdominal muscles in expiration.

Functions of accessory muscles (Fig. 3.20):
- *Sternocleidomastoid muscle* during inspiration, produce upward movement of clavicles (and 1st rib) in patient with COPD, mainly those patient with flattened diaphragm and unfavorable lung mechanics. Upward movement of clavicle >5 mm is the sign of severe obstructive lung disease
- *Scalene muscles* attach cervical spine to 1st and 2nd ribs. They assist with intercostal muscles in raising the rib cage
- *Accessory expiratory muscles* help in:
  - ❖ Primarily in exhalation providing additional push
  - ❖ In inspiration by easing inspiratory recoil following expiration.

Inspection areas other than the chest:
- *Neglected pyorrheal teeth* may produce necrotizing aspiration pneumonia

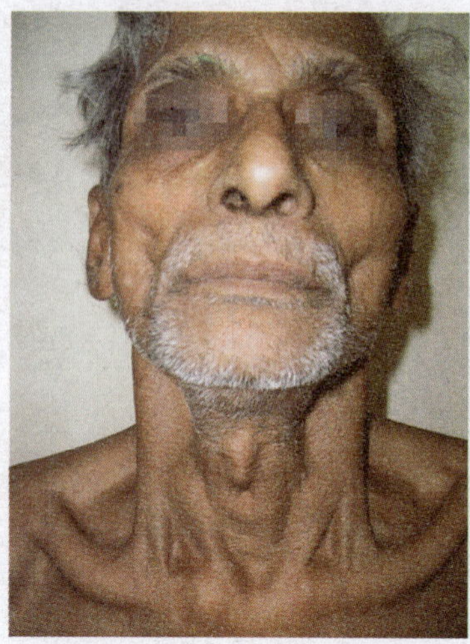

FIG. 3.20 Accessory muscles of respiration

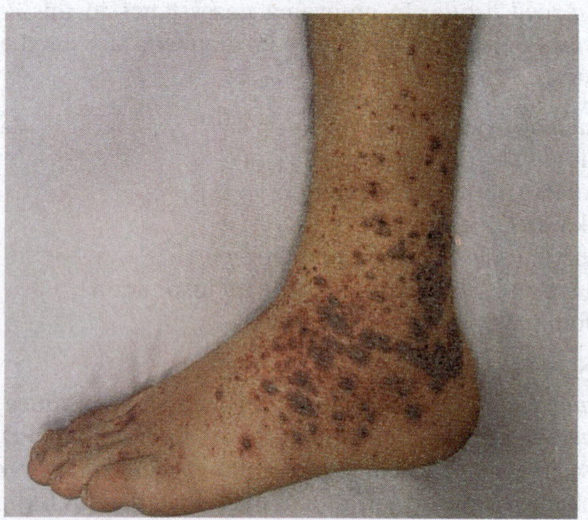

FIG. 3.21 Vasculitis

- *Lacerated tongue* suggest convulsive episodes, may produce aspiration pneumonia
- *Pursuing the lips during expiration indicates* chronic obstructive pulmonary disease
- *Changes in consciousness or confusion* indicates carcinoma lung metastasize to brain, or carbon dioxide retention
- *Sarcoidosis in the skin* the probability of pulmonary sarcoidosis

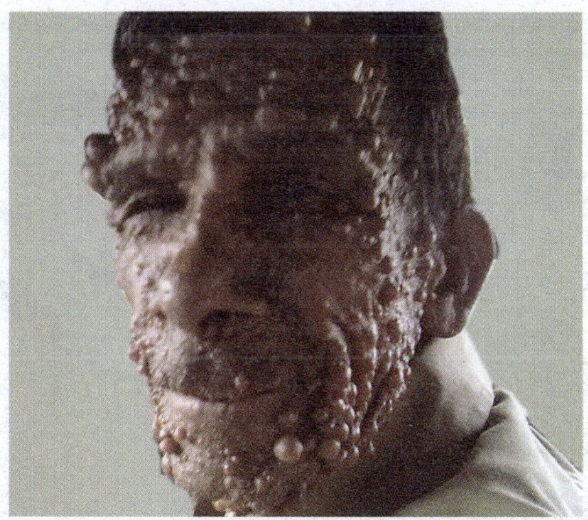

FIG. 3.22 Neurofibroma

- *Petechiae in the skin* indicate systemic vasculitis (Fig. 3.21)
- *Skin lesion in neurofibromatosis* may signify solitary pulmonary nodule (Fig. 3.22)
- *Minute skin abscess* may be a source of future lung abscess
- *Distinct scar on the antecubital veins in case of drug addict* may signify the source of lung abscess
- *Erythema nodosum, erythema multiforme* may complicate sarcoidosis, histoplasmosis, and coccidioidomycosis
- *Presence of Horner's syndrome unilateral ptosis, miosis, anhidrosis,* indicates carcinoma of lung at the pulmonary sulcus with involvement of ipsilateral sympathetic nervous system
- *Puffy face, neck, eyelids along with dilated veins on the shoulder, upper arm, neck and thorax* indicate superior vena cava syndrome (Fig. 3.19).

■ Palpation

Trachea

It can be assessed by its shift and mobility.

Value of Tracheal Shift

- It reflects mediastinal shift
- Associated with other methods (percussion and auscultation), it helps proper interpretation.

Method of detection of tracheal deviation (Fig. 3.23):
- Patient is asked to sit up and lean forward, head straight or lie down on bed

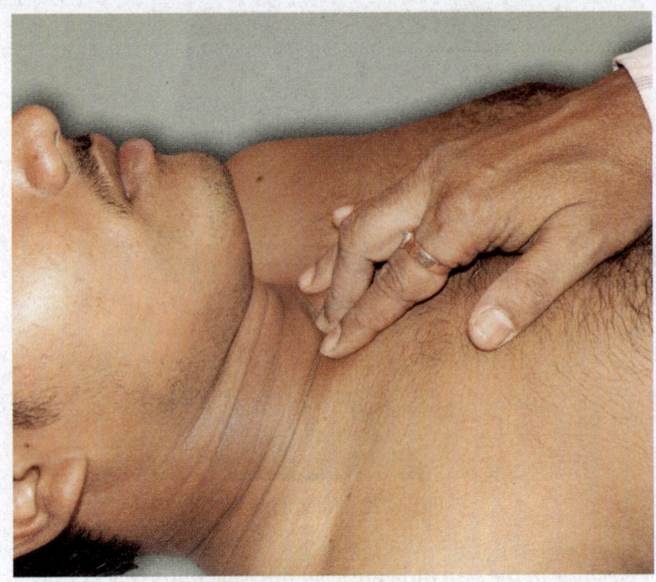

FIG. 3.23 Palpation of trachea

- Hand should be kept by the side of the bed
- Place the tip of index finger in the fossa in between medical end of sternocleidomastoid and lateral wall of the trachea
- Compare the depth of the fossa on both sides of trachea
- If there is shift, then it is typically towards smaller fossa.

Causes of tracheal shift
- *Towards the side of lesion:*
  - ❖ Pulmonary fibrosis
  - ❖ Collapse of lung.
- *Away from side of lesion:*
  - ❖ Pleural effusion
  - ❖ Pneumothorax
  - ❖ Superior mediastinal mass—lymphoma, carcinoma.
- *Downward displacement:* In chronic airflow obstruction during inspiration. This may greatly reduce the space between cricoid's cartilage and suprasternal notch.

Assessment of Mobility of Trachea

- *Induced mobility:* It can assessed by pushing the trachea side to side
  Indicates mediastinal fibrosis from:
  - ❖ Mediastinitis
  - ❖ Tumor.

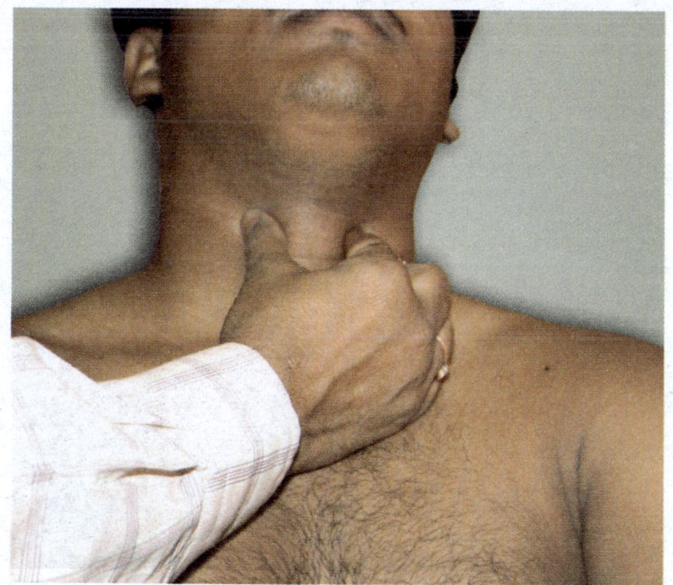

FIG. 3.24   Oliver's sign

- *Spontaneous mobility:* It can be detected as rostrocaudal tracheal tug synchronous with each heart beat. It indicates the aneurysm of aortic arch.

Oliver's Sign

It is downward displacement of cricoid cartilage coincides with each heart beat.

To detect it (Fig. 3.24):
- Ask the patient to sit up
- Grasp the cricoid cartilage and apply the upward pressure by thumb and index finger
- A downward movement with each heart beat indicates aneurysm of aortic arch.

Because aortic arch overrides left main bronchus, with each ejection it pulls the left bronchus downwards and thus the trachea.

Causes

- Aneurysm of aortic arch
- Mediastinal tumor
- COPD.

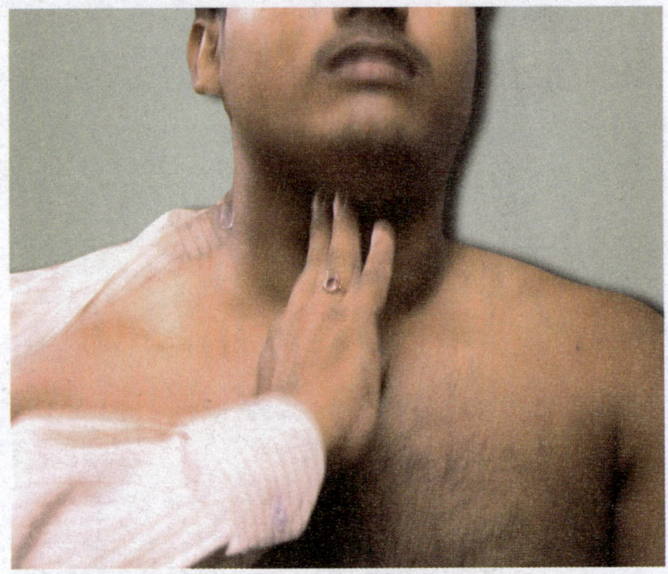

FIG. 3.25 Cardarelli's sign

Cardarelli's Sign (Fig. 3.25)

Press gently the thyroid cartilage and push it towards left side. This shits of trachea and increases the contact between left main bronchus and the aorta. Thus helping to feel the transverse pulsation over trachea—in case of aortic arch aneurysm.

Campbell's Sign (Fig. 3.26A)

Downward displacement of thyroid cartilage during inspiration >2.5 inches—indicates COPD.

- This is an accurate predictor of severe airflow obstruction
- It correlates with duration of symptoms
- It correlates with reduction in FEV1.

Laryngeal Height (Fig. 3.26B)

It is the distance between the top of thyroid cartilage and the suprasternal notch.

Value of laryngeal height:
- If the height is <4 cm, then it is predictive of postoperative pulmonary risk.
- It is a strong predictor of obstructive lung disease. If maximum height of larynx is <4 cm, then it indicates marked hyperinflation of chart.

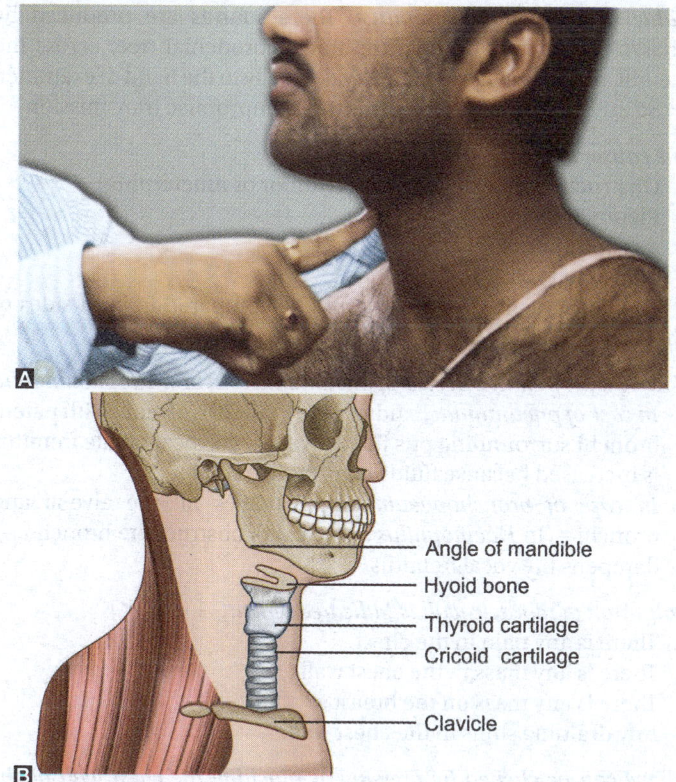

FIGS 3.26A AND B (A) Campbell's sign; (B) Laryngeal height measurement (Campbell's sign)

Tracheal auscultation: It recognize:

- *Stridor wheeze:* Present during inspiration should not be confused with true wheezes—which is expiratory or inspiratory and expiratory
- *Expiratory wheeze:* Louder over the trachea, it reflects expiratory adduction of vocal cords. This should prompt laryngoscopy because these patients present with refractory asthma.

Vocal tactile fremitus: It is Latin term. It is a palpable thrill produced by patients' voice.

Detection: This can be detected by placing the hand over the various part of chest in different intercostal spaces, then feel the thrill that is transmitted whenever patient is asked to say 99 or 1, 2, 3.

These digits are of choice because, there are low pitched notes; and low pitched voices better pass the alveolar air filter and produce stronger tactile fremitus.

Value of vocal tactile fremitus: There sounds are produced by pharynx, transmitted down the tracheobronchial tree, across the pleural, pleural cavity and chest wall, finally to the hand of examiner.

So any abnormality along this way compromise transmission.

The causes are:
- Obstruction in distal bronchus (tumor or mucus plug)
- Pleural effusion
- Pneumothorax
- Thickened skin.

The vocal tactile fremitus should be compared in both sides of chest and in same areas on both sides.

Vocal tactile fremitus in case of pneumonia and bronchopneumonia:
- *In case of pneumonia:* Exudates are limited to alveoli, with patent bronchi surrounding pus filled alveoli—so vocal tactile fremitus is increased because fluids behaves like solid
- *In case of bronchopneumonia:* Exudates fill the alveoli and bronchi—(In *Haemophilus influenzae*), obstruct the bronchus—dampens the vocal fremitus.

Palpation of thoracic wall is indicated when:
- There is any pain in the chest
- There is any mass in the chest wall
- There is any mass on the breast
- Any draining sinus in the chest wall.

Above can be elicited by pressing or pinching the chest wall or the muscle:
- *Palpate soft tissue* for tenderness, crepitus
- *Palpate intercostals spaces* for local tenderness, hematoma
- *Palpate costochondral junctions and costal cartilages* for tenderness, swelling, and mobility
- *Palpate the ribs* for point tenderness, swelling, bone crepitus remote pain on compression
- *Palpate xiphisternal joint* for tenderness.

Assessment of Expansion of Hemithoraces

It confirms abnormal respiratory dynamics suspected during inspection:
- Observing flaring of nostrils
- Pursed-lip respiration
- Asynchrony of chest expansion
- Asynchrony of abdominal movements
- Use of accessory muscles.

Unilateral lag in palpation is usually seen:
- Pneumonic consolidation
- Pneumothorax
- Pleural effusion
- Fibrosis.

Bilateral lag in excursion indicative of:
- Airflow obstruction
- Neuromuscular disease.

Testing excursion of upper thorax (Fig. 3.27):
- Place the hand on each side of the neck with palms against the anterior thoracic wall
- Curl the fingers firmly over the superior edge of the trapezii
- Push the palm downwards against the skin until the palms of both hands firmly lie in the infraclavicular fossae
- Then extend the thumb of both hands, so that both of them touch at the midline at the end of full expiration
- Upper four ribs move forwards with inspiration. So during deep inspiration both the thumb diverge from the midline in equal distance and the palms move freely with the chest and fingers firmly anchor the chest wall
  - ❖ *In case of asynchrony:* The thumbs of the affected side move little than unaffected side.
  - ❖ *In case of synchrony:* Both the thumbs move same distances from the midline.
  - ❖ *In case COPD:* Thumbs of both sides' movements are little.

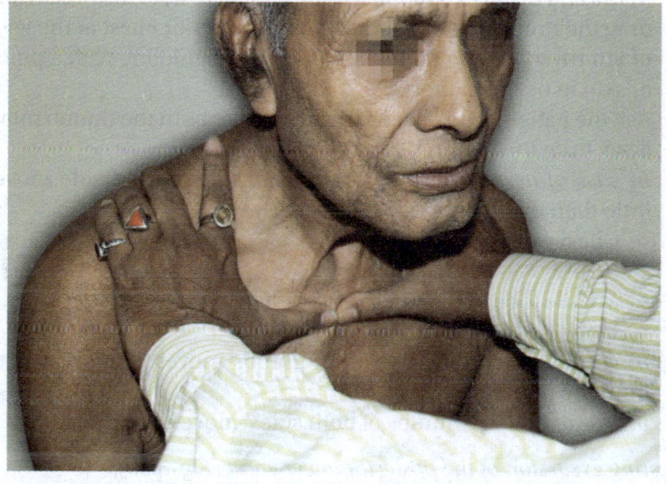

FIG. 3.27 Excursion of upper thorax

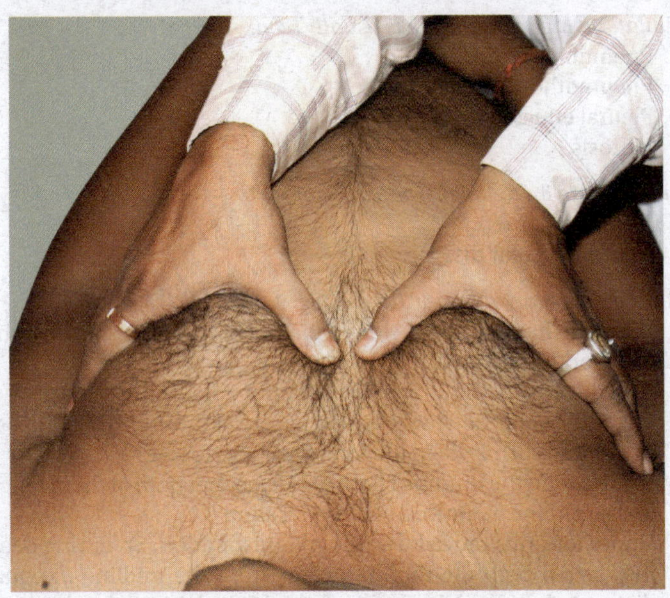

FIG. 3.28 Extension of anterior middle thorax

Testing excursion of the anterior middle thorax (Fig. 3.28):
- With your fingers in the axilla and the thumbs abducted, place your both palms on the anterior chest wall
- Drag the thumbs of both the hands towards the midline. Ask the patient to take full expiration
- At the end of full expiration ask the patient to hold the breath and drag the thumbs in the midline on the anterior chest at the level of 6th rib so that both of them touch at the midline with a pinch of skin in between them
- Ask the patient to take deep breath, so that both the thumb move away from the midline
- *In case of asynchrony:* The thumbs of the affected side moves little than unaffected side indicating lesion:
  - ❖ Chest wall
  - ❖ Pleura
  - ❖ Middle lobe of the lung
  - ❖ Lingual of left lung.
- *In case of synchrony:* Both the thumbs moves same distances from the midline
- *In case of COPD:* Thumbs of both sides' movements are little.

Testing excursion of the posterior lower chest (Fig. 3.29):
- Ask the patient to sit with back towards you

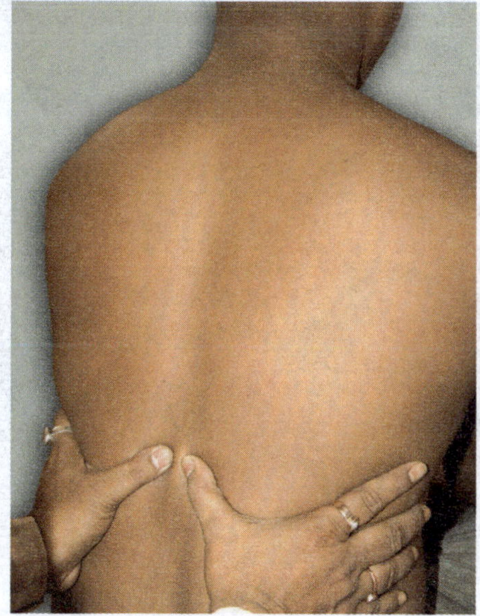

FIG. 3.29   Extension of posterior lower chest

- Place your hand on the sides of the chest with forefingers towards axilla one or two ribs below the inferior angle of scapula and both the thumbs abducted and extended towards the midline on the posterior chest wall
- Ask the patient to exhale fully and hold the breath so that both the thumbs are pulled medially towards the midline over the vertebral spines and touch with a pinch of a skin in between them
- Ask the patient to take deep breath. Watch the movement of the thumbs from the midline
- *In case of asynchrony:* The thumbs of the affected side moves little than unaffected side indicating lesion in the:
  - ❖ Chest wall
  - ❖ Pleura
  - ❖ Lower lobe of the lung.
- *In case of synchrony:* Both the thumbs moves same distances from the midline
- *In case COPD:* Thumbs of both sides' movements are little.

Testing excursion of the costal margin (Fig. 3.30):
- Ask the patient to lie in supine position
- Place your hand on the lower part of the chest with the extended thumbs along the inferior edge of the costal margins and thumbs abducted to touch with each other at the end of full expiration

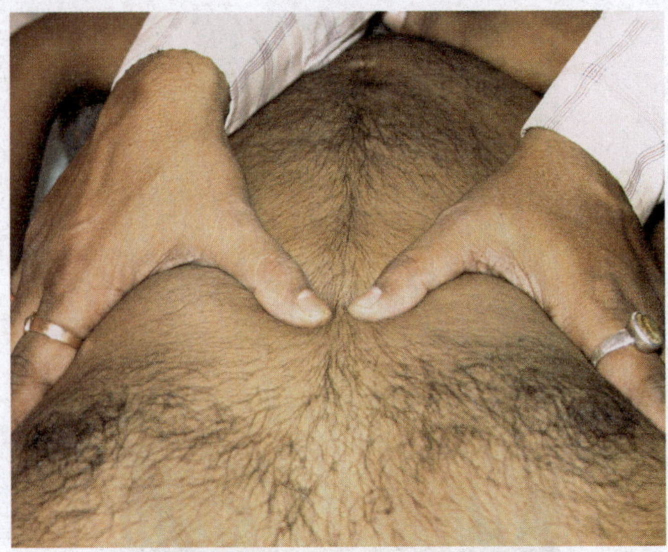

FIG. 3.30 Extension of costal margin

- With respiration, watch the divergence of the thumbs
- *In case of asynchrony:* The thumbs of the affected side move little than unaffected side, indicating lesion in:
  - ❖ Dome of diaphragm
  - ❖ Pleura.
- *In case of synchrony:* Both the thumbs move same distances from the midline
- *In case of COPD:* Thumbs of both sides' movements are little.

Vibratory palpation of the lung and pleura (Figs 3.31A and B)

Mechanism of production of vibration: During speech patient' vocal cord set-up a vibration in the bronchial air column that are conducted to the chest wall through the lung tissue. This vibration can be palpated by palpatory method as described here:

- Ask the patient to sit
- Ask the patient to speak 'one' or 'three'
- Apply palmar bases of the fingers of one hand to the interspaces. Alternatively ulnar surface of hand and finger may be used
- At the same time, both sides of the chest should be examined by the same hand, e.g. left infraclavicular fossa followed by right infraclavicular fossa
- When lower thorax has been reached, use ulnar surface of your hand to confirm the point where the fremitus is lost. In absence any type of pleural lesion, it dictates the position of lung bases.

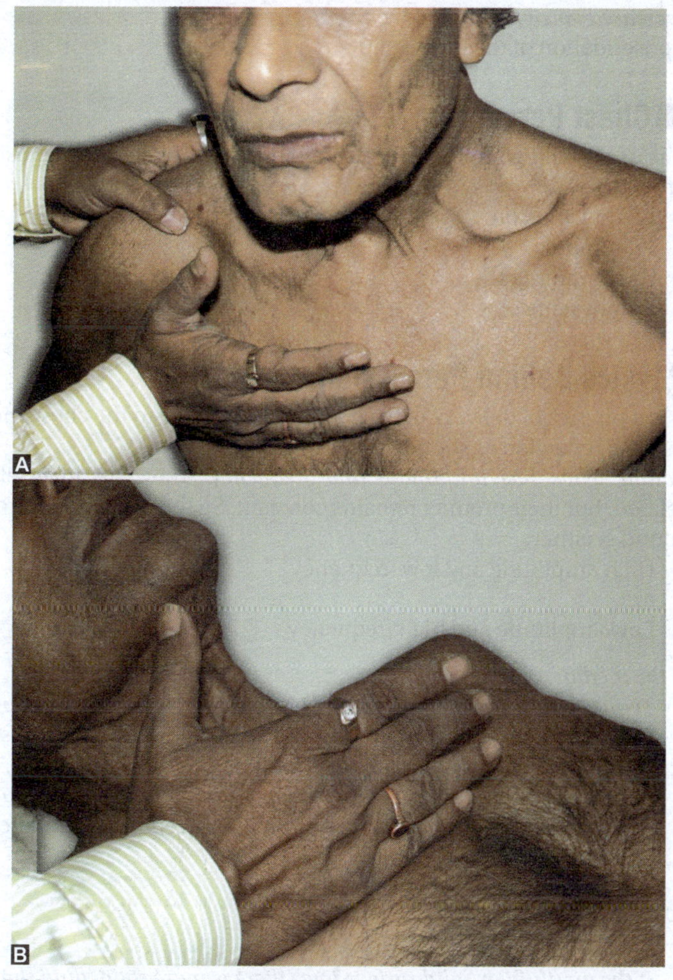

FIGS 3.31A AND B (A) Vibratory palpation of lung, (B) Vibratory palpation of lung and pleura

Normal variation in vocal fremitus:
- Normal intense fremitus in the parasternal region in the right 2nd intercostals space closest to bronchial bifurcation
- Interscapular region near the bronchi produces increased fremitus
- High-pitched voice produce unsatisfactory vibration.

Diminished vocal fremitus:
- Blockage of the airways
- Fluid or air in the pleural cavity
- Fibrosis of the pleura.

Increased vocal fremitus:
Consolidation of the lung

Chest Percussion

It is useful and complements auscultation in differential diagnosis of:

- Pleural effusion
- Pneumonia
- Pneumothorax
- Emphysema.

Physics Behind Percussion

It is a physics of delivery of fixed amount of energy to the chest and its back reflection as sound.

Sound wave has amplitude and frequency: They are inversely related, but their product remains constant. So the characteristic of sound is either:

- High amplitude and low frequency
  or
- Low amplitude and high frequency

If the media:

- *Tissue rich in air and poor in solid (high air/solid ratio):* Percussion note have high amplitude and low frequency—so sound is resonant, typical of normal lung
- *If air is more abundant than normal (very high air/solid ratio),* percussion note has greater amplitude and very low frequency character is tympanic, typical of:
  - ❖ Pneumothorax
  - ❖ Emphysema
  - ❖ Big blebs.
- *If the air/fluid or solid ratio is low (there is more solid/fluid than air):* Percussion note has low amplitude and high frequency. So the sound becomes dull or soft—sometimes so soft, that light percussion technique may even fail to elicit anything audible.

  So light percussion technique is used to identify the areas of resonances and areas of silence. So dull note identify:

- Consolidation
- Pleural effusion
- Collapse.

General Rules for Percussion

- Percuss the back in sitting position and percuss the anterior chest in sitting or supine position

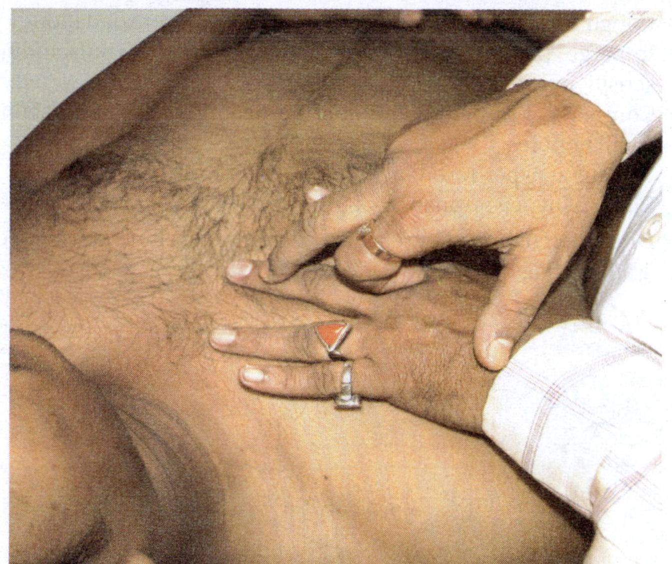

FIG. 3.32   Method of percussion

- When the patient is ill and unable to sit, he must be examined in right or left lateral decubitus positions
- All the examinations must be done from the right side
- Both sonorous and definitive percussion are applied to the back.

Current Technique of Indirect Percussion (Fig. 3.32)

- Lay pleximeter finger (middle finger) of the left hand in right handed examiner on the intercostal space (not on the rib)
- To avoid dampening, distal interphalangeal joint only can be touched to skin
- The rest of the fingers are lifted off the chest wall
- The blow is then delivered by middle finger of right hand, flexed as hammer at 90° angle, brought down over distal interphalangeal joint of left hand
- Tap should be gentle; it allows better detection of percussion note
- Tap should be delivered by using wrist, as a fulcrum
- After delivery, percussion finger should be lifted from pleximeter.

Value of Indirect Percussion

- A normal percussion note sometimes occurs in diseased lung
- Percussion note complements auscultation in differential diagnosis of consolidation, atelectasis, pneumothorax, pleural effusion

- Cough with fever, unilateral dullness suggests consolidation
- In large pleural effusion, percussion note has outstanding sensitivity
- Comparison of percussion is of no or little value in detecting small nodules
- Unilateral hyper-resonance—pneumothorax
- Bilateral hyper-resonance—airflow obstruction COPD.

Direct percussion of the clavicle as pleximeters for assessment of lung apices (Figs 3.33A and B).

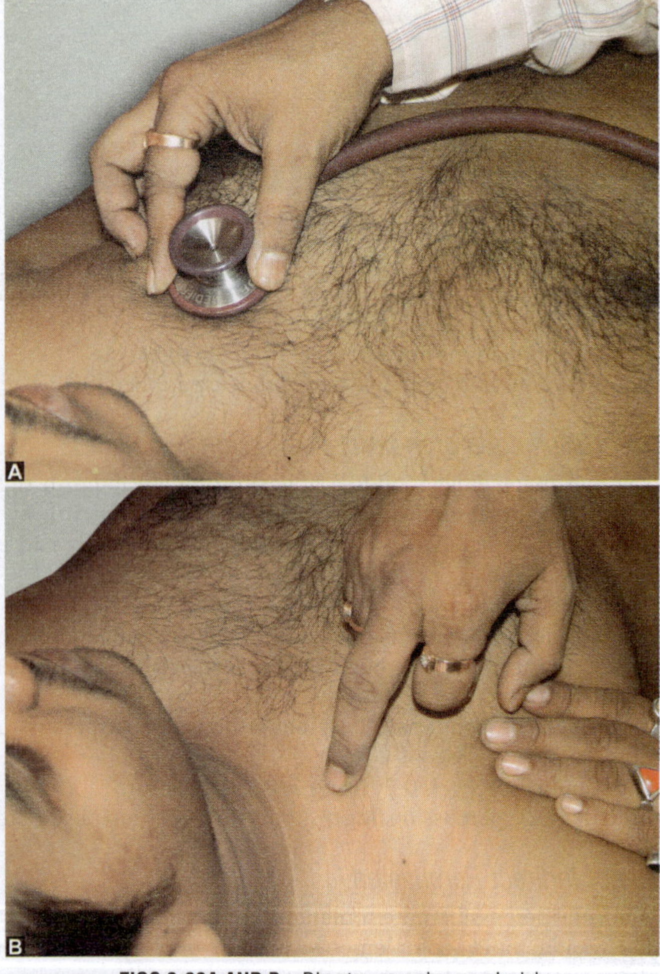

FIGS 3.33A AND B   Direct percussion on clavicle

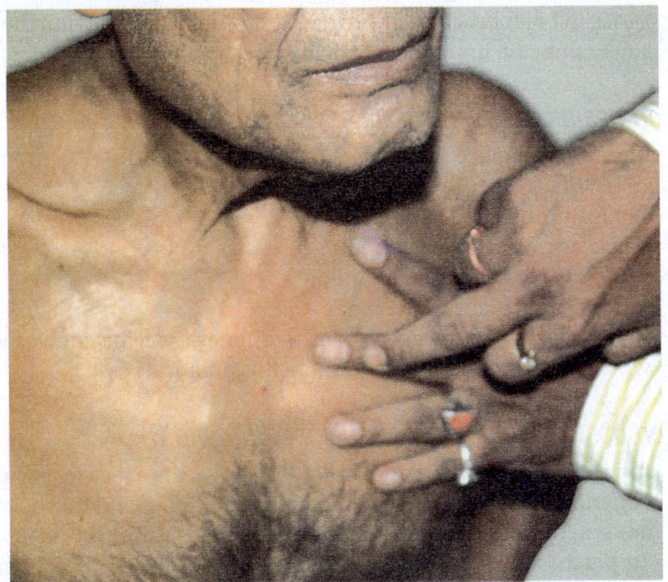

FIG. 3.34 Percussion of anterior lung

Percussion of the Anterior Lung (Fig. 3.34)

- These procedures call for sonorous percussion
- Ask the patient to sit with arm of both hands abducted with hand to rest on the hips, so that anterior and lateral aspect of the chest accessible
- Start from under the clavicles, compare the interspaces of both sides sequentially
- Extend the percussion downward up to the region of hepatic dullness on the right side and Traube's semilunar space on the left side
- An entire anterior region except cardiac area is resonant.

Percussion of Hepatic Dullness

- Upper aspect of dullness produces a transverse area of dullness from 4th to 6th intercostals spaces in the right mid clavicular line
- Since a wedge-shaped of lung tissue is present in between the chest wall and upper border of liver, transition of resonance to dullness up to 6th interspace is gradual.

Percussion of Gastric Tympany

- Normally gastric air bubbles produces tympany in the area, known as Traube's semilunar space

- Since left diaphragm is lower, upper border of gastric tympany is lower than the upper border of liver.

Percussion of Splenic Dullness

- This is the space in between left 9th and 11th ribs in the midaxillary line
- It may be obscured by:
  - ❖ Gastric or colonic tympany
  - ❖ Gastric or colonic solid or fluid
  - ❖ Left sided pleural effusion.
- In case of splenomegaly, area of dullness will be increased, which creates attention to examine this organ.

Percussion of Lung Apices (Figs 3.35A and B)

- Apices of the lungs extend slightly above the clavicle having widened areas at the sternal and clavicular end, and narrowest areas at the shoulder top—named as Kronig's isthmus
- To percuss the right supraclavicular fossa, your left thumb will be pleximeter
- For the left supraclavicular fossa, your left arm will be put around the patient's back of the neck, and the left middle finger will be curled over the trapezius muscle into the fossa
- Fibrosis of the lung narrows, sometimes obliterate the site, producing dullness over that area.

Percussion of the Posterior Lung (Figs 3.36A and B)

- Ask the patient to sit with arms folded in front of the body, shoulder to be kept forward and spine will be in antiflexed position
- Percussion should be started from the top and gradually downward towards bases
- Percussion areas will be in between the scapular bones in the paravertebral areas
- Percussion should be compared bilaterally in the symmetrical zones sequentially to compare the intensity of resonance
- Zone of resonance ends at the level of 9th rib on the right, a little below on the left.

Percussion of the Posterior Lung Bases

- During normal respiration inferior edge of the right lung is at 8th intercostals space and that of left lung is at 9th rib
- Transition between the lung resonance and muscle dullness is a wedge-shaped area, it requires light percussion to elicit it
- At quiet respiration mark the level of lower lung edge

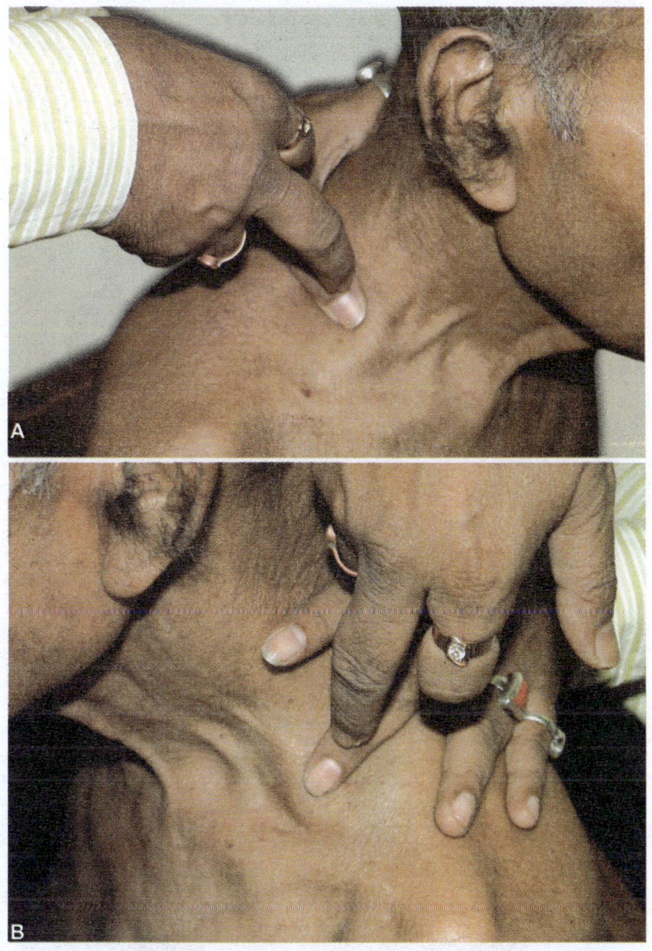

FIGS 3.35A AND B   (A) Percussion of right lung apex; (B) Percussion of left lung apex

- At the end of full inspiration, ask the patient to hold his breath, again percuss the level in the same method
- Measure the distance. Normally, the base should move downward at about 5 to 6 cm
- In chronic obstructive lung disease, this measurement will be <2 cm.

Definitive percussion: In the examination of chest, this type of percussion is required to outline the borders between the lung resonance and liver dullness, gastric tympany, lumbar muscles below the lung bases.

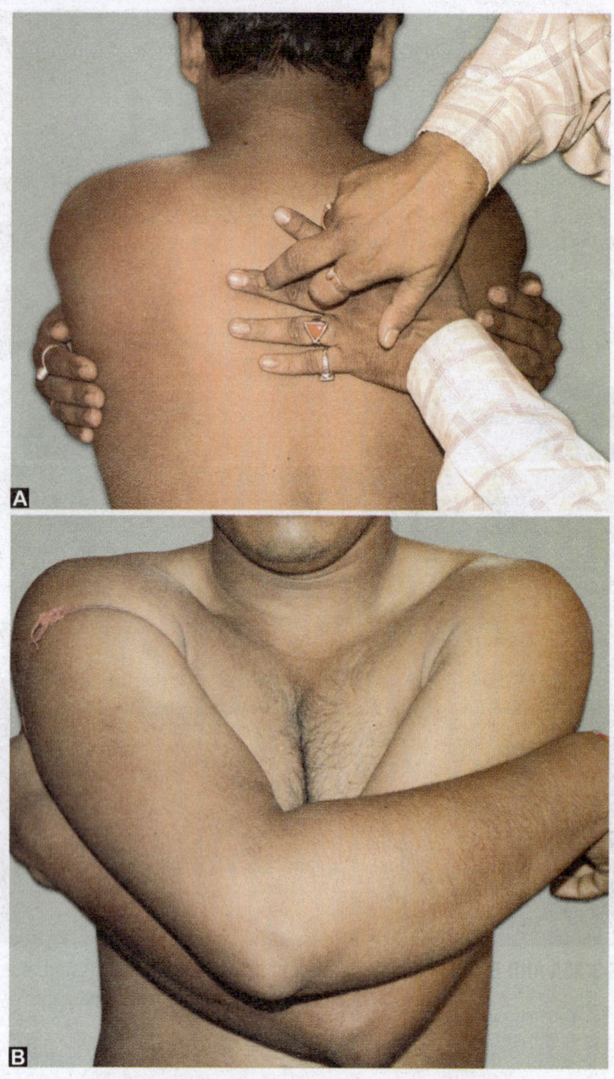

FIGS 3.36A AND B   Percussion of posterior lung

Auscultatory percussion (Fig. 3.37): It is a modified variety of topographic percussion. In this mode, detection of sounds can be done by stethoscope.

Role of Auscultatory Percussion in Detection of Pleural Effusion

- Patient has to be seated, stethoscope placed in the back 3 cm below the 12th rib

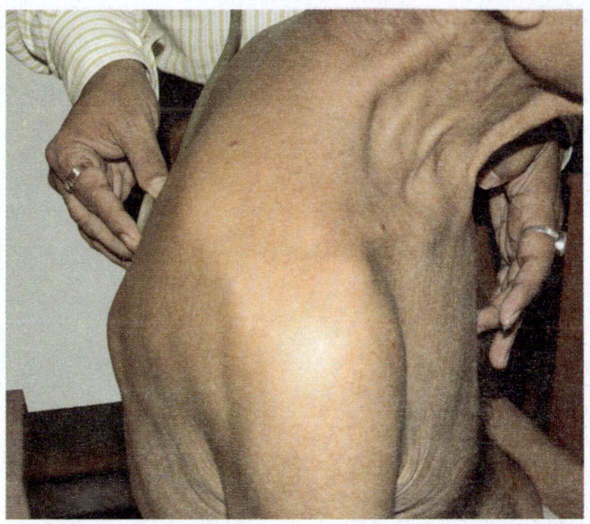

FIG. 3.37 Auscultatory percussion

- The chest is then percussed downwards and posteriorly from apex to base
- A change is percussion note from loud to dull that is localized over the 12th rib—indicates the presence of pleural fluid.

Another Method of Auscultatory Percussion

- Physician taps lightly with distal tip of one finger over the manubrium sterni
- At the same time the physician listening with the stethoscope over symmetrical location on the posterior wall
- Sound, generated travels uninterrupted through the lungs reaches opposite chest wall in a symmetrical fashion
- Any asymmetry in sound intensity is considered a sign of lung disease.

Auscultation

Major types of lung sounds (respiratory sounds) are described as:

Lung Sounds

Breath Sounds

- Vesicular breath sound
- Bronchovesicular breath sound
- *Bronchial sound:*
  - ❖ Tracheal breath sound
  - ❖ Cavernous breath sound

- ❖ Tubular breath sound
- ❖ Amphoric breath sound.

Adventitious sound
- *Discontinuous sounds:*
  - ❖ *Crackles:*
    - Early
    - Mid
    - Late
    - Posture induced.
- *Continuous sounds:*
  - ❖ Wheeze
  - ❖ Rhonchi.
- *Vocal sounds:*
  - ❖ Bronchophony
  - ❖ Whispering pectoriloquy
  - ❖ Ego phony
  - ❖ EA changes.

Procedure of auscultation of the lungs and pleura (Figs 3.38 to 3.41):
- Patient should be examined in a quiet room at normal or warm temperature to avoid muscle shivering
- Patient should be in sitting position. In case of serious patient, he should be examined in recumbent position by turning him from side to side
- Ask the patient to take breath deeply and slightly forcefully than usual. Watch, whether the patient heave and puff irregularly make noise from, the mouth.

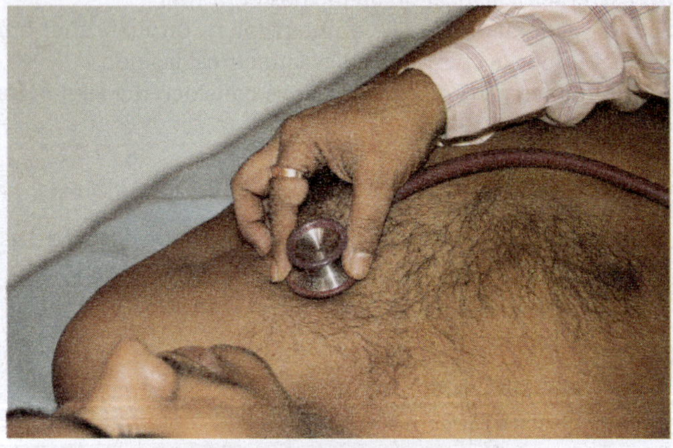

FIG. 3.38 Auscultation of anterior chest

- Start auscultation anterior and posterior lung from above downwards and compare the both right and left side simultaneously and sequentially
- Watch any change in character of breath sound and any added sound.

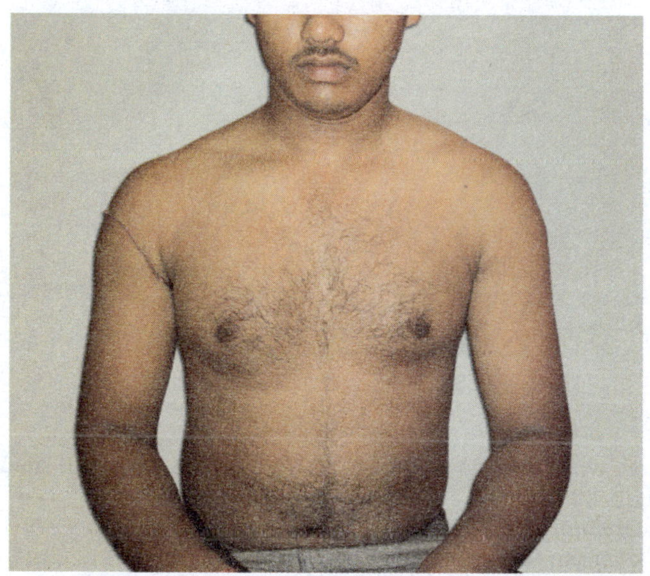

FIG. 3.39   Position of patient during auscultation of anterior chest

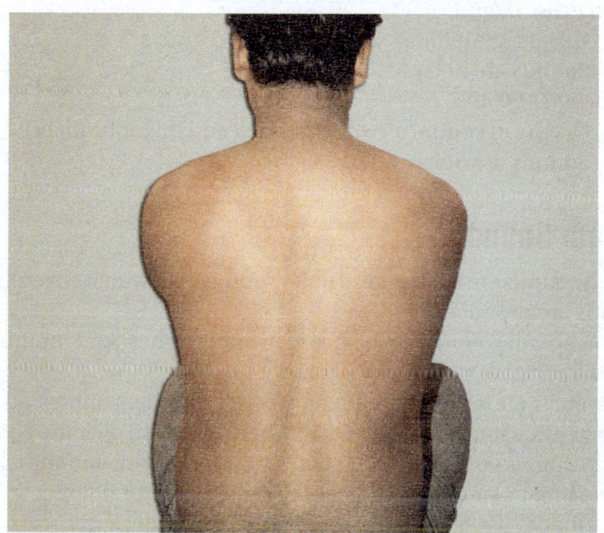

FIG. 3.40   Position of the patient during auscultation of posterior chest

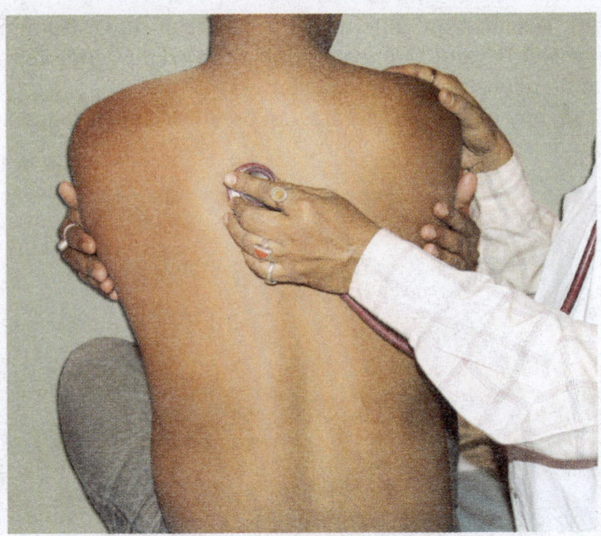

FIG. 3.41 Auscultation of posterior chest

Three types of airflow in lungs are responsible for breath sounds (Fig. 3.42):
1. *Laminar flow:*
    ❖ Occurs in peripheral airways including alveoli
    ❖ Airflow is very slow
    ❖ Some sounds are silent and some are noisy.
2. *Vorticose flow:*
    ❖ Occurs in medium-sized bronchial airways
    ❖ Sounds are noisy.
3. *Turbulent flow:*
    ❖ Occurs in central airways (trachea and major bronchi)
    ❖ Sounds are noisy.

Breath Sounds

Breath sounds are background noisy sounds over which adventitious sounds are produced.

The breath sounds can be heard over both chest and mouth. But the differences on character of the sounds are:
- Alveolar air is a high frequency filter, so it filters almost all high frequency sounds >2000 Hz. So when it is heard over the chest — it becomes very soft, soften than sounds head over mouth
- The breath sounds heard over the mouth is not filtered, so high frequency sound remains and heard in a louder way.

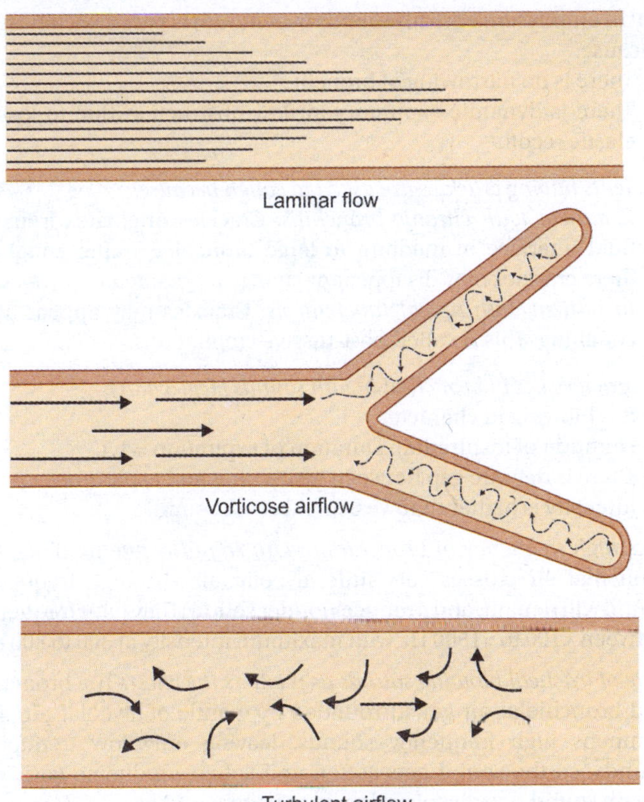

FIG. 3.42   Types of airflow

Value of comparing breath sounds at the mouth with those over the chest:

- *Breath sound heard at the mouth* by unaided ear have an intensity that is directly proportional to degree of airflow obstruction
- *Breath sound heard on the chest* by stethoscope have an intensity that is inversely proportional to airflow obstructions, i.e. as airflow obstruction is increased, breath sounds become distant.

Intensity of inspiratory breath sounds heard over the mouth can differentiate emphysema from chronic bronchitis and bronchial asthma, since last two conditions directly correlates with:

- Increased airway resistance
- Reduced FEV1 (forced expiratory volume in 1 seconds)
- Reduced peak expiratory airflow.

But in emphysema breath sounds over mouth is paradoxically quiet because:

- There is no narrowing of bronchi
- There is dynamic expiratory airflow obstruction due to loss of elastic recoil.

Patients having crackles are asked to cough because:
- *It patient with chronic bronchitis:* Crackles originates from air fluid interface of medium to large bronchi. So after coughing there crackles may disappear or change its character
- *In patient with apical tuberculosis:* Crackles may appear after coughing. This is called post-tussive crepitations.

Characteristics of bronchial breath sounds (Fig. 3.43A):
- It is blowing in character
- Duration of inspiration: Duration of expiration = 1:1
- There is definite gap between inspiration and expiration
- Intensity is higher than vesicular breath sound.

This high frequency of bronchial breath sound is due to: Since the bronchial air crosses very little alveolar air, the high frequency sound will remain, and produces louder sound. They have frequency between <100 to >1500 Hz with maximum intensity at 300 to 800 Hz.

Fate of tracheal blowing sounds as it enters the chest: The bronchial and bronchiolar air get surrounded by mantle of alveolar air, that dampens high frequency sounds, leaving only low frequency sounds, so the sound gets soften and soften producing vesicular breath sound—so alveolar air acts as low-pass filter.

The characteristics of vesicular breath sound (Fig. 3.43B):
- It is resulting in character
- It is low frequency sounds (100–500 Hz)
- Length of expiration is one third of length of inspiration
- No gap between inspiration and expiration.

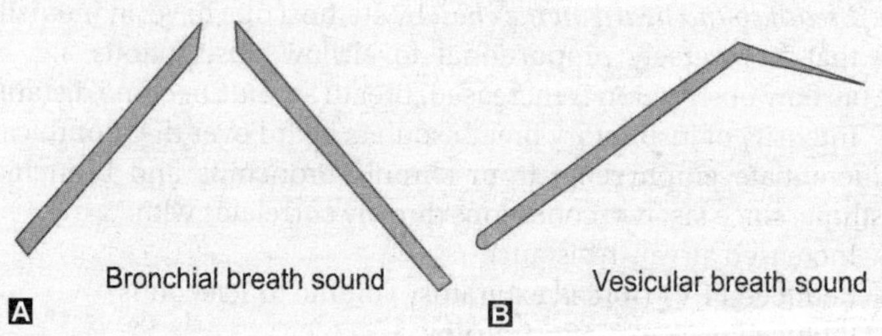

FIGS 3.43A AND B Types of breath sounds

So vesicular breath sound is originated in bronchi and bronchioles modified and filtered by alveolar air.

The following conditions where alveoli cannot filter the air:
- *When alveolar air is replaced by:*
  - ❖ Pus—pneumonia
  - ❖ Serum—pulmonary edema
  - ❖ Blood—alveolar hemorrhage.
- *When alveolar air can be squeezed out:*
  - ❖ Alveolar collapse.

So in above cases, air in bronchi or bronchioles; cannot be filtered by alveolar air, hence high frequency sound remains and heard over the chest as bronchial breath sound.

The length of expiratory component is one-third of the length of inspiratory component, because: Expiratory component is low pitch in intensity, hence, the last two-thirds of total length is entirely absent.

Character of vesicular breath sound varies with age, e.g.:
- In children (up to age 9), it is high pitched than adults
- In adult, vesicular breath sound is louder than elderly.

The causes are:
- Different resonance of small thoraces in children, leading to less power in low frequencies for children breath sound
- In elderly patient there is increase in muffling of air due to progressive emphysema
- Smaller radius of children's airways may be responsible for high turbulence of air and loudness of vesicular breath sound.

In healthy lung vesicular breath sound is absent in: Two narrow areas, corresponding anteriorly and posteriorly to the trachea and central bronchi (Para scapular areas)—here vesicular breath is replaced by bronchovesicular breath sound (Fig. 3.11).

The breath sound in pneumothorax is absent or distant, because:
- Reduced sound production due to diminished airflow in collapsed lung
- Reduced sound transmission due to cushion of air in pleural space.

The breath sound in pleural effusion is absent because:
- Reduced sound production due to collapsed lung
- Reduced sound transmission due to presence of fluid in pleural space.

So the above conditions can be differentiated by percussion—in pneumothorax, it is hyper-resonant to tympanic, in pleural effusion it is story dull.

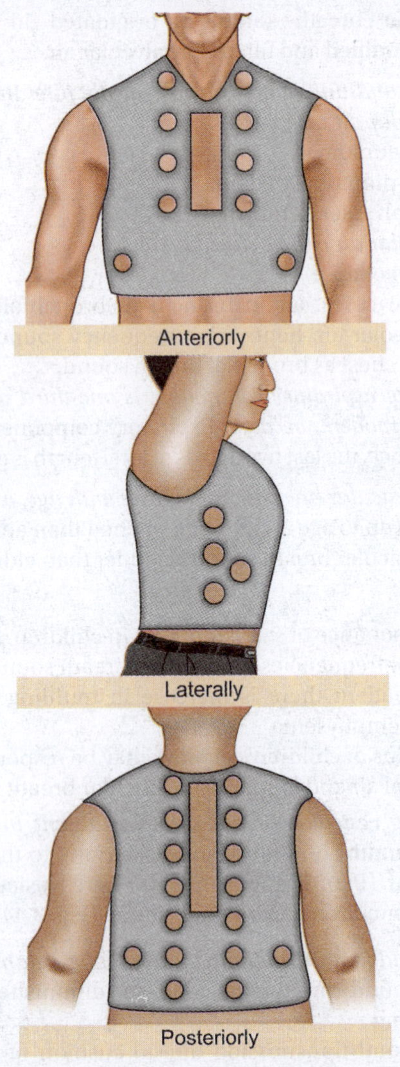

FIG. 3.44 Sites of absent vesicular breath sound

The intensity of vesicular breath sound is decreased in:
- COPD
- Hyperventilation following exercise
- Endotracheal tube in misplaced or displaced to right major bronchus producing obstruction to left main stem bronchus.

Provided the following conditions are ok:
- Chest wall thin (not obese)
- No air or fluid in pleural space

- No respiratory muscle weakness.

Breath sound intensity (BSI) is the best bedside predictors of chronic obstructive lung disease.

This can be measured in the following ways:
- Ask the patient to sit up and inspire from residual volume fast and deep, same time breathing through the mouth, produces loud breath sound as possible.
- Auscultation should be done in:
  ❖ Anterior zone
  ❖ Axillary zone
  ❖ Posterior bases.
- *Quantify the inspiratory component of vesicular breath sound:*
  ❖ 0—Absent
  ❖ 1—Barely audible
  ❖ 2—Faint but definitely audible
  ❖ 3—Normal
  ❖ 4—Louder than normal.
- *Sum of intensities of sound recorded in each area generates BSI score:* The score rangers from 0 to 24 total in 6 areas, i.e. 0 to 4 in each of 6 areas
- During scoring, adventitious sounds (rhonchus, wheeze, or crepitations) should be disregarded, because, there sounds being louder, may overestimates BSI.

Values of Breath Sound Intensity

BSI correlates with:
- Forced expiratory volume in 1 second (FEV1)
- FEV1/FVC.
  ❖ BSI score <9—strongly suggest obstruction
  ❖ BSI score >15—argues against obstruction.

In patient with positive metacholine test, reduced BSI is typical of asthma. This is an excellent tool for monitoring bronchial provocation.

As the obstructions to airflow increases, the intensity of breath sound becomes louder.

Mechanism of reduced BSI in COPD:
- Reduced sound production—due to diminished airflow—is more explratory than inspiratory
- Reduced sound transmission due to parenchymal destruction and air-trapping.

Best bedside predictor of severity of airflow obstruction
Forced expiratory time (FET): This can be measured in following ways:

- Ask the patient to take deep breath and exhale it as quickly as possible and forcibly
- At the same time put your bell of stethoscope over the patient's suprasternal notch
- Measure the forced expiratory time to the nearest half seconds
- *Results:*
    - ❖ FET >6 seconds—corresponds to $FEV1_1/FVC$ <40 percent
    - ❖ FET <5 seconds—corresponds $FEV1_1/FVC$ >60 percent.

Bronchial Breath Sound

- *In normal healthy individual:* In posterior right upper chest—where right lung is continuous with trachea through 1st thoracic vertebra—normal bronchial breath sound can be heard.
- *In other areas of lung:* Bronchial breath sound is always pathological, until proved otherwise.

Bronchial breath sound in case of consolidation
Consolidation: It is the replacement of alveolar air by mantle of solidified lung tissue but the bronchi remain patent to transmit high frequency sounds. Consolidation occurs in following two ways:
1. *Alveolar collapse:* It may be due to pleural effusion or pneumothorax but not severe enough to compress bronchi.
2. *Alveolar fluid filling:*
    - ❖ Pus—pneumonia
    - ❖ Blood—alveolar hemorrhage
    - ❖ Fluid—alveolar edema.

Patient presents with fever, cough and presence of bronchial breath sound—strongly favor pneumonia.
Depth of consolidated lung from the chest surface to generate bronchial breath sound: Consolidation and/or fibrosis must extend 4 to 5 cm from the hilum towards chest surface (where large bronchi are located). So the breath sounds containing high frequencies coming from the large bronchi resemble tracheal sounds.

Difference between bronchial breath sound due to collapse and fluid-filled alveoli:
- Bronchial breath sound due to collapse is not associated with crackles
- Bronchial breath sound due to fluid filled alveoli is associated with crackles.

Most common cause of bronchial breath sounds unaccompanied by crackles
Pleural effusion: Fluid-filled half hemithorax presents with:
- *Upper third of chest:* Vesicular breath sound—reflects normal aeration

- *Middle third of chest:* Tubular breath sound—reflects compressed alveoli but patent airways
- *Lower third of chest:* Breath sound is absent—due to compression of alveoli and airways by pleural fluid accumulation.

Bronchial breath sound due to cardiac tamponade
Ewart's sign: Posterior dullness due to percussion and bronchial breath sounds—between tip of left scapula and vertebral column due to compressive atelectasis caused by distended pericardial sac.

Bronchial breath sound due to mitral stenosis
It occurs in Ortner's syndrome of mitral stenosis. It occurs due to squeezing of left main bronchus by enlarged left atrium, which in turn causes:
- Compression of left recurrent laryngeal nerve between aortic arch and pulmonary artery (resulting hoarseness and bitonal voice)
- Left lower lobe atelectasis (posterior dullness and bronchial breath sounds)
- Dysphagia (esophageal impingement).

Amphoric breath sound: It is a metallic quality bronchial breath sound—high-pitched, loud and resonant. It occurred in bronchus opens into a cavity, very large cyst or blebs.
Cavernous breath sound: It occurs when large bronchus opens into a cavity. It occurs in tuberculous cavity draining into large bronchus. This breath sound means blowing sound blowing through a cave.

Bronchovesicular Breath Sound

- It is a combination of both vesicular and bronchial breath sound
- It can be heard in parasternal and parascapular areas of normal people from third to sixth intercostals space.

Three characteristics of bronchovesicular breath sounds:
1. Like tubular breath sound long and well-preserved expiration, (Inspiration:Expiration = 1:1).
2. Like vesicular breath sound lack of silent phase between inspiration and expiration.
3. They are soft and low-pitched, like vesicular breath sound and harsh, and loud like tubular breath sound.

The peculiar bronchovesicular breath sound is due to peculiar transmission of the sound: First it produces turbulent flow in large and central airways.

Then it crosses a thin mantle of alveolar air before reaching to chest piece of stethoscope. Hence tracheal sounds undergo some physical changes before going to chest piece.

Clinical significance of bronchovesicular breath sounds:
- In healthy person, parasternal and parascapular areas anteriorly and posteriorly
- Early consolidation
- Thin pleural effusion, partially compressing alveoli but not the bronchi.

Adventitious Sounds

- These sounds are normally absent in respiratory cycle, but becomes superimposed on underlying bronchial or vesicular breath sounds when the lung will be diseased
- These sounds may be:
  - Discontinuous (if lasting <250 msec)
  - Continuous (if lasting >250 msec).

Discontinuous sounds—is crackles—replacing British term—'Crepitations' and French term 'rales'.

Crackles can be described by following characteristics:
- *Number:* Scanty or profuse
- *Predominant frequency:*
  - High-pitched (fine)
  - Low pitched (coarse).
- *Amplitude:*
  - Loud
  - Faint.
- *Timing during inspiration:*
  - Early
  - Mid
  - Late.

Mechanism of production of adventitious sound:
Adventitious sounds are produced by vibration of respiratory structures and pleura. This may occur in four ways:

1. *Rupture of fluid films or bubbles (Fig. 3.45):* When air flows through central bronchi-coated with thin secretions, air-fluid interface causes rupture of fluid films and bubbles, producing crackles—discontinuous sounds.
   Disease: Acute and chronic bronchitis.
2. *Sudden equalization in inter-airway pressure (Fig. 3.46):* The small airways those are partially collapsed due to interstitial pressure or scarring, suddenly open up due to equalization of intra-airway pressure, producing fine crackles, these are also discontinuous sounds.
   Diseases: Interstitial pressure produces producing partial collapse of distal airways due to:
   - Pus—pneumonia

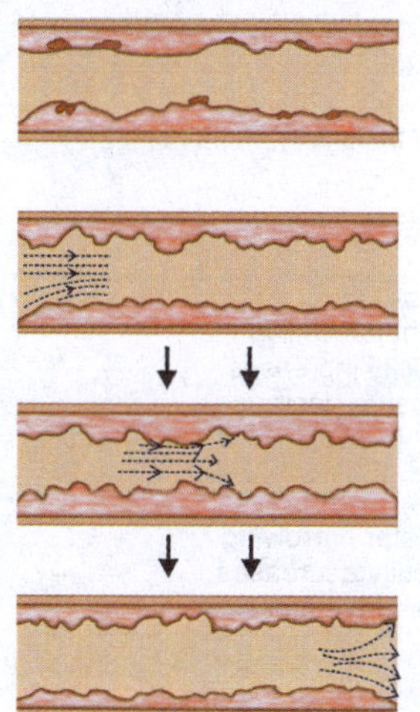

FIG. 3.45   Rupture of fluid films or bubbles

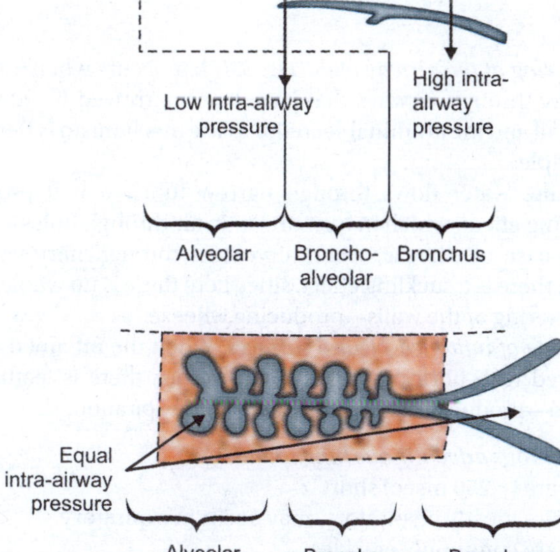

FIG. 3.46   Sudden equalization intra-airways pressure

- ❖ Serum—pulmonary edema
- ❖ Blood—pulmonary hemorrhage
- ❖ Pulmonary fibrosis.

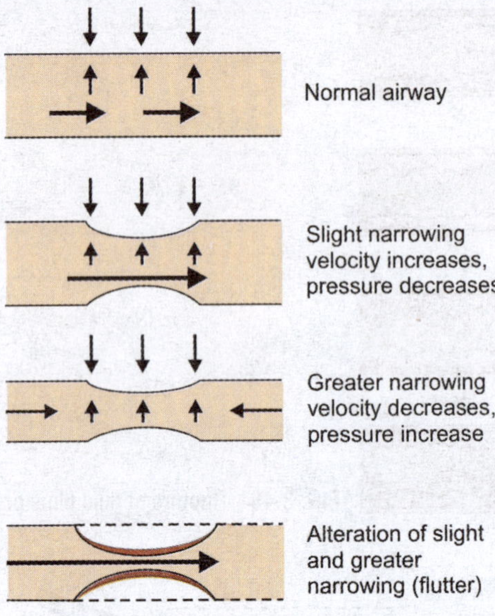

FIG. 3.47 Fluttering of airway wall

3. *Fluttering of the airway wall (Fig. 3.47):* It occurs when air flows rapidly through airways that have been narrowed by edema of the wall and intraluminal secretions. The mechanism is Bernoulli principle:

   If the water flows through narrow tube, then it produces suckling effect, which in turn draws-in air through holes.

   In case of wheeze, when air passes through narrowed airways, there is a suckling effect, since here there is no whole, there is fluttering of the walls—producing wheeze.

4. *Rubbing of inflamed pleural surfaces:* When the inflamed pleura covered with fibrin rub against each other, there is leather like sound—produced during inspiration and expiration.

Discontinuous adventitious lung sounds:
- They are (< 250 msec) short
- They are mostly inspiratory, may occur in expiratory
- They are commonly crackles.

Production of Wheeze

When luminal narrowing occurs, air must flow with greater velocity through the constricted regions to maintain constant flow rate.

According to Bernoulli principle, increased air velocity leads to decrease in air pressure, thus allowing external pressure to further collapse the airway.

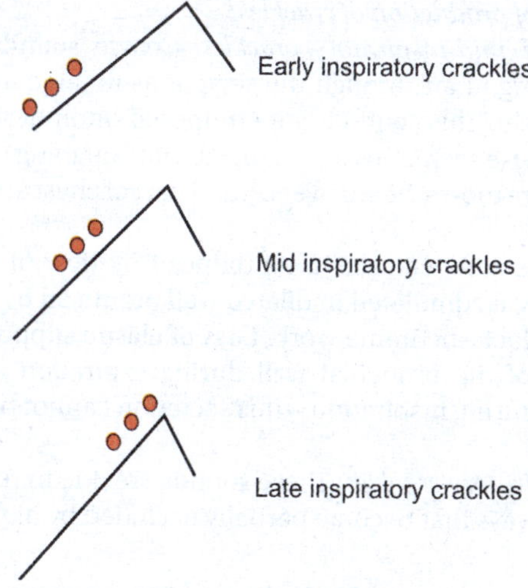

FIG. 3.48 Types of crackles

The process beings to reverse when, the pressure inside the airway begins to increase and reopen the lumen, so the airway well-beings to flatter producing wheeze.

The underlying breath sound during crackles

Production or presence of type of breath sounds during crackles depends upon type of crackles (Fig. 3.48):

- *Early and mid inspiratory crackles* are associated with vesicular breath sound
- *Late inspiratory crackles* are associated with bronchial or vesicular breath sounds.
  - ❖ *Fluid-filled alveoli:* Produces late inspiratory crackles and bronchial breath sound
  - ❖ *Fluid-filled interstitum:* Produces late inspiratory crackles and bronchial breath sound
  - ❖ *Scarring of interstitum:* Produces late inspiratory crackles and vesicular breath sound.

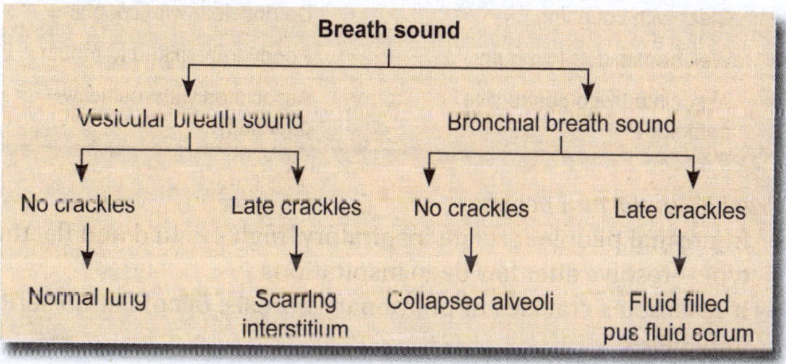

Mechanism of production of crackles:
- *Early and mid-inspiratory crackles:* Coarse sounds produced by bubbling of air through the secretions in large and medium size bronchi. This sound is superimposed on underlying breath sound. These secretions are changed with coughing

  They are mostly heard over central part of chest anteriorly and posteriorly.

  Brochiectatic crackles are produced by flow of air through secretions accumulated in dilated wall produced by destruction of musculoelastic frame work. Loss of elastic support produces collapse of the bronchial wall during expiration and sudden open up during inspiration—this secretion cannot be cleared by coughing.
- *Late inspiratory crackles:* These sounds are due to re-opening of distal airways that become partially occluded by high interstitial pressure.

Since the two ends of semicollapsed bronchi have different air way pressure (high at central, low at distal), inspiratory sudden reopening of the partially collapsed airways produces equalization of intra-airway pressure, thus a 'pop'.

This high interstitial pressure behind them is due to, scarring of interstitium or fluid, pus or blood in interstitial spaces (pulmonary edema, pneumonia, pulmonary hemorrhage).

Regional differences of late inspiratory crackles: In posterior lung bases—due to region of high interstitial pressure, gravity can easily collapse the bronchi—producing late inspiratory crackles.

Characteristics of early, mid and late inspiratory crackles:

Early and mid inspiratory	Late inspiratory
Coarse	Fine
Low pitched	High pitched
Scaly	Profuse
Gravity independent	Gravity dependent
Do not change with posture	Change with posture
Clear with coughing	Do not clear with coughing
Well transmitted to mouth	Poorly transmitted to mouth
Associated with obstructive pathology	Associated with restrictive pathology

Crackles in normal people:
- In normal people it is late inspiratory, high pitched and fleeting type—resolve after few deep inspirations
- It resembles crackles of pulmonary fibrosis, occurs at posterior lung bases

- It indicates reopening of atelectatic lung unit, which occurs in normal healthy adult after a deep inspiration
- It occurs in person, recumbent for prolonged period of time
- It can be detected by electronic stethoscope in 92 percent people. Late inspiratory crackles may occur in early and mid inspiratory period, but the hallmark is it must be present until late inspiration.

Late inspiratory crackles occur in:
- Idiopathic pulmonary fibrosis
- Asbestosis
- Sarcoidosis (5–20%).

These are rarely present in:
Granulomatous diseases
- Tuberculosis
- Allergic alveolitis
- Eosinophilic granuloma.

Areas of late inspiratory crackles:
- *Idiopathic pulmonary fibrosis:* Lower lobe location and sub-pleural searing
- *Sarcoidosis.* Upper lobe location
- *Asbestosis:* At the bases—first centrally, followed by postero-laterally.

Correlation with disease severity:
- *Number of crackles:* Correlates with severity of asbestosis
- *Absence of crackles:* Eliminates diagnosis of interstitial pulmonary fibrosis.

Correlation with idiopathic pulmonary fibrosis:
- *In milder case:* Crackles are late inspiratory and gravity dependent limited to bases in upright patients
- *As the disease progresses:* It becomes pan-inspiratory with predominant late inspiratory—present in spite of change in posture eventually they reach apical region.

Crackles in expiration: Ten percent cases crackles occurs during expiration.
- *In obstructive lung disease (bronchitis and bronchiectasis):* They are coarse, early expiratory, gravity in dependent and profuse, and decrease with coughing
- *In restrictive lung disease—(pulmonary fibrosis), connective tissue disease:* They are:
    - ❖ Fine
    - ❖ Mid and early expiratory
    - ❖ Gravity dependent
    - ❖ Scanty
    - ❖ Cannot decrease with coughing.

Mechanisms of production of late expiratory crackles:
- High interstitial pressure tends to collapse the small airways
- Inspiratory traction would snap the airways open, creating a pop during late inspiration
- In early expiration, there is closing of lumen once again, which reopens again in late expiration.

Importance of late expiratory crackles: Number of expiratory crackles correlates with reduction in diffusion capacity.

Continuous Adventitious Sound

Rhonchi: Musical sound produced by flow of air through narrowed bronchi—due to edema and/or mucus plug.
- Expiratory
- May occur in inspiratory phase, even throughout respiratory cycle, but never in inspiratory phase only
- If high pitched—called wheeze (dominant frequency >400 Hz)
- It is called continuous because according to American Society Guidelines they should last >250 msec.

Monophonic and polyphonic wheeze:
- *Monophonic wheeze:*
  - Contains single or multiple tones starting and ending at different times
  - This can be produced by a tumor almost completely obstructing bronchi.
- *Polyphonic wheeze:*
  - Contains several notes starting and ending at different times.
  - It occurs in healthy people at the end of full expiration, which must be forceful
  - In asthma—narrowing of multiple airways produce typical polyphonic wheeze
  - In polyphonic wheeze its pitch can be determined by its lowest (fundamental) frequency.

Mechanism of production wheeze: When air flows through narrowed bronchi, there is sucking effect on the bronchial wall by pulling it inward, thus initiates flutter by closing and opening— this fluttering of bronchial wall produces wheeze. This fluttering depends upon:
- The mass
- Elasticity of the bronchial wall
- Tightness of narrowing
- Rate of gas flow through it.

Physical principle behind wheeze productions:
The Bernoulli principle: It suggests—local drop in intra-airway pressure when airflow at high velocity through it.

As the velocity of airflow will be increased, intra-airway pressure decreases, eventually drop in pressure will be severe enough to collapse the airway.

Again collapsed airway reduces the airflow; airway reopens, fluttering cycles starts—repeating it again and again.

So wheeze is not produced by vibration of air, but by vibration of bronchial walls.

Continuous adventitious lung sounds (CALS) are divided into 4 categories:

1. *Expiratory polyphonic CALS:*
   - Multiple musical tones
   - Heard during expiration
   - It has constant frequency
   - Same duration
   - Summation of frequency of all tones produce polyphonic sound
   - It occurs in:
     - Bronchial asthma
     - People at the end of forceful expiration.
2. *Random monophonic CALS:*
   - Single or multiple musical tones
   - Heard throughout respiration
   - It has variable frequency
   - Variable duration
   - High-pitched hissing quality—often referred as multiple monophonic wheezes
   - It occurs in status asthmaticus—heard throughout chest
   - It occurs in expiration or throughout the cycle.
3. *Fixed monophonic CALS:*
   - Single musical tone
   - Constant frequency
   - Long duration
   - Produced by vibration of partially obstructed bronchus by tumor, inflammation, secretions, and foreign body
   - Change in posture eliminate or soften the sound
   - It may be the earliest findings in endobronchial lesion.
4. *Sequential inspiratory CALS:*
   - It is late inspiratory squeaks associated with late inspiratory crackles
   - It is associated with common interstitial lung diseases, e.g.:
     - Pulmonary fibrosis
     - Allergic alveolitis
     - Bronchiolitis obliterans.
   - It in high pitched.

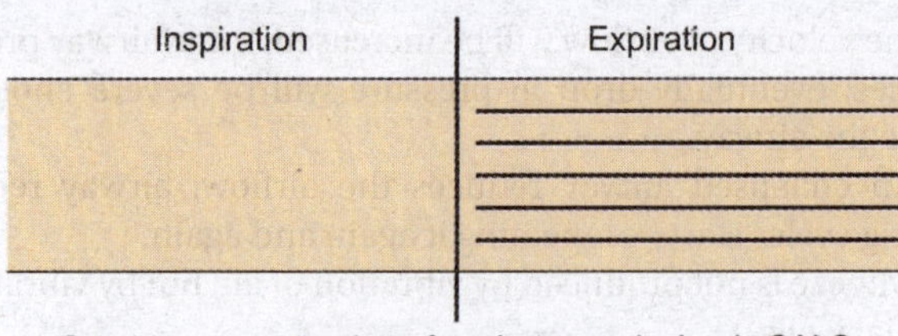

Graphic representation of expiratory polyphonic CALS

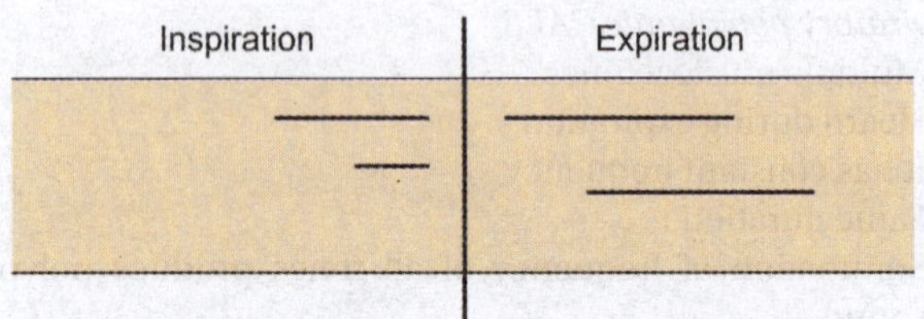

Graphic representation of random monophonic CALS

FIG. 3.49 Graphic representation of CALS

Graphical representation of CALS: It can be represented by bars:
- Pitch can be represented by height of the bar (Vertical localization of the bar above the respiratory cycle)
- Loudness can be represented by thickness of the bar
- Duration can be represented by length of the bar
- Timings can be represented by position in respiratory cycle (Fig. 3.49).

Presence of wheezing rule in or not bronchial narrowing:
- *In normal people* forced expiratory maneuver produces wheezing. So forced expiration has no value in unmasking subclinical asthma. So it has very low specificity and low sensitivity in bronchial asthma
- Weak expiratory flow remains totally silent while passing through quite narrowed bronchi.

Thus presence of wheezing does not rule in bronchial narrowing and its absence does not exclude it.

Underlying breath sound in asthmatic patient
Since breath sound depends upon degree of narrowing of bronchi, so following types of breath sounds can be heard:
- Increase in frequency of underlying breath sounds—it is the earliest manifestations of bronchospasm even before the appearance of wheeze
- As the airway becomes narrower, breath sound become soften
- Opposite effect occurs during bronchodilator therapy

- Softening of breath sounds may be the earliest manifestation of bronchoprovocation.

Relationship of wheeze with severity of obstruction:
- Longer the duration of wheeze, severe the obstruction
- Higher the pitch of wheeze, severe the obstruction
- T_w/T_{tot} (proportion of respiratory cycle occupied by wheeze) is inversely proportional to FEV1 in severe obstruction.

The course of status asthmaticus based on auscultation:
- *In mild asthma:*
  - ❖ Site of obstruction in the central airways
  - ❖ Bronchial wall fluttering produces random monomorphic wheezes transmitted upwards (to the mouth) and downward (to the chest wall).
- *In worse asthma:*
  - ❖ Site of obstruction is peripheral airways
  - ❖ Airflow in small airways is too slow to cause major fluttering
  - ❖ Sound generated in monomorphic wheezes—low pitches—barely audible on the chest and barely transmitted to mouth.
- *In status asthmatics:*
  - ❖ *Airflow obstruction is due to:*
    - Bronchial wall edema
    - Mucus plug
    - Bronchial smooth muscle spasm.
  - ❖ Airflow obstruction starts in central airways
  - ❖ It is first expiratory
  - ❖ Wheeze in monomorphic CALS.

Subsequently:
- Airway fluttering moves to peripheral airways
- Airflow is so slow, that it fails to generate vibrations.
  So the chest becomes silent paradoxically.

Relationship with pulsus paradoxus
Pulsus paradoxus has a direct relation with hypercapnia in children with status asthmaticus, so acts as indirect monitor of hypercapnia.

Clinical conditions associated with wheezes:
- Laryngomalacia, tracheomalacia or bronchomalacia
- Infections (croup, whooping cough, laryngitis, tracheobron-chitis)
- Laryngeal and tracheal tumor
- Tracheal stenosis
- Vocal cord dysfunction
- Asthma
- COPD
- Bronchiolitis obliterans

- Interstitial fibrosis
- Hypersensitive pneumonitis
- Pulmonary edema.

Stridor:
- High pitched
- Inspiratory
- It indicates upper airway obstruction
- Louder over the neck.

In case of tracheal stenosis: Tracheal narrowing <5 mm—producing stridor.

Pleural Rub

- It is caused by friction of both inflamed pleural surface (both visceral and parietal) against each other
- It is grating in character
- It is heard during both in inspiratory and expiratory phases:
    - In inspiration, it is faster and louder
    - In expiration, it is longer.
- Sometimes, it may be in inspiratory phase
- It is not changed with coughing or change of posture
- It can be increased with pressure with diaphragm of stethoscope
- It is localized to small area only
- It is sometimes palpable.

Differences between Crackles and Pleural Rub

Crackles	Pleural rub
• It is cracking in character	• It is grating in character
• It is usually inspiratory	• It is heard in both phases
• It can be changed with coughing and posture	• It cannot be charged with coughing or change of posture
• No relation with pressure with stethoscope	• It is increased with pressure of diaphragm of stethoscope
• It cannot be palpable	• It can be palpable

Differences between Wheeze and Pleural Rub

Wheeze	Pleural rub
• It is musical sound	• It is grating in character
• It is heard in expiration	• It can be heard in both phases or in inspiratory phase only
• It is a continuous sound	• It is interrupted sound

Differences between pericardial and pleural rub:
By holding the breath if rub persist, it is pericardial.
   If rub disappears, it is pleural.

Natural history of pleural rub:
- Normally, pleura are lined by single layer of mesothelial cells. This layer is lubricated by thin film of fluid, so that during normal respiration the pleural surfaces glide on each other silently
- During pleural inflammation, pleural surface are lined by fibrin and inflammatory/neoplastic cells, as a result the roughened pleural surfaces rub against each other during respiration producing grating sound—pleural rub
- As the fluid accumulates in the pleural space, pleural surfaces are separated, pleural rub disappear
    So pleural rub in pathgnomonic of pleural inflammation.
- Noninflammatory effusions such as nephritic syndrome, CCF, cirrhosis are not associated with pleural rub.

Most common causes of pleural rub:
- *Inflammation:*
    ❖ Infective—pneumococcal, staphylococcal, gram –ve bacteria
    ❖ Noninfective—collagen vascular disease.
- *Neoplastic conditions:*
    ❖ By direct invasion
    ❖ By producing inflammation.
- Pulmonary embolism
- Parapneumonic pleuritis.

Transmitted Voice Sounds

This sounds are produced in larynx, they are abnormally transmitted to chest in certain diseases—providing a valuable clue.

Type of transmitted voice sounds are:
- *Bronchophony:* This is heard over the chest areas remote from either bronchi or larynx—but as clear heard as over central bronchi or larynx
- *Pectoriloquy:* The sound heard is clear and intelligible words over the chest in the form of either:
    ❖ Whispering (whispering pectoriloquy)
    ❖ Speaking (spoken pectoriloquy).
- *Egophony:* Goat-like bleating sound produced by patient's voice, heard over the areas of consolidation
- *E to A change:* A variant of egophony.

Significance of this maneuver: It suspects abnormal sound transmission along the tracheobronchial tree across the lungs when suspecting consolidation.

Mechanism of voice sound produced and transmission:
Normally voice sounds are produced by vibration of vocal cords. They then transmitted upwards towards mouth and downwards towards chest wall. The alveolar air acts as low-pass filter, eliminating high frequency sounds (>3000 Hz) and most of low frequency sounds (100–300 Hz) reach the chest wall. This filter also eliminates high frequency components of vowels so called formants.

Because recognition of vowels is essential for comprehension of words, elimination of formants by the normal lung, hence voice sounds heard on the chest wall is low pitched, unintelligible, mumbles.

But in case of consolidation—solid lung (fluid or solid) can transmit higher frequencies, so transmitted vowels become louder, clear and intelligible.

Mechanism of E to A change:
Consolidation extending from chest wall to tracheobronchial tree produce E to A change.

Less extensive consolidation of a pulmonary nodule would not create a bridge enough to cause egophony.

The most common causes of consolidation:
- Filling of alveoli with:
  - ❖ Pus
  - ❖ Fluid
  - ❖ Blood.
- *Pleural effusion:* Fluid must be thick enough to collapse of alveoli and but not enough to compress the bronchi.

The exception is—patient with collapsed bronchi or obstructed bronchi still manages to transmit high frequency sound through lung parenchyma directly.

Transformation of E to A in vocal resonance in consolidated lung:
- E is a mixture of high and low frequencies—high frequencies are 2000 to 3500 Hz and low frequencies are 100 to 400 Hz range

  A is a mixture of high and low frequencies—low frequencies are higher than the low frequencies of E (600 Hz).
- When E and A are heard over the chest, none of their high frequencies will come across, regardless the lung consolidation, the consolidated lung can transmit higher frequency sound better than normal lung (close to 1000 Hz instead of 400 Hz). It cannot transmit the highest frequencies such as, 2000 to 3500 Hz, typical of E.

  So, consolidated lung can transmit low frequency sound, i.e. 600 Hz of A better, but cannot transmit high frequency sound (2000–3500 Hz) characteristic of E.

  Hence, E becomes A as do other vowels.

Mechanisms of production of whispering pectoriloquy
Whispering consists of high frequency sounds—so they are not transmitted in the aerated lung, but becomes audible when alveolar air is lost (due to consolidation).

Disease	Trachea	Fremitus	Percussion note	Breath sound	Adventitious sound	Vocal resonance
• Normal	Midline	Normal	Resonant	Vesicular	Late-inspiratory crackles at bases (resolved with deep breath)	Absence
• Consolidation (pneumonia hemorrhage)	Midline	Increased	Woody dul	Bronchial (tubular)	Late inspiratory crackles	Increased
• Pulmonary fibrosis	Midline	Increased	Dull	Bronchovesicular	Late inspiratory crackles	Absent
• Bronchiectasis	Midline	Normal	Resonant	Vesicular	Mid inspiratory crackles	Absent
• Bronchitis	Midline	Normal	Resonant	Vesicular	Early inspiratory crackles	Absent
• Large pleural effusion	Shifted to opposite side	Decreased or Absent	Stony dull	Absent over effusion bronchial above effusion	Rub above effusion	Egophony above effusion absent above effusion

Contd...

Contd...

Disease	Trachea	Fremitus	Percussion note	Breath sound	Adventitious sound	Vocal resonance
• Pneumothorax	Shifted to opposite side	Absent	Tympanic	Absent	Absent	Absent
• Alelectasis (patent bronchi)	Shifted to same side	Increased	Woody dull	Bronchial	Absent	All present
• Atelectasis (plugged bronchi)	Shifted to same side	Absent	Woody dull	Absent	Absent	Absent
• Emphysema	Normal midline	Decreased	Hyper-resonant	Vesicular breath sound with prolonged expiration	Usually absent	Absent
• Status asthmaticus	Midline	Decreased	Hyper-resonant	Vesicular	Inspiratory/expiratory wheeze	Absent

Cardiovascular System

Gross Anatomy

Heart

- *Situation:*
  - ❖ In middle mediastinum in between 3rd, 4th and 5th ribs and sternum anteriorly, vertebrae posteriorly and diaphragm inferiorly
  - ❖ Apex in left 5th intercostals space, a little inside left mid clavicular line and touches the anterior wall.
- *Shape:* Resembles a truncated cone, one and half times of the closed fist of a man
- *Size:* 12 cm × 9 cm
- *Weight:*
  - ❖ *In male:* 320 ± 75 g
  - ❖ *In female:* 275 ± 70 g.

There are four chambers of the heart:

1. Right atrium
2. Right ventricle
3. Left atrium
4. Left ventricle.

Apex of the Heart [External Features of the Heart (Fig. 4.1)]

- Directed anteriorly and to the left formed by inferolateral surface of the left ventricle
- Located posterior to the left 5th intercostals space in adult, 9 cm from the median plane
- It is the place where a sound of mitral valve closure is maximally heard.

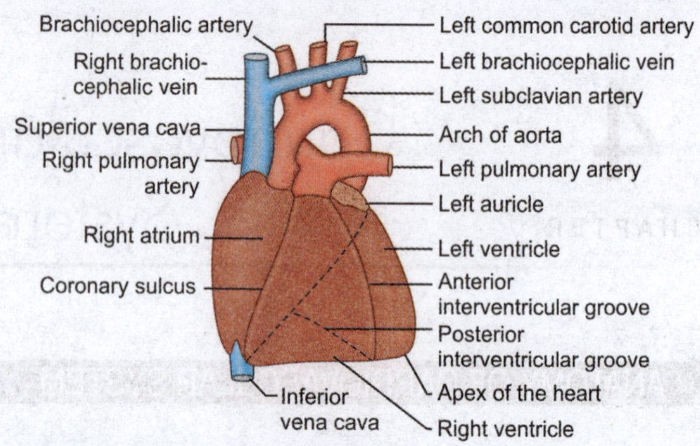

FIG. 4.1 External features of the heart (anterior view)

Base of the Heart [External Features of the Heart (Fig. 4.2)]

- It is the posterior aspect of the heart
- It is formed mainly by left atrium and lesser contribution of right atrium
- It is separated from the bodies of vertebrae by:
  - ❖ Pericardium
  - ❖ Oblique pericardial sinus
  - ❖ Esophagus
  - ❖ Aorta.
- Extends superiorly up to bifurcation of pulmonary trunk and inferiorly up to coronary groove
- It receives pulmonary veins on the right and left side of left atrium
- It receives superior and inferior vena cavae on superior and inferior ends of right atrium.

Four surfaces:
1. *Anterior surface:* Mainly by right ventricle.
2. *Diaphragmatic (inferior) surface:* Mainly by left ventricle and part of the right ventricle.
3. *Left pulmonary surface:* Mainly by left ventricle.
4. *Right pulmonary surface:* Mainly by right atrium.

Borders:
- Right vertical border is formed by right atrium extending from superior vena cava to inferior vena cava
- Left oblique border is formed by left auricle and left ventricle
- Inferior horizontal border is formed by right ventricle and small portion of left ventricle

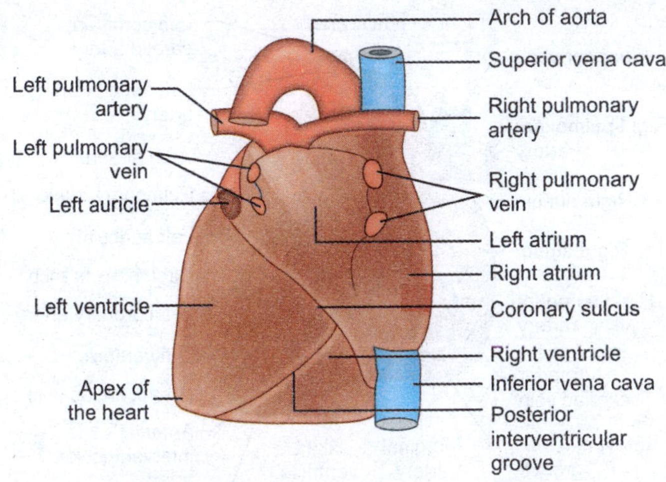

FIG. 4.2 External features of the heart (posterior view)

- Superior border is formed by:
  - ❖ Right and left atria and auricles on anterior view
  - ❖ Ascending aorta, pulmonary trunk emerge from superior border
  - ❖ Superior vena cava enters right atrium on right side
  - ❖ Posterior to the aorta and pulmonary trunk and anterior to superior vena cava, this border forms the inferior border of transverse pericardial sinus.

External Features of the Heart

External View [External Features of the Heart (Figs 4.3 and 4.4)]

View from the front

- Front surface of the heart is mostly right ventricle. Having a chink of right atrium on its right and left ventricle on its left
- Right atrium is separated from right ventricle by right atrioventricular sulcus, also called coronary sulcus, containing right coronary artery and a great vein of the heart that drains into right atrium by coronary sinus
- Right ventricle is separated from left ventricle by interventricular sulcus containing left anterior descending artery.

View from below—base of heart (Fig. 4.5)

- Inferior surface, mostly diaphragmatic surface, is formed by:
  - ❖ Largely left ventricle (2/3rd)
  - ❖ To a small extent right ventricle (1/3rd)

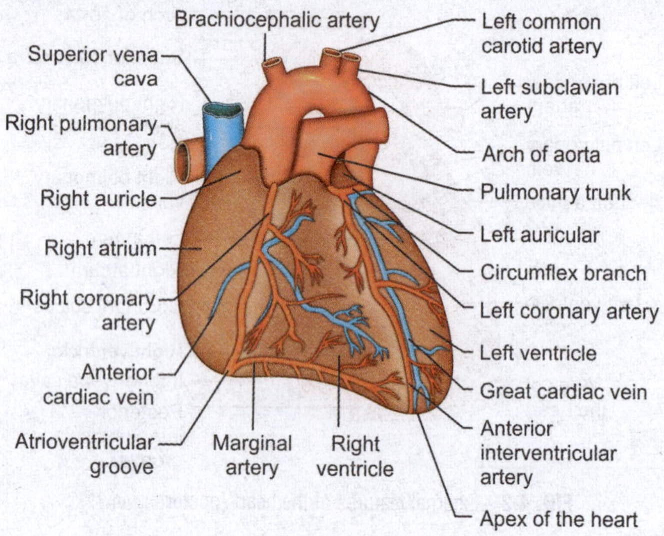

FIG. 4.3 Anterior surface of the heart and great vessels

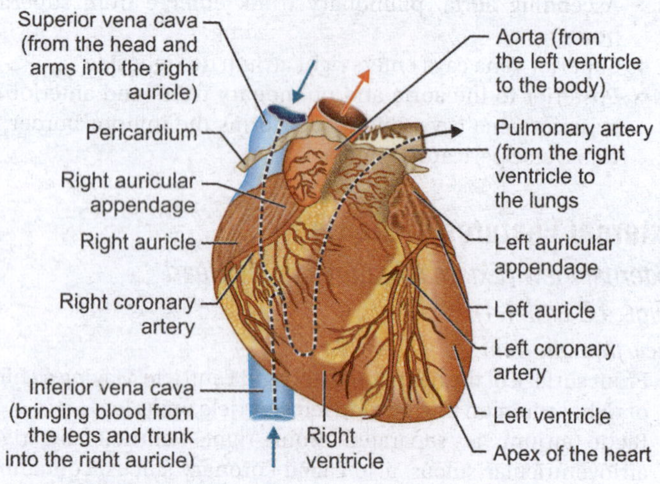

FIG. 4.4 External features of the heart (view from front)

- Sometimes it is called posterior wall
- Coronary sulcus meets posterior interventricular sulcus.

View from behind—external feature of heart (Fig. 4.6)
- Left ventricle is separated from right ventricle by posterior interventricular groove—containing posterior interventricular branch of right coronary artery running towards apex

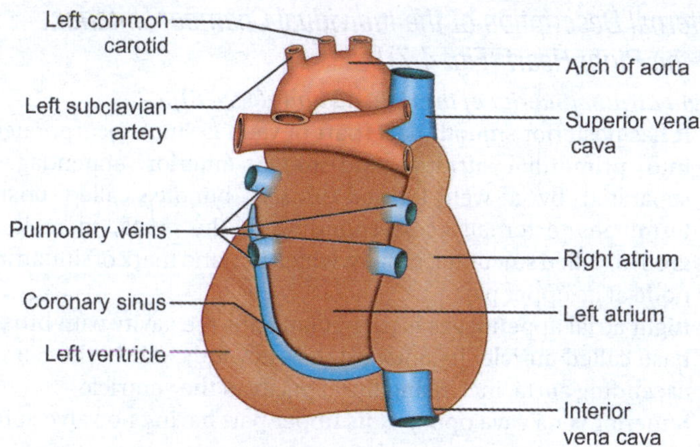

FIG. 4.5   Base or posterior surface of heart

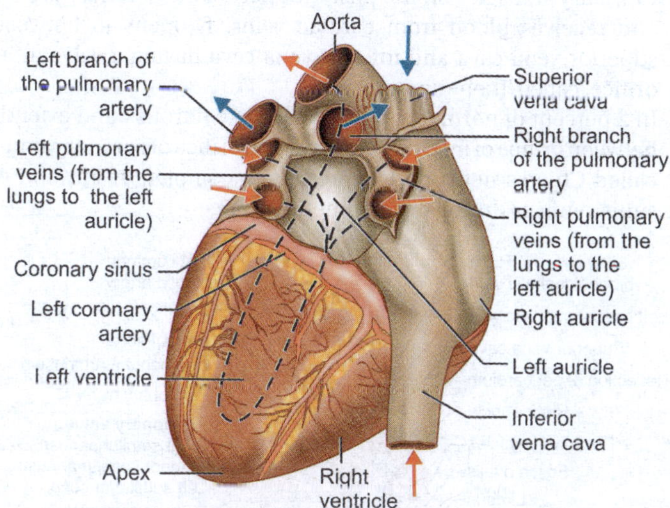

FIG. 4.6   External features of heart (view from behind)

- Side of the heart facing spinal column—composed of left ventricle
- Left atrium is separated from left ventricle by posterior atrioventricular sulcus containing left circumflex branch of left coronary artery.

Internal Description of the Individual Chamber [Interior of the Right Heart (Fig. 4.7)]

Right atrium [interior of the right atrium (Fig. 4.8)]

- It has posterior smooth part (part of venous sinus incorporated into primordial atrium) and rough anterior appendages, separated by a well formed muscle bundle, called crista terminalis, externally corresponding to the crista, there is a groove, called sulcus terminalis, which is a land mark of sinuatrial node at its upper part
- Right atrial appendages is triangular, joins the cavity with broad base called auricle. Its apex extends upwards and to the left of ascending aorta, increasing the capacity of the ventricle
- Superior vena cava opens at its upper part having no valve at its orifice
- Inferior vena cava opens at its lower end having a rudimentary valve at its orifice (Eustachian valve)
- Coronary sinus lies on the posterior part of the coronary groove and receives blood from cardiac veins. It opens in between superior vena cava and inferior vena cava having a valve at its orifice, called Thebesian valve
- In 2 percent of normal people—a lace like fibrous band extends between orifice of inferior vena cava and orifice of coronary sinus, called Chiari's network. It represents incomplete resorption of sinus venosus during development.

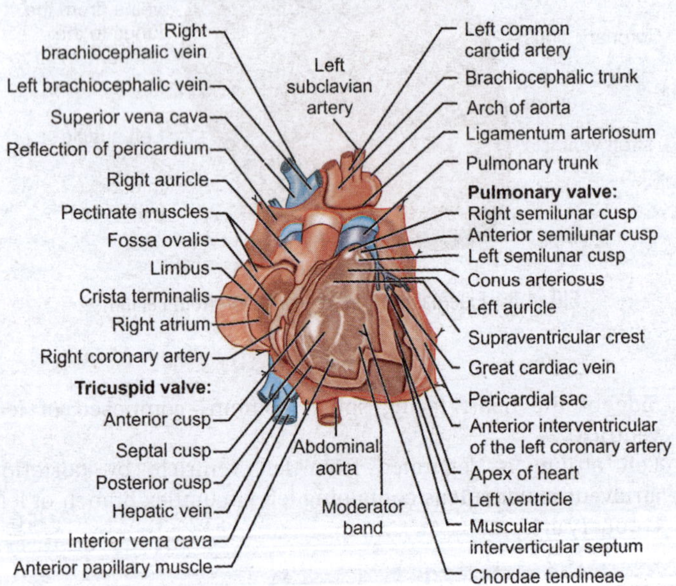

FIG. 4.7 Interior of the right heart

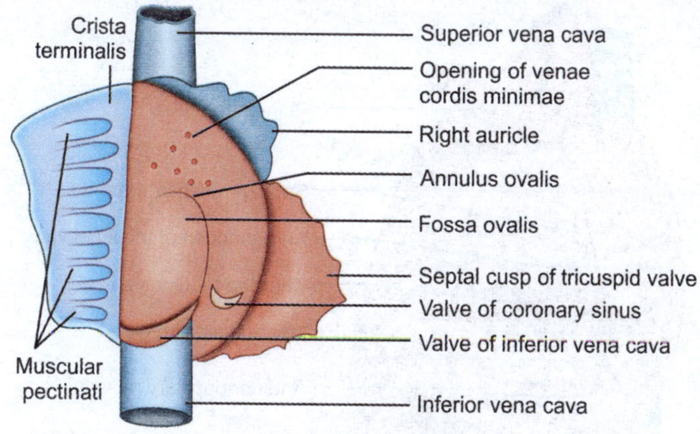

FIG. 4.8   Interior of right atrium

- On the right atrial septal surface, at the site of foramen ovale, there is depression, called fossa ovalis, which is a communication between right and left atria during fetal life. It has a prominent rim, called limbus
- In the floor of the fossa there is flap valve, which is sufficiently large to close the fossa ovalis
- In 25 percent of people, flap valve may not join limbus superiorly. In that condition, a probe can pass through it to left atrium. This is called patent foramen ovale
- *Triangle of Koch:* It is bounded anteriorly by base of septal cusp of tricuspid valve, behind by coronary sinus and above by tendon of todaro—a fibrous ridge extending from a fibrous body to the left horn of inferior vena cava. AV node lies in this triangle
- *Torus aorticus:* Bulge on the anterosuperior part of septum formed by:
  - ❖ Bulging of a posterior aortic cusp
  - ❖ Bulging of right coronary cusp of the aortic root.

Right Ventricle [Interior of the Right Ventricle (Fig. 4.9)]

Inlet component
- Tricuspid valve—located posterior to the body sternum at the level of 4th and 5th intercostals space
- Septomarginal trabeculation, a coarse muscle ridge on its septal surface, extending from ventricular septum to the base of anterior papillary muscle
- Another trabeculation extends from septomarginal trabeculation to the anterior papillary muscle, then to parietal wall. It is called moderator band. It contains right branch of AV bundle. It prevents over distension of ventricle

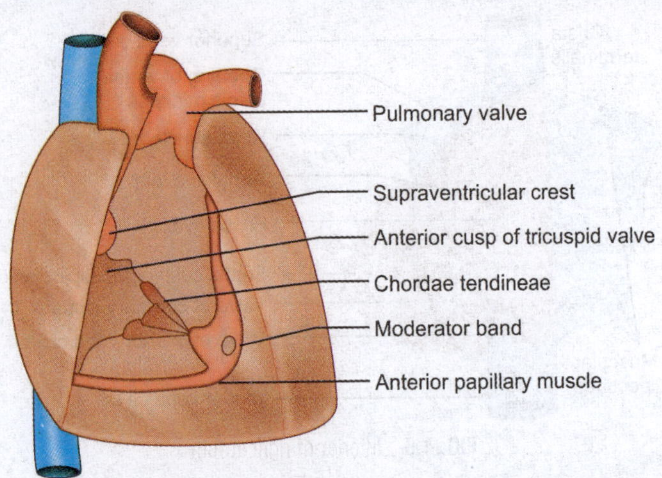

FIG. 4.9 Interior of right ventricle

- Inlet and outlet component is separated by a muscle ridge called supraventricular crest.

Outlet component
- It forms superior portion of right ventricle. Shape is conical
- Apex of infundibulum has pulmonary orifice having three semilunar cusp
- Free edge of each cusp has thickening at its center called Nodule Arantii.

Apical trabecular part—it is much coarser than that of left ventricle.

Left Atrium [Interior of the Left Side of the Heart (Fig. 4.10)]

- Quadrangular chamber—posterior most part of the heart
- Its wall is thicker than wall of the right atrium
- It is smooth walled and receives two openings of pulmonary veins on either side having no valve at their orifice. But atrial muscle extends towards pulmonary orifice for 1 to 2 cm and acts as a sphincter, which lessens the reflux during atrial contraction
- Left atrial appendage is much smaller than that of right atrium, it is not marked by any crista internally or sulcus externally
- Inter atrial septum slopes posteriorly and to the left
- Septal wall has left atrial part of fossa ovalis known as fossa lumanta. It has no rim or limbus
- Its appendage projects anteriorly and overlaps infundibulum of left ventricle.

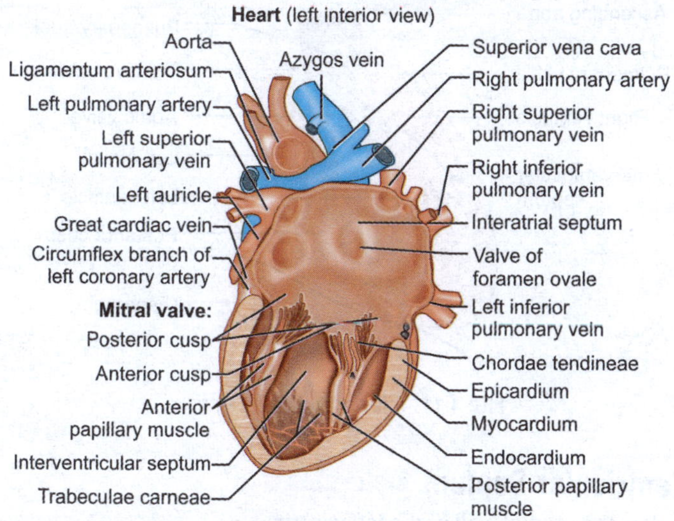

FIG. 4.10   Interior of the left side of the heart

Left Ventricle [Interior of the Left Ventricle (Fig. 4.11)]

- Its apex projects anteriorly, inferiorly and to the left
- Its wall is 8 to 15 mm thick; but apex is often thin (1–2 mm).

Inflow component

- Anteromedial leaflet of mitral valve extends from posteromedial wall of the septum to the anteromedial wall of the left ventricle. It separates the left ventricular cavity into inflow tract and outflow tract
- Mitral orifice is elliptical, guards the left atrioventricular orifice
- Inflow tract is funnel shaped; contains mitral apparatus, which direct the flow of blood anteriorly, inferiorly and to the left.

Outflow component

- It is conical shaped, smooth walled, nonmuscular supero-anterior outflow part of aortic vestibule leading to aortic orifice and aortic valve
- It is bounded by:
  - ❖ Inferior surface of anteromedial mitral cusp
  - ❖ Left ventricular free wall
  - ❖ Ventricular septum.
- Aortic orifice is surrounded by a fibrous ring to which right, left and posterior cusps are attached
- It directs the blood flow anteriorly and superiorly making an angle of 90° with the inflow tract towards ascending aorta
- Aortic orifice is guarded by three semilunar cusp.

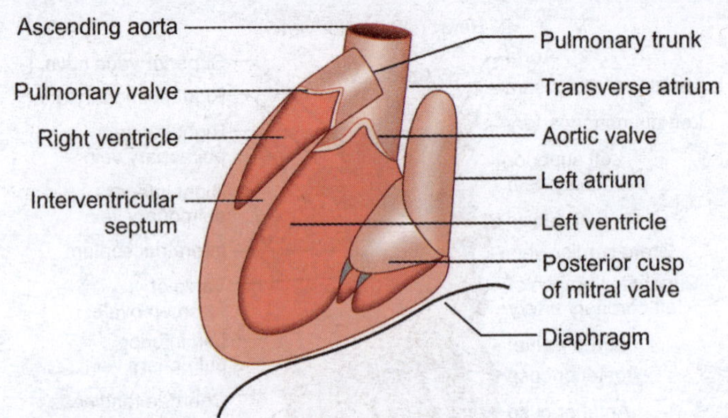

FIG. 4.11 Interior of the left ventricle

Ventricular Septum

- It is the medial wall of the left ventricle
- It is mostly muscular, the membranous part is present superiorly between coronary and noncoronary cusp and in contact with mitral and tricuspid annuli
- Membranous part forms the fibrous skeleton and supports the atrioventricular musculature
- Tricuspid valve is more apically placed than the mitral valve
- Septal cusp of tricuspid valve divides the ventricular septum into atrioventricular and interventricular component
- Septal cusp of tricuspid valve separates the inflow part of right ventricle from outflow part of left ventricle
- Posterior wall of the infundibulum beneath the pulmonary valve is not a part of septum. It separates infundibulum from the outside of the heart
- With increasing age, septum becomes sigmoid and inter-ventricular component of the membranous part increases.

Apical Part of Ventricle

Extensive fine trabeculation more than the right ventricle is present here.

Left Ventricular Free Wall

Valves [Valves of the Heart (Figs 4.12 and 4.13)]

Mitral valve (Fig. 4.14)

- It is present posterior to sternum at the level of 4th costal cartilage
- Annulus size is 4 to 6 square cm

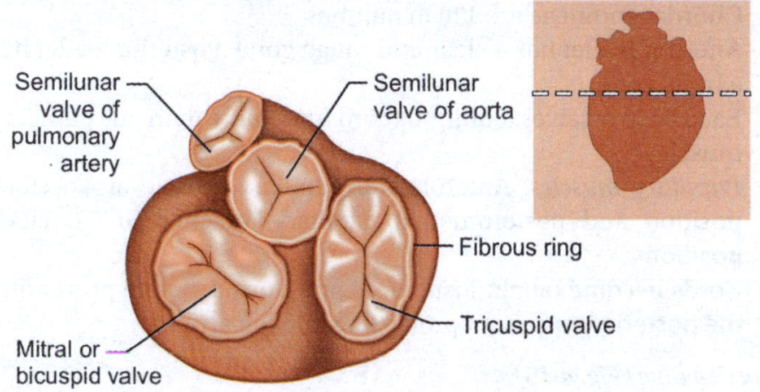

FIG. 4.12 Valves of the heart

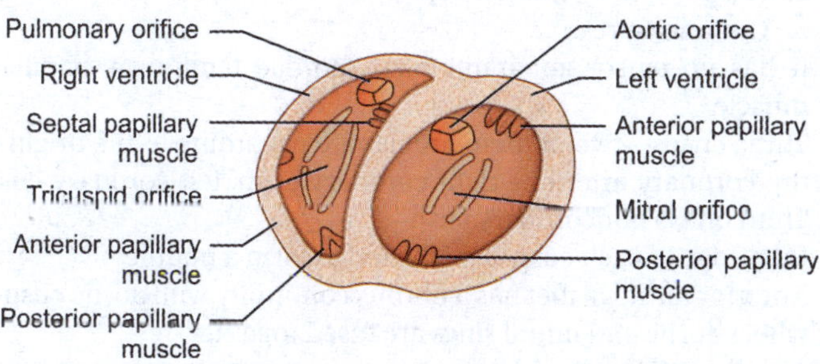

FIG. 4.13 Trans-section through ventricles showings valves of the heart

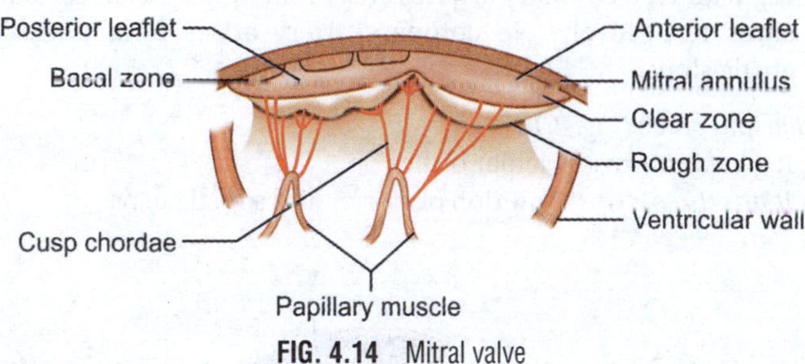

FIG. 4.14 Mitral valve

- *Two leaflets:* Anterior or aortic leaflet and posterior or mural leaflet
- They are separated by anterior and posterior commeasures
- Posterior leaflet is C shaped, scalloped, attached with 2/3rd of annular circumference
- Anterior leaflet triangular, sail shaped, it has a fibrous continuity with aortic valve leaflet

- Chorda tendineae are 120 in number
- Anterior leaflet has a clear and rough zone. Posterior leaflet has a basal zone
- Each cusp receives tendinous cord from more than one papillary muscle
- *Papillary muscles:* Anterolateral papillary muscle at 4'o clock position and posteromedial papillary attached at 7'o clock positions
- Cords become taught just before and during systole preventing the posterior cusp from prolapsing into left atrium.

Aortic valve (Fig. 4.15)
- It has three components:
  1. Annulus
  2. Cusps
  3. Commeasures.
- It has no tensor apparatus like, chordae tendineae, papillary muscle
- Three cusps—two of them are named according to the origin of the coronary arteries—right coronary cusp, left coronary cusp. Third one is noncoronary cusp
- Free edge of each cusp is thickened to form a nodule
- Anterior mitral leaflet has a fibrous continuity with aortic cusp—where aortic and mitral rings are fused together
- Annulus—2.5 square cm
- Aortic sinus is the dilated space in between dilated aortic wall and each cusp of the valve
- Right and left coronary arteries arise from right and left coronary sinus respectively. No coronary artery arises from posterior aortic sinus.

Tricuspid valve (Fig. 4.16)
- It guards atrioventricular orifice
- *It has three cusps:* Anterior, posterior and septal cusps

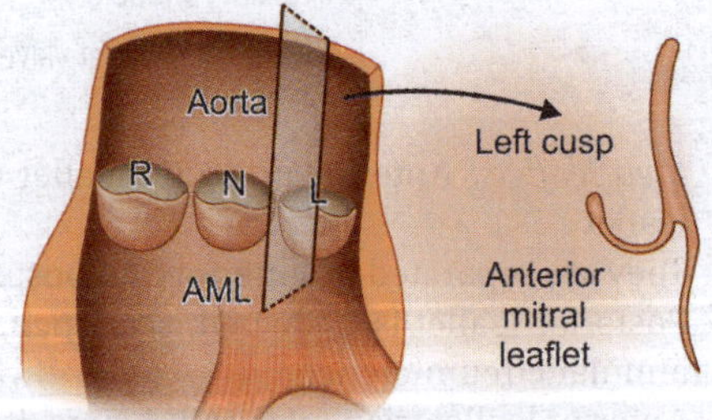

FIG. 4.15 Structure of aortic valve

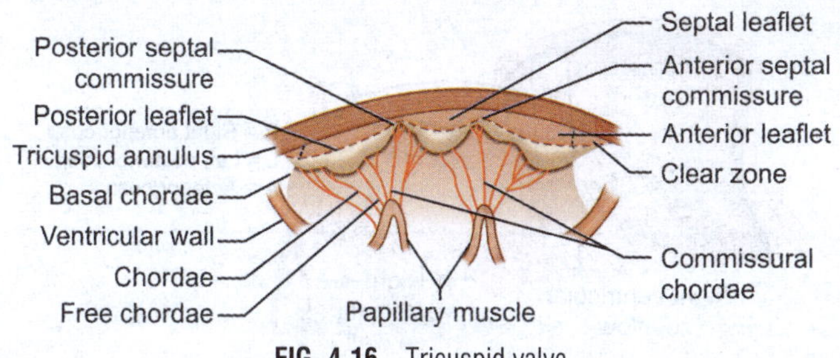

FIG. 4.16 Tricuspid valve

- Their bases are attached to the AV ring. Chordae tendineae are attached to free edges of ventricular surfaces of the cusps like parachute
- Since chordae are attached to the adjacent sides of the cusps—they prevent:
  - ❖ Separation of cusps
  - ❖ Inversion of the cusps
  - ❖ Prolapse of the cusps into right atrium
  - ❖ Backflow of blood from right ventricle into right atrium during forceful ventricular contraction.
- Papillary muscles are triangular in shape with their apices attached to the more than one cusp through the attachment with the chordae
- Papillary muscles contract before the start of right ventricular contraction.

Pulmonary valve (Fig. 4.17)
- It is present at the apex of conus arteriosus at the level of 3rd intercostal space
- It has three cusps—anterior, right, and left cusp, concave superiorly
- Pulmonary sinus is the space between dilated wall of the trunk and the cusp of the pulmonary valve. Blood present in the pulmonary sinus prevent the cusps from sticking the wall of the pulmonary trunk.

Arterial Supply of the Heart

Heart is supplied by the coronary arteries lie deep to the epicardium embedded in fat. They are two in number.

Right Coronary Artery (Arterial Supply of the Heart— Fig. 4.18)

- *Origin:* From right coronary sinus at the posterior part of ascending aorta

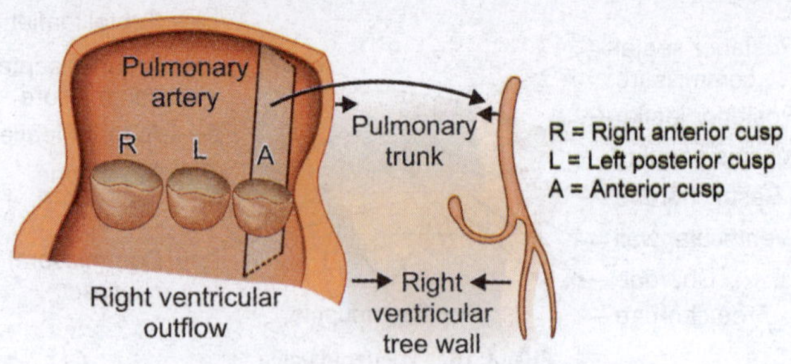

FIG. 4.17   Structure of pulmonary valve

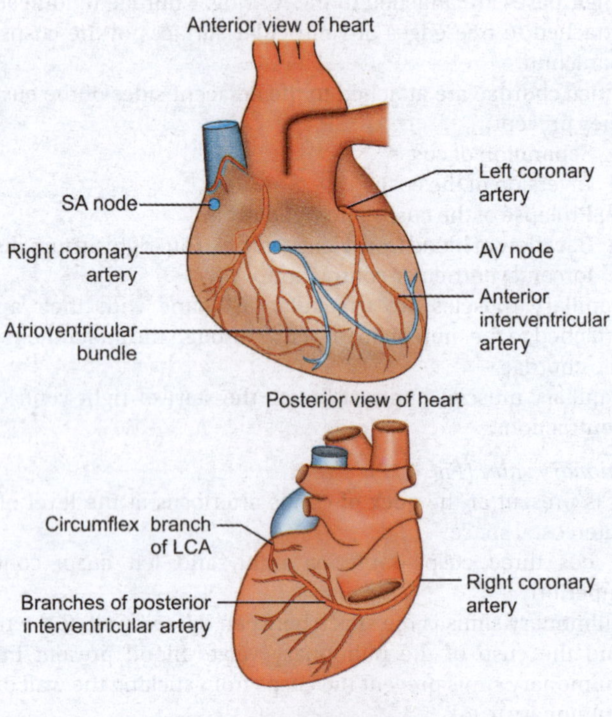

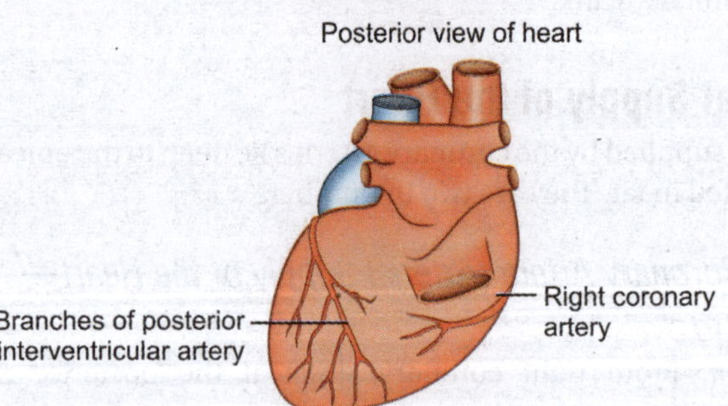

FIG. 4.18   Arterial supply of the heart

- *Courses:* It runs along the anterior coronary sulcus—descends anteriorly and to the left along the sulcus, it winds round the posterior border of the heart and turns on the posterior aspect of the heart, runs upwards till it reaches the crus of the heart—junction of the septa and walls of the members of the heart and terminates by anastomosing with branches of the left coronary artery
- *Branches:*
  - ❖ *Conus artery:* First branch of right coronary artery, supplying the infundibulum of the right ventricle. In 50 percent of cases, it may originate from separate ostium in right coronary sinus (third coronary artery)
  - ❖ *Sinoatrial nodal branch:* Second branch of the right coronary artery, runs along the anterior surface of right atrium to superior vena cava to penetrate SA node. In 50 percent of cases it may originate from left coronary artery
  - ❖ *Right marginal branch:* Supplies most of the right ventricle
  - ❖ Apical branches
  - ❖ *AV nodal branch:* Supplies AV node
  - ❖ *Posterior interventricular branch:* It descends along the posterior interventricular groove towards the apex of heart and supplies to both ventricles (diaphragmatic part of left ventricle)
  - ❖ Posterior descending arterial (PDA) branch supplies posteroinferior 1/3rd of the ventricular septum
  - ❖ Posterolateral left ventricular (PLV) branches supply posterolateral portion of the left ventricle.

Left Coronary Artery

- *Origin:* It arises from left anterior coronary sinus
- *Courses:* It passes in between left pulmonary trunk and left auricle and divides into two branches:
  1. Left circumflex artery
  2. Left anterior descending artery.

Left circumflex artery

- Small branch, after its origin it follows the coronary sulcus on the left border of the heart to the posterior surface of the heart
- It terminates in the posterior coronary sulcus before reaching the crus and anastomosing with branches of right coronary artery.

Branches

- *In right coronary artery dominant circulation:*
  - ❖ Left atrium (1–2 branches)
  - ❖ Lateral free wall of left ventricle (1–2 obtuse marginal branches).

- *In left coronary artery dominant circulation:*
  - ❖ In 40 percent of cases—SA node
  - ❖ Left arterial branches
  - ❖ Obtuse marginal branches
  - ❖ Posterior left ventricular branches
  - ❖ Posterior descending artery.

Left anterior descending artery
Origin and courses
- This artery runs along the anterior interventricular groove towards the apex
- It winds round the inferior border of heart and anastomose with posterior interventricular branch of right coronary artery.

Branches
- 2 to 6 diagonal branches—supplies anterolateral wall of left ventricle
- 3 to 5 septal branches—supply the interventricular septum.

Angiographic Divisions of Coronary Arteries

Left anterior descending (LAD) artery
- Proximal LAD—between origin and 1st diagonal branch
- Mid LAD—between 1st and 2nd diagonal branch
- Distal LAD—beyond 2nd diagonal branch.

Left circumflex artery
- Proximal left circumflex artery—between origin of left circumflex artery (LCA) and origin of 1st obtuse marginal branch
- Mid left circumflex artery—between of 1st and 2nd obtuse marginal branch
- Distal left circumflex artery—portion beyond the origin of 2nd obtuse marginal branch.

Right coronary artery
- Proximal right coronary artery—from its origin in right coronary sinus and origin of right ventricular branch
- Mid right coronary artery—between the origin of right ventricular branch and posterior descending artery
- Distal right coronary artery—portion distal to origin of posterior descending artery.

Venous Drainage of the Heart (Fig. 4.19)

Heart is mainly drained by following three veins:

Coronary Sinus

- This is wide venous channel runs from left to right along coronary sinus

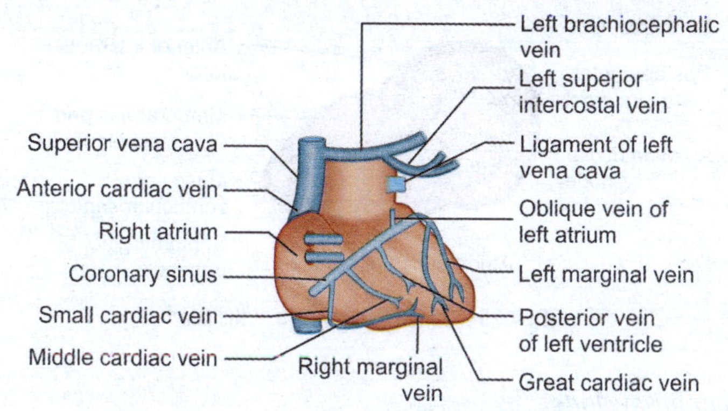

FIG. 4.19   Venous drainage of the heart

- It is 2 to 3 cm long
- Finally coronary sinus opens into inferoposteromedial aspect of right atrium between the orifice of inferior vena cava and septal leaflet
- A rudimentary valve—Thebesian valve present at the coronary sinus orifice
- It receives blood from the following veins:
  - ❖ Great cardiac veins
  - ❖ Oblique vein of left atrium
  - ❖ Posterior vein of left ventricle
  - ❖ Middle cardiac vein
  - ❖ Small cardiac vein.

Anterior Cardiac Veins

- They drain the anterior right ventricular wall
- It directly drains into right atrium.

Thebesian Veins (Venae Cordis Minimi)

- Drain the myocardium
- Directly drains into right atrium.

Conduction System of the Heart (Fig. 4.20)

This impulse conductive system coordinates cardiac cycle. It consists of cardiac muscle cells and specialized conducting fibers for initiating impulses and conducting the impulses through the heart. The conduction system consists of:

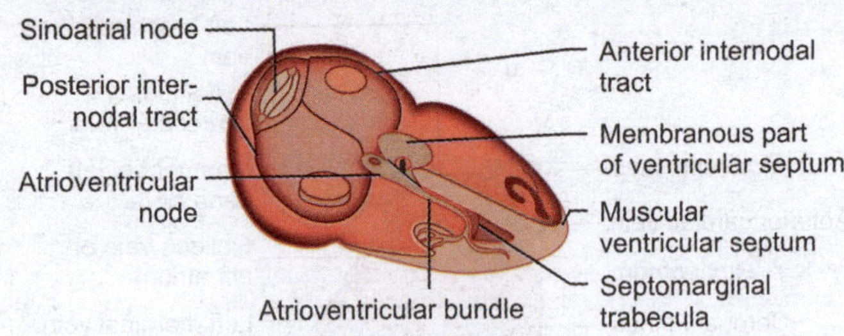

FIG. 4.20 Conduction system of the heart

Sinoatrial Node

- This is called pacemaker of the heart
- 10 to 12 mm long and 1 mm thick
- Situated in the subepicardial area in the terminal groove at the junction of superior vena cava and right atrium
- Vascular supply—60 percent from right and 40 percent from left coronary arteries.

Internodal Tract of Right Atrium

They conduct impulses from SA to AV node.

- *Anterior internodal tract (Bachmann-James):*
  - ❖ It connects anterosuperior part of SA node curved around in front of superior vena cava.
  - ❖ It divides into two bundles of fibers:
    1. One enters into right atrium
    2. The other enters AV node on anterosuperior margin.
- *Middle internodal tract (Wenckebach):*
  - ❖ It leaves posteroinferior margin of SA node
  - ❖ It joins the AV node on the superior margin, after running along the posterior margin of internodal septum.
- *Posterior internodal tract (Thorel):*
  - ❖ It leaves posteroinferior margin of SA node
  - ❖ It runs along the margin of crista terminalis
  - ❖ It joins AV node on posterior margin.

Atrioventricular Node

- *Transitional cell zones:* It is outer layer of AV node
- It lies subendocardially at the apex of triangle of Koch
- Its size is $1 \times 3 \times 5$ mm
- Blood supply—AV nodal artery—from right coronary artery (80–90%) and left circumflex artery (10–15%)
- AV node is susceptible to injury during tricuspid annuloplasty or plication procedure in Ebstein anomaly

- From electrophysiological point of view, AV node can be subdivided into three parts:
  1. *AN region:* Consist of transitional groups present in the upper portion of the nodes.
  2. *N region:* Here the cells consist of transitional cells and mid nodal cells.
  3. *NH region:* It consists of lower nodal cells. It is the anterior portion of bundle.

Bundle of His

- It arises from distal portion of AV node
- It travels along the membranous part of ventricular septum
- It travels through the central fibrous body, so closely:
  - ❖ Related to annuli of tricuspid, mitral and aortic valves.
    So in operative procedure involving the above valves or membranous part of ventricular septum—the bundle is liable to be injured.
- In normal heart, AV bundles run along posteroinferior rim of membranous septum
  In case of AV discordance, it runs along anterosuperior rim of membranous septum.
- At the crest of muscular septum AV bundle bifurcates into right and left bundles
- *Blood supply:* From perforators of left anterior descending coronary artery.

Bundle Branches

- *Right bundle branch:* It arises from distal portion of bundle of His in the form of cord like structure, travels along the septal and moderator bands towards anterior tricuspid papillary muscles
- *Left bundle branch:* It is broad fenestrated sheet—present in subendocardial area. It progresses like fan like structure
  It has two divisions: Thin anterosuperior and thick postero-inferior fascicles.
  Recent study shows, it is trifascicular structure.
  Blood supply of bundle branches:
  Septal perforators of:
  - ❖ Left anterior descending artery
  - ❖ Posterior descending coronary artery.

Terminal Purkinje Fibers

- These connect the lower end of bundle of His to endocardial surface of both ventricles in the form of interweaving network

- These fibers are connected in the papillary muscles at the base of the ventricles.

Physiology of the Heart and Great Vessels

Left ventricles contracts
↓
To the aorta
↓
To the arterioles
↓
To the capillaries
↓
To the venules
↓
To small veins
↓
To superior and inferior vena cava
↓
To the right atrium
↓
To the right ventricle
↓
To the pulmonary artery
↓
To the pulmonary capillaries
↓
To the pulmonary veins
↓
To the left atrium
↓
To the left ventricle

Veins, right side of the heart and pulmonary arteries capillaries are known as high capacitance vessels, because:

- In normal person, 80 percent of blood is stored here, but when required, blood is released by venous vasoconstriction
- In case of blood transfusion, 99 percent of total transfused blood remains in low pressure system and 1 percent circulates through high pressure system.

Central venous pressure, measured in right atrium, is 4 to 12 cm of water. It is good indicator of blood volume.

Cardiac output: Stroke volume × heart rate.

Stroke volume = Amount of blood ejected during each ventricular contraction. Normally it is 70 mL

Heart rate = 72 beats per minute in normal individual.

Minute volume = Amount of blood ejected by left ventricle in one minute, i.e.

Minute volume = Stroke volume × heart rate.

Normal value = 70 × 72 = 5000 mL per minute.

Cardiac index = Minute volume expressed in relation to body surface area in square meter.

Normal adult body surface area is 1.734 square meter and normal minute volume is 5 liter/minute, so cardiac index = 2.8 ± 0.3 liters per square meter of body surface area per minute.

Distribution of blood volume ejected by left ventricle per minute

Liver	Kidney	Skeletal muscles	Brain	Heart	Skin, bones GI tract
30%	26%	18%	16%	4%	6%
1500 mL	1300 mL	900 mL	800 mL	200 mL	300 mL

Type of Blood Flow in the Artery

- *Streamline flow:* In this type of flow, layer in contact with arterial wall does not move or moves very slowly. Central layer moves very fast, in between the above layers, rest of the layers move progressively increasing rate from periphery to center
- *Turbulent flow:*
  - ❖ This flow occurs above critical level
  - ❖ This type of flow produces sounds.

Volume of Blood Flow Depends upon Various Factors

- *Pressure gradient:* It is the pressure difference between the two ends of blood vessels: $P_g = P_1 - P_2$

P_1	P_2	P_1	P_2	P_g
Aorta	Vena cava	120	0	120
Aorta	Aorta	120	100	20
Proximal end of arteries	Distal end of arterioles	100	30	70
Arterial end of capillaries	Venus end of capillaries	30	15	15
Proximal end of venules	Distal end of venules	15	10	5
One end of vein	Other end of vein	10	0	10
One end of vena cava	Other end of vena cava	0	–2	–2

- *Peripheral resistance:* This is the resistance of the conduit provided against the flow of blood. According to the Poiseuille's law of resistance:

$$R = 8Ln/\pi r^4.$$

Where R = resistance, L = length of the vessel, r = radius of the vessel, n = viscosity of blood.

Radius is important variable, because radius is raised to fourth power.

Resistance in circulation occurs in series or parallel:

❖ When resistance occurs in series, total resistance (R_T is the sum of individual resistances, i.e. $R_T = R_1 + R_2 + R_3 +$ -----.

❖ When resistance arranged in parallel, e.g. in organ system of systemic circulation, individual resistance contributes as reciprocal, e.g.

$$1/R_T = 1/R_1 + 1/R_2 + 1/R_3 +$$ ------.

Here, total resistance is much less than for serial resistance.

Physiologically, most of the resistance is offered at the arteriolar level, because of sympathetic tone.

Causes of vasoconstriction at the arterial level

❖ *Local control:*
  • Internal blood pressure
  • Endothelin I.
❖ *Neural control:* Sympathetic nerve.
❖ *Hormonal control:*
  • Epinephrine
  • Angiotensin II
  • Vasopressin.

Causes of vasodilation at the arterial level

❖ *Local control:*
  • Hypoxia
  • Carbon dioxide, hydrogen ion
  • Adenosine
  • Osmolarity
  • Bradykinin
  • Nitric oxide
  • Eicosanoids.
❖ *Neural control:* Neurons responsible for release of nitric oxide.
❖ *Hormonal control:* Atrial natriuretic peptide.

• *Blood viscosity:* It is the friction of blood volume provided to the arterial wall. Resistance is directly related to the blood viscosity. Blood viscosity is governed by:
  ❖ Number of cell in the blood
  ❖ Plasma protein, mainly albumin.

• *Diameter of blood vessels:* Blood flow is directly related with diameter of blood vessels
  ❖ Aorta has maximal diameter and capillary has minimal diameter
  ❖ Cross-sectional area of vessels are gradually increased in arterioles and capillaries.

Cross-sectional area of an individual branch is small, but total cross-sectional areas of total branches are greater than that of parent vessel, e.g.

- Cross-sectional area of aorta is 4 square cm
- Cross-sectional areas of capillaries are 2500 square cm.

- *Velocity of blood flow:* It is the rate at which blood flows through the particular region of the body
  - Large arteries—50 cm/sec
  - Small arteries—5 cm/sec
  - Arteries—0.5 cm/sec
  - Capillaries—0.05 cm/sec
  - Venules—0.10 cm/sec
  - Small veins—1.0 cm/sec
  - Large veins—2.0 cm/sec.

Velocity of blood flow depends upon
  - Viscosity of blood
  - Cardiac output.
  - Cross-sectional area of blood vessels.

Circulation time: It is the time taken for the blood to travel through a part of circulation or whole circulatory system.

Blood pressure: It is the lateral pressure given by column of blood on the arterial wall. It consists of:

- *Systolic pressure:* It is the maximal pressure exerted on the wall of the vessel during ventricular systole. Normal value is 120 to 140 mm Hg
- *Diastolic pressure:* It is the minimum pressure in arteries during ventricular diastole. Normal value is 60 to 80 mm Hg
- *Pulse pressure:* It is the difference between systolic and diastolic blood pressure. Normal value is 40 mm Hg
- *Mean blood pressure:* It is the sum of diastolic blood pressure and one-third of pulse pressure. Normal value is 80 + 13 – 93 mm Hg.

Physiological variation of blood pressure
- *Age:* Blood pressure is progressively increased as the age advances
- *Sex:*
  - In premenopausal women, blood pressure is 5 mm Hg, less than male of same age
  - In postmenopausal period, blood pressure is same in male and female of the same age.
- *BMI:* If BMI is high, blood pressure will be raised
- *Diurnal variation:*
  - In early morning and in the evening, blood pressure is low
  - It is maximum at noon.
- *Sleep:* During sleep, blood pressure is 15 to 20 mm Hg less than that present during day time. But in case of dream during sleep, blood pressure is slightly increased

- *Postprandial time:* Blood pressure is increased postprandially
- *Emotion:* During anxiety or disturbed mood or Type I personality, blood pressure will be increased due to release of adrenaline
- *Exercise:*
  - ❖ During moderate exercise, systolic blood pressure is increased by 20 to 30 mm Hg, due to increase in cardiac output, but diastolic pressure is unaltered due to unaltered peripheral resistance
  - ❖ During severe exercise, systolic blood pressure is increased by 40 to 50 mm Hg, but diastolic blood pressure will be low due to decreased peripheral resistance.

Summary of factors that determine systemic arterial pressure shown by algorithm (Flow chart 4.1).

Control Blood Pressure

- *Baroreceptor mechanism:*

Increase in blood pressure
↓
Stimulation of baroreceptor
↓
Impulse conduction via IXth and Xth cranial nerves
↓

↓ Sympathetic outflow to heart and great vessels	↑ Parasympathetic outflow to heart and great vessels
↓	↓
Decreased cardiac output Dilatation of blood vessels	Bradycardia
↓	↓
Decrease in blood pressure	Decrease in blood pressure

- *Chemoreceptor mechanism:*

Decreased arterial blood flow
↓
Development of hypoxia, hypercapnea
↓
Stimulation of chemoreceptor
↓
Impulse travels to vasoconstrictor center
↓
Blood pressure is increased

- *Renal rennin-angiotensin mechanism:*

Decrease in arterial blood pressure
↓

FLOW CHART 4.1   Summary of factors that determine systemic arteries pressure

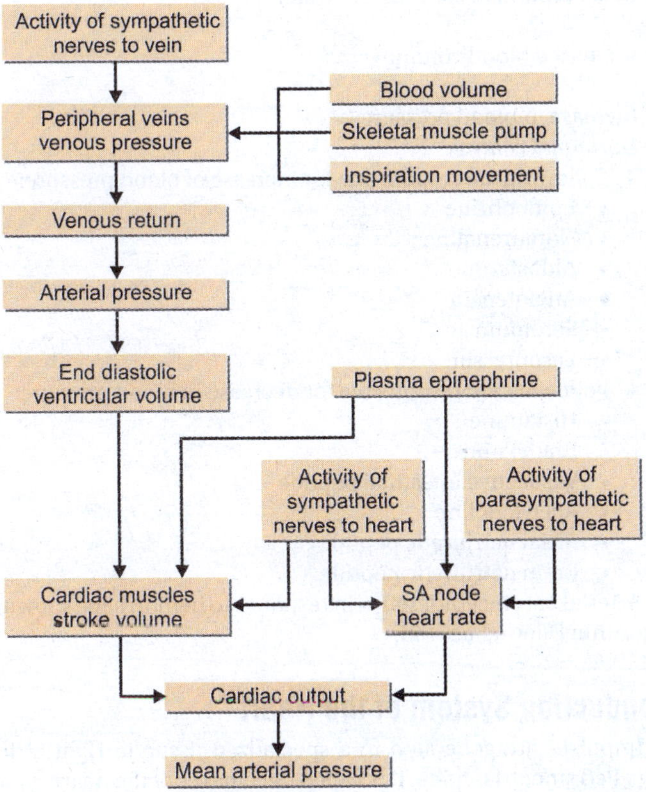

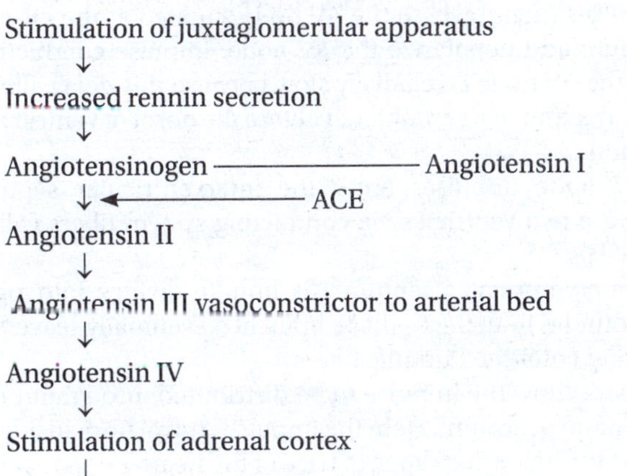

Stimulation of juxtaglomerular apparatus
↓
Increased rennin secretion
↓
Angiotensinogen ———————— Angiotensin I
↓ ←———————— ACE
Angiotensin II
↓
Angiotensin III vasoconstrictor to arterial bed
↓
Angiotensin IV
↓
Stimulation of adrenal cortex
↓

Release of aldosterone

↓

Reabsorption of sodium and water

↓

Increased blood volume

↓

Increase in blood pressure

- *Hormonal control:*
  - ❖ Following are responsible for increase of blood pressure:
    - Epinephrine
    - Noradrenaline
    - Aldosterone
    - Angiotensin
    - Serotonin
    - Vasopressin.
  - ❖ Following are responsible for decrease in blood pressure:
    - Histamine
    - Bradykinin
    - Vasoactive intestinal peptide
    - Acetylcholine
    - Atrial natriuretic peptide
    - Brain natriuretic peptide.

Arterial baroreceptor reflex in response to hemorrhage shown by algorithm (Flow chart 4.2).

Conduction System of the Heart

- Impulses are generated in a specialized tissue in right atrium called sinoatrial node. It is called pacemaker of the heart
- The impulses are conducted through three internodal fibers
- The impulses then travel to the AV node situated at the base of right atrium and depolarize the AV node. Impulse conduction through the AV node is relatively slow because this delay allows atrial contraction to be completed before the onset of ventricular contraction
- From AV node impulses enter the interventricular septum between the two ventricles via conducting system fibers called bundle of His
- Within interventricular septum His bundle divides into right and left bundle branches—these branches eventually leave the septum and enter the Purkinje fibers
- These fibers allow the impulse to be distributed throughout the ventricular myocardium. Here the impulses travel from inside to outside of the heart from apex to base of the heart
- These impulses spread simultaneously to both ventricles, so that both the ventricles contract more or less simultaneously

FLOW CHART 4.2 Arterial baroreceptor reflex in response to hemorrhage

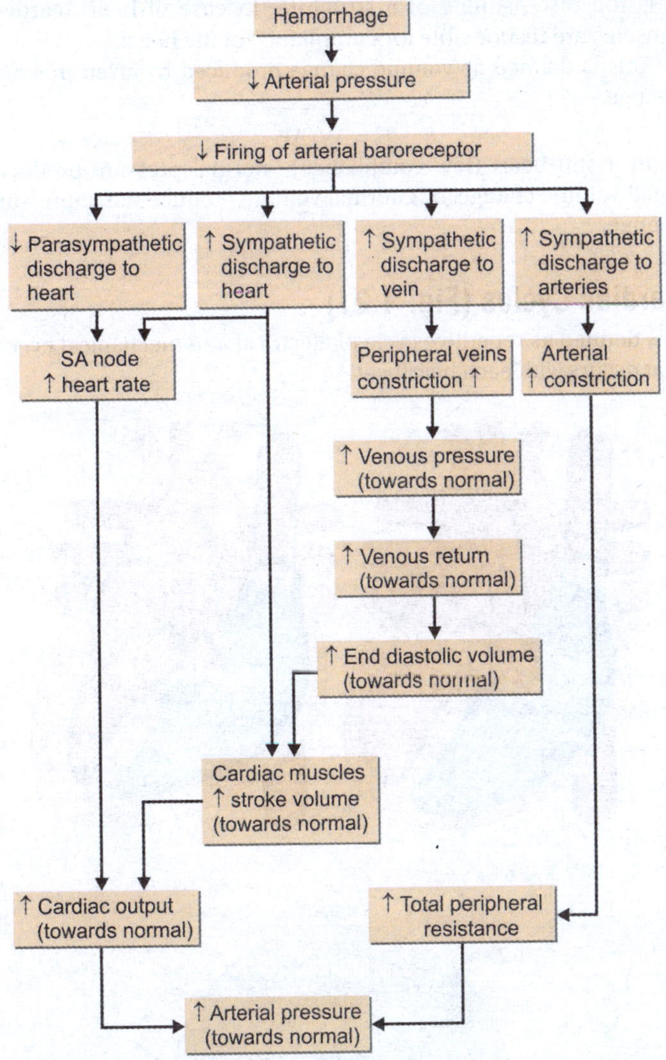

- Velocity of impulses in different parts of conduction system:
  - Atrial muscle fibers—0.3 meter/sec
  - Internodal fibers—1.0 meter/sec
  - AV node—0.05 meter/sec
  - Bundle of His—0.12 meter/sec
  - Purkinje fibers—4.0 meter/sec
  - Ventricular muscle fibers—0.5 meter/sec.

Compliance

It is the distensibility of a structure. In case of heart, cardiac muscles are responsible for compliance of the heart.

This is defined as volume change produced by given pressure change.

$$C = \Delta V/\Delta P.$$

In a stiff heart (low compliance)—normal pressure produces small volume change, but normal volume produces large pressure change.

Cardiac Cycles (Fig. 4.21)

It is defined as repetitive cycle of electrical and mechanical events that occurs with each heartbeat.

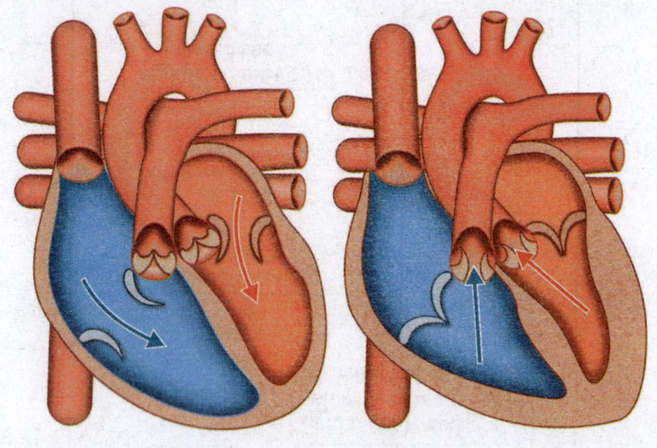

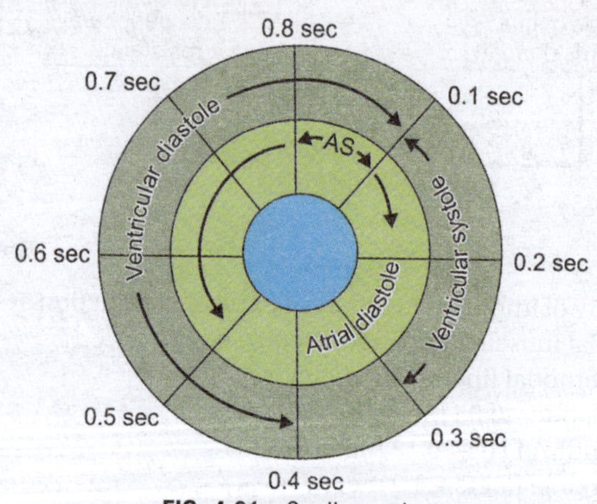

FIG. 4.21   Cardiac cycles

Electrical events precede the mechanical events due to entry of calcium in myocytes, during cardiac action potentials. ECG can be correlated with mechanical events.

- 'P' wave precedes atrial contraction
- During 'PR' interval, there is conduction through the AV node and ventricular conduction
- 'QRS' complex precedes ventricular systole
- 'T' wave of ventricular repolarization precedes ventricular relaxation.

Mechanical events can be divided broadly into two events:
1. *Systole:* It can be described under two headings:
     i. *Isovolumetric contraction:* 0.05 sec
    ii. *Ejection phase:* 0.22 sec.
2. *Diastole:* It can be described under five headings:
      i. *Protodiastole:* 0.04 sec
     ii. *Isovolumetric relaxation:* 0.08 sec
    iii. *Rapid filling phase:* 0.11 sec
     iv. *Slow filling phase:* 0.19 sec
      v. *Last phase of atrial systole:* 0.11 sec.
   Total mechanical event is 0.8 second.

Description of events will be started with atrial contraction
- *Atrial contraction:*
  ❖ It is last rapid filling phase
  ❖ It contributes 10 percent of ventricular filling at rest. But during exercise, passive ventricular filling gradually decreases, atrial contraction phase increases up to 30 percent of ventricular filling
  ❖ Intra-atrial pressure increases with little increase in ventricular pressure
  ❖ Atrial contraction produces 4th heart sound.
- *Isovolumetric contraction period:*
  ❖ In this phase, ventricular muscle contracts, in such a way that muscle tension increases, but no change in the length of muscle fiber
  ❖ As the ventricular intracavitary pressure increases, AV valves are closed, producing 1st heart sound
  ❖ As the semilunar valves are already closed, ventricular muscle tension increases without any change in the length of muscle fiber
- *Ejection phase:* When left ventricular intracavitary pressure exceeds that of aorta (80 mm Hg) and when right ventricular intracavitary pressure exceeds that of pulmonary artery (10 mm Hg), semilunar valves open and the blood column are ejected from both ventricles into aorta and pulmonary artery respectively

- ❖ In early rapid ejection phase, large amount of blood are ejected from both the ventricles
- ❖ In late slow ejection phase, small amount of blood is ejected (0.09 seconds)
- ❖ Stroke volume at rest is 80 mL 47 mL/square meter body surface area. End systolic volume at rest (EDV) is 40 mL/square meter. So ejection fraction at rest (SV/EDV) is 0.67.
- *Protodiastole:*
  - ❖ As the ventricular intracavitary pressure decreases and when the pressure falls below that of aorta or pulmonary artery, semilunar valves of both the ventricles close, producing 2nd heart sound
  - ❖ It is the beginning of diastolic phase.
- *Isometric relaxation phase:*
  - ❖ In this phase, ventricular muscles relax with decrease in tension, but no change in the length of muscle fibers
  - ❖ Ventricles contract as closed cavities
  - ❖ Aorta, meanwhile is filed due to suction effect, created by lowering of valve plane during ejection.
- *Rapid filling phase:*
  - ❖ As the intracavitary pressure of both ventricles decrease gradually, so that they fall below right and left atrial pressure, AV valves open
  - ❖ Seventy percent of filling take place during this phase
  - ❖ Rushing of blood in to the ventricles produce the 3rd sound.
- *Slow filling phase:* In this phase, 20 percent of ventricular filling occurs at slow phase.

Duration of Cardiac Cycle Decreases at the Cost of Diastole

Pressures in different cardiac chambers

Area	Systolic (mm Hg)	Diastolic (mm Hg)
Left atrium	7–8	0–2
Right atrium	5–6	0–2
Left ventricle	120	5
Right ventricle	25	2–3
Aorta	120	80
Pulmonary artery	25	7–8

Ejection fraction: It is defined as a portion of end diastolic volume that has been ejected into aorta with each beat.

$$\text{Ejection fraction} = \frac{\text{Stroke volume}}{\text{End diastolic volume}}$$

$$= \frac{\text{End diastolic volume} - \text{End systolic volume}}{\text{End diastolic volume}}$$

Capillary pressure: It is the pressure of blood column in the wall of a capillary.

Normal value: Arterial end—30 to 32 mm Hg.

Venous end: 15 mm Hg.

In kidney: Capillary pressure—60 mm Hg.

In lung: Pulmonary capillary pressure—7 mm Hg.

Capillary pressure is responsible for:
- Exchange of various substances between blood and interstitial fluid
- Filtration in kidney
- Gaseous exchange in lung between blood and alveoli.

SYMPTOMS RELATED TO CARDIOVASCULAR SYSTEMS

Main cardinal symptoms are:
- Chest pain
- Palpitation
- Syncope
- Breathlessness
- Cough (see chapter 3 Respiratory System, for details)
- Hemoptysis
- Claudication.

Chest Pain

Discomfort in the anterior chest above the epigastrium but below the mandible.

Regarding pain chest, the following questions are to be asked to the patient:
- Character of pain
- Site of pain
- Onset of pain
- Radiation of pain
- Duration of pain
- Intensity of pain
- Aggravating factors
- Relieving factors
- Associated phenomenon, if any.

Causes of chest pain according to intensity of pain and site of pain:
- *Life-threatening causes:*
  - *Cardiac causes:*
    - Acute coronary syndrome:
      - Stable angina
      - 'ST' elevated myocardial infarction (STEMI)
      - Non 'ST' elevated myocardial infarction (NSTEMI).
    - Acute pericarditis
    - Aortic dissection.
  - *Pulmonary causes:*
    - Pulmonary embolism
    - Pulmonary infarction
    - Tension pneumothorax.
  - *Gastroesophageal causes:*
    - Esophageal rupture
    - Esophageal spasm
    - Corrosive poisoning.

- *Nonlife-threatening causes:*
  - ❖ *Cardiac causes:*
    - *Ischemic causes:*
      - – Aortic stenosis
      - – Hypertrophic obstructive cardiomyopathy
      - – Severe systemic hypertension
      - – Severe pulmonary hypertension
      - – Severe aortic regurgitation.
    - *Nonischemic causes:*
      - – Mitral valve prolapse syndrome
      - – Chronic pericarditis.
  - ❖ *Gastrointestinal causes:*
    - Gastroesophageal reflux disease
    - Peptic ulcer disease
    - Esophageal spasm.
  - ❖ *Pulmonary causes:*
    - Pneumonia
    - Pleurisy.
  - ❖ *Neuromuscular skeletal causes:*
    - Thoracic outlet syndrome
    - Degenerative joint disease of cervical or thoracic spine
    - Costochondritis (Tietze's disease)
    - Herpes zoster infection of the chest.
  - ❖ *Systemic causes:*
    - Anemia
    - Hypoxia.
  - ❖ *Psychological causes:*
    - Anxiety
    - Depression
    - Cardiac psychosis.

Description of Pain According to Types

Anginal Pain

- *Character:* Dull, pressure like, suffocating, squeezing, sensation of heavy weight in the chest. Anginal pain does not vary with:
  - ❖ Respiration
  - ❖ Position
  - ❖ Palpitation.
- *Site:* Central or left side of the chest, occasionally diffuse. Pain above the mandible or below the epigastrium is very uncommon Pain localized to an area less than one finger tip in size and radiation to lower extremities is not an anginal pain.
- *Duration:* Last for 2 to 5 minutes (not more than 15 minutes)

- *Radiation:* It is often referred to corresponding dermatomes (C8 to T4), i.e. left shoulder, inner aspect of left arm, forearm, neck, jaw, epigastrium, occasionally to the right side of the chest, and right arm. Occasionally, site of radiation of chest pain denotes or excludes specific coronary arteries:
  - ❖ Left-sided chest pain with radiation to left arm—denotes involvement of left coronary artery
  - ❖ Epigastric pain, radiating to neck or jaw—excludes left anterior descending artery.
- *Onset:* During physical exertion, emotional stress, elevation of left arm above the shoulder
- *Mode of onset:*
  - ❖ Progressively increasing pain, reaching the peak instantaneously
  - ❖ Low threshold in the morning. So in the morning, any type of activity may produce pain, but during the day time, this type of activity may not start pain due to progressively increasing threshold of pain as the day progresses.
- *Relieving factors:* Anginal pain usually is relieved with rest, or after taking nitroglycerin tablets
- *Other types of presentation of anginal pain:*
  - ❖ Shortness of breath—discomfort in mid chest
  - ❖ Discomfort at any sites—the sites of radiation. Abdominal gaseous discomfort, like, belching, nausea, diaphoresis.
- *Angina is stable, if:*
  - ❖ It occurs only with provocations
  - ❖ It has been occurring for last two months
  - ❖ It is symptomatically stable.

Unstable angina can be presented in any of the following ways:

- *Rest angina:*
  - ❖ Occurs, when the patient is at rest
  - ❖ It is prolonged for more than 20 minutes
  - ❖ Occurs within a week of presentation with anginal symptoms
  - ❖ At night it may occur when the diastolic blood pressure decreases to lower levels—nocturnal angina.
- *New onset angina:*
  - ❖ Angina at rest having CCSC III severity
  - ❖ Onset within 2 months of initial presentation of anginal symptoms.
- *Increasing angina:* Started as stable angina, but changes its orientation like:
  - ❖ More frequent
  - ❖ Longer than 15 minutes
  - ❖ Progressively increasing severity of chest pain to CCSC class III.

Linked angina
- *It is a type of anginal δ pain, where there is:*
  - ❖ Typical history of angina
  - ❖ Definite history of coronary artery disease
  - ❖ It occurs after gastrointestinal factor, such as, stooping after heavy meals.

Grading of anginal pain by Canadian Cardiovascular Society classification system:

CLASS I	A. Ordinary physical activity, like, walking, climbing stairs do not cause angina. B. Angina pectoris occurs with strenuous, rapid and prolonged exertion.

CLASS II	A. Slight limitation of ordinary activity.
	B. Angina occurs on:
	  1. Walking or climbing stairs rapidly.
	  2. Walking uphill.
	  3. Walking or climbing stairs after meals, in cold wind, under emotional stress or during after few hours after awakening.

CLASS III	A. Marked limitation on ordinary activity.
	B. Angina occurs on:
	  1. Walking one or two blocks on the level.
	  2. Climbing one flight in normal condition and in normal pace.

CLASS IV	A. Inability to carry out any physical activity without discomfort. B. Angina may be present at rest.

Pain of Myocardial Infarction (Fig. 4.22)

- *Character:* Crushing type, as if elephant is standing.
- *Site:* Substernal or left side of the chest.
- *Duration:* It persists for hours, till treatment is started, although pain is absent in diabetic and elderly individual.
- *Radiation:* It is often referred to corresponding dermatomes (C8 to T4), i.e. left shoulder, inner aspect of left arm, forearm, neck, jaw, epigastrium, occasionally to the right side of the chest and right arm. Occasionally, site of radiation of chest pain denotes or excludes specific coronary arteries:
  - ❖ Left-sided chest pain with radiation to left arm—denotes involvement of left coronary artery
  - ❖ Epigastric pain radiating to neck or jaw—excludes left anterior descending artery.
- *Onset:*
  - ❖ It may be very severe from onset
  - ❖ There may be preceding history of stable or unstable angina or both.

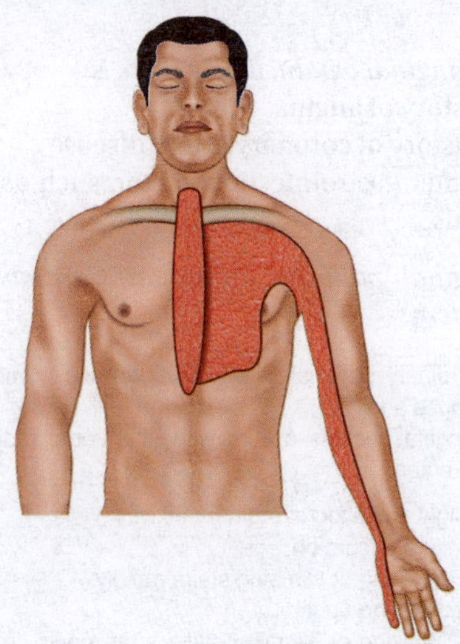

FIG. 4.22 Distribution of pain in myocardial infarction

- *Relieving factors:*
  - ❖ Pain can be relieved by sedation only
  - ❖ Failure of rest and nitroglycerin to relieve pain.
- *Associated symptoms:* Sweating, palpitation, syncope, dyspnea, vomiting
- *Pain may be absent in:*
  - ❖ Elderly
  - ❖ Diabetic
  - ❖ Women.

Pain of Mitral Valve Prolapse (Fig. 4.23)

- *Character:* Angina like pain, may be like neurocirculatory asthenia
- *Duration:* More than hours
- *Associated symptoms:* Palpitation, fatigue, postural hypotension.

Pain of Acute Pericarditis

- *Character:* Knifelike, sharp
- *Site:* Central, more often left sided
- *Duration:* It may be present for minutes to hours
- *Radiation:* To trapezius ridge and neck, shoulder tip, occasionally jaw and left arm
- *Exacerbation:*
  - ❖ Deep breathing
  - ❖ Thoracic motion

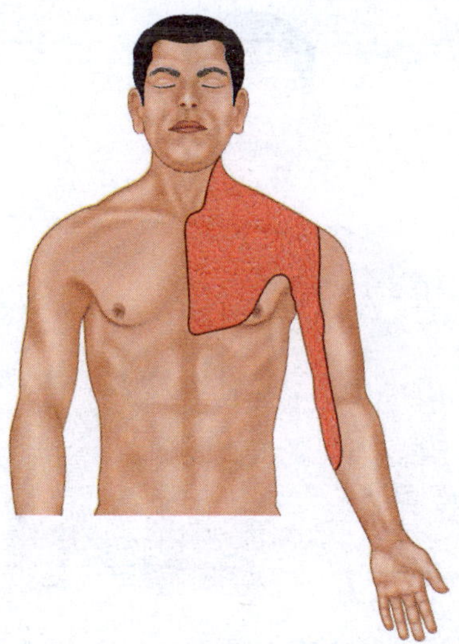

FIG. 4.23   Distribution of pain in mitral valve prolapse

- ❖ If associated congestive failure is present.
- *Relieving factor:* Leaning forward
- *Associated symptoms:*
  - ❖ Fever of myocarditis
  - ❖ Congestive cardiac failure.

Pain of Aortic Dissection (Fig. 4.24)

- *Site:* It is present according to site of dissection:
  - ❖ When chest pain is present anteriorly, ascending aorta is involved in 98 percent of cases
  - ❖ When chest pain is present in the interscapular region, descending aorta is involved in 90 percent of cases.
- *Following history may be present:*
  - ❖ Congenital disease, like Marfan's syndrome
  - ❖ *Trauma:*
    - • Blunt trauma to the chest
    - • Direct trauma to the aorta
    - • *Iatrogenic trauma:* Transarterial catheterization, intra-aortic balloon pump.
- *Duration:* Persists for hours till intervention
- *Character:* Acute sharp, stabbing, ripping in nature
- *Radiation:* It migrates according to site of dissection:
  - ❖ Chest pain radiates to neck, throat, jaw and face—ascending aorta is involved
  - ❖ Pain in back radiates to abdomen or lower limb—descending aorta will be involved.

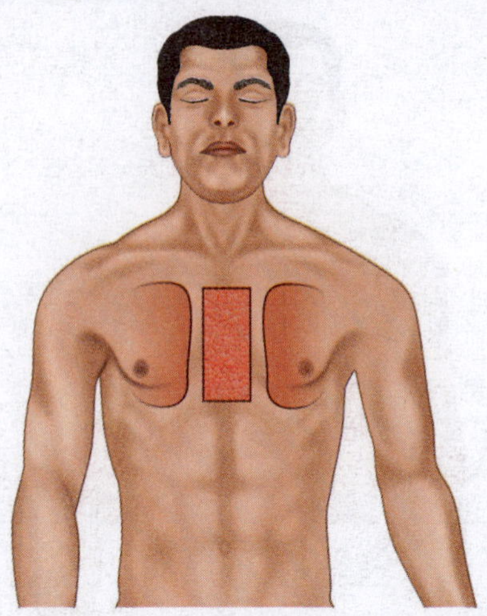

FIG. 4.24 Site of interscapular pain in aortic dissection

- *Associated symptoms:*
  - ❖ *Syncope:* If it ruptures into pericardial space
  - ❖ Heart failure due to aortic insufficiency, due to proximal dissection of aorta
  - ❖ Syncope due to cerebral hypoperfusion
  - ❖ Myocardial infarction due to involvement of coronary ostium.

Chest Pain due to Pulmonary Embolism

- *Site:* Anterior chest according to site of obstruction of pulmonary vein
- *Character:* Pleuritic in nature
- *Radiation:* No radiation
- *Onset:* Acute in nature
- *Duration:* It may persist for minutes to hours
- *Associated symptoms:* Dyspnea, tachypnea, hypotension, and hemoptysis
- *History suggestive of pulmonary embolism:*
  - ❖ Deep vein thrombosis
  - ❖ Recent surgery
  - ❖ Prolonged immobilization
  - ❖ Malignancy
  - ❖ Oral contraceptive pill
  - ❖ Pregnancy
  - ❖ Hypercoaguable state

* ❖ Congestive cardiac failure
* ❖ Prolonged travel.

Pleuritic chest pain from infection of lung producing pneumonia can be differentiated by high fever, cough with rusty sputum production.

Chest Pain due to Gastrointestinal Causes

* *Pain due to esophagitis of reflux origin:*
  * ❖ *Site:* Starts at epigastric region or in retrosternal region
  * ❖ *Character:* Burning type, squeezing, aching type
  * ❖ *Radiation:* If it starts at epigastric region, it may radiate to back, retrosternal region, occasionally to left shoulder, left arm and forearm
  * ❖ *Aggravating factors:* It aggravates:
    * After meals
    * In recumbent position after heavy meals
    * Increased abdominal pressure by:
      – Bending
      – Coughing
      – Squatting.
  * ❖ *Relieving factor:*
    * Antacids
    * Nitroglycerinc.
  * ❖ *Associated symptoms:* Hoarseness of voice due to repeated clearing of throat
  * ❖ *Supportive history of:*
    * Acid regurgitation
    * Water brush due to acid reflux to the throat
    * Caffeine, alcohol abuse
    * Heavy meal consumption
    * Cigarette smoking.

  Esophageal reflux may lower the threshold of development of angina.
* *Pain due to esophageal spasm:*
  * ❖ *Site:* Retrosternal
  * ❖ *Radiation:* to back
  * ❖ *Onset:* Severe at onset
  * ❖ *Character:* Stabbing in nature
  * ❖ *Duration:* Last for seconds to hours
  * ❖ *Aggravating factor:* Following intake of meals
  * ❖ *Relieving factors:* Relieved by nitroglycerin
  * ❖ *Associated symptoms:*
    * Dysphagia
    * Weight loss
    * Hematemesis.

❖ *Supportive evidence:*
- Barium swallow shows motility problems
- Manometry shows:
  - Increased esophageal resting pressure
  - Increased resting pressure at lower esophageal sphincter.

Chest Pain due to Pleural Disorder

- *Character:* Stabbing in nature
- *Radiation:* No radiation
- *Duration:* Persists for minutes to hours
- *Site:* Area of involvement
- *Aggravating factors:* Respiration, movement of chest wall
- *Relieving factors:*
  - ❖ Lying down on the same side
  - ❖ Holding breath at the end of deep inspiration to prevent friction between parietal and visceral pleurae.

Chest Pain due to Pneumothorax

- *Onset:* Acute
- *Intensity:* Very severe at the onset
- *Radiation:* No radiation
- *Site:* At the localized area
- *Aggravating factor:* Movement of the chest
- *Associated symptoms:* Dyspnea, cough
- *History:* Trauma to chest, violent cough, iatrogenic procedure.

Chest Pain due to Musculoskeletal System Disorders

- *Site:* Area is localized, chest wall, or thoracic spine
- *Character:* Pricking in nature
- *Duration:* Several hours to several days
- *Radiation:* No radiation
- *Aggravating factors:*
  - ❖ Deep inspiration
  - ❖ Postural movements
  - ❖ Movement of upper limbs
- *Relieving factor:* Pain killer and rest
- *Intensity:* Low intensity
- *History:* Trauma, injury, strenuous exercise.

Pain of Thoracic Inlet Syndrome

- Pain associated with paresthesia
- Distribution along the ulnar side of arm and forearm

- *Aggravated by:*
  - ❖ Abduction of the affected arm
  - ❖ Lifting heavy weight
  - ❖ Elevating the arm above shoulder.

Chest Pain due to Herpes Zoster

- *Character:* Lancinating or shooting in character
- *Radiation:* Along the corresponding dermatome
- *Duration:* It persists for more than hours
- *Associated phenomenon:* Characteristic vesicles along the affected dermatome.

Chest Pain due to Tietze Syndrome

- Aching pain
- Anterior chest pain
- Localized swelling and tenderness over costal cartilage, costochondral joints and costosternal junction
- No radiation
- Resolves spontaneously
- Aggravated by coughing, sneezing
- No muscle tenderness.

Pericardial scratch syndrome

- Sudden onset
- Scratch, sharp needle like, jabbing pain
- Short lasting
- It may recur.

Functional Chest Pain

- Pain off and on
- It may persist for several hours.
- *Associated symptoms:*
  - ❖ Anxicty
  - ❖ Dizziness
  - ❖ Depression
  - ❖ Tingling and numbness in the extremities.

Pain Radiates from Back of the Neck to the Left Shoulder and Left Arm: Cervical Spondylosis

Pain in the nipple and around the apex radiation to left lower chest

- Cervical (lower) or cervicodorsal osteoarthritis
- Acid-peptic disorder.

Differentiating features of cardiac chest pain from noncardiac chest pain

Cardiac	Noncardiac
Ischemic origin	Nonischemic origin
Characteristics of pain	**Characteristic of pain**
Squeezing	Sharp
Burning	Stabbing
Heaviness	Aggravated by respiration
Location of pain	**Location of pain**
Substernal	Left submammary area
Across mid thorax	Left hemithorax
Radiation to jaw, left shoulder, inner arm, back, interscapular area	Localization by one finger
	Back pain, suggestive of aortic dissection
Provocating factors	**Provocating factors**
Exercise	Specific body motion
Emotion	Position of the body
Stress	Immobilization
Cold weather	Deep respiration
Duration	**Duration**
Minutes	Seconds
	Hours without any myocardial damage

Questions to be Asked in Case of Angina

- Any pain during exertion, e.g. walking rapidly, climbing upstairs?
- The site of chest pain?
- Whether it becomes worse in cold weather?
- Whether it becomes worse after a big meal?
- Is it bad enough to stop you from exercise?
- Does it go away after taking rest?
- Whether similar pain occurs during or after excitement?

■ Palpitation

Definition: Subjective awareness of one's own heart beat, often with perception of some types of heart rhythm irregularity, acceleration or both. It is not due to forceful contraction of the heart, as in case of aortic stenosis, pulmonary stenosis, severe systemic and pulmonary hypertension.

Causes of Palpitation

Cardiac Causes

- *Valvular heart diseases:*
  - ❖ Aortic stenosis
  - ❖ Mitral regurgitation
  - ❖ Aortic regurgitation
  - ❖ Mitral valve prolapses
  - ❖ Prosthetic heart valves.
- *Ischemic heart diseases:*
  - ❖ Stable or unstable angina
  - ❖ Myocardial infarction
  - ❖ Ventricular aneurysm—complication of infarction.
- *Congenital cyanotic heart diseases:*
  - ❖ *Increase pulmonary blood flow:*
    - • Total anomalous pulmonary venous connection
    - • Transposition of great vessels.
  - ❖ *Arrhythmogenic:*
    - • Ebstein anomaly
    - • After mustard operative procedure.
- *Congenital acyanotic heart diseases:*
  - ❖ *With shunt:*
    - • Atrial septal defect
    - • Ventricular septal defect.
  - ❖ *Arrhythmogenic:* Right ventricular arrhythmogenic dysplasia.
- *Cardiac muscle disease:* Hypertrophic obstructive cardio-myopathy.

Noncardiac Causes

- *Hyperkinetic circulation:*
  - ❖ Anemia
  - ❖ Fever
  - ❖ *Endocrinological overactivity:*
    - • Thyrotoxicosis
    - • Pheochromocytoma.
  - ❖ *Endocrinological hypoactivity:* Hypoglycemia.
- *Drugs:*
  - ❖ Caffeine
  - ❖ Alcohol (holiday heart syndrome)
  - ❖ Nicotine
  - ❖ Cocaine
  - ❖ Sympathomimetics
  - ❖ Digitalis
  - ❖ Tricyclic antidepressants

- ❖ *Vasodilators:*
  - Nitrates
  - Calcium channel blockers.
- *Psychogenic:*
  - ❖ Anxiety neurosis
  - ❖ Depressive psychosis
  - ❖ Manic depressive psychosis.

Different Types of Arrhythmias Producing Palpitation

- *Extrasystoles:*
  - ❖ Atrial
  - ❖ Ventricular.
- *Supraventricular tachycardia:*
  - ❖ Extrasystoles
  - ❖ Atrial flutter.
- Paroxysmal supraventricular tachycardia
- Paroxysmal atrial fibrillation
- Sinus tachycardia due to fever, thyrotoxicosis
- Arrhythmias due to tea, coffee or alcohol intake.

The following enquiries to be done to diagnose the patients:
- *How long this problem persists?*
  - ❖ *If persists for weeks, months or years:* It indicates:
    - Congenital cyanotic heart disease
    - Congenital acyanotic heart disease
    - Valvular heart disease
    - Hyperkinetic circulatory states
    - Lone atrial fibrillation.
  - ❖ *If it originates recently (hours to days):* It indicates acute or subacute cardiopulmonary process, here patient may experience shortness of breath or chest pain.
- *In which circumstances it has been started?*
  - ❖ During physical activity—catecholamine induced arrhythmias
  - ❖ Clusters of palpitations in 24 hours period:
    - Ectopic beats at the bed time—when patient tries to fall asleep and distracting from all stimuli
    - Tachyarrhythmia occurring in the middle of the night, interrupting sleep—suggestive of episodes of vagally mediated atrial fibrillation.
  - ❖ *Palpitation occurs with assumption of upright posture:* Tachycardia secondary to postural orthostatic tachycardia syndrome:
    - Occurs in dysautonomic conditions
    - Occurs in young female.

- *How it will start and stop?*
  - ❖ Heart rate increases abruptly and ends abruptly—pathologic tachycardia
  - ❖ Heart rate increases gradually and decreases gradually—sinus tachycardia
  - ❖ Overlap occurs—where paroxysmal supraventricular tachycardia starts suddenly but partially overlapped by sinus tachycardia—due to arrhythmia related catecholamine discharge.
- *Where the rhythm is regular or irregular:* To diagnose it, ask the patient to tap on the table the rate at which the heart pumps during the attack
  - ❖ *This might clearly indicate:*
    - Whether the rate is truly rapid or not
    - How fast the rate is?
  - ❖ *If the rhythm is irregular:*
    - Supraventricular ectopic
    - Ventricular ectopic
    - Atrial tachyarrhythmia with rapid irregular ventricular response.
- *Persistence of episode duration:* Whether the episode lasts for seconds, minutes or hours?
  Fleeting episodes—do not require urgent treatment, if there is no associated heart disease.
- *How frequently this symptom occurs?* Whether the symptoms occur at interval of hours to days or months to years
- *Whether the patient aware of the palpitation:*
  - ❖ *In few advanced arrhythmias*—patient may be totally unaware
  - ❖ *In long standing atrial fibrillation*—patient may feel discomfort and palpitation occurs only during exertion or excitement
  - ❖ Patient may be totally unaware of symptoms, when lies down on the left side and fall asleep
  - ❖ Thin built person is aware of own heart block
  - ❖ *Awareness of skipped beat*—when palpitation lasts for instance
  - ❖ *Premature beat*—may be described as floating sensation in the chest
  - ❖ *Pounding sensation*—due to paroxysmal tachycardia
  - ❖ *Sensation of stop beating*—may be due to compensatory pause following ectopic beat
  - ❖ *Regular rapid palpitation*—due to sinus tachycardia, supraventricular tachycardia or paroxysmal tachycardia
  - ❖ *Irregular rapid palpitation*—due to atrial flutter, atrial fibrillation, atrial tachycardia with varying block.
- *Relieving factor:* Vagal maneuvers, such as stooping, breath holding, terminate paroxysmal supraventricular tachycardia

- *Associated symptoms:*
  - ❖ *Chest pain:* If associated with angina, myocardial infarction, pulmonary embolism with or without infarction, bronchial asthma
  - ❖ *Syncope:* If associated with heart block, ventricular arrhythmia, pulmonary hypertension, orthostatic hypertension, dysautonomic response, Stokes-Adams attack, hypoglycemia, pheochromocytoma
  - ❖ *Breathlessness:* If associated with myocardial infarction with shock, left ventricular failure, severe aortic stenosis
  - ❖ *Weakness and fatigue:* If associated with congestive cardiac failure, severe aortic stenosis
  - ❖ *Polyuria:* Paroxysmal supraventricular tachycardia, paroxysmal atrial fibrillation
  - ❖ *Throbbing in the neck:* Aortic stenosis
  - ❖ *Diarrhea:* If associated with thyrotoxicosis, irritable bowel syndrome, hypokalemia induced arrhythmia
  - ❖ *Deafness:* If associated prolonged QT syndrome.

Cardiac History

- Presence of ischemic heart disease or prior history of myocardial infarction—may be associated with ventricular or supraventricular beats
- Presence of suspected or known case of congestive cardiac failure on the basis of hypertension
- Presence of history of right or left ventricular dysfunction with atrial fibrillation—produce atrial arrhythmia
- Presence of mitral valve disease—may present with atrial arrhythmia
- In absence of organic heart disease—isolated atrial or ventricular beat producing palpitation. If it is sustained, it may represent as:
  - ❖ Paroxysmal supraventricular tachycardia in younger or middle aged persons
  - ❖ Paroxysmal atrial fibrillation or atrial flutter—in middle aged or elderly person.

History of Arrhythmia

- Past history of radiofrequency ablation—suggest the recurrence of arrhythmia
- History of paroxysmal atrial fibrillation in patient with left ventricular dysfunction and prior symptomatic premature ventricular complexes
- History of implantation cardiac pacemaker or implantable cardioverter defibrillator—it may produce paroxysmal

ventricular complexes with 1:1 retrograde conduction. This is called pacemaker syndrome

- History of implantation of dual chamber pacemaker or defibrillator, may produce pacemaker mediated endless loop tachycardia
- History of use of pacemaker device with internal sensor, it may produce overdrive ventricular pacing so during the period of inactivity, it may produce inappropriately rapid heart beating.

Family History

- Family history of sudden death gives rise to suspicion of familial inherited arrhythmogenic disorder, e.g.
  - ❖ Long QT syndrome
  - ❖ Brugada syndrome
  - ❖ Catecholamine mediated polymorphic ventricular tachycardia
    All above usually produce ventricular tachycardia—it may be associated with lightheadedness, presyncope or syncope.
- Familial history of loan atrial fibrillation may be inherited.

History Related to Endocrine Disorders

- History of hyperthyroidism (iatrogenic or endogenous) may produce sinus tachycardia, paroxysmal atrial fibrillation
- History suggestive of pheochromocytoma—headache, diaphoresis, pallor.

History of Drug Use

- History of intake of bronchodilator therapy, over the counter sympathomimetic agent for cold symptoms
- Drug producing prolonged QT syndrome (Torsade De Pointes)
- History of intake of tea, coffee, alcohol, herbal substances (cocaine, amphetamine)
- History of intake of thyroid replacement therapy.

Patient with palpitation refers to emergency department
- *Palpitation with:*
  - ❖ New onset syncope
  - ❖ New onset or worsening of chest pain or dyspnea.
- *Recent onset palpitation with lightheadedness may be with:*
  - ❖ Drug induced prolonged QT syndrome
  - ❖ Inherited prolonged QT syndrome—catecholamine induced ventricular tachycardia, Brugada syndrome, arrhythmogenic right ventricular dysplasia.

- *Sustained supraventricular tachycardia with:*
  - ❖ Hypotension
  - ❖ Chest pain
  - ❖ Dyspnea
  - ❖ Lightheadedness.
- *Atrial flutter or fibrillation with:*
  - ❖ Hypotension
  - ❖ Chest pain
  - ❖ Dyspnea
  - ❖ Light headedness
  - ❖ Ventricular rate 120 beats/minute
  - ❖ Onset clearly within 48 hours regardless of rate
  - ❖ Onset of uncertain duration with known stroke or other thromboembolic events (no history of receiving anti-coagulant therapy)
  - ❖ Sustained ventricular tachycardia
  - ❖ Non sustained ventricular tachycardia with:
    - Unexplained syncope
    - New onset or worsening of chest pain
    - Dyspnea
    - *Organic heart disease:*
      Asymptomatic ventricular tachycardia with:
      - Organic heart disease
      - Prolonged QT syndrome
      - Brugada syndrome
      - Induction of exercise
      - Rate >120 beats/minute.

■ Syncope

Definition: Sudden transient loss of consciousness and postural tone with subsequent spontaneous recovery.

Presyncope: Feeling of awareness of impending faint—it may or may not progress to overt syncope—depending on whether the cause has been eliminated or not.

Causes of Syncope

Neurally Mediated Syncope

- *Vasovagal, neurocardiogenic syncope:*
  - ❖ *Precipitating factors:*
    - Prolonged standing
    - Hypovolemia due to dehydration
    - Fear
    - Severe pain
    - Sight of blood

- Strong emotion
- Instrumentation
- No cause.
- ❖ *Predisposing factors:*
  - Fatigue
  - Warmth
  - Eye surgery
  - Dental surgery.
- ❖ *Prodromal symptoms:* This phase usually lasts for 30 to 60 seconds followed by syncope. In few cases this phase may not be present, in that case syncope occurs suddenly without any warning:
  - Patient becomes unsteady, feels bad, confused, yawn
  - Ringing in ears
  - Visual disturbances—dimness of vision, seeing of spots
  - Associated symptoms—nausea, warmth, vomiting, facial pallor, and diaphoresis.
- ❖ *Syncopal episode:* Patient develops hypotension, bradycardia, seizure like activity (involuntary muscle jark), 3 phases are:
  1. *First phase:* Increase in heart rate and blood pressure due to increase in sympathetic tone.
  2. *Second phase:* Consisted of decrease in heart rate and blood pressure, occasionally asystole of more than 20 seconds—producing syncopal attack due to increase in parasympathetic tone.
  3. *Third phase (recovery phase):* This occurs when the patient is in supine position.
- *Situational syncope:*
  - ❖ *Micturition syncope:* It occurs in young men, in the early morning immediately after rising from the bed.
    - *Predisposing factors:*
      - Fatigue
      - Decreased intake of food
      - Alcohol intoxication
      - Urinary tract infection
      - Bladder neck obstruction.
    - *Provocating factors:*
      - Decreased sympathetic tone results in decreased peripheral vascular resistance, which produces lowering of blood pressure
      - Alcohol intoxication producing autonomic dysfunction
      - During micturition, sudden decompression of the bladder, if superadded by any type of straining to relieve bladder neck obstruction
      - In elderly individual, autonomic dysfunction producing orthostatic hypotension.

All of the above produce decreased cardiac output

↓

Increase in sympathetic tone
Increase myocardial contractility
Increase in heart rate

↓

Stimulation of cardiopulmonary mechanoreceptors

↓

Decrease in sympathetic tone and
increase in parasympathetic tone

↓

Vasodilation and bradycardia

↓

Syncope

❖ *Defecation syncope:* It occurs in elderly individual, who goes to defecate just after rising from the bed.
  - Predisposing factors:
    - Fatigue
    - Decreased food intake
    - Alcohol intake
    - Mechanical obstruction in the rectum
  - Provocating factors:
    - During rectal, vaginal examination
    - During giving enema
    - During manual evacuation of rectum.

  All the above factors produce syncope in similar methods as like micturition syncope.
❖ *Swallowing syncope:*
  - Predisposing factors:
    - Structural abnormalities of the esophagus:
      - Achalasia cardia
      - Stricture of esophagus
      - Esophageal tumor
      - Diffuse esophageal spasm.
    - Cardiac status:
      - Acute myocardial infarction
      - Sino atrial block
      - High degree AV block.

    During swallowing and immediately after swallowing (aggravated by mechanical obstruction)

    ↓

    Stretching of the esophageal wall

    ↓

    Stimulates the mechanoreceptors on the esophageal wall

    ↓

Decreased sympathetic tone and
increase in parasympathetic tone
↓
Hypotension and
bradycardia
↓
Syncope

❖ *Cough syncope:* This occurs in elderly individual during forceful coughing.
  - *Predisposing factors:*
    - Alcohol intake
    - Smoking
    - History of chronic obstructive lung disease
    Sudden forceful coughing
    ↓
    - Increase in intrathoracic pressure
    ↓
    Decreased venous return to the heart
    ↓
    Decreased cardiac output
    ↓
    Stretching of the pulmonary mechanoreceptors
    ↓
    Increase in sympathetic tone producing reflex tachycardia and increase in ventricular contraction
    ↓
    Stimulation of the mechanoreceptors on the cardiac wall
    ↓
    Decrease in sympathetic tone and increase in parasympathetic tone
    ↓
    Hypotension and bradycardia
    ↓
    Syncope
    - Increase in intrathoracic pressure
    ↓
    Increase in pressure of subarachnoid space
    ↓
    Increase in cerebrovascular resistance
    ↓
    Reduction of cerebral flow
    ↓
    Syncope

- ❖ *Valsalva syncope:*
  - *Predisposing factors:*
    - Athesclerotic heart disease
    - Sick sinus syndrome
    - Elderly individual.

    In patient with above predisposing conditions
    ↓
    Increase in intrathoracic pressure of the heart
    ↓
    Decrease venous return to the heart
    ↓
    Decrease cardiac output and decrease in arterial blood pressure
    ↓
    Reflex increase in sympathetic tone and increase in myocardial contractility
    ↓
    Tachycardia and increased cardiac output
    ↓
    Stimulation of mechanoreceptors on the cardiac wall
    ↓
    Decrease in sympathetic tone and increase in parasympathetic tone
    ↓
    Hypotension and bradycardia
    ↓
    Syncope

- ❖ *Diver's syncope:* Here the predisposing factors are:
  - Hypoxia
  - Diving reflex induced reflex bradycardia and vasodilatation, which produces syncope.

- ❖ *Postprandial syncope:* Provocating factors:
  - Elderly individual
  - Impaired autonomic activity
  - Release of gastrointestinal peptides.

    Half to one hour after taking meal

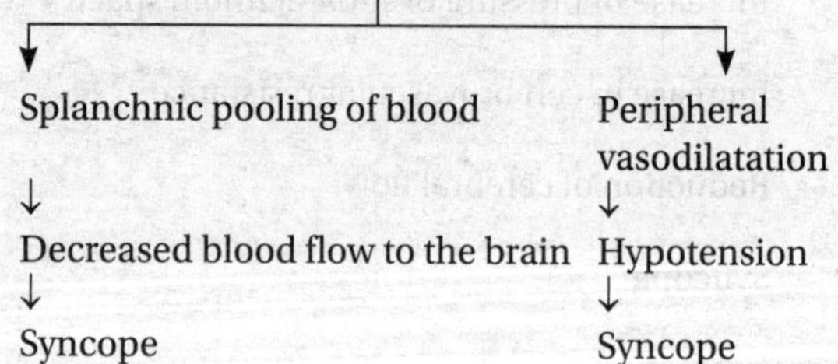

- *Carotid sinus syncope:* It occurs in individual with hypersensitive carotid sinus
  - ❖ *Provocating factors:*
    - Waring tight collar around the neck
    - Shaving around the neck
    - Sudden turning of the head.
  - ❖ *Predisposing factors:* For carotid sinus syncope:
    - Coronary artery disease
    - Thymus
    - Enlarged lymph nodes
    - Parotid tumor
    - Thymic tumor
    - Thyroid tumor.
  - ❖ *Carotid sinus hypersensitivity:*
    - Sinus node dysfunction
    - AV node dysfunction.

Triggering of the baroreceptors in the internal carotid artery above the bifurcation of the common carotid artery.

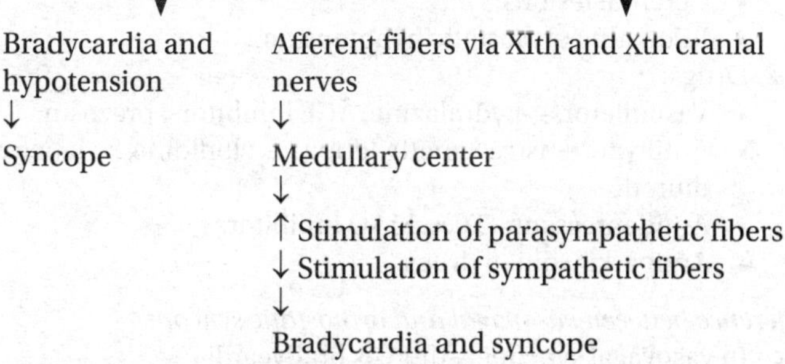

Carotid sinus hypersensitivity may be of:
Bradycardia predominant (cardioinhibitory)—extreme sinus bradycardia, sinoatrial block, asystole more than 3 seconds.

Hypotension predominant (vasodepressor)—decrease blood pressure by more than 50 mm Hg, but no bradycardia.

Mixed type—combination of bradycardia and hypotension.

- *Orthostatic hypotension:* It can be diagnosed by documentation of 20 mm Hg, or more decrease in systolic blood pressure, and/or >10 mm Hg, of diastolic blood pressure during initial 5 minutes after the patient in upright position. As a result:
  - ❖ Blurring of vision
  - ❖ Lightheadedness
  - ❖ Pallor.

Blood circulation to the brain is decreased, resulting in syncope.

Pathophysiology of syncope:
Aggravating factors:
❖ After arising in the morning
❖ After taking heavy meal
❖ After heavy exercise.

When the patient will be in recumbent position, venous return to the heart increases, perfusion to the brain increases, syncope disappears.

Causes of orthostatic hypotension:
❖ Blood volume depletion:
  • Blood loss
  • Fluid loss.
❖ Venous pooling:
  • Prolonged standing
  • Pregnancy.
❖ Neurogenic causes:
  • Autonomic dysfunction
  • Tabes dorsalis, syringomyelia
  • Autoimmune diseases
  • Cerebral lesions
  • Idiopathic orthostatic hypotension.
❖ Drugs:
  • Vasodilators—hydralazine, ACE inhibitors, prazosin
  • Antihypertensive—methyldopa, clonidine, labetolol, diuretic
  • Antidepressant—TCA, MAO inhibitors
  • Antiparkinsonian drugs.

Difference between vasovagal and orthostatic syncope
❖ In vasovagal syncope—there is bradycardia
❖ In orthostatic syncope—there is tachycardia.

Cardiac Abnormalities

Structural Abnormalities

● *Left ventricular outflow tract obstruction:*
  ❖ Aortic stenosis (Fig. 4.25):
    In the face of fixed cardiac output, during exercise and heavy exertion, cardiac output is not increased and peripheral resistance is decreased
    ↓

    Excessive increase in intraventricular pressure
    ↓

    Excessive stretching of left ventricular wall
    ↓

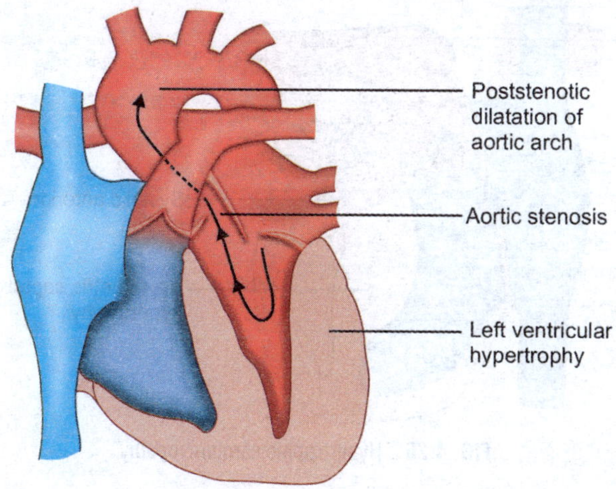

FIG. 4.25   Aortic stenosis

Stimulation of left ventricular mechanoreceptors (Bezold-Jarisch reflex)

↓

Inhibition of sympathetic tone and stimulation of parasympathetic tone (through cardiac vagal afferent)

↓

Hypotension and bradycardia

↓

Syncope

- Decreased myocardial perfusion due to diminished coronary perfusion produce cardiac pain
- Ventricular arrhythmias, atrial fibrillation, paroxysmal AV block produce syncope.

❖ Hypertrophic obstructive cardiomyopathy (Fig. 4.26)
  The causes of syncope:
  - Stimulation of left ventricular mechanoreceptor produces worsening of left ventricular outflow tract obstruction
  - Decreased myocardial perfusion
  - Any type of straining, like, coughing, valsalva maneuver, increase outflow tract obstruction, produce hypotension. As a result, there is diminished circulation to the brain producing syncope.

- *Left ventricular inflow tract obstruction:*
  ❖ Mitral stenosis (Fig. 4.27)
    - Diminished left ventricular filling

↓

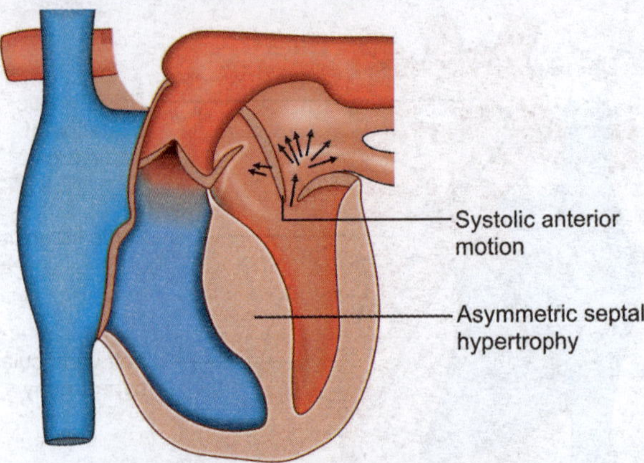

FIG. 4.26 Hypertrophic cardiomyopathy

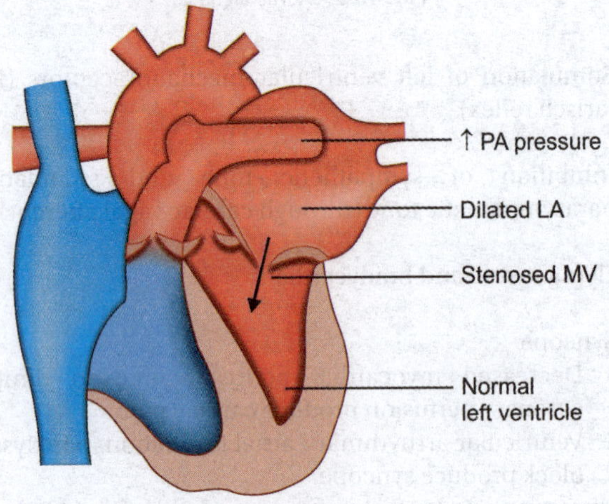

FIG. 4.27 Mitral stenosis

Low cardiac output
↓
Hypotension
↓
Low circulation to the brain
↓
Syncope

- *Atrial fibrillation produces syncope by:*
  - Low atrial kick
  - By embolism.
- In severe mitral stenosis, the pulmonary hypertension.

- ❖ Left atrial myxoma
  Diminished left ventricular filling
  ↓
  Decreased cardiac output
  ↓
  Syncope
- *Right ventricular outflow tract obstruction:*
  - ❖ Pulmonary hypertension
  - ❖ Pulmonary stenosis
  - ❖ Pulmonary embolism with >50 percent of pulmonary vascular bed obstruction.
- *Pathophysiology:*
  - ❖ Low cardiac output—produces hypotension, syncope.
  - ❖ As a result of increased right ventricular filling pressure
    ↓
    There is stimulation of mechanoreceptors
    ↓
    Decreased sympathetic tone and
    increased parasympathetic tone
    ↓
    Hypotension and bradycardia
    ↓
    Syncope
  - ❖ In Fallot tetralogy with right to left heart shunt—deoxygenated blood will go to brain, producing syncope due to tissue hypoxia.
- *Ischemic heart disease:*
  - ❖ In case of anterior wall myocardial infarction:
    - • Sudden pump failure
      ↓
      Hypotension
      ↓
      Decreased perfusion to the brain
      ↓
      Syncope
    - • Arrhythmias
      ↓
      Syncope
  - ❖ In inferior wall myocardial infarction
    ↓
    Stimulation of left ventricular baroreceptors
    ↓
    Increased parasympathetic tone and
    decreased sympathetic tone
    ↓

Hypotension

↓

Syncope
- ❖ Myocardial ischemia
- ❖ Mechanical complications—mitral regurgitation, ventricular septal defect, and ventricular wall rupture
- ❖ Cardiac tamponade due to thrombolysis, anticoagulant therapy
- ❖ Prolonged immobilization
- ❖ Aortic dissection.
- *Arrhythmias:*
  - ❖ Tachyarrhythmias:
    - Atrial arrhythmias—eighty percent cause of syncope. Normally PSVT does not produce syncope, but, if the following factors are associated with PSVT, may produce syncope:
      - Advanced age
      - Rate >200/minute
      - Associated organic heart disease, e.g. hypertrophic obstructive cardiomyopathy, aortic stenosis, pulmonary stenosis, pulmonary hypertension
      - WPW syndrome with rapid conduction over accessory pathways
    - Sustained monomorphic ventricular tachycardia
    - Prolonged ventricular repolarization syndrome
      Congenital:
      - L-G-L syndrome
      - Brugada syndrome (ST segment elevation in precordial leads—V_1, V_2 and V_3 with incomplete or complete right ventricular block)
      - Familial catecholaminergic polymorphic ventricular tachycardia
      - Arrhythmogenic right ventricular dysplasia with ventricular arrhythmias.
    - Hypertrophic obstructive cardiomyopathy with minimal cardiac hypertrophy may develop sustained ventricular tachyarrhythmia
    - Drugs induced long QT syndrome—arrhythmogenic drugs:
      - Quinidine
      - Procainamide
      - Flecainide
      - Amiodarone
      - Sotalol.

Pathophysiology:
- Marked tachycardia >150 beats/minute

↓

Decrease in diastolic filling

↓

Decrease in cardiac output

↓

Hypotension

↓

Syncope
- Vigorous ventricular contraction

↓

Stimulation of ventricular mechanoreceptors

↓

Hypotension

↓

Syncope

- *Bradyarrhythmias:* Thirty percent of cardiac causes of syncope.
  - ❖ *Severe sinus bradycardia:*
    - Increased vagal tone
    - Eye surgery
    - Intracranial tumor
    - Mediastinal tumor
    - Myxedema.
  - ❖ *Sick sinus syndrome:*
    - Sinus arrest
    - Exit block.
  - ❖ *Heart block:*
    - AV block with escape rhythm or ventricular arrhythmias
    - Complete heart block producing Stoke-Adams syndrome.
      In congenital heart block, due to normal ventricular rate, syncope dose not occur.
  - ❖ *Pacemaker and implantable cardiac defibrillator syncope produce due to:*
    - Pacemaker malfunctioning
    - Pacemaker syndrome.

Neurological Syncope

- *Cerebrovascular:*
  - ❖ *Vertebrobasilar artery:*
    Atherosclerotic occlusive disease

    ↓

    Diminished perfusion of medullary center

    ↓

Prodromal symptoms, like, vertigo, dysarthria, alexia.

↓

Syncope →

❖ *Subclavian steal syndrome:* Due to occlusive disease of subclavian artery proximal to origin of vertebral artery

❖ *Aortic arch syndrome:* Occlusive disease of origin of brachiocephalic artery, in aortic arch

❖ Cervical spondylosis.

- *Reflex mediated:*

❖ *Glossopharyngeal neuralgia:* Paroxysmal pain in oropharynx, tonsillar fossa, base of the tongue.

Precipitating factors:

- Swallowing
- Chewing
- Coughing.

Above pain is sent via afferent nerve to medulla

↓

Efferent pathway through Xth cranial nerve

↓

Asystole →
Bradycardia

↓

Syncope →

- *Metabolic disturbances:*

❖ *Hypoglycemia:* When blood sugar is <40 mg%. This is associated with:

- Confusion
- Tremor
- Salivation
- Hyperadrenergic state
- Hunger
- Patient is on insulin or hypoglycemic.

During attack:

- Not associated hypotension
- Syncope persists even when the patient is in supine position
- Does not resolve until blood glucose level is restored to normal.

❖ *Hypoadrenalism:*

- Suspected, when long-term therapy with steroid is suddenly discontinued
- Stigmata of adrenal insufficiency.

- *Psychiatric disturbances:*
  - ❖ *Psychiatric disorders associated with syncope:*
    - Anxiety neurosis
    - Panic disorder
      They produce hyperventilation, which leads to cerebral vasoconstriction and loss of consciousness.
    - Major depression
    - Alcohol abuse
    - Somatization disorders.
  - ❖ *Complex interaction between psychiatric disorder and syncope:* Depression, stress, psychosocial disorder may provoke arrhythmia or myocardial infarction.
  - ❖ *Repeated syncope may precipitate psychiatric disorder:*
    - Panic disorder
    - Anxiety.

Deduction of cause from the history
- *New onset of syncopal attack without prodromal event:*
  - ❖ Fluid loss from dehydration
  - ❖ Blood loss due to gastrointestinal hemorrhage
  - ❖ In case of female, blood loss due to menorrhagia, ruptured ectopic.
- *Sudden onset without prodromal event:* Cardiac arrhythmia
- *Sudden onset of syncope with prodrome:* (Pain, nausea, diaphoresis) in association with precipitating factor, pain, extreme emotion, bad sight—vasovagal syncope
- Loss of consciousness after prolonged standing—vasovagal syncope
- Loss of consciousness immediately after standing—orthostatic hypotension
- Loss of consciousness during episode of cough—cough syncope
- Loss of consciousness during micturition—micturition syncope
- Loss of consciousness following swallowing or defecation—swallowing or defecation syncope
- *Loss of consciousness following due to alcohol abuse:*
  - ❖ History of orthostatic hypotension due to impaired vasoconstriction
  - ❖ History of micturition syncope.
- *Loss of consciousness following:*
  - ❖ Shaving around the neck
  - ❖ Waring tight collars
  - ❖ Neck rotation
    Carotid sinus syncope.

- *Syncope associated with exertion:*
  - ❖ Aortic stenosis
  - ❖ Hypertrophic obstructive cardiomyopathy
  - ❖ Exercise induced tachycardia.
- *Syncope associated arm exercise:* Subclavian steal syndrome
- Loss of consciousness associated with head-up tilt testing in athlete—vasovagal syncope
- Syncope associated with exertional chest pain—anomalous origin of coronary artery
- *Syncope associated with:*
  - ❖ Physical exertion—mainly swimming
  - ❖ Emotional stress
  - ❖ In response to sudden unexplained aquastic stimuli—sound of alarm clock or telephone.

Associated Symptoms

- Associated with palpitation—cardiac origin
- Associated with brain stem findings—dysarthria, vertigo Ataxia, visual disturbance—vertebrobasilar insufficiency
- Postevent confusion—seizures
- Loss of consciousness associated with headache:
  - ❖ Migraine
  - ❖ Seizure.
- Associated with throat or facial pain:
  - ❖ Glossopharyngeal neuralgia
  - ❖ Trigeminal neuralgia.

Differentiating features between seizures and syncope

Clinical features	Syncope	Seizures
• Loss of consciousness precipitated by pain, micturition, exercise, pain, defecation, stressful events	+	−
• Sweating, nausea, before and during meals	+	−
• Aura	−	+
• Tongue biting	−	+
• Myoclonic jerks	+/−	++
• Disorientation after events	−	+
• Slowness in returning to consciousness	−	+
• Unconsciousness >5 minutes	−	+

Causes of Syncope According to the Age

- *Less than 30 years:*
  - ❖ Situational syncope
  - ❖ Alcohol abuse

  - ❖ Undiagnosed seizures
  - ❖ Cardiac syncope:
    - HOCM
    - Coronary artery anomalies
    - WPW syndrome
    - Long QT syndrome.
- *Middle aged (30–65 years):*
  - ❖ Neurally mediated syncope
  - ❖ Structural or arrhythmogenic cardiac syncope.
- *Elderly (>65 years):*
  - ❖ Neurally mediated syncope
  - ❖ Structural or arrhythmogenic cardiac syncope
  - ❖ Situational syncope
  - ❖ Carotid sinus hypersensitivity
  - ❖ Orthostatic hypotension
  - ❖ Drugs—antihypertensive medication, antidepressants.

Family History

- Family history of sudden death (including accidental drowning):
  - ❖ IIOCM
  - ❖ Arrhythmogenic right ventricular dysplasia
  - ❖ Long QT syndrome
  - ❖ Brugada syndrome
  - ❖ Catecholaminergic polymorphic ventricular tachycardia.
- Male gender >54 years, three or fewer episodes of syncope of 6 seconds or shorter duration, without warning before syncope—ventricular tachycardia or atrioventricular block.

Drug history
- *Antihypertensive medication:*
  - ❖ Doxazosin
  - ❖ Clonidine
  - ❖ Hydralazine
  - ❖ Prazosin
  - ❖ ACE inhibitors
  - ❖ ARB receptor blockers.
- Antidepressant drugs.
- *Others:*
  - ❖ Morphine
  - ❖ Phenothiazine
  - ❖ Calcium channel blockers
  - ❖ Nitroglycerin
  - ❖ Amiodarone
  - ❖ Aggressive antidiuretic therapy.

- *Drugs prolonging QT:*
  - Sotalol
  - Quinidine
  - Procainamide
  - Disopropamide
  - Amiodarone
  - Noncardiac drugs:
    - Macrolide antibiotics
    - Tricyclic antidepressant
    - Phenothiazines
    - Methadone
    - Antihistaminics
    - Cisapride.

Pregnancy

- In third trimester of pregnancy, in supine position due to compression of inferior vena cava or aorta by enlarged uterus
- In known cardiac disease, patient having history of palpitation, arrhythmias, exertional syncope, and pathologic murmur.

■ Claudication

From History

- History of cramping pain and weakness occurs with exercise and relieved by rest for 5 minutes or by slowing the pace of walking
- One can deduce the level and extent of the disease by considering the location and severity of discomfort
  Since pain is usually manifested one segment below the areas of stenosis:
  - Buttock pain—aortic or iliac artery disease
  - Thigh muscle pain—femoral artery disease
  - Calf muscle pain—popliteal artery disease
  - Calf, ankle and foot—tibiofemoral artery disease
  - Foot—pedal vessels.
- Amount or duration of exercise—should be asked, because amount of exercise to precipitate pain is inversely related to the extent of narrowing of vessels
- History of rest pain—it is classically defined as severe nocturnal pain or a burning sensation that begins over the metatarsal heads or heels and relieved by movement or dependency—it is sign of severe ischemia
- History of pain in buttock, thigh, calf and leg—increased during climbing stairs, better with rest—arterial disease

- History of taking sleep with legs hanging by the side of the chair—arterial disease.
- History of pain in the buttock and thigh with erectile dysfunction—aortoiliac disease.

Causes

- *Arterial causes:*
  - ❖ Atherosclerotic disease
  - ❖ Peripheral embolism
  - ❖ Burger disease
  - ❖ Aortic aneurysm
  - ❖ Coarctation of aorta.
- *Venous causes:* It shows the following features:
  - ❖ Venous outflow obstruction involving iliac vein
  - ❖ Peripheral embolism
  - ❖ History of burning discomfort of the limb with activity
  - ❖ *Relieved by:*
    - Leg elevation
    - Rest.
- *Nonvascular causes:*
  - ❖ *Neurogenic claudication:* It shows the following features:
    - Due to impingement of spinal cord by osteophytes or spinal stenosis
    - Pain occurs simply after assumption of upright posture
    - Ache in the thigh, hip and buttock and associated with numbness.
    - Pain aggravated by:
      - Assumption of upright posture
      - Walking
        Walking downstairs—because spine held in upright, thus increasing spinal pressure.
    - Pain is relieved by:
      - Stooping
      - Forward flexion
      - Sitting
      - Riding bicycle
      - Walking upstairs.
- *Compartment syndrome:* Occurs in athlete with hypertrophied muscles with impaired venous outflow
- *Neuropathic pain:* It shows the following features:
  - ❖ They occur in the distribution of dermatome
  - ❖ This pain is aggravated by exercise
  - ❖ This pain is relieved by change of posture that relieves pressure on a peripheral nerve.

Breathlessness (Fig. 4.28)

Definition: Awareness of own respiratory effort or sensation of one's own breathing.

Main pathogenesis of dyspnea depends on the calculation of dyspnea index, which can be calculated as percentage of pulmonary reserve:

$$\frac{[\text{Maximum voluntary ventilation (MVV)}-\text{Pulmonary ventilation (PV)}]}{\text{Maximum voluntary ventilation (MVV)}} \times 100$$

Dyspnea occurs when the dyspnea index is below 60 percent.

Maximum voluntary ventilation may be defined as maximum volume of air that can be expired or inspired in one minute. It depends upon:

- Strength of the respiratory muscles. It has to work against:
  - ❖ Elastic resistance of the lung and the chest wall—normal value is 0.13 liter/cm of water. It means lung and the thoracic wall increase by 0.13 liter when the increase in airway pressure will be 1 cm of water.
  - ❖ Airway resistance—maximum resistance occurs from trachea up to 7th generation of bronchial division (normal value—1.5 to 2 cm of water).
  - ❖ Viscosity resistance.

Pulmonary Ventilation

It is the amount of air inspired or expired by normal lung in one minute.

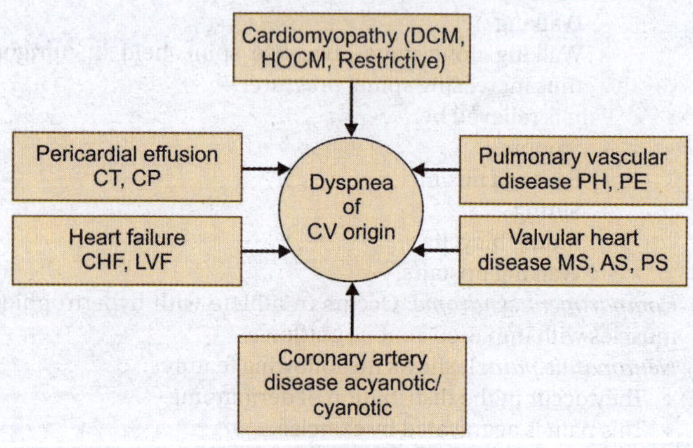

FIG. 4.28 Breathlessness

Pulmonary ventilation (PV) = Tidal volume (TV) × Respiratory rate (RR).

If, tidal volume = 500 mL per breath. And respiratory rate = 12/minute.

Pulmonary ventilation = 6 liter/minute.

Pulmonary ventilation may be increased by:
- *Juxta:* Pulmonary receptor (present in between alveolar epithelium and capillary endothelium) stimulated by:
  - ❖ Pulmonary edema
  - ❖ Pulmonary capillary congestion
  - ❖ Increased amount of fluid in interstitial area.
- *Hypoxemia:* Due to ventilation/perfusion mismatch

  Alveolar ventilation per breath = Tidal volume – Dead space.

  If, tidal volume = 500 mL and dead space = 150 mL.

  So, alveolar ventilation = 500 – 150 = 350 mL per breath.

  So, minute alveolar ventilation = 350 × 12 = 4200 mL per minute.

  Pulmonary blood flow = 5 liter per minute.

  V/P = 4.2/5 = 0.84.

  So, decreased V/P ratio means:
  - ❖ Decreased alveolar ventilation:
    - Bronchial asthma
    - Pleural effusion
    - Pneumothorax
    - Emphysema
    - Pulmonary edema due to congestive failure.
  - ❖ Increased pulmonary blood flow with normal alveolar ventilation—congenital cyanotic heart disease.
- *Acidosis:* It may be due to:
  - ❖ Respiratory acidosis with Type II respiratory failure in case of:
    - Bronchial asthma
    - Emphysema
    - Pneumonia.

    In this case, high PCO_2 stimulates chemoreceptor in carotid and aortic bodies, which in turn, stimulates medullary respiratory center, and produces increase rate and depth of breathing.
  - ❖ Metabolic acidosis—due to:
    - Different types of ketoacidosis
    - Renal failure.

In this case, high H^+ ion stimulates chemoreceptor in carotid and aortic bodies, which in turn stimulates medullary respiratory center, increases respiratory rate and depth of breathing, and wash out CO_2 and H^+ ion.

Causes of Breathlessness

- *Cardiac cause—any cause producing congestive heart failure:*
  - ❖ *Systolic dysfunction:*
    - Ischemic cardiomyopathy
    - Nonischemic cardiomyopathy.
  - ❖ *Diastolic dysfunction:*
    - Hypertensive heart disease
    - HOCM
    - Restrictive cardiomyopathy.
  - ❖ *Valvular heart diseases:*
    - Mitral stenosis
    - Acute mitral regurgitation
    - Aortic stenosis.
  - ❖ *Coronary artery disease:*
    - Papillary muscle dysfunction
    - Left ventricular systolic dysfunction
    - Left ventricular diastolic dysfunction
    - Myocardial infarction.
  - ❖ *Pericardial disease:*
    - Acute pericarditis
    - Cardiac tamponade.
  - ❖ *Pulmonary causes:*
    - Pulmonary thromboembolism
    - Pneumonia
    - Bronchial asthma
    - Pneumothorax
    - Upper airway obstruction:
      - Vocal cord paralysis
      - Endobronchial tumor
      - Foreign body in the trachea.
    - ARDS, a manifestation of SARS.
  - ❖ *Skeletal abnormalities:* Severe kyphoscoliosis
  - ❖ *Neuromuscular disease:* Myasthenia gravis
  - ❖ *Congenital heart diseases:*

Right to left heart shunt

↓

This produces hypoxemia

↓

This activates respiratory control center through the stimulation of chemoreceptors in the carotid bodies

↓

Increases ventilation

  - ❖ *Left to right heart shunt:*

If it is sufficiently large

↓

It produces left ventricular volume overload

↓

Left ventricular systolic dysfunction
If blood flow through the pulmonary vasculature

↓

Adverse pulmonary vasculature remodeling

↓

Pulmonary hypertension

↓

Stimulation of stretch receptor

↓

V/Q mismatching

↓

Dyspnea

❖ *Drugs:*
  - Beta blockers—produces bronchospasm
  - Steroids aggravate heart failure
  - Digoxin in HOCM
  - Diuretics in pericardial disease
  - Anticoagulants in pericardial effusion in case of renal failure.

New York Heart Association classification of heart failure

Grade I	No symptom at rest Dyspnea only on vigorous exertion
Grade II	No symptom at rest Dyspnea on moderate exertion
Grade III	May be mild symptom at rest Dyspnea at mild exertion Severe dyspnea on moderate exertion
Grade IV	Significant dyspnea at rest Severe dyspnea on mild exertion Patient is often bed bound

Questions to be asked for evaluation of breathlessness
- Whether the patient ever feels shortness of breath?
- Whether it occurs with exertion?
- How much the patient can do work before becoming breathless?
- Whether the patient even awakes up being gasping for breath?
- Whether he uses to sit up by the side of the bed to take fresh air?
- How many numbers of pillows the patient takes during going to bed?
- Whether breathlessness starts in walking the floor?
- If so, after how many meters of walk, breathlessness will be started?

- Whether breathlessness occurs during climbing upstairs? If so, after how many steps?
- Whether any cough or wheeze is present during breathlessness?

Evaluation of a Patient Presenting with Dyspnea

- *Mode of onset:*
  - ❖ *Acute onset:*
    - Acute bronchoconstriction
    - Acute pulmonary edema
    - Pulmonary embolism
    - Tension pneumothorax
    - Foreign body obstruction in upper airway
    - Psychogenic.
  - ❖ *Acute on chronic:*
    - Mitral stenosis—patient may develop atrial fibrillation, after prolonged immobilization.
    - Angina may suddenly turns into acute myocardial infarction, mainly in diabetic patient.
    - Patient with myocardial infarction may suddenly develop ventricular rupture or rupture chordae tendineae.
    - Patient with chronic renal failure may suddenly develop dyspnea due to:
      - Sudden fluid overload
      - Hemopericardium
      - Hyperkalemia.
  - ❖ *Chronic:*
    - Mitral regurgitation
    - Aortic stenosis
    - Aortic regurgitation
    - Chronic obstructive lung disease
    - Interstitial pulmonary fibrosis.
- *Duration of breathlessness:*
  - ❖ Longer duration (more than 5 years)—in mitral stenosis
  - ❖ Shorter duration of dyspnea—in aortic stenosis, coronary artery disease.

Paroxysmal nocturnal dyspnea: This type of dyspnea usually is Grade III NYHA classification.

At night after peaceful sleep of 2 to 3 hours sudden onset of dyspnea

↓

Relieved after assuming upright position, sitting by the side of the bed with hanging legs

↓

Patient develops sweating, coughing with expectoration of mucoid or pink frothy sputum

Causes:
- ❖ Mitral stenosis
- ❖ Coronary artery disease.

PND disappears when right ventricular failure appears.

Mechanism of development of paroxysmal nocturnal dyspnea:
- ❖ In mitral stenosis
  ↓
  Increase in left atrial pressure
  ↓
  Increase in pulmonary venous pressure
  ↓
  Increase in pulmonary capillary pressure
  ↓
  Exudation of fluid into interstitial spaces
  ↓
  Permeation of fluid into alveoli
  ↓
  Development of pulmonary edema
  ↓
  Development of PND
- ❖ Absorption of edema fluid into venous system during supine position
  ↓
  Increase venous return to the heart
  ↓
  Increase right atrial pressure
  ↓
  Increase right ventricular pressure
  ↓
  Increase pulmonary arterial pressure
  ↓
  Increase arterial end capillary pressure
  ↓
  Accumulation of fluid into interstitial spaces
  ↓
  Exudation of fluid into alveoli producing pulmonary edema
  ↓
  Development of PND

Causes of nocturnal dyspnea:
- Bronchial asthma—usually starts at 4 to 5 am in the morning preceded by a bout of cough
- Patient with chronic obstructive lung disease may develop respiratory distress in supine position, because of:
  - Diminished ventilatory drive
  - Pressure of the abdominal contents to the diaphragm, which ascends and compromises the thoracic cavity
  - In obese person tongue fall back

- Obesity—due to:
  - Elevation and upward movement of the diaphragm due to pressure of the abdominal contents increases intrathoracic pressure and decreases thoracic compliance
  - Reflux of intragastric contents into the esophageal cavity through thy lax lower esophageal sphincter, and enters into the trachea.
- Postnasal drip in case of common cold and associated with cough
- Recurrent pulmonary emboli
- Anxiety neurosis.

Orthopnea: Dyspnea occurs in supine position, relieved by erect position.

Common causes are:
- Acute left ventricular failure
- Bronchial asthma
- Congestive heart failure
- Gross ascites
- Constrictive pericarditis
- Fluid overload in chronic renal failure.

Platypnea: Dyspnea occurs in upright position, relieved by supine position. The causes are:
- Ball valve thrombus
- Left atrial myxoma.

The above two produce obstruction to flow through the mitral valve in upright posture, so there is increase in left atrial pressure, and produce dyspnea.

But in supine position, the thrombus or tumor leave the orifice, increase the flow through the mitral valve, relieve dyspnea.

Trepopnea: Dyspnea occurs in lateral position, relieved by change in position.

- *Relieving factors:*
  - ❖ *Relieved by rest:* Coronary artery disease.
  - ❖ *Drugs:*
    - Nitroglycerin, beta blockers—CAD
    - Diuretics—CCF, LVF
    - Digoxin—In rapid ventricular response.
  - ❖ *Positions:*
    - Upright position—Bronchial asthma PND
    - Supine position—Left atrial myxoma, thrombus
    - Squatting position—Tetralogy of Fallot.

- *Associated symptoms:*
  - ❖ *Cough:*
    - May precede dyspnea—chronic obstructive lung disease
    - Respiratory cause—pneumonia
    - Cardiac cause may produce cough.
  - ❖ *Fever:*
    - Pleural effusion
    - Pneumonia
    - Infected bronchiectasis
    - Lung abscess
    - Subacute bacterial endocarditis
    - Winter bronchitis in mitral stenosis
    - Pulmonary tuberculosis, CAD.
  - ❖ *Cyanosis:*
    - Congenital cyanotic heart disease
    - COPD with Type II respiratory failure.
  - ❖ *Edema:*
    - Congestive heart failure
    - COPD
    - Angioneurotic edema.

■ Hemoptysis

Coughing of blood is called hemoptysis.
- *Congenital:*
  - ❖ Eisenmenger syndrome
  - ❖ Rupture of AV fistula.
- *Acquired:*
  - ❖ Mitral stenosis
  - ❖ Pulmonary embolism
  - ❖ Pulmonary infarction
  - ❖ Pulmonary edema
  - ❖ Rupture of bronchopulmonary AV fistula.
- *Drugs:*
  - ❖ Anticoagulant
  - ❖ Oral contraceptives.

Evaluation of a Patient with Hemoptysis

- *Duration, frequency and recurrence of hemoptysis:*
  - ❖ Mitral stenosis
  - ❖ Tuberculosis
  - ❖ Chronic bronchitis
  - ❖ Bronchiectasis.

- *Quantity of hemoptysis:*
  - ❖ *Small quantity:*
    - Mitral stenosis
    - Eisenmenger syndrome
    - Pulmonary infarction
    - Rupture of bronchopulmonary fistula.
  - ❖ *Massive quantity:*
    - Rupture of pulmonary arteriovenous fistula
    - Rupture of aortic aneurysm into bronchopulmonary artery.

Association
- *Chest pain:*
  - ❖ Pulmonary embolism
  - ❖ Pulmonary infarction
  - ❖ Rupture of aortic aneurysm.
- *Breathlessness:*
  - ❖ Pulmonary edema
  - ❖ Mitral stenosis
  - ❖ Rupture of aortic aneurysm
  - ❖ Eisenmenger syndrome (Fig. 4.29).
- *Type of sputum:*
  - ❖ *Pink frothy sputum:* Pulmonary edema.
  - ❖ *Blood tinged sputum:*
    - Mitral stenosis
    - Pulmonary embolism.
  - ❖ *Gray sputum:* Chronic obstructive pulmonary disease
  - ❖ *Fetid sputum:* Lung abscess
  - ❖ *Large amount:* Bronchiectasis
  - ❖ *Yellowish green:* Pulmonary infarction.

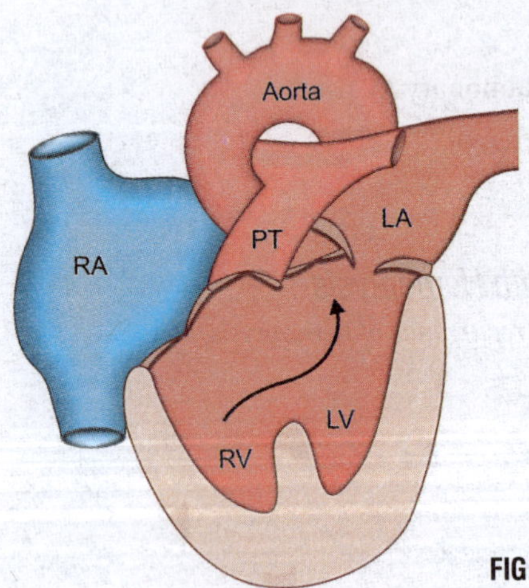

FIG. 4.29 Eisenmenger complex

- *Weight loss:* Ca lung, recurrent pulmonary infarction
- *Drugs:*
  - ❖ Oral anticoagulant
  - ❖ OCP
  - ❖ Immunosuppressive drugs.
- *Hoarseness of voice.*

Causes

- *Compression of recurrent laryngeal nerve by:*
  - ❖ Dilated right atrium
  - ❖ Dilated pulmonary artery
  - ❖ Aortic aneurysm.
- Myxedema
- Trauma to trachea due to intubation producing laryngitis.

CARDIOVASCULAR SYSTEM EXAMINATIONS

Main features of cardiovascular system examination are:
- General appearance of the patients
- Arterial pulse
- Jugular venous pressure
- Precordial area inspection
- Precordial area palpation
- Precordial percussion
- Precordial area auscultation.

Body Appearance and Facies

Anasarca—congestive cardiac failure.

Frightened, orthopneic, struggling, diaphoretic look—pulmonary edema.

Tall stature, long slender extremities, arm span exceeds patient's height, loss of subcutaneous fat—Marfan's syndrome (Figs 4.30A and B). These patient may present with signs of:
- Mitral valve prolapses
- Aortic dissection
- Aortic dilation.

Long extremities, kyphoscoliosis, pectus carinatum—Homocystinuria, may present with signs of arterial thromboembolism.

Tall stature, long extremities—Klinefelter's syndrome (Fig. 4.31), may present with the signs of:
- Atrial septal defect
- Ventricular septal defect
- Patent ductus arteriosus
- Tetralogy of Fallot.

Tall stature, thick extremities, club-shaped hands, thickened lips, frontal bossing—Acromegaly (Figs 4.32A to C), this patient may present with the signs of:
- Hypertension
- Cardiomyopathy
- Conduction defect

Short stature, webbed neck, low hair line, small chin, wide spaced nipples, sexual infantilism—Turner syndrome (Fig. 4.33). This patient may present with signs of:
- Coarctation of aorta
- Pulmonary valvular stenosis.

Short stature—Dwarfism (Fig. 4.34). This patient may present with the features of:
- Atrial septal defect
- Common atrium.

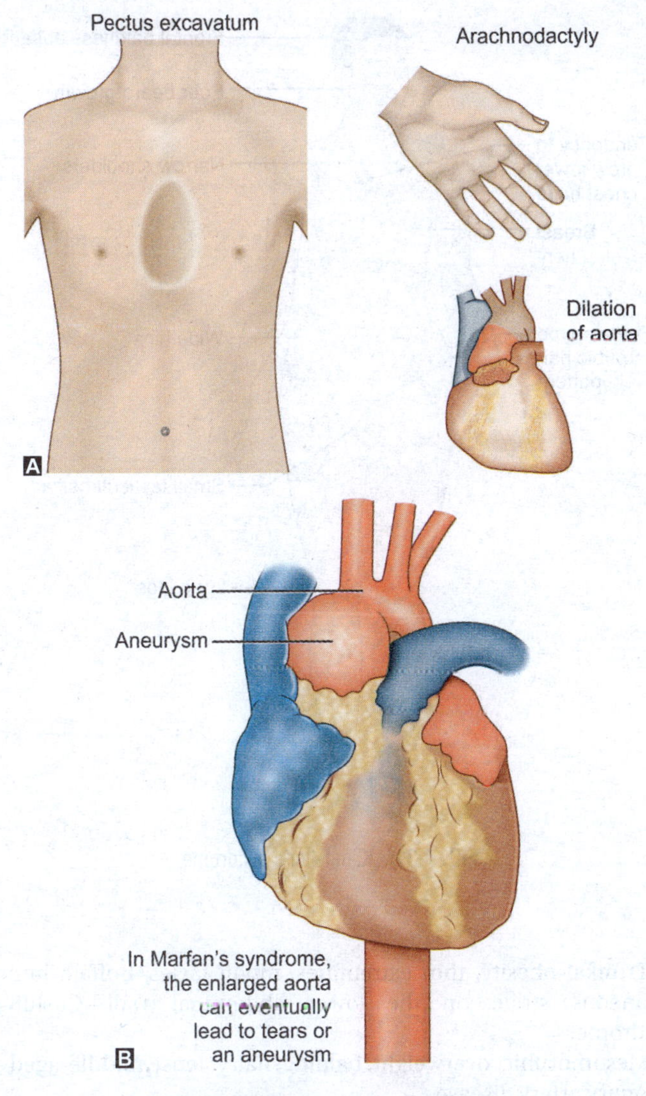

FIGS 4.30A AND B Marfan's syndrome

Morbid obesity, somnolence—Obstructive sleep apnea syndrome.
This patient may present with the features of:
- Hypoventilation
- Pulmonary hypertension
- Cor pumonale.

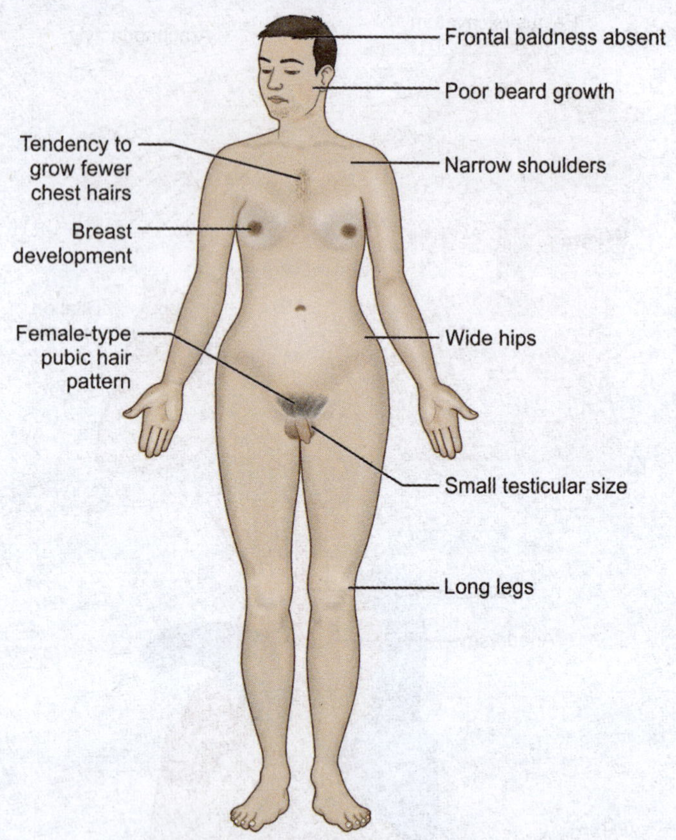

FIG. 4.31   Klinefelter's syndrome

Trunkal obesity, thin extremities, moon facies, buffalo hump, cutaneous striae on the lower abdominal wall—Cushing's syndrome.

Mesomorphic, overweight, balding, hairy, tense middle-aged — coronary artery disease.

Hammer toes, pes cavus—Friedreich ataxia, having the features of:
- Hypertrophic cardiomyopathy
- Angina
- Sick sinus syndrome

Straight lower back—Ankylosing spondylitis, having the features of:
- Aortic regurgitation
- Congenital heart block.

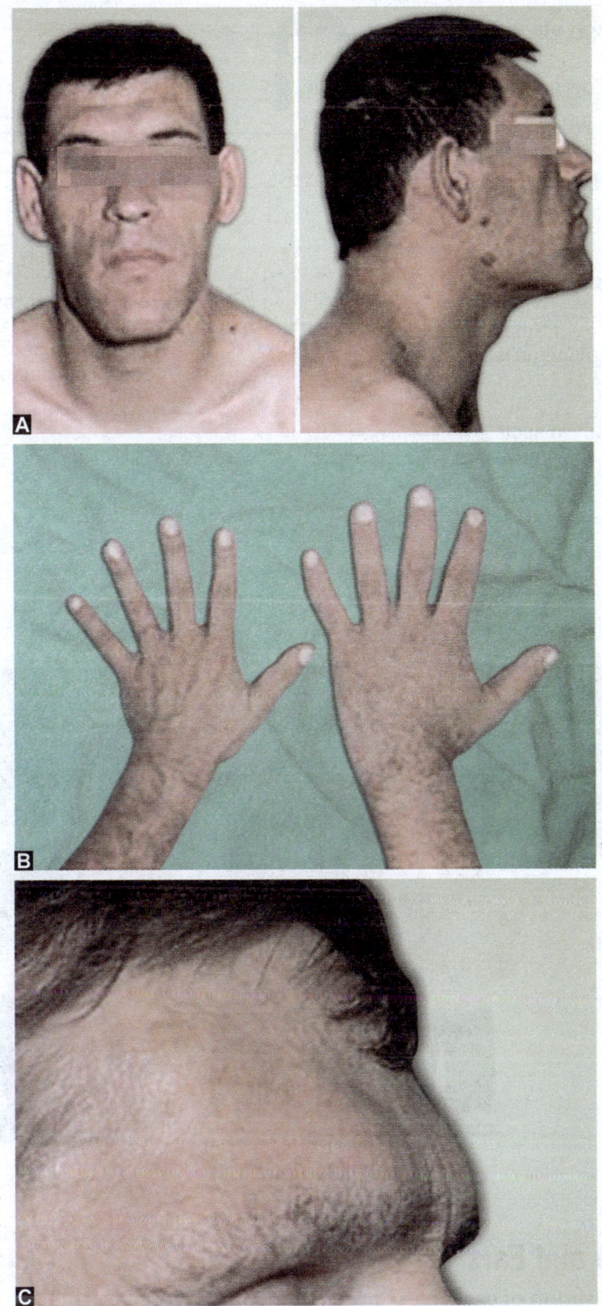

FIGS 4.32A TO C   (A) Acromegaly facial features; (B) Acromegaly hands; (C) Brow protrusion

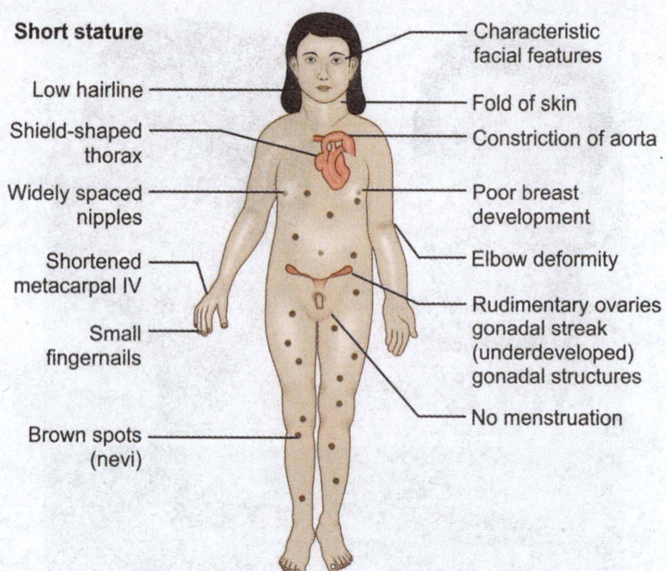

FIG. 4.33 Turner syndrome

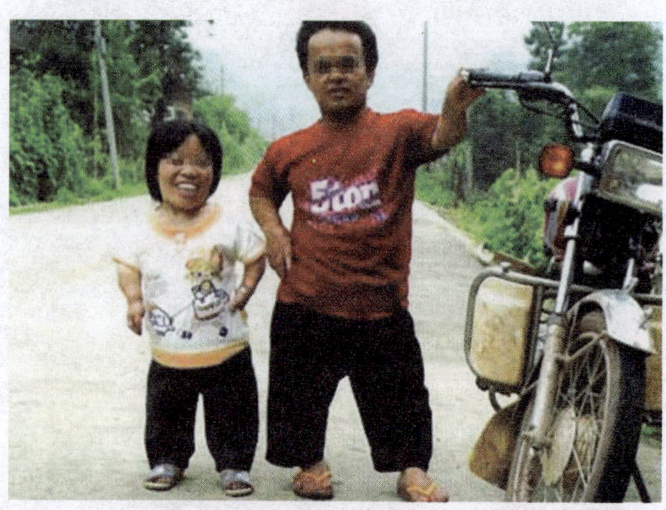

FIG. 4.34 Dwarfism

Face and Ears

- Pulsation of ear lobes—tricuspid regurgitation
- Nodding of head (De Musset's sign)—aortic regurgitation
- Round chubby face—congenital pulmonary stenosis

- Webbed neck, low set ears, hypertelorism, pigmented moles—Turner syndrome
- Unilateral lower facial weakness in infant—Cardiofacial syndrome
- Elfin facies (small chin, malformed teeth, wide set eyes, baggy cheeks, blunt and upturn nose) (Fig. 4.35):
  - ❖ Congenital pulmonary stenosis
  - ❖ Supravalvular aortic stenosis.
- Premature aging:
  - ❖ Progeria (Fig. 4.36)
  - ❖ Werner's syndrome.

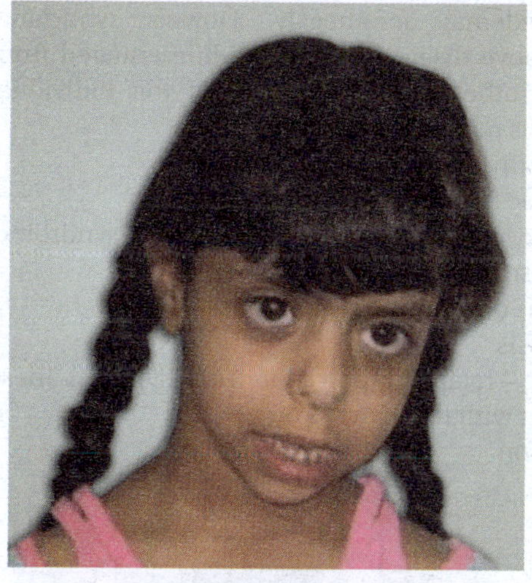

FIG. 4.35   Elfin facies

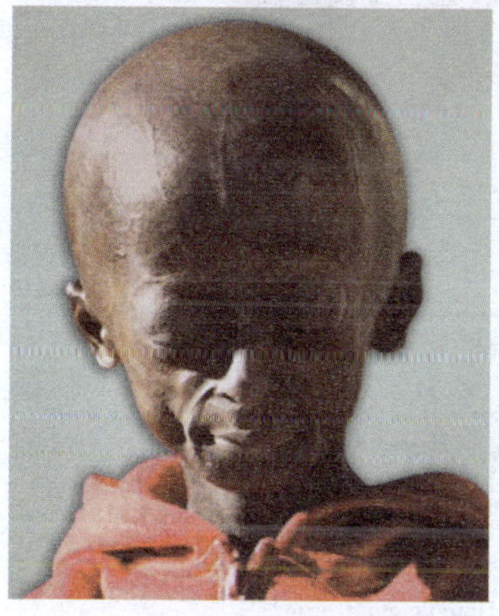

FIG. 4.36   Progeria

- Drooping of eyelids, expressionless face, bilateral cataract, receded hairline—Steinert's disease, may present with:
  - ❖ Conduction defect
  - ❖ Mitral valve prolapes.
- Slanting eyes, increase epicanthic fold, protruding tongue, saliva dribbling, small ears, flat nasal bridge, short nose—Down's syndrome, may present with—endocardial cushion defect (Fig. 4.37)
- Puffy face, thickened lips, loss of lateral part of eye brow, protruding tongue, thickened and dry skin—myxedema. This case may present with the features of:
  - ❖ Pericardial effusion
  - ❖ Coronary artery disease.
- Macroglossia—myxedema, acromegaly, Down's syndrome, amyloidosis. The above diseases are to be differentiated from each other by the other specific features of the individual diseases. Amyloidosis patient may present with:
  - ❖ Restrictive cardiomyopathy
  - ❖ Congestive cardiac failure.
- Recurrent and paroxysmal facial flushing—Carcinoid syndrome, this patient may present with features of:
  - ❖ Tricuspid stenosis or tricuspid regurgitation
  - ❖ Pulmonary stenosis.
- Saddle shaped nose—relapsing polychondritis, syphilis. These patients may present with the features of:
  - ❖ Aortic regurgitation
  - ❖ Aortic aneurysm.

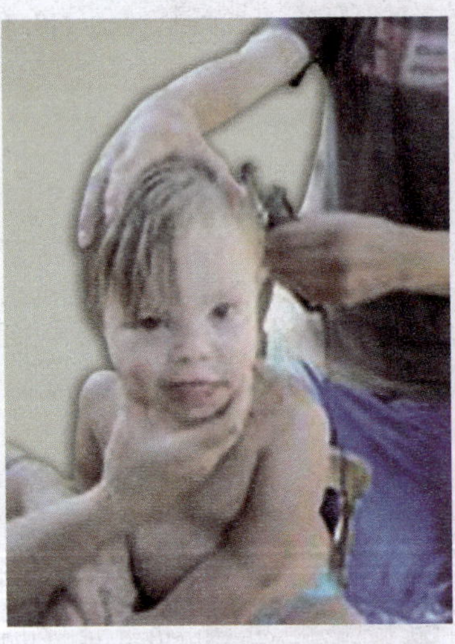

FIG. 4.37 Down's syndrome

- Tightening of skin, telangiectasia, fish mouth appearance, differential pigmentation—scleroderma, may present with:
  - ❖ Pericarditis
  - ❖ Myocarditis
  - ❖ Pulmonary hypertension.
- Malar flush—Mitral stenosis
- Gargoylism—Hurler syndrome, may present with (Fig. 4.38):
  - ❖ Mitral valve disease
  - ❖ Aortic valve disease.
- Diagonal ear lobe crease—coronary artery disease, may present with the features of coronary artery disease
- Narrow palpable fissure, hypoplastic mandible, small upper lip—fetal alcohol syndrome, may present with the features of (Figs 4.39A to D):
  - ❖ Atrial septal defect
  - ❖ Ventricular septal defect.

Gesture, Gait and Stance

- *Levine's sign:* Clenched fist over the chest of the patient—acute myocardial infarction (Fig. 4.40)
- Preference of squatting—Tetralogy of Fallot
- Ataxic gait—Tertiary syphilis—associated with:
  - ❖ Syphilitic aortic regurgitation
  - ❖ Aortic regurgitation.
- Waddling gait with lumbar lordosis and pseudohypertrophy of calves:
  - ❖ Hypertrophic cardiomyopathy
  - ❖ Pseudoinfarction in ECG.

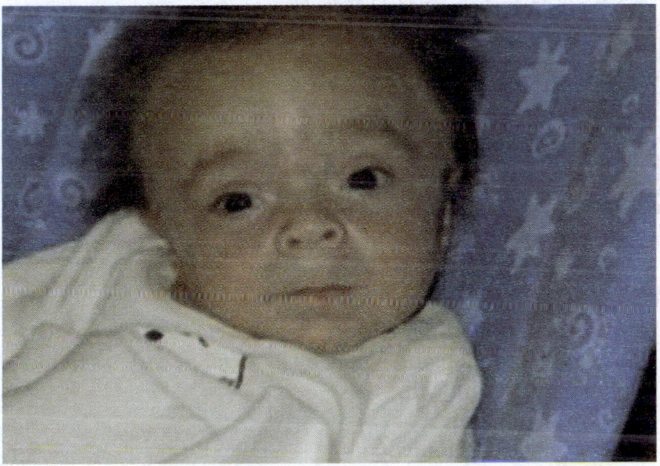

FIG. 4.38   Hurler syndrome

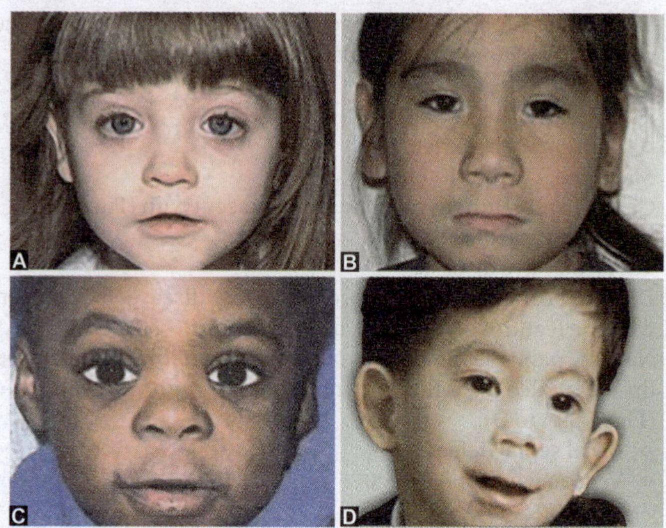

FIGS 4.39A TO D Fetal alcohol syndrome facial pictures

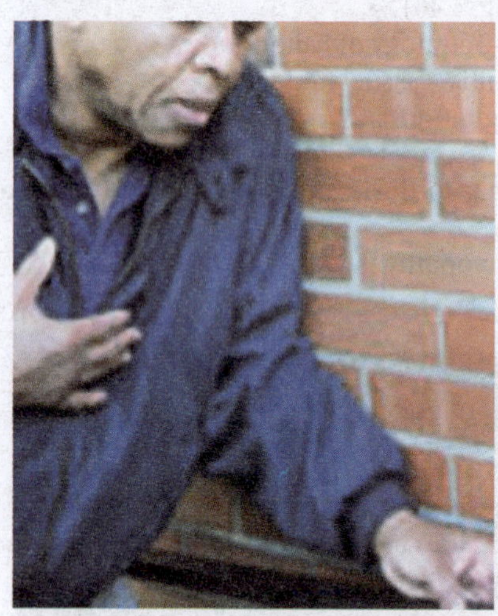

FIG. 4.40 Heart attack

Eyes

- Xanthelasma—coronary artery disease (Fig. 4.41)
- Enlarged lacrimal gland—may be associated with—sarcoidosis, which may present with:
  - ❖ Conduction defect
  - ❖ Restrictive cardiomyopathy
  - ❖ Cor pulmonale.

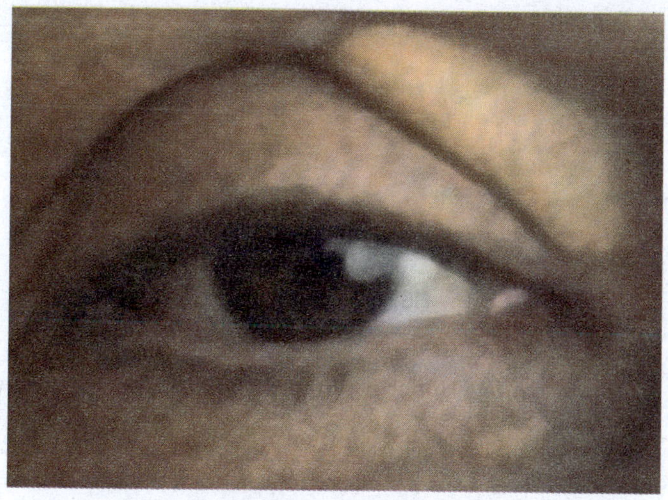

FIG. 4.41 Xanthelasma

- Cataract, deafness—Rubella syndrome, which may be associated with:
  - ❖ Patent ductus arteriosus
  - ❖ Pulmonary artery stenosis.
- Proptosis and staring look—high central venous pressure
- Lid lag, stare, exophthalmos—hyperthyroidism, which may be associated with:
  - ❖ Angina
  - ❖ Tachycardia
  - ❖ High output failure.
- Conjunctival patches—endocarditis
- Bluesclera (Fig. 4.42)—osteogenesis imperfacta—may be associated with aortic regurgitation
- Brushfield's spots (small whitish spots on the periphery of iris)—Down's syndrome, which may be associated with endocardial cushion defect
- Fissure in iris—coloboma—may be associated with total anomalous pulmonary venous return
- Dissociated lens—Marfan's syndrome
- Retinal changes:
  - ❖ Hypertension
  - ❖ Diabetes.
- Roth spot—infective endocarditis
- *Arcus Juvenilis:* Yellowish white ring in the outer margin of cornea—dyslipidemia
- *Arcus senilis:* Grayish-white crescent, or circle seen on the outer margin cornea—old eye

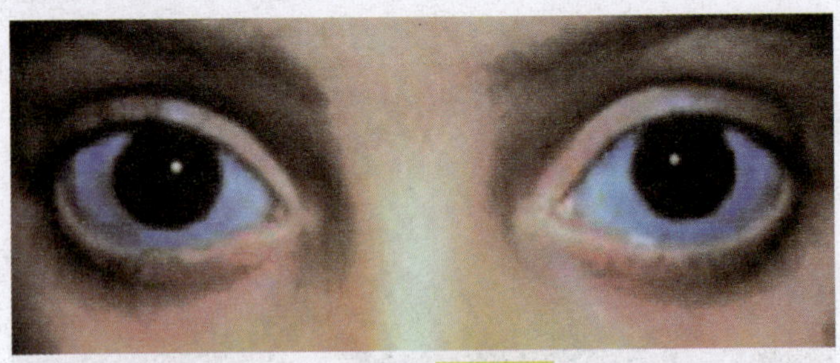

FIG. 4.42 Bluesclera

- *Corneal clouding:* Hurler syndrome, type IV and VI mucopoly-saccharidosis
- *Hypertelorism:* Distance between two eyes is more than the size of one eye:
  - Noonan syndrome—PS
  - Turner syndrome—coarctation of aorta
  - William's syndrome—AS or PS
  - Hurler syndrome—valvular regurgitation
- *Exophthalmos:*
  - Thyrotoxicosis—may be associated with lid lag or lid retraction—hyperdynamic circulation
  - Pulsatile exophthalmos—TR.
- *Ptosis:*
  - External ophthalmoplegia, pigmentary retinopathy, myocardial disease, heart block
  - Klippel–Feil syndrome.
- *Pallor:* Anemia
- *Nystagmus:* Friedreich's ataxia—may be associated with kyphoscoliosis, HOCMSA nodal artery occlusion
- *Argyll Robertson pupil:* In neurosyphilis—may be associated with aortic regurgitation.

Extremities

- *Central cyanosis with clubbing:*
  - Right to left shunt
  - Pulmonary arteriovenous fistula
  - Inferior vena cava drainage into left atrium.
- *Differential cyanosis with clubbing:*
  - Patent ductus arteriosus with pulmonary hypertension
    Reverse shunt limits the cyanosis and clubbing of feet but spares the hands.
- *Tight tapered and contracted fingers, ischemic ulcers and hypoplastic nails—scleroderma, may be associated with:*

- ❖ Pericarditis
- ❖ Restrictive cardiomyopathy
- ❖ Pulmonary hypertension.
- *Arachnodactyly, hyperextensable joints (knee, wrist and fingers), flat feet—Marfan's syndrome, may be associated with:*
  - ❖ Aortic aneurysm
  - ❖ Aortic regurgitation.
- *Ulnar deviation of hands:*
  - ❖ Pericarditis
  - ❖ Myocarditis
  - ❖ Valvular heart disease.
- *Hyperemicthener and hypothener eminences:* Liver disease
- *Reversal of differential cyanosis and clubbing:* Transposition of great vessels—aorta originates from right ventricle
- *Sudden pain, pallor and coldness:* Peripheral embolization
- *Osler nodes (Figs 4.43A and B):* (Swollen, tender, raised pea shaped lesions in finger pads, palms and soles)—subacute bacterial endocarditis
- *Janeway lesion (Fig. 4.44):* (Small nontender erythematous or hemorrhagic lesion on the palm and sole)—subacute bacterial endocarditis
- *Raynaud's phenomenon* in scleroderma
- *Simian line in the palm (single palmar crease)—Down's syndrome, which may be associated with:*
  - ❖ ASD
  - ❖ VSD.
- *Pedal edema:* Congestive cardiac failure.

Skin

- *Jaundice:* Hepatic congestion
- *Cyanosis:* Right to left heart shunt
- *Pallor or anemia:* High output failure
- *Bronzing of skin:* Hemochromatosis, may be associated with restrictive cardiomyopathy
- *Telangiectasia:*
  - ❖ Rendu-Osler-Weber disease
  - ❖ Pulmonary arteriovenous fistula.
- *Neurofibroma (Fig. 4.45):* Café-au-lait spot, axillary freckles (Crowe's sign)—von-Recklinghausen's disease
- *Symmetric vitiligo of distal extremities:* Hyperthyroidism
- *Butterfly rash (Fig. 4.46)—systemic lupus erythematosus, which may be associated with:*
  - ❖ Endocarditis
  - ❖ Myocarditis
  - ❖ Pericarditis.

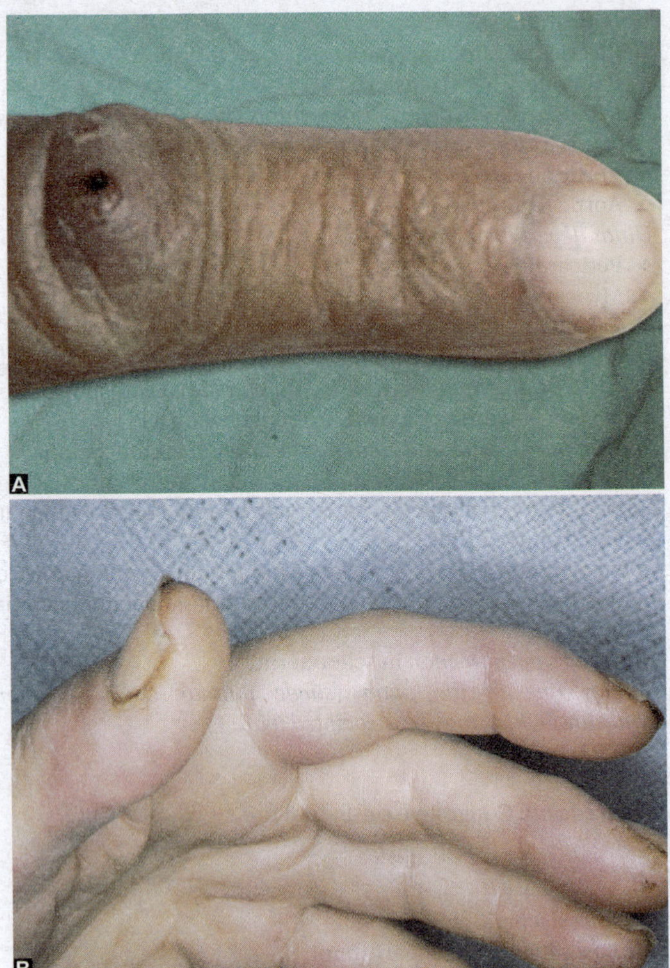

FIGS 4.43A AND B   (A) Osler nodules hand; (B) Osler nodes

- *Purplish discoloration of eye lids—dermatomyositis (Fig. 4.47), which may be associated with:*
  - ❖ Cardiomyopathy
  - ❖ Heart block
  - ❖ Pericarditis.
- *Macules and nodules in the skin:*
  - ❖ *Sarcoidosis:*
    - • Cardiomyopathy
    - • Heart block.
- *Xanthoma:* Hyperlipidemia

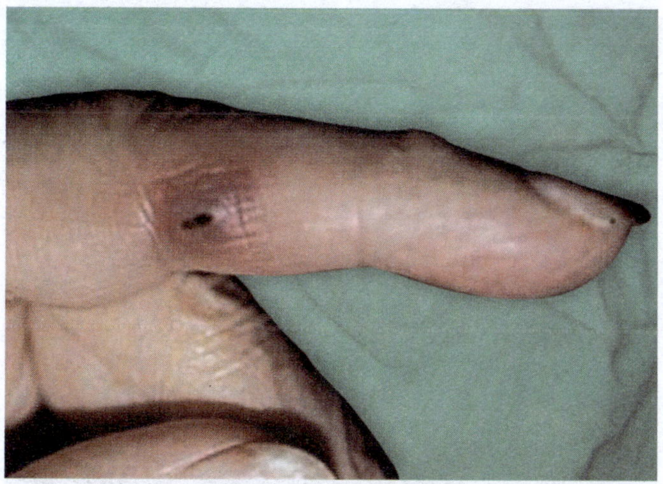

FIG. 4.44   Janeway lesion

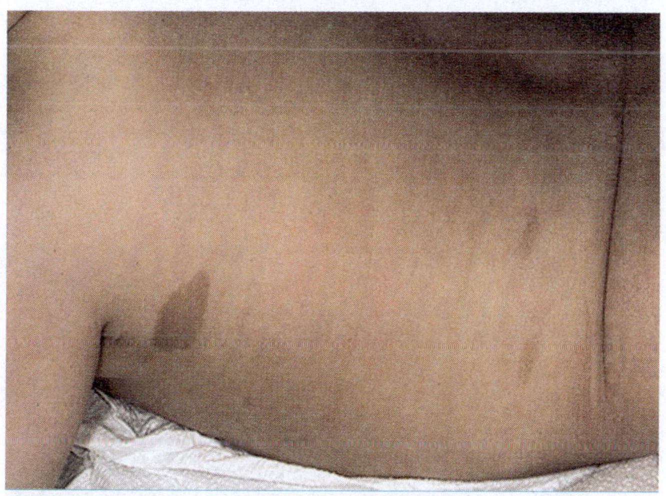

FIG. 4.45   Café-au-lait spot

- *Hyperextensible skin:*
  - ❖ *Ehlers-Danlos syndrome (Fig. 4.48)*
    - Mitral valve prolapse.
- Coarse, shallow, dry skin and sparse hair—hyperthyroidism
- *Skin nodules (Sebaceous adenoma), shagreen patches and periungual fibroma Tuberous sclerosis (Fig. 4.49):*
  - ❖ Rhabdomyoma of heart
  - ❖ Arrhythmias.

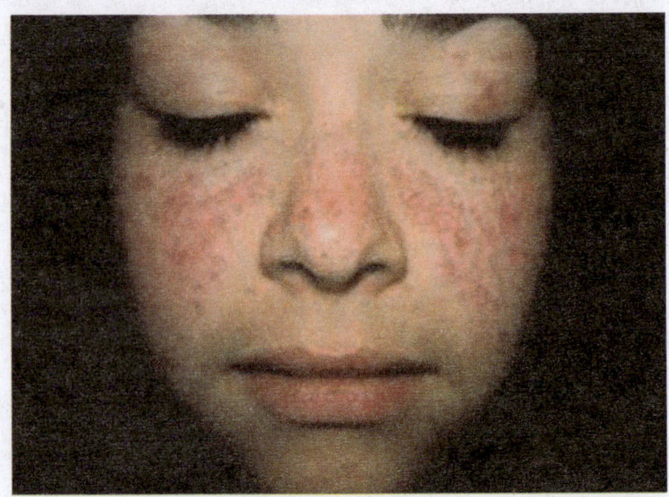

FIG. 4.46 Butterfly rash

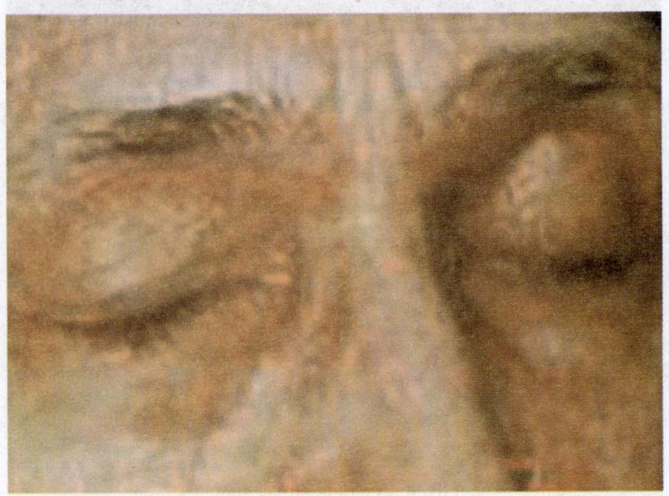

FIG. 4.47 Purplish discoloration of the face in dermatomyositis

Thorax and Abdomen

- *Thoracic bulge:*
  - ❖ Atrial septal defect
  - ❖ Ventricular septal defect.
- *Straight back syndrome—loss of normal thoracic kyphosis:* Mitral valve prolapse syndrome

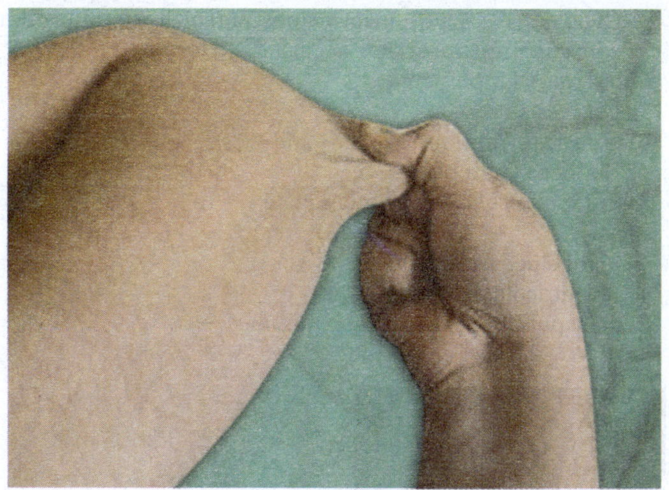

FIG. 4.48   Ehlers-Danlos syndrome

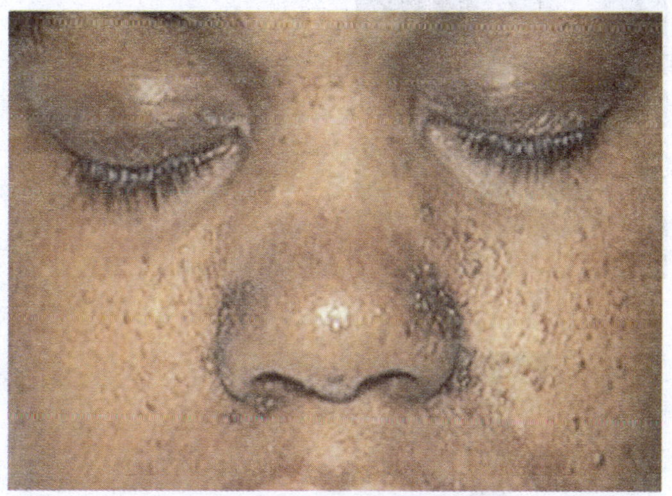

FIG. 4.49   Tuberous sclerosis

- *Pectus carinatum, kyphoscoliosis:*
  - ❖ Marfan's syndrome
  - ❖ Noonan syndrome.
- *Pectus excavatum:*
  - ❖ Homocystinuria
  - ❖ Ehlers-Danlos syndrome
  - ❖ Rickets

- ❖ Cobblers (Fig. 4.50)—in lower most part of the sternum due to constant pressure of shoe against it.
- *Barrel chest:* Emphysema
- *Shield chest:*
  - ❖ Turner's syndrome (Figs 4.51 and 4.52)
  - ❖ Noonan syndrome.
- *Severe kyphoscoliosis:* Cor pulmonale
- *Ascites:*
  - ❖ Right-sided heart failure
  - ❖ Biventricular failure
- Hepatic pulsation—tricuspid syndrome

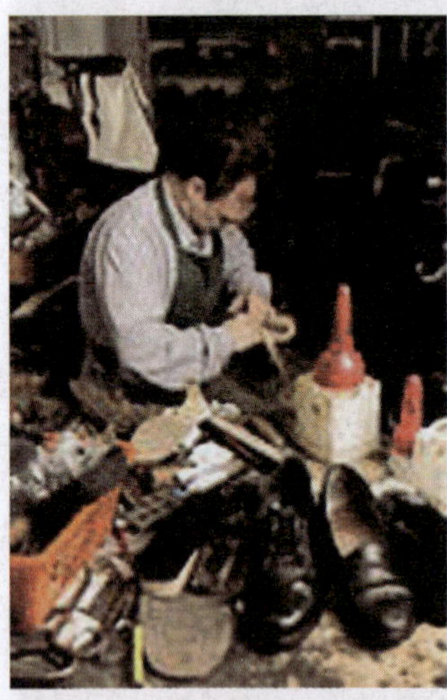

FIG. 4.50 Cobbler

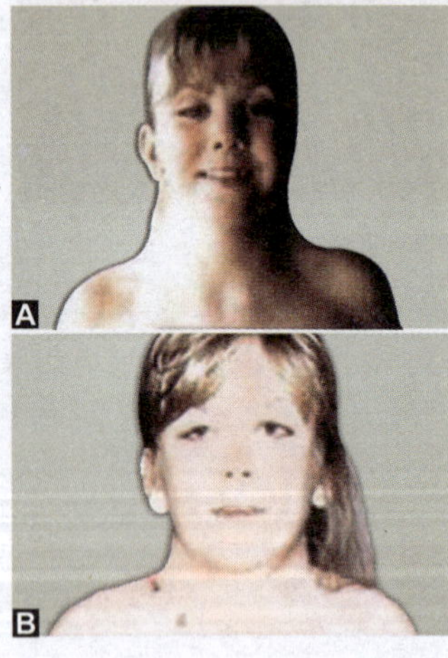

FIGS 4.51A AND B Neck turner

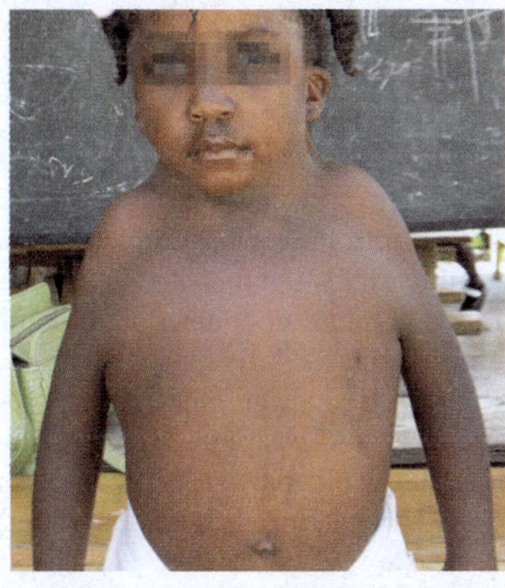

FIG. 4.52 Turner's syndrome

- Positive abdominojugular reflux—congestive heart failure
- Muscular thorax with thin lower limbs—coarctation of aorta
- Bulging of right upper syndrome—aortic aneurysm.

Abnormalities of Breast

- *Male gynecomastia—unilateral or bilateral:*
  - ❖ Digitalis toxicity
  - ❖ Klinefelter's syndrome.
- Female hypomastia—mitral valve prolapse
- *Wide-spaced nipples:*
  - ❖ Turner's syndrome
  - ❖ Noonan syndrome.

Arterial Pulse

Aim Behind Palpation of Arterial Pulse

- Arteries of both side must be palpated and compared to detect asymmetries, suggestive of:
  - ❖ Embolic occlusion
  - ❖ Thrombosis
  - ❖ Atherosclerosis
  - ❖ Dissection
  - ❖ Extrinsic occlusion.
- Arteries of upper and lower extremities simultaneously examined to detect any delay, suggestive of—aortic coarctation
- To detect any arterial waveform—central arteries should be examined, e.g.
  - ❖ Carotid
  - ❖ Brachial
  - ❖ Femoral.

Method of Palpating Arteries

- Right radial pulse of the patient can be best felt by fingers of examiner's left hand—used to asses (Fig. 4.53)
  - ❖ Heart rate
  - ❖ Heart rhythm
  - ❖ Compare the radial pulses of both hands simultaneously to detect the pulse volume timing or any delay
  - ❖ Simultaneous feeling of radial and femoral pulses of the same side to detect any radiofemoral delay.
- *Brachial pulse (Fig. 4.54):* Right pulse can be best palpated by using the thumb of right hand of examiner applied to the flexor aspect of the elbow just medial to biceps tendon and other fingers cupped back behind the elbow. Thumb is used to detect the character of the pulse
- *Carotid pulse (Fig. 4.55):*
  - ❖ Right carotid artery must be located by the tip of the thumb of examiner against the patient's larynx and give firm and gentle pressure directing backwards, so that, the artery can be best palpated against precervical muscles
  - ❖ Carotid pulse can be felt from behind by curling the fingers around the sides of the neck.

  This artery can be used to detect pulse character, e.g.:
  - ❖ Aortic stenosis
  - ❖ Hypertrophic obstructive cardiomyopathy.
- *Femoral pulse (Fig. 4.56):* Patient must be in lying down position with groin area exposed. Examiner's thumb or fingers should be

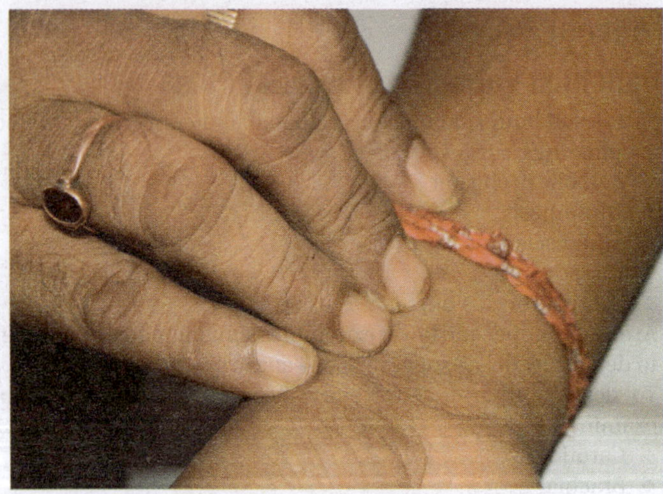

FIG. 4.53   Right radial pulse

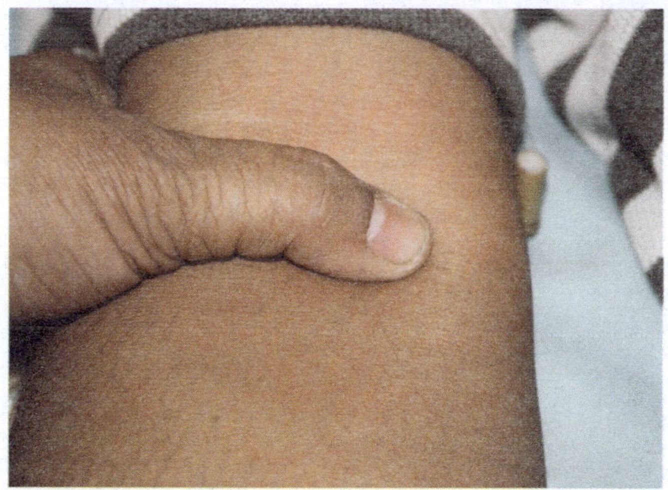

FIG. 4.54   Brachial pulse

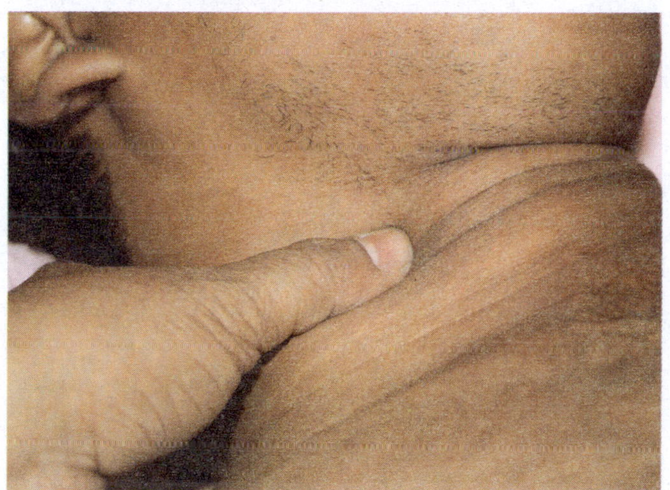

FIG. 4.55   Carotid pulse

placed directly above the superior pubic ramus midway between pubic tubercle and anterior superior iliac spine

- *Popliteal pulse (Fig. 4.57):* This artery is present deep in popliteal fossa. Patient must be lying down position with knee slightly flexed. The fingers of one hand are used to press the tips of the fingers of the other hand into popliteal fossa, so that, this artery can be felt against the back of the knee joint. This artery is usually palpated to evaluate intermittent claudication

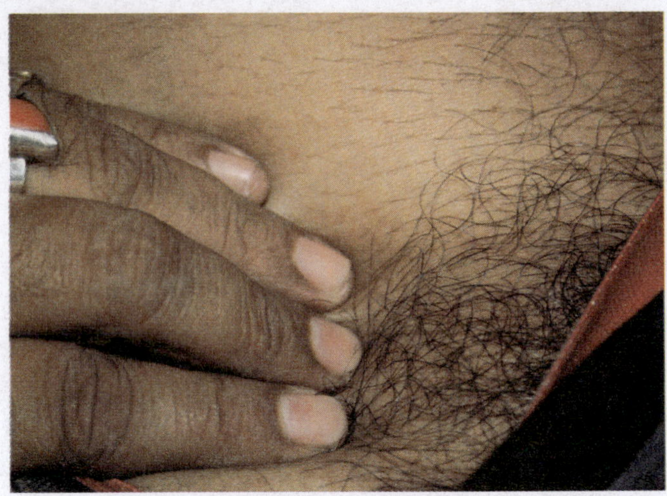

FIG. 4.56 Femoral pulse

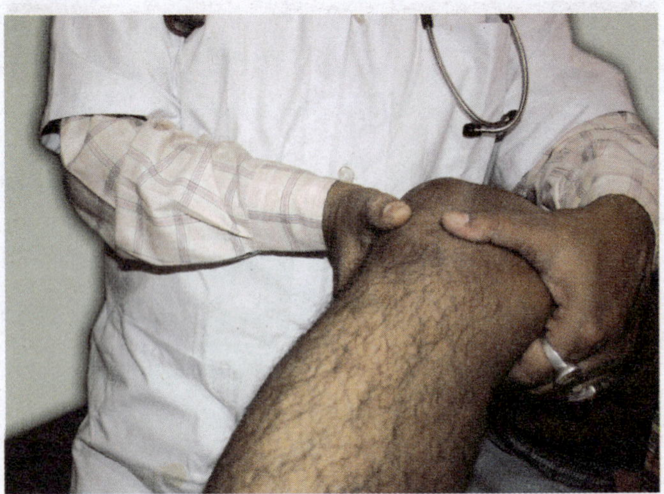

FIG. 4.57 Popliteal pulse

- *Tibialis posterior (Fig. 4.58):* This artery can be palpated with fingers cupped around the ankle joint posterior to medial malleolus
- *Arterial dorsalis pedis (Fig. 4.59):* This artery can be palpated with fingers aligned along the dorsum of the foot lateral to extensor hallucis longus tendon. This artery is usually palpated to see adequacy of the circulation

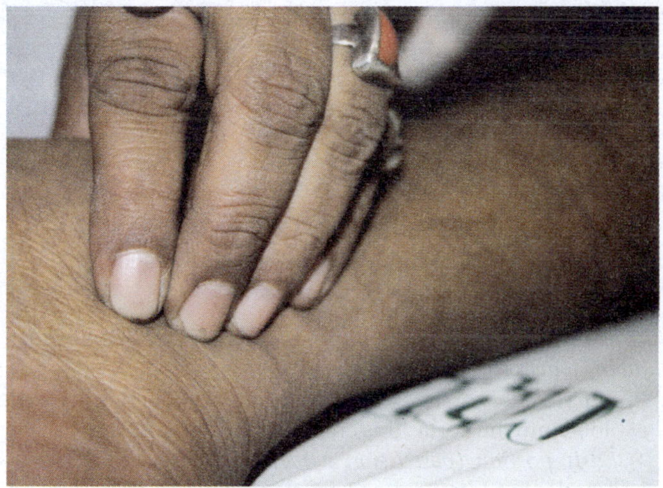

FIG. 4.58 Tibialis posterior

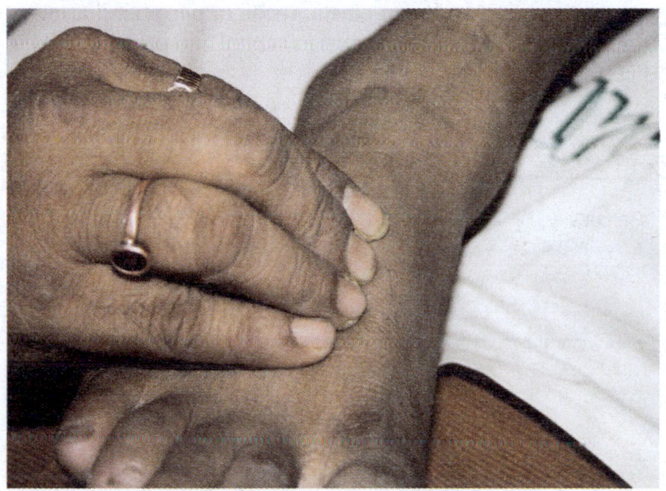

FIG. 4.59 Arterial dorsalis pedis

Major attention in peripheral arteries is detect increase in amplitude or upstroke, velocity, because the percussion wave transmitted downward from heart along the aorta begins to merge with the secondary waves that revert back from peripheral arteries. As a result of fusion, the pulse amplitude becomes higher as compared with central arteries and the waves become taller.

The following things must be evaluated in arterial pulse:
- Rate
- Rhythm
- Volume
- Contour
- Speed of upstroke
- Speed of downstroke
- Stiffness of arterial wall
- Presence of palpable shudder
- Presence of bruit or transmitted murmur.

Characteristics of normal pulse—normal pulse comprises of following waves (Fig. 4.60):
- *Primary systolic wave:* This wave is generated by ejection of blood into the aorta. This consists of:
  - *Early portion (percussion wave):* This reflects discharge of blood into central aorta by left ventricular ejection
  - *Mid and late portion (tidal wave):* Reflects movement of blood from central to peripheral aorta.
- *Dicrotic wave:* It is due to elastic recoil of peripheral arteries of the arteries. (Pulse wave pattern in central and peripheral arteries Fig. 4.61).

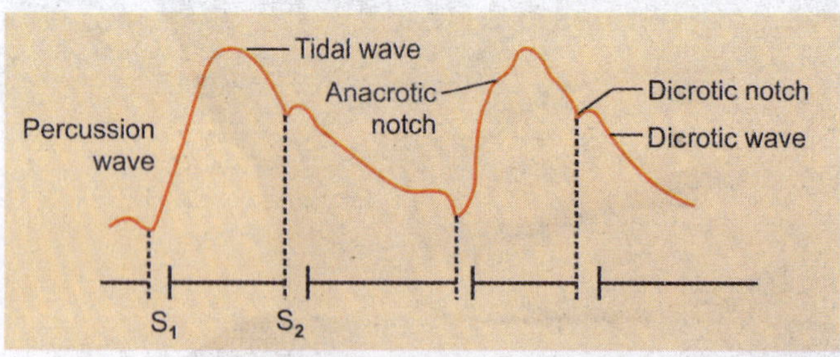

FIG. 4.60 Characteristic of normal pulse

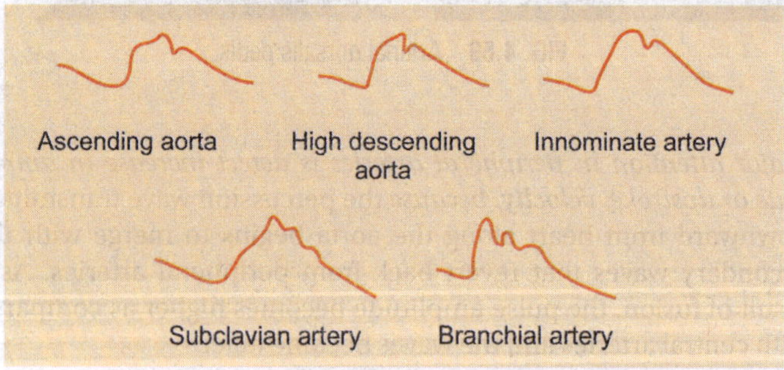

FIG. 4.61 Pulse wave in central and peripheral arteries

In ascending aorta:
- Pulse wave rises rapidly to a rounded dome with a small notch on upstroke, occasionally felt but frequently recorded
- Descending limb is less steep interrupted by a notch, produced by closure of aortic valve
- This is immediately followed by slight rise and then gradual declining in pressure.

In peripheral arteries: As the pulse wave gradually progresses downward, e.g.
- Carotid artery at 30 msec
- Brachial artery at 60 msec
- Femoral artery at 75 msec
- Radial artery at 80 msec.

In these arteries, the waves are distorted, because:
- Distortion of pulse wave forms
- Different rates of waves in different arteries
- Changes in the vessel wall
- Distortion of reflected waves.

As a result:
- Ascending wave becomes steeper
- Tidal wave will be less significant
- Anacrotic notch disappears
- Steep diacrotic notch will be replaced by smoother ones and appears later.
- So the pulse felt peripherally are the summation of forward and reflected waves.

The examination of arterial pulse can be measured according to the following scale:
- Grade 0—No pulse on palpation
- Grade 1+—Feeble pulse
- Grade 2+—Diminished as compared to other side
- Grade 3+—Normal pulse
- Grade 4+—Bounding pulse.

Rate: Normal sinus rate
- Just after birth to 1 week—140/minute
- During 6th year—100/minute
- After puberty—80/minute.

Increased rate (Fig. 4.62A)
- *Physiological:*
  - ❖ Childhood
  - ❖ Exercise
  - ❖ Anxiety
  - ❖ Emotional stress.

- *Pathological, not related directly to cardiac disease:*
  - ❖ Fever
  - ❖ Thyrotoxicosis
  - ❖ Anemia
  - ❖ Beriberi.
- *Pathological, related to drug and drugs of intoxication:*
  - ❖ Epinephrine
  - ❖ Atropine
  - ❖ Amyl nitrate
  - ❖ Nicotine
  - ❖ Alcohol.
- *Cardiac cause:*
  - ❖ Supraventricular tachycardia
  - ❖ Atrial flutter
  - ❖ Atrial fibrillation
  - ❖ Ventricular tachycardia
  - ❖ Ventricular fibrillation.

Decreased rate (Fig. 4.62B): Sinus bradycardia—rate <60/minute.

Causes of sinus bradycardia

- *Physiological causes:*
  - ❖ Trained athlete
  - ❖ Deep sleep.
- *Pharmacological causes:*
  - ❖ Acetylcholine
  - ❖ Diltiazem
  - ❖ Verapamil
  - ❖ Digoxin
  - ❖ Beta blocker.
- *Cardiac causes:*
  - ❖ Carotid sinus hypersensitivity
  - ❖ Sick sinus syndrome
  - ❖ Second degree heart block
  - ❖ Complete heart block (Fig. 4.63).

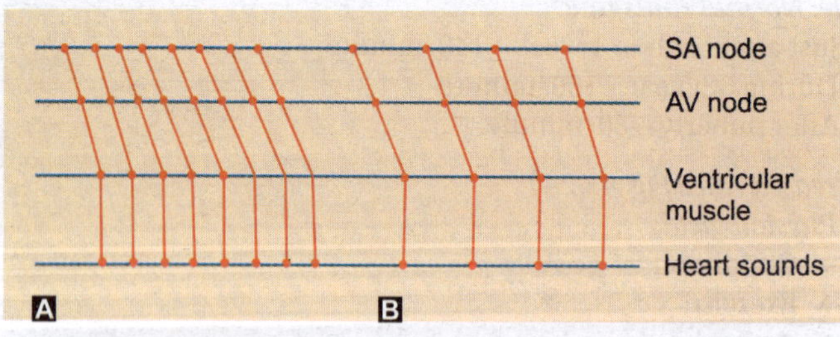

FIGS 4.62A AND B   (A) Sinus tachycardia; (B) Sinus bradycardia

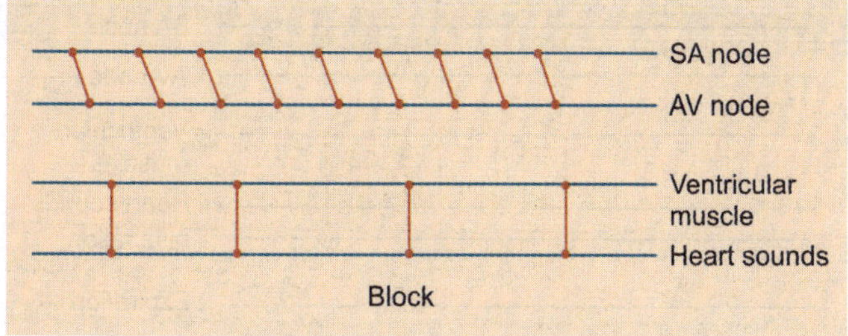

FIG. 4.63   Complete heart block

- *Noncardiac causes:*
  - ❖ Myxedema
  - ❖ Increased intracranial pressure
  - ❖ Hypothermia
  - ❖ Obstructive jaundice
  - ❖ First week of typhoid fever
  - ❖ Viral fever
  - ❖ Gram negative sepsis.

Rhythm

This is defined by palpation of pulse at definite interval. This can be:
- *Regularly irregular:*
  - ❖ *Sinus arrhythmia (Fig. 4.64):* It is present when variation between the longest and shortest P-P interval is more than 0.12 second
    - • Variation with respiration
    - • Common in children.
  - ❖ *Pulsus bigeminus, pulsus trigeminus:*
    - • Exercise
    - • Alcohol
    - • Digoxin
    - • Structural cardiac diseases.
- *Irregularly irregular rate (Fig. 4.65)*
  - ❖ Multifocal atrial tachycardia
  - ❖ Atrial fibrillation
  - ❖ Atrial flutter with varying block
  - ❖ Recurrent atrial or ventricular ectopic (Fig. 4.66).
- *Pulse deficit:* This is defined by difference between pulse rate and heart rate
  - ❖ If the difference is >6/minute—atrial fibrillation
  - ❖ If the difference is <6/minute—premature ventricular contraction.

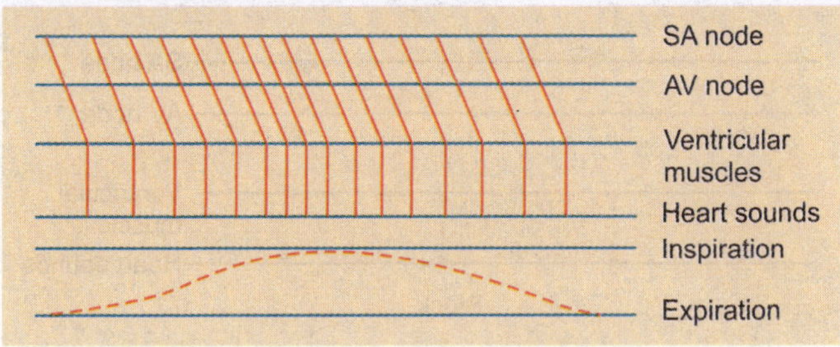

FIG. 4.64   Sinus arrhythmia

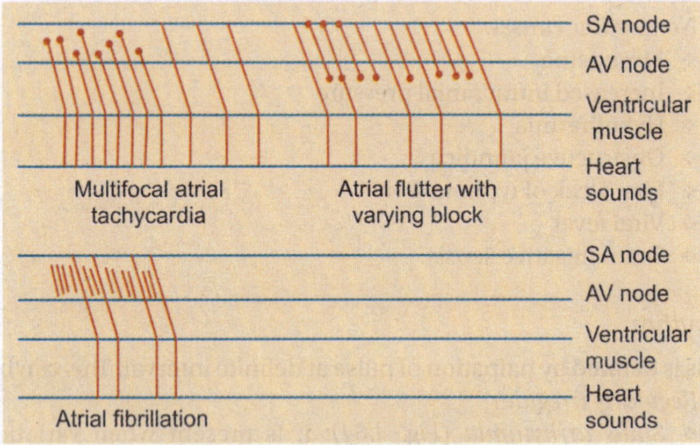

FIG. 4.65   Irregularly irregular rate

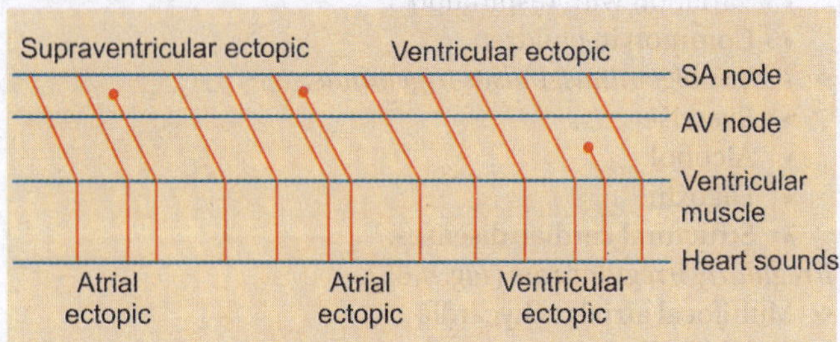

FIG. 4.66   Ectopic beats

Best technique to evaluate brachial pulse.
First obliterate the brachial pulse.
Slowly release the pressure over the brachial artery until you feel the pulse.

At this point you measure amplitude and contour of the brachial pulse.

Character of pulses (Fig. 4.67)
- *Pulsus tardus:* Slow rise with delayed peak—aortic stenosis
- *Pulsus parvus:* Low volume pulse—it occurs in:
  - ❖ Left ventricular outflow tract obstruction—aortic stenosis
  - ❖ Diminished left ventricular obstruction—dilated cardiomyo-pathy
  - ❖ Diminished left ventricular filling—mitral stenosis.

Difference between pulsus tardus and pulsus parvus
- *In pulsus parvus:* Volume is small but upstroke is normal
- *In pulsus tardus:* Upstroke is delayed e.g. aortic stenosis.

In arterial atherosclerosis—due to thickening of arterial wall the upstroke is brisk, hence pulsus tardus is not delayed. In aortic stenosis, there is apical—carotid artery delay or brachioradial delay.

Correlation between pulsus tardus and severity of aortic stenosis: If left ventricular function is good—rate of slow rise correlates with severity of aortic stenosis.

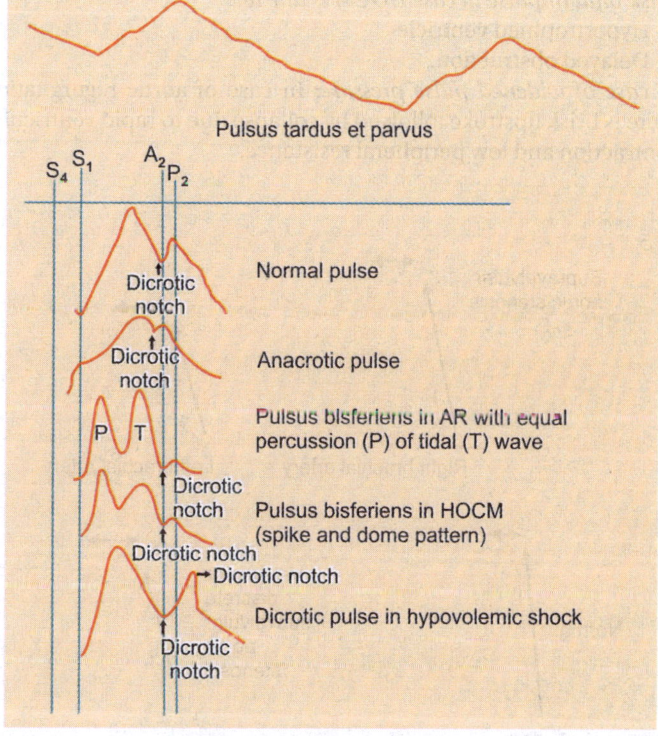

FIG. 4.67   Character of pulses

If left ventricle is failing—pulsus tardus occurs with mild aortic stenosis.

Presence of pulsus tardus indicates pressure gradient between the aorta and left ventricle is >70 mm Hg.

Difference between valvular and supravalvular aortic stenosis (Fig. 4.68)

In supravalvular aortic stenosis:
- Right brachial artery shows normal pulse
- Left brachial artery shows pulse of valvular aortic stenosis.

In subvalvular aortic stenosis:
- Arterial pulse is brisk
- Systolic pulse is double.

Significance of brisk arterial upstroke—significance of brisk arterial upstroke depends upon normal and widened pulse pressure.

In case of normal arterial pressure: Simultaneous emptying of left ventricle to high pressure bed (aorta) or low pressure bed (left atrium in mitral regurgitation, right ventricle in case of ventricular septal defect) produce brisk arterial upstroke.

Brisk bifid impulse in case HOCM is due to:
- Hypertrophied ventricle
- Delayed obstruction.

In case of widened pulse pressure: In case of aortic regurgitation there is brisk upstroke followed by collapse due to rapid ventricular contraction and low peripheral resistance.

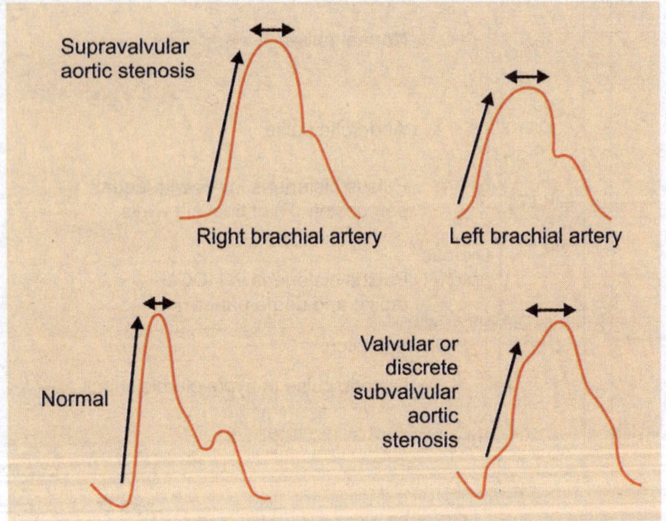

FIG. 4.68 Valvular or discrete subvalvular and supravalvular aortic stenosis

In case of hyperkinetic states:
- Anemia
- Fever
- Beriberi
- Pregnancy
- Thyrotoxicosis
- AV fistula
- Cirrhosis
- Paget's disease
- Patent ductus arteriosus
- Anxiety.

Pulsus Paradoxus

Exacerbation in fall of systolic blood pressure during quiet-inspiration as evidenced by pulse amplitude despite normal and regular rhythm. If systolic blood pressure decreases more than 12+–2 mm Hg during inspiration—denotes pulsus paradoxus.

Pulsus paradoxus can be best detected in radial and brachial artery if inspiratory systolic pressure drop >20 mm Hg.

Peripheral arteries (wrist is better than the arm or neck) are best suited for detecting pulsus paradoxus.

Although palpable, best detection can be done by sphygmo-manometer.

The pulsus paradoxus occurs in:
Pathological:
- Pregnancy
- Extreme obesity
- Student's paradox
- COPD
- Pericardial tamponade
- Massive pulmonary embolism
- Restrictive cardiomyopathy.

Pathophysiology of pulsus paradoxus (Flow chart 4.3)
Normally during inspiration fall in intrapericardial pressure in –3 to –6 mm Hg, which increase right ventricular transmural pressure and venous return.

Method of measurement of pulsus paradoxus
- Stand by the side of the patient in such a way that you can monitor respiratory movement of the patient and column of sphygmomanometer cuff simultaneously
- Ask the patient to take normal breath, because deep breathing may produce abnormal paradoxus
- Inflate the cuff to such a point, so that no sound can be heard (20 mm Hg above systolic blood pressure)

FLOW CHART 4.3 Pathophysiology of pulsus paradoxus

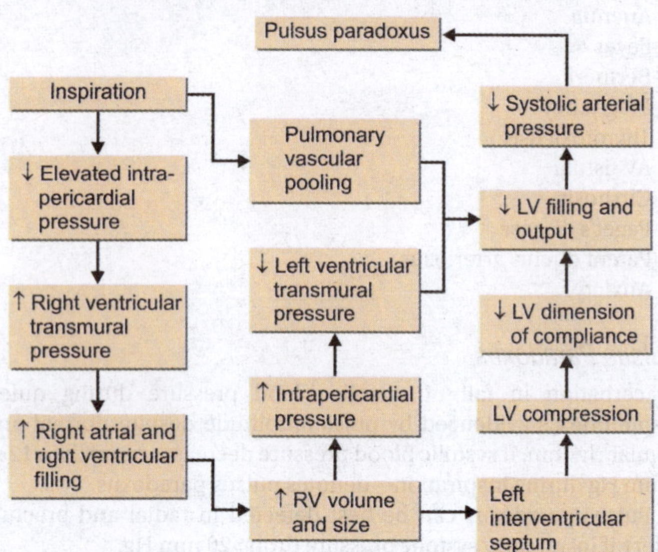

- Start deflating the cuff very slowly to such a position, when Korotkoff sounds start hearing during expiration. Measure the point by stopping deflation of the cuff
- Restart deflating very slowly until Korotkoff sound is heard both during inspiration and expiration. Record the point
- The difference between these two above systolic readings is called pulsus paradoxus.

Values to be remembered in pulsus paradoxus
- Age of puberty—pulsus paradoxus is 12+-2 mm Hg
- Age of driving—pulsus paradoxus may be normal up to 16 mm Hg
- Age of drinking—between 16 and 21 mm Hg pulsus paradoxus has been reported in:
  ❖ Pulmonary embolism
  ❖ Right ventricular failure
  ❖ Right ventricular infarction
  ❖ Severe congestive heart failure.

In cardiac tamponade: Large collection of pericardial fluid produces intrapericardial pressure greater than intracardiac diastolic pressure. This:
- Prevents adequate filling of the heart and ventricular ejection
- Creates a situation where cardiac chambers start competing for limited intrapericardial space—as a result there is major respiratory swings in:

- ❖ Swings in ventricular septum
- ❖ Systolic blood pressure
- ❖ Ventricular filling.

Characteristics of pulsus paradoxus in cardiac tamponade: It is >12 mm Hg in 100 percent of cases.

If it is >20 mm Hg, it can be palpated in brachial or radial artery.

Beck's triad: It is a triad described by Dr Clade Beck:
- Hypotension
- Distended neck veins
- Small and quiet heart

It is found in advanced cases, but tetrads are better tools for diagnosis. It includes addition of pulsus paradoxus.

False negative pulsus paradoxus in cardiac tamponade
- *Isolated right heart tamponade:* It occurs in:
  - ❖ Chronic heart failure. Who are on hemodialysis
  - ❖ Loculated pericardial effusion.

    In above cases pericardial bag is too asymmetric to produce competition between two ventricles.
- In aortic regurgitation, during inspiration, left ventricle is filled up from aorta, prevent development of pulsus paradoxus. So, patient with aortic dissection (patient who have both AR or cardiac tamponade)—present without pulsus paradoxus
- *Large atrial septal defect:* Normal inspiratory increase in systemic venous return is counterbalanced by decreased left to right shunt, result in minimal change in right ventricular volume
- *Elevated left ventricular diastolic pressure:* In severe left ventricular dysfunction, left ventricular pressure is very high. So ipsilateral shift of ventricular septum will not occur during inspiration
- *Disease of bony thorax:* It prevents mobility of chest wall during respiration.

Pulsus paradoxus in air flow obstruction: In status asthmaticus, hyperinflation of chest produces excessive inspiratory pooling of blood, producing greater drop in systolic blood volume.

This form of pulsus paradoxus depends upon respiratory effort and rate, so it is not a sensitive indication.

In status asthmaticus, pulsus paradoxus is >10 mm Hg.

If it is more than 20 mm Hg, FEV1 < 0.5 to 0.7 L.

Diseases causing pulsus paradoxus >10 mm Hg
- *Lung causes:*
  - ❖ Bronchial asthma
  - ❖ Status asthmaticus
  - ❖ Tension pneumothorax.

- *Cardiac causes:*
  - ❖ Cardiac tamponade
  - ❖ Pericardial effusion
  - ❖ Constrictive pericarditis
  - ❖ Restrictive cardiomyopathy
  - ❖ Pulmonary embolism
  - ❖ Right ventricular failure
  - ❖ Right ventricular infarction.
- *Extracardiac causes:*
  - ❖ Anaphylactic shock
  - ❖ Hypovolemic shock
  - ❖ Volvulus of stomach
  - ❖ Diaphragmatic hernia.

Reverse pulsus paradoxus: This occurs in:
- *Hypertrophic obstructive cardiomyopathy (HOCM):* The wall of the heart is very stiff so that the cavity is not adequately filled
- *Left ventricular failure on positive pressure ventilation:* PPV moves the left ventricular wall during systole, so stroke volume will be increased during inspiration
- *Isorhythmic dissociation:* Atrial activity precedes ventricular activity during inspiration and follow ventricular activity during expiration.

Pseudopulsus paradoxus: In isorythmic dissociation—due to increased respiratory rate, P wave is positioned before QRS—producing synchronization of atrioventricular contraction. So, strictly adheres to guidelines of pulsus paradoxus:
- Palpate in all accessible arteries
- Avoid deep inspiration during palpation
- No irregularity of cardiac action.

Kussmaul sign: This is inspiratory increase in venous distension. This occurs in:
- Tricuspid stenosis
- Superior venacaval syndrome
- Right ventricular hypertrophy
- Right ventricular infarction
- Constrictive pericarditis
- Pulmonary emboli
- Pulmonary hypertension.

Pulsus Alternans (Fig. 4.69)

This denotes alternate strong and weak arterial pulse volume despite regular heart rate and rhythm. This indicates:

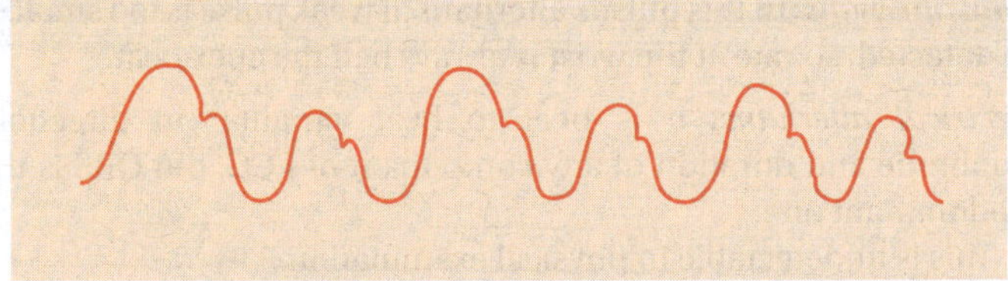

FIG. 4.69   Pulsus alternans

- *Severe left ventricular dysfunction with:*
  - ❖ Worsening ejection
  - ❖ Higher pulmonary capillary pressure
  - ❖ S3 gallop.

This occurs in:
- Ischemia
- Valvular heart disease
- Cardiomyopathy
- Hypertension.

Methods of measuring pulsus alternans
- Wrap the blood pressure cuff around the arm
- Inflate the cuff till the sound will disappear
- Slowly deflate the cuff until you hear the first Korotkoff sound
- At this time only the stronger ejections produce the sound
- Further deflate the pressure cuff till the weaker ejections becomes detectable, it produce doubling of the sound. The difference in systolic blood pressure between stronger and weaker ejections are usually 15–20 mm Hg
- Finally ask the patient to take deep breath or suddenly assume upright positions. This may help to elicit pulsus alternans.

Mechanism of pulsus alternans: Two schools of thought:
1. *Contractility school of thought:* There is bit to bit variation in left ventricular diameter—leads to cycling of weaker and stonger ejections. As a result there is pulse to pulse variation.
2. *Hemodynamic school of thought:* According to this school, variation in ejection fraction is due to changes in systolic and diastolic duration.

If systolic duration increases, ejection fraction lengthens—producing high volume of pulse. As a result, diastolic duration shortens, so diastolic ventricular filling time decreases and next ejection fraction is diminished, producing weak volume pulse.

In next cycle, diastolic filling time increases, so next ejection fraction is higher, producing high volume in pulse.

Total alternans: In this pulsus alternans, if weak pulse is too small to be detected, so rate at the wrist is always half the apex beat.

Electrical alternans: It is beat to beat variation in direction, amplitude and duration of any componant of ECG, but QRS is the predominant one:

- This is undetectable in physical examination
- It may coexist with pulsus alternans
- It may be associated with:
    - ❖ COPD
    - ❖ Pericardial effusion
    - ❖ Cardiac tamponade.

Pulsus Bigemini

It denotes beats occur in pairs (with different strength)—rhythm is irregular.

Doubled peaked pulse: It denotes two palpable beats per cycle:
- First peak occurs in systole
- *Second peak occurs either in systole:*
    - ❖ Pulsus bisferiens
    - ❖ Bifid pulse.
- *Second peak occurs in diastole:* Diacrotic pulse.

Pulsus bisferiens: It denotes—two palpable peaks of equal strength. It has:
1. Large amplitude.
2. Quick upstroke/down stroke.

Method of detection of bisferiens pulse
- Light but firm pressure on large central artery
- It can be detected by blood pressure cuff, as a closely split Korotkoff sounds.

Significance of pulsus bisferiens: It occurs:
In mild-to-moderate aortic regurgitation with or without aortic stenosis.

In high output states. It can be detected as:
- *Double Korotkoff sounds:* Heard in systolic blood pressure measurement
- *Traube's pistol shot sound:* It can be heard in femoral artery giving light pressure by diaphragm over the artery with mild artery compression distal to stethoscope. This sound may be:
    - ❖ Single—pistal shot sound
    - ❖ Double—Traube's femoral double sound
    - ❖ Tripple sound.

Duroziez's murmur
- This can be elicited over the central artery—femoral or brachial
- Apply gradual but firm compression over femoral artery by diaphragm. This produces:
  - Systolic murmur (normal)
  - Diastolic murmur (aortic regurgitation).
- *False negative may occur in:*
  - Mild disease
  - Concomitant aortic stenosis
  - Inadequate ventricular filling (mitral stenosis)
  - Inadequate ventricular emptying (concomitant mitral regurgitation)
  - Obstruction to waveform transmission (coarctation of aorta).
- *False positive occur in:* High output condition—in these conditions—murmur is continuous, like AV fistula
- Double murmur of high output state and aortic regurgitation is the result of forward flow

  Whereas the double murmur of PDA and AV fistula is the result of forward and reverse flow.

  The above can be differentiated by:
  - Pressing the artery at cephalad edge of diaphragm- increases the forward flow murmur
  - Pressing the artery at caudal edge of diaphragm—increases the reverse flow murmur.

Mechanism of bisferiens pulse: Trough between two peaks is due to venturi effect caused by rapid blood flow.

This will pull the artery wall inward producing transient arrest in flow.
- In turn it will stop Bernoulli effect
- Restart the flow
- Produce the second peak.

Prognostic significance of bisferiens pulse: It indicates large stroke volume—it may disappear in left ventricular dysfunction.

Bifid Pulse

It classically occurs in HOCM. Unless there is severe obstruction to outflow, it can be palpated in carotid artery, it can detected in tracing.

Mechanism of bifid pulse: Its first peak is due to systolic emptying of left ventricle.
- Trough is due to obstruction to outflow
- Second peak is due to another emptying of left ventricle.

Dicrotic Pulse

It denotes:

- One peak is in systole
- Second peak is in diastole, as an accentuation of secondary wave
- This pulse can be felt in carotid—it is probably due to a rebound of blood against closed aortic valve, causing secondary wave—it is due to elasticity of arterial wall, hence it occurs in elastic arteries felt in young patient, never over the age of 45 years
- It can be differentiated from pulsus bisferiens and bifid pulse by its:
  - Diastolic filling
  - Longer interval between peaks.

Significance of dicrotic pulse
It suggests:

- Low cardiac output
- Increased systemic vascular resistance.

It occurs in:

- Congestive cardiomyopathy
- Pericardial tamponade
- First week of typhoid fever
- Myocarditis.

In case of low cardiac output—primary wave cannot be recognized, hence feeling of secondary wave is obvious.

Carotid shudder

- It is palpable thrill at the peak of carotid pulse
- It occurs in:
  - Aortic stenosis
  - Aortic regurgitation
  - Aortic stenosis with regurgitation.

Anacrotic Pulse

This is the combination of low volume (parvus) and slow upstroke (tardus) and there is an anacrotic notch on the ascending limb.

This type of pulse is not palpable but can be seen in tracings.

Hyperkinetic Pulse (Fig. 4.70)

It denotes:

- Large volume due to increased stroke volume
- Rapid upstroke—due to increased velocity of contraction.

This type of pulse is also known as pulsus celer.

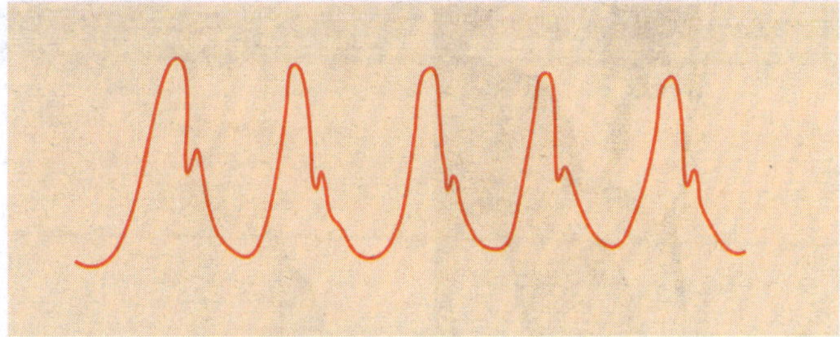

FIG. 4.70 Hyperkinetic pulse

Causes of hyperkinetic pulse
With wide pulse pressure:
- Fever
- Anemia
- Thyrotoxicosis
- Anxiety
- Beriberi
- Exercise
- Paget's disease
- AV fistula.

With normal pulse pressure:
- Simultaneous opening of left ventricle to high pressure bed
- Simultaneous opening of left ventricle to low pressure bed (mitral regurgitation) or in right ventricle (in ventricular septal defect).

Corrigan's Pulse
- It denotes bounding and collapsing pulse
- It occurs in aortic regurgitation
- It is also called water hammer pulse.

Water hammer: It is a Victorian toy, half filled with water or mercury in vacuum. Since solids or liquids fall at same rate in vacuum, inversion of tube causes precipitous fall of fluid or solid hitting the glass with brisk jalt.

Method of detection of Corrigan's pulse (Figs 4.71A and B)
Elevate the patient's arm, while at the same time feel the radial pulse with the palm.

Rising the arm above the heart's level reduces the intraradial diastolic pressure, collapses the vessel and facilitates the palpability of the subsequent systolic thrust.

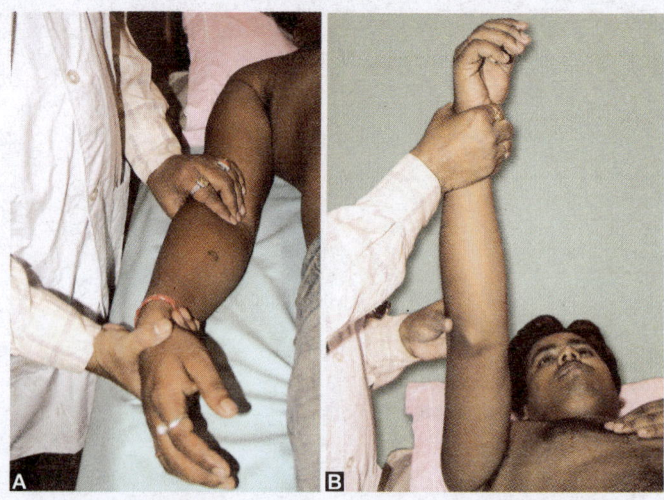

FIGS 4.71A AND B   Method of detection of Corrigan's pulse

Pulsus Durus (Durus 'Hard' in Latin)

Pulse is so hardened that it is difficult to compress.

- It occurs in atherosclerosis
- It is associated with Osler's node.

Method of compressibility of the arterial pulse to predict the arterial blood pressure

- Palpate the radial artery with fingers of yours left hand
- At the same time compress the brachial artery with the thumb of your right hand
- Press the brachial artery gradually till radial artery is impalpable:
  - ❖ If pressure is mild, systolic blood pressure probably is 120 mm Hg
  - ❖ If pressure is intermediate, systolic blood pressure is 120–160 mm Hg
  - ❖ If pressure is high, systolic blood pressure is >160 mm Hg.

Carotid bruit

It can be heard:

- By placing the bell of the stethoscope on the neck
- Room must be quiet
- Auscultation from just behind the upper end of thyroid cartilage to immediately below the angle of the jaw.

Other findings mimicking carotid bruit

- *Systolic heart murmur:* These are only transmitted to the neck Hence they are much louder in precordium than in the neck.

- *Venous hum:*
  - ❖ Innocent murmur caused by flow in the internal jugular vein
  - ❖ They are continuous but loudest in diastole
  - ❖ It can be only heard during sitting position.

Carotid bruit occurs in:
- 20 percent of children younger than 15 years of age
- 2.5 percent—between 45 and 54 years of age
- 8.2 percent—above 75 years of age
- AV fistula in hemodialysis patients.

Significance of carotid bruit in asymptomatic ambulatory patient
- In 50 years aged person it is associated with increased risk of cerebrovascular accident or ischemic heart disease
- This increased incidence or risk decreases sharply with age, nonexistent among people older than 75 years.

Other Special Signs of Aortic Regurgitation

Eye signs
- *Landolfi's sign:* Contraction and dilatation of the pupil in systole and diastole respectively
- *Becker's sign:* It is evidenced by prominent retinal artery pulsation.

Head and neck signs
- *De Musset's sign:* It can be described as simultaneous nodding of the head with each heart beat
- *Corrigan's sign:* It can be described as dancing of the carotid
- *Müller's sign:* It can present as pulsation of the uvula
- *Minervini's sign:* The tongue depressor moves up and down when the tongue is lightly depressed
- *Logue's sign:* It is a pulsation of the sternoclavicular joint when AR is associated with aortic dissection.

Upper limb
- *Locomotor brachialis:* It is worm-like visible pulsation of the brachial artery
- *Quincke's sign:* It is visible capillary pulsation as evidenced by alternate blanching and reddening in the nail bed seen by transmitting light on the finger tips. It can be visualized in the lips also
- *Palfrey's sign:* It is the pistol shot sound heard over the radial artery.

Lower limb
- *Traube's sign:* Pistal shot sound heard over the femoral artery due to sudden distension of the arterial wall

- *Duroziez's sign:* It consists of:
    - ❖ *Systolic murmur:* A forward murmur heard by pressing the femoral artery 2 cm above the stethoscope—due to powerful contraction of LV and increased stroke volume
    - ❖ *Distolic murmur:* A backward murmur heard by pressing the femoral artery 2 cm below the stethoscope, due to arterial recoil and back flow.

Abdomen
- *Rosenbach's sign:* It is evidenced by pulsation of the liver
- *Gerhard's sign:* It is the pulsation of the spleen
- *Dennison's sign:* Pulsation in the cervix in female.

Blood Pressure

Blood pressure is divided into diastolic and systolic blood pressure.
Systolic blood pressure: Highest intrarterial pressure produced by left ventricular systole.
Diastolic blood pressure: Lowest intra-arterial pressure just prior to left ventricular systolic event.

Various Blood Pressure Sound According to the Phases

These are called Korotkoff sound.

These sounds are aquastic notes heard during the process of deflation of blood pressure cuff. These include:
- *Phase 1:* First appearance of low frequency tapping sound
- *Phase 2:* Softer and longer sound
- *Phase 3:* Crisper and louder sound
- *Phase 4:* Muffling of sound
- *Phase 5:* Complete disappearance of sound.

Production of Korotkoff Sound

- Systolic sound is produced by sudden reopening of the already collapsed artery during gradual deflation of blood pressure cuff, when the pressure of the cuff is below the level of blood pressure of the patient
- Diastolic sound is produced when the arterial wall is completely opened.

Blood pressure should be measured more than once because:
- Record the blood pressure twice and take the average
- If diastolic reading differs more than 5 mm Hg between two measurements, take third time measurement
- Initially measure the blood pressure of both arms, then take the arm having higher blood pressure

- When indicated, take the blood pressure of lower extremities (in sitting and supine positions)
- Blood pressure should be measured once in both upper extremities by two observers working simulteneously and then switch over.

Blood pressure values between two arms
- Normally, difference of systolic blood pressure 10–15 mm Hg
- If the difference is >20 mm Hg—it indicates subclavian artery obstruction, whose etiologies varies according to clinical settings.
  - ❖ In acute conditions:
    Aortic dissection (in case of proximal involvement it is associated with aortic regurgitation).
  - ❖ In chronic case—Subclavian steal syndrome—in this case blood is stolen from vertebral artery and driven to subclavian artery. This patient will present with vertigo, hemiparesis, ataxia, visual disturbance.

Factors not affecting the blood pressure
- Menstruation
- Chronic caffeine ingestion
- Phenylephrine nasal spray
- Sleeves under the cuff
- Self inflation the cuff
- Bell versus diaphragm
- Room temperature
- Working hours
- Discordance gender
- Discordance race.

Methods of Measuring Blood Pressure (Fig. 4.72)

- Patient should be kept in quiet room (feet flat on the floor and back supported against the chair)
- His or her bared arm should be kept on the side of the table in such a position that the mid point of the upper arm at the level of the heart
- Circumference of the bare arm at the mid point between acromian and olecranon will be measured with tape
- Bladder inside the cuff should encircle 80 percent of the arm in adult and 100 percent in children
- Palpate the brachial artery and place the bladder in such a position so that the mid line of the bladder is over arterial pulsation

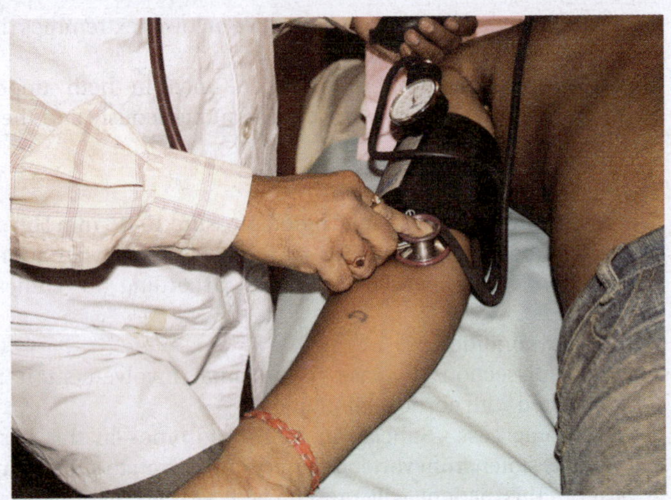

FIG. 4.72 Method of measuring blood pressure

- Wrap the cuff tightly around the upper arm. Loose application results over estimation of the blood pressure
- Lower edge of the cuff should be 1 inch above the ante cubital fossa—so that the diaphragm can be placed
- Inflate the cuff to 70 mm Hg then increase by 10 mm Hg per increment, while palpating the radial pulse
- Note the pressure at which radial pulse is disappeared and the pressure at which the radial pulse will reappear
- Palpatory method is useful to
  - ❖ For preliminary approximation of systolic BP
  - ❖ As it ensures adequate level of inflation for actual auscultatory measurement
  - ❖ As it avoids underinflation of cuff in patient with auscultatory gap
  - ❖ As it avoids over inflation in those with low BP.
- Place the stethoscope over the brachial artery above and medial to ante cubital fossa below the edge of the cuff and hold it firmly in place
- Inflate the bladder rapidly to 20–30 mm Hg above the level previously governed/determined by palpation
- Deflate the bladder by 2 mm Hg/second, while listening for the appearance of Korotkoff sounds
- Then the bladder should be deflated and wait for muffling of sounds (Phase IV) and disappearance of sound (Phase V)
- Systolic and diastolic pressure should be recorded and round off to nearest 2 mm Hg

- Measurement should be repeated after at least 30 seconds and two recordings should be arranged.

Factors Affecting the Blood Pressure

- *Examinee:*
  - ❖ *Increase in blood pressure:*
    - Soft Korotkoff sound
    - Missed auscultatory gap
    - Diastolic blood pressure
    - Pseudohypertension
    - White coat reaction to physician
    - Paretic arms
    - Anxiety
    - Acute caffeine ingestion
    - Acute smoking
    - Acute ethanol ingestion.
  - ❖ *Decrease in blood pressure:*
    - Soft Korotkoff sound
    - Recent meal
    - Missed auscultatory gap
    - High stroke volume
    - Shock.
- *Examiner:*
  - ❖ *Increase in blood pressure:*
    - Hearing impairment
    - Expectation bias.
  - ❖ *Decrease in blood pressure:*
    - Impaired hearing
    - Expectation bias
    - Reading next lowest 5 10 mm Hg.
- *Examination:*
  - ❖ *Increase in blood pressure:*
    - Cuff is too small and narrow
    - Cuff not centered
    - Cuff over clothing
    - Elbow too low
    - Cuff too loose
    - Too short rest period
    - Back unsupported
    - Arm unsupported
    - Too fast deflation
    - Cold season
    - Rapid measurement.

❖ *Decrease in blood pressure:*
  • Elbow too high
  • Left versus right arm
  • Resting period is too long
  • Too rapid deflation
  • Excessive bell pressure
  • Leak bulb
  • Low mercury level.

Variability of blood pressure
- Standard deviation between visit is 5–12 mm Hg for systolic and 6–8 mm Hg for diastolic blood pressure
- Between visits the blood pressure fluctuation is higher than within the visit blood pressure fluctuation
- According to Joint National Committee on prevention, detection, evaluation and treatment of high blood pressure recommends repeat measurement.
  ❖ Within two months for Stage 1 hypertension
  ❖ Within one month for Stage 2 hypertension
  ❖ Within one week for Stage 3 hypertension
  ❖ Immediate evaluation for Stage 4 hypertension.

Equipment error for measuring blood pressure
- *Wrong cuff size:*
  ❖ Shorter cuff overestimate blood pressure
  ❖ Longer cuff under estimate blood pressure.
- Aneroid instrument sometimes goes out of calibration.

Auscultatory gap
- It is mainly found in elderly with hypertension
- It consists of temporary disappearance of Korotkoff sound after the systolic reading followed by reappearance of the sound just before diastolic values
- Auscultatory gap may underestimate the blood pressure reading unless simultaneous radial artery is palpated
- It is more common in females
- It is associated with atherosclerotic plaques in carotid artery
- It is associated with arterial wall stiffness.

Difference between values of direct and indirect blood pressure measurement
- Korotkoff Phase 1 sound appears 4–15 mm Hg below the systolic blood pressure
- Korotkoff Phase 5 sound disappears 4–6 mm Hg above the diastolic blood pressure
- *Physician's inaccuracy:*
  ❖ British doctor always measures once only

❖ In some patient, blood pressure measured in physician's chamber is higher than their ambulatory value. This is called "white coat reaction" occurs in 10–40 percent borderline uncorrected or borderline hypertensive patients.
This white coat reaction is more common in female.

Blood pressure can be felt by palpatory method in:
- Radial artery
- Brachial artery.
  Diastolic blood pressure can be determined by palpatory method in brachial artery below the cuff, by:
  The point at which sudden decrease in volume and peak makes the pulse less bounding.

Systolic blood pressure difference between palpatory and auscultatory method
Palpatory values is 7 mm Hg lower than auscultatory value.

Definition of Blood Pressure
- Risk of cardiovascular disease begins at 115/75 mm Hg
- Risk is doubled with each increment of 20 mm Hg of systolic blood pressure and 10 mm Hg. Diastolic blood pressure.
- *According to Joint Committee Guidelines:*
  - ❖ 119/79 mm Hg or below—normal blood pressure
  - ❖ 120–139/80–89 mm Hg—pre-hypertension.
  - ❖ 140–159/90–99 mm Hg—stage I hypertension.
  - ❖ ≥160/≥100 mm Hg—stage II hypertension.

Prehypertensive patients may develop overt hypertension, if there is no lifestyle modification. It includes:
- Weight reduction
- DASH diet (Dietary approaches to stop hypertension).

Pseudohypertension
Elevated indirect recording of blood pressure in patient whose intra-arterial blood pressure measurement is normal.

In shock, high peripheral vascular resistance tightens the arteries to such a point that systolic and diastolic blood pressure cannot be measured. So this leads to gross under estimation.

Significance of pseudohypertension
- Myocardial infarction
- Pneumonia in intensive care setting.

Osler's Maneuver
- First inflate the cuff to obliterate the radial pulse
- Then feel the radial artery

- This maneuver is positive when the artery remains palpable as a firm tube.

Significance of positive Osler sign

Palpation of an artery in absences of pulses—is a sign of atherosclerosis. In this case both systolic and diastolic blood pressure can be over estimated. It is called pseudohypertension.

Malignant hypertension
- A level of hypertension with one or more end organ damage, e.g.
  - ❖ Renal function
  - ❖ Retinal function
  - ❖ Left ventricular failure
  - ❖ Myocardial infarction
  - ❖ Cerebrovascular accident.
- This may occur with blood pressure 180/120 mm Hg. Sometimes there is no organ damage with this high blood pressure
- Sometimes in very high blood pressure, patient may not show signs of end organ damage.

Mean arterial blood pressure
[Systolic blood pressure + 2(Diastolic blood pressure)]/3.

Pulse pressure: Systolic blood pressure—diastolic blood pressure.

Wide pulse pressure: Where the pulse pressure is >50 percent of systolic blood pressure.

Causes of wide pulse pressure: It occurs in high output states, where there is increase stroke volume, low peripheral vascular resistance.

This occurs in:
- Fever
- Anxiety
- Anemia
- Thyrotoxicosis
- Beriberi
- Peget's disease
- Exercise
- Pregnancy
- Aortic regurgitation
- Patent ductus arteriosus
- Cirrhosis.

In aortic regurgitation, pulse pressure more than 80 mm Hg. It is moderate to severe regurgitation.

Wide pulse pressure in one extremity—cause is arteriovenous fistula.

Branham Sign

It is typical bradycardia after the compression of the AV fistula. It is due to inhibition of Bainbridge reflex—operates continuously in patient with large fistulas.

In large fistula
↓ ↓

High right atrial pressure
↓

Increased right atrial stretching
↓

Compensatory tachycardia through:
a. Inhibition of vagal influence
b. Sympathetic acceleration.

In pulmonary embolism
↓

Bainbridge reflex
↓

Supraventricular tachycardia.

Test for Branham's sign
- Inflate the cuff over the limb having AV fistula. Heart rate will slow down
- Upon deflation of the cuff, there is compensatory tachycardia due to reopening of AV fistula

Narrow pulse pressure: When the pulse pressure is <25 percent of systolic pressure. Common causes are:
- *Decreased left ventricular filling:*
  - ❖ Constrictive pericarditis
  - ❖ Cardiology.
- *Decreased left ventricular stroke volume:*
  - ❖ Aortic stenosis
  - ❖ Tachycardia.

Hill's Sign

It is an exaggerated difference in systolic pressure between upper and lower extremities.
- Normal physiologic difference is 12+–
  mm Hg
- If the difference is >60 mm Hg—it is highly specific
- If it is >20 or <40 mm Hg—it is pathologic.

It occurs in severe aortic regurgitation and any hyperdynamic state. This Hill's sign is positive in indirect recording. But in direct recording, there is no discrepency.

Methods of performing Hill's sign:
- Measure systolic pressure in lower extremity—rapping the cuff around the calf and palpate artery dorsalis pedis or posterior tibial artery
- Measure systolic pressure in upper extremity
- Normally legs have higher systolic pressure than upper extremity.

Ankle–Brachial Pressure Index

It asses chronic lower extremity ischemia.

Methods of measuring ankle-brachial pressure (ABP):
- Patient must be in supine position
- Measure brachial pressure by handheld Doppler
- Measure lower extremity systolic blood pressure of both artery dorsalis pedis an posterior tibial artery—whichever is higher, take the value
- Divide the selected highest ankle pressure by highest brachial systolic pressure
- *Value:*
  - Normal value—0.97–1.1.
  - If it is <0.97—it is due to angiography ally proven occlusion or stenosis
  - If it is 0.5–0.8—it is due to claudication
  - If it is <0.5—pain at rest
  - If it is <0.2—associated with ischemia or gangrene.

Fallacies of ABP:
- Since it only measures the ankle systolic pressure—it cannot detect distal occlusion due to microemboli or plaques
- ABPI may be falsely elevated in Monckeberg's sclerosis—medial wall calcification in diabetic patient.

Valsalva maneuver
It measures the autonomic control (both sympathetic and vagal) over cardiovascular system—controlling heart rate, systolic pressure and venous return—all are the results of respiratory swings of intrathoracic pressure.

Valsalva maneuver consists of two periods (Fig. 4.73)
- *Held (strain) period:* Ask the patient to full inspire and then forcefully expire against closed glottis for 10 seconds, by either:
  - Placing a fist to the abdomen, while the patient is in supine position and ask him to give strain against it
  - Ask the patient to blow against an aneroid manometer at a constant pressure of 40 mm Hg. Following things will be happened:

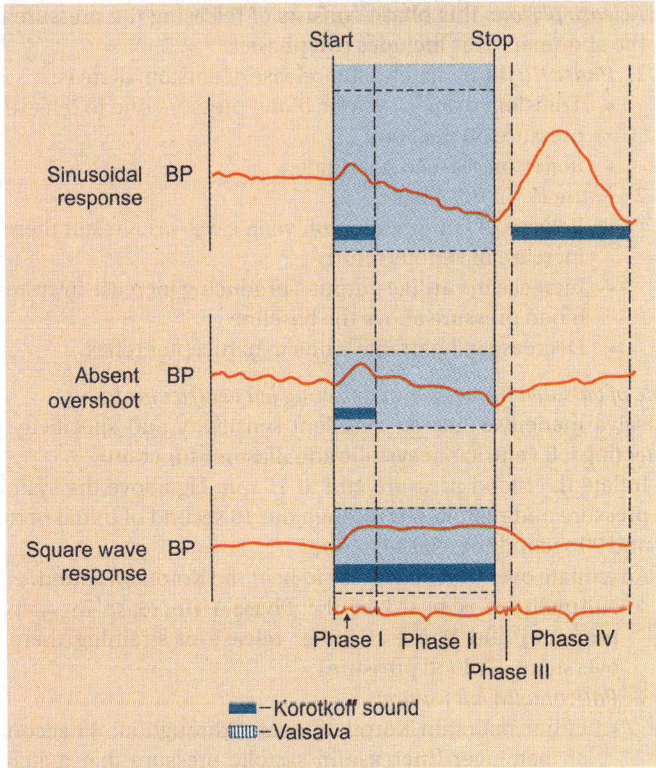

FIG. 4.73   Blood pressure response to valsalva maneuver in normal individual

- Phase I: At the onset:
  - Increase in systolic pressure due to aortic compression
  - Decrease in heart rate due to reflex bradycardia (baroreceptor activation)
- Phase II:
  - Decrease in venous return due to compression of vena cava (straining induced)
  - Decrease in cardiac output producing decrease in systolic pressure—due to fall in aortic pressure
  - Secondary increase in heart rate due to baroreceptor activity.

All the above phases are due to:
- Decrease in venous return due to increase in intrathoracic pressure
- Decrease in cardiac output
- Reduction in left ventricular diameter.

- *Release period:* This phase consists of releasing the pressure on the abdomen. This includes two phases:
  1. *Phase III:* Immediately after release of tension, there is:
     - Transient drop in systolic blood pressure due to release of pressure on the aorta
     - Reflex increase in heart rate.
  2. *Phase IV:* In this phase:
     - Release of compression on vena cava—as a result there is increase in venous return
     - Increase in cardiac output—producing increase in systolic blood pressure above the baseline
     - Decrease in heart rate—due to barocepter reflex.

Role of valsalva maneuver in detecting left ventricular failure

Valsalva maneuver has an excellent sensitivity and specificity in detecting left ventricular systolic and diastolic function:

- Inflate the blood pressure cuff to 15 mm Hg above the systolic pressure and maintain it through out 10 second of initial period and 20 seconds of release period
- Auscultate over brachial artery to hear the Korotkoff sound:
  - ❖ Normally, it is heard in the Phase I (increase in systolic pressure) and Phase IV (after release of straining there is overshoot of blood pressure)
  - ❖ *Patient with left failure:*
    - Either maintain Korotkoff sound throughout 40 seconds of maneuver (increase in systolic pressure that matches intrathoracic pressure)—square wave response
    - Or, fail to overshoot the systolic pressure in Phase IV during release period—due to failing of left ventricle to increase systolic output after hypotension induced by straining.

Diagnostic use of valsalva maneuver

- Identification of congestive heart failure
- Enhancement of murmur of HOCM and mitral valve prolapse.

Therapeutic use of valsalva maneuver

- Interrupting supraventricular tachycardia (by increasing vagal tone)
- Helping the patient with multiple sclerosis, whose bladder is flaccid and cannot empty fully
- Diminishing chest pain in patient with coronary artery disease
- Avoiding premature ejaculation.

PRECORDIAL MOVEMENT OF IMPULSE

Apical Area of Chest

It is the area of chest where definite cardiac thrust is left. It is due to brisk movement of left ventricle against chest wall.

In disease condition—additional precordial impulse can be felt, reflecting mechanical events of ventricles, atria, large vessels.

The following precordial are usually left (Fig. 4.74)
- Apical area or apex (left fifth intercostal space in left mid clavicular line)
- Two basilar areas in right and left intercostal spaces reflecting aortic of pulmonary areas respectively
- Left lower parasternal areas—reflecting right ventricular and right atrial projections
- Sternoclavicular area
- Epigastric area
- Ectopic areas.

Right ventricular impulses can be felt in:
- *Normally:*
  - ❖ Child
  - ❖ Chest having narrow anteroposterior diameter.
- Pathologically—right ventricular hypertrophy.

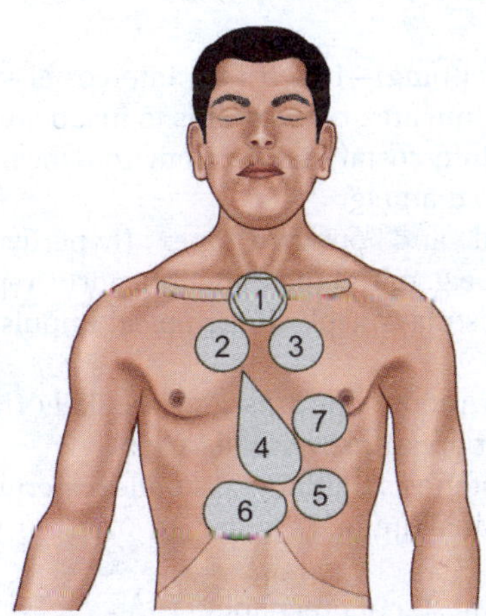

FIG. 4.74 Cardiovascular pulsation can be felt in following areas. (1) Sternoclav icular area; (2) Aortic area; (3) Pulmonary area; (4) Left parasternal area; (5) Apical area; (6) Epigastric area, (7) Ectopic area

Methods of Assessing Precordial Impulses

- *First inspection:* The apical, basilar, left parasternal and other areas of chest on front sides—it requires, project tangential light to visualize retractions and outward motion
- *Second inspection—palpation:*
  - ❖ Major areas must be palpated in supine position. Localize:
    - Site of palpable impulse
    - Evaluation of force.
  - ❖ Then palpate the apical area with patient in left lateral position, this may detect:
    - Otherwise under detectable apical impulse
    - Palpable S_3 and S_4.
  - ❖ Basilar areas should be palpated with sitting posture and leaning forward:
    - During holding breath after full inspiration
    - During holding breath after full expiration.
  - ❖ Use palm to detect—heaves or lifts
  - ❖ Use proximal metacarpals to identity thrills
  - ❖ Use finger pads to detect various abnormalities.

The precordial events can be timed by:
- Palpating carotid simultaneously
- Simultaneously ausculting for S_1 and S_2.

Description of Apical Impulse

- *Location:*
  - ❖ Normal (tapping)—in left fifth intercostal space in left mid clavicular line area corresponds to just below the nipple—in 4th or 5th intercostal space <10 cm from the midline, confined to <3 cm in diameter
  - ❖ Downward and outward apex (hyperdynamic)—volume overloads, e.g. mitral regurgitation, aortic regurgitation POA, VSD, AV fistula—displace the apical impulse downwards of outwards
  - ❖ Apex beat mores upwards and medially (heaving)—in left ventricular pressure overloads, e.g.:
    - Aortic stenosis (initially) systemic hypertension
    - Abdominal tumor
    - Ascites
    - Last trimester of pregnancy
    - Severe AI
    - Severe MI of ischemic origin.

- *Size:*
  - ❖ Normal apical impulse—size of dime
  - ❖ Anything larger than nickel, quarter or old silver dollar—should be abnormal
  - ❖ Diameter >4 cm specific for cardiomegaly.
- *Duration and training:*
  - ❖ Normal apical impulse—tapping—never passes midsystole —normal, mitral stenosis
  - ❖ Heaving apical impulse—sustained, continuous into S_2 or beyond:
    - Pressure overload
    - Volume overload
    - Cardiomyopathy.

  Differentiation of above conditions can be done:
  - ❖ In patient with no murmur—cardiomyopathy with low ejection fraction
  - ❖ In patient with systolic murmur—ejection—consider pressure overload from aortic stenosis
  - ❖ In patient with diastolic murmur—volume overload—aortic regurgitation.
- *Amplitude:* This denotes force, not the length of impulse
  - ❖ *Hyperdynamic impulse:* It is forceful enough to lift the examiner's finger, it occurs in:
    - Volume overload:
      - VSD
      - AI
      - Left ventricular aneurysm.
    - Normal subject with very thin chest
    - General pathological conditions:
      - Thyrotoxicosis
      - Anemia
      - Beriberi.
    - Retraction of lung due to fibrosis or collapse.
- *Contour:*
  - ❖ Single—normal
  - ❖ Double or triple apical impulse:
    - Hypertrophic obstructive cardiomyophy
    - Left ventricular aneurysm.

Abnormal Apical Movements

- *Double apical impulse occurs in:*
  - ❖ *Left ventricular wall dyskinesia due to:*
    - Ischemia
    - Aneurysm.
  - ❖ Hypertrophic obstructive cardiomyopathy.

The impulses denote:
Systolic—one is due to initial left ventricular contraction and second one is due to overcome the outflow tract obstruction by the septum.

In case of triple apical impulse, third one is presystolic—due to strong atrial contraction.

- *Precordial apical impulse:* It is a palpable fourth heart sound—due to reduced left ventricular compliance—due to:
  - ❖ Ischemia
  - ❖ Pressure load (aortic stenosis or systemic hypertension).

  In aortic stenosis—S_4 denotes to presence of significant gradient between left ventricle and aorta.

  It may be associated with palpable thrill at right 2nd intercostal space.

- *Early diastolic apical impulse:* It is equivalent to S_3—usually impalpable. It indicates—dilated left ventricle. It may occur in:
  - ❖ Mitral regurgitation
  - ❖ Left ventricular failure.

  It may be associated with sustained apical impulse.

  Significance of precordial movement in lower left sternal areas:
  - ❖ Sustained movement just after S_1 sound reflect—pressure or volume load in right ventricle
  - ❖ Sustained movement that begins late in systole, reflect—mitral regurgitation with dilatation of left atrium
  - ❖ Hyperdynamic movement:
    - Thin chest
    - Sternal malformation
    - High output state
    - Atrial septal defect.

Retracting Apical Impulse

This movement is just opposite to normal apical impulse, i.e. inward movement during systole and outward movement during diastole.

The above impulses can be corroborated by:
- Auscultation
- Carotid artery pulsation.

Causes of retracted apical impulse (Skoda's sign):
- Constrictive pericarditis
- Tricuspid regurgitation. Rocking movements of the chest with retraction at the apex in systole (occupied enlarged right ventricle) and bulging of the xyphoid area or epigastric area (occupied by right atrium). Associated findings are as follows:
  - ❖ Palpable P_2—due to pulmonary hypertension
  - ❖ Left parasternal heaves—due to enlarged right ventricle

❖ Occasionally right ventricular impulse in epigastric area
❖ Pulsatile liver—synchronous with each systole.

Heart Sounds

The normal heart sounds are:
- First heart sound
- *Second heart sound:*
  ❖ Pulmonary component
  ❖ Aortic component.

Hemodynamic Characteristics of Cardiac Cycle

Cardiac cycle starts with atrial contraction (S_4)
↓
This completes ventricular diastolic filling
↓
Electrical activation and contraction of the ventricles
↓
Pressure in ventricle is more than the pressure in atria
↓
Closing of atrioventricular valves
↓
There is gradual increase in contraction of ventricles (isometric contraction) when both AV valves and semilunar valves are closed
↓
A point will be reached when the pressure in the ventricles will be more than the pressure in the aorta and pulmonary artery
↓
As a result semilunar valves open
↓
As a result of isotonic contraction of the ventricles, they eject the blood into the aorta or the pulmonary artery
↓
At a point of time pressure in the ventricles will be lower than the aorta or the pulmonary artery
↓
There are closures of the semilunar valves
↓
Phase of isometric relaxation of ventricles will be started, as a part of diastole
↓
Diastole is always longer than the systole, till heart rate reaches 120/minute.

First heart sound is generated by closure of AV valves. Following two characteristics are valuable for S_1:

1. Intensity
2. Splitting.

Differentiation of S_1 from S_2
- Areas of greatest intensity are different (S_2 in basilar and S_1 in apical area)
- *Timing:*
  - ❖ Beginning of short interval for S_1
  - ❖ Beginning of long interval for S_2.
- *Pitch:*
  - ❖ S_1 is low pitched
  - ❖ S_2 is high pitched.

Significance of S_2 being louder than S_1
- S_2 is louder than S_1 (in pulmonary and systemic hypertension)
- S_2 is normal, S_1 is softer.

■ Inspection

Abnormalities of Breast
- Male gynecomastia—unilateral or bilateral
  - ❖ Digitalis toxicity (toxic effect)
  - ❖ Klinefelter's syndrome.
- Female hypomastia—mitral valve prolapse.
- *Wide-spaced nipples:*
  - ❖ Turner's syndrome
  - ❖ Noonan's syndrome.

Visibility of Vessels on the Chest (Front and Back)
- Visible veins with direction of flow above downwards—superior vena caval obstruction (Fig. 4.75)
- Visible vein with direction of flow below upwards—inferior vena caval obstruction
- Visible collateral vessels in interscapular, infrascapular regions or posterior intercostals spaces—suggest coarctation of aorta. This can be demonstrated—when asking the patient to stand and bend forwards with his both hands hanging down on both sides—Suzman's signs (Fig. 4.76).

Precordium
- Precordial prominence with ICS bulging without involvement of ribs—pericardial effusion
- Precordial bulging with involvement of ribs—cardiac involvement due to right ventricular dilatation of long duration

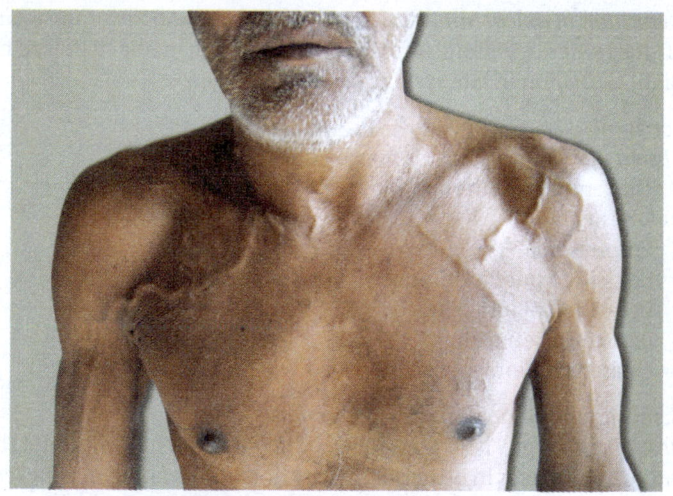

FIG. 4.75   Superior venacaval obstruction

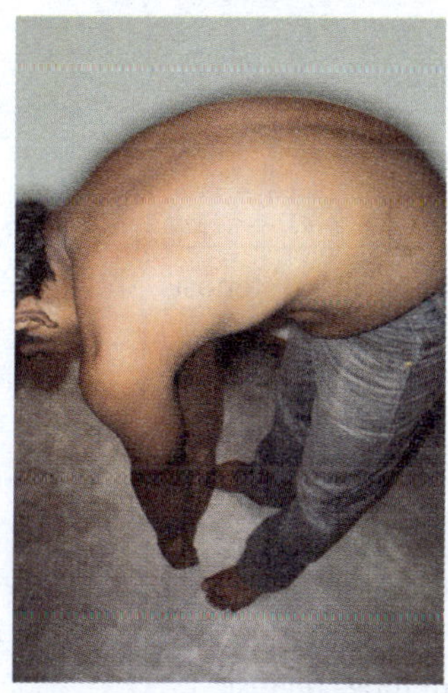

FIG. 4.76   Suzman's sign

- Precordial bulging but heart is not diseased:
  - ❖ Skeletal deformities
  - ❖ Emphysema
  - ❖ Bronchogenic carcinoma.
- *Ossification:*

	Start	*Completion*
Manubrium—	Puberty	25th year
Body of sternum—	Puberty	25th year
Xyphoid process—	3rd year	40th year
Manubriosternal joint—		60th year

Definition of apical impulse: It is the outermost and lowermost part of chest where a definite impulse is felt in systole medial followed by slight retraction in late systolic event.

Locations
Absent apical impulse: This may be due to:
- Thick muscular thorax
- Obesity
- Emphysema
- Left-sided pneumothorax
- Left-sided pleural effusion
- Pericardial effusion
- Dilated cardiomyopathy.

Below lateral retraction of apical impulse
Broadbent's sign: It is a systolic indrawing of left 10th and 11th intercental spaces in posterior axillary line. This is found in adhesive pericarditis.

Displacement
Lateral displacement:
- Scoliosis
- Straight back syndrome
- Right-sided pleural effusion
- Right-sided preumothorax
- Left lung fibrosis or collapse
- Right ventricular hypertrophy due to mitral stenosis
- LVH due to MI or AI.

Downward displacement: Aortic aneurysm.

Right-Sided Apical Impulse

- Dextrocardia
- Left-sided pneumothorax
- Left-sided pleural effusion
- Congenital heart disease
- Right-sided pulmonary fibrosis or lung collapse
- Scoliosis.

Pulsations in left 2nd intercostal space is due to:
- Pulmonary hypertension
- Aneurysmal dilatation of pulmonary artery
- Pulmonary artery dilatation
- Increased pulmonary blood flow
- Hyperdynamic circulation
- Retraction of left lung.

Pulsation of right 2nd intercostal space:
- Aortic aneurysm
- Aortic regurgitation.

Pulsations in sternoclavicular area:
- *Pulsation at sternoclavicular joint:*
  - ❖ Aortic aneurysm
  - ❖ Aortic dissection
  - ❖ Aortic regurgitation—syphilitic
  - ❖ Right-sided aortic arch.
- *Pulsation in suprasternal notch:*
  - ❖ Aneurysm of aorta
  - ❖ Thyroidea ima artery.
- *Pulsation in supraclavicular area:*
  - ❖ Aneurysm of aorta
  - ❖ Anomalous origin of right subclavian artery
  - ❖ Kinked right carotid artery.

Left Parasternal Pulsation

Site
- Right ventricular inflow portion—present underneath left 4th and 5th intercostal spaces (mid to lower left sternal edge)
- Right ventricular outflow portion present underneath left 3rd intercostal space.

Visibility
- Normally not visible
- *Physiologically:* Thin built patient
  - ❖ Patient of pectus excavatum.
- *Right ventricular pressure overload:*
  - ❖ Pulmonary stenosis
  - ❖ Pulmonary hypertension
  - ❖ Pulmonary embolism.
- *Right ventricular volume overload:*
  - ❖ Tricuspid regurgitation
  - ❖ Atrial septal defect
  - ❖ Ventricular septal defect.
- *Anterior motion of right ventricle:* Mitral regurgitation in absence of pulmonary hypertension
- In case of myocardial infarction involving septal wall due to bulging of septum into right ventricle.

Epigastric Pulsation

- Right ventricular hypertrophy due to pressure or volume overload

- Right ventricular pulsation due to downward displacement of right ventricle in case of chronic obstructive pulmonary disease
- In case of thin built individual normal aortic pulsation
- Aortic aneurysm of descending aorta
- In case of tricuspid regurgitation—systolic pulsation—correlated with heart sound
- In case of tricuspid stenosis—during diastolic phase, right atrial contraction against closed valve produces diastotic pulsation in liver area.

Ectopic Pulsation

In other than apical area:
- *Left ventricular pulsation:*
  - ❖ Left ventricular aneurysm due to myocardial infarction
  - ❖ Dyskinesia of left ventricle.
- *Left atrial pulsation:* Mitral regurgitation—hugely dilated left atrium.

Palpation of the Precordium

- *Chest wall for direction of flow of veins:*
  - ❖ If the flow is above downwards—superior vena caval obstruction.
  - ❖ If the flow is below up wards—inferior vena caval obstruction.
- *Precordium for localized tenderness:*
  - ❖ Costochondral junction tenderness
  - ❖ Acute myositis
  - ❖ Acute pericarditis.
- *Precordium for palpation of heart sounds—thrill and rubs:* Method of palpation of heart sounds—thrill:
  - ❖ Patient should be in supine position
  - ❖ Examiner should examine the patient from his right side
  - ❖ Upper trunk is elevated at 30°—should in left lateral position—so heart will more laterally and toward the wall
  - ❖ Areas of the hand responsible for cardiac palpations (Fig. 4.77):
    - Palm of the hand and ventral surface of proximal metacarpals:
      - Ejection sounds
      - Valve closure sound
      - Mitral valve opening sound
      - Thrill.
    - By light pressure of fingertips:
      - Third heart sound
      - Fourth heart sound.

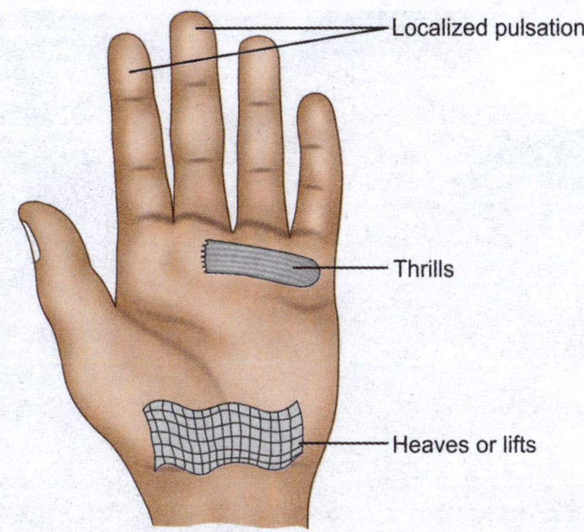

FIG. 4.77 Areas of examiner's hand for precordial pulsation

- Occasionally, by placing palm of right hand on the precordium and at the same time, placing the left hand on the back of the chest forcing forward. Heaves or lift can be palpated.

Palpation of Apex Beat (Figs 4.78 and 4.79)

Size and extent (displacement)
- Normal apical impulse
- Displacement
- Multiple cardial impulse.

In hypertrophic obstructive cardiomyopathy (HOCM), late systolic bulge, produces double apical impulse.

Character of Apical Impulse

- *Tapping:* Mitral stenosis
- *Hyperdynamic—volume overload:*
  - ❖ *Cardiac causes:*
    - Aortic regurgitation
    - Mitral regurgitation—increase in duration and amplitude of excursion
    - Ventricular septal defect
    - Atrial septal defect
    - Arteriovenous fistula.
  - ❖ *Systemic causes:*
    - Fever
    - Anemia

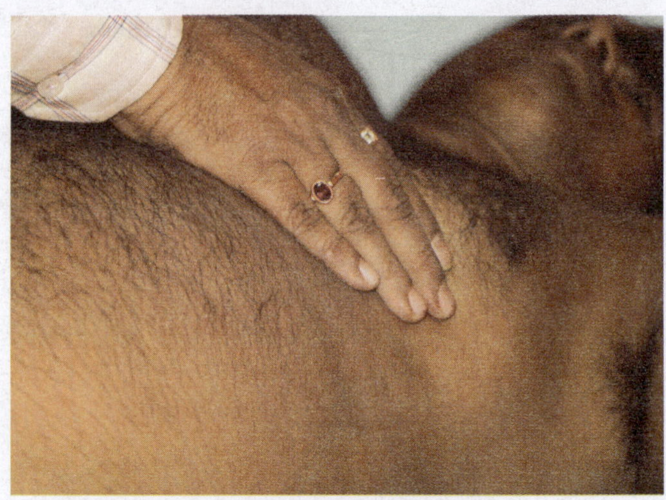

FIG. 4.78 Palpation of apex beat

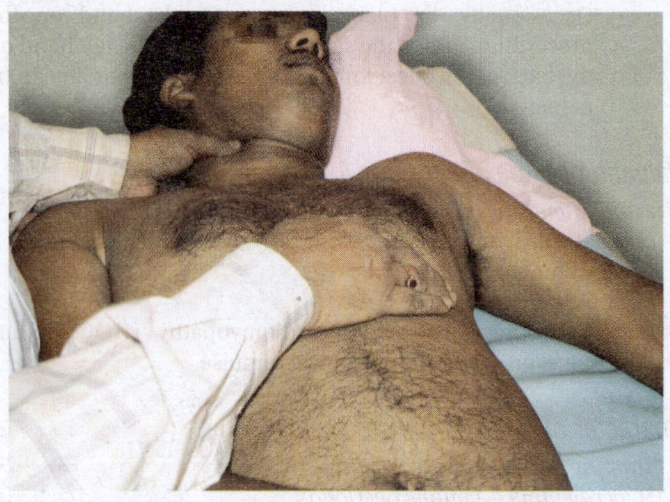

FIG. 4.79 Palpation of apex beat in left lateral position

- Beriberi
- Thyrotoxicosis.

● *Heaving—Due to pressure overload:*
  - ❖ Aortic stenosis
  - ❖ Systemic hypertension
  - ❖ HOCM
  - ❖ Aortic regurgitation

sustained in duration of excursion—due to increased duration of left ventricular ejection against resistance.

Palpable Third Sound

Third heart sound (left ventricular)
It is low frequency sound due to rapid ventricular filling phase:
Normally not palpable. But it can be palpable by light palpation with fingertips in expiration at the apex:

- *Physiologic:*
  - ❖ Children
  - ❖ Pregnancy.
- *Systemic:*
  - ❖ Thyrotoxicosis
  - ❖ Anemia.
- *Cardiac:*
  - ❖ Chronic mitral regurgitation
  - ❖ Left ventricular failure.

Fourth heart sound (left ventricular)
This is low frequency sound produced by forceful atrial contraction against noncompliant left ventricle, i.e. with elevated left ventricular end diastolic pressure—>15 <18 mm Hg (normal value <12 mm Hg).

It is not normally palpable. But it may be palpable at the apex.
The causes are:

- Aortic stenosis
- Systemic hypertension
- HOCM
- Acute mitral regurgitation.

Palpable 1st heart sound: Due to mitral stenosis.

Palpable opening snap—is due to pliability of mitral valve leaflet—heard and radiates to lower left sternal edge in early diastole.

Tumor plop—early diastolic sound—due to left atrial myxoma.

Palpable ejection sound—high frequency sound—occurs in systolic phase—due to opening of pliable aortic bicuspid valve—felt in apex more than right 2nd intercostals space.

Palpable pulmonary ejection sound—palpable in left 2nd inter-costals space.

But ejection sound of dilated aortic root may be palpated in right 2nd intercostals space.

Palpability of Thrill

- *Diastolic thrill:* Mitral stenosis—thrill may be palpated in (Figs 4.80A and B):
  - ❖ Apical area
  - ❖ If not palpable in supine position, it can be palpable in left lateral position and intensified in forced expiration.

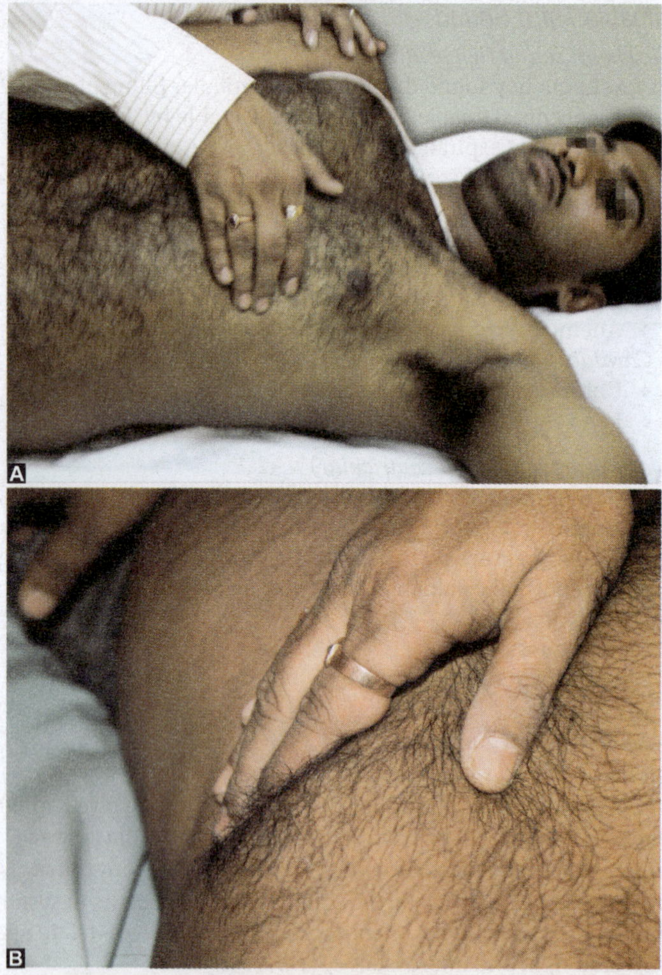

FIGS 4.80A AND B Diastolic thrill palpation in mitral stenosis: (A) Supine (B) Left lateral position

- *Systolic thrill:*
  - *Mitral regurgitation:* Palpated in (Fig. 4.81)
    - Apical area
    - Increased in expiration and forceful coughing
    - Increased left lateral position.
  - *Aortic stenosis (see Fig. 4.91)*
    - Right 2nd intercostals space
    - Radiated to carotid artery and towards apex

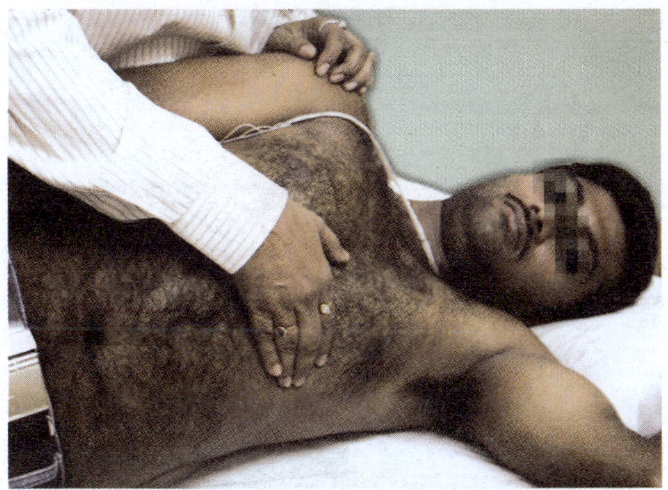

FIG. 4.81   Systolic thrill (MI) in left lateral position

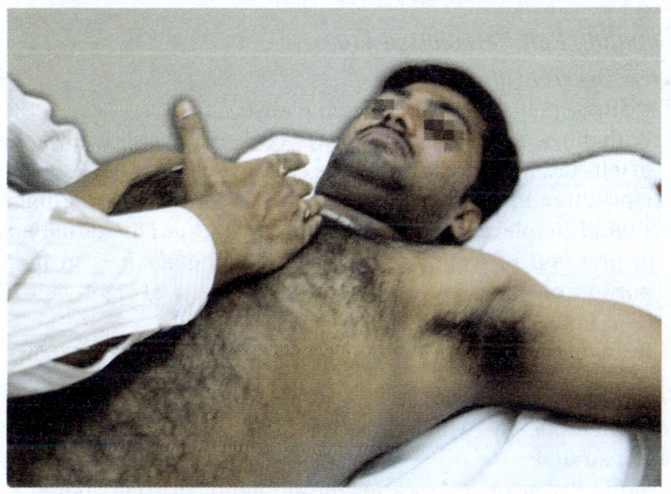

FIG. 4.82   Palpation of thrill in left 3rd and 4th ICS

- Intensified in forced expiration
- In sitting position and leaning forward.
- ❖ *VSD (Fig. 4.82):* At left 3rd and 4th intercostals space on left sternal edge.
- *Pericordial rub (Fig. 4.83):* Palpable in sitting position and leaning forward.

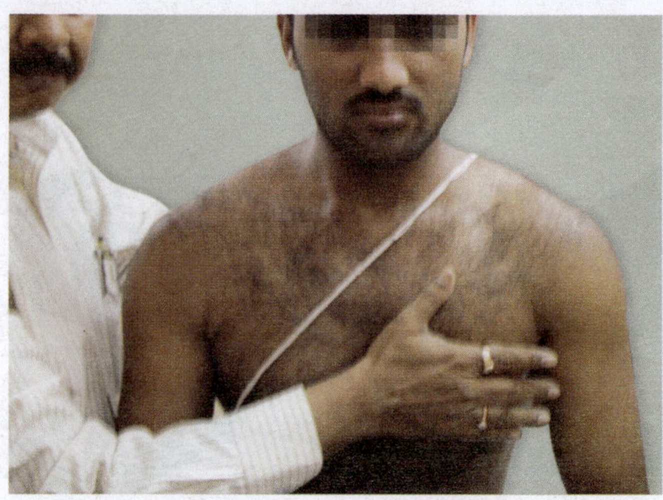

FIG. 4.83 Palpation of precordial rub

Palpating Left Parasternal Area

Left parasternal lift

This can be palpated in the following ways:

- With the heel of the hand and wrist cocked upwards in lower half of left sternal edge during end of expiration (Fig. 4.84)
- First three tips of the fingers (index, middle, and ring finger) should be placed at 3rd, 4th, and 5th ICS at left sternal edge during end of expiration—it detects—whether it is in inflow portion of right ventricle or outflow portion of right ventricle (Fig. 4.85A)
- By ulnar border of the hand on left parasternal area (Fig. 4.85B)

Gradation of parasternal lift

Two methods by which gradation of parasternal lift can be demonstrated:

- *Subjective method:* Assessing the amplitude of excursion
- *Objective method:* Assessing duration of parasternal lift.

Grade I parasternal lift (Fig. 4.86)

- *Subjective:* Light object (pencil) keeping it on parasternal area—it is to be seen, how much amplitude of excursion occurs
- *Objective method:* Duration less than 1/3rd of systolic phase.

Causes

- Childhood, young adult
- Thin chest.

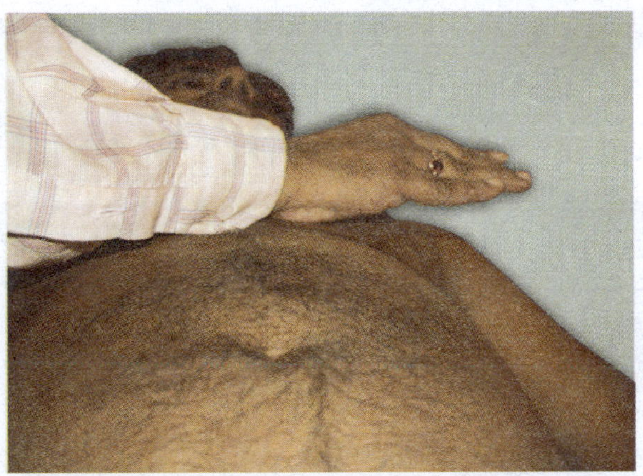

FIG. 4.84   Palpation of left parasternal area—I

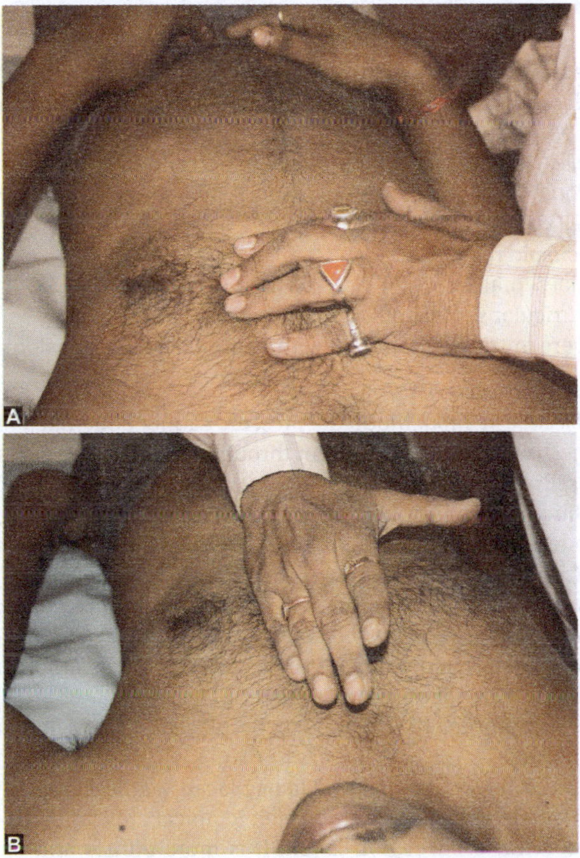

FIGS 4.85A AND B   Palpation of left parasternal area—II

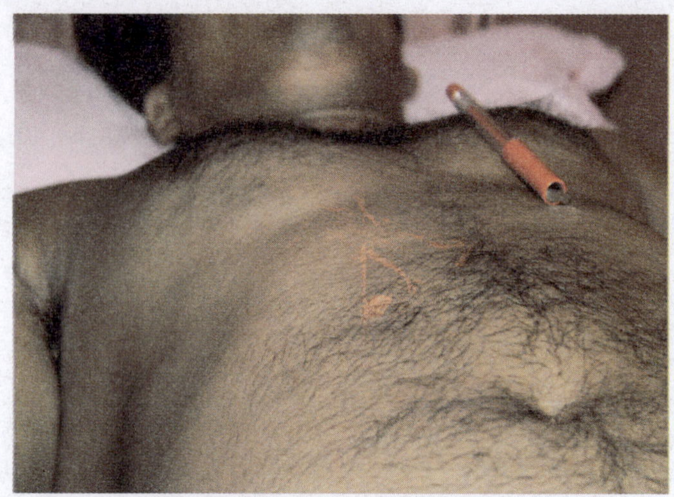

FIG. 4.86 Grade I parasternal lift

Grade II parasternal lift
- *Subjective method:* Moderate counter pressure can obliterate the amplitude of lift
- *Objective method:* More than 50 percent of systole but not throughout systole (well sustained).

Causes: Volume overload:
- Tricuspid regurgitation
- Atrial septal defect
- Ventricular septal defect
- Severe mitral regurgitation with pulmonary hypertension.

Grade III parasternal lift
- *Subjective method:* Moderate pressure cannot obliterate PSL
- *Objective method:* It is present throughout the period of systole.

Causes: Pressure overload:
- Pulmonary stenosis (moderate to severe)
- Moderate-to-severe pulmonary hypertension due to severe mitral stenosis or VSD.

Parasternal lifts in case of severe mitral regurgitation can be diagnosed by following methods (Figs 4.87A and B):
- Simultaneous palpation of apex and the parasternal area is mandatory to identify the type of PSL
  - ❖ Ulnar border of left hand to be placed at lower left sternal border
  - ❖ Index finger of right hand to be placed at apical area
  - ❖ Usually, first heart sound is felt in apical area followed by lift of parasternal region is felt. It is more diffuse and of short duration.

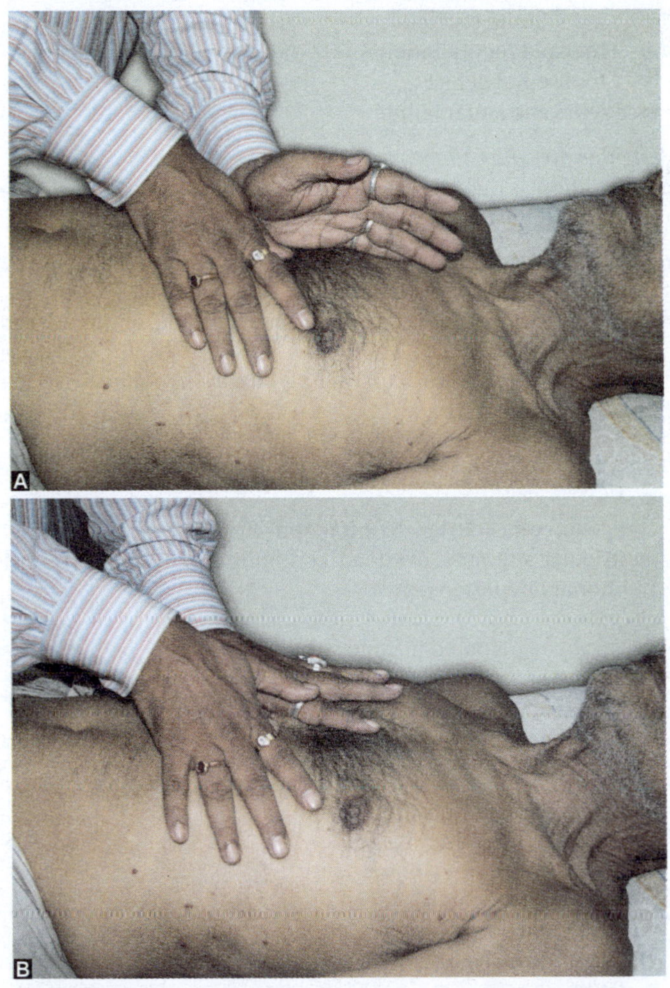

FIGS 4.87A AND B   Simultaneous palpation of apex and left parasternal area

- Simultaneously placing of index finger of right hand at the apex and index finger of left hand on left PSL.

Palpable right sided S$_3$
- Due to rapid right ventricular filling phase
- It can be felt in epigastric region or lower left sternal edge in supine and right lateral position
- It is present during forced inspiration, disappears during expiration.

- *Causes:* Volume overload
  - ❖ Tricuspid regurgitation
  - ❖ Atrial septal defect
  - ❖ Right ventricular failure.

S_4 (right ventricular 4th heart sound)
Same position as right ventricular S_3—pulmonary hypertension and pulmonary stenosis.

Palpation of lower left sternal area (tricuspid area)
- *Palpation of low frequency sound:*
  Position: Patient should be in supine position or right lateral position
  Sound: S_3—rapid ventricular filling phase—in volume overload condition:
  - ❖ Tricuspid regurgitation
  - ❖ ASD
  - ❖ VSD.

  S_4—forceful atrial contraction—in patient with right ventricular pressure overload condition—pulmonary stenosis, pulmonary hypertension.
- *Palpation of high frequency sound:* Opening snaps of tricuspid valve can be palpated in epigastrium
- *Palpation of thrill:*
  - ❖ In patient with tricuspid stenosis—diastolic thrill
  - ❖ In patient with tricuspid regurgitation—systolic thrill.

Palpation of aortic area (Fig. 4.88)
- *Site:* Right 2nd intercostal space
- *Sound:* High frequency sounds.
  - ❖ *Ejection sound:*
    - Aortic stenosis
    - Dilated aortic root
    - Congenital aortic stenosis—more readily palpable at apex.
  - ❖ *Palpable A_2:*
    - Systemic hypertension
    - Dilated aortic root
    - Congenital aortic stenosis
    - Congenital cyanotic heart disease—when aorta is anterior to pulmonary trunk.

Palpation of pulmonary area (Fig. 4.89)
- *Site:* Left 2nd intercostal space
- *Sound:*
  - ❖ *Pulmonary ejection sound*—in pulmonary stenosis
  - ❖ *Palpable P_2*—in pulmonary hypertension—may be heard in left sternal edge or apex.

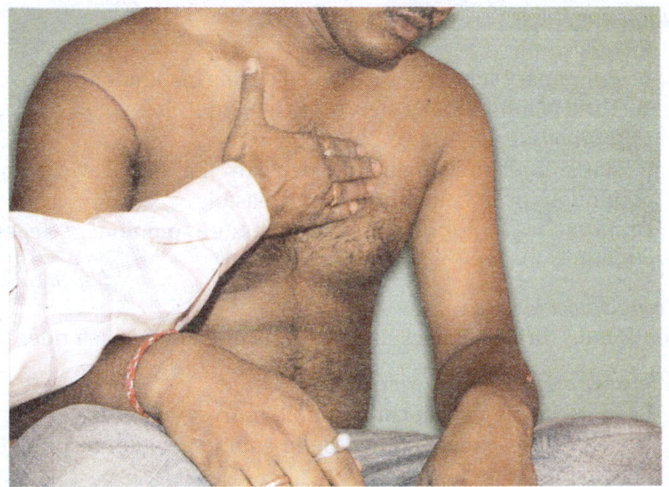

FIG. 4.88   Palpation in aortic area

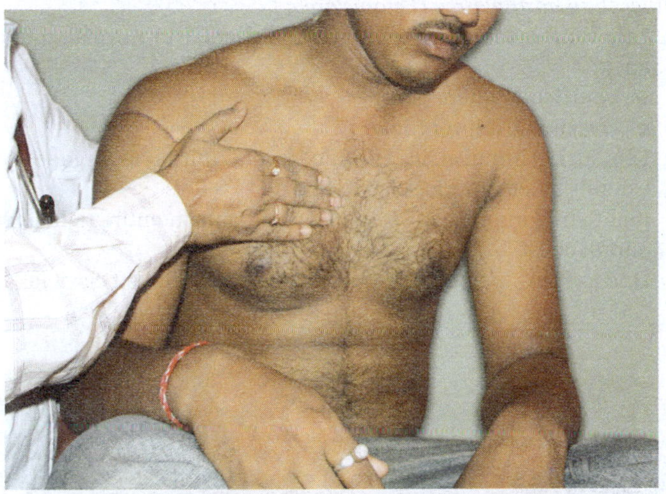

FIG. 4.89   Palpation in pulmonary area

Thrill

It can be described as a sensation the body of purring cat.

Aortic area

- *Systolic thrill:* This is due to presence of aortic stenosis exacerbated during expiration
- *Diastolic thrill:* Due to dilated aortic root in Marfan's syndrome

Pulmonary area
- *Systolic thrill:*
    - ❖ Pulmonary stenosis exacerbated during inspiration
    - ❖ Thrill of infundibular stenosis in left 3rd ICS.
- *Continuous thrill:* PDA:
    It starts in systole, palpable beneath the left clavicle and continuous over S_2. It proceeds into diastole
- *Graham-Steell murmur* of high pressure pulmonary regurgitation.

Sternoclavicular area
Continuous thrill of Blalock–Taussig shunt operation on left ride.

Epigastric area (Figs 4.90 and 4.91)
- By index finger just beneath zyphoid process—for RV
    Palpation—patient should be in supine position respiration held in inspiration.
- Aortic pulsation—for aortic aneurysm, aortic regurgitation
- Hepatic pulsation—in tricuspid regurgitation.

Other than normal area (Ectopic areas)
- Left ventricular impulse above and medial to normal cardiac apex:
    - ❖ Ventricular aneurysm
    - ❖ Dyskinetic left ventricle
- Left atrial impulse in chronic severe mitral regurgitation—extends to left anterior chest, left axilla
- Right atrial impulse in severe TR—palpable in entire right lower part of chest
- Due to POA—palpable ectopic impulse beneath left clavicle.

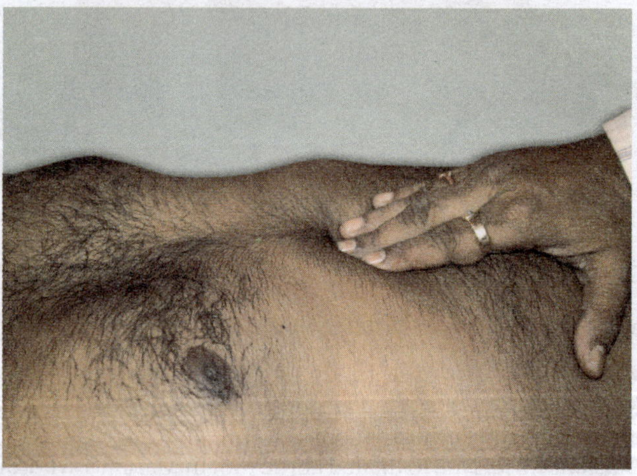

FIG. 4.90 Palpation in epigastrium

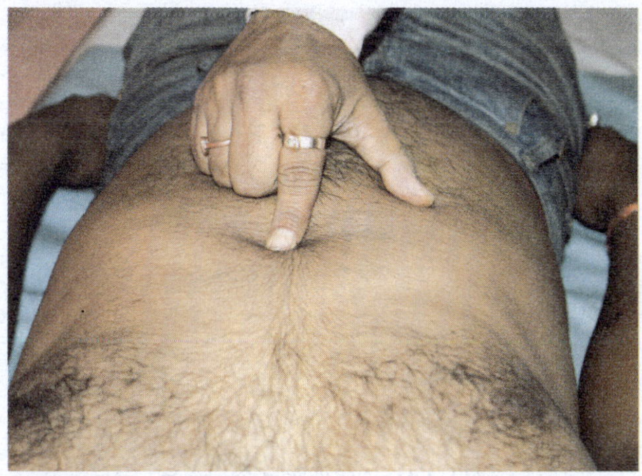

FIG. 4.91 Palpation in epigastrium with the help of index finger

Percussion

Percussion is not usually done in cardiological examination, but for following conditions, percussion should be done:
- To determine the size and shape of the heart
- To determine the border of the heart
- To determine the right atrium, right ventricle and pulmonary area
- To determine situs inversus.

Percussion may be of:
- *Direct percussion*—on sternum and clavicles
- *Indirect percussion*—using plexor—percussion finger and pleximeter—the finger on which plexor is being percussed
- *Auscultatory percussion (Fig. 4.92)*
  - ❖ *Method:*
    - Place the stethoscope on the sternum just above xiphi sternum
    - Scratch the skin lightly by finger of other hands from axillary area towards sternum. So, at which point soft scratch becomes suddenly intense, this detects cardiac border of that side.
  - ❖ *To detect:* Cardiac borders.

Percussion is usually done in the following conditions:
- *Right border of the heart (Figs 4.93A and B)*
  - ❖ First detect upper border of liver dullness by percussion along the right mid-clavicular line from above downwards
    It is usually detected in right 5th intercostal space in right MCL.

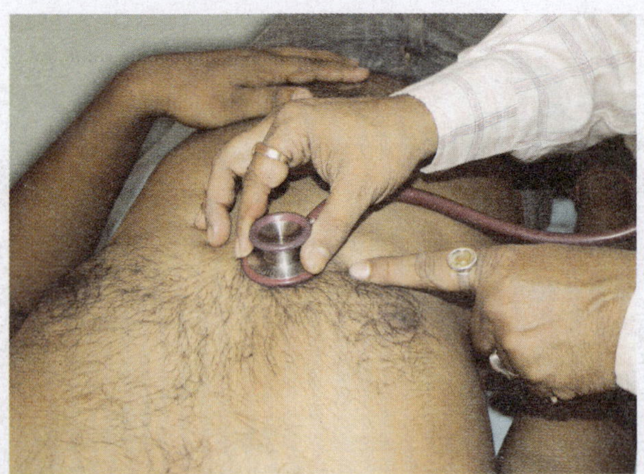

FIG. 4.92 Auscultatory percussion

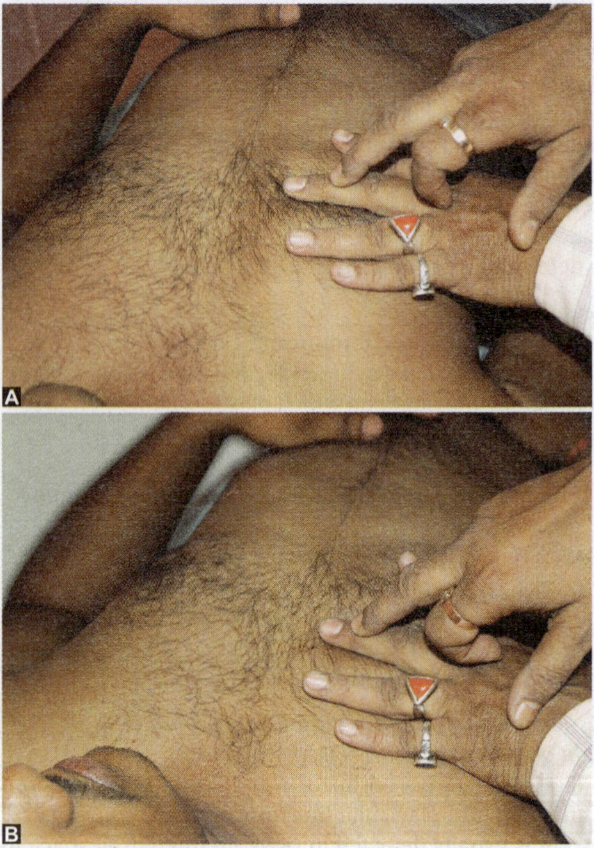

FIGS 4.93A AND B Right border of heart percussion

❖ From just above one space start percussion towards right side of sternum at right angle to the right border of heart

Normally, right cardiac border corresponds to right sternal border.

The cardiac border is progressed >1 cm from right sternal margin, it indicates:

❖ Mediastinal tumor
❖ Right atrial enlargement
❖ Pericardial effusion.

- *Left border of heart (Fig. 4.94):* Starts percussion from left axilla towards left cardiac border

When the dullness is reached—it detects left cardiac border—corresponds to cardiac apex.

But in the following conditions, the left cardiac border does not correspond to apex:

❖ Left ventricular aneurysm—apex beat is upward and medial to left border
❖ Pericardial effusion—apex beat in medial to lateral border
❖ If left cardiac border is >3.5 cm from the mid sternal line, it indicates enlarged left atrial appendages.

- *Percussion of aortic area (Fig. 4.95):* Normally right 2nd intercostals space—aortic area—is resonant. But in following conditions it is dull:

❖ Pericardial effusion
❖ Aortic aneurysm
❖ Mediastinal widening due to tumor.

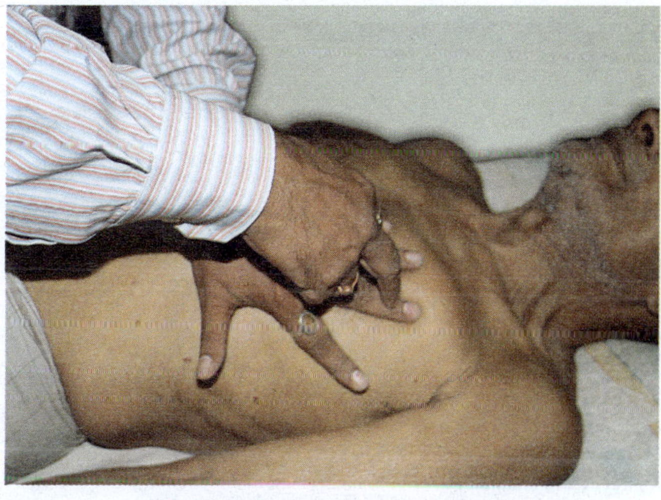

FIG. 4.94 Cardiac left border percussion

- *Percussion in pulmonary area (Fig. 4.96):* Normally left 2nd intercostal space (pulmonary area) to resonant. But in the following conditions it is dull:
  - ❖ Pericardial effusion
  - ❖ Patent ductus arteriosus
  - ❖ Dilated pulmonary artery.
- *Direct percussion on the sternum (Fig. 4.97):* It should be done to detect pathology of mediastinum:
  - ❖ Superior mediastinum
  - ❖ Middle mediastinum.

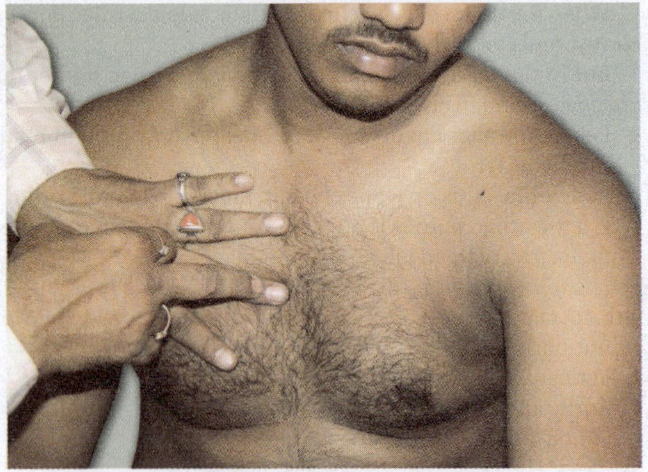

FIG. 4.95   Percussion in aortic area

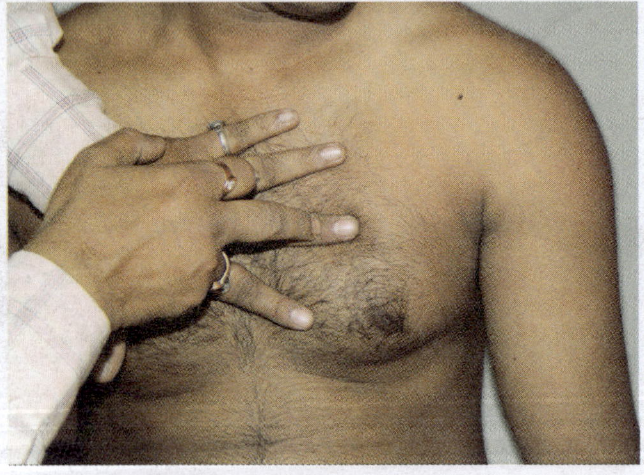

FIG. 4.96   Percussion in pulmonary area

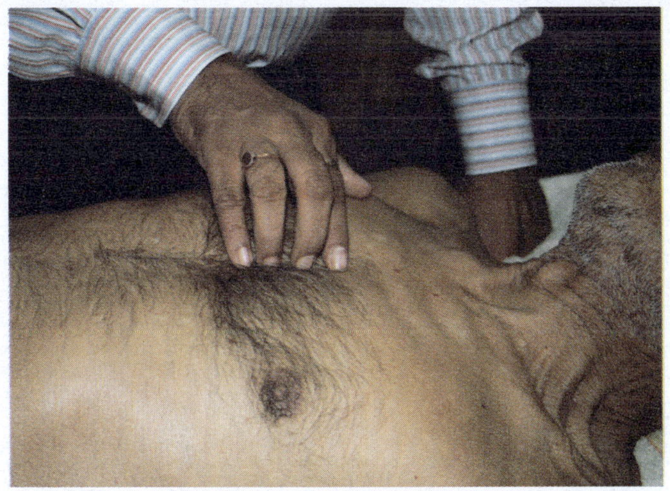

FIG. 4.97 Direct sternal percussion

In case of superior mediastinum the following conditions may produce dullness in upper sternum:
❖ Aortic aneurysm
❖ Mediastinal tumor.

In case of middle or inferior mediastinum, the following conditions may produce dullness in lower sternum:
● Pericardial effusion
● Right ventricular hypertrophy
● Mediastinal mass.

Rotch's Sign

● First defect upper border of liver dullness
● Next, detect right border of heart along the right sternal edge
● The lines parallel to the above borders cross at angle, which is called cardiohepatic angle.

If the angle is obtuse—it is due to pericardial effusion—it correlates with dullness in right 2nd intercostals space.

Determination of situs inversus
● Detect—liver dullness
● Detect—gastric fundus (Fig. 4.98)
  ❖ Normally fundal resonance is on left side and liver dullness is on the right side of the body
  ❖ If, fundal resonance is on the right side of liver dullness is on the left side of the body—it indicates situs inversus.

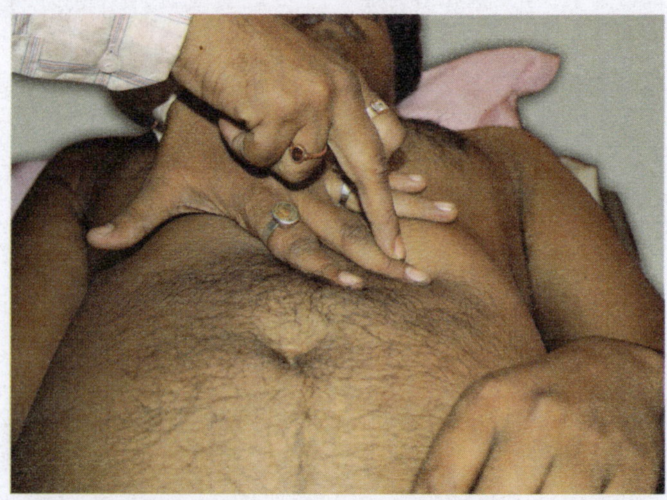

FIG. 4.98 Detection of gastric fundus

Auscultation

Principles based on which auscultation method will be described:
- Human ear capability—20–20000 Hz
- Human ear sensitivity—1000–5000 Hz
- Human auditory activity—1000–2000 Hz
- Most cardiovascular sounds and murmur—30–1000 Hz.

If human acoustic sensitivity <1000 Hz, low intensity sounds and murmur will be missed.

Cardiac sounds are usually described in the following heads:
- Loudness—it correlates with amplitude and intensity of sounds
- Pitch of sounds—it correlates with frequency of sounds.

Four types of sounds and murmurs are described according to frequency:
- *Low frequency (25–125 cycles per seconds):*
  - ❖ *The sounds are:*
    - Third heart sound
    - Fourth heart sound
    - Pericardial knock.
  - ❖ *The murmurs are:*
    - Mid diastolic murmur of mitral stenosis
    - Mid diastolic murmur of tricuspid stenosis.
- *Mid frequency (126–300 cycles per seconds):*
  - ❖ Sounds are not present
  - ❖ *Murmurs—rough flow murmurs:*
    - Innocent systolic murmur
    - Physiological murmur.

- *High frequency (>300 cycles per seconds):*
  - ❖ *The sounds are:*
    - Aortic and pulmonary components of 2nd sound
    - Opening snap
    - Ejection sound.
  - ❖ *Murmurs are soft and blowing murmurs:*
    - Murmur of mitral regurgitation
    - Murmur of tricuspid regurgitation
    - Murmur of aortic regurgitation
    - Cooing murmur of papillary muscle dysfunction.
- *Mixed frequency* combination of high and medium frequency.
  - ❖ *The sound:* First heart sound
  - ❖ *Murmur:* Harsh in character.
    - Murmur of aortic stenosis
    - Murmur of pulmonary stenosis
    - Murmur of ventricular septal defect.

Factors Affecting the Auscultation of Cardiac Areas

- *From the patient's side:*
  - ❖ *Chest wall:*
    - Thin—chest helps in clear auscultation
    - Thick chest wall—muffles the sounds.
  - ❖ Obese patient
  - ❖ Breast size—in case of female
  - ❖ Chronic obstructive pulmonary disease.
- *Examination room:* If noise in the room >35 decibel, it hampers normal hearing of cardiac sounds.
  Normal noise of examination room is 60–70 decibel.
- *Noise of atmosphere:*
  - ❖ Sounds of traffic
  - ❖ Sounds of construction
  - ❖ Sounds of talk between peoples.
- *From doctors sides:*
  - ❖ Bad diaphragm of stethoscope
  - ❖ Age related otosclerosis—producing hearing loss.

Areas to be ausculated for detection of heart sounds and murmur
- *Apical area:* Mitral area
- *Tricuspid area:* 4th and 5th intercostals space adjacent to left sternum
- *Pulmonary area:* Left 2nd intercostal space
- *Aortic area:* Right 2nd intercostal space
- *Over the carotid:* Radiation of murmur of:
  - ❖ Aortic valve disease
  - ❖ Carotid bruit in atherosclerotic disease.

- *Axilla to hear the murmur radiation in case of:* Mitral valvular regurgitation
- *Back:*
  - ❖ *Interscapular area:*
    - Murmur of coarctation of aorta—descending aorta
    - Aneurysm of aorta.
  - ❖ Collateral circulation
  - ❖ *Over the spine:*
    - Murmur of coarctation of descending aorta
    - Aneurysm of aorta.
- *Right side of chest:* Dextrocardia
- *Epigastric region:* For tricuspid regurgitation murmur
- *Peripheral arterial sites:* Over femoral arteries—for aortic regurgitation, murmur radiation—Duroziez murmur.

Identification of Sounds

- S_1 or first heart sound—signifies onset of ventricular systole
- S_2 or 2nd heart sound—signifies onset of ventricular diastole
- Simultaneous palpation of carotid artery pulse can detect systolic and diastolic phases.

Position of patients
- Supine and left lateral position—S_1—mitral valve (Figs 4.99A and B)
- Supine position—S_1—tricuspid valve (Fig. 4.100)
- Sitting position with leaning forward—aortic and pulmonary component of 2nd sound (Figs 4.101 and 4.102).

Maneuvers to alter the intensity of heart sounds and murmur
- Alteration in depth of respiration
- Isometric exercise
- Position of patient—in standing and squatting position
- Valsalva maneuvers, Müller maneuver
- Pharmacological maneuver (amyl nitrite).

Basic Heart Sound (Fig. 4.103)

First Heart Sound

Intensity of 1st heart sound depends upon:
- Presence of pleural effusion, pericardia effusion
- Transmission through chest wall—whether thin or obese or muscular
- Position of mitral valve leaflet at the onset of ventricular systole. It depends on:

    Duration of PR interval, i.e. difference in timing between atrial and ventricular contraction.

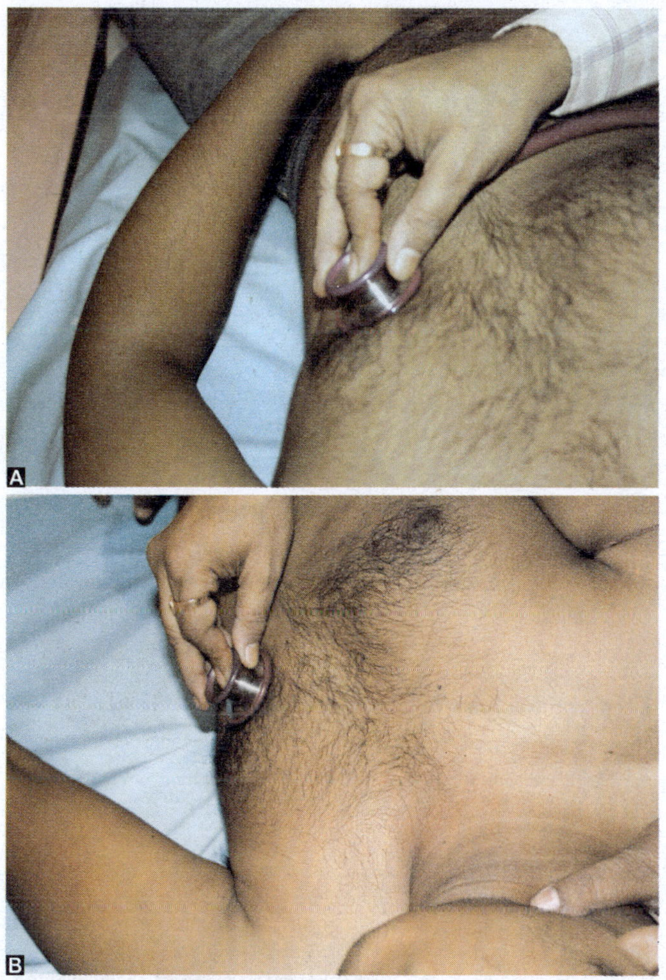

FIGS 4.99A AND B   Auscultation of 1st heart sound (Mitral area)

Normal PR interval = 140–200 ms.

If PR interval <140 ms—position of mitral valve leaflets are furthest apart at the onset of ventricular systole, so speed of closure, is high producing loud 1st heart sound.

If PR interval >200 ms—mitral valve leaflets already start closing during atrial relaxation, less separation of leaflets at the onset of ventricular contraction, so S_1 will be soft.

- *Venous return to left atrium if:*
  - *Less:* Less amount of blood will go to LV, so leaflets are furthest apart during onset of ventricular contraction, producing loud

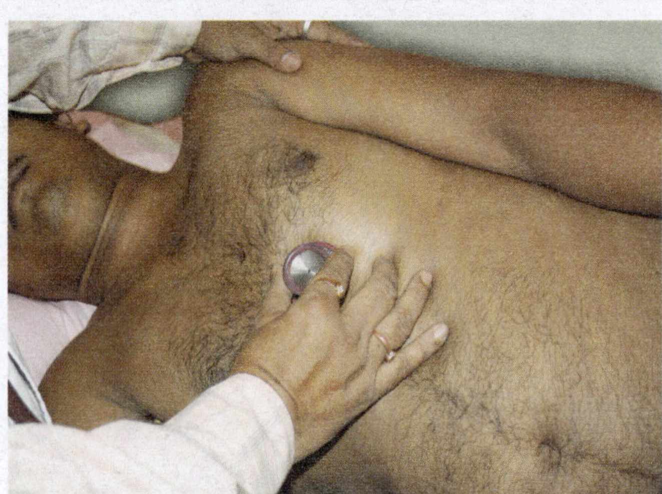

FIG. 4.100 Auscultation of tricuspid area

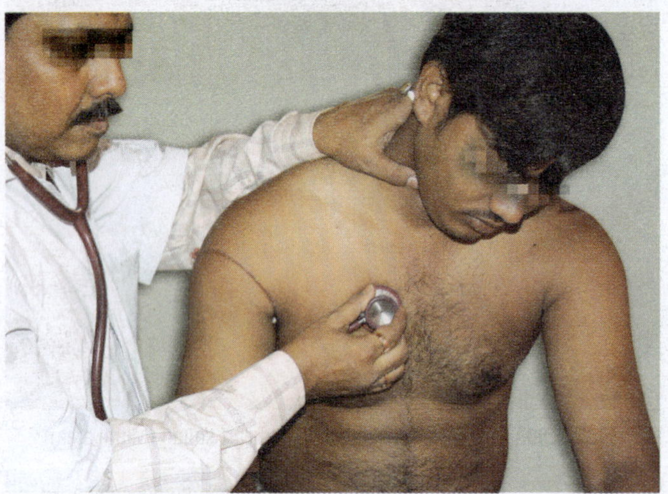

FIG. 4.101 Auscultation in aortic area

S_1 and soft S_4. If large amount of blood will go to LV by vigorous atrial contraction.

❖ *High:* Leaflets become closure at the onset of ventricular systole producing soft S_1 and loud S_4.

- *Structural integrity of mitral valve:*
  ❖ Whether mitral valve is pliable or calcified or thickened
  ❖ Whether leaflet tissue is damaged by infection.
- Size of the AV orifice.

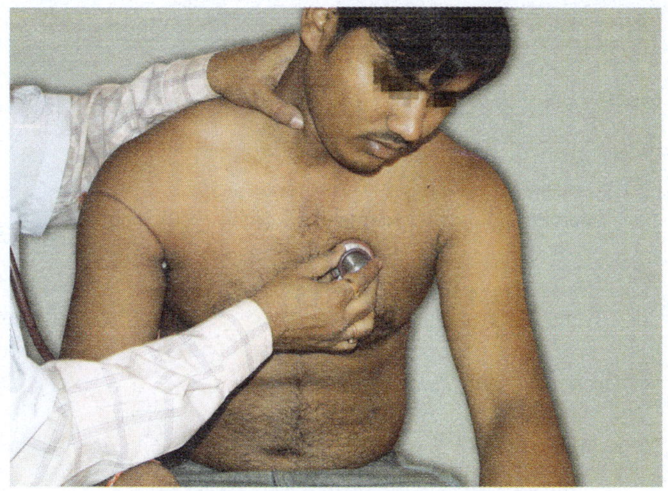

FIG. 4.102 Auscultation in pulmonary area

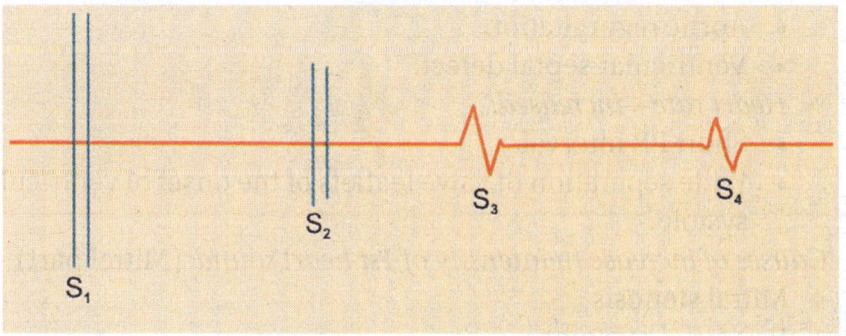

FIG. 4.103 Basic heart sounds

- *Ventricular contraction status. It depends upon:* Size of LA-LV pressure gradient
  - ❖ *Increased ventricular contractility depends upon:*
    - Exercise
    - Anemia
    - Thyrotoxicosis
    - Pregnancy
    - Pheochromocytoma
    - AV fistula.

  Heart rate—it increases intensity of heart sound due to:
    - Shortened PR interval (Figure 4.104 showing relation of S_1 with PR interval)
    - Wide open valve due to high flow through shortened diastole.

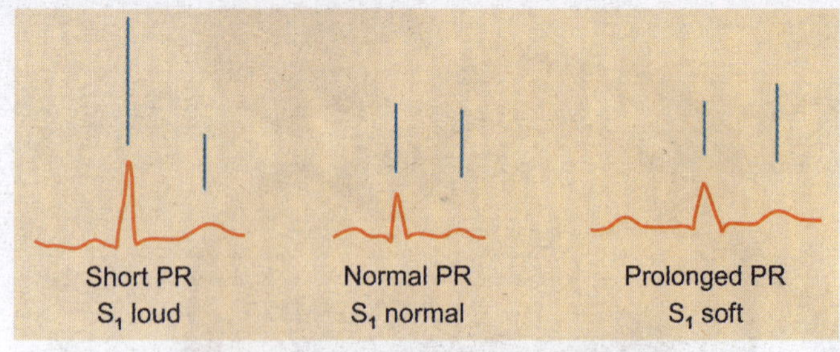

FIG. 4.104 Relation of S_1 with PR interval

❖ *Decreased ventricular contractility:*
- MI
- Myocarditis
- Dilated cardiomyopathy
- Ventricular aneurysm.

❖ *Loss of isometric ventricular contraction phase:*
- Mitral regurgitation
- Aortic regurgitation
- Ventricular septal defect.

❖ *Heart rate—increased:*
- Short PR interval
- Wide separation of valve leaflets of the onset of ventricular systole.

• *Causes of increase in intensity of 1st heart sound:* (Mitral part)
- ❖ Mitral stenosis
- ❖ Left atrial myxoma
- ❖ Hyperkinetic circulatory states
- ❖ Exercise
- ❖ Mitral valve prolapose.

In case of tricuspid valve
- Tricuspid stenosis
- Right atrial myxoma
- ASD.

Causes of decreased intensity of 1st heart sound
- Mitral regurgitation (severe)
- Severe aortic regurgitation
- Calcified valve
- Cardiomyopathy
- Myocarditis
- Left bundle branch block.

Variable intensity of 1st heart sound
- Atrial fibrillation
- Atrial flutter with varying block
- Atrial tachycardia with varying block
- Ventricular tachycardia with varying block.
  Normal gap between mitral component and tricuspid component of 1st heart sound is 0.02–0.03 ms.
  If the gap is >0.03 ms—the separate sound can be heard in lower left sternum.

Wide split of 1st heart sound is due to:
- Complete right bundle branch block
- Ebstein's anomaly—sail sound due to:
  - ❖ Delayed activation.
  - ❖ Increased right atrial pressure.

Reverse splitting of 1st heart sound (T_1 component heard before M_1):
- Complete left bundle branch block
- Idioventricular rhythm originating from RV
- Right ventricular pacing
- Right ventricular ectopic
- Right mitral stenosis
- Large left atrial myxoma.

Second Heart Sound

This sound is composed of two components:
1. Aortic valve closure sound—A_2
2. Pulmonary valve closure sound P_2

The areas where the above sound can be heard
- Aortic valve closure sound (A_2) is best heard in right 2nd intercostal space, it can also be heard in pulmonary area as well as at the apex
- Pulmonary valve closure sound (P_2) is best heard in left 2nd intercostal space.

Characteristics of 2nd heart sound
- It is louder, high frequency, duration is 0.11 sec.
- A_2 occurs earlier than P_2 because:
  - ❖ Right ventricle ejection starts earlier and longer than that of left ventricle ejection, resulting P_2 occurring after A_2
  - ❖ Hangout interval—this is the difference between cross-over of pressure and actual closure (Fig. 4.105).
    This hangout interval in case of left side (difference between left ventricular pressure and aortic pressure) is 30 msec.

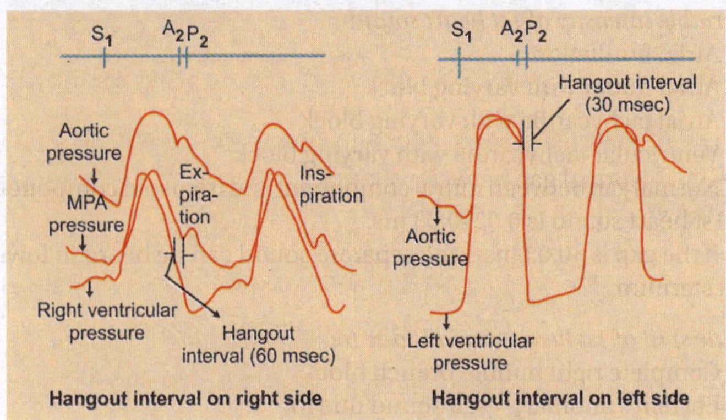

FIG. 4.105 Hangout interval

The hangout interval in case of right side (difference between right ventricular and mean pulmonary artery pressure) is 60 msec.

Since hangout interval in case of right side is more than that of left side, hence P_2 is late than that of A_2.

- A_2 coincides with incisura of aortic pressure
  P_2 coincides with incisura of pulmonary valve closure
- A_2 is louder than P_2, because there is high pressure in aorta than that in pulmonary artery
- *S_2 is louder than S_1 because:*
  ❖ Decreased elasticity of semilunar valve and aorta
  ❖ Low blood volume in arteries acts as vibrating mass.

  Since, low inertia of small amount of blood may produce intense vibration on the arterial wall, hence, intensity of 2nd heart sound is louder than first heart sound.
- *Variation with respiration:*
  ❖ *During inspiration:* Increased venous return to the right side of the heart, produces increased stroke volume, and prolongs the duration of right ventricular cardiac output. So P_2 component of 2nd heart sound is delayed
  ❖ *During expiration:* Intrathoracic pressure is positive, hence less amount of blood will enter the right side of the heart, so right ventricular stroke volumes is decreased. On the other hand, left ventricular stroke volume is large duration of left ventricular stroke volume is increased. So the gap between A_2 and P_2 will be decreased.
- *Variation with position:*
  ❖ In recumbent position, large amount of venous blood will enter the right side of the heart in inspiratory phase of respiration, it lengthens right ventricular systole, thus widens

the splitting of S_2—prolonging the P_2 component (A_2 - P_2 = >30 msec)

❖ *In upright position:* In expiration, venous return to the heart is decreased, shortens the right ventricular ejection times, shortens the physiological split of S_2.

Normal gap between A_2 and P_2 is 30 msec.

During expiration, gap between A_2 and P_2 is <30 msec, so 2nd sound is usually heard as single sound.

During inspiration the gap between A_2 and P_2 is >30 msec, so there is splitting of 2nd sound.

Mechanism of split (Fig. 4.106)
- *During inspiration:*
  ❖ *In right side of heart:* Increase in venous return to right atrium is increased:

↓

Right ventricular volume is increased

↓

Increased right ventricular stroke volume

↓

Increased pulmonary vascular bed capacitance

↓

Increases hangout interval between right ventricular pressures and mean pulmonary arterial pressure

↓

Delay in closure of pulmonary valve
  ❖ *In left side of the heart:* During inspiration:
  Increased pooling of blood in pulmonary vascular bed

↓

Decreased amount of blood will go to left atrium

↓

Decreased amount of blood will enter left ventricle

↓

Decreased left ventricular stroke volume

↓

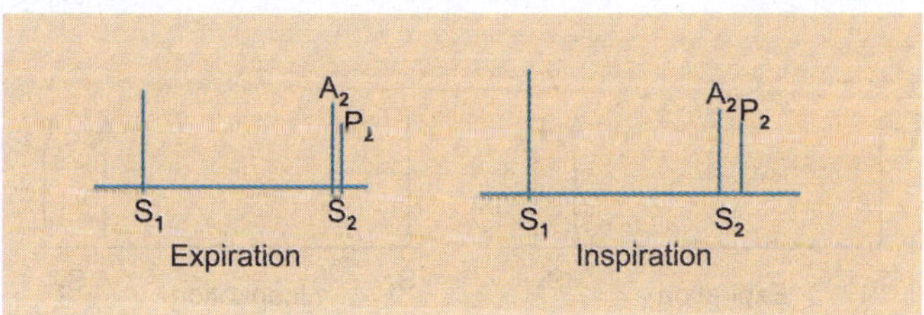

FIG. 4.106 Normal physiological splitting of 2nd heart sound

Decreased hang out time in between left ventricular pressure and aortic pressure

↓

Early occurrence of A_2

- *During expiration:*
  - ❖ *In right side of the heart:*
    Increase in intrathoracic pressure

    ↓

    Decrease venous return to the right side of the heart

    ↓

    Decrease right ventricular stroke volume

    ↓

    Decrease hang out interval between right ventricular pressure and mean pulmonary pressure

    ↓

    Early closure of pulmonary valve
  - ❖ *In left side of the heart:*
    Increased intrathoracic pressure

    ↓

    Increased volume of blood will go to left atrium

    ↓

    Left ventricle

    ↓

    Increased hangout interval between left ventricular pressure and aortic pressure

    ↓

    Delayed closure of A_2

So net result is:
During inspiration: There is increase in physiological split.
During expiration: There is single 2nd heart sound.

Now, the splitting of 2nd heart sound may be abnormal, when expiratory split occurs in both supine and upright position.

The abnormal splitting of S_2 may be:
- *Persistent physiological splitting:* Wide physiological splitting (Fig. 4.107)

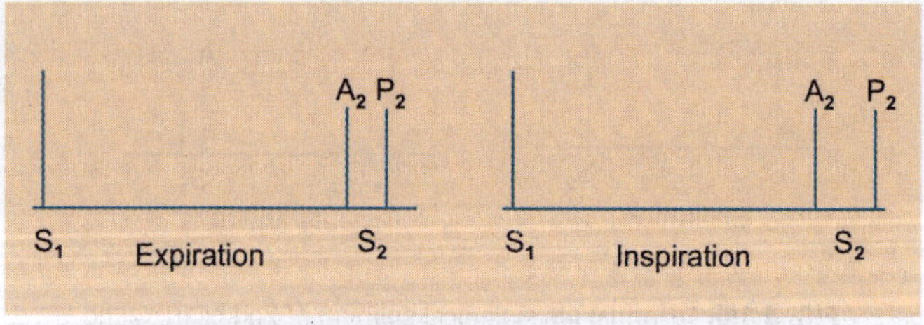

FIG. 4.107 Wide physiological splitting of 2nd heart sound

❖ *Delayed closure of pulmonary valve:*
- Electrical abnormalities in heart:
  - Complete right bundle branch block
  - Left ventricular pacing
  - Left ventricular ectopic.
- Mechanical obstruction to right ventricular systole:
  - Pulmonary stenosis
  - Pulmonary hypertension with right ventricular failure
  - Pulmonary embolism
  - ASD.
- Early aortic valve closure:
  - Mitral regurgitation
  - Ventricular septal defect—uncomplicated.

In above two cases, during left ventricular contraction large amount of blood enter into left atrium (in case of MS) and right ventricle (in case of VSD).

Narrowed physiological splitting (Fig. 4.108)
- In pulmonary hypertension:
  Increased impedance to right ventricular emptying
  $\downarrow$

  There is no inspiratory lengthening of right ventricular systole
  $\downarrow$

  Early closure of pulmonary valve
  $\downarrow$

  Decreased splitting or no splitting of 2nd sound.
- Diseased semilunar valve of either side may produce A_2 and P_2 singly
- *Emphysema:* During inspiration—due to hyperinflation of lung—pulmonary component of the 2nd sound is muffled. But during expiration, this phenomenon is less pronounced.

- *Wide and fixed splitting of 2nd heart sound:* This means the splitting between A_2 and P_2 is wide and fixed in both inspiratory or expiratory phases

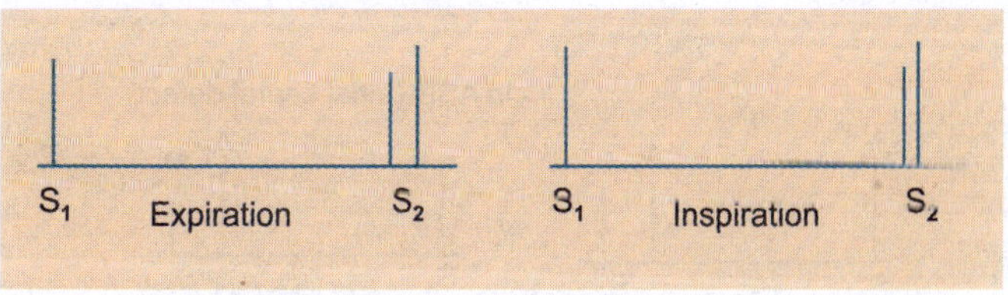

FIG. 4.108 Narrow physiological splitting of 2nd heart sound

The split is wide because of the following reasons:

Delay in right ventricular ejection time due to:

* Prolonged right ventricular contraction
* Increased hang out time.

The split is fixed because:

* This split is not decreased with valsalva maneuver
* There is no delay in inspiration because of no change in right ventricular filling and stroke volume during inspiration.

The causes of fixed wide split of 2nd heart sound:

* Ostium secundum type of atrial septal defect
* Total anomalous pulmonary venus connection
* Severe impedance to right ventricular filling, e.g. pulmonary stenosis, massive pulmonary embolism. These patients cannot cope with increase venous return during inspiration, so they maintain fixed wide splitting during respiration.

  In ASD (atrial septal defect) the split is fixed and wide.

The causes of wide split in ASD are (Fig. 4.109):

* Prolonged right ventricular ejection time
* Increase hangout time
* Right bundle branch block.

The causes of fixed split in ASD:

* During inspiration, increased venous return produces prolonged right ventricular stroke volume and ejection time.

  At this time there is no left to right stunt through ostium secundum.
* *During expiration:* Venus return to the right side of heart is decreased. So accordingly right ventricular volume should be decreased. But in atrial septal defect, there is left to right atrial shunt through secundum, so it maintains normal right ventricular stroke volume and minimizes the respiratory variation.
* Due to increased pulmonary vascular capacitance, no addition decrease of pulmonary vascular impedance during inspiration, so no inspiratory delay of P_2.

* *Reverse or paradoxical splitting:* Here aortic component closes later than P_2. So it may be due to:

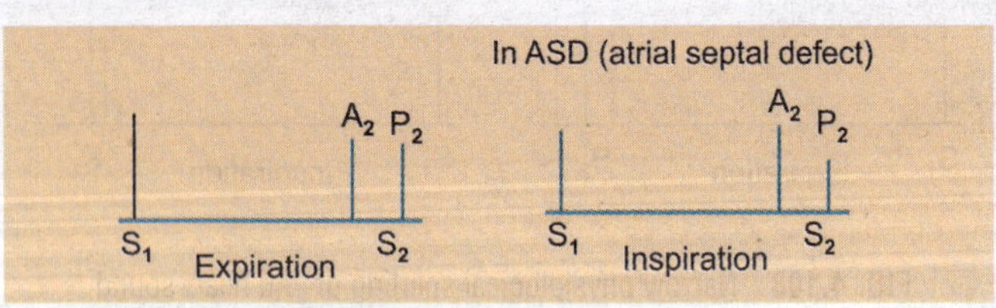

FIG. 4.109   Wide and fixed split

- ❖ *Delayed aortic valve closure:*
  - Complete left bundle branch block
  - Right ventricular ectopic
  - RV pacing
  - Aortic stenosis
  - Systemic hypertension
  - Cardiomyopathies
  - Myocarditis
  - Ischemic heart disease.
- ❖ *Early closure of pulmonary valve:*
  - Tricuspid regurgitation
  - Right atrial myxoma
  - Type B WPW syndrome.

Three types of reverse splitting
- *Type I reverse splitting (Fig. 4.110):* Here:
  - ❖ During inspiration—single S_2
  - ❖ During expiration—split occurs reverse sequence, i.e.—A_2 following P_2—due to prolonged left ventricular electro-mechanical systole
- *Type II reverse splitting (Fig. 4.111):* Here:
  - ❖ Normal inspiratory splitting
  - ❖ Expiratory splitting in reverse sequence.
- *Type III reverse splitting:* Here:
  - ❖ Single sound in both phases of respiration
  - ❖ A_2 and P_2 interval <20 msec with reverse sequence during expiration.
- *Single second heart sound:* Absence of split in both phases of respiration—when the gap between aortic and pulmonary sound is <30 msec. The causes are:
  - ❖ Type III reverse splitting
  - ❖ *Absent P_2:*
    - Old age >60 years
    - Emphysema
    - Obesity
    - Chest wall thickened

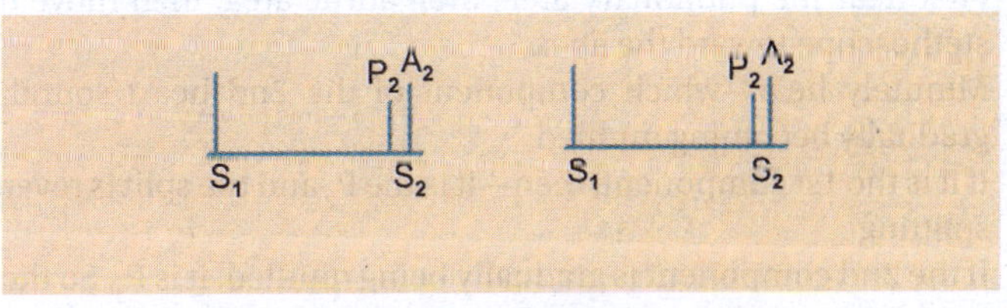

FIG. 4.110 Reverse splitting of S_2 (Type I)

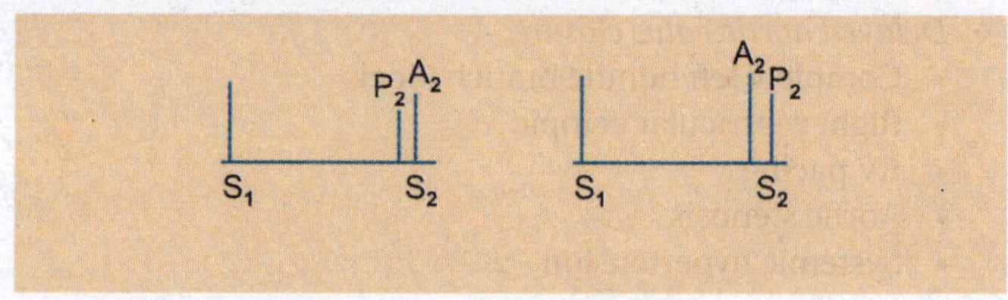

FIG. 4.111   Reverse splitting of S₂ (Type II)

- Serve pulmonary stenosis
- Pulmonary valve atrosia
- Fallot's tetralogy
- Severe aortic stenosis
- Single left ventricle
- Double outlet right ventricle.

- *When aortic or pulmonary component is inaudible:*
  - ❖ Severe aortic stenosis
  - ❖ Aortic atresia
  - ❖ Severe pulmonary stenosis
  - ❖ Conditions producing delay in A_2 producing reverse splitting but the interval between P_2 and A_2 is <30 seconds.

Intensity of 2nd heart sound depends upon
- Status of the valves
- Flow across the valve
- Pressure in the vessels—increased pressure produces ↑ P_2
- The size of vessels beyond the valve:
  - ❖ If it is increased—it produces loud P_2
  - ❖ If it is decreased—it reduces intensity of P_2.

Differentiation of two components of S_2

Aortic component can be heard in aortic areas, pulmonary areas and apex.

Pulmonary component—can be heard in pulmonary area only, since it is too soft to be heard in other areas.

So to detect A_2 and P_2:
- First hear the pulmonary area, then aortic area, then move the stethoscope toward the apex
- Minutely hear—which component of the 2nd heart sound is gradually becoming muffled
- If it is the 1st component, then—it is the P_2 and the split is reverse splitting
- If the 2nd component is gradually being muffled, it is P_2. So there is no reverse splitting.

Causes of increased intensity of pulmonary component of 2nd heart sound:
- Pulmonary hypertension
- *Hyperdynamic circulation:*
  - ❖ Fever
  - ❖ VSD
  - ❖ ASD
  - ❖ Dilatation of pulmonary artery
  - ❖ Chest wall—thin.
- Loss of thoracic kyphosis.

Causes of increased intensity of aortic component:
- Systemic hypertension
- Dilatation of ascending aorta—in syphilis, ankylosing spondylosis—associated with increased flow through the valve
- Aneurysm of ascending aorta
- Congenital heart disease—bicuspid aortic valve.

Causes of decreased intensity of pulmonary component:
- *Causes other than the heart:*
  - ❖ Chest wall
  - ❖ Obesity
  - ❖ COPD
- *Cardiac cause:*
  - ❖ Tetralogy of Fallot
  - ❖ Pulmonary atresia
  - ❖ Dysplastic pulmonary valve
  - ❖ Pulmonary stenosis.

Causes of decreased intensity of aortic component:
- Severe aortic stenosis—diminished mobility or calcification
- Valvular aortic regurgitation.

Grading of intensity of pulmonary component

Grade	Area of loudness	Systolic pressure in pulmonary artery
I	P_2 intensity like that of A_2 in pulmonary area	30–49 mm Hg
II	P_2 intensity more than that of A_2 in pulmonary area palpable P_2 in pulmonary area	50–75 mm Hg
III	P_2 is very loud and can be heard beyond the pulmonary area palpable P_2	>75 mm Hg

'Tambour' S_2: It indicates ringing and loudness of the sound.
It is caused by: Dilatation of aortic root in:
- Syphilis—Potain's sign
- Marfan's syndrome
- Dissecting aneurysm of ascending aorta   Harvey's sign.

Extra sounds: These can be divided into:
- Diastolic sounds—these are snaps, plops, knock
- Systolic sounds—early, mid and late systolic.

Diastolic sounds are the following (Fig. 4.112):
- *Third heart sound:* Low pitched and soft—early diastolic
- *Fourth heart sound:* Low pitched and soft—late diastolic
- *Opening straps:* High pitched and loud—early diastolic
- *Pericardial knock:* High pitched and loud—early diastolic
- *Tumor plop:* Medium pitched—early diastolic.

Mechanism of production of S_3—third heart sound:
There are several theories regarding production of third heart sound. These are:
- *Ventricular theory:* Sudden and abnormal deceleration of left ventricular flow during the phase of rapid ventricular filling producing entire cardiovascular system into vibrations
- *Impact theory:* According to this theory, ventricular mechanism can be recorded in ventricular cavity of apex ventriculogram.

But the S_3—heard from chest wall—is not the passive transmission of ventricular mechanism to the chest wall.

It is the combination of impact of chest wall and heart. This depends on:
- Size of heart
- Decreased space in between chest wall and heart
- The movement of heart in thoracic cavity
- Thickness of chest wall—obese, emphysema, etc.
- Phase of respiration

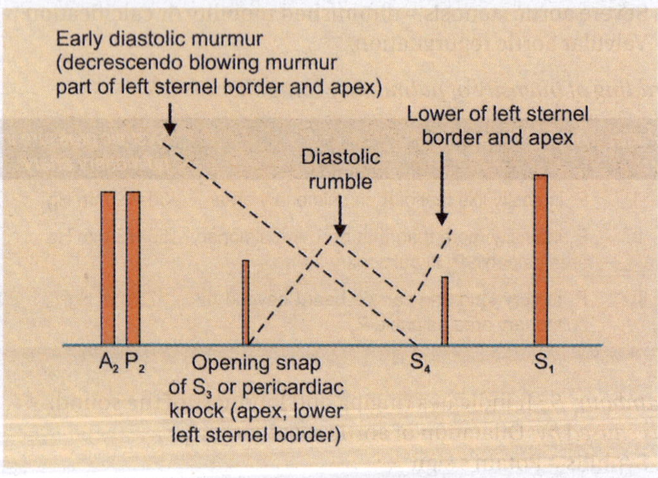

FIG. 4.112 Diastolic sounds

- Position of the body during examination, e.g.
  - ❖ Left lateral decubitus for left ventricular S_3
  - ❖ Supine position for right ventricular S_3.

Third heart sound occurs in two conditions:
1. *Physiological:*
   - ❖ 120–200 msec after aortic sound
   - ❖ Early diastolic sound
   - ❖ Low pitched, soft
   - ❖ It can be heard with bell of stethoscope and with light pressure on the apical area
   - ❖ Patient should be in left lateral decubitus position, it brings left ventricle nearer to chest wall
   - ❖ The sound is usually heard during expiratory phase of respiration
   - ❖ It coincides with 'y' descent of Jugular venous curve.

Causes of physiological third heart sound
- Child
- Young adult male <40 years, female <50 years
- In athletes—if associated with bradycardia—it is due to increased left ventricular filling caused by high cardiac output in patients with bradycardia

  In patients with >40 years of age, slowing of ventricular relaxation leads to delayed diastolic filling—responsible for disappearance of third heart sound. Hence it's presence at this age is always pathological.
- In 80 percent of pregnant woman—increased sympathetic tone produces rapid circulation and tachycardia (hyperkinetic heart syndrome).

  Bell of stethoscope is usually used to hear third heart sound because it fillers all extraneous sounds and makes low pitched 3rd heart sound more detectable.

  Again, if too much pressure is applied with the bell during auscultation, it will be transformed into diaphragm, making 3rd heart sound inaudible. Hence light pressure should be given with bell during hearing of 3rd heart sound.

Third heart sound occurs in early diastole because:
Third heart sound occurs during rapid ventricular filling phase. Again rapid ventricular filling phase starts at the onset of diastole as soon as AV valve opens. Eighty percent of blood from atrium will enter into ventricle.

Last 20 percent of blood will enter in later phase of diastole and at the time of active atrial contraction, which is responsible of fourth heart sound (S_4).

Pathological third heart sound:
- It occurs in mid-diastole—140–160 msec after A_2
- It occurs in mid diastolic phase.

Causes of third heart sound
- *Hyperkinetic circulatory states:* Anemia, fever
- *Valvular heart disease:*
  - ❖ Mitral regurgitation
  - ❖ Tricuspid regurgitation.
- *Congenital heart disease:*
  - ❖ Ventricular septal defect
  - ❖ Atrial septal defect
  - ❖ Patent ductus arteriosus
  - ❖ TAPVC.
- Myocarditis—dilated cardiomyopathy
- Ischemic heart disease.

Difference between physiologic S_3 and pathologic S_3
- Pathologic S_3 is softer, low pitched, associated with gallop
- Duration may be longer.

Pathologic S_4 is softer because of reduced ventricular contractility. This may produce tachycardia.

Sometimes low pitched diastolic murmur may follow pathologic third heart sounds because:

This sound is produced by sudden rush of blood through atrioventricular valves—occurs in case of ventricular dysfunction or increased transmitral flow, in case of mitral regurgitation.

This condition is purely pathological.

The conditions producing ventricular overload responsible for third heart sound:

- *Intracardiac shunt:* VSD:

  ASD is not responsible for production of S_3, because in case of left to right intra-atrial shunt, less blood will flow through transmitral area, on the other hand, most blood will flow through tricuspid valve, which is less likely to produce right sided S_3.

- *Intravascular shunt:* PDA

- *Mitral regurgitation:* S_3 is louder and high pitched, occurs due to rush of flow through mitral valve.

S_3 in mitral regurgitation does not indicate heart failure but may indicate the severity of the regurgitation.

In case of aortic regurgitation, third heart sound more indicate left ventricular failure.

Gallop: It is nothing but triple lift like the cadence of the horse. There are three types of gallop:

1. Ventricular gallop (Fig. 4.113)—produced by S_1, S_2 and S_3.
2. Protodiastolic gallop (Fig. 4.114)—produced by S_4, S_1 and S_2.

3. Summation gallop—produced by summation of S_3 and S_4 (S_3 + S_4) = S_7 in association with S_1 and S_2 in case of sinus tachycardia, when ventricular systolic time is shortened.

Causes of summation gallop:
- Hypertensive heart failure
- Hypertrophic cardiomyopathy
- First degree AV block.

The summation gallop may resemble mid diastolic rumble—easily palpable.

This can be diagnosed by slowing the heart rate by cautious carotid massage.

Quadruple rhythm: This is the combination of:
S_3, S_4, S_1, S_2—this occurs in patient with:
- Ventricular aneurysm
- Cardiomyopathy
- Left ventricular failure.

Hemodynamic effect of S_3
This depends upon mechanism of its generation:
- *Increased ventricular preload (diastolic overload):*
  - ❖ Atrial pressure is decreased
  - ❖ Cardiac index, ejection fraction increased.
- *Ventricular dysfunction (systolic):*
  - ❖ Cardiac index—decreased
  - ❖ Ejection fraction <30 percent
  - ❖ Left atrial pressure, pulmonary wedge pressure, pulmonary capillary pressure—increased.

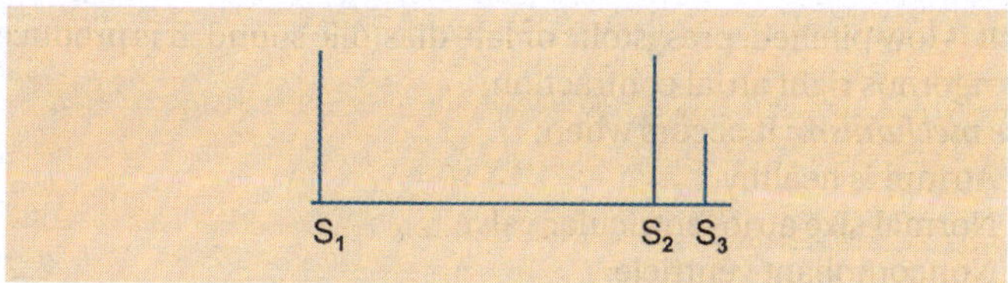

FIG. 4.113   Ventricular gallop

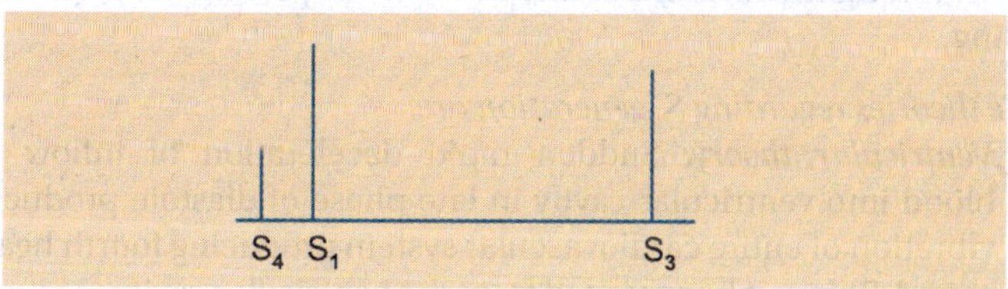

FIG. 4.114   Protodiastolic gallop

Clinical implication of S_3:
- Its presence predicts poor systolic dysfunction (left atrial pressure)
- It's absence dictates ejection fraction >30 percent
- It's presence in patient with mitral regurgitation—signifies its severity
- In case of noncardiac surgery, S_3—predicts postoperative mortality due to cardiac failure or infarction
- Its presence in patient with congestive cardiac failure and elevated jugular venous pressure—predicts worse outcome
- In myocardial infarction:
  - ❖ In early stage it may appear, but may resolve within a matter of days or weeks
  - ❖ If it persists for weeks—it may predict—large myocardial damage, cardiac failure.

Causes of right ventricular third heart sound:
- Increased flow across the tricuspid valve
- Increased impedence to right ventricular emptying, e.g. pulmonary embolism, cor pulmonale.

Differentiation between opening snap and third heard sound

S_3	Opening snap
• Low pitched, softer	• High pitched, louder
• Heard with bell	• Heard with diaphragm
• Heard at the apex	• Heard in lower left border of sternum

Fourth Heart Sound

S_4: It is low pitched, presystolic or late diastolic sound. It is produced by vigorous right atrial contraction:

The mechanism: It occurs when:
- Atrium is healthy
- Normal size atrioventricular valve
- Noncompliant ventricle.

In case of noncompliant ventricle, vigorous atrial contraction in necessary for large amount of blood to enter into left ventricular cavity through atrioventricular orifice. It is >25 percent of ventricular filling.

The theories regarding S_4 generation are:
- *Ventricular theory:* Sudden rapid deceleration of inflow of blood into ventricular cavity in late phase of diastole produces vibration of entire cardiovascular system producing fourth heart sound. This can be recorded from the ventricular cavity

- *Impact theory:* According to this theory, dynamic impact of heart and chest wall produces fourth heart sound, heard from the chest wall.

Sites and recognition of fourth heart sound
- *Left ventricular fourth heart sound:*
  - ❖ This is heard at the apex
  - ❖ Bell of the stethoscope has to be used
  - ❖ Pressure should be gentle
  - ❖ Patient should be in left lateral position
  - ❖ Should be heard in expiratory phase
  - ❖ Any maneuver, that increases the venous return, increases the intensity of S_4
  - ❖ S_4 is also increased with hand grip in sitting up position and coughing.

  Differentiation from first heart sound:
  - ❖ S_4 will be obliterated with pressure applied with the bell but S_1 does not
  - ❖ S_4 will be accentuated by hand grip during sitting up position
  - ❖ Any maneuver that increases venous return to the heart, e.g.—supine position may accentuates the S_4.
- *Right ventricular fourth heart sound:*
  - ❖ This is usually heard at lower left sternal border
  - ❖ Patient should be in supine position
  - ❖ Accentuated during inspiratory phase
  - ❖ This correlates with 'a' wave of Jugular venous wave. So S_4 may be audible in right jugular vein.

Causes of fourth heart sound
- *Physiological:* In elderly person >60 years of age, may be due to:
  - ❖ Hypertrophy—as a result of hypertension.
  - ❖ Fibrosis—as a consequence of myocardial ischemia.
- *Pathological:* This may be present in:
  - ❖ *Excessive rapid late diastolic filling due to:* Hyperkinetic circulation:
    - Anemia
    - AV fistulas
    - Acute valvular regurgitation:
      - Acute mitral regurgitation
      - Acute aortic regurgitation
      - Acute tricuspid regurgitation.

    In acute valvular regurgitation:
    - Left ventricle is noncompliant due to volume overload
    - Left atrium is not dilated, produces forceful atrial contraction.

But in chronic valvular regurgitations:
- Left ventricle will be dilated and compliant
- Left atrium will be dilated, hence force of contraction will be diminished
- In few cases atrial fibrillation will be present, so in that case there will be no contraction
- If associated mitral stenosis, atrial contraction cannot be transmitted to ventricle.

❖ *Left ventricular pressure overload:*
- Left side of the heart:
  - Systemic hypertension
  - Aortic stenosis
  - Hypertrophic obstructive cardiomyopathy.
- Right side of the heart:
  - Pulmonary hypertension
  - Pulmonary stenosis.

S_4 is due to increased left ventricle—aortic pressure gradient (presystolic gradient > 70 mm Hg, left ventricular end diastolic pressure ≥13 mm Hg).

❖ *Ischemic heart disease:*
- Myocardial ischemia—producing angina pectoris may be due to vessel occlusion or vessel spasm
- Myocardial infarction—producing:
  - Fibrosis
  - Aneurysm.

Differentiation of S_4 from split S_1:
- Split S_1—varies with respiration
- Best heard with diaphragm
- Attenuate or soften after standing
- S_1 can be heard on left border or sternum.

Differentiation from ejection sound:
- Ejection sounds are usually heard with diaphragm
- These sound are best heard in sitting position leaning forward
- These sounds vary respiration
- These sounds cannot be palpable.

Heart Sound in Different Conditions (Fig. 4.115)

Opening Snap (Fig. 4.116)

It is a diastolic sound occurs in early part of diastole due to opening of atrioventricular valves. Normally these do not produce any sound during opening. But if the valves are thickened, deformed, they may produce snap sound during opening.

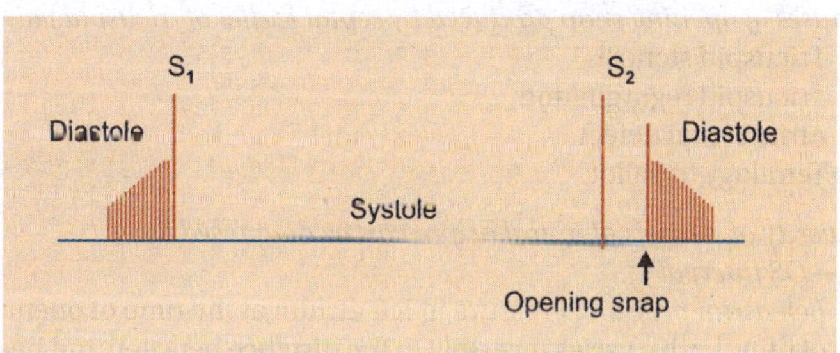

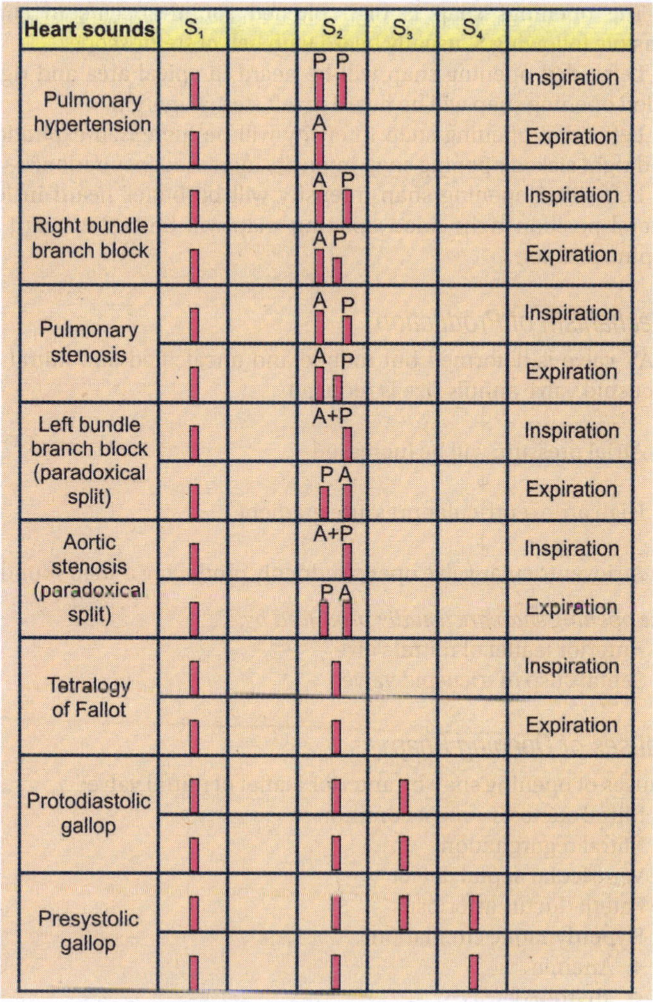
Heart sounds
S1
S2
S3
S4
Pulmonary hypertension
P P
A
Inspiration
Expiration
Right bundle branch block
A P
A P
Inspiration
Expiration
Pulmonary stenosis
A P
A P
Inspiration
Expiration
Left bundle branch block (paradoxical split)
A+P
P A
Inspiration
Expiration
Aortic stenosis (paradoxical split)
A+P
P A
Inspiration
Expiration
Tetralogy of Fallot
Inspiration
Expiration
Protodiastolic gallop
Presystolic gallop

FIG. 4.115 Heart sounds in different cardiac disease

S1
S2
Diastole
Diastole
Systole
Opening snap

FIG. 4.116 Opening snap

The openings snap is high pitched sound—occurs in early diastole following S_2 usually heard with bell of stethoscope.

Left sided opening snap will be heard in apical area and right sided opening snap will be heard in left sternal margin.

Left sided opening snap intensity will be increased expiration and right sicked opening snap intensity increased inspiration.

Left sided opening snap intensity will be better heard in left lateral position right sided opening snap will be better heard in supine position.

Mechanism of Production

If AV valve is deformed but mobile and uncalcified and mitral or tricuspid valve annuls size is reduced

↓

Atrial pressure will be increased

↓

High atrioventricular pressure gradient

↓

Atrioventricular valve opens suddenly producing a snap sound

The opening snap are usually produced by:
- Anterior leaflet of mitral valve
- Septal cusp of tricuspid valve.

Causes of Opening Snap

Causes of opening snap by anterior leaflet of mitral valve:
- Mitral stenosis—most common
- Mitral regurgitation
- Ventricular septal defect
- Patent ductus arteriosus
- Hyperdynamic circulation:
  - ❖ Anemia
  - ❖ Thyrotoxicosis
  - ❖ Beriberi.

Causes of opening snap produced by septal leaflet of tricuspid valve:
- Tricuspid stenosis
- Tricuspid regurgitation
- Atrial septal defect
- Tetralogy of Fallot.

Severity of stenosis of mitral orifice can be diagnosed by:
A_2—OS interval
- *Left atrial pressure:* Pressure in left atrium at the time of opening of mitral valve varies inversely to the distance between 2nd heart sound and opening snap.

- ❖ If LAP is increased to 15 mm Hg—the distance between A_2 and OS will be 120 msec—mild type
  - ❖ If LAP is 20 mm Hg—this distance will be 60 to 80 msec—moderate type.
  - ❖ If LAP is 25 mm Hg—this distance will be <60 mm.
- *Heart rate:*
  - ❖ In bradycardia—the distance will be increased
  - ❖ In tachycardia—the distance will be decreased.
- *Hypertension:* Left ventricular systolic pressure will take time to decrease below the left atrial pressure. So the distance will be increased
- In coronary artery disease, due to left ventricular dysfunction, left ventricular end diastolic pressure will be remain increased, so atrioventricular pressure gradient will be low and A_2—OS—distance will be increased
- *In aortic regurgitation:* There is early closure of aortic valve, so A_2—OS—distance will be increased
- *Stiffness of mitral valve leaflet:* If mitral valve leaflet will be stiffened, the mobility of the cusps will be decreased as a result A_2—OS—distance will be increased.

Decreased intensity of opening snap:
- Calcified mitral valve
- Associated mitral regurgitation
- Congestive cardiac failure
- Dilated left ventricle—where left ventricular wall is being pushed away from the chest wall
- Pulmonary hypertension—producing low flow of blood through mitral orifice
- *Noncardiac causes:*
  - ❖ Emphysema
  - ❖ Obesity.

Tumor Plop (Fig. 4.117)

- It occurs due to left or right atrial myxoma
- They arise from interatrial septal long stock
- Tumor plop is early diastolic sound
- It is high frequency sound
- This sound in case of left side of heart, can be heard in the apical area and in case of right side of heart, can be heard in left lower sternum
- The intensity is variable and varies with body position. From supine to standing position tumor suddenly blocks the AV orifice, i.e. it occurs at the maximal diastolic descent of the myxoma

FIG. 4.117 Tumor plop

- In case of right-sided atrial myxoma, there is diastolic rumble, holosystolic murmur of tricuspid regurgitation, prominent 'a' wave in Jugular venous pulse with rapid y descent, elevated Jugular venous pressure.

Pericardial Knock

Characteristics of knock:
- It is of sharp, high pitched early diastolic sound
- It is usually heard by bell of stethoscope
- Position—supine
- Site—left sternal border
- Phonocardiographically—it is heard 0.1 to 0.2 sec after A_2.

Mechanism of production of sound
It is produced due to sudden cessation of rapid ventricular filling.

Confusions with the following sounds
- Third heart sound
- Opening snap.

The cause of pericardial knock
- Chronic calcific pericarditis
- Chronic constrictive pericarditis.

The following features—which are associated the above pericarditis that can differentiate them from third heart sound or opening snap:
- Inspiratory fullness of neck vein—present in more or less half of the patients
- Systolic retraction of apex (Broadbent's sign) due to contact with calcific and fibrotic pericardium
- Pulsus paradoxus—occurs in 40 percent of patients
- Deep 'X' and 'Y' descent in jugular venous pulse. 'Y' descent is due to impairment of ventricular filling only at the end of diastole—Friedreich's sign

- Hepatomegaly—congestive
- Engorged neck vein
- Pedal edema
- Anasarca.

Systolic Sound

Ejection sound (Fig. 4.118): This is high pitched sound—originates in early parts of systole.

Origin of sound mechanism

Ejection sound originates from:

- In case of noncardiovascular causes—it results from hyperdynamic circulation, e.g. fever, thyrotoxicosis
- In case of cardiovascular cause, it originates from:
  - Valvular cause—either from aortic or pulmonary valves—caused by abrupt doming of semilunar valves followed by opening of thickened valve.
  - Vascular cause—this is due to opening movement of the leaflet that resonate the arterial trunk.

Causes of ejection sound

- *Valvular ejection sound:*
  - *Aortic valve:*
    - Aortic stenosis
    - Bicuspid aortic valve.
  - *Pulmonary valve:*
    - Pulmonary stenosis
    - Tetralogy of Fallot.
- *Vascular ejection sound:*
  - *Increased postvalvular pressure:*
    - Systemic hypertension
    - Pulmonary hypertension.
  - *Increased blood flow through the valve:*
    - *Hyperdynamic circulation:* Anemia, fever, thyrotoxicosis
    - Atrial septal defect—pulmonary ejection sound
    - Aortic regurgitation.

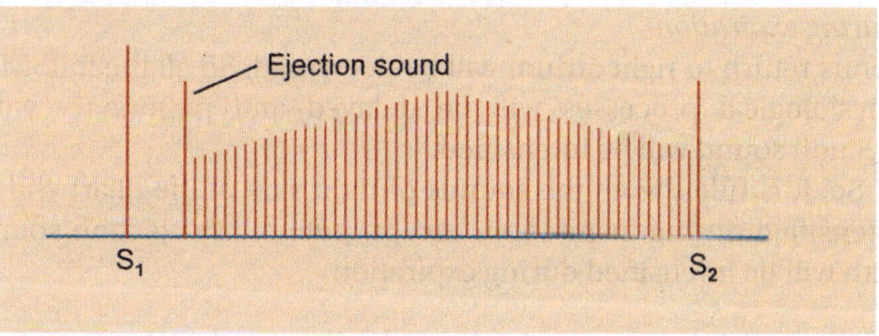

FIG. 4.118   Ejection sound

✦ *Dilatation of vascular structure beyond the valve:*
- Idiopathic dilatation of aorta or pulmonary artery
- Aortic aneurysm.

Ejection sound may be accompanied by murmur occasionally due to, bicuspid aortic valve with relative stenosis.

This bicuspid stenotic aortic valve is accompanied by post-stenotic dilatation of aorta, intensify the ejection sound.

Character of ejection sound (Fig. 4.119)
- *Aortic sound:*
  - ✦ It is discrete, high pitched sharp sound
  - ✦ If is heard at the aortic area (right 2nd and 3rd intercostal space, it may be heard at the apex, occasionally this sound may be heard in apex only)
  - ✦ Patient should sit and lean forward
  - ✦ Sound will be heard with the diaphragm of stethoscope
  - ✦ This sound does not vary with respiration.
- *Pulmonary sound:*
  - ✦ This sound should be heard in left 2nd and 3rd intercostal space.
  - ✦ This sound is intensified during expiration because:

    During inspiration—venous return to the right atrium is increased

    ↓

    Large volume of blood enter into right ventricle

    ↓

    Right ventricular end—diastolic pressure is increased (RVEDP)

    ↓

    RVEDP will be above pulmonary artery diastolic pressure

    ↓

    There will early opening of pulmonary valve

    ↓

    The early appearance of pulmonary valve ejection sound and this premature opening makes the pulmonary ejection sound soften.

During expiration
Venus return to right atrium will be decreased. So all the following physiological processes will be delayed and pulmonary valve ejection sound will be intensified.

So, it is rule the all the sounds of right side of the heart will be intensified during inspiration, except, pulmonary ejection sound, with will be intensified during expiration.

Significance of aortic ejection sound
Aortic ejection sound only can be heard in valvular aortic stenosis, not in subvalvular aortic stenosis or supravalvular aortic stenosis or hypertrophic obstructive cardiomyopathy.

Significance of intensity of aortic ejection sound
Aortic ejection sound signifies that:
- Aortic valve cusps are not fibrotic or calcified
- Aortic valve leaflets are mobile
- In elderly patient, stenosed valves are less pliable.

Aortic vascular ejection sound
- This sound is localized to the aortic area cannot be heard at the apex
- Second heart sound is normal split and loud
- It occurs on the upstroke of aortic pressure curve.

Pulmonary vascular ejection sound
- This sound is heard at pulmonary area, may be heard lower down the sternum
- Pulmonary component of 2nd sound is loud and 2nd sound is narrow split.

Nonejection Sound

Mid-systolic click (Fig. 4.119)
Character of the sound:
- High pitched, short clicky sound
- Timing—mid-systolic
- Site—over the apex and lower left sternum
- Best heard with diaphragm of stethoscope
- Intensity is variable with various maneuvers.

Causes of mid-systolic click
- Mitral valve prolapse
- Tricuspid valve prolapse.

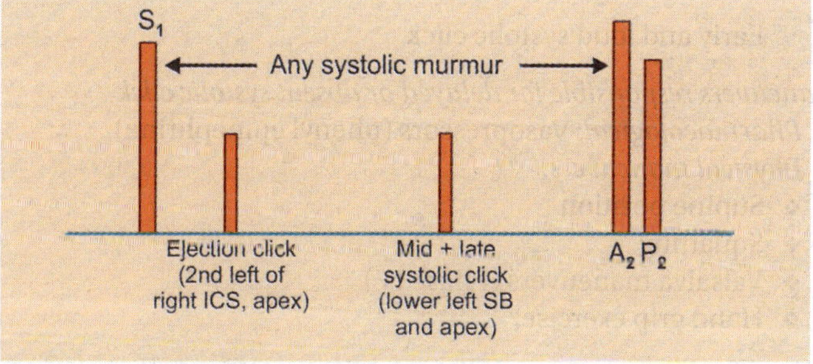

FIG. 4.119   Ejection sound (Mid-systolic click)

Mechanism of producing of sound
- Backward ballooning of prolapsed mitral valve leaflet
- Sudden stretching of chordae tendinae.

But occasionally, papillary muscle contract to prevent stretching of chordae and present prolapse of leaflet into right atrium. So only ballooning of leaflet may produce mid-systolic dick.

Occasionally mid-systolic check may merge with first heart sound, in that case:
- Loud first heart sound
- Hollow systolic murmur.

The Maneuvers Responsible for Loud and Early Systolic Click

Impact of postural changes on systolic click in MVP (Fig. 4.120)
- *Pharmacological drugs:*
  - ❖ Amyl nitrite.
  - ❖ Nitroglycerin

    The above two drugs decrease peripheral resistance

    ↓

    Left ventricular end diastolic volume will be decreased

    ↓

    Size of left ventricle will be decreased

    ↓

    There is early and greater degree of prolapse

    ↓

    Ejection click is closure to S_1 and loud
- *Physical maneuvers:*
  - ❖ Standing
  - ❖ Valsalva maneuvers (Phase II)

    The above two maneuvers reduces venous return to the heart

    ↓

    Left ventricular EDV will be decreased

    ↓

    Size of left ventricle will be decreased

    ↓

    Early and loud systolic click

Maneuvers responsible for delayed or absent systolic click
- *Pharmacological:* Vasopressors (phenyl epinephrine)
- *Physical maneuvers:*
  - ❖ Supine position
  - ❖ Squatting
  - ❖ Valsalva maneuvers (Phase IV)
  - ❖ Hand grip exercise.

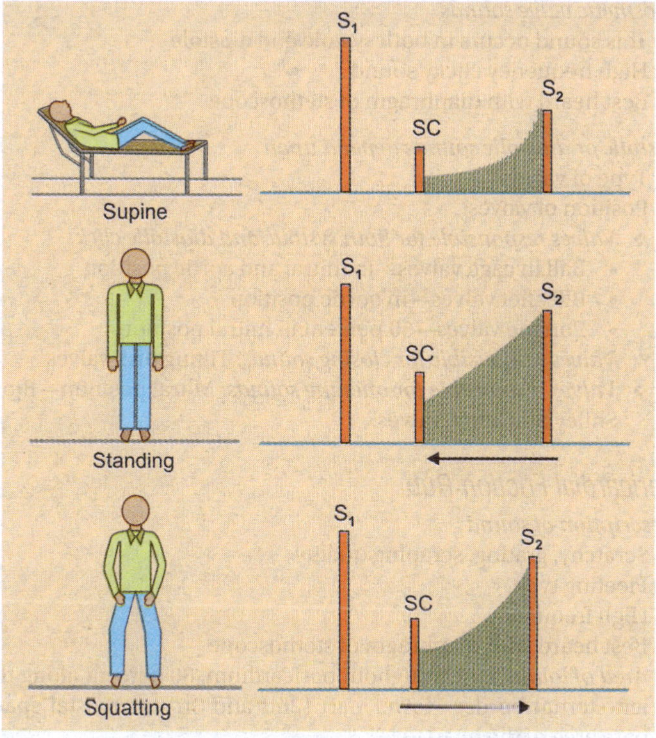

FIG. 4.120   Impact of postural changes on systolic click

All above procedures—increase peripheral resistance

↓

LVEDV—will be increased

↓

Left ventricular size will be increased

↓

Mitral valve leaflet prolapse will be decreased

↓

Systolic click will be delayed or absent

Means-Lerman scratch

- This is systolic grety sound
- Heard over the pulmonary area
- Sounds increased during expiration
- The diseases responsible are:
  - ❖ Thyrotoxicosis
  - ❖ Hyperdynamic circulation
    - Fever
    - Anemia.

Prosthetic valve sounds
- This sound occurs in both systole and diastole
- High frequency clicky sound
- Best heard with diaphragm of stethoscope.

Systolic or diastolic sounds depend upon
- Type of valves
- Position of valves:
  - ❖ *Valves responsible for both systolic and diastolic click:*
    - Ball in cage valves—in mitral and aortic position
    - Bileaflet valves—in aortic position
    - Porcine valves—50 percent in mitral position.
  - ❖ *Valves responsible for closing sounds:* Tilting disk valves
  - ❖ *Valves responsible for opening sounds:* Mitral position—Bjork Shiley Sri Chitra Valves.

Pericardial Friction Rub

Description of sound
- Scratchy, grating, scraping quality
- Fleeting type
- High frequency
- Best heard with diaphragm of stethoscope
- *Area of loudness:* Throughout pericardium, 80 percent along the left sternal border—lower part (2nd and 3rd intercostal space bare area of the heart)
- Vary from site to site—in terms of maximal intensity
- *Heard in both phases of respiration: During, deep inspiration:* Inspiratory descent of diaphragm

↓

Both layers of pericardium are stretched

↓

Two inflamed layers of pericardium are being rubbed against each other more intensely

↓

Inspiratory exacerbation of pericardial rub
During expiration, the heart is closure to chest wall and there is stretching of pericardium due to left ventricular volume overload as a result of increased venous return to left ventricle

↓

Pericardial layers are being rubbed between them

↓

Production of pericardial rub
- Pericardial rub intensity is increased when the patient will sit up, lean forward; rest on elbows and knees—because in this position, contact between visceral and parietal pleura will be increased.

There are two components of pericardial rub:
1. Systolic component—due to ventricular contraction
2. Diastolic component—has two parts:
   i. In early diastole—in rapid ventricular filling phase
   ii. Late diastole—in atrial contraction phase.

But during auscultation:
- Systolic component is always heard
- Occasionally early diastolic component may be heard, so if any diastolic component is not heard—it is the late diastolic component, i.e. atrial contraction phase.

Differentiation of pericardial rub from pleural rub:
Ask the patient to hold his breath—first during inspiration and then during expiration.
- In case of pleural rub—it will be absent
- In case of pericardial rub at least systolic phase must be present, or both phases may be present.

Causes of pericardial rub
Pericarditis—acute or subacute:
- If may be localized:
  - Traumatic
  - Postmyocardial infarction.
- If may be diffuse:
  - Bacterial
  - Uremia
  - Connective tissue disease
  - Radiation.

In case of acute myocardial infarction—if pericarditis will develop—it suggests:
- Large area of infraction
- Low ejection fraction
- Large vessel coronary artery disease
- Chance of development of large numbers of complications.

Pericardial rub cannot exclude pericardial effusion or pericardial tamponade
One fourth case of pericardial tamponade, pericardial rub can occur because, parts of pericardium rub against each other, while other parts of pericardium is filled up with large amount of pericardial fluid.

Heart Murmur

Definition: Murmur can be defined as turbulent flow of blood having varying intensity, frequency, duration and shape, which can be detected by diaphragm of bell of stethoscope.

Relation of Murmur with Heart Sounds and Timing

To create murmur the following abnormalities are necessary:
- *Structural abnormalities:*
  - ❖ *Abnormal size:* As the orifice becomes smaller, the turbulence of blood flow will be greater and the intensity of murmur will be louder
  - ❖ *Abnormal shape of the orifice:* As the orifice becomes irregular; the turbulence will be greater
  - ❖ *Edge of the orifice:* As the edge of the orifice is sharper, the turbulence of blood flow and intensity of the murmur will be higher and louder respectively.
- *Viscosity of blood:* As the viscosity of blood decreases, the turbulence of blood flow will be increased and murmur will be louder.

The consequences of turbulence of blood flow, which ultimately produce murmur:
- Vortices of blood column while passing through the narrowed orifice produces vibration on the lateral wall of blood vessels by hitting the walls
- Turbulence of blood flow produces a jet which will hit the cardiac wall and wall of blood vessels producing murmur
- Turbulence of blood flow produces an eddy current adjacent to the surroundings and produces vibration of surrounding soft tissue structures
- Turbulence of blood flow produces microbubble in blood column, which is responsible of musical murmur
- Jet of blood flow, pulls the wall of blood vessels producing 'Bernoulli's effect', which in turn produces vibration of vessel walls.

The following factors are responsible for production of murmur:
- High flow through narrowed orifice
- Forward flow or antegrade flow through narrowed orifice
- Backward flow through narrowed orifice.

Areas to be examined for auscultation of heart sounds and murmur:
- *Left ventricle* → Mitral area → Left 3rd to 5th intercostal spaces 2 cm medially to anterior axillary line, it may be 2 cm laterally to anterior axillary line:
  - ❖ *Sound to be heard:*
    - First heart sound
    - Aortic component of 2nd heart sound
    - Third heart sound
    - Fourth heart sound
    - Opening snap
    - Pericardial knock.

- ❖ *Murmur to be heard:*
  - Mitral stenosis
  - Mitral regurgitation
  - Aortic stenosis
  - Aortic regurgitation
  - Idiopathic hypertrophic subaortic stenosis
  - Austin flint murmur.
- *Right ventricle* → Tricuspid area:
  - ❖ *Site:* Lower left sternum 2 cm medially or laterally in 3rd to 5th intercostals space.

  In case of right ventricular hypertrophy, it may be displaced laterally towards apex, may be in apical area.
  - ❖ *Sounds to be heard:*
    - Right ventricular third heart sound
    - Right ventricular fourth heart sound
    - Opening snap of tricuspid stenosis.
  - ❖ *Murmur to be heard:*
    - Tricuspid stenosis
    - Tricuspid regurgitation
    - Ventricular septal defect
    - Pulmonary regurgitation.
- *Aortic area:*
  - ❖ *Site:* Second right intercostal space near sternal edge extends across the manubrium sterni to left 2nd intercostals space
  - ❖ *Sound to be heard:*
    - Aortic component of 2nd heart sound
    - Aortic ejection click
  - ❖ *Murmur to be heard:*
    - Aortic stenosis
    - Aortic regurgitation
    - Aortic flow murmur.
- *Pulmonary area:*
  - ❖ *Site:* Left 2nd intercostal spaces adjacent to sternum in intraclavicular area

  Posterorly at the level of T_4, 2–3 cm on either side of spine
  - ❖ *Sounds to be heard:*
    - Pulmonary component of 2nd heart sound
    - Pulmonary ejection click.
  - ❖ *Murmur to be heard:*
    - Pulmonary stenosis
    - Pulmonary regurgitation
    - Pulmonary flow murmur
    - Patent ductus arteriosus.

- *Left atrium:*
  - ❖ *Site:* At the level of left scapular tip in between axillary line and spine
  - ❖ *Murmur to be heard:* Mitral regurgitation.
- *Right atrium:*
  - ❖ *Site:* Right 4th to 5th intercostals space 2 cm right to sternal margin
  - ❖ *Murmur to be heard:* Tricuspid regurgitation.
- *Noncardiac area—descending thoracic aorta:*
  - ❖ *Site:* T_2 - T_{10}, 2 to 3 cm on either side of spine
  - ❖ *Murmur to be heard:*
    - Coarctation of aorta
    - Aortic aneurysm
    - Aortic stenosis.

Murmur can be Described According to the Following Characters

Murmur and relation with heart sounds and timing (Fig. 4.121)

- *Timing of murmur:* This can be:
  - ❖ *Systolic murmur:* Begins after S_1 and ends before or merge with S_2

    This can be classified according to the time in systolic interval:
    - Early systolic—these are mainly flow related murmur, i.e. benign systolic murmur—depends upon the pressure gradient—so maximal during early part of systole
    - Mid systolic—present in mid part of systole
    - Late systolic—occurs in late part of systole
    - Pan systolic or holosystolic—starts just after first heart sound and merge or occasionally extends beyond 2nd heart sound—regurgitant murmur.
  - ❖ *Diastolic murmur:* This murmur begins after 2nd heart sound and ends before 1st heart sound

    This can be classified according to the time in diastolic interval:
    - Early diastolic—starts immediately after 2nd heart sound it is usually semilunar regurgitant murmur
    - Mid diastolic murmur
    - Late diastolic murmur.

    Sometimes mid diastolic murmur may extend up to 1st heart sound due to presystolic accentuation as a result of forceful atrial contraction.
  - ❖ *Continuous murmur:*
    - This murmur is present in systole and diastole without interruption

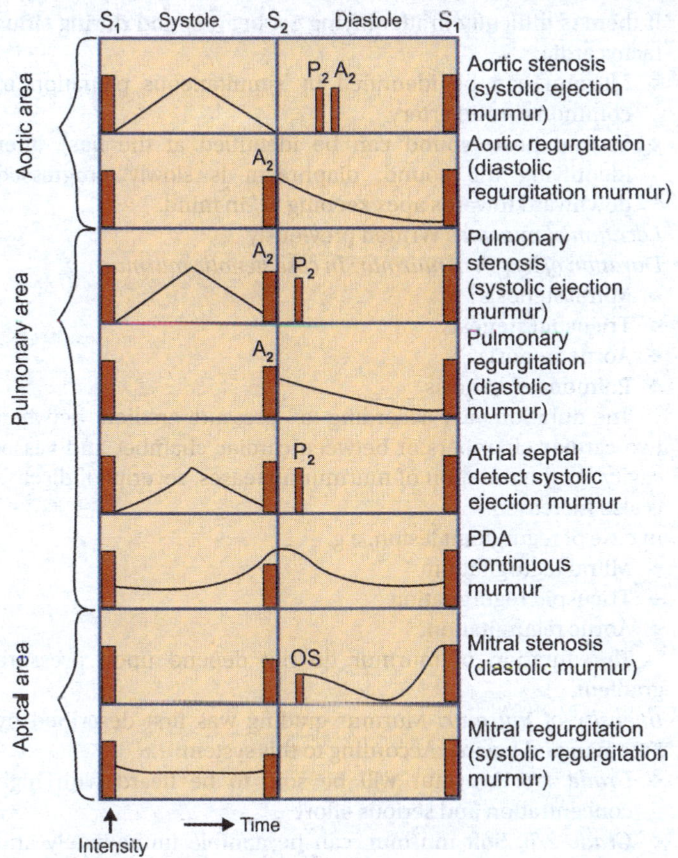

FIG. 4.121   Heart sounds and murmur in different cardiac conditions

- It does not respect the systolic and diastolic bound areas of cardiac cycle
- This murmur depends upon the pressure gradient
- It originates outside the heart.

In normal heart rate: Systolic time is shorter than diastole. The murmur can be heard easily.

In sinus tachycardia: Murmur identification is difficult. In this case—carotid sinus massage may slower the heart rate and reveals the murmur and help to differentiate the whether systolic diastolic.

In case of extra systole: The immediately following beat is separated by compensatory pause—during this pause only murmur can be identified.

If there is difficulty in identifying 1st heart sound during sinus tachycardia:

- ❖ Murmur can be identified by simultaneous palpation of common carotid artery
- ❖ Second heart sound can be identified at the base after identifying the sound, diaphragm is slowly progressed downward towards apex keeping 'S_2' in mind.

- *Location of murmur:* Written previously
- *Duration of length of murmur: In case stenotic murmur, e.g.*
  - ❖ Mitral stenosis
  - ❖ Tricuspid stenosis
  - ❖ Aortic stenosis
  - ❖ Pulmonary stenosis.

  The duration vary according to—pressure gradient between two cardiac chambers or between cardiac chamber and vessel cavity. As the duration of murmur increases, severity of disease is also increased.

  In case of regurgitant lesion, e.g.
  - ❖ Mitral regurgitation
  - ❖ Tricuspid regurgitation
  - ❖ Aortic regurgitation.

  The duration of murmur do not depend upon pressure gradient.

- *Intensity of murmur:* Murmur grading was first described by Freeman and Levine. According to this system:
  - ❖ *Grade 1/6:* Murmur will be soft, to be heard with high concentration and serious effort
  - ❖ *Grade 2/6:* Soft murmur, can be audible immediately and with every beat
  - ❖ *Grade 3/6:* Murmur easily audible and loud
  - ❖ *Grade 4/6:* Murmur is very loud, associated with palpable thrill
  - ❖ *Grade 5/6:* Murmur is so loud, that it can be heard by placing the edge of diaphragm of stethoscope on the chest
  - ❖ *Grade 6/6:* Exceptionally loud murmur that can be heard, when the diaphragm of stethoscope is not in contact with the chest.

  Factors affecting the intensity of murmur:
  - ❖ *Noncardiac cause:*
    - *Distance between the diaphragm of stethoscope and origin of murmur—increase in:*
      - Obesity
      - Highly muscular body
      - Emphysema

- Left sided pleural effusion
- Pericardial effusion.
- *Distance decreases in:* Thin chest wall.
❖ *Cardiac cause:*
  - *Flow related:*
    - Hyperdynamic states, e.g. anemia, fever, etc. Large amount of blood flow through narrowed orifice—producing increase in intensity
    - Hypokinetic states—small amount of blood flows through the narrowed orifice—producing decrease in intensity.
  - *Orifice dimension related:* If orifice progressively narrows in diameter, same amount of blood flows with progressively increasing intensity.
- *Character of murmur:* The character of murmur depends upon pressure gradient between two cardiac chambers:
  ❖ *High pressure gradient between two cardiac chambers:*
    - Regurgitant murmur (>300 Hz)
      - Aortic regurgitation—soft murmur (Fig. 4.122)
      - Mitral regurgitation—blowing murmur
      - Papillary muscle dysfunction—musical quality.
    - Stenotic murmur originates in semilunar valves:
      - Aortic stenosis
      - Pulmonary stenosis.
  All above produces harsh murmur.
  ❖ *Low pressure gradient between two cardiac chamber between atrium and ventride through atrioventricular valve:*
    - Mitral stenosis
    - Tricuspid stenosis.
  All above produce diastolic rumble (30–100 Hz).
- *Configuration of murmur:* The shape is not clinically useful and cannot be detected clinically by auscultation.
Type of shape of murmur can be detected by phonocardiogram.

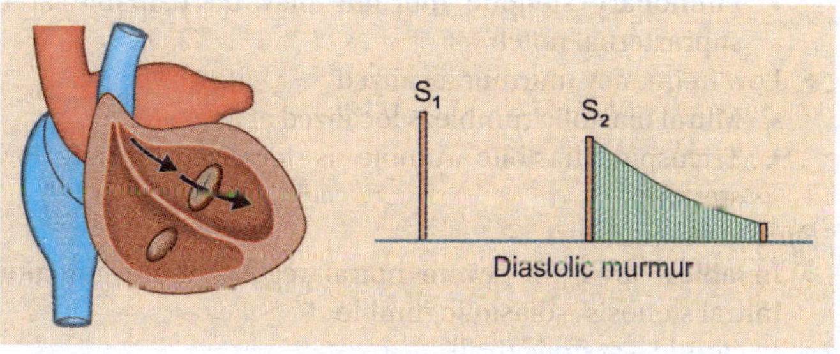

FIG. 4.122 Regurgitant murmur

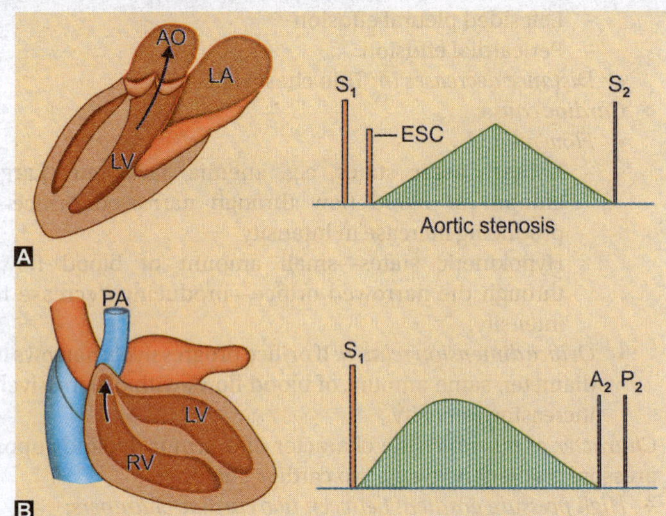

FIGS 4.123A AND B (A) Aortic stenosis; (B) Pulmonary stenosis

- ❖ Crescendo murmur—aortic stenosis, pulmonary stenosis
- ❖ Decrescendo murmur—aortic regurgitation
- ❖ Crescendo-decrescendo (diamond shaped) murmur:
  - Aortic stenosis (Fig. 4.123A)
  - Pulmonary stenosis (Fig. 4.123B).
- ❖ *Plateau murmur:*
  - Mitral regurgitation (Fig. 4.124A)
  - Tricuspid regurgitation (Fig. 4.124B).
- ❖ *Presystolic accentuation:* Atrial contraction in mitral stenosis
- ❖ *Late systolic accentuation:* Mitral stenosis (Fig. 4.125).
- *Radiation of murmur:*
  - ❖ High frequency murmur radiates upwards
    - Aortic stenotic murmur radiates to carotid
    - Mitral regurgitation murmur radiates to axilla
    - Pulmonary stenotic murmur may be palpable at the suprasternal notch.
  - ❖ Low frequency murmur localized
    - Mitral diastolic rumble is localized at apex
    - Tricuspid diastolic rumble is localized at left lower sternum.

Functional murmurs
- ❖ In apical area—in severe mitral regurgitation—functional mitral stenosis—diastolic rumble
- ❖ In carotid—systolic thrill
  Causes: Severe aortic regurgitation producing functional aortic stenosis.
- ❖ *In pulmonary area:* Diastolic rumble.

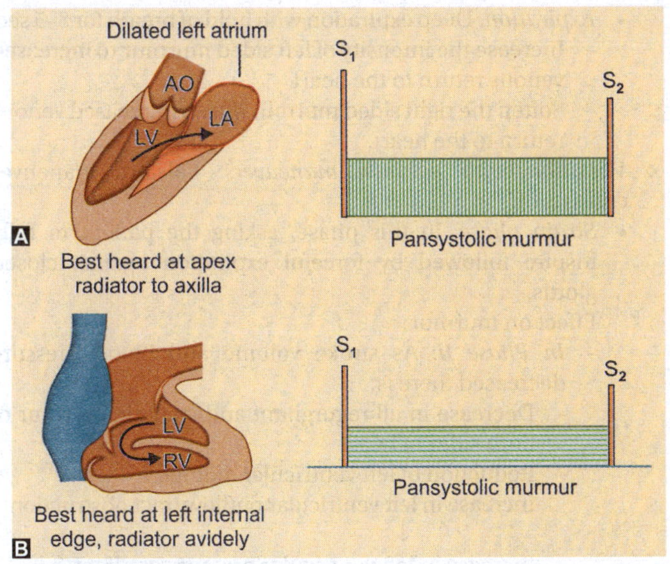

FIGS 4.124A AND B   (A) Mitral regurgitation; (B) Tricuspid regurgitation

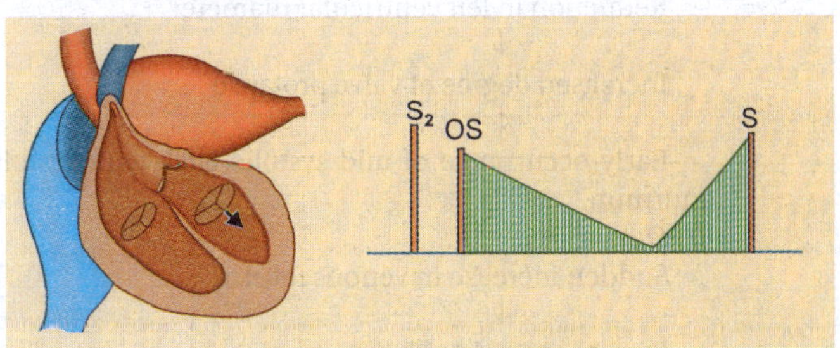

FIG. 4.125   Mitral stenosis

Cause:
- ❖ Severe pulmonary regurgitation producing functional pulmonary stenosis
- ❖ Atrial septal defect.
- ● *Variation with different maneuvers:*
  - ❖ *Variation with respiration:*
    - • Inspiration
      - – Deep inspiration with hold of breath for 3 to 5 seconds—increases right sided murmur due to increase venous return to the heart
      - – Deep inspiration—soften the left sided murmur due to venous pooling by the lungs.

- *Expiration:* Deep expiration with hold of breath for 3–5 sec.
  - Increase the intensity of left sided murmur to increased venous return to the heart
  - Soften the right sided murmur due to decreased venous return to the heart.
- ❖ *Variation with valsalva maneuvers:* Valsalva maneuver consists of:
  - *Strain phase:* In this phase, asking the patient to fully inspire followed by forceful expiration against closed glottis.
    Effect on murmur:
    - *In Phase II:* As stroke volume and blood pressure decreased there is:
      - Decrease in all regurgitant and stenotic murmur of both sides of heart
      - Reduction of left ventricular diameter
        Increase in left ventricular outflow tract obstruction
        ↓
        Increase in left ventricular pressure gradient
        ↓
        Increased intensity of systolic murmur in HOCM
      - Reduction in left ventricular diameter
        ↓
        Increased degree of valve prolapse
        ↓
        Early occurrence of mid systolic click with systolic murmur.
    - *II. During Phase III:*
      Sudden increase in venous return
      ↓
      - Increase in right sided murmur.
      - Decrease in left sided murmur.
    - *During Phase IV:*
      During to increase in cardiac output
      ↓
      - Left sided murmur intensity returns to normal or may be increased.
- ❖ *Müller's maneuver:* This consists of:
  Forceful inspiration against closed glottis:
  All right sided murmur decreased in intensity.
- ❖ *Variation with postural changes:*
  - Lying down, leg rising in supine position (Fig. 4.126):
    Increases venous return to the heart
    ↓

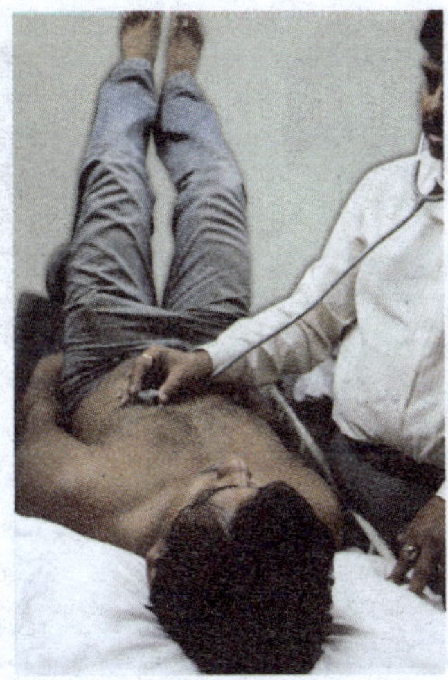

FIG. 4.126   Auscultation in lying down with leg raised position

Increase in right ventricular diameter and volume initially followed by increase in LV stroke volume

↓

- Softens the murmur of HOCM and MVPS (mid systolic click, late SM).
- Increases the intensity of murmur of pulmonary and aortic stenosis.
- Increases murmur of MR and TR, VSD.
- Rapid standing after 30 seconds of squatting or supine position:

Sudden drop of after load and preload

↓

Decreases the ventricular volume and diameter

↓

- Increases the intensity of HOCM and MVPS
- Decrease stenotic and regurgitant murmur.
- Squatting position (Fig. 4.127):

It increases preload by squeezing the blood from abdominal veins to chest.

Increases after load by compressing femoral and inguinal arteries

↓

Increases ventricular volume and diameter.

- Decreases the intensity of HOCM and MVPS
- Increased systolic and diastolic stenotic murmur, e.g. AS, PS, MS, TS.

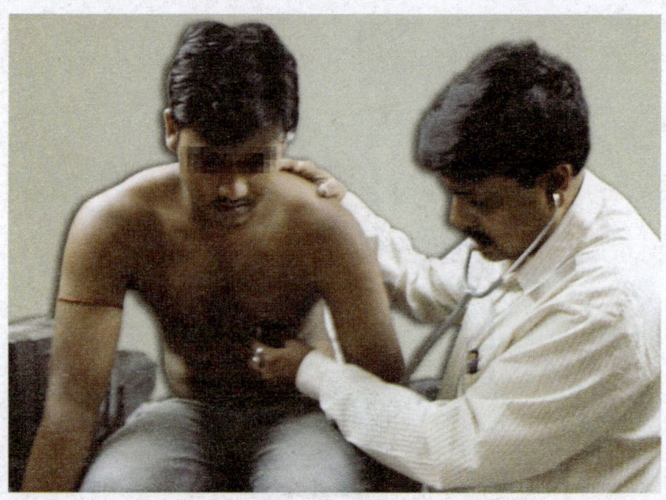

FIG. 4.127 Auscultation in squatting position

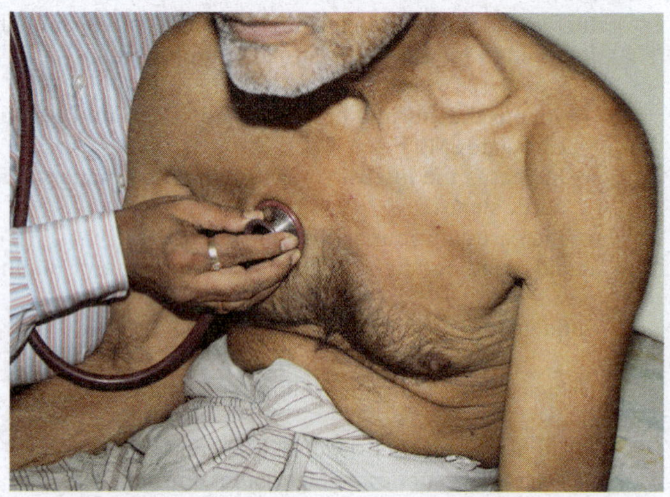

FIG. 4.128 Auscultation in sitting up and lean forward

- Sitting up and lean forward:
  Heart base comes close the chest wall (Fig. 4.128).
  - Diastolic murmur of PR and AR are more readily audible.
- Lying in left lateral position (Fig. 4.129):
  - Apical part of heart comes close to the chest wall.
  - Heart rate slightly increases.

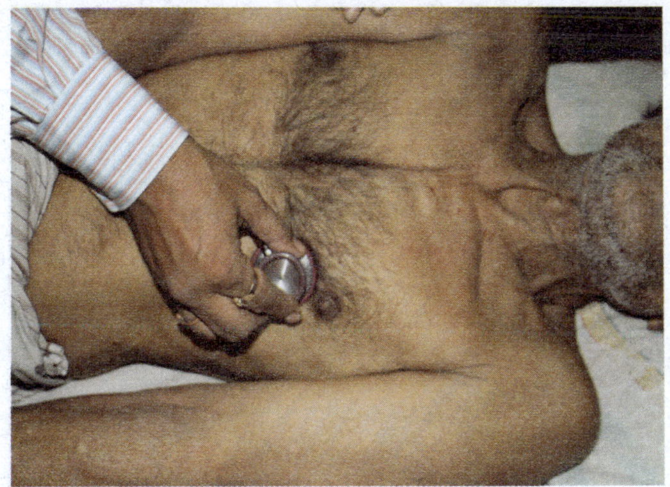

FIG. 4.129   Auscultation in left lateral position

Result:
- Diastolic rumble of MS and autin flint murmur are heard more easily
- Early occurrence of mid systolic click and last systolic murmur—due to tachycardia.

Isometric Exercise

Method: Isometric hand grip can be done by:
- By pressing the ball simultaneously with both hands (Fig. 4.130)
- By locking the cupped fingers of both hands into grip and then trying to make them apart (Fig. 4.131).

The following physiological changes occur:
- Increase in peripheral vascular resistance
- Increase in blood pressure
- Increase in cardiac output
- Increase in heart rate.
  - ❖ Increase in blood pressure
    Increase in intensity of murmur of (due to increase in systemic vascular resistance):
    - Aortic regurgitation
    - Mitral regurgitation
    - VSD.
  - ❖ Increase in cardiac output
    ↓
    Increase in intensity of diastolic rumble of mitral stenosis

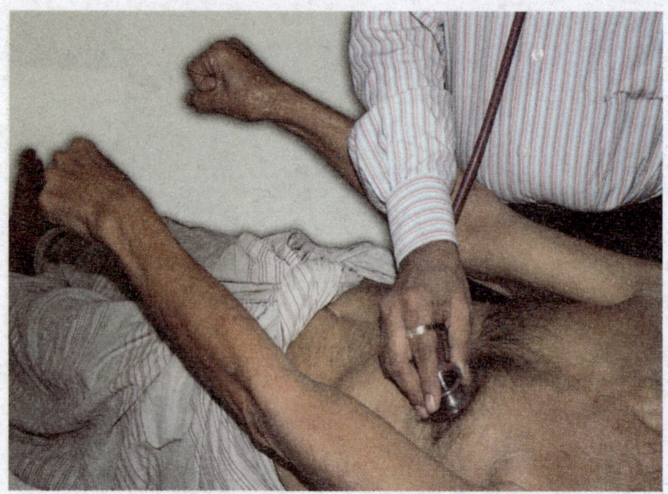

FIG. 4.130   Isometric hand grip method

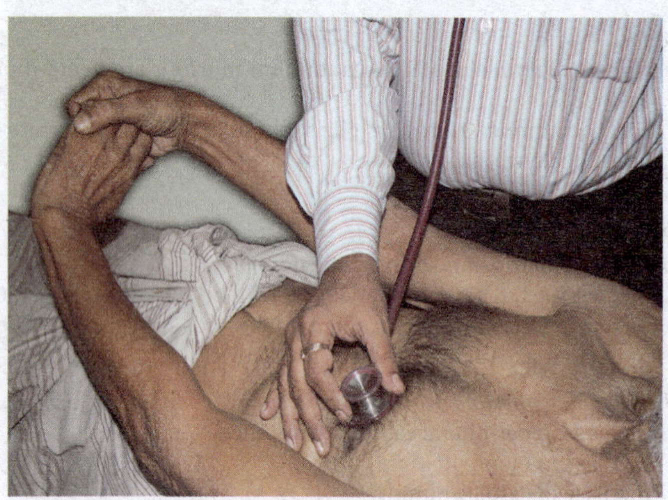

FIG. 4.131   Locking the cupped fingers in isometric hand grip method

❖ Increase in blood volume in left ventricle and increase in size of left ventricular cavity

↓

Soften the systolic murmur of HOCM.
Delay in ejection click and late systolic murmur of MVPS.

Pharmacological Agents

Amylnitrate inhalation: A guaze mixed with amyl nitrate has to be inhaled by taking deep breath for 30–60 seconds.

Physiological changes
- *Phase I:*
  - ❖ Systemic vascular resistance will be diminished due to peripheral vasodilatation
  - ❖ Systemic blood pressure will be decreased.
- *Phase II:*
  - ❖ Reflex tachycardia due to stimulation of barorecepter
  - ❖ Increase in cardiac output.

In Phase I—systemic vascular resistance diminished

$$\downarrow$$

Diminised intensity of:
- ❖ Aortic regurgitation
- ❖ Mitral regurgitation
- ❖ Austin fint murmur of aortic regurgitation
- ❖ Diastolic murmur of PDA
- ❖ Pulmonary regurgitation
- ❖ Small VSD.

Due to increase in cardiac output in Phase II:
Increase in:
- Systolic murmur in aortic stenosis and pulmonary stenosis
- Diastolic murmur in mitral stenosis and tricuspid stenosis
- Functional systolic murmur
- Systolic murmur tricuspid regurgitation.

Due to decrease in left ventricular size:
- Increase in murmur of HOCM
- Early occurrence of mid systolic click and late systolic murmur.

Intravenous Administration of Phenylephrine

Method
Intravenous administration of 0.3 to 0.5 mg of phenylephrine.

Physiological changes
- Increase in peripheral vascular resistance and blood pressure
- Reflex bradycardia
- Decrease in cardiac output.

Increase in blood pressure—produces increase in:
- Aortic regurgitation—diastolic murmur and Austin flint murmur. Increase in intensity of murmur

- Systolic murmur of aortic stenosis—no change in intensity
- Systolic murmur of pulmonary stenosis—no change in intensity.

In case of premature beat:
If there is a full compensatory pause. The following events will occur:
The following physiological changes will occur:
- Decrease in peripheral vascular resistance due to longer time available for the blood to rum into peripheral arteries
- Higher left ventricular blood volume
- Increased cardiac contractility.
  In case of systolic murmur of aortic stenosis:
  Transvalvular pressure gradient will be increased
  ↓
  Increase in intensity of aortic stenosis murmur

In case regurgitant murmur through AV orifice
There are usually two outlets in case of ejection chamber:
- Antegrade to aorta (high pressure site)
- Retrograde to atrium (low pressure site).

Now, in case of premature beat with long compensatory pause—
Blood of aorta will be flowed to the periphery
↓
Decrease in vascular resistance in aorta
↓
Increase in pressure gradient between aorta and left ventricular cavity
↓
Large amount of blood will flow into aorta
On the other hand resistance offered by the left atrium is more than that offered by aorta in case long compensatory pause
↓
So less proportion of blood with enter into left atrium
↓
So there is no change or decrease in intensity of mitral regurgitant murmur

Functional Murmur

This is produced by turbulence during ejection of blood into great vessels of no clinicopathological significance.

Functional murmur can be found in:
- Children (40–50%), rare below 2 years of age
- Normal—86 percent
- Elderly individual
- Pregnant women
- Exercise.

In children—the following physiological causes are responsible for production of functional murmur:

- High flow velocity
- Faster circulation time
- Angulations of great vessels.

Pathological noncardiac causes of functional murmur

- Anemia
- Fever
- Beriberi
- Thyrotoxicosis.

The following are the causes of high stroke volume, which are responsible for functional murmur:

- *Shunt—left to right shunt:* Heard over the base:
  - ❖ Atrial septal defect
  - ❖ Ventricular septal defect
  - ❖ Patent ductus arteriosus.
- *Valvular defect:* Bicuspid aortic valve heard in right 2nd or 3rd intercostals space.

  The following are the causes, responsible for high flow velocity, functional murmur:
  - ❖ Dilatation of aortic root.
  - ❖ Dilatation of pulmonary root.
  - ❖ Aortic sclerosis—aorta—dilated and tortuous.

Character of functional murmur

- Systolic
- Soft
- Ejection systolic, grade 3/6
- Located at the base
- Normal split 2nd heart sound
- Disappears with sitting, standing, or straining.

But functional murmur may be:

- Diastolic
- Continuous.

Difference from pathologic murmur

Pathologic murmur has associated extra findings:

- Symptom related to cardiac disease
- Extra sound
- Thrill
- Abnormal arterial pulses
- Abnormal venous pulses
- ECG
- Chest X-ray
- *Second golden rule:* Abnormal 2nd heart sound

- *Character of murmur:*
  - ❖ Holosystolic or late systolic murmur is pathologic
  - ❖ Diastolic murmur is pathologic
  - ❖ Continuous murmur is pathologic.

Mechanism of production of functional murmur

- *Systolic murmur:* Caused by vigorous ejection of blood into great vessels. There can be heard at bases like, aortic area, or pulmonary area

  But since, left ventricle generates higher pressures than the right, systolic murmur can be heard mainly in aortic area.
- *Continuous murmur:*
  - ❖ Venus hum
  - ❖ Mammary soufflé. This caused by: Turbulence in flow in great veins or great arteries.
- *Diastolic murmur:* This is mainly due to rapid ventricular filling, but has:
  - ❖ No abnormal pressure gradient
  - ❖ No structural abnormalities
  - ❖ No hemodynamic abnormalities

  This murmur is usually very rare, hence, diastolic murmur is usually regarded as pathologic, unless proved otherwise.

Description of functional murmur

Still's murmur: Quiet essential innocent, soft, low pitched, mid systolic murmur having musical quality, heard over middle or lower left sternal border, radiates often to right upper sternal edge—grade 3/6 intensity, flow through aortic valve. It occurs in children 2–5 years of age.

Cause of Still's murmur: No known cause:

- But it may be due to smaller surface area of ascending aorta relative to body surface area
- Children have higher peak velocity in ascending and descending aorta

Pulmonary ejection systolic murmur: This is counter part of still's murmur.

- Systolic ejection murmur due to flow across the pulmonary valve
- Heard in mid to upper left sternal border with diaphragm of stethoscope
- P_2 is normal with normal split
- Heard in thin adolescent chest—Pectus excavatum or straight back syndrome
- Loud in supine position, fades upon standing and sitting.

Supraclavicular arterial bruit

- It is due to ejection—turbulence in aortic arch
- It is heard above the clavicles
- Louder on the right due to brachiocephalic branching.

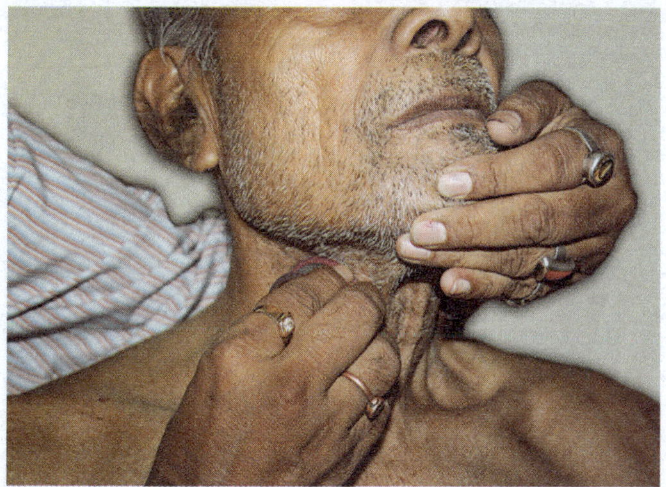

FIG. 4.132 Method of elicitation of venous hum

Venous hum (Fig. 4.132)
- Functional murmur, due to turbulent flow in internal jugular vein
- Continuous, more in diastole, high pitched, associated with palpable thrill
- It can be heard on the right side of the neck, just above the clavicle, occasionally over sternal or parasternal areas—right of left
- Patient will sit up with head turned on left side—30°–60° left ward
- Sound is aggravated by sitting up position
- Sound will be decreased by:
  ❖ Valsalva maneuver
  ❖ Pressure over vein just distal to vein.

Mechanism of production of venous hum: Mild compression of internal jugular vein by transverse process of atlas, in patient with:
- Strong cardiac output
- Increased venous flow.

Venus hum can be abolished by digital compression of internal jugular vein with head in neutral position (Fig. 4.133).

Found in:
- Normal children—31–60 percent
- Young adult—25 percent
- Pathological causes:
  ❖ Hyperkinetic circulatory states
  ❖ Intracranial AV fistula with bruit over skull
  ❖ Compression of jugular vein by fascia or bony structure in neck.

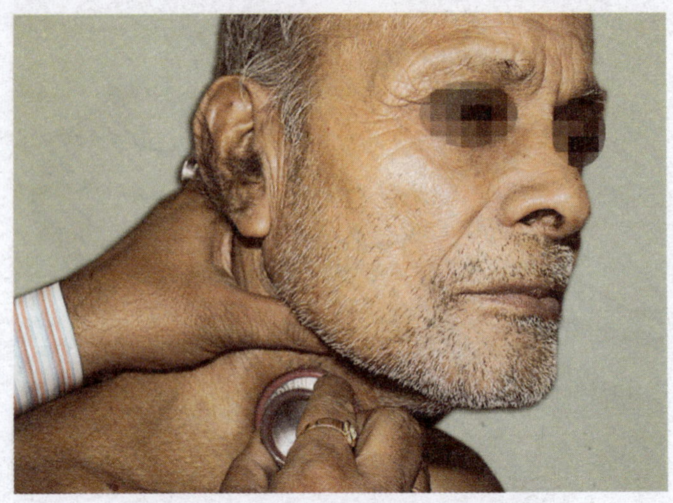

FIG. 4.133   Method of abolition of venous hum

Mammary Soufflé
- This is usually heard over both breast, in late pregnancy
- Disappears during lactation
- Heard over internal mammary arteries
- It is systolic—diastolic murmur, medium to high pitched
- It can be obliterated by pressure over the area maximally
- Mid pressure over the breast augments the murmur.

Common ejection systolic murmur in adult in:
Aortic sclerosis:
- Age—two fold higher risk for each 10 years increase in age
- Male sex
- Smoker
- History of hypertension
- Hypercholesterolemia.

Causes of aortic sclerosis murmur
- Degenerative changes in aortic valve
- Dilatation of aortic root:
  - ❖ Diffuse—tortuous or dilated aorta
  - ❖ Localized—calcific spur protruding into the lumen—creating turbulence in blood flow.

Prognosis of aortic sclerosis: Increased risk of:
- Myocardial infarction
- Angina
- Cardiac failure
- Stoke.

Gallavardin phenomenon in aortic stenosis
In some patient, aortic stenosis—this is evidence of dissociation of systolic murmur into two components:
1. Aortic systolic like murmur—harsh medium pitched murmur heard in right parasternal areas, radiating to carotid
2. Mitral regurgitation like murmur—high pitched, musical murmur, heard best at the apex. This can be misinterpreted as MR.

Bernheim phenomenon: It consists of interaction of right and left ventricle alteration of action of one ventricle impairs the function of other ventricle. So, if left ventricle hypertrophies or dilates, the right ventricle will be compressed, resulting in impaired filling of right ventricle.
This phenomenon is mainly due to:
- Impaired expansibility of pericardium
- Right ward shift of interventricular septum
- Pulmonary hypertension due to increased left ventricular filling pressure.

Reverse Bernheim phenomenon: This is evidenced by left ward shift of interventricular septum, which is caused by right ventricular volume or pressure overload.
This produces following abnormalities:
- Decrease in left ventricular size
- Decrease left ventricular contractility
- Decrease left ventricular compliance
- Decrease left ventricular ejection fraction
  Hence there will be left ventricular diastolic dysfunction.

Chest examination in patient with cardiovascular disease
Auscultation of lung reveals:
Crepitations—during inspiration—sign of pulmonary edema.
In mild heart failure—this crepitations will be confined to lower zones, posteriorly.
May be evidence of bilateral pleural effusion.

Abdominal examination in patient with cardiovascular disease:
- *Liver enlargement:*
  - ❖ *Enlarged tender liver—due to:*
    - Biventricular failure
    - Right ventricular failure
    In above both conditions:
    Raised right ventricular pressure
    ↓
    Raised right atrial pressure
    ↓
    Impaired hepatic venous outflow
    ↓
    Congestive enlarged tender liver, smooth surface

- ❖ *Enlarged pulsatile liver:*
  Tricuspid incompetence

  ↓

  Enlarged tender pulsatile liver—transmitted impulse from right ventricle
- *Splenomegaly:*
  - ❖ Enlarged congestive splenomegaly due to passive congestion due to right ventricular failure
  - ❖ Enlarged, tender splenomegaly due to immune response in subacute bacterial endocarditis.
- *Ascites:* It results from:
  Congestive heart failure
  Constrictive pericarditis.
- *Auscultation of bruit:* By diaphragm of stethoscope—2.5 cm lateral and superior to umbilicus—for renal artery stenosis—in patient with resistant hypertension.

Aorta

It is the peripheral conducting system starting from heart, as ascending aorta, then arch of aorta, then going downwards as descending aorta, which is named as thoracic aorta, when in thorax, then in abdomen as abdominal aorta. So the aorta is described in following manner:

- *Ascending aorta:* It includes aortic root, contains the sinus of valsalva. It gives rise to two branches:
  - i. Right coronary artery
  - ii. Left coronary artery.
- *Arch of aorta:* It gives rise to following branches:
  - ❖ Brachiocephalic artery
  - ❖ Left common carotid artery
  - ❖ Left subclavian artery.
- *Descending aorta:* Thoracic portion:
  - ❖ Intercostal vessels
  - ❖ Anterior spinal artery
- *Abdominal aorta:*
  - ❖ Splenchnic arteries
  - ❖ Renal artery
  - ❖ Bifurcation to common illiac arteries.

Aorta has three layers
1. *Intima:*
   - ❖ Inner most layer
   - ❖ This layer is liable to be damaged.

2. *Media:* This is middle layer consists of:
   - ❖ Elastic tissue
   - ❖ Smooth muscles of varying amounts.
3. *Adventitia:*
   - ❖ It is the outer most layer
   - ❖ It provides nourishment to the outer half of the wall.

Physiology of Aorta

- When ventricle contracts during systole, the kinetic energy developed is stored as potential energy in the distended aortic wall
- During ventricular diastole, this potential energy will be reverted back to kinetic energy, which is evidenced by elastic recoil of the wall
  This flow will be maintained in forward direction.
- Pressure receptors in ascending aorta—response to pressure in aorta.
  This pressure receptors send signals to vasomotor centers in brain
  When blood pressure will be elevated
  Reflex response lowers the heart rate

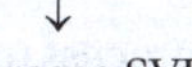

Decrease SVR

Dissecting aneurysm
General survey:
- Hypertension—may be as a cause—or as a complication —when dissection involves renal artery and perpetuates hypertension
- Hypotension—when dissection involves aortic root and subsequently develops hemopericardium and cardiac tamponade
- Pseudohypotension—when dissection involves subclavian artery with resultant compression of vessel
- Pressure difference between right and left arm—if blood flow is compromised in one limb
- Ascending aortic aneurysm—may involve aortic valve and produces diastolic murmur of aortic regurgitation
- Descending thoracic aortic aneurysm—may be palpated in the chest wall
- Descending abdominal aortic aneurysm—may be palpated, mainly in elderly above the age of 60 years.
  The characteristic pulsation is present at the level of umbilicus. It can be palpated between thumb and index fingers.

Aortic dissection: This is defined as tear in intima results in separation of intima from the aortic wall (media) resulting in formation of a false lumen:

Aortic dissection—classification: Anatomical.
- *Stanford:*
  Type A: Dissection involving ascending aorta.
  Type B: Dissection not involving ascending aorta.
- *DeBakey (Fig. 4.134):*
  Type I: Entry port—ascending aorta.
  Extension—to aortic arch and beyond.
  Type II: Confined entirely to ascending aorta.
  Type III: Entry port—in descending aorta.
  (distal to left subclavian artery).
  extends distally or proximally.

Classification according to duration
- Acute—less than 2 weeks
- Chronic—>2 weeks.

Aortic aneurysm
- Abdominal and femoral bruit.
- *Physical survey:*
  - ❖ Livedo reticularis
  - ❖ Painful blue toes
  - ❖ Hypertension
  - ❖ Renal insufficiency.
- Palpation of aneurismal dilatation from xiphoid process to below the umbilicus palpation should be gentle
- If tender on palpation sign of impending rupture
- *Falacies in palpation:*
  - ❖ Accurate size cannot be estimated
  - ❖ In obese patient, it is difficult to palpate.

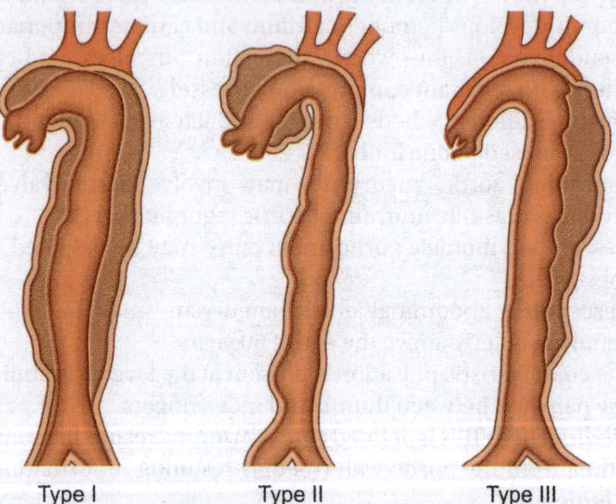

FIG. 4.134 DeBakey classification of aortic dissection

Diameter of aortic aneurysm
In case of abdominal aortic aneurysm:
- Diameter ranges from 0.2 cm to more than 3 cm/year
- Majority enlarge at rate of 2.6 cm/year.

According to Laplace's law
Wall tension (WT) = Transmural pressure (TP) × radius (r)

When radius will increase

↓

Wall tension will increase at a given blood pressure

↓

Perpetuation of increase in radius (r)

↓

Progressive increase in growth of aneurysm

Claudication: Cramping pain, discomfort, and fatigue on buttock, thigh or calf musculature—precipitated by exercise relieved by rest or standing.

If stenosis is progressively severe, pain will occur at rest, tissue ulceration or gangrene.

Two types of ischemia to limbs:
1. *Critical limb ischemia:* It can be defined as progressively increasing atherosclerotic narrowing of vessels compromising the blood flow distal to narrowing, producing—rest pain, ulcers or gangrene.
2. *Acute limb ischemia:* It is defined as acute and abrupt ischemia— threatening the viability of limbs.

Pulse Volume Recordings

Method
- Blood pressure cuffs are placed at the thigh, calf, ankle, midfoot and toe
- Changes in volume of respective cuff during cardiac cycle, identifies the presence of arterial stenosis which can be evidenced by:
  - Changes in pulse contour.
  - Changes in amplitude of cuff volume.

This can be helpful in:
- Diabetic patient with foot ulcer
- Suspected arterial calcification.

Physical examination
- Pulsation of peripheral pulses
- Auscultation of bruits in:
  - Abdomen
  - Bilaterally in groin
  - Carotid arteries.

- Palpation of aneurysm in:
    - ❖ Abdominal aorta
    - ❖ Popliteal arteries
    - ❖ Carotid arteries.
- Signs of lower extremity arterial insufficiency:
    - ❖ Coolness
    - ❖ Dry skin
    - ❖ Pallor
    - ❖ Scaling
    - ❖ Worsening of pain and blanching by elevation of legs.

    Sign of 'P' → Pain, pallor, pulselessness, paresthesia and paralysis.

Deep vein thrombosis
Site:
- Mainly lower extremity
- May involve upper extremity, mesenteric and pelvic veins.

Pathogenesis: It includes:

Virchow's triad:
- Stasis
- Hypercoagulability
- Injury to vessel wall.

Symptoms
- Pain
- Swelling.

Signs
- Warmth
- Tenderness
- Erythema
- Cyanosis
- Gangrene
- *Homans sign:* Dorsiflexion of ankle of 30 flexion at ankle elicits pain in calf muscles
- *Laurels sign:* Worsening of pain coughing and sneezing
- *Lowenberg sign:* Worsening of pain in affected leg after inflation of sphygmomanometer in each calf.

5

CHAPTER

Gastroenterology and Urinary System

Digestive systems have:
- *Specific structures:*
  - ❖ *Digestive tract:*
    - Oral cavity
      ↓
    - Pharynx
      ↓
    - Esophagus
      ↓
    - Stomach
      ↓
    - Small intestine
      ↓
    - Large intestine
  - ❖ *Accessory organs:*
    - Liver → secretes bile
    - Gallbladder → stores bile
    - Pancreas → secretes numerous enzymes and bicarbonates
    - Salivary glands → secretes amylase lipase.
- *Specific functions:*
  - ❖ Digestion of food → aided by enzymes and bicarbonates
  - ❖ Absorption of digested food → through portal circulation → through lymphatics
  - ❖ Homeostatic regulation of calcium, iron and phosphates
  - ❖ Elimination of undigested food
  - ❖ Secretion of enzymes and bicarbonates
  - ❖ Movement of digestive tract to propel the food from stomodeum to proctodeum.

Secretion of enzymes and movement of GI tract are controlled by:
- Hormones.
- Nerve plexuses.

Mouth and Oral Cavity

Oral cavity (Fig. 5.1) is formed by:
- Cheek—on two sides.
- *Roof – formed:*
  - ❖ Anteriorly by hard palate
  - ❖ Posteriorly by soft palate. From its posterior border—a cone-shaped musculature—called uvula—hangs posteriorly. Its function is to prevent spillage of food into nasal area.
- Floor formed by fleshy tongue.

Anterior Portion of Cheeks End in Lips

Lips

It is the door of oral cavity—covered:
- Externally by skin
- Internally by squamous mucous membrane
- In between—there is orbicularis oris muscles.

Inner surface of lip is attached to gum by fold of mucous membrane—labial frenulum.

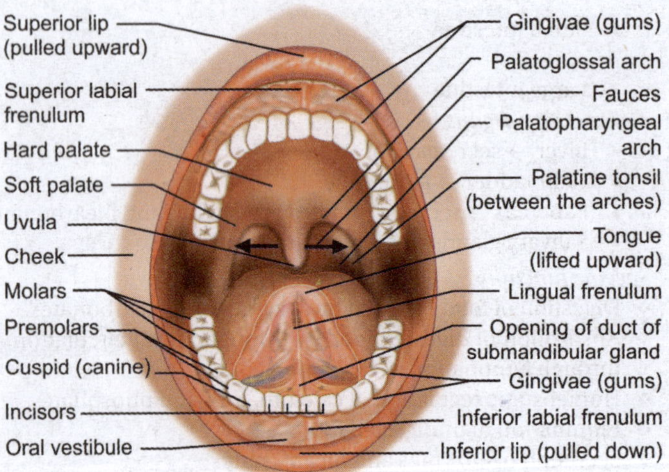

FIG. 5.1 Oral cavity

Actions

- The muscles of lips and cheeks help in keeping the food between upper and lower teeth.
- These muscles help in speech
  Palate—separates oral cavity from nasal cavity.
  Actions—it helps to chew and breathe at the same time.

Action of uvula and soft palate
During swallowing, soft palate and uvula are drawn superiorly; close the nasopharynx and prevents the swallowed food and liquid from entering into nasal cavity.

Two arches:
1. *Palatoglossal arch:* Anteriorly extends to the sides of base of tongue
2. *Palatopharyngeal arch:* Posteriorly extends to the sides of pharynx.

Two tonsils:
1. *Palatine tonsils:* Present in between two arches.
2. *Lingual tonsils:* Present at the base of tongue.

Salivary Glands

These are divided into two types:
1. *Major salivary glands:*
   - ❖ *Parotid glands (Fig. 5.2):*
     - Located inferior and anterior to the ears
     - It secretes saliva through parotid duct in the oral cavity opposite the upper 2nd molar tooth (Stensen's duct).
   - ❖ *Submandibular glands (Fig. 5.3):*
     - Present in floor of the mouth medial and inferior to mandible body

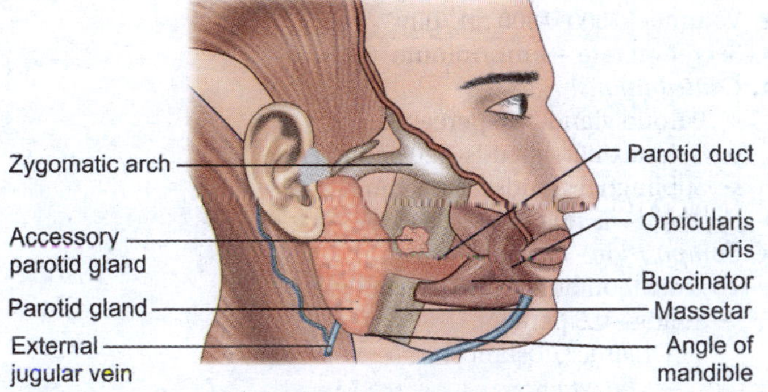

FIG. 5.2   Parotid glands

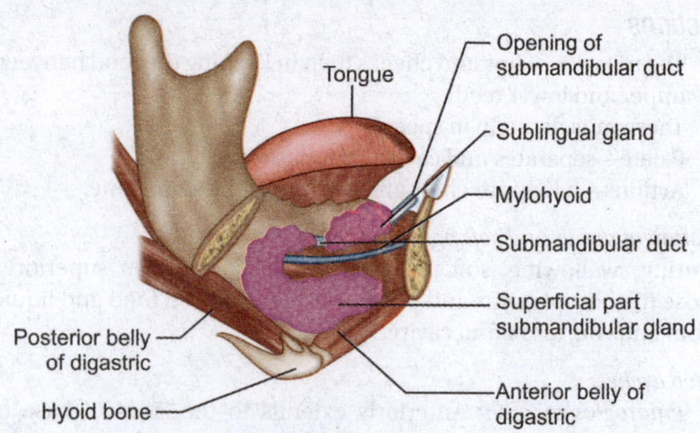

FIG. 5.3 Submandibular glands and sublingual glands

- Duct of submandibular gland (Wharton's duct) runs under the mucosa on either side of midline in the floor of the mouth and opens lateral to frenulum lingual.
- ❖ *Sublingual glands (Fig. 5.3):*
  - Present beneath the tongue and superior to submandibular glands
  - Sublingual ducts opens onto floor of the mouth.
2. *Minor glands:*
  - ❖ Lingual glands—situated on the posterior ⅓rd of tongue
  - ❖ Lingual serous glands—located near the vicinity of taste buds (circumvallate papillae and filiform papillae)
  - ❖ Buccal glands present between mucous membrane and buccinator muscle
  - ❖ Labial glands—beneath the mucous membrane around orifice of the mouth
  - ❖ Palatal glands—beneath mucous membrane of soft palate.

Salivary secretion composition
- Volume—1000–1500 mL/day
- Secretion rate—1 mL/minute
- *Contributions:*
  - ❖ Parotid gland—70 percent
  - ❖ Submaxillary glands—20 percent
  - ❖ Sublingual glands—5 percent.
- Reaction—acidic pH—6.35–6.85
- *Composition:*
  - ❖ Water contains—99.5 percent
  - ❖ Solids—0.5 percent
    - Organic substance:
      - *Enzymes:*
        - Amylase

- Maltase
- Lingual lipase
- Secretory IgA
- Kallikrein
- Lysozyme
- Lactoferrin
- Carbonic anhydrase
- *Other organic substances:*
  - Blood group antigen
  - Amino acids
  - Nonprotein nitrogen
- *Inorganic substances:*
  - *Gases:*
    - Oxygen
    - Carbon dioxide
    - Nitrogen

Functions of saliva
- *In propulsion and digestion:*
  - ❖ Food is moistened and dissolved by saliva, chewed, masticated by teeth and tongue and a bolus is formed
  - ❖ Sensation of taste—food particles are dissolved by saliva and stimulates taste buds.
  - ❖ *Digestion:*
    - Amylase (in acid medium) converts starch to maltose
    - Maltase (in acid medium) converts maltose to glucose
    - Lingual lipase (in acid medium) converts triglycerides of milk fat into fatty acid and diacylglycerol.
- *Cleaning and protective functions:*
  - ❖ Due to constant flow of saliva—food debris, epithelial cells, and foreign particles will be washed out.
  - ❖ *Lysozymes—kills bacteria:*
    - *Staphylococcus*
    - *Streptococcus*
    - *Brucella*
  - ❖ Antimicrobial property—neutralizes toxic substances like tannin
  - ❖ Mucin protects mucous membrane of oral cavity
  - ❖ IgA has antibacterial and antiviral actions
  - ❖ Lactoferrin has antibacterial property.
- *Saliva:* It moistens and lubricates the parts of mouth and helps in speech.
- *Excretory functions:*
  - ❖ It secretes inorganic substances like mercury, thiocyanate, lead, and potassium iodide
  - ❖ It excretes some virus like mumps, rabies

- ❖ It excretes glucose in diabetes mellitus
- ❖ It excretes large amount of urea in nephritis.
- *Regulation of body temperatures:* In human being this function is not known.

Teeth (Figs 5.4A and B)

There are two sets of teeth in human being in lifetime:

1. *Deciduous teeth:*
   - ❖ Incisors—2/2 $10 \times 2 = 20$ teeth
   - ❖ Canine—1/1
   - ❖ Deciduous molar—2/2.
2. *Permanent dentition formula:*
   - ❖ Incisor—2/2
   - ❖ Canine—1/1 $16 \times 2 = 32$ teeth
   - ❖ Premolar—2/2
   - ❖ Molar—3/3

Above dentition formula represents:

- Type of teeth
- Number of teeth
- Position of teeth

Functions of teeth:

- Incisors—for cutting the food
- Canines—for tearing the food
- Molar—for grinding the food.

According to number of cusp molars are divided into:

- Premolars—have two cusps—bicuspid
- Molars—have three cusps—tricuspids.

A tooth is divided into three portions:

1. *Crown:* This portion is above the level of gums. It is covered by enamel. This protects tooth from acids and alkali.
2. *Neck:* Constricted portion between crown and root.
3. *Root:* It consists of one, two, or three projections embedded into socket.

Tongue (Fig. 5.5)

- It is accessory organ of digestive system.
- It is divided into two symmetrical halves by a medline septum.
- *Each half consists of:*
   - ❖ *Extrinsic muscles*—originate from outside the tongue. These are:
      - Genioglossus
      - Hyoglossus
      - Styloglossus.

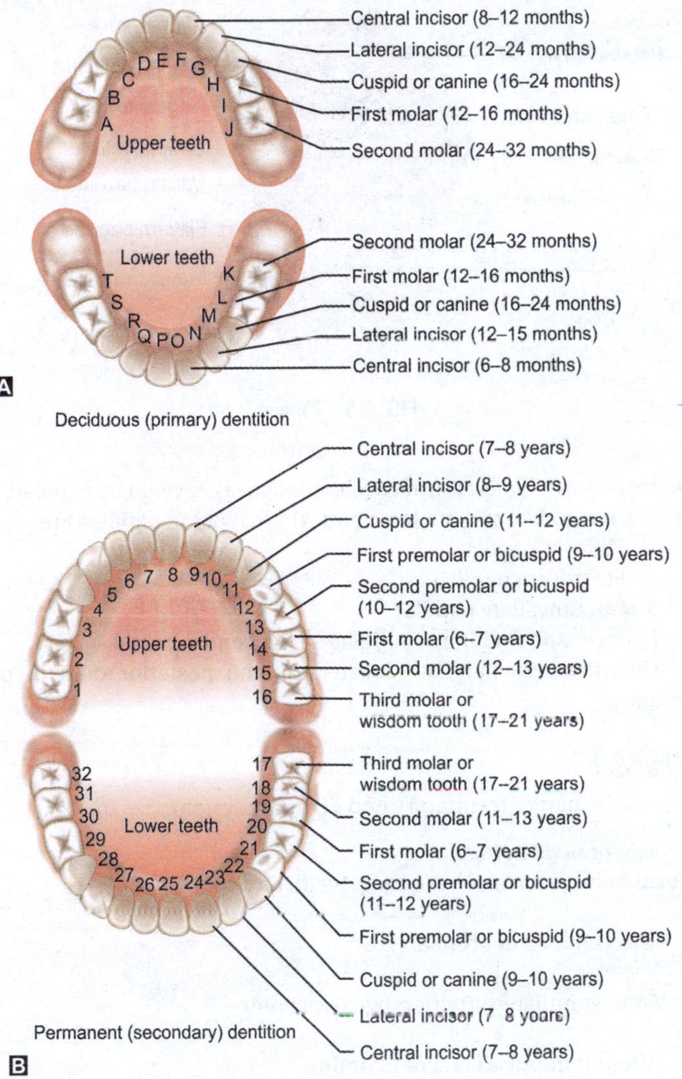

FIGS 5.4A AND B   Teeth

Extrinsic muscle actions:
- Side to side movement of tongue
- In and out movement of tongue
- Forms floor of mouth
- Keep the tongue in position.

❖ *Intrinsic muscles:* They originate and terminate in the connective tissues of the tongue.

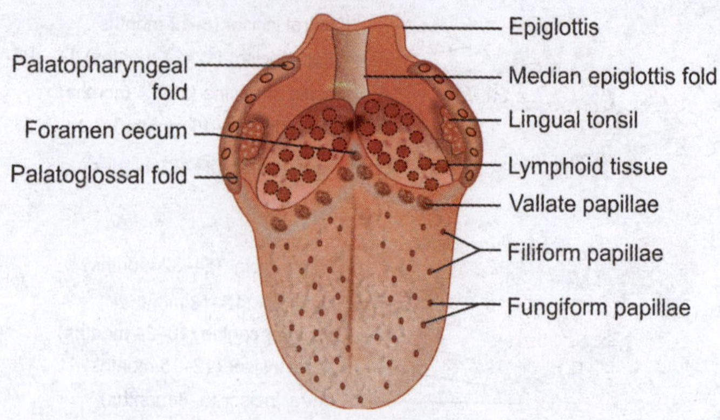

FIG. 5.5 Tongue

- Dorsum and lateral surface of the tongue is covered by papillae.
- Many papillae contain taste bud. Three types of papillae are:
  1. Filiform papillae
  2. Fungiform papillae
  3. Circumvallate papillae

Filiform and fungiform papillae—cover entire dorsal surface

Circumvallate papillae—located on the posterior dorsum of tongue.

Pharynx

This is the part of respiratory and digestive system.

Process of swallowing:
Focal bolus is formed by tongue, teeth, and saliva.
↓
This is forced to oropharynx.
↓
Food stimulates oropharyngeal receptors.
↓
Afferent impulses is sent to brain.
↓
As result of efferent response the following processes progressed:
- Soft palate and uvula move upward to close nasopharynx.
- Larynx is pulled upward and forward under the tongue to close glottis with the help of epiglottis.
↓
Food bolus processes through laryngopharynx.
↓
Fold bolus enters esophagus.

Then respiratory pathways reopen and breathing resumes.

Esophagus (Fig. 5.6)

- Length—10 m (25 cm)—joins pharynx with stomach.
- Greater part present in thorax.
- It enters the abdomen through right crus of diaphragm. Abdominal part length is 0.5 inch.
- Lower end of esophagus is narrowed—called gastroesophageal sphincter.

Artery supply: Branches of left gastric artery.

Nerve supply: Anterior and posterior gastric nerves.

Functions

- Esophagus propels the food bolus into stomach through peristalsis
- *The closure of sphincter is under vagal control:* It is augmented by gastrin.

Reduced by:

- Secretin
- Cholecystokinin
- Glucagon.

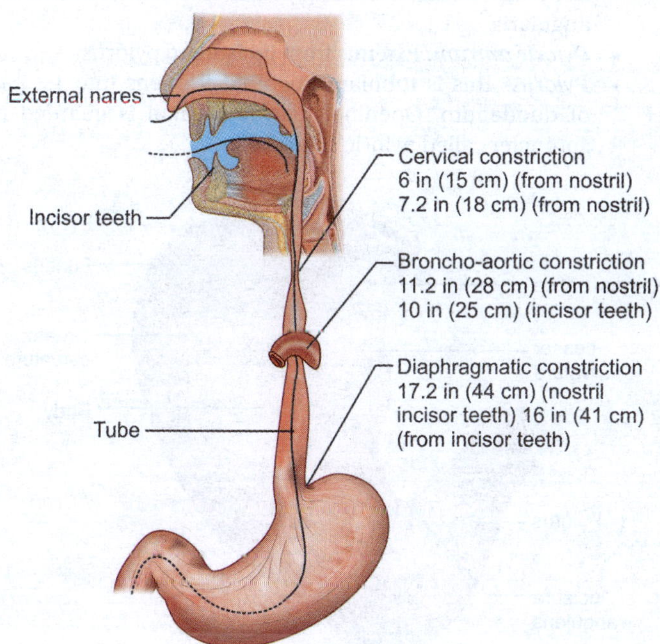

FIG. 5.6 Three constrictions of esophagus

■ Stomach

- It is situated in the upper part of abdomen—joins esophagus with duodenum.
- It extends from beneath left costal margin to epigastric region.
- *Parts of the stomach (Fig. 5.7):*
  - ❖ *Two openings:*
    1. Cardiac opening
    2. Pyloric opening.
  - ❖ *Two curvatures:*
    1. Greater curvature
    2. Lesser curvature.
  - ❖ *Two surfaces:*
    1. Anterior surface
    2. Posterior surface.
  - ❖ *Two shape:*
    1. Steer-horn stomach—transversely arranged in short, obese person
    2. J-shaped stomach—elongated vertically in tall, thin person.
  - ❖ *Parts (interior):*
    - *Fundus:* It is full of gas—it is above and left to cardia
    - *Body:* Extends from cardiac orifice to the level of incisura angularis
    - *Pyloric antrum:* Extends from incisura to pylorus
    - *Pylorus:* This is tubular structure—it opens into 1st part of duodenum. Opening of pyloric canal is guarded by sphincter called pyloric sphincter.

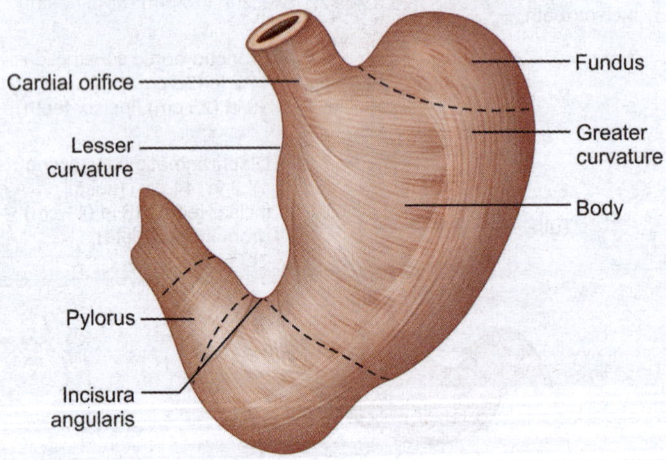

FIG. 5.7   Parts of the stomach

Cut Section and Histology of Stomach (Fig. 5.8)

- Outer layer—formed by peritoneum
- Muscular layers—consist of three muscular layers:
  1. Inner oblique
  2. Middle circular layer
  3. Outer longitudinal layers.
  Auerbach's plexus—present between longitudinal and circular muscle layer.
- Submucus layer—contains Meissner's plexus.
- *Inner mucus layer:* It is lined by mucus secreting glands.

Gastric glands—consist of three types of exocrine gland cells (Fig. 5.9)

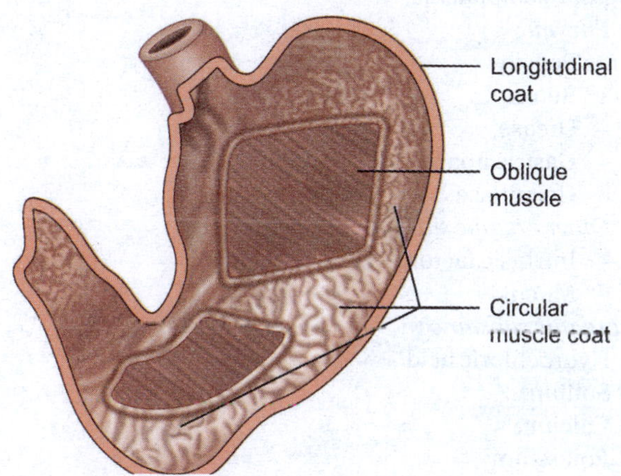

FIG. 5.8   Histology of stomach

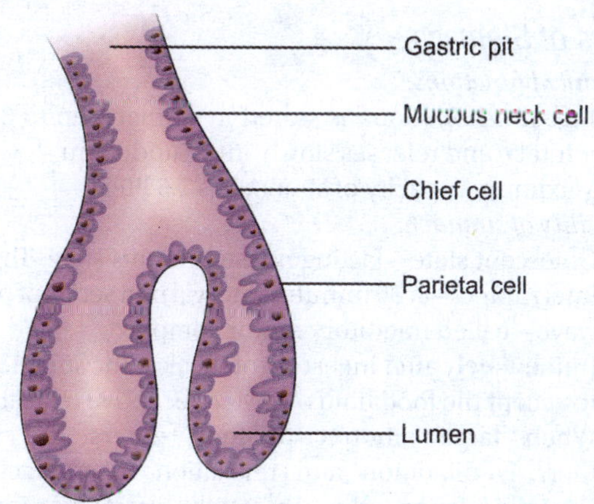

FIG. 5.9   Gastric glands

Those secrete their product into stomach lumen:
- Mucous neck cells—secretes mucus
- Parietal cells—secretes hydrochloric acid
- Chief cells—produces pepsinogen and gastric lipase
- Enterochromaffin cells or Kulchitsky cells—secretes serotonin
- Enterochromaffin like cells—secretes histamine
- G cells—present in pyloric antrum—secrete gastrin into circulation.

Gastric Juice

- Water—99.5 percent
- Solid (0.5%). It consists of:
  - ❖ *Organic components:*
    - *Enzyme:*
      - Pepsin
      - Renin
      - Urease
      - Gastric lipase
      - Gelatinase.
    - *Other organic substances:*
      - Intrinsic factor
      - Mucus.
  - ❖ *Inorganic substances:*
    - Hydrochloric acid
    - Sodium
    - Calcium
    - Potassium
    - Bicarbonate
    - Chloride.

Functions of Stomach

- *Mechanical functions:*
  - ❖ *Storage function:* Food is stored in stomach up to 3–4 hours after intake and releases slowly into duodenum.
    Maximum capacity of stomach is 1.5 liters.
  - ❖ *Motility of stomach:*
    - Quiescent state—fasting phase is in this state. This state is interrupted—at 90 minutes interval by a series of peristaltic wave—called migratory motor complex
    - Immediately after ingestion of meals—the stomach relaxes to accept the food bolus—called receptive relaxation
    - When large amount of food enters the stomach, there is dilatation and relaxation of stomach—called accommodation—this indirectly increases intragastric pressure.

Receptive relaxation and accommodation are controlled by vagovagal reflex.

- As food ingestion is completed and proximal stomach exhibits slow and sustained contraction, which propels the food towards pylorus. This is called tonic contraction. This contraction is determined by intragastric pressure
- Antral systole—It is rhythmic contraction of distal part of stomach, which help in mixing of gastric juice with food bolus to reduce particle size
- Retro propulsion—by which food is bringing back from pyloric orifice to stomach cavity—this helps to break the food particles
- Food is processed into liquid suspension in gastric juice called chyme.

Peristaltic wave pushes the suspension at 1 mL per wavy contraction into the duodenum. Particle size should be 0.5–2 mm to pass through pyloric channel.

- *Digestive function:*
Hydrochloric acid activation
$$\downarrow$$

- ❖ Pepsin $\longrightarrow$ Protein $\longrightarrow$ Proteoses, peptones, polypeptides
$$\uparrow$$
Acid medium
Acid medium
$$\downarrow$$

- ❖ Gastric lipase $\longrightarrow$ Triglyceride $\longrightarrow$ Fatty acid and glycerols
Acid medium
$$\downarrow$$

- ❖ Gastric amylase $\longrightarrow$ Starch $\longrightarrow$ Dextrin and maltose
Acid medium
$$\downarrow$$

- ❖ Gelatinase $\longrightarrow$ Gelatin $\longrightarrow$ Peptides
Acid medium
$$\downarrow$$

- ❖ Urease $\longrightarrow$ Urea $\longrightarrow$ Ammonia

Formation and secretion of hydrochloric acid (Fig. 5.10)

In parietal cells:

- Carbon dioxide is produced by:
  - ❖ Metabolic activities in cells
  - ❖ Some amount is derived from blood.
- CO_2 combines with water to form carbonic acid, in presence of enzyme called carbonic anhydrase.
- Carbonic acid is immediately broken down into hydrogen ion and bicarbonate ion.

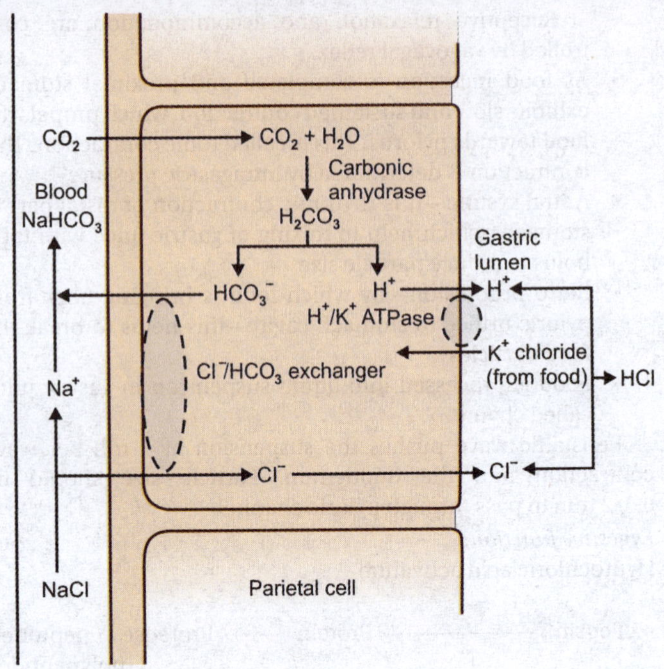

FIG. 5.10 Method of hydrochloric acid secretion in parietal cell

- Hydrogen ion is actively pumped into stomach lumen by H^+/K^+ATPase—in exchange of K^+—derived from food
- Chlorine ion uptake into oxyntic cells from extracellular fluid occurs via Cl^-/HCO_3 ion exchange—at basolateral membrane. HCO_3^- is released into interstitial fluid then to gastric vein, hence, gastric venous blood becomes alkaline. This is known as alkaline tide.

Actions of hydrochloric acid
- Activates pepsinogen to pepsin
- Kills some pathogenic bacteria
- Maintains acid medium in stomach, which is necessary for several enzymes for their actions.

Two components of acid secretions
1. At low secretion, rate—gastric juice mainly resembles interstitial fluid
2. At high secretion rate—gastric juice mainly composed of hydrochloric acid.

So changes in composition of gastric fluid according to secretion rate can be explained by two component model:

1. *Oxyntic component—fluid contains:* 140 mEq HCl, 20 mM.K^+, 5 mM of Na^+ and 165 mM of Cl^-
2. *Nonoxyntic component:* It is collective secretion of all other cells types.

Factors stimulating secretions of hydrochloric acid
- *Neural stimulation*—by vagal nerve—release acetylcholine, which stimulates ach receptors on oxyntic cells
- *Hormonal stimulation:*
  - Gastrin—stimulates gastrin receptors on oxyntic cells
  - Histamine—stimulates histamine receptors on oxyntic cells.

Factors inhibiting secretions of hydrochloric acid:
- Secretin
- Gastric inhibitory polypeptide
- Peptide YY
- PGE_2—produced locally in the stomach—inhibitors of histamine receptors on oxyntic cells through inhibiting production of cyclic AMP.

Phase of Gastric Secretion

I. *Cephalic phase:* This phase consists of secretion of gastric juice in response to neural stimulation—cephalic phase. This phase is regulated by two types of reflexes:

1. *Unconditioned reflex:* This is inborn reflex.

   Presence of food in the mouth

   ↓

   Stimulates the taste buds of the tongue and other receptors in the mouth

   ↓

   Afferent impulses pass through glossopharyngeal nerve and facial nerve

   ↓

   To appetite center present in amygdala and hypothalamus

   ↓

   From here, efferent impulses through dorsal nucleus of vagus and vagal efferent nerve fibers to the wall of stomach

   ↓

   Acetylcholine is secreted at vagal efferent nerve endings

   ↓

   Stimulates gastric glands

   ↓

   Increase the secretion.

2. *Conditioned reflex:* This reflex is being initiated by previous experiences.

Sight, smell and hearing of food
↓

- Stimulates afferent ending of eye, ear, and nose to cerebral cortex.
- Thinking of food stimulates the cerebral cortex directly.
↓

From cerebral cortex, impulses pass through dorsal nucleus of vagus
↓

Vagal efferent nerve fibers to stomach wall
Acetylcholine is released from nerve receptors
↓

Stimulates gastric glands
↓

Increase secretions.

II. *Gastric phase:* This phase is started when food enters the stomach. The stimulation, responsible are:
- ❖ Distension of stomach
- ❖ Mechanical stimulation of gastric mucosa by food
- ❖ Chemical stimulation by food substances.

The controllers are:
- ❖ *Nervous control:* Two types of control:
  1. *Local reflex:*
     Food in stomach
     ↓

     This stimulates local myenteric plexus
     ↓

     Release of acetylcholine from these nerve fibers
     ↓

     Stimulates gastric glands further
     ↓

     Large quantity of gastric juice is being released
     Stimulates G cells to secrete gastrin.
  2. *Vagovagal reflex:*
     Food in stomach
     ↓

     Impulses pass through afferent nerve of vagus
     ↓

     To brainstem
     ↓

     Efferent impulses pass through motor fibers of vagus to stomach
     ↓

     Release of large amount of gastric juice.

* *Hormonal controls:* Gastrin hormone is secreted by G cells in pyloric glands of stomach and upper small intestine

Food in stomach

↓

Stimulation of local myenteric reflex and vagovagal reflex

↓

Release neurotransmitter (gastrin releasing peptide)

↓

Stimulates G cells to release gastrin.

↓

Stimulates the secretion of pepsinogen and HCl. By gastric glands.

III. *Intestinal phase:* This phase starts when food enters the intestine. This phase consists of:

* *Local control:* (Initial stage)

Chymes in the intestine.

↓

Stimulates duodenal mucosa

↓

Release of gastrin

↓

To stomach through blood

↓

Increased secretion of gastric juice.

* *Later stage of intestinal phase:* In this phase—complete stop of gastric juice secretion. This inhibition is done through two factors:

i. *Enterogastric reflex:*

Distension of intestinal lumen

or

Chemical or osmotic irritation of intestinal mucosa

↓

Through local my enteric reflex and vagal reflex

↓

Inhibition of gastric juice secretion.

ii. *GI hormones:* The following hormones are released from intestinal mucosa, inhibiting gastric acid secretion:
   - Secretin—secreted by presence of acid in duodenum
   - Cholocystokinin—by presence of fat and amino acid in duodenum.
   - Gastric inhibitory polypeptide—by glucose and fat
   - VIP—by acid in duodenum
   - Peptide YY—by fat in duodenum.

IV. *Interdigestive phase:* Due to gastrin hormone, a small amount of gastric juice is being secreted in interdigestive phase.

Pepsin

It is the active state produced from two types of pepsinogens:

i. *Type one pepsinogen:* Secreted in oxyntic gland area

ii. *Type two pepsinogen:* Secreted in pyloric gland area.

When acidic pH below 5

↓

Pepsinogen auto activated to pepsin

↓

Once active pepsin is present it auto stimulates pepsinogen through positive feedback manner.

Stimulation of pepsinogen secretion

- Acetylcholine from vagus nerve
- Acid sensitive reflex—this ensures when hydrogen ion is available for conversion to pepsin.

Arterial Supply of Stomach (Fig. 5.11)

- Left gastric artery from celiac axis.
- Right gastric artery from hepatic artery
- Right gastroepiploic artery from gastroduodenal branch of hepatic artery
- Left gastro epiploic artery from splenic artery
- Short gastric artery from splenic artery.

Nerve Supply of Stomach

Parasympathetic fibers from right and left vagus nerve.

- *Anterior vagal trunk:*
  - ❖ Formed mainly by left vagus nerve
  - ❖ It enters the abdomen along anterior surface of esophagus.

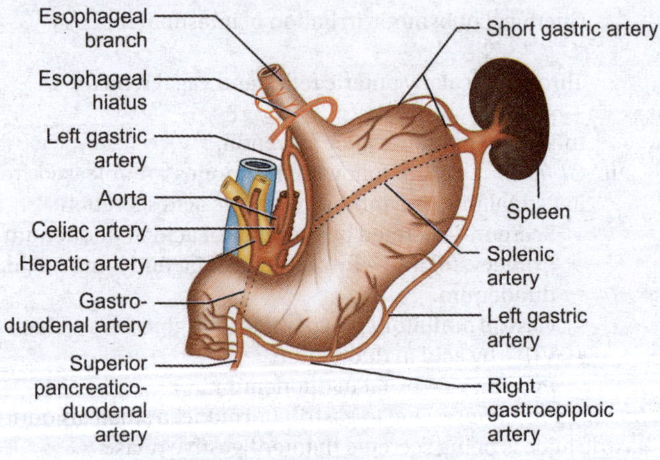

FIG. 5.11 Arterial supply of stomach

* ❖ Trunk—is divided into branches—that supply anterior surface of stomach
* ❖ A large hepatic branch—gives off a branch to pylorus.
* *Posterior vagal trunk:*
  * ❖ Formed by right vagus nerve
  * ❖ It enters abdomen along the posterior surface of esophagus
  * ❖ It divides into branches that supply posterior surface of stomach.

Lymphatic Supply of Stomach

Lymphatic vessels follow the arteries—drain into:
* Left and right gastric nodes
* Left and right gastroepiploic nodes
* Short gastric nodes.
  All the above nodes ultimately drain into celiac nodes.

Small Intestine

Small intestine consists of three parts:

Duodenum

It originates from pylorus—10 inches long consists of 4 parts (Fig. 5.12):

1. *1st part (2 inch):* It ascends from gastroduodenal junction and overlapped by liver and gallbladder. It is present at the level of L_1
2. *2nd part (3 inch):* It runs vertically downwards and curves around the pancreas

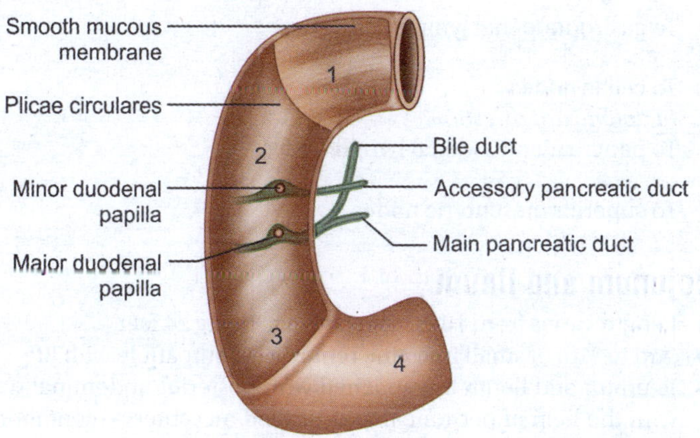

FIG. 5.12   Duodenum

On its posteromedial aspect, half way down there is common opening of bile duct and pancreatic duct, named as hepatopancreatic ampulla (ampulla of vater). This opening is guarded by sphincter of oddi.

Occasionally accessory pancreatic duct, if present, opens into the duodenum a little higher up the major papilla—this is minor papilla.

3. *3rd part (4 inch):* It runs horizontally and to the left along the inferior border of pancreas in front of vertebral column
4. *4th part (1 inch):* It ascends upwards and to the left to end in duodenojejunal junction—here this junction is held by a peritoneal fold called ligament of Treitz.

Mucous Membrane

- In 1st part it is smooth
- In 2nd to 4th part—this is thrown into numerous circular folds plica circularis
- At major duodenal papilla there is nodular elevation.

Arterial Supply

- *Upper half supplied by:* Superior pancreaticoduodenal artery, branch of gastroduodenal artery
- *Lower half supplied by:* Inferior pancreaticoduodenal artery branch of superior mesenteric artery.

Lymphatic Supply of Duodenum

Lymph vessels follow the arteries—divide in two directions:
1. *In upward direction:*
   To pancreaticoduodenal lymph nodes
   ↓
   To gastroduodenal lymph nodes
   ↓
   To celiac nodes
2. *In downward direction:*
   To pancreaticoduodenal lymph nodes
   ↓
   To superior mesenteric nodes.

Jejunum and Ileum

- Length varies from 10–33 feet, average being 24 feet
- ⅓rd to ⅔rd of small intestine removal is compatible with life
- Jejunum and ileum are attached with posterior abdominal wall with the help of peritoneal fold—called mesentery—containing following structures:
  ❖ Entry and exit of superior mesenteric vessels

- ❖ Lymph nodes draining small intestine
- ❖ Autonomic nerve fibers.

Jejunum can be distinguished from ileum in following points:
- Jejunum coiled in upper part of peritoneal cavity
  Ileum coiled in lower part of peritoneal cavity
- *Jejunum is wider bored, thickened wall due to:*
  - ❖ Permanent infolding of mucous membrane
  - ❖ Plicae circularis
  - ❖ Closely set loops.
    Ileum is small bored, widely separated.
- Mesentery containing jejunum attached to posterior abdominal wall above the aorta
  Ileal mesentery attached below and right to the aorta.
- Jejunal vessels produce one or two arcades with infrequent branches to intestine
  Ileal vessels have 3 to 4 arcades—having short numerous vessels.
- *Fat disposition:*
  - ❖ In jejunal mesentery—they are deposited at the root—scanty near intestinal wall
  - ❖ In case of ileal mesentery—fat are distributed through out.
- Lymphoid aggregates are more numerous on the antimesenteric border of ileum.

Arterial Supply
- Mainly by superior mesenteric artery
- Ilio-colic artery—supplying lowest part of ileum.

Histology of Small Intestine
The wall of small intestine is composed of:
- *Mucosa:* Simple columnar epithelium contains following types of cells:
  - ❖ Absorptive cells—absorb small intestinal nutrients
  - ❖ Goblet cells—secrete mucus
  - ❖ Cells lining the cervices form intestinal glands (crypts of Lieberkühn)—secrete intestinal juice
  - ❖ Paneth cells—secrete lysozyme—capable of phagocytosis
  - ❖ Enteroendocrine cells—these consist of:
    - S cells—secrete secretin
    - OCK cells—cholecystokinin
    - K cells—secrete GIP—gastric inhibitory polypeptide.
- Submucosa
- *Lamina propria:* Contain:
  Mucosa-associated lymphoid tissue:

- ❖ Solitary lymphatic nodules—numerous in distal part of ileum
- ❖ Aggregated lymphatic nodule (Payer's patches)—present in ileum.
- *Muscularis mucosae:* Contains smooth muscles—arranged in two layers:
  - i. Outer, thinner, longitudinal layer
  - ii. Inner, thicker, circular layer.

Special Structures in Intestine

- *Circular folds or plica circulares:* Folds of mucosa and sub-mucosa—present from 2nd part of duodenum to mid portion of ileum.

  It increases the surface area for absorption.
- *Villi (Tuft of hair):* These are folds of mucosa— 0.5–1 mm long, finger like projections. Each projection is composed of:
  - ❖ Mucous membrane
  - ❖ *Lamina propria containing:*
    - An arteriole
    - A venule
    - A lacteal.

    Food chyme absorbed through mucosa—enter into blood and lymphatic.
  - ❖ *Microvilli:* Projections of apical free membrane of absorptive cells—viewed from light microscope—these can be seen as fuzzy outline called, brush border.
    - These increase the surface area of absorption
    - These contain a large number of enzymes.

Functions of Small Intestine

Motility Functions

Three functions:

1. Mixing of food stuffs digestive enzymes and secretions
2. Distribution of food chyme along the intestinal mucosa to enhance absorption
3. Propulsion of food chyme in aboral direction.

Two types of intestinal motility during fed state

1. Segmentation contractions—consists of constant form and reform of a segment—it helps in mixing of luminal contents
2. Peristalsis helps in movement of bolus aborally.

Sometimes process of food segmentation and peristalsis continue simultaneously but segmentation is faster in upper small intestine.

So alternative classifications of small intestinal movement
- Tonic contraction of sphincters
- Rhythmic phasic contractions—small peristaltic contractions and segmentations
- Giant migratory contractions—powerful peristaltic contractions.

Digestion in small intestine
Secretions of small intestine are called succuss entericus.
   Volume—1800 mL/day
   Reaction—alkaline
   pH—8.3.

Succuss entericus
- Water—99.5 percent
- Solid—0.5 percent
  - *Inorganic substances:*
    - Sodium
    - Calcium
    - Potassium
    - Chloride
    - Bicarbonate
    - Phosphate
    - Sulfate.
  - *Organic substances:*
    - *Enzymes:*
      - *Proteolytic:*
        - Aminopeptidase
        - Dipeptidase
        - Tripeptidase
      - *Lipolytic:* Lipase
      - *Amylolytic:*
        - Sucrase
        - Lactase
        - Maltase
        - Dextrinase
        - Enterokinase
    - *Other organic substances:*
      - Mucus
      - Intrinsic factor
      - Defensins.

Digestion of food by following enzymes of succus entericus:
- Peptidase › Peptides → Amino acids
- Sucrase → Sucrose → Fructose + glucose
- Maltase → Maltose → Glucose – 2 molecules
- Lactase → Lactose → Galactose + glucose
- Dextrinase → Dextrin, maltose and maltotriose → Glucose
- Intestinal lipase → Triglyceride › Fatty acid.

Protective Functions

- Mucus protects the intestinal wall.
- Defensins, secreted by Paneth cells has antimicrobial actions.

Activation of enzymes
Enterokinase, activates trypsinogen secreted by pancreatic trypsin.

Hematopoietic Functions

Vitamin B_{12} bound to protein
↓
Released in stomach cavity by the action of pepsin.
↓
Formation of complex of vitamin B_{12} with haptocorrin secreted by saliva and gastric juice
↓
Pancreatic proteolytic enzymes hydrolyzes haptocorrin to liberate vitamin B_{12} —to be available in intestine
↓
Vitamin B_{12} blinds with intrinsic factor
↓
This complex is absorbed in distal ileum

Carbohydrate absorption: This is absorbed as monosaccharides:
- Glucose and galactose transport via Na^+ coupled cotransporter SGLF-1
- Further by facilitated diffusion across the brush border membrane, via GLUT-5.

Protein absorption: They are absorbed as amino acids:
- Levo-amino acids are absorbed via Na^+ cotransporter
- Dextroamino acids are absorbed by facilitated diffusion.

Fat absorption
- Medium chain fatty acids—freely diffuses from intestinal lumen into the blood without modification
- Long chain fatty acids are absorbed in following steps:
  LCFT dissolve in micelles to become hydrophilic
  ↓
  They diffuse through unstirred fluid layer in intestinal surface
  ↓
  LCFT here escapes from micelles and enters the enterocyte by diffusion
  ↓
  Enterocyte converts LCFT to triglyceride within smooth ER
  ↓
  Triglyceride complexes with apo lipoprotein in ER
  ↓

Golgi apparatus delivers lipoprotein complexes in large vesicles called chylomicrons

↓

Chylomicrons are transported across basolateral membrane by exocytosis

↓

From there chylomicrons pass to lymphatic vessels, because of their large size, they cannot enter blood vessels

↓

Chylomicrons enters the venous blood where lymphatic channels drain into venous system

↓

The action of enzyme lipoprotein lipase of endothelial origin release fatty acid from chylomicrons

↓

Fatty acid are stored in adipose tissue, muscle cells.

Vitamin Absorption

- Fat soluble vitamin enters the micelles and are absorbed by enterocyte by simple diffusion
- Water soluble vitamin are absorbed by carrier mediated transport but very slowly.

Absorption of water and minerals: In small intestine:

- Na^+ ion is absorbed actively
- Glucose, amino acid and other substances are absorbed by means of sodium co-transport
- Water absorption across the intestinal wall depends upon the osmotic pressure of intestinal context
- Chlorides are absorbed in exchange of bicarbonate
- Iron and calcium are absorbed in upper part of small intestine.

Large Intestine

Large intestine can be differentiated from small intestine by following points:

- *Tenia coli:* Three thickened band of longitudinal muscle fibers
- Appendix
- Haustra
- Caliber of large intestine.

Large intestine has following parts:

Cecum

- It is blind part of intestine—connects terminal ileum to ascending colon.

- It has a blind fingerlike pouch called appendix—a vestigial organ—attached on the posteromedial aspect—interior to ileo-cecal junction—Appendix is attached with a short triangular mesentery—meso-appendix.
- Cecum is present in right iliac fossa—it has no mesentery.

Blood supply
- Cecum is supplied by ileocolic artery
- Appendix is supplied by appendicular artery
- Branch of superior mesenteric vein drains blood from cecum and appendix.

Nerve supply
- Sympathetic nerve supply from T_{10} to T_{12}.
- Parasympathetic nerve supply through vagus nerve.

Ascending Colon

- This extends from cecum to under surface of liver, present in right paracolic gutter retroperitoneally
- It is separated from anterolateral abdominal wall by greater omentum
- It turns to the left to join tranverse colon at right colic flexure.

Blood supply
- Ileocolic arteries
- Right colic arteries.

Venus supply
- Ileocolic vein.
- Right colic vein
- Nerve supply—superior mesenteric plexus.

Transverse Colon

- It extends from right to left colic flexure (splenic flexure)
- Splenic flexure is more acute, less mobile and more superior
- This is the most mobile part
- Splenic flexure is attached with diaphragm by phrenicocolic ligament.

Arterial supply
- Middle colic artery—proximal 2/3rd.
- Left colic artery—distal 1/3rd.
Venous drainage: Branches of superior mesenteric vein.

Nerve supply
- Superior mesenteric plexus
- Inferior mesenteric plexus

Both the plexus supplies sympathetic and parasympathetic nerve fibers.

Descending Colon

- It starts from splenic flexure and continuous with sigmoid colon
- It is present retroperitoneally in left paracolic gutter.

Sigmoid Colon

- It is 'S' shaped, links descending colon with rectum
- It extends from left iliac fossa to third sacral segment
- Three *tinea* ends at recto sigmoid junction.
- It has long mesentery—called—sigmoid meso colon—for which sigmoid colon has considerable freedom of movement.

Blood supply
Sigmoidal artery—branch of inferior mesenteric artery.

Nerve supply

- *Sympathetic nerve supply from:*
    - Lumbar part of sympathetic trunk
    - Superior mesenteric plexus
    - Periarterial plexus.
- *Parasympathetic nerve supply from:* Pelvic splanchnic nerves—via inferior hypogastric plexus.

Rectum (Fig. 5.13)

- 5 cm long tube begins as a continuation of sigmoid colon at S_3
- It follows the curve of sacrum ends infront of coccyx continuous with anal canal
- Lower part of rectum is dilated to form rectal ampulla
- Peritoneum covers anterior and lateral surface of upper third, anterior surface of middle third, but lower third is devoid of peritoneum.

Blood supply

- Superior, middle and inferior rectal arteries
- Superior rectal vein to inferior mesenteric vein
  Middle rectal vein to internal iliac vein
  Inferior rectal vein to pudendal vein.

Nerve supply
Sympathetic and parasympathetic plexus from interior hypogastric plexus.

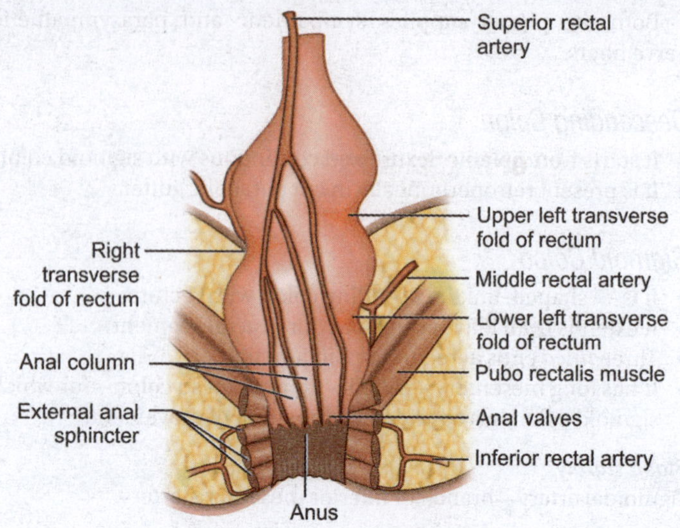

FIG. 5.13   Rectum and blood supply

Anal Canal

- 1.5 cm long canal—continuation of rectum—ends in anus
- Except defecation, lateral wall get apposed
- Upper half—lined by columnar epithelium—it is thrown into longitudinal anal folds, which join at lower end by semilunar folds called anal valves.

Artery supply
Superior rectal artery, branch of inferior mesenteric artery.

Venus supply
- Superior rectal vein, branch of inferior mesenteric vein
- Portal vein.

Lower half of anal canal—lined by stratified squamous epithelium—it merges gradually with perianal epidermis at the anus.

Arterial supply
Inferior rectal artery, branch of internal pudendal artery.

Venus drainage
Inferior rectal vein, branch of internal pudendal vein.
Anal canal has two sphincters:
1. *Internal sphincter:* Composed circular muscle coat at upper part of canal.
2. *External sphincter:* It has three parts:
    1. *Subcutaneous part:* Encircles lower end of canal.

2. *Superficial part:* It is attached with coccyx behind and perineal body in front.
3. *Deep part:* Encircles upper end of canal.

Physiology of Large Intestine

I. *Movements of large intestine:* Two types of movement:
1. *Mixing movements:* This is segmentation contraction—large circular constriction—occurs at regular distance. This is more rapid in left colon than right colon, it tends to slow the movement, so allow more time for complete absorption of fluid from feces.
2. *Mass movement:* This movement ends in anus called giant migrating type of contraction occurs 3–5 times per day.
   Each movement move fecal contents 20 cm or more aborally.

II. *Secretion of large intestine:*
   ❖ *Composition:*
   - Water—99.5 percent
   - Solid—0.5 percent
     - Organic substances
     - Inorganic substances
   ❖ Secretion is alkaline due to large quantity of bicarbonate.
   ❖ Mucin—in large intestine, lubricate the mucosal wall so that:
   - It facilitates the movement of faces
   - It prevents damage of mucosa by faces—by chemically and mechanically
   - Large intestine excretes mercury, lead, bismuth, and arsenic through feces
   - Bowel flora in large intestine synthesizes folic acid, vitamin B_{12}, and vitamin K.

Spleen

- It is situated in left hypochondrium, rest on left colic flexure, behind the stomach, under the diaphragm.
- It is largest lymphoid organ in the body.
- Spleen is surrounded by peritoneum except at hilum, where splenic artery and vein enter and exit respectively.
- It is 12 cm long and 7 cm wide along splenic axis.
- *It has two ligaments:*
  1. Linorenal ligament—joins with kidney
  2. Gastrosplenic ligament—joins with stomach.
- *Parenchyma of spleen composed of:*
  ❖ *Red pulp:* Consists of venous sinus, cord like structures, e.g. RBC, macrophages, and mesenchymal cells.

❖ *White pulp:* It has central artery surrounded by splenic corpuscles formed by lymphatic sheath containing lymphocytes and macrophages.

Functions of Spleen

- *Red blood cell production:*
  In hepatic stage—spleen produces RBC along with liver.
  In myeloid stage—spleen produces RBC along with liver and bone marrow.
- Destruction—RBC, lymphocytes, thrombocytes are destroyed by spleen. Fragile RBC (life span 120 days) are usually destroyed—during passage through capillaries.
- Defense function—spleen removes microorganism and other foreign body by phagocytosis.
- Spleen forms antibody—spleen contains 25 percent of T lymphocytes and 15 percent of B lymphocytes.

Liver (Figs 5.14 and 5.15)

- It is largest organ in the body—weight—1.3 kg.
- It is situated beneath the diaphragm in right hypochondrium and epigastrium.
- Liver has four lobes and two ligaments.
  - ❖ Right and left lobes are separated by falciform ligament anteriorly.
  - ❖ Inferiorly, caudate lobe present near inferior vena cava. Quadrate lobe present adjacent to gallbladder.
    - • Falciform ligament extends from liver to anterior abdominal wall.
    - • Ligamentes teres extends from falciparum ligament to diaphragm.

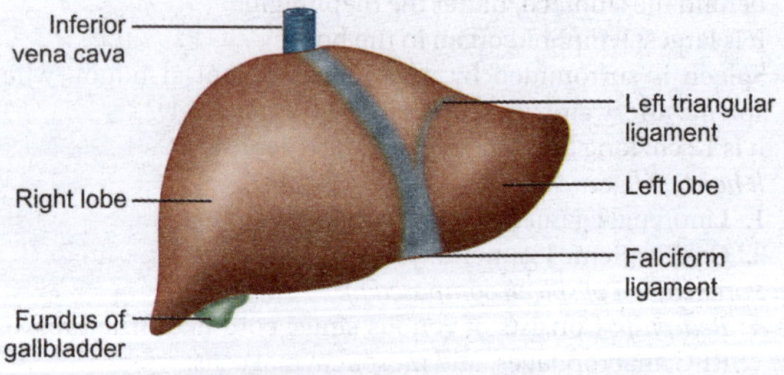

FIG. 5.14 Liver from front

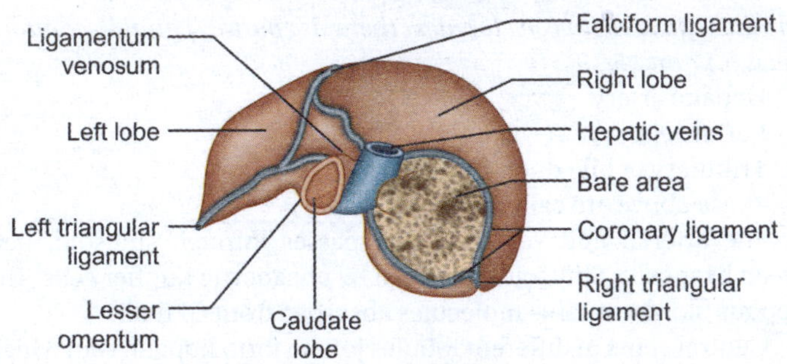

FIG. 5.15   Liver from behind

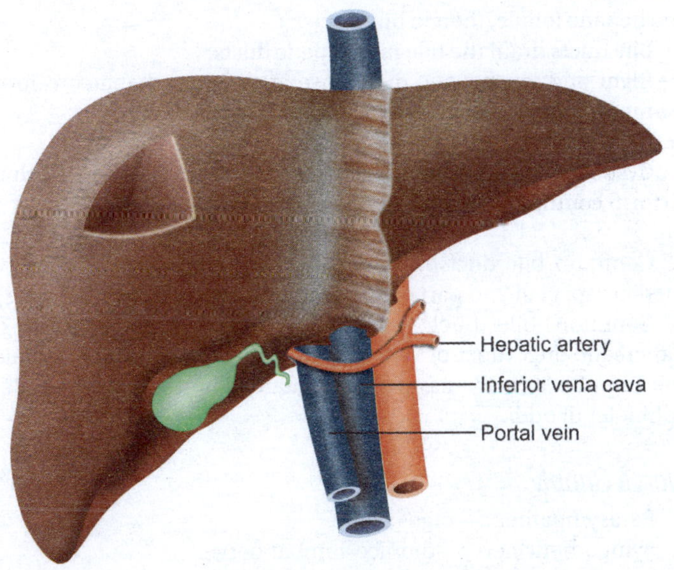

FIG. 5.16   Porta hepatis

- Porta hepatis (Fig. 5.16)—It is hilum of liver present on postero inferior surface between caudate lobe and quadrate lobe. It contains:
  - ❖ Right and left hepatic ducts with common hepatic duct anteriorly.
  - ❖ Right and left branches of hepatic artery, in the middle portal vein posteriorly.
  - ❖ Sympathetic and parasympathetic nerve fibers.
    Liver is made up of liver lobules—hexagonal in shape.
    At the center of lobule—there is central vein, branch of hepatic vein.

In the space between lobules there is portal canals—contains (Figs 5.17 and 5.18)
- Hepatic artery
- Portal vein
- Tributary of bile duct.

These above are called—portal triad.

The arterial and venous blood passes through sinusoid, between liver cells. Sinusoids are lined by phagocytic Kupffer cells. The venous blood contains molecules absorbed from GI tract.

Central veins of different lobules join to form hepatic vein which drains into inferior venacava.

Bile is secreted into biliary canaliculi, located within each hepatic plate. Biliary canaliculi drain into bile ductules at the periphery of the hepatic lobule, then to bile ducts.

Bile ducts drain the bile into hepatic ducts.

Right and left hepatic ducts fuse at the porta hepatis to form common hepatic duct.

↓

Cystic duct from gallbladder—fuses with common hepatic duct to form common bile duct at 4 cm above the duodenum.

↓

Common bile duct passes behind the duodenum to open on medial aspect of 2nd part of duodenum at a papilla.

Common bile duct termination joins the termination of pancreatic duct (duct of Wirsung) in a dilated common vestibule, the ampulla of vater—its opening is guarded by a sphincter—called sphincter of oddi.

Nerve Supply

- Parasympathetic—vagus nerve.
- Sympathetic nerve—thoraco-lumbar nerve.

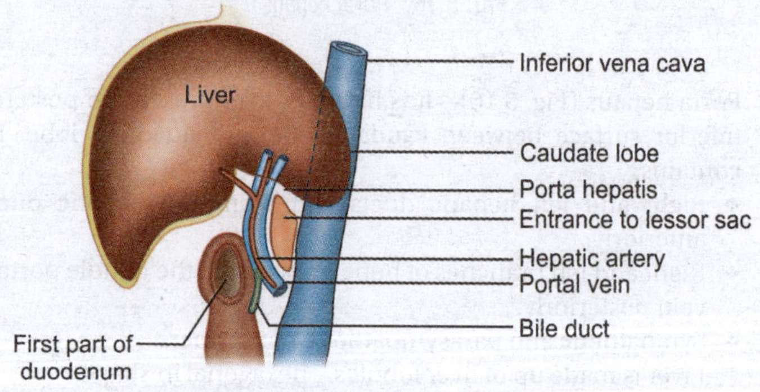

FIG. 5.17   Structure at the porta hepatis

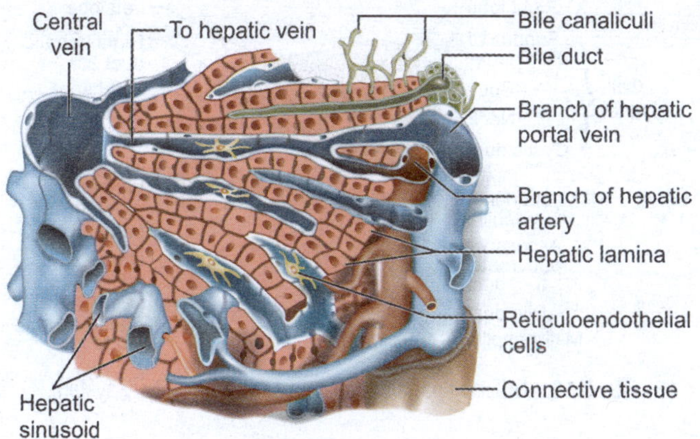

FIG. 5.18 Histology of liver

Diagram of blood flow in the liver

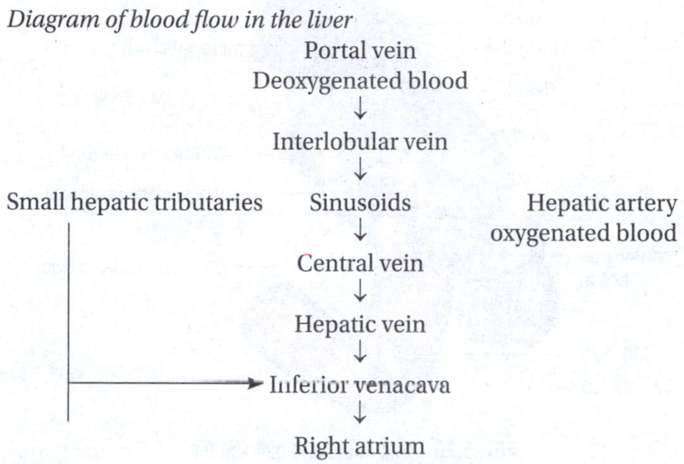

Gallbladder (Figs 5.19 and 5.20)

- It acts as bile concentrator.
- It acts as bile reservoir.
- It lies in between right lobe and quadrate lobe of liver.
- It is close to the duodenum and transverse colon.
- It has three parts:
  1. Fundus
  2. Body
  3. Neck—continuous with cystic duct.

A pouch just ventral to gallbladder neck called Hartmann's pouch—gallstones may be lodged here.

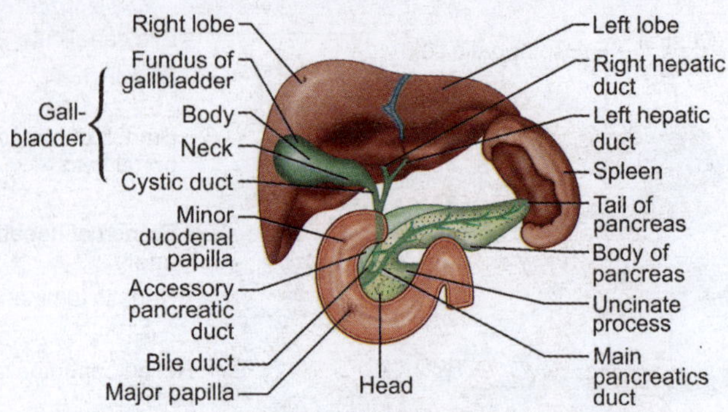

FIG. 5.19 Different parts of hepatico pancreaticobiliary system

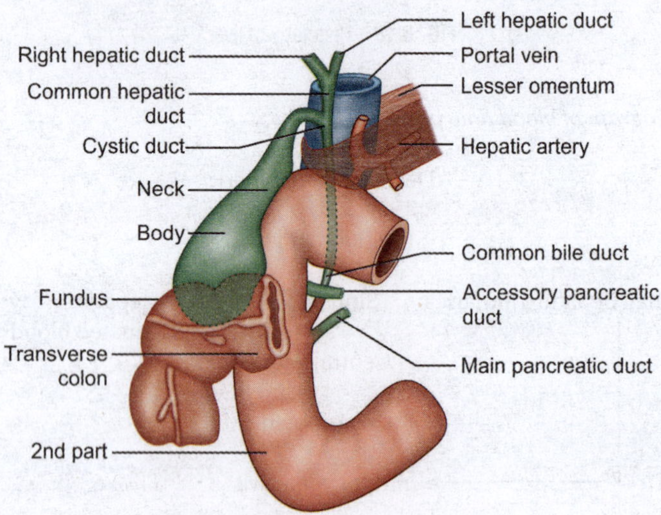

FIG. 5.20 Bile ducts and gallbladder

Blood Supply to Gallbladder

There is a triangle—Calot's triangle bounded by:

- Inferior margin of liver
- Cystic duct
- Common hepatic duct.

Cystic artery lies in the triangle—this is also accompanied by veins.

Small veins pass from gallbladder through its bed directly into tributaries of right portal vein within the liver.

Bile Salt Formation

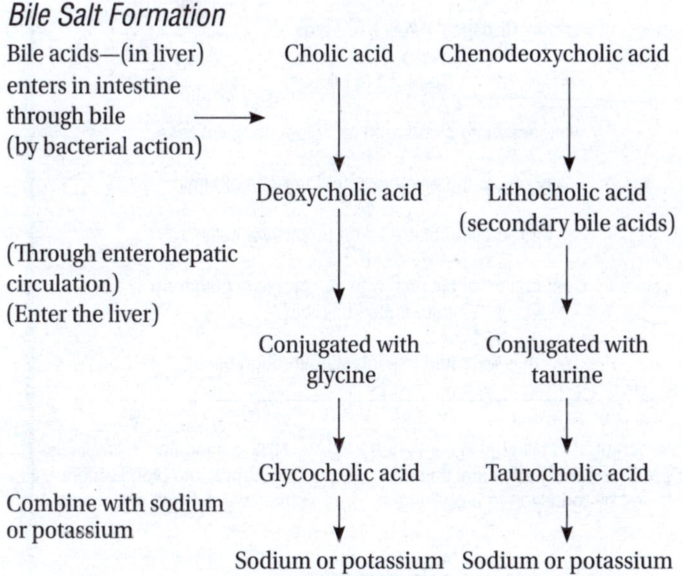

Functions of Bile Salts

- Absorption of fat
- Bile salt stimulates bile secretion in liver.
- Bile salt acts as cholagogue.
  ↓
  Stimulates the secretion of cholecystokinin.
  ↓
  Cholecystokinin stimulates the contraction of gallbladder.
- Laxative → induces peristaltic movement producing defecation
- Emulsification of fat and helps in digestion
- It keeps the lecithin and cholesterol in solution and prevents stone formation.

Formation of Bile Pigment

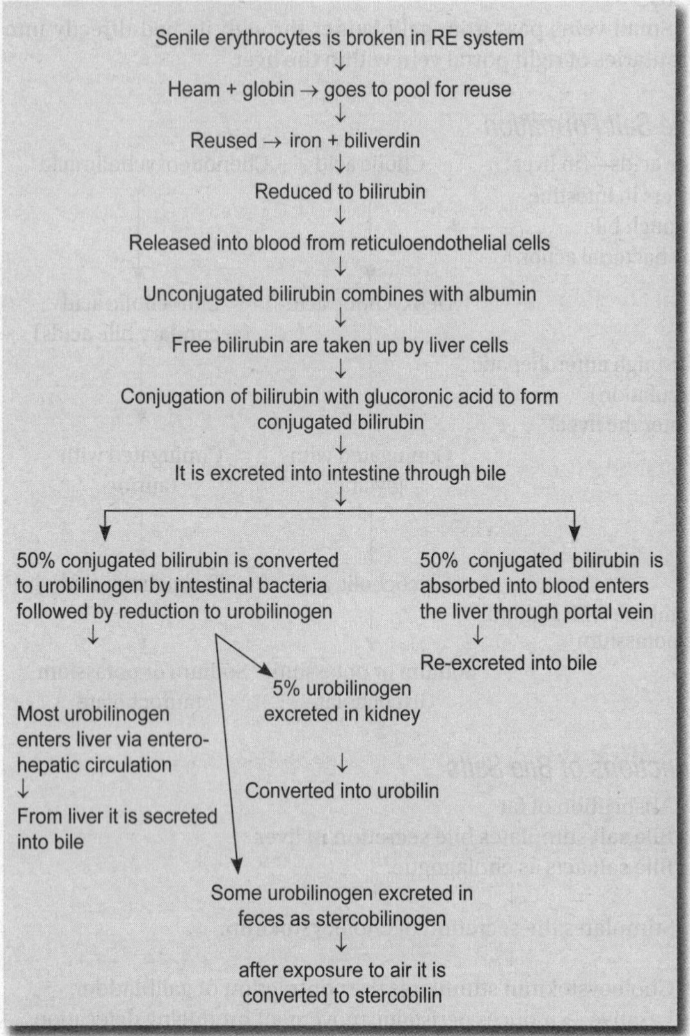

Function of Liver

- *Metabolic function:* Liver carries out carbohydrate, protein, and fat metabolism.
- *Storage function:* Liver stores glycogen, fat, iron, folic acid, Vitamin A, B_{12}, D.
- *Excretory function:* Liver excretes—bile pigment, cholesterol, bacterial toxin, heavy metals like lead, arsenic, bismuth.

- *Secretion:* Liver secretes—bile salts, bile pigment, fatty acid, lecithin, cholesterol.
- *Synthesis:* Liver synthesizes—protein, clotting factors, complement factors, hormone binding proteins.
- *Destroying function:* Liver destroys senile RBC.
- Liver generates heat during metabolic functions.
- Inactivation of hormones and drugs.
- *Function of reticuloendothelial system of liver:*
  - ❖ Foreign bodies—like bacteria, antigen—swallowed and digested.
  - ❖ Production—liver—interleukins, tumor necrosis factors.
  - ❖ Removal of toxin properly of harmful substances—detoxification.

Function of Gallbladder

- Storage of bile
- Secretion of mucin to lubricate the motion of chyme
- Concentration of bile by absorption of water and electrolytes except potassium
- Alteration of pH of bile to less alkaline
- Due to concentration capacity, it maintains a pressure.

Pancreas

- It is a combination of both exocrine and endocrine glands.
- It is situated retroperitoneally in upper abdomen in epigastrium and left upper quadrant.
- *Pancreas is divided into four parts:*
  1. *Head:*
     - Situated in the concavity of duodenum.
     - It has an uncinate process—extending to the left.
  2. *Neck:* It is a constricted portion joining head with body.
  3. *Body:* It runs to the left across the midline, triangular in cross-section.
  4. *Tail:* It runs in the linorenal ligament, and comes in contact with hilum of the spleen.

- *Pancreatic duct:* It opens into 2nd part of duodenum on major duodenal papilla. It drains whole of pancreas.
- *Accessory duct:* It drains upper part of head and drains into minor duodenal papilla.
- *Blood supply:*
  Artery: Superior and interior pancreaticoduodenal artery.
  Vein: Superior and interior pancreaticoduodenal vein.
- *Nerve supply:* Sympathetic and parasympathetic nerves.

Physiology

Pancreas has three functions:

1. *Exocrine functions:* Secretions of enzymes.
2. *Endocrine functions:* Secretions of hormones.
3. Secretion of bicarbonates.

Secretion of enzymes:

Pancreatic juice volume—500–800 mL/day, alkaline.

Enzymes are composed of the following:

- *Proteolytic enzymes:*

                               Proteins

  ❖ Trypsinogen ———→ Trypsin ———→ Proteose and peptides.
                ↑
           Enterokinase

             Proteins

  ❖ Chymotrypsin ———→ Peptides.
               Proteins

  ❖ Carboxypeptidase ———→ Amino acids.
                  Peptides
          RNA

  ❖ Nuclease ———→ Mononucleotides
         DNA
       Elastin

  ❖ Elastase ———→ Amino acids.
        Collagen

  ❖ Collagenase ———→ Amino acids.

All the above are activated by trypsin.

- *Amylolytic enzymes:*

              Starch

Pancreatic amylase ———→ Dextrin and Maltose.

- *Lipolytic enzymes:*

            Triglyceride

  ❖ Pancreatic lipase ———→ Monoglycerides and fatty acids.
           Phospholipids

  ❖ Phospholipase A ———→ Lysophospholipid.
     ↑

  Activated by trypsin
     ↓   Lysophospholipids

  ❖ Phospholipase B ———→ Phosphoryl choline and fee fatty
                                   acids

            Phospholipids

  ❖ Bile salt activated lipase ———→ Lysophospholipids
    │

  Cholesterol esters Triglycerides ———→ Fatty acids and
     ↓   Monoglycerides

  Cholesterol + fatty acids

Secretion of Bicarbonates

- Secretion of HCO_3^- into ductal lumen via Cl^-/HCO_3^- exchange mechanism
- To maintain adequate Cl^- supply for cell, Cl^- comes out of the cells via chloride channel
- H^+ ion is actively transported into blood in exchange of Na^+ ions
- Loss of Na^+ and HCO_3^- from the blood, there is some disturbance in osmotic equilibrium to maintain normal equilibrium, water leaves the blood and enters the ductal lumen
- Bicarbonate combines with water to form bicarbonate solutions.

Secretion of enzymes and prevention of pancreatic auto digestions
- Enzymes are sequestrated in membrane—bound vesicles during synthesis
- Enzymes are produced as inactive precursors called zymogens
- Zymogens granules are released into small intestine through exocytosis
- In the intestine enzymes are activated:
  Trypsinogen are activated to active trypsin by enterokinase
  Other proteolytic enzymes are activated by trypsin
  So, pancreatic acinar cells do not come in contact with activated enzymes, as a result the cells are not autolysed.

Regulation of Pancreatic Secretions
- Cephalic phase—nervous phase (conditioned reflex—small, right and hearing of food)
  (Unconditioned reflex—food in mouth)
  ↓
  Stimulate vagus nerve
  ↓
  Stimulates secretion of pancreatic juice
- Gastric phase
  Food in stomach
  ↓
  Stimulates the secretion of gastrin
  ↓
  Secretion of pancreatic juice.
- Intestinal phase
  Food chyme intestine
  ↓
  Secretion of secretin and cholecystokinin
  ↓   ↓
  Stimulate recreation   Stimulate secretion
  of bicarbonate   of enzymes

Cephalic and gastric phase controlling gastric acid secretion

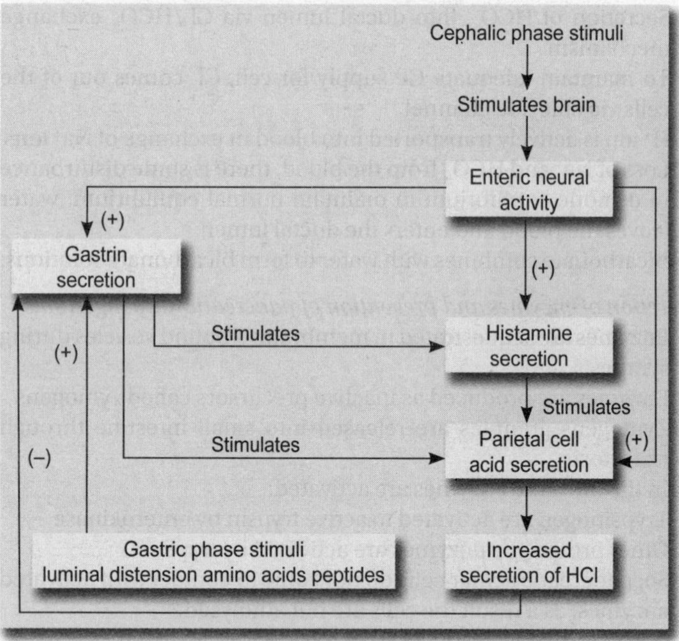

Intestinal phase inhibiting gastric emptying

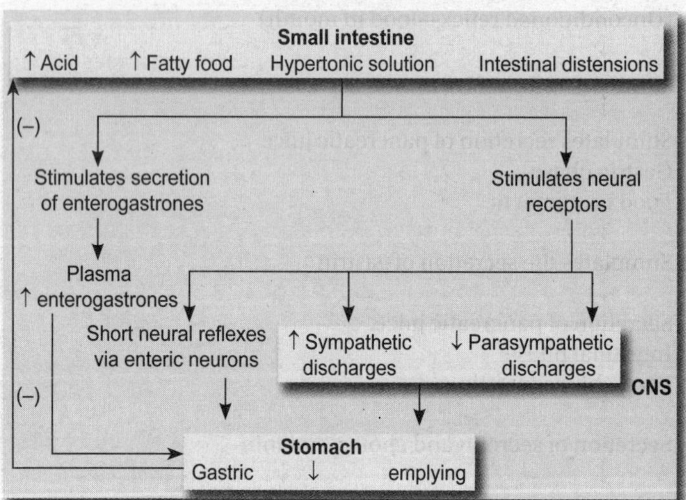

Hormonal regulation of pancreatic bicarbonate recreation

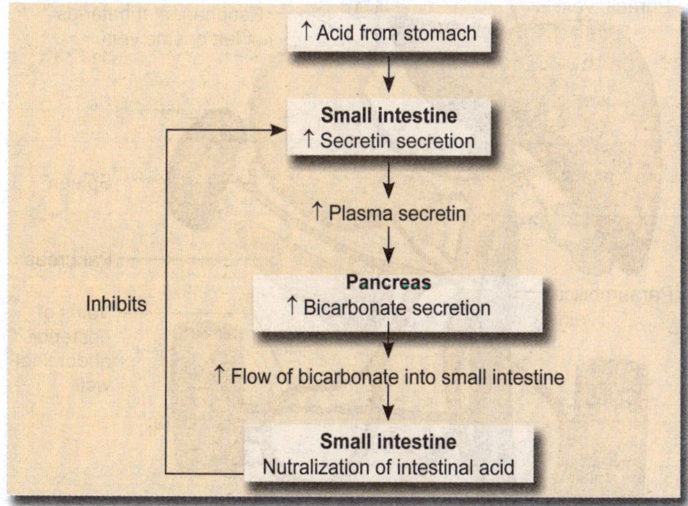

Regulation of bile entry into small intestine

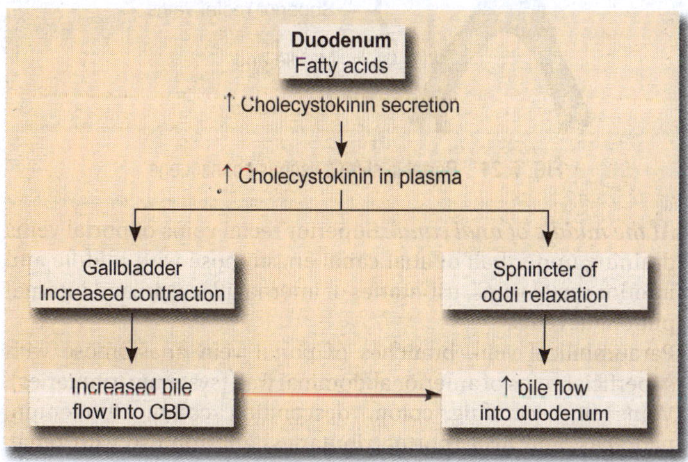

Porto Systemic Circulations (Fig. 5.21)

- *At the lower third of esophagus:* Esophageal branches of the left gastric vein (portal tributary) anastomose with the esophageal veins draining middle third of esophagus draining into azygos vein.

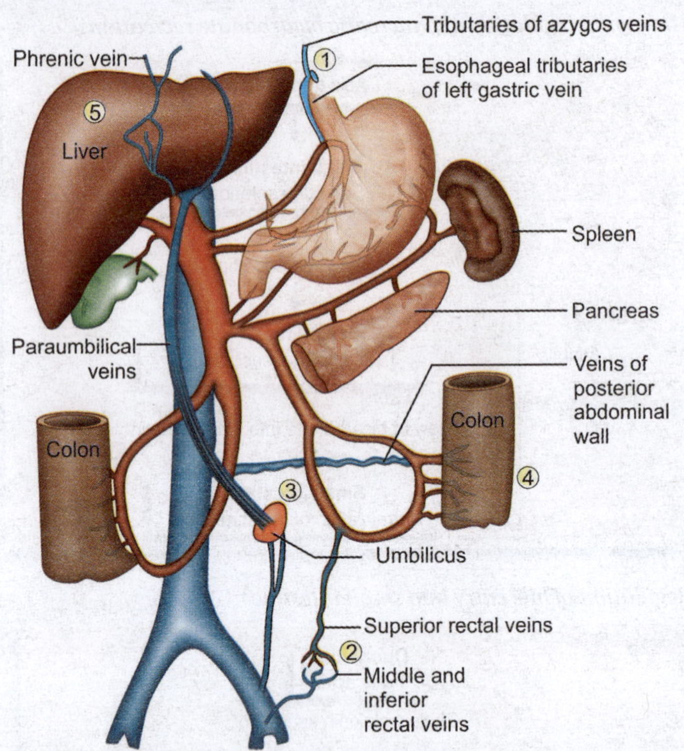

FIG. 5.21 Portal systemic venous connections

- *At the middle of anal canal:* Superior rectal veins of portal veins draining upper half of anal canal anastomose with middle and inferior rectal veins, tributaries of internal iliac vein and internal pudendal veins.
- Paraumbilical vein, branches of portal vein anastomose with superficial veins of anterior abdominal wall (systemic tributaries).
- Veins of ascending colon, descending colon, duodenum, pancreas, and liver (portal tributaries) anastomose with renal, lumbar, and phrenic veins (systemic tributaries).

Kidney—Anatomy and Physiology (Figs 5.22A and B)

Position: Two kidneys—each lies on either side of vertebral column in the abdominal cavity at the level of 12th thoracic vertebrae to 3rd lumbar vertebrae.

Size: Each kidney 11.25 cm long × 5.5 to 7.5 cm wide × 2.5 cm thick.

Medial surface of kidney is concave called hilum through which renal artery enters, renal vein and ureter exit.

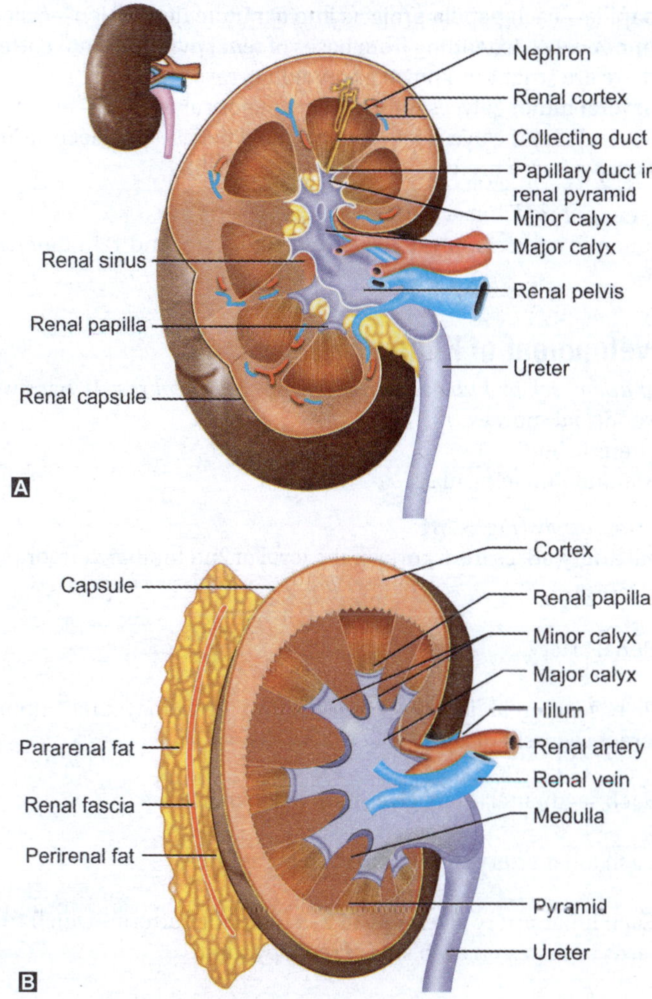

FIGS 5.22A AND B   Cross-section of kidney

Left kidney lies slightly higher than the right (because the left lobe of the liver is smaller than the right).

Both kidneys—are embedded retroperitoneally by retroperitoneal pad of fat and fibrous capsule.

Kidney is divided into two parts
1. *Outer portion—cortex:* It contains:
   ❖ Tuft of capillaries.
   ❖ Convoluted tubules.
2. *Inner portion—renal medulla:* It contains series of triangular masses—called pyramids. Apex of each pyramid is called renal

papilla—each papilla projects into a minute depression—called minor calyx. Extending from bases of renal pyramids into cortex there are striations known as medullary rays.

Several minor calyces unite to form major calyx.

Several major calyces join to form renal pelvis—it collects urine and drains it into ureter.

Nerve supply of kidneys
Autonomic nerve supply derived from 10th, 11th, and 12th thoracic nerve.

Development of Kidney

Permanent set of kidneys derived from metanephros: It has two mesodermal sources:
1. Ureteric bud.
2. Matanephrogenic mass.

Arterial supply (Fig. 5.23)
Renal artery arises from aorta at the level of 2nd lumbar vertebra.

Aorta
↓
Renal artery
↓

Five segmental arteries enters hilum of kidney and supply different segment of kidney
↓

Each segmental artery gives rises to lobar arteries
↓

Each lobar artery supplies to each pyramid
↓

Each lobar artery given rise to 2–3 interlobar arteries which run towards to cortex on each side of renal pyramid
↓

At the junction of cortex and medulla interlobar arteries give rise to arcuate arteries—these branches arch over the base of the pyramid
↓

Arcuate arteries give rise to several interlobular arteries ascend the cortex
↓

Each interlobular artery gives rise to afferent glomerular arteriole
↓

Glomerulus
↓

Efferent arteriole.

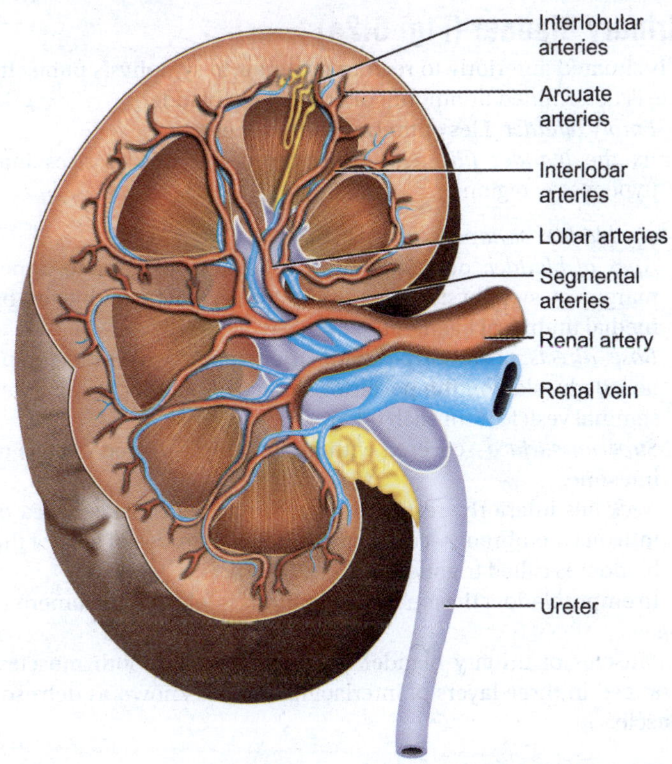

FIG. 5.23   Arterial supply in kidney

Ureter (Fig. 5.22)

Two ureters: Each ureter is a hollow muscular tube that extends from kidney to posterior surface of urinary bladder.

Each ureter is 25 cm in length—have three constrictions along its course:

- At the junction of renal pelvis with ureter
- Where it crosses pelvic brim
- Where it enters the bladder wall. Rental pelvis is the expanded upper end of ureter.

Blood supply

- Upper end—by renal artery
- Middle portion—by testicular or by ovarian artery
- Lower portion in the pelvis by—superior vesicle artery.

Nerve supply

Renal, testicular or ovarian, and hypogastric plexuses.

Urinary Bladder (Fig. 5.24)

It is situated anteriorly to rectum posterior to symphysis pubis. Its size is determined by amount of urine in the bladder.

- *Empty bladder:* Lies entirely within the pelvis.
- *As the bladder fills with urine:* Its upper border rises into hypogastric regions.

Empty bladder's shape is that of pyramid:

- *Apex of bladder,* points anteriorly and lies posterior to upper margin of symphysis pubis—it is connected to umbilicus by medial umbilical ligament.
- *Base directs* posteriorly—shape triangular. Two vas deferens lie side by side on the posterior surface of bladder, it separates seminal vesicle from each other.
- *Superior surface*—covered with peritoneum—related to coils of intestine.
- *Neck* lies inferiorly, rests on upper surface of prostate. Area of mucous membrane—covering the internal surface of base of the bladder is called trigone.

In empty bladder the mucous membrane is folded into numerous rugae.

Muscles of urinary bladder is composed of smooth muscles, arranged in three layers of interlacing bundles known as detrusor muscle.

Nerve supply of urinary bladder

- *Sympathetic fibers* from T_{12}, L_1, L_2 innervate trigone, ureteral openings, and blood vessels of urinary bladder.

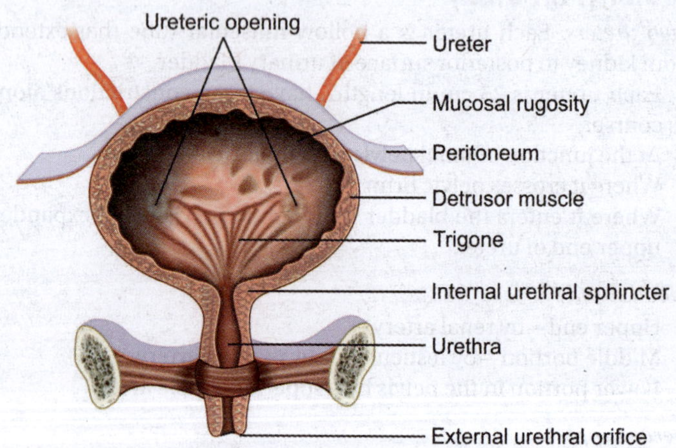

FIG. 5.24 Urinary bladder

- *Parasympathetic fibers* from S_2, S_3, S_4 innervates detrusor muscles.
- Special stretch receptors—responds to bladder distension and relay sensory impulses to brain, via pelvic splanchnic nerve.

Basic Structure of Nephron

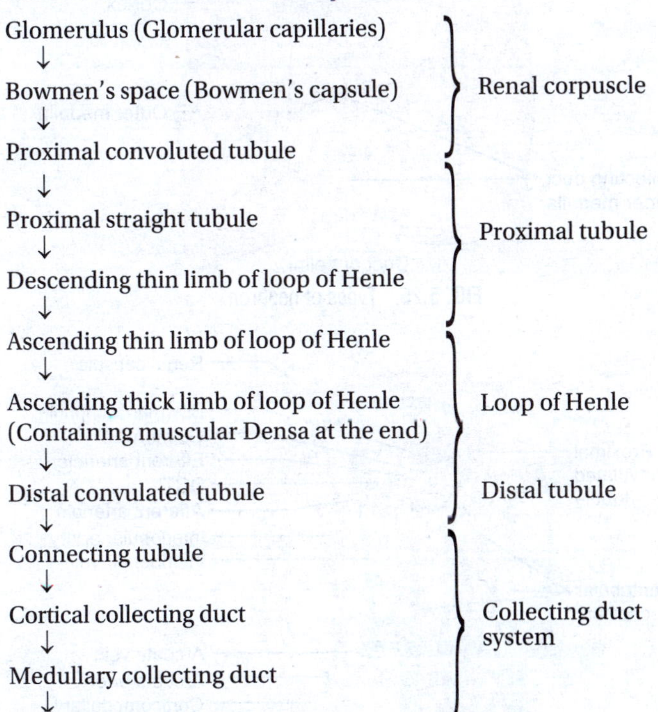

Two Types of Nephron (Fig. 5.25)

1. *Cortical type (Fig. 5.26):*
   - ❖ Glomeruli lie in cortex
   - ❖ Loop of Henle is short.
2. *Juxtamedullary type (Fig. 5.27):*
   - ❖ Glomeruli lie in deep cortex
   - ❖ Loop of Henle are long—extends all the way to renal papilla
   - ❖ They reabsorb higher proportion of glomerular filtrate than cortical nephron.
   - ❖ They are salt conserving—so in case of decreased effective circulatory volume, higher proportion is directed to juxtamedullary nephron.

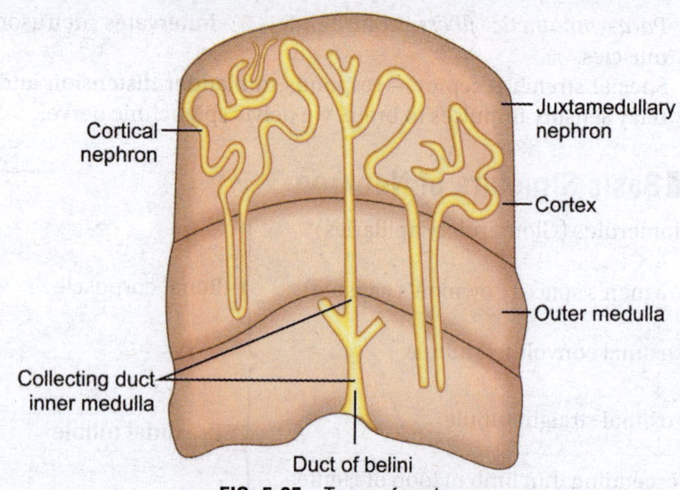

FIG. 5.25 Types of nephron

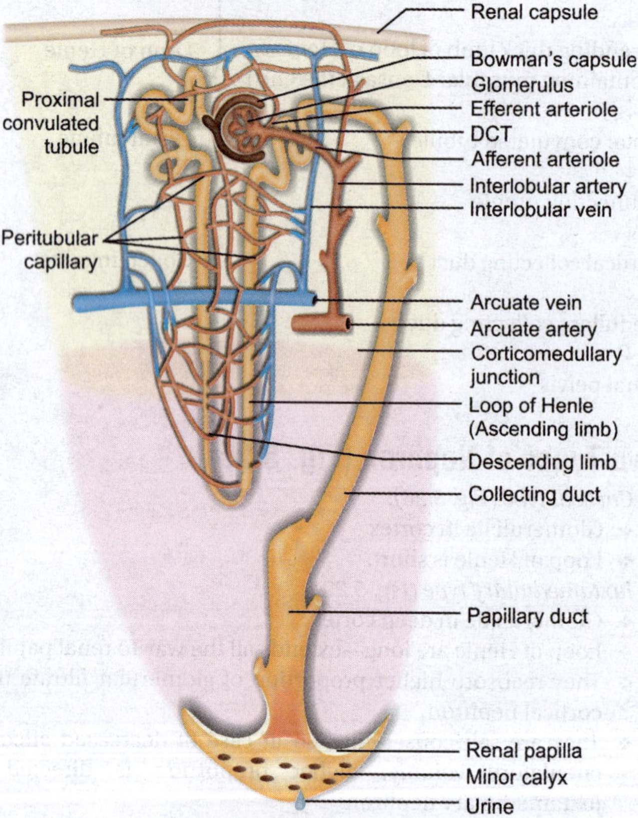

FIG. 5.26 Cortical nephron

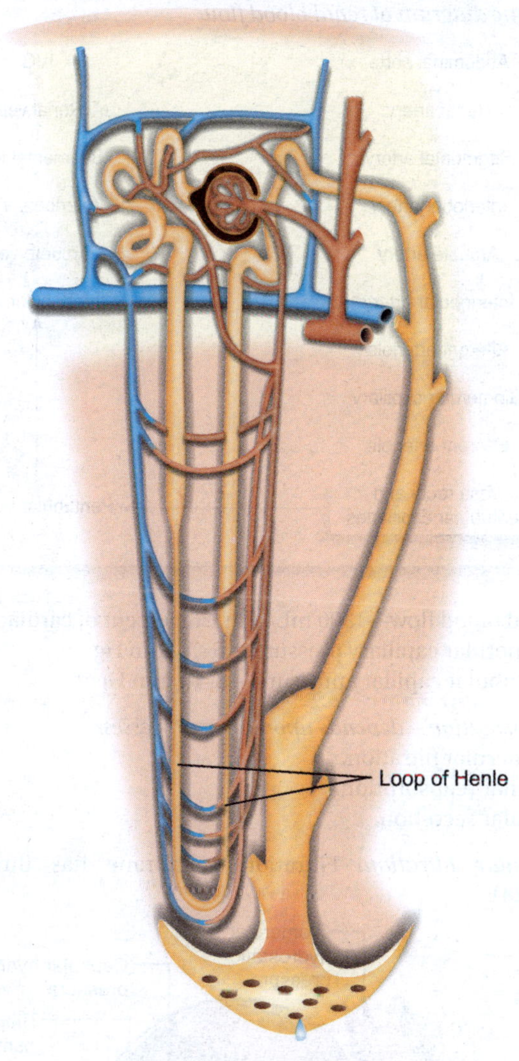

FIG. 5.27 Juxtaglomerular nephron

Schematic diagram of renal blood flow

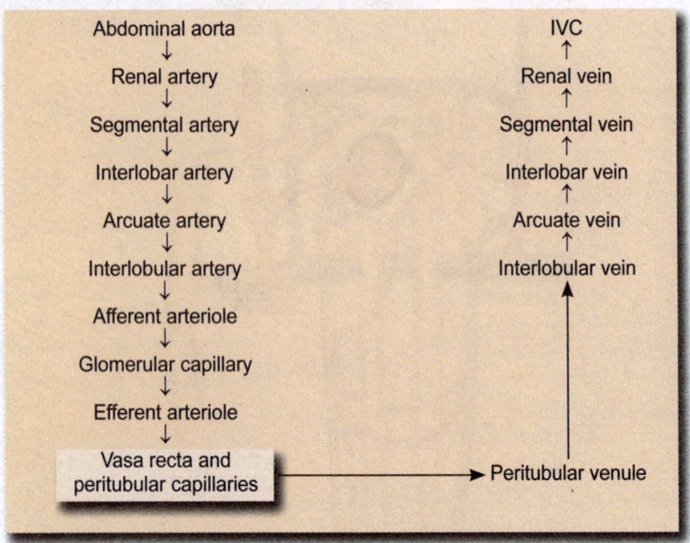

- Renal blood flow—1300 mL/min, 26 percent of cardiac output.
- Glomerular capillary pressure— 6–70 mm Hg.
- Peritubular capillary pressure— 8–10 mm Hg.

Urine formation—depends upon three processes:
1. Glomerular filtration.
2. Tubular reabsorption.
3. Tubular secretion.

Glomerular filtration: Filtration membrane has three layers (Fig. 5.28):

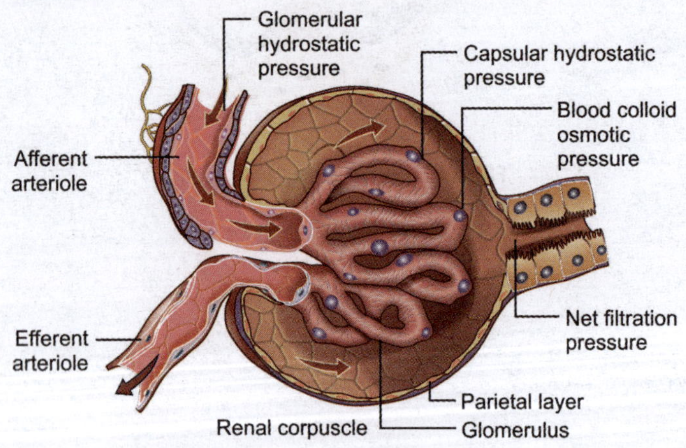

FIG. 5.28 Bowman's capsule

1. Glomerular capillary membrane
2. Basement membrane
3. Epithelial layer of Bowman's capsule.
- *Glomerular filtration rate* = 125 mL/min = 180 liters/day.
- *Filtration fraction* = Ratio of glomerular filtration rate:
  - ❖ Renal plasma flow in percentage
  - ❖ Normal = 15–20 percent.

Pressures responsible for glomerular filtration
- *Glomerular capillary pressure:* 45–70 mm Hg—pressure exerted by blood in capillary.
- *Colloid osmotic pressure:* It is the pressure exerted by glomeruli— it opposes glomerular capillary pressure. It is 25 mm Hg.
- *Hydrostatic pressure in Bowman's capsule:* It is the pressure exerted by the filtrate in Bowman's capsule. It opposes glomerular capillary pressure. It is 15 mm Hg.

So,

Net filtration pressure:

Glomerular capillary pressure – (Colloid osmotic pressure + Hydrostatic pressure in Bowman's Capsule)

– 60 – (25 ׀ 15) – 20 mm Hg.

$$\text{Filtration co-efficient} = \frac{\text{GFR per mm of Hg}}{\text{Net filtration pressure}}$$

– 125 mL/20 mm Hg = 6.25 mL/mm Hg.

Factors affecting glomerular filtration rate (Fig. 5.28)
- Renal blood flow
- Glomerular capillary pressure
- Colloid osmotic pressure
- Bowman's capsule's hydrostatic pressure
- Constriction of afferent arteriole—reduces blood flow to glomerular capillaries—it in turn reduces GFR
- Constriction of efferent arteriole—increases GFR due to stagnation of blood in capillaries
- Systemic arterial pressure.
- Sympathetic stimulation.

↓

Release of neurotransmitter substance (nor adrenaline)

↓

More constriction of efferent arterioles than afferent arterioles.

↓

Increased filtration of substances in early phase. But in later phase due to stagnation of blood in capillary, no fresh blood enters the capillary.
- *Surface area of capillary membrane:* It is decreased in some renal diseases—so there is reduction in GFR.

- *Permeability of capillary membrane:* It is decreased in:
  - ❖ Hypoxia
  - ❖ Toxic agents
  - ❖ Lack of blood supply.
- *Hormones:*
  - ❖ *Increases GFR:*
    - Atrial natriuretic peptide
    - Brain natriuretic peptide
    - PGE_2
    - Dopamine
    - CAMP.
  - ❖ *Decreases GFR:*
    - Angiotensin II
    - Endothelin
    - Nor adrenaline
    - PDGF.
    - Platelet-activating factor.
- *Tubuloglomerular feedback:* Tubuloglomerular feedback is controlled by macula densa situated in the terminal portion of thick ascending limb, close to afferent arteriole.

Increase in GFR
↓
Increased concentration of sodium chloride in renal tubule
↓
Detection of it by maculo densa
↓
Release of adenosine from ATP
↓
Causes constriction of afferent arteriole by adenosine receptor
↓
Blood flow through glomerulus will be decreased
↓
Decrease in glomerular filtration rate.

Tubular Reabsorption

It is the reabsorption of water and other solute from filtrate back into blood.

Selective Reabsorption

Because a tubular cell reabsorbs water and substances according to the need of the body, e.g. glucose, amino acid, and vitamins are absorbed completely.

Mechanism of Reabsorption

- *Active reabsorption:* It means reabsorption of solutes against electrochemical gradient. The molecules reabsorbed are:
  - ❖ Sodium
  - ❖ Calcium
  - ❖ Potassium
  - ❖ Phosphates
  - ❖ Sulfates
  - ❖ Bicarbonates
  - ❖ Glucose
  - ❖ Amino acids
  - ❖ Ascorbic acid
  - ❖ Uric acid
  - ❖ Ketone bodies.
- *Passive absorption:* It means absorption of solutes along the electrochemical gradient.
  The substances responsible are:
  - ❖ Chloride
  - ❖ Water
  - ❖ Urea.

Sites of absorption (Fig. 5.29)

- *Transcellular route:*

Transport of substances from tubular lumen into tubular cell through apical surface

↓

Transport of substances from tubular cell into interstitial fluid

↓

Transport from interstitial fluid into capillary.

- *Paracellular route:*

Transport of substances from tubular lumen into interstitial fluid present in lateral intercellular spaces through tight junction.

↓

Transport of substances from interstitial fluid into capillary.

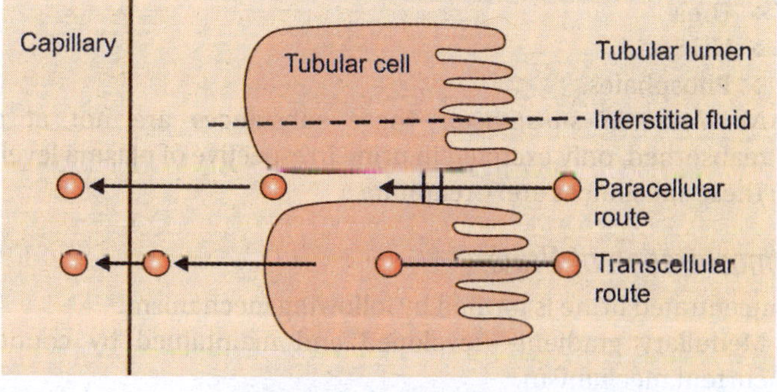

FIG. 5.29 Routs of absorption

Sites of absorption:
- *From proximal tubule:*
  - ❖ 7/8th portion of filtrate will be absorbed.
  - ❖ Substances reabsorbed are:
    - Glucose
    - Amino acid
    - Sodium
    - Potassium
    - Calcium
    - Bicarbonates
    - Amino acid
    - Chloride
    - Uric acid
    - Phosphate
    - Water.
- *Substances absorbed from loop of Henle:*
  - ❖ Sodium
  - ❖ Chloride.
- *From distal tubule:*
  - ❖ Sodium
  - ❖ Calcium
  - ❖ Bicarbonate
  - ❖ Water.

Threshold Substances

- *High threshold substances:* These substances do not appear in urine in normal circumstances.
  These are:
  - ❖ Glucose
  - ❖ Amino acid
  - ❖ Acetoacetic acid
  - ❖ Vitamins.
- *Low threshold substances:* These substances usually appear in urine in normal circumstances. These are:
  - ❖ Urea
  - ❖ Uric acid
  - ❖ Phosphates.
- *Nonthreshold substances:* These substances are not at all reabsorbed, only excreted in urine irrespective of plasma level. These substances are: Creatinine.

Concentration of Urine

Concentrated urine is formed by following mechanism:
- Medullary gradient—developed and maintained by counter current mechanism.
- Secretion of ADH.

Counter current mechanism: It includes:
- Counter current multiplier
- Counter current exchanger.

Counter current multiplier (Fig. 5.30)
Loop of Henle acts as multiplier in case of juxtamedullary nephron because loop extends up to deeper parts of medulla.

Mechanism
- Sodium, chloride and other solutes are reabsorbed from ascending limb of loop of Henle—so osmolarity of medullary interstitium progressively increased from above downwards, so that osmolarity of inner medulla is higher than that of outer medulla.

  The osmolarity of urine in ascending limb is progressively decreased from below upwards.
- Due to concentration gradient, sodium, and chlorides are reabsorbed from medullary interstitium into descending limb of loop of Henle along the concentration gradient via hair pin bend.

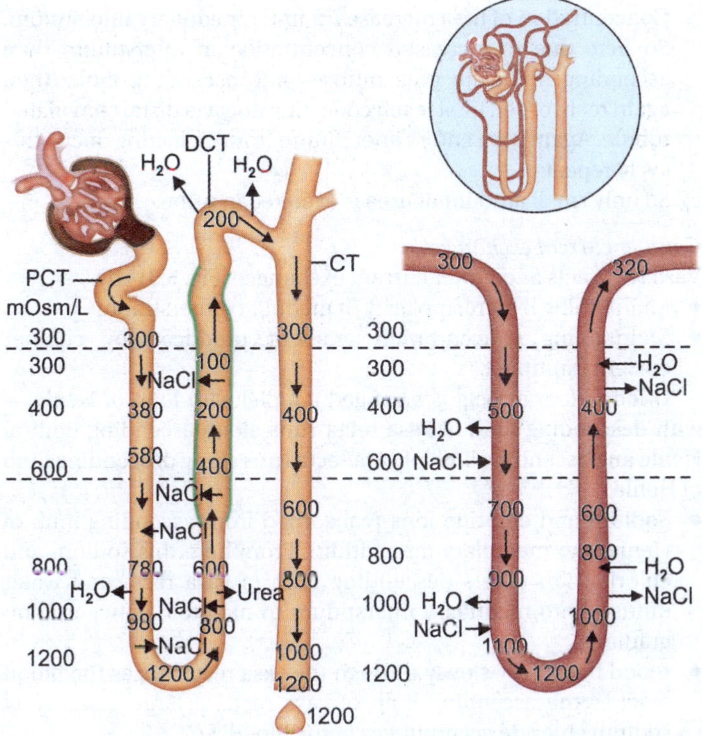

FIG. 5.30 Counter current multiplier

- Sodium and chloride ions are repeatedly recalculated between ascending limb and descending limb, only small amount will be excreted in urine.
- In addition, there is constant and regular addition of sodium and chloride into descending limb of loop of Henle by constant filtration.

So constant reabsorption of sodium and chloride ions from ascending limb into medullary interstitium and addition of new sodium and chloride ions into filtrate increase or multiply the osmolarity of medullary interstitial fluid. Hence, it is called counter count multiplier.

Other factors responsible for increase in hyperosmolarity of medullary interstitial fluid:

- Reabsorption of sodium ion from the medullary part of collecting duct—increases the osmolarity
- Urea is completely filtered in glomeruli. Since, it is not absorbed in any part of renal tubule, it reaches the collecting duct and concentration of urea increases in collecting direct. Now along the concentration gradient urea diffuses into inner part of medullary interstitium—increases osmolarity of inner medulla. Concentration of urea increases in inner medullary interstitium. So here due to increased concentration in interstitium than ascending limb, the urea diffuses into ascending limb. Then again reabsorbed urea reach collecting duct via distal convulated tubule. Again urea enters interstitium from collecting duct—this cycle repeats.

So only small amount of urea is excreted in urine.

Counter current exchanger

Vasa recta acts as counter current exchanger (Fig. 5.31) by:

- Maintaining hyperosmolarity of medullary interstitium
- Maintaining concentration gradient produced by counter current multiplier.

U loop of vasa recta is arranged parallel with loop of Henle — with descending limb of vasa recta runs along ascending limb of Henle and ascending limb of vasa recta runs along descending limb of Henle.

- Sodium and chloride ions reabsorbed from ascending limb of Henle into medullary interstitium. From here this sodium and chloride ion enters descending limb of vasa recta and water diffuses into medullary interstitium to maintain concentration gradient.
- Blood flows very slowly through the vasa recta. So, as the blood reaches the ascending limb of vasa recta, a large quantity of sodium chloride accumulates in the blood. So,
  - ❖ Sodium and chloride ion diffuses into medullary interstitium.

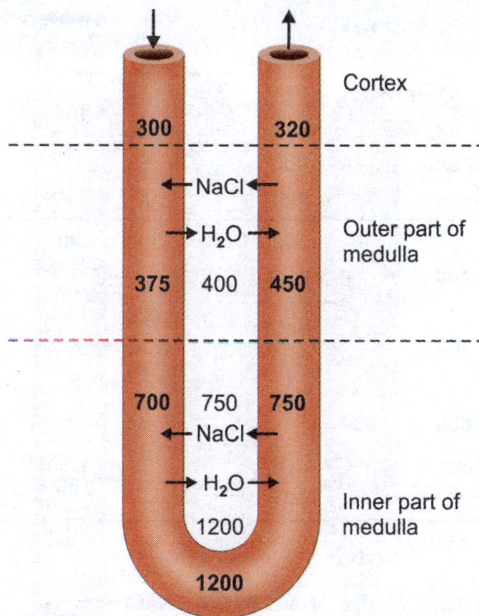

FIG. 5.31   Vasa recta counter current exchanger

- ❖ Water is reabsorbed from medullary interstitium into ascending limb of vasa recta.

Thus vasa recta

- Retains sodium chloride in medullary interstitium.
- Reabsorbs water.

Thus hyperosmolarity of medullary interstitium is maintained.

Recycling of urea occurs through vasa recta in similar mechanism as sodium chloride recycles.

Role of ADH

It helps in concentration of urine (Figs 5.32 and 5.33).

Normally distal convulated tubule and collecting duct are impermeable to water.

But in presence of ADH these ducts and DCT are permeable to water, resulting in water reabsorption. This method of reabsorption is called facultative reabsorption.

Summary of Urine Concentration

- Osmolarity of filtrate in Bowman's capsule—300 mOsmol/L.
- Osmolarity of filtrate in PCT is 300 mOsmol/L.
- Osmolarity of urine in thick descending limb—450–600 mOsmol/L.

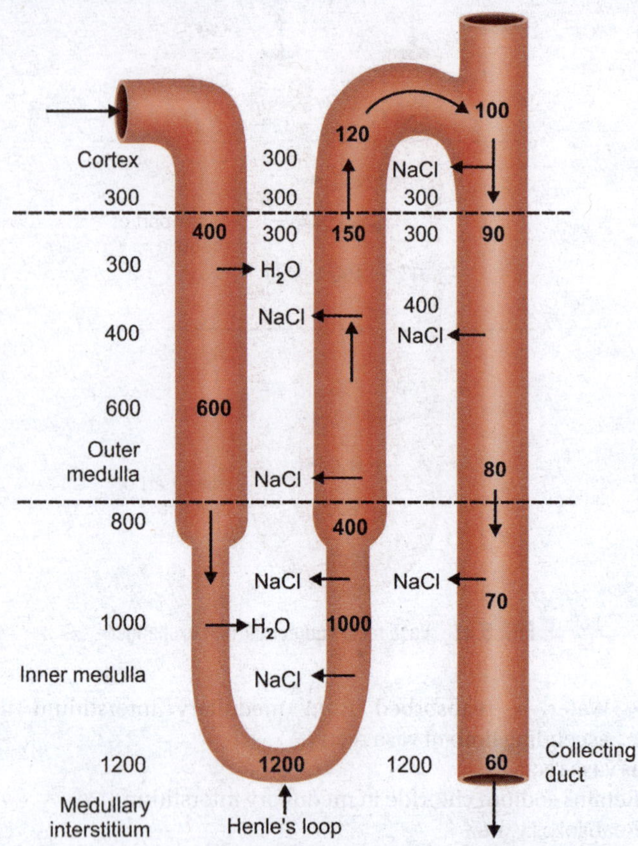

FIG. 5.32 Mechanism of formation of dilute urine

- Osmolarity of urine in thin descending limb—1000–1200 mOsmol/L.
- Osmolarity of urine in the ascending limb—400 mOsmol/L.
- Osmolarity of urine in thick ascending limb—150–200 mOsmol/L.
- Osmolarity of urine in DCT and CT in presence of ADH—1200 mOsmol/L.

Functions of nerve supplying the urinary bladder and sphincters

	Detrusor muscle	Internal sphincter	External sphincter	Function
• Sympathetic nerve	Relaxation	Constriction	Not supplied	Filling of urinary bladder
• Parasympathetic nerve	Contraction	Relaxation	Not supplied	Emptying of bladder
• Somatic nerve	Not supplied	Not supplied	Constriction	Voluntary control of micturition

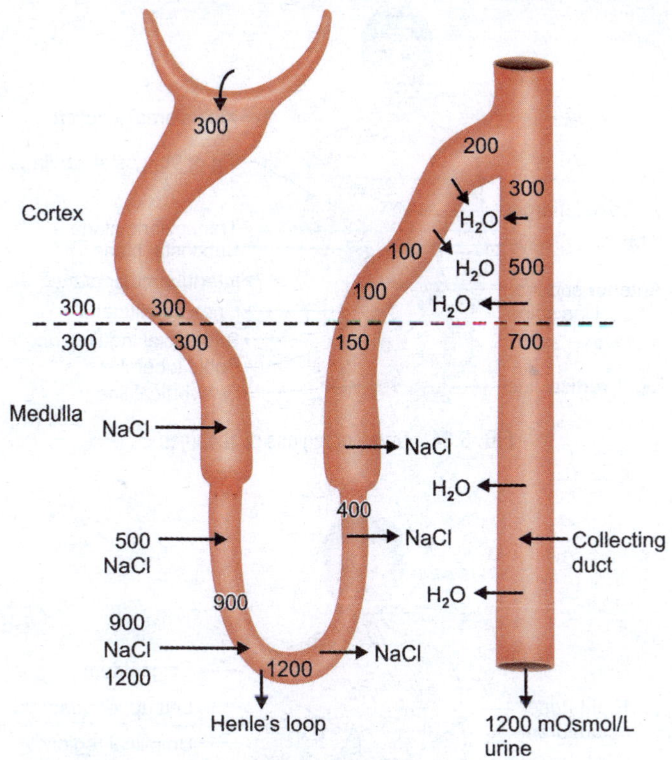

FIG. 5.33   Role of ADH in the formation of concentrated urine

SYMPTOMS AND PHYSICAL EXAMINATION

For descriptive purpose abdominal cavity is divided into nine regions by four imaginary lines (Fig. 5.34):

1. Two vertical imaginary lines drawn extending from right and left midclavicular lines to right and left midinguinal ligaments respectively.
2. Two horizontal imaginary lines drawn at right angles to above lines—one at costal margins and other at the level of superior iliac spines.

The regions are (clockwise):

- Right hypochondrium.
- Epigastric region.
- Left hypogastric region.
- Right lumbar region.
- Umbilical region.
- Left lumbar region.

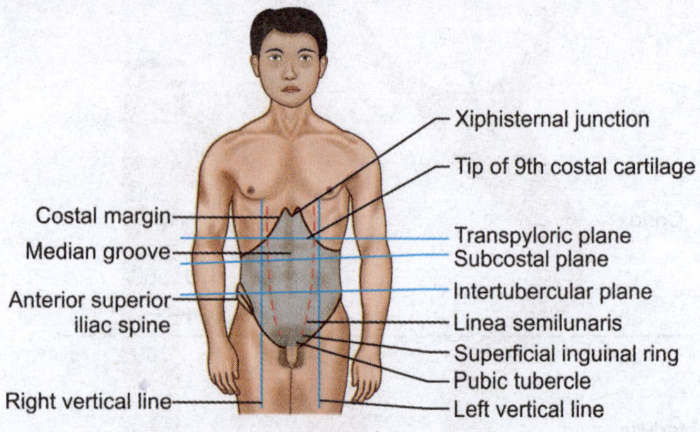

FIG. 5.34   Different regions of abdomen

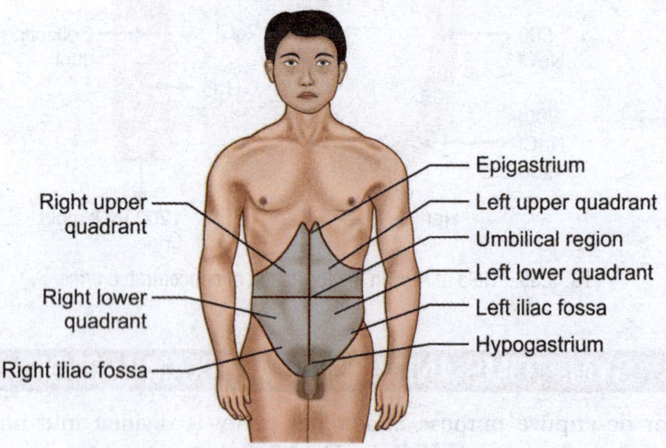

FIG. 5.35   Surface landmark of anterior abdominal wall

- Right inguinal region or right iliac fossa.
- Suprapubic region.
- Left iliac fossa.

For description purpose, abdominal cavity is divided into four quadrants—by two imaginary lines (Fig. 5.35)
They cross the umbilicus perpendicularly to divide the abdomen into four quadrants:

1. *Right upper quadrant:*
   - Right lobe of liver
   - Gallbladder
   - Pylorus

 ❖ Duodenum
 ❖ Head of pancreas
 ❖ Right kidney—upper pole
 ❖ Right adrenal gland
 ❖ Ascending colon distal part
 ❖ Proximal part of transverse colon
 ❖ Hepatic flexure.

2. *Right lower quadrant:*
 ❖ Cecum
 ❖ Proximal part of ascending colon
 ❖ Appendix
 ❖ Right ovary
 ❖ Right fallopian tube
 ❖ Right kidney—lower part
 ❖ Right ureter
 ❖ Right spermatic cord.

3. *Left upper quadrant:*
 ❖ Left lobe of liver
 ❖ Stomach
 ❖ Body and tail of pancreas
 ❖ Spleen
 ❖ Distal portion of transverse colon
 ❖ Proximal portion of descending colon
 ❖ Upper pole of left kidney
 ❖ Left adrenal gland
 ❖ Splenic flexure.

4. *Left lower quadrant:*
 ❖ Left colon—distal portion
 ❖ Sigmoid colon
 ❖ Left kidney lower pole
 ❖ Left ureter
 ❖ Left ovary
 ❖ Left fallopian tube
 ❖ Left spermatic cord.

The symptoms related to gastrointestinal systems:
- Abdominal pain
- Nausea and vomiting
- Constipation
- Diarrhea
- Jaundice
- Mass
- Hematemesis
- Malena
- Rectal bleeding
- Itching.

Abdominal Pain

According to the onset of pain—it may be acute or chronic.

Acute Abdominal Pain

- *According type of onset:*
  - *Sudden, severe, and localized:*
    - Cholecystitis—right upper quadrant
    - Pancreatitis—epigastrium
    - Perforated gastric ulcer—epigastrium
    - Ruptured ectopic pregnancy—lower quadrant.
  - *Sudden, severe, and diffuse:*
    - Mesenteric infarction
    - Perforated peptic ulcer—later on
    - Ruptured abdominal aortic aneurysm—back, flank.
- *Course of pain:*
  - Pain—gradually increases and subsides spontaneously—gastroenteritis.
  - Pain progresses and remits overtime—renal, biliary, intestinal obstruction.
  - *Progressive with time:*
    - Acute appendicitis
    - Acute diverticulitis.
  - Catastrophic onset—aortic aneurysm, peptic perforation.
- *Location (Fig. 5.36):*
  - Periumbilical early later localized to right lower quadrant—appendicitis
  - *Epigastric:*
    - Gastritis
    - Pancreatitis
    - Peptic perforation.

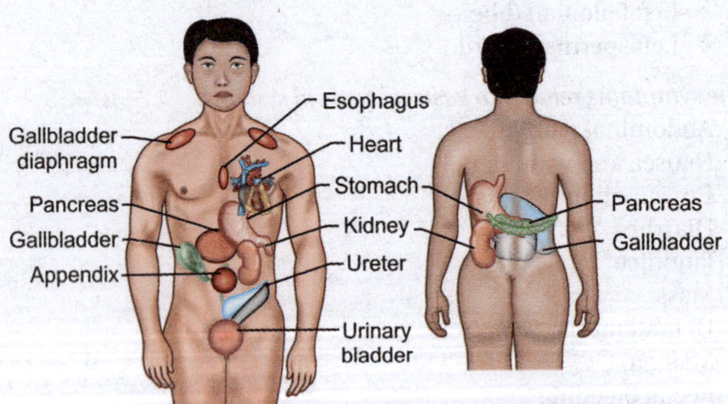

FIG. 5.36 Referred pain in skin area from viceral pain

- ❖ Right upper quadrant pain—acute cholecystitis
- ❖ Left lower quadrant—acute diverticulitis
- ❖ *Periumbilical area—diffuse:*
  - Mesenteric infarction
  - Small bowel obstruction
  - Acute gastroenteritis.
- ❖ *Lower quadrant—diffuse:*
  - Pelvic inflammatory disease
  - Ruptured ectopic pregnancy
- ❖ Retrosternal—esophagitis.
- *Character of pain:*
  - ❖ Diffuse early—localized late—appendicitis
  - ❖ Localized early, diffuse later—perforated peptic ulcer
  - ❖ *Localized:*
    - Cholecystitis
    - Pancreatitis
    - Diverticulitis
    - Ruptured ectopic pregnancy.
  - ❖ *Diffuse:*
    - Small bowel obstruction
    - Mesenteric infarction
    - Ruptured abdominal aortic aneurysm.
- *Description of pain:*
  - ❖ *Aching:*
    - Appendicitis
    - Diverticulitis
    - PID
  - ❖ *Spasmodic:*
    - Cholecystitis
    - Renal colic
    - Intestinal obstruction
  - ❖ *Burning:*
    - Gastritis
    - Peptic perforation
  - ❖ *Agonizing pain:*
    - Mesenteric infarction
    - Ruptured ectopic.
- *Radiation of pain:*
  - ❖ Radiation to right shoulder, scapula—cholecystitis
  - ❖ Radiation to back—pancreatitis
  - ❖ Radiation to upper thigh—pelvic inflammatory disease.
- *Aggravating and alleviating factors:*
  - ❖ Patient becomes motionless—peritoneal inflammation due to any cause
  - ❖ Patient tosses up on the bed to get a comfortable position—renal colic

- ❖ Diet—containing fatty food—biliary colic
- ❖ Postprandial pain—gastric ulcer, mesenteric infarction
- ❖ Pain in lying down positions, relieved by stooping posture—pancreatitis
- ❖ Flexion of knees—peritonitis
- ❖ Flexion of right thigh—(right psoas muscle)—appendicits
- ❖ Flexion of left thigh—(left psoas muscle)—diverticulitis.
- *Associated symptoms:*
  - ❖ Projectile vomiting—gastric outlet obstruction
  - ❖ Nausea vomiting—gastritis, pancreatitis, biliary colic
  - ❖ Feculent vomiting—small bowel obstruction
  - ❖ Hematemesis following retching and vomiting—esophagitis
  - ❖ Hematuria, dysuria—renal colic
  - ❖ Associated loose motion—occasionally blood—gastroenteritis
  - ❖ Weight loss—usually not present.

Chronic Abdominal Pain

This pain is defined as constantly or intermittently occurring over last 6 months.

In this type of pain—except the onset and severity—other description is similar for all type of pain described above.

Cause of Recurrent and Chronic Abdominal Pain

- *Inflammatory:*
  - ❖ Appendicitis
  - ❖ Celiac disease
  - ❖ Inflammatory bowel disease
  - ❖ Primary sclerosing cholangitis
  - ❖ Eosinophilic gastroenteritis.
- *Vascular:*
  - ❖ Mesenteric ischemia
  - ❖ Celiac artery involvement
  - ❖ Superior mesenteric artery syndrome.
- *Metabolic:*
  - ❖ Diabetic
  - ❖ Familial Mediterranean fever
  - ❖ Porphyria.
- *Neuromuscular:*
  - ❖ Anterior cutaneous nerve entrapment syndrome
  - ❖ Slipping rib syndrome
  - ❖ Thoracic nerve radiculopathy
  - ❖ Myofascial pain syndrome.

- *Others:*
  - ❖ Abdominal malignancy
  - ❖ Gall stones
  - ❖ Endometriosis
  - ❖ Hernias
  - ❖ Lactose intolerance.
  - ❖ Postoperative abdominal adhesions.
- *Functional gastrointestinal disorders:*
  - ❖ Irritable bowel syndrome
  - ❖ Functional dyspepsia
  - ❖ Functional abdominal pain syndrome
  - ❖ Sphincter of oddi dysfunction.

Slipping rib syndrome
- Unilateral sharp lancinating pain in subcostal region—followed by protracted aching sensation.
- Hypermobility of costal cartilage at the anterior end of false 8, 9 and 10th rib.
- Slipping of the affected rib behind the superior adjacent rib during abdominal muscular contraction.
- Key to the diagnosis is hooking maneuver done by clinician—Examiner hooks underneath the patient's lowest ribs—produces pain with an audible pop or click.

Abdominal Pain: Pain Characteristics

- *Inflammation of parietal peritoneum:*
  - ❖ *Quality*—boring, acting
  - ❖ *Location*—area of peritoneum exposed
  - ❖ *Intensity*—this depends upon:
    - Type of material
    - Amount of material
    - Duration of exposure
    - Type of exposure
      - Sterile acid—small amount but sudden release—produces more pain than same amount of feculent material
      - Blood or urine may produce pain if—the amount is high or onset is rapid
      - Pancreatic juice containing enzymes may produce server pain than the same amount of bile.
      - Bacterial contamination is less severe than contamination bacterial toxins.
  - ❖ *Aggravating factors*—changes in tension of peritoneum
    - Any type of body movements like, cough, sneezing increase spasm of abdominal musculature.

- Any type of body movements mainly of abdomen— produce intense abdominal pain because of abdominal muscle guard.
- ❖ *Tonic spasm of abdominal musculature:*
  - Localized spasm of abdominal musculature, which is related to:
    - Site of contact
    - Amount of material
    - Rate at which the peritoneum is exposed
  - In case of retrocecal appendix or perforated peptic ulcer releasing fluid in lesser sac may not produce any intense pain.
- *Hollow viscous obstruction:*
  - ❖ *Character*—Colicky— exacerbations and remissions
  - ❖ *Localization*—depends upon organ of obstruction:
    - Periumbilical in case of small intestine
    - Infraumbilical in case of large intestine
    - Right upper quadrant in biliary colic
    - *Epigastrium:*
      - in case of CBD dilatation
      - in case of carcinoma head of pancreas
    - Suprapubic pain—obstruction to urinary bladder
    - Server suprapubic pain and flank pain—obstruction of intravesicle portion of ureter
    - Pain at costovertebral angle—obstruction at pelviureteric junction
    - Flank pain—obstruction to ureter, inflammed colon
  - ❖ *Referred pain:* Depends upon the organ involved
    - Radiation to lumbar region—colonic obstruction
    - Radiation to right scapular tip or right posterior region of thorax—biliary colic.
    - Radiation to upper part of lumbar sign—obstruction to CBD.
    - Radiation to penis, scrotum, inner aspect of thigh— obstruction of intravesicle portion of ureter or calculus in urinary bladder.
    - Radiation to groin—pain pelviureteric junction.
- *Vascular disturbances:*
  - ❖ *In case of mesenteric arterial obstruction:*
    - At the onset, pain is mild to moderate, continuous, occasionally cramping in nature—due to hyperperistalsis
    - *In late stage:* Continuous diffuse pain, occasionally associated. Muscle guard—no radiation
  - ❖ *Rupture of abdominal aortic aneurysm:*
    - Intense, excruciating pain in abdomen
    - Radiation to flank, genitalia, or sacral region.

- *Pain from abdominal wall:*
  - ❖ Pain is constant
  - ❖ Increases with respiration, prolonged standing
  - ❖ Localized pain—may have hematomas in rectus sheath due to anticoagulant therapy.

Referred Pain to Abdomen

- *Lower lobe pneumonia:* Diaphragmatic pleurisy—in right or left upper quadrant of abdomen.
- *Referred pain of thoracic spine:* Pain in upper abdomen with abdominal muscle guard.
- *From spine:*
  - ❖ Pain along the involved dermatome
  - ❖ Lancinating pain
  - ❖ Pain is increased by:
    - • Cough
    - • Sneeze
    - • Any type of strain
  - ❖ Hyperesthesia of involved dermatomes.
- *From testicle:*
  - ❖ Pain in lower abdomen above symphysis pubis
  - ❖ Dull acting in character
  - ❖ Not definitely localized.

Metabolic Abdominal Crises

- Diffuse acute abdominal pain leading to unnecessary laparotomy—acute pancreatitis
- *Acute abdominal pain:*
  C1-esterase deficiency
  Familial Mediterranean fever
- Colicky abdominal pain—lead intoxication
- Nonspecific acute abdominal pain—diabetes
- Intense pain and rigidity of abdominal muscles and back muscles—black widow spider bites.

Neurological Origin

- *Sensory nerve involvement:*
  - ❖ Character—burning
  - ❖ Radiation—along the distribution of nerve
  - ❖ Provocation—touch, temperature, palpation
  - ❖ Relieving factor—no physical movement.
- *Pain along spinal root:*
  - ❖ Character—lancinating type
  - ❖ Timing—recurrent

- ❖ No relation food, abdominal distension
- ❖ Radiation—along the dermatomes
- ❖ Aggravating factors—movement of spine
- ❖ Lancinating pain on touch.

Functional Causes

- No specific pattern of pain
- Recurrent abdominal colicky pain with alternate constipation and diarrhea
- Aggravation by stress.

◼ Vomiting

Pathophysiology of Vomiting

The mechanism of vomiting includes:

- *The trigger areas arise from different sites:*
  - ❖ *Gastrointestinal tract:*
    - Pharynx
    - Stomach
    - Small intestines
    - Bile ducts.
  - ❖ *Nongastrointestinal tract:*
    - Kidney and ureter
    - Urinary bladder
    - Vestibular apparatus (motion sickness)
    - Coronary arteries
    - Peritoneum
    - Testicles
    - Pregnancy
    - Cortex
    - Brainstem
    - Cerebellum.
- *Afferent pathways:*
  - Vogel afferents
  - Sympathetic afferents.
- *Receptors include:*
  - ❖ Stimulation of 5-hydroxytryptamine—3 receptors
    ↓
    Release of dopamine
    ↓
    Stimulates dopamine receptors D_2 in emetic center
    ↓
    Activates emesis.

This reflex can be inhibited by:
- $5HT_3$ antagonists
- D_2 receptor antagonist.

❖ Histamine H_1 receptors, muscarinic receptors M_1 receptors—present in vestibular nucleus and tractus solitary nucleus —responsible for motion sickness and pregnancy related emesis.

This reflex can be inhibited by:
- Anti H_1 receptors
- Anti M_1 receptors.

❖ Canabinoid receptors present in dorsal vagal nucleus

Inhibits emesis

It also modulates $5HT_3$ channels.

❖ Neurokinin 1 receptors present in prostema and solitary nucleus.

Binds to P substance and part of terminal emetic pathways
Inhibitors of NK1 or NK1 antagonists reduce emesis centrally and peripherally.

- *Centrally chemoreceptor trigger zone (CTZ)* located in the area of prostema on the floor of 4th ventricle.

Activates emetic center.

- As a result of efferent impulses from vomiting center—the following sequences of emesis occur as a result of activation of cerebral cortex:
  - ❖ Stomach relaxes concomitantly
  - ❖ Antral peristalsis is inhibited
  - ❖ Small intestinal peristalsis is inhibited.

So, nausea starts
- Spasmodic contraction of diaphragm
- Spasmodic contraction of intercostal muscles
- Closure of glottis.

Retching Starts

Vomiting starts when:
Somatic and visceral components act simultaneously:
- Brisk contraction of diaphragm and abdominal muscles
- Relaxation of esophageal sphincter
- Forceful retrograde propulsion of jejunum pushes the enteric contents into stomach, then towards mouth.

Protective reflexes are also activated simultaneously:
- Soft palate is raised to prevent the gastric content from entering into nasopharynx

- Inhibition of respiration for a moment
- Glottis is closed to prevent pulmonary aspiration.

This vomiting may be complicated by:
- Hypersalivation
- Cardiac dysrhythmia
- Passage of gas per rectum.

Nausea is an unpleasant subjective sensation of impending vomiting in the epigastrium or throat.

Retching consists of spasmodic and abortive respiratory movements with closed glottis.

It may start with nausea.

It may culminate with vomiting.

Vomiting is the forceful expulsion of gastric or intestinal content through mouth.

Regurgitation: It is effortless reflux of gastric contents into the esophagus, may be into mouth but not associated with forceful expulsion of gastric contents.

Causes of Vomiting

- *Abdominal causes:*
  - ❖ *Mechanical obstruction:*
    - Gastric outlet obstruction
    - Small bowel obstruction.
  - ❖ *Motility disorder:*
    - Achalasia cardia
    - Other esophageal dysmotility
    - Chronic intestinal psudo-obstruction.
  - ❖ *Inflammatory causes:*
    - Acute gastritis
    - Acute cholecystitis
    - Acute appendicitis
    - Acute pancreatitis
    - Acute hepatitis
    - Acute mesenteric ischemia
    - Active duodenal ulcer
    - Peritonitis
    - Ulcerative colitis
    - Crohn's disease.
  - ❖ *Malignant causes:*
    - Esophageal carcinoma
    - Gastric carcinoma
    - Pancreatic carcinoma
    - Peritoneal carcinomatosis.

- *Infection:*
  - ❖ *Acute gastroenteritis:*
    - Bacterial
    - Viral.
  - ❖ *Nongastrointestinal:*
    - Meningitis
    - Systemic infections.
- *Metabolic causes:*
  - ❖ Diabetic ketoacidosis
  - ❖ Diabetes mellitus
  - ❖ Hyperthyroidism
  - ❖ Hyperparathyroidism
  - ❖ Hypoparathyroidism
  - ❖ Pregnancy
  - ❖ Acute intermittent porphyria
  - ❖ Addison disease.
- *Nervous system causes:*
  - ❖ Disorder of autoimmune nervous system.
  - ❖ *Hydrocephalus:*
    - Increased intracranial pressure
    - Low pressure hydrocephalus.
  - ❖ *Intracerebral lesions:*
    - Subdural hematomas or abscesses
    - Intracerebral infarction
    - Intracerebral hemorrhage
    - Intracerebral abscess
    - Subarachnoid hemorrhage.
  - ❖ *Labyrinthine disorders:*
    - Labyrinthitis
    - Meniere's disease
    - Motion sickness.
  - ❖ Meningitis.
  - ❖ Demyelinating disorders.
- *Other causes:*
  - ❖ Eating disorders
  - ❖ Ethanol abuse
  - ❖ Hypervitaminosis A
  - ❖ Postvagotomy
  - ❖ Functional disorders.

Acute Vomiting—Causes

- *Acute gastric outlet obstruction:*
  - ❖ *Consequence of peptic ulcer disease:*
    - Pylorospasm
    - Ulcer with severe surrounding edema
    - Marked deformity of duodenal bulb.

- ❖ Gastric volvulus
- ❖ Paraesophageal hernia
- ❖ *Sequelae of acute on chronic pancreatitis:*
  Producing duodenal, less commonly pyloric obstruction:
  - Pancreatic mass
  - Pancreatic phlegmon
  - Pancreatic necrosis.
- ❖ Malignancy of stomach, pancreas, rarely duodenum.
- *Acute intestinal obstruction:*
  - ❖ Stool impaction in intestine
  - ❖ Incarcerated hernia
  - ❖ *Neoplasm of distal duodenum or proximal jejunum:*
    - Leiomyoma
    - Adenocarcinoma
    - Lymphoma
    - Carcinoid.
- *Intestinal infarction:* Due to sudden vascular obstruction.
- *Extraintestinal causes:*
  - ❖ Myocardial infarction
  - ❖ Renal colic
  - ❖ Biliary colic
  - ❖ Testicular torsion
  - ❖ Intraperitoneal inflammatory conditions:
    - Appendicitis
    - Acute pancreatitis
    - Bowel perforation.
- *Drugs:*
  - ❖ Cancer chemotherapy
  - ❖ NSAID
  - ❖ Cardiovascular drugs—digitalis, antiarrhythmics
  - ❖ Levodopa
  - ❖ Theophylline.
- *Metabolic:*
  - ❖ Diabetic ketoacidosis
  - ❖ Hypercalcemia
  - ❖ Hyponatremia.
- *Toxin:*
  - ❖ Bacterial toxins—staphylococcal
  - ❖ Alcoholism.
- *Neurological:*
  - ❖ Cerebrovascular accident producing sudden increase intra-cranial pressure
  - ❖ Migraine
  - ❖ Meningitis producing raised ICP.
- Postoperative.

Chronic or Relapsing Vomiting

Above all are the causes of chronic vomiting having following few differences and some additional causes:

- *Partial intestinal obstruction:*
  - ❖ All above causes of intestinal obstruction in early phase may produce partial intestinal obstruction
  - ❖ Mechanical or ischemic stricture of small intestine
  - ❖ Intestinal pseudo-obstruction due to motility disorders of small intestine.
- *Motility disorder of gastrointestinal tract:*
  - ❖ Diabetic gastroparesis
  - ❖ Chronic intestinal pseudo-obstruction.

    In neuropathic gastroparesis—repeated vomiting evening empty stomach.

    In partial gastric outlet obstruction—repeated vomiting—having food containing vomitus.
- *Neurological:*
  - ❖ Migraine without aura or no family history of headache
  - ❖ Hydrocephalus or lesion compressing emetic center
    - *Vomiting may be or may not be associated with weight loss:*
      - *Associated with weight loss:*
        - Esophageal carcinoma
        - Gastric carcinoma—anorexia or early satiety
        - Achalasia cardia
          Associated history
          i. Nocturnal regurgitation and aspiration
          ii. Vomiting after large amount of meal
          iii. Dysphagia to liquid
        - Esophageal stricture—dysphagia to solid and liquid

        Not associated with weight loss:
        - *Esophagitis—with or without ulceration:* Associated with:
          i. Retrosternal burning
          ii. Water brush
          iii. Acid regurgitation
        - *Pharyngeal pouch:* Regurgitation of undigested food—longtime after ingestion of meal or in lying down position.
    - *Vomiting occurs in the morning in empty stomach and emission of saliva as vomitus:*
      - Pregnancy
      - Toxins
      - Drugs
      - Metabolic disorders (diabetes mellitus, uremia)

- – Psychological cause
- – Exclusive nocturnal postnasal drip.
- *Vomiting occurs shortly after intake of food:* Vomitus contains undigested or partially digested food:
  - – Partial gastric outlet obstruction
  - – Long standing achalasia cardia
  - – Zenker's diverticulum
  - – Gastroparesis
  - – Small intestinal obstruction—associated symptoms may be—abdominal pain—cramping type, weight loss, anorexia.
- *Vomiting after fatty meals—acute:* Cholecystitis—may be associated with abdominal pain
- *Vomiting—vomitus is feculent:*
  - – Small intestinal obstruction
  - – Paralytic ileus peritonitis
  - – Long standing gastric outlet obstruction
- *Vomiting not associated with nausea:* Increased intra-cranial pressure due to:
  - – Tumor
  - – Abscess
  - – Infarction
- *Vomiting with abdominal pain and fever:*
  - – Food poisoning
  - – Acute appendicitis
  - – Renal—acute pyelonephritis
  - – Urinary tract infection
  - – Jaundice—due to infective hepatitis
  - – Pelvic inflammatory disease
  - – Toxic shock syndrome—associated symptoms may be skin rash, confusion, hypotension, myalgia
  - – Occasionally pneumonia affecting lower lobe—irritating the diaphragm.
- *If vomiting is associated with abdominal pain, but not associated with fever:*
  - – Gastric, intestinal neoplasm
  - – Renal colicky pain—due to kidney stones
  - – Ruptured ectopic pregnancy
  - – Small intestinal obstruction
  - – Mesenteric vein occlusion
  - – Acute myocardial ischemia
  - – Abdominal cancer pain
  - – Diabetic ketoacidosis
  - – Lead poisoning

- Acute intermittent porphyria
- Hypercalcemia
- Pheochromocytoma.

- *Vomiting may associated with headache in following conditions:*
  - Migraine
  - *Increased intracranial tension due to:*
    - Tumor
    - Abscess
    - Benign intracranial hypertension
    - Cerebral infarction
    - Hemorrhagic stroke
    - Meningitis
  - Malignant hypertension
  - Acute glaucoma
  - Drugs
  - Hypervitaminosis A
  - Alcohol intoxication.

Questions to be asked regarding vomiting:
- When mainly vomiting occurs?
- Diurnal variation of vomiting.
- Is the vomiting worse in the morning?
- What is the content of vomitus?
- What is the taste of vomitus?
- Is there any relation with posture?
- Is there any history of associated symptoms?
  - ❖ Weight loss
  - ❖ Headache
  - ❖ Abdominal pain
  - ❖ Diarrhea.
- History of any drug intake.

Symptoms Related to Esophageal Diseases

Dysphagia

It is defined by difficulty in deglutition.

It indicates malfunction of esophagus starting from pharynx to lower esophageal junction.

Mechanism of dysphagia

- *This swallowing mechanism includes:* Primary and secondary peristaltic contractions of esophagus transport solid and liquid from mouth to stomach within 10 seconds.

- ❖ If peristaltic contractions fail to progress, bolus will be stucked in esophagus and distends the lumen
- ❖ In few patients, low amplitude wave fails to clear the esophagus
- ❖ In few patients, disordered contractions of esophagus produce dysphagia.
- *Mechanical obstruction of esophageal lumen:* It depends upon:
  - ❖ Degree of luminal obstruction
  - ❖ Type of food ingested
    In case of minimal obstruction, large bolus of food, poorly chewed food may produce dysphagia.
  - ❖ In case of gastroesophageal reflux disease:
    - If there is associated stricture—there is dysphagia
    - In absence of stricture, some sensory perception may produce dysphagia, though the food is cleared off.

Two types of dysphagia

Oropharyngeal dysphagia: Inability to propel the food bolus from hypopharyngeal area to upper esophagus through upper esophageal sphincter is called oropharyngeal dysphagia. These patients present with any of the following:

- History of recurrent manual impacted food lodgement
- Drooling of saliva at the corner of mouth
- Nasal intonation of voice
- History of dryness of mouth produced by—medications, salivary dysfunction
- Swallowing associated with gurgling noise
- Hoarseness of voice—due to recurrent.
  Laryngeal nerve dysfunction or intrinsic muscle disease.

Causes are:
- *Neuromuscular causes:*
  - ❖ Manometric dysfunction of UES
  - ❖ Muscular dystrophy
  - ❖ Myasthenia gravis
  - ❖ Polymyositis and dermatomyositis
  - ❖ Thyroid dysfunction
  - ❖ ALS
  - ❖ Multiple sclerosis.
- *Structural causes:*
  - ❖ Zenker's diverticulum
  - ❖ Proximal esophageal web
  - ❖ Prior surgery
  - ❖ Postradiotherapy
  - ❖ Carcinoma.

Esophageal dysphagia
Causes are:
- *Motility disorders (Neuromuscular):*
  - *Primary disorder:*
    - Achalasia cardia
    - Diffuse esophageal spasm
    - Nut-cracker esophagus.
  - *Secondary disorders:*
    - Chagas disease
    - GERD
    - Collagen vascular disease.
- *Mechanical disorders:*
  - *Intrinsic:*
    - Esophageal carcinoma
    - Barrett's esophagus
    - Corrosive stricture
    - Esophageal ring
    - Esophageal diverticula
    - Eosinophilic esophagitis.
  - *Extrinsic:*
    - Mediastinal mass
    - Osteophytes.

Questions to be asked to diagnose in esophageal dysphagia:
- Type of food or liquid producing symptoms.
- Whether dysphagia is intermittent or progressive.
- Any associated symptoms, e.g. heart burn, acid regurgitation.
- *Dysphagia to solid and liquid: Achalasia cardia*—associated symptoms:
  - Regurgitation of undigested food at night
  - Weight loss
  - Vomiting not with every meals.
- *Dysphagia with crushing retrosternal pain, increasing sensitivity to hot and cold:* Diffuse esophageal spasm.
- *Dysphagia with heart burn*—scleroderma—associated features may be cough, inhalation of fluid, tight skin.
- *Severe dysphagia:* Peptic stricture—associated history of reflux.
- *Dysphagic to solid to start with mechanical obstruction, when progressive:*
  - Dysphagia to solid and liquid
  - Weight loss, anorexia
  - Regurgitation of liquid—oropharyngeal carcinoma.
- *Episodic and nonprogressive dysphagia—esophageal web. on Schatzki's ring:*
  - This may at first starts with hurried meal; often with alcohol.
  - It can be resolved by taking large quantity of fluid.

- ❖ The offending food may be dry bread or steak. Hence called steakhouse syndrome.
- ❖ It can recur after weeks or months.
- ❖ Later on, the interval between the episodes gradually shorten.
- ❖ History of iron deficiency anemia.
- *Dysphagia with history of caustic ingestion:* True lye stricture.
- *History of lump sensation in throat, regurgitation of undigested food, bulging of neck during drinking, recurrent aspiration:* Pharyngeal pouch.
- *History of lump sensation in throat, anxiety:* Globus hystericus.
- *History of progressive difficulty in swallowing, cough precipitated by swallowing in later phase:* Myasthenia gravis.
- *History of nasal intonation of voice, small spastic tongue:* Pseudobulbar palsy.
- *History of dysphagia, hoarseness, flaccid fasciculating tongue—involvement of other cranial nerve:* Bulbar palsy.

Odynophagia

This can be defined as painful dysphagia starting from—retrosternal pain during swallowing to stabbing or piercing pain radiating to back, so that, the patient cannot swallow a drop of liquid or saliva.

Causes of odynophagia
- *Caustic:*
  - ❖ Acid
  - ❖ Alkali.
- *Pill induced esophagitis:*
  - ❖ Aspirin
  - ❖ Potassium iodide
  - ❖ Bisphosphonates.
- *Infection:*
  - ❖ *Virus:*
    - Epstein—Barr virus
    - Cytomegaly virus
    - Herpes simplex
    - HIV.
  - ❖ Bacterial
  - ❖ *Fungal:*
    - *Candida albicans*
    - Histoplasma.
- Reflux esophageal.
- Early esophageal carcinoma.

Globus Sensation

This can be defined as feeling of lump, tightness in between meals—relieved by swallowing solid or liquid.

Causes:
- Esophageal distension—can produce this—in spite of normal UES function.

    Again mental stress can increase UES pressure not associated with Globus sensation.
- Documentation of esophagitis.
- GERD.
- *Psychological disorders:*
  - Anxiety
  - Panic disorders
  - Somatization disorder
  - Depression.

Hiccough

This occurs due to combination of:
- Glottic closure
- Diaphragmatic contractions.

Causes:
- Idiopathic—mostly.
- *Gastroenterological:*
  - GERD
  - Achalasia
  - Gastroparesis
  - Peptic ulcers.
- Uremia
- Large meal
- Infections.

Chest Pain

Other than cardiac cause, esophagus is the 2nd most common site of chest pain.
- Character—squeezing or burning.
- Site—substantial or retrosternal.
- Radiation—to back, neck, jaw, arms, or laterally.
- Duration—ranges from minutes to hours or occurs intermittently over several days.
- *Aggravating factors:*
  - Ingestion of hot or cold liquids
  - Emotional stress.

- Relieving factors—antacids, sublingual nitroglycerin.
- Associated symptoms.

Causes of Chest Pain

- *Due to stimulation of chemoreceptor:* Acid, pepsin, or bile.
  - ❖ Gastroesophageal reflux disease
  - ❖ Bile reflux.
  All above produce esophagitis.
- *Due to stimulation of mechanoreceptors produced by distension:*
  - ❖ Esophageal spasm
  - ❖ Nut-cracker esophagus
  - ❖ Achalasia cardia.
  Here chest pain occurs due to:
  Sustained longitudinal esophageal smooth muscle contraction.
- *Stimulation of temperature receptors:*
  - ❖ *Ingestion of hot and cold liquids:* This produces esophageal aperistalsis and dilatation—this dilatation stimulates the stretch receptors
  - ❖ Acute food impaction
  - ❖ Ingestion of carbonated beverages
  - ❖ Dysfunction of belching reflex.
- *Psychiatric disorder:*
  - ❖ Anxiety neurosis
  - ❖ Panic disorder
  - ❖ Depression.

Heart Burn

Burning sensation arising from stomach radiating upto esophagus producing retrosternal burn—it then radiates to back and rarely to arms.

The heart burn may relieved by:
- Antacids
- Baking soda
- Milk.

Aggravating factors of heart burn—that should be asked during history taking. These are:
- *Decreasing the lower esophageal sphincter pressure:*
  - ❖ Sugar
  - ❖ Carminatives
  - ❖ Onions
  - ❖ High fatty acid

- ❖ Nicotine
- ❖ Smoking.
- *Irritating the inflamed lower esophageal mucosa:*
  - ❖ Citrus product
  - ❖ Tomato-based food
  - ❖ Spicy food (all above have high acidity and high osmolarity)
  - ❖ Alcohol
  - ❖ Coffee
  - ❖ Soft drinks
  - ❖ Obesity.
- *Lying on right lateral position.*
- *Maneuvers producing increase in abdominal pressure:*
  - ❖ Straining
  - ❖ Forward bending
  - ❖ Lifting heavy objects
  - ❖ Isometric exercise
  - ❖ Running.
- *Emotions:*
  - ❖ Anxiety
  - ❖ Fear
  - ❖ Depressions—all these decrease visceral sensitivity threshold.
- *Drugs:*
  - ❖ *Producing decrease in LES pressure:*
    - • Theophylline
    - • Calcium channel blocker.
  - ❖ *Imitating inflamed esophagus:*
    - • Aspirin
    - • NSAID
    - • Bisphosphonates.

Regurgitation

It can be defined by appearance of bitter or acidic fluid, food, bilious material in the mouth, which can be effortless. This will be aggravated at night.

Water Brush

Sudden appearance of salty clear fluid in the mouth. This is secreted from salivary gland as a result of protective vagally mediated reflex from lower esophagus.

Regurgitation may be distinguished from rumination. Rumination is nothing but rechewing of recently ingested pleasant food, not sour or bitter by taste, not associated with retching.

Extra Esophageal Symptoms

The symptoms produced by microaspiration of stomach contents into upper or lower respiratory tracts:

- Asthma
- Sore throat
- Hoarseness of voice
- Globus sensation
- Laryngitis
- Pulmonary fibrosis—the following history to be taken in patient with esophageal symptoms as well as upper and lower respiratory tract symptoms:
  - ❖ Any history of bronchial asthma and on bronchodilator therapy because bronchodilator dilates lower esophageal sphincter and helps in gastroesophageal reflux
  - ❖ Wheezing in adulthood who has no history of allergic asthma
  - ❖ History of nocturnal cough or wheezing
  - ❖ Wheezing worsened by meals, or exercise or in supine position
  - ❖ History of sore throat, excessive salivation, burning sensation in throat, hoarseness is voice.

Dyspepsia

Dyspepsia—means difficult digestion. It means a heterogeneous group of disorders centering upper abdomen and they include:

- Epigastric pain
- Postprandial abdominal distension
- Early satiety
- Nausea
- Vomiting
- Heart burn.

According to Rome III criteria, dyspepsia originates from gastroduodenal region. According to this consensus committee only the following four symptoms are specific for gastroduodenal regions.

- *Postprandial fullness:* Unpleasant sensation in upper abdomen perceived after taking full meals.
- *Early satiety:* Feeling of fullness of stomach just after start taking foods, so patient cannot finish his meal.
- *Epigastric pain:* This is defined as pain originating in upper abdomen in between umbilicus and lower sternum, having no relation with food.
- *Epigastric burning:* This refers to unpleasant sensation of heat in epigastric region.

Associated Symptoms

- *Upper abdominal bloating sensation:* This refers to tightness in upper abdomen, but other causes of visible abdominal distension should be ruled out.
- *Nausea:* Sensation of some unpleasant thing, which is need to be expelled out.
- *Vomiting:* Forceful expulsion of gastric content associated with contraction of abdominal and chest muscles. It may be associated with retching.
- *Belching:* Expelling of air out of stomach or esophagus.

Causes of Dyspepsia

- *Luminal gastrointestinal tract:*
  - ❖ Gastroesophageal reflux disease
  - ❖ Gastric or duodenal ulcers
  - ❖ Gastric or esophageal neoplasm
  - ❖ Gastric infection
  - ❖ Gastroparesis
  - ❖ *Inflammatory gastric disorders:*
    - Crohn's disease
    - Sarcoidosis
    - Eosinophilic gastroenteritis
  - ❖ Irritable bowel syndrome
  - ❖ Food intolerance.
- *Pancreatic disorder:*
  - ❖ Chronic pancreatitis
  - ❖ Pancreatic neoplasm.
- *Biliary disorder:*
  - ❖ Cholelithiasis
  - ❖ Choledocholithiasis
  - ❖ Sphincter of oddi dysfunction.
- *Nongastrointestinal disorders:*
  - ❖ Myocardial ischemia
  - ❖ Congestive cardiac failure
  - ❖ Hyperparathyrodisim
  - ❖ Adrenal insufficiency
  - ❖ Thyroid disease
  - ❖ Renal insufficiency.

So history should be taken accordingly:
- Relation with meals
- Relation with dietary factors
- If loose motion is present—number of motions, consistency of stools—whether it is acute or chronic

- Associated symptoms—anemia, weight loss, dysphagia.
- Associated thyroid disorders.

■ Diarrhea

Normally small intestine and large intestine absorb 99 percent of water secreted endogenously (9–10 liter/day), from salivary gland, stomach, liver, and pancreas.

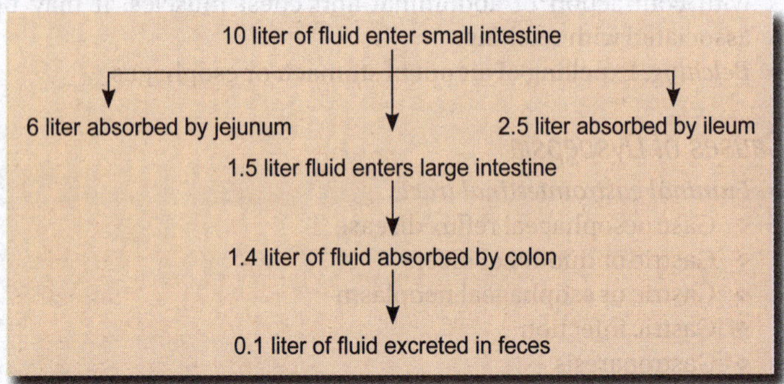

So diarrhea means excess excretion of fluid through stool. This can occur in following two ways:

1. *Secretary diarrhea:* It means excessive secretion of fluid into small intestine. It may be:
   - *Due to exogenous toxin* (Cholera)
   - *Endogenous toxin*—due to carcinoid syndrome:
     Above two produce inflammation of the intestinal mucosa. Increasing secretion and release of vasoactive peptides, 5HT, histamine, etc.
   - *Due to disordered transport*—abnormal ion transporter, cholera diarrhea
   - *Intestinal resection*—due to diminished area or site of absorption
   - *Mesenteric ischemia*—due to loss of vascularity, which is mainly responsible for absorption
   - *Intestinal hurry through*—due to vagotomy—the time required for electrolyte and water absorption is very short.

2. *Osmotic diarrhea:*
   - *Due to poor absorption of osmotically active substances:*
     - Magnesium
     - Lactose—due to intestinal brush border lactase deficiency.

Diarrhea clinically classified according to following criteria:

- *According to time course:*
  - *Acute diarrhea:* <4 weeks:
    - Due to bacterial cause or viral cause—<1 week
    - >7 days—protozoal cause.

* ❖ Chronic diarrhea >4 weeks—*Yersinia* or *Aeromonas* in immunocompetent person.
* *According to volume:*
  * ❖ If patient has left sided colonic inflammation or motility disorder—stool volume—small, recurrent, painful and sense of incomplete evacuation.
  * ❖ If patient has right sided colonic inflammation or motility disorder—stool volume large, painless.
  * ❖ If patient has normal stool volume—painless or painful. Occasionally related to food intake or stress—irritable bowel syndrome.
* *According to pathophysiology:* Osmotic diarrhea from secretary diarrhea.
  * ❖ In secretary diarrhea—stool is watery, stool matter is less
  * ❖ In osmotic diarrhea—stool is less watery, stool matter is large—in case of fasting, osmotic diarrhea is less.
* *According to stool characteristics:*
  * ❖ Watery due to defect in water absorption from intestinal wall.
  * ❖ Secretary—due to reduced electrolytic absorption or increased electrolyte secretion
  * ❖ Osmotic—due to poor absorption of osmotically active substance.

So during history taking following questions are to be asked:

In case of watery diarrhea:

* History of traveling abroad recently, no history of contamination of water or food—Traveller's diarrhea.
* History of large amount watery diarrhea, fever, vomiting—cholera.
* History of child below 5 years—automatic resolution of loose motion—Rota viral diarrhea.
* History of recent antibiotic therapy—antibiotic associated diarrhea:
  * ❖ History of intake of pastry, meat, vomiting, fever—Staphylococcal or *Bacillus cereus* poisoning
  * ❖ If associated with cramping abdominal pain—*Clostridium perfringens*
  * ❖ If associated intake of stored, canned food—suggestive of botulism
  * ❖ It history of intake of rotten egg, meat from poultry—and associated fever, headache—suggestive of *Salmonella typhimurium*.

In case of bloody diarrhea:

* History of recurrent bloody diarrhea >4 weeks, abdominal pain, weight loss, associated signs of vitamin deficiency—Crohn's disease.

- History of recurrent moderate to server bloody diarrhea (>4–8 stools/day) fever, cramping abdominal pain, urgency to defecation—ulcerative colitis.
- History of recurrent cramping abdominal pain—postprandially, loose motion—may be associated with blood—ischemic colitis.
- History of blood and mucus with stool, sense of incomplete evacuation, urgency to defecation—colorectal carcinoma.
- History of recurrent left abdominal pain, fever, diarrhea, middle aged patient—diverticular disease.
- History of cramping abdominal pain, fever, blood mucus—
  Shigella dysentery.
  Campylobacter.
  Entamoeba histolytica.
  Enteroinvasive *E. coli*.
- If above is associated with hemolysis, hematuria—hemolytic uremic syndrome.

Recurrent but no blood in stool, no systemic manifestation like fever:
- History of cramping abdominal pain, large voluminous stool, weight loss, nutritional deficiencies—malabsorption
- History of long time laxative abuse, antibiotic—drug induced.
- History of prolonged constipation is aged persons, followed by loose fluid like stool—recurrent and in small amount—fecal impaction with spurious diarrhea.
- History of recurrent flushing, loose motion, bronchial wheezing, abdominal pain—carcinoid syndrome.
- History of heat intolerance, tremor, palpitation, loose motion—thyrotoxicosis.
- History of diarrhea—intermittent, postural hypotension, impotence, urinary retention—high blood sugar.
  Diabetes.

In case of diarrhea (acute) following questions are to be asked:
- Onset of diarrhea
- Duration of diarrhea
- Number of bowel movements per day
- Is there any relation with food?
- Consistency of stool
- Smell of stool
- Any blood with stool.
- Any associated abdominal pain, weight loss, nausea or vomiting.
  Bloody diarrhea—may be associated with:
  ❖ Shigellosis.
  ❖ Amebiasis.
  ❖ Toxic.

In case of chronic diarrhea following questions are to be asked:
- Duration of diarrhea
- Consisting—watery, semisolid
- Commencement of diarrhea
- If there any alternate constipation with diarrhea—diverticulitis
- Color of stool
- Number of motions per day
- Is there any relation with particular food like wheat, flour, milk?
- Is there any associated abdominal pain, weight loss, anorexia, nausea, vomiting?
- If the stool is mixed with mucus, undigested food?
- Is there anytime of the day during which stool becomes loose?
  - ❖ Loose stool—from left colon
  - ❖ Watery stool—protein loosing enteropathies, inflammatory bowel diseases
  - ❖ Floating stool—malabsorption syndrome
  - ❖ More diarrhea in the morning—irritable bowel syndrome.

■ Constipation

Definitions of constipation vary among the patient and doctors.

According to patient constipation means passage of hard stool and painful straining during passage of hard stool.

According to doctor—less than three motion per week.

So decoding to definition (maintained by doctor) motions may not be hard or painful.

Definition: At least 12 weeks in preceding 12 months having two or more of following features:
- Straining during >1 in 4 defecations
- Lumpy or hard stool in >1 in 4 defecations
- Sensation of incomplete evacuation in >1 in 4 defecations
- Sensation of anorectal obstruction/blockade in >1 in 4 defecation
- Manual maneuvers in >1 in 4 defecations
  (Digital evacuation)
  and <3 defecation/week.

Acute constipation may be due to:
- Physical inactivity
- Decrease intake of fiber
- Use of antimotility agent
- Pain during defecation
- Malignancy.

So to standardize the definition, Rome III criteria of functional constipation—two or more of the following criterias must be present:
- Straining during at least 25 percent of defecation
- Lumpy or hardy stools in at least 25 percent of defecation

- Sensation of incomplete evacuation for at least 25 percent of defecation
- Sensation of anorectal blockage at least 25 percent of defecation
- Manual maneuvers (digital evacuation, supports of pelvic floor) to facilitate 25 percent of defecation
- Fewer than three defecations per week

When abdominal pain is predominant symptom—irritable bowel syndrome will be diagnosis, as like intermittent large stool unrelated to laxative.

Classification of Functional Constipation

- *Normal transit constipation:*
  - ❖ Incomplete evacuation
  - ❖ Abdominal pain is not predominant features.
- *Slow transit constipation:*
  - ❖ Infrequent motion <1 motion/week
  - ❖ No urge to defecate
  - ❖ No response or very poor response to laxative, or fiber
  - ❖ Associated symptoms—fever, malaise.
- *Defecatory disorders:*
  - ❖ Infrequent defecation
  - ❖ Manual removal of stool
  - ❖ Frequent straining required.

Causes of Constipations

- *Disorders of anorectum and pelvic floor:*
  - ❖ *Rectocele*—bulging or displacement of anterior wall of rectum.
  - ❖ *Descending perineum syndrome:* Pelvic floor descends greater extent than normal (1–4 cm) during straining during defecation, so rectal expulsion is difficult.

    Anorectal angle becomes widened due to pelvic floor weakness. As a result rectum becomes more vertical and prolapse may occur.
  - ❖ *Diminished rectal sensation:* Urge to defecate depends upon:
    - Amount of distension of rectal wall
    - Rate of distension
    - Tension of rectal wall circular muscle
    - Size of rectum.

    Few patients feel the pain of rectal distension but fail to defecate till maximum amount of distension will occur.
  - ❖ *Rectal prolapse:* Variable protrusion of rectum through anus.
  - ❖ *Solitary rectal ulcer syndrome:* Mucosal hyperemia with ulcer seen on the anterior wall of rectum, due to:

- Chronic straining
- Rectal prolapse and paradoxical contraction of pubo-rectalis muscle
- Impairment of rectal blood flow producing ischemia.
- *Systemic disorders:*
  - ❖ Hypothyroidism—pain, flatulence, constipation
  - ❖ Diabetes mellitus due to autonomic neuropathy.
  - ❖ *Hypercalcemia:*
    - Hyperparathyroidism
    - Paraneoplastic syndrome
    - Sarcoidosis.
- *Nervous causes:*
  - ❖ Loss of conscious control
  - ❖ *Parkinson's disease:*
    - Inability to relax striated muscles of pelvic floor on defecation
    - Slow colonic transit
    - Paradoxical anal sphincter contraction on defecation
    - Weak abdominal muscle contraction.
  - ❖ *Multiple sclerosis:*
    - Viceral neuropathy
    - Decreased compliance of colon
    - Disease of lumbosacral spinal cord
    - Pelvic floor and anal sphincter dysfunction.
- *Spinal cord lesions:*
  - ❖ *Above sacral segments:* Upper motor neuron lesion:
    - Slow colonic transit
    - Sensation of rectal distension—diminished.
  - ❖ *Lesion of sacral cord, conus medullaris, cauda equina— produce severe constipation:*
    - Diminished progression of movement of left colon
    - Spasticity of anal canal
    - Loss of perineal sensations may extend to anal canal, so rectal sensation may be diminished
    - High rectal tone.
- *Structural disorder of the colon, rectum, anus, and pelvic floor:*
  - ❖ *Disorder of smooth muscles:*
    - Congenital and acquired myopathy of colon producing colonic pseudo-obstruction
    - Autosomal dominant—hereditary internal and external sphincter myopathy
    - Progressive systemic sclerosis
    - Mytonic dystrophy—megacolon, abnormal anal sphincter function.

- ❖ *Disorder of enteric nerves:*
  - Congenital aganglionosis or hyperganglionosis.
  - *Acquired neuropathies:*
    - Chagas disease due to infection with *Trypanosoma cruzi*
    - *Paraneoplastic syndrome:*
      - Lung carcinomas
      - Carcinoid tumors
      - Neuropathy of unknown cause.
- *Medication:*
  - ❖ Opioid for remitting chronic pain
  - ❖ Antispasmodic
  - ❖ Calcium supplements
  - ❖ TCA
  - ❖ Phenothiazines
  - ❖ Long-term neuroleptics
  - ❖ Antiparkinsonian drugs.
- *Psychogenic disorders:*
  - ❖ Depression
  - ❖ *Eating disorders:*
    - Anorexia nervosa
    - Bulimia.
  - ❖ Denied bowel movements.

Questions to be asked during interrogation:
- Duration of constipation
- Frequency of bowel movement
- Amount of stool
- Color of stool
- Consistency of stool
- Whether associated with blood or mucus
- Whether constipation is associated with loose motion
- Whether stool is associated with expulsion of gas
- Associated symptom—malaise, pain during straining, anorexia, abdominal pain, weight loss, rectal bleeding
- Whether manual expulsion of stool?
- Associated feature of:
  - ❖ Hypothyroidism—cold extremity, sleeps
  - ❖ Lung related symptoms—cough, chest pain, hemoptysis, breathlessness
  - ❖ Feature of carcinoid tumors—flushing, abdominal pain—recurrent, palpitation.
- Recent change in caliber of stool
- Onset—long duration—IBD
- New onset—structural

Family history
- Hypothyroidism
- Colon cancer.

Dietary habit
- Daily fiber and fluid consumption history
- Whether breakfast is skipped or not—if breakfast is skipped, there will be constipation, because postprandial increase in colonic motility is greatest after breakfast.
- Whether patient regularly ingest caffeine or caffeinated coffee—it stimulates colonic motility.

Past medical history
- Obstetrics history, surgical history
- Neurological history
- Trauma to spinal cord.

Drug history
- Antiparkinsonian drugs.
- Over the counter laxatives, herbal medications—frequency, duration of intake.

Society history
- Sexual abuse
- Physical abuse
  May suggest irritable bowel syndrome.

Intestinal Gaseous Distension

Intestinal gas formation depends upon:
- Gas production
- Gas consumption
- Movement of gas in intestine
- Diffusion of gas between intestine and blood.

Volume of gas in intestine depends upon balance between:
- *Input of gas:*
  - Swallowing
  - Bacterial fermentation
  - Chemical reactions
  - Diffusion from blood.
- *Output of gas:*
  - Belching
  - Bacterial consumption
  - Absorption by blood
  - Evacuation.

Volume in healthy adult: 200 mL.

Gas is uniformly distributed in six spaces:
1. Stomach
2. Small intestine
3. Ascending colon
4. Transverse colon
5. Descending colon
6. Pelvic colon.

The gases are:
- Oxygen
- Carbon dioxide
- Nitrogen
- Hydrogen
- Methane.

Clinical problems related to gas in intestine
- *Expulsion of gases:*
  - ❖ *Repetitive eructation due to:*
    - Inadvertent swallowing of air into hypopharynx either
      - Immediately expelled or
      - Enters into stomach—which may be entered with swallowing into stomach—producing vicious cycle.
    - Associated emotional stress
  - ❖ *Voluminous flatus:*
    - Diet rich in fermentable residues
    - Carbohydrate malabsorption—due to lactase deficiency —or wheat malabsorption
    - Swallowed air may be expelled
  - ❖ *Excessive odoriferous flatus:* Sulfur containing gas—diets:
    - Excessive production of sulfate reducing flora
    - Excessive sulfate containing substrate—(cruciferous vegetables, some amino acids).

  Usually these gases are absorbed. So if amount of these gases is very high or rapid colonic transit time, these gases are expelled per anum.
- *Impaired gas expulsion:*
  - ❖ *Abdominal bloating:* This refers to subjective sensation of swelling of abdomen, abdominal pressure or excessive gas and objective sensation—by increase in abdominal girth.

    The relationship between abdominal gas and distension is complex and mainly based on altered motility.

    Patient with irritable bowel syndrome—complains of bloating sensation postprandially due to:
    - Excessive production due to intestinal bacterial over-growth
    - Malabsorption.

- *Pneumatosis cystoides intestinalis:* Gas-filled cysts in the wall of small bowel, colon or both—due to excessive accumulation of H_2—due to:
  - Excessive production
  - Decreased consumption.

History should be taken in following manner:
- When gas does occur?
- Whether this gas is associated with diet?
- Quality of diet—high carbohydrate or protein.
- Whether patient is sensitive to wheat, milk?
- How the gas is expelled—orally or rectally?
- If during abdominal bloating, no gas is expelled, whether it is associated with abdominal distension or cramping abdominal pain.
- If bloating is associated with diet, which ingredient of the diet is responsible for it.

Fecal Incontinence

Fecal incontinence is defined by involuntary passage of fecal matter through anus.

The severity ranges from unintentional elimination of fecal fluid during passage of flatus to involuntary complete evacuation of bowel contents.

The causes of fecal incontinence:
The anorectal unit is responsible for fecal incontinence.
- Normally the angle between rectum and anus is 90° at rest.
- With voluntary squeeze, the angle becomes acute—70°.
- During defecation, angle becomes obtuse—110°.

Anal sphincter—internal anal sphincter and external anal sphincter—IAS responsible for—70 to 85 percent of normal resting sphincter pressure, remainder by EAS.

Principal nerve to anorectum is pudendal nerve.

The mechanism and causes are:
- *Anorectal and pelvic floor structural defect:*
  Causes:
  - Anal sphincter muscle—hemorrhoidectomy, obstetrics injury
  - Puborectalis muscle—trauma, aging
  - Pudendal nerve—obstetrics injury, surgical injury, excessive straining
  - Nervous system, spinal cord—diabetes mellitus, multiple sclerosis, stroke
  - Rectum—prolapse, radiation, IBS.

- *Anorectal floor functional abnormality:*
  - ❖ Impaired rectal sensation—CNS disorder, ANS disorder
  - ❖ Fecal impaction—dyssynergia.
- *Alteration of stool characteristics:*
  - ❖ Increased volume, loose stool—IBD, IBS, bile salt mal-absorption, drugs, laxatives.
- *Others:*
  - ❖ Abnormal cognitive function—aging, dementia
  - ❖ Psychosis—willful soiling
  - ❖ Drugs—antidepressant, caffeine
  - ❖ Food intolerance—fructose, lactose, wheat.

Following history should be taken for evaluation of anal incontinence:
- When this incontinence starts? Whether it is passive?
- Duration of incontinence.
- During which time it is occurring?
- Severity of incontinence.
- Whether stool is loose or hard.
- Any history of fecal impaction.
- Coexisting—loose motion, inflammatory bowel disease drug abuse.
- Drug history—caffeine, antipsychotic drugs.
- Past history—spine surgery, urinary incontinence, CVA.
- History of intake of lactulose, fructose, wheat.
- History of hemorrhoidectomy, obstetrics history, trauma to muscles. Obstetrics history includes—use of forceps, perineal tears, defective repair of tears.
- Whether incontinence is associated with fecal fluid matter.

So above detailed history may facilitate the recognition of following types of incontinence:
- Passive fecal incontinence with involuntary passage of flatus —impaired rectoanal reflexes with or without sphincter dysfunction.
- In spite of active attempt to retain fecal matter in rectum, it is expelled involuntarily:
  - ❖ Disruption of sphincter function
  - ❖ Low rectal capacity.
- Fecal seepage after bowel movement, normal evacuation and continence:
  - ❖ Impaired rectal sensation
  - ❖ Incomplete bowel evacuation.

Gastrointestinal Bleeding

Gastrointestinal bleeding means:

- Hematemesis
- Melena
- Hematochezia
- Positive nasogastric lavage
- Occult blood in stool.

Bleeding is severe when there is:

- Decrease in hematocrit value—at least 6 percent or
- Transfusion of at least 2 units of packed RBC.

Hematemesis—means vomiting of blood—the color depends upon:

- Amount of bleeding
- Speed of bleeding
- Duration of bleeding
- Site of bleeding.

If amount of bleeding is large, on-going bleeding—the color is bright.

If bleeding is of some duration or site is in stomach and small to moderate amount—the color will be black.

Hematemesis indicates bleeding from esophagus, stomach or duodenum.

Melena: It means black tarry stool due to degredation of blood to acid hematin by gastric acid.

One bout of melena require at least 50–100 mL of blood and time should be 8 hours.

Melena indicates bleeding from upper gastrointestinal tract up to proximal colon.

Hematochezia: It means fresh bleeding per rectum—it indicates:

- On going bleeding from UGI tract
- On going bleeding from small intestine
- Distal rectal bleeding
- Anorectal bleeding.

Obscured bleeding: It means bleeding from anywhere in GI tract, not apparent by endoscopic evaluation, only occult blood test is positive.

Suspected source of bleeding elicited from patient's history:

- *History of:*
  - ❖ Recurrent epistaxis
  - ❖ Malignant lesion in nose or nasopharynx
  - ❖ Any prior radiation of nasopharynx.
  - *Source*: Bleeding from nasopharynx.

- History of hemoptysis, associated with fever, when past history of tuberculosis or branchiectasis.
  Source: Lung.
- History of heart burn, acidity, odynophagia gastroesophageal reflux disease .
  Trauma—during nasogastric tube intubations.
  Alcohol abuse.
  Past history—peptic ulcer.
  Source: Gastric ulcer.
- History of dysphasia weight loss.
  Source: Esophageal cancer.
- History of severe vomiting followed by hematemesis alcohol abuse.
  Mallory-Weiss tear.
- History of jaundice, alcohol abuse, ascites,
  Past history of liver disease, anorexia, vomiting—
  Esophageal variceal rupture or portal hypertensive gastropathy.

Epigastric Discomfort

- *History of ingestion of NSAID*
  Past history of peptic ulcer—diagnosed endoscopically—duodenal ulcer or gastric ulcer.
- *Pain abdomen—mainly after taking food*
  Early satiety: Occasional vomiting
  Aged male or female: Gastric cancer.
- *History operation around biliary tract*
  Liver biopsy
  History of percutaneous cholangiopancreatography
  Angiography: Hemobilia.
  Endoscopic sphincterotomy: Trauma at ampulla.
- *History of unexplained bleeding*
  History of multiple polyp in small intestine.
  Vomiting and pain abdomen.
  Weight loss: Small intestinal malignancy.
- *History of postprandial abdominal pain—periumbilical region*
  History of cardiovascular disease
  Bleeding per rectum: Ischemic colitis.
- *Sudden change in bowel habit*
  Passage of frank blood mucus per rectum.
  Weight loss.
  Family history of colonic malignancy: Colonic carcinoma.
- *History of passage of blood and mucus per rectum*
  Bloody diarrhea—numbers 4–12 times per day.
  Family history of IBD: Ulcerative colitis.

If this is associated with abdominal pain: Suggestive of Crohn disease.

- *History of pain in anal region mainly after defecation*
  Hematochezia, blood mixed with stool: Anal fissure.
- *History of bleeding per rectum*
  Passage of large amount blood after defecation:
  History of chronic constipation: Hemorrhoids.
- *Pain in abdomen*
  Bleeding per rectum
  History of radiation in abdomen: Radiation enteritis radiation proctitis.

Followings are the factors indicating poor prognosis in upper gastrointestinal bleeding:

- *From history:*
  - ❖ Age >60 years
  - ❖ History of onset of bleeding in hospital
  - ❖ History of comorbid illness like, cardiovascular disease, chronic lung disease, chronic kidney disease.
  - ❖ History of multiple transfusion—already given.
- *From physical examination diagnostic procedures:*
  - ❖ Shock
  - ❖ Orthostatic hypotension
  - ❖ Higher lesser curvature gastric ulcer (adjacent to left gastric artery).
  - ❖ Posterior duodenal bulb ulcer (adjacent to gastroduodenal artery).
  - ❖ Endoscopically visible vessels at the base of the ulcer.

Causes of Upper Gastrointestinal Bleeding

- Peptic ulcer
- Esophageal varices
- Gastric varices
- Erosive esophagitis
- Gastric cancer
- Mallory-Weiss tear
- Gastric erosions
- Angioma
- No cause found.

Causes of Lower Gastrointestinal Bleeding

- Diverticulosis
- Colonic polyp
- Infections colitis
- Ischemic colitis
- Ulcerative colitis

- Postpolypectomy
- Rectal ulcer
- Hemorrhoids
- Anal fissure
- Radiation colitis.

Lower gastrointestinal bleeding patient is usually >70 years, they may present with:
- Painless hematochezia
- Positive occult blood test
- Anemia
- Sudden and heavy bleeding
- Bleeding—may be episodic
- Bleeding may be present after passage of hard stool
- Painful defecation with bleeding.

Following questions to be asked to patient of rectal bleeding:
- For how many days or months patient is having rectal bleeding?
- Whether blood is mixed with stool or after passage of stool?
- If blood is coming after passage of stool:
  - ❖ Whether it is drop by drop?
- Whether the blood is coming in streak on the surface of the stool?
- Is there any change in bowel habit?
- Is there any pain during defection?
- Is there any tenesmus—painful, continued and ineffective straining at stool—causes may be space occupying lesion in distal rectum and anus?

Obscure occult gastrointestinal bleeding—means when occult blood test is positive—but no visible blood in stool.

Fecal blood loss is 0.5 to 1.5 mL/day.

These patients are usually asymptomatic, main presenting features are symptoms related to anemia like breathlessness, vertigo, weakness, tinnitus, etc.

Or these patients can be diagnosed—on routine investigation.

Rock all score of gastrointestinal bleeding:
- *Pre-endoscopic criteria:*

Criteria	Score (0)	Score (1)	Score (2)	Score (3)
• Age (years)	<60	60–79	≥80	–
• Shock	SBP>100 HR<100	SBP>100 HR>100	SBP<100 HR>100	–
• Comorbidity	None	–	Cardiac disease, any other major comorbidity	Renal failure. Liver failure. Disseminated malignancy

Initial score—(pre-endoscopy) maximum 7.
Initial score— 0 – regarded low risk

- *Postendoscopy criteria:*

Criteria	Score (0)	Score (1)	Score (2)	Score (3)
• Endoscopic diagnosis	Mallory-Weiss tear or no lesion	All other diagnosis	Malignancy of UG tract	–
• Major stigmata of recent hemorrhage	None or dark spot only		Blood in UGI tract. adherent; clot visible vessels	–

Full Rock all score (after endoscopy):
Maximum—11, Full rock all score 2—low risk.
   The above score predicts mortality.

Glasgow—Blatchford Scoring System

Admission risk marker	Criteria	Score
• Blood urea—nitrogen (mmol/L)	≥6.5–<8	2
	≥8.0–<10	3
	≥10–<25	4
	≥25	6
• Hemoglobin (dg/L) for men	≥12–<13	1
	≥10–<12	3
	<10	6
• Hemoglobin (dg/L) for women	≥10–<12	1
	<10	6
• Systolic blood pressure (mm Hg)	100–109	1
	90–99	2
	<90	3
• Pulse	>10	1
• Melena	Present	1
• Syncope	Present	2
• Hepatic disease	Present	2
• Cardiac failure	Present	2

Score – 0   Low risk.

This scoring system predicts:
- Need for intervention
- Identification of patients with low risk of bleeding

Iron Deficiency Anemia with Bleeding

In case of young menstruating women with iron deficiency anemia-first exclude menstrual cause—followed by GI cause.

But in case of postmenopausal women with iron deficiency anemia—1st exclude:

- Gastrointestinal cause, pulmonary lesions, urinary tract lesions.
- Malabsorption (celiac disease, gastric atrophy, gastric bypass surgery).
- CRF.
- Hemolysis.

Jaundice (Fig. 5.37)

Jaundice is defined by yellowish discoloration of upper bulbar conjunctiva and mucous membrane and urine due to deposition of pigmented metabolite bilirubin or excretion of conjugated bilirubin in urine respectively.

Bilirubin Metabolism

Bilirubin—hydrophobic, tetrapyrrole ring.
It is derived from:

- Breakdown of hemoglobin from senescent erythrocytes.
- Premature destruction of newly formed erythrocytes (ineffective erythropoiesis).

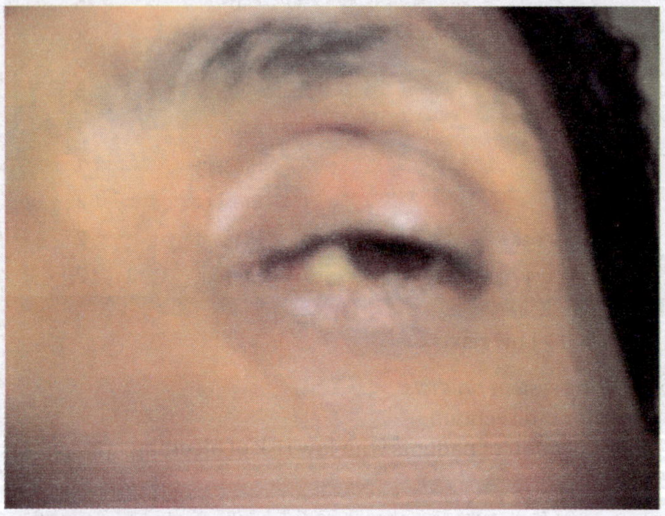

FIG. 5.37 Jaundice

- Breakdown of hem proteins—catalyses and cytochrome
  - ❖ Free human globin
  - ❖ Haptoglobin bound hemoglobin.
  - ❖ Methemalbumin

    Haem
    ↓← Haem oxygenase   in reticuloendothelial cells
    Biliverdin   in spleen, liver, and bone
                          marrow
    ↓← Biliverdin reductase
→ Bilirubin
    ↓

It circulates in blood bound with albumin
    ↓

Bilirubin is taken up across sinusoidal membrane of hepatocytes by carrier uptake mechanism
    ↓

Bilirubin enters the endoplasmic reticulum by cytosolic binding proteins.
    ↓

Bilirubin is conjugated with UDP-glucuronic acid by enzyme UDP-glucoronyl transferase
    ↓

Bilirubin becomes conjugated into water soluble form
    ↓

Conjugated bilirubin excretes into biliary canaliculi through apical membrane of hepatocytes—by ATP—dependent—pump (80% in diglucuronide form, 20% in monoglucuronide form).
    ↓

Conjugated bilirubin is excreted into intestine through bile. ←

50 percent bilirubin	50 percent conjugated bilirubin
↓← Intestinal bacteria.	is absorbed in the blood
Free bilirubin	and enters the liver through
↓← Intestinal bacteria.	enterohepatic circulation
Urobilinogen	↓

90 percent of urobilinogen Resecreted into bile.
Some urobilinogen excreted in urine.
    ↓

After exposure to air urobilinogen is converted to urobilin.
→ Some urobilinogen
    ↓

Stercobilinogen → excreted into feces → converted to stercobilin.

- ❖ Normal bilirubin level in the blood: 0.8–1.0 mg/dL.
- ❖ When bilirubin contents is more than 3 mg percent—clinical jaundice.
- ❖ When bilirubin level >1.0–<3 mg percent—anicteric jaundice.

Causes of Hyperbilirubinemia

- **Disorder of bilirubin metabolism:** (Isolated)
  - ❖ *Unconjugated hyperbilirubinemia:*
    - Increased bilirubin production:
      - Ineffective erythropoiesis
      - Transfusion of blood
    - Decreased hepatocellular uptakes:
      - Gilbert's syndrome
      - Drugs
    - Decreased conjugation:
      - Gilbert's syndrome
      - Crigler-Najjar syndrome
      - Physiological disease of newborn
      - Drugs—antiviral drugs
  - ❖ *Conjugated hyperbilirubinemia:*
    - Dubin-Johnson syndrome
    - Rotor syndrome.
- **Liver disease:**
  - ❖ *Hepatocellular dysfunction:*
    - Acute or subacute hepatocellular injury
    - Reye syndrome
    - Chronic hepatocellular disease.
  - ❖ *Intrahepatic cholestasis:*
    - Infiltrative disorder
    - Cholestatic injury
    - Others:
      - Benign intrahepatic cholestasis
      - Cholestasis of pregnancy
      - Drugs—estrogen, anabolic steroid
      - Paraneoplastic syndrome
      - Benign postoperative cholestasis.
- **Obstruction to bile ducts:**
  - ❖ Choledocholithiasis
  - ❖ *Disease of bile ducts:*
    - Inflammation:
      - Primary solerosing cholangitis
      - Cholangiopathy
      - Postsurgical stricture
    - Neoplasm—cholangiocarcinoma.

- ❖ *Extrinsic compression:*
  - • Neoplasm:
    - – Lymphadenopathy
    - – Pancreatic carcinoma
    - – Hepatocellular carcinoma
    - – Lymphoma.
- ❖ Pancreatitis
- ❖ Vascular enlargement.

In broad sense the following history is important in differentiating liver disease from biliary tract disease:
- Fever chill and rigor.
- Occasionally only rigor.
- Colicky abdominal pain.
- Progressively increasing jaundice.
- Itching.
- Past history of biliary surgery.
- Old age.
- History of pregnancy.

Suggestive of Liver Disease

Following symptoms are suggestive of hepatic disease:
- *Anorexia:*
  - ❖ Viral hepatitis
  - ❖ Malignancy of liver, colon, pancreas.
- Weight loss more than 10 pounds—neoplastic disorder.
- Fever with chills, headache, and myalgia—viral hepatitis A.
- Chill with fever, right quadrant pain—biliary tract disease.
  - ❖ Choledocholithiasis
  - ❖ Ascending cholangitis.
- *Arthritis:*
  - ❖ Hepatitis
  - ❖ Collagen vascular disease
  - ❖ Primary sclerosing cholangitis
  - ❖ Sarcoidosis.
- *History of rash:*
  - ❖ Hepatitis
  - ❖ Collagen vascular disease.
- *Pruritis:*
  - ❖ Cholestatic phase of liver disease
  - ❖ Intrahepatic cholestasis
  - ❖ Extrahepatic cholestasis.
- History of blood transfusion—viral hepatitis.
- Intravenous drug abuser—hepatitis C.
- *Sex:*
  - ❖ Anal intercourse—risk of hepatitis B and hepatitis C
  - ❖ Multiple sexual partners in 1 year

- ❖ Intercourse with prostitute—hepatitis B and C virus
- ❖ Intercourse with hepatitis B or C positive person.
- *Changes in smell:*
  - ❖ Decreased sense of smell   Hepatitis A
  - ❖ Perception of unpleasant smell   Hepatitis A
- *Changes in taste:*
  - ❖ Decreased sense of taste (hypogeusia)—hepatitis A virus
  - ❖ Perception of unpleasant taste (dysgeusia)—hepatitis A
- Health care personal—hepatitis C.
- Medication—over the counter drugs—produces:
  F: Fever
  A: Arthritis
  R: Rash
  E: Eosinophilia.
- Detail history of alcohol abuse.
- Detail history of abdominal pain.
- History of inflammatory bowel disease and fever right upper quadrant pain—primary sclerosing cholangitis.
- History of different type of drugs abuse—drug induced hepatitis:
  - ❖ ATD drugs
  - ❖ Pain killer
  - ❖ Anabolic steroid.

Anorexia: This means loss of appetite. This occurs in any system involvement:

- Gastrointestinal disease
- Renal failure
- Liver failure
- Heart failure
- Lung disease—cancer, tuberculosis
- Anorexia nervosa.

Weight loss:

Causes:

- *Depression:* History of loss of concentration, mood disorder, sleep disorder.
- *Thyrotoxicosis:* Tremor, heat intolerance, diarrhea, palpitation, tremor.
- *Advanced malignancy:* Progressive weight loss, hemoptysis, rectal bleeding, hematemesis, change in bowel habit. Progressive vomiting, headache, neurological deficit.
- *Diabetes:* History of diabetic symptoms.
- *Addison's disease:* History of vertigo, hyperpigmentation, lethargy, weakness.
- *Chronic pancreatitis:* Abdominal pain, insulin sensitive diabetes mellitus. Loose motion, postprandial abdominal pain.

The following questions to be asked to detect weight loss:
- How is his appetite—increased, normal or decreased.
- Amount of meals—in each session—breakfast, lunch, and dinner.
- Associated symptoms—nausea, vomiting, diarrhea, cough, abdominal pain, fever, bleeding per rectum, hemoptysis, dysphagia.
- Any associated features of thyrotoxicosis.
- Any history of acid ingestion.

Symptoms Related to Urinary System

Frequency of Micturition

Normal adult micturates 4–5 times per day. Frequency of micturition depends upon:
- Fluid balance
- Renal functions
- Presence of irritation of genitourinary tract.

Causes:
- *Congenital:*
  - Small bladder capacity
  - Ureterovesical reflux
  - Meatal stricture.
- *Inflammation:*
  - Urethritis
  - Cystitis
  - Prostatitis
  - Appendicitis—irritating urinary bladder.
- *Mechanical:*
  - Pelvic floor relaxation
  - Cystocele
  - Rectocele.
- *Traumatic:*
  - Bladder stone
  - Urethral stone
  - Ureteral stone
  - Instrumentation in urethra or urinary bladder.
- *Malignancy:*
  - Carcinoma
  - Carcinoma of rectum.
- *Neurogenic:*
  - Spinal cord lesion
  - Cauda equina lesion
  - Autonomic neuropathy.

Frequency of Micturition with Polyuria

In adult male—volume is 500 mL, in case of female—little less. Average output = 1200 mL/day. This volume depends upon:
- Type of fluid intake
- Insensible loss (sweating)
- Sensible loss (vomiting, diarrhea)
- Increased osmotic load (diabetes)
- Medications
- Decreased concentrating ability.

Causes of polyuria:
- *Congenital:* Renal tubular acidosis.
- *Endocrine:*
  - Diabetes mellitus
  - Nephrogenic diabetes insipidus
  - Central diabetes insipidus.
- *Interstitial:* Interstitial nephritis.
- *Metabolic:* Hypercalcemia, hypokalemia.
- *Psychogenic:* Psychogenic polydipsia.

Nocturia

Normally adult male does not micturate at night, unless the following causes are present:
- High intake of alcohol or caffine containing liquid.
- *Edematous state:*
  - Cardiac failure
  - Renal failure
  - Nephrotic syndrome
  - Hepatic failure.
    In above conditions the fluid is mobilized in recumbent state into vascular spaces.
- In recumbent state—in female, posthysterectomy with pelvic floor relaxation.
- Metabolic—diabetes mellitus.

Urinary Incontinence

Involuntary passage of urine is called urinary incontinence. When it is induced by straining:
- Coughing
- Sneezing
- Laughing—it is called stress incontinence.

Causes with pathophysiology:
- Abnormal function of detrusor muscles—urge incontinence.
- Inadequate sphincter function—stress incontinence.

- Excessive bladder filling—due to bladder neck obstruction—overflow incontinence.
- Damage to nerve supply to bladder—neurogenic bladder—overflow incontinence.
- Idiopathic—benign prostatic hyperplasia, cystocele, urethrocele, prostatic carcinoma.
- Inflammation—urethritis, cystitis.
- Neurogenic—stroke, spinal cord injury, autonomic neuropathy.

Difficulty in Micturition

Effortless relaxation of bladder and co-coordinated contraction of detrusor muscles produces normal micturition.

So, difficulty in micturition—may be hesitancy in micturition, i.e. delay between attempting to initiate urination and actual flow of urine.

The following are the causes:
Idiopathic: Benign prostatic hyperplasia, chronic prostatitis.
- Obstruction—bladder neck obstruction, urethral stricture—urethral valve, bladder stone.
- Neoplastic—urethral carcinoma, prostatic carcinoma. Uterine fibroid or carcinoma cervix producing pressure from outside.
- Neurologic—autonomic neuropathy, spinal cord trauma, myelitis, syringomyelia.

Dysuria

Straining or burning sensation during micturition. It may occur with:
- *Inflammation:* Cystitis, urethritis, prostatitis.
- *Mechanical:* Bladder stone.

Inflammation breaks bladder and urethral epithelium—submucosa is exposed to acidic urine—resulting pain in penis in male and urethra in female.

Anuria and Oliguria

Decreased urine formation or absent urine formation measured in bladder due to:
- Decline in glomerular filtration rate
- Decrease in renal blood flow
- Intrarenal or ureteral obstruction.

Oliguria is defined as urine volume:
<500 mL per day or <30 mL per hour. Or, less than 0.5 mL/kg of body weight/hour.

Anuria is defined as urine volume less than 100 mL/day.

Anuria or oliguria occurs: In advanced stage of renal dysfunction.
Anuria mostly occurs in:
- Urinary tract obstruction—bilaterally
- Acute cortical necrosis
- Good-pasture syndrome.

Oliguria and anuria both can occur in:
- Prerenal cause—hypovolemia, shock
- *Renal cause:*
  - ❖ Congenital—sickle cell crisis
  - ❖ Infectious—septicemia, pyelonephritis, hemorrhagic fever
  - ❖ Immunological cause—good-pasture syndrome, microscopic polyangiitis, polyarteritis nodosa, SLE, systemic sclerosis
  - ❖ Endrocrinological—hyperparathyroidism
  - ❖ Drugs—aminoglycosides, NSAIDs
  - ❖ Toxins—myoglobin, radiologic contrast material, heavy metals—copper, bismuth, mercury, carbon tetrachloride. Paraldehyde, ethylene glycol
  - ❖ *Mechanical:* Trauma, burn, hematomas, methemoglobinemia, defective blood transfusion with mismatched blood.
- *Postrenal:* Renal calculi, tumor, cyst.
  Cervical cancer producing bilateral ureteral obstruction.

Discoloration of Urine

Normal urine color is yellow due to presence of urochrome.

Depending upon the concentration, the yellow color will vary—increased in concentrated urine and decreased in dilute urine.

True color change may occur due to substances filtered from blood or arising from urinary tract.

The color of urine and causes of change in urine color:
- *Colorless:*
  - ❖ Normal
  - ❖ Diabetes insipidus
  - ❖ Large amount of fluid intake
  - ❖ Chronic glomerulonephritis.
- *White cloudy:*
  - ❖ Phosphates in alkaline urine (cloudiness disappears after addition of acid)
  - ❖ Epithelial cells
  - ❖ Bacteria
  - ❖ Pus
  - ❖ Chyle.

[This can be separated from milk in urine by centrifugation]
  - ❖ Chyle is homogeneously distributed
  - ❖ Milk-fat is distributed at the top.

- *Yellow-colored urine:*
  - ❖ Concentrated normal urine
  - ❖ Pyridium
  - ❖ Tetracycline
  - ❖ Bilirubin.
- *Orange:*
  - ❖ Pyridium
  - ❖ INH
  - ❖ Urobilinogen
  - ❖ Cathartic—senna
  - ❖ Hemoglobin.
- *Red-colored urine:*
  - ❖ Cathartic, red in alkaline urine, colorless in acid urine
  - ❖ Rifampicin
  - ❖ Beet
  - ❖ Aniline dyes
  - ❖ Hemoglobin
  - ❖ Myoglobin
  - ❖ Porphyrin
  - ❖ Phenolphthalein.
- *Blue green:*
  - ❖ Bilirubin—yellow froth
  - ❖ *Pseudomonas* infection.
- *Black brown:*
  - ❖ Bilirubin (yellow froth)
  - ❖ Acid hemolysis (in standing urine)
  - ❖ Phenol (black in large quantities)
  - ❖ Methemoglobin.
- *Brown black:* After standing:
  - ❖ Porphyrin (change in exposure to sunlight)
  - ❖ Melanin (change in exposure to sunlight)
  - ❖ Homogentisic acid (changes from bacterial alkalization of urine).
- *Cola-colored urine:* Acute poststreptococcal glomerulo- nephritis.

Hematuria

Two types of hematuria:

1. *Microscopic hematuria:*
   - ❖ Which is defined by >4 erythrocytes per HPF, on a spunned urine.
   - ❖ It can be detected by microscopic or chemical examination of urine.

2. *Macroscopic hematuria:*
   - Sufficient red blood-cells to change the color of urine to red—always above 10000 cells per mL
   - It can be detected during micturition.

Hematuria can be distinguished from hemoglobinuria or myoglobinuria:
In freshly voided urine collected within 1 hour after complete bladder emptying
   RBC can be identified in hematuria, but not in hemoglobinuria or myoglobinuria.
   Glomerular or nonglomerular bleeding can be identified in following manner.

Glomerular bleeding should be suspected if any of the following are present:
- Dysmorphic erythrocytes
- Erythrocytes with mean corpuscular volume <72 fl
- Red blood cell cast with concomitant proteinuria >1 g/day.

Nonglomerular proteinuria can be characterized by:
- Presence of isomorphic erythrocytes
- Erythrocytes with mean corpuscular volume >72 fl
- Absence of red blood cell cast.

Time of hematuria during micturition can differentiate sites of bleeding:
- Visible hematuria at the start of micturition and subsequent clearing of urine—urethral bleeding—"Initial hematuria".
- Visible hematuria at the end of micturition called "Terminal hematuria"—indicates, bleeding from bladder or prostate.
- Presence of RBC cast and cola-colored urine—Glomerular sites.
- Visible hematuria with episodes of pharyngeal infection—or exercise—IgA nephropathy.
- Presence of blood clot—ureteric, cystic bleeding—never glomerular bleeding.

Causes of hematuria
- *Congenital:*
  - Polycystic kidney disease
  - Sickle cell disease.
- *Acquired:*
  - *Infection:*
    - Urethritis
    - Cystitis
    - Acute pyelonephritis
    - Pyelitis
    - Prostatitis.

❖ *Traumatic:*
  - Urethral stricture
  - Stone
  - Instrumentations
  - Trauma
  - Sudden decompression of bladder in case of acute retention of urine
  - Exercise
  - Radiation.
❖ *Neoplastic:*
  - Urethral, bladder, ureteral carcinoma
  - Hypernephroma
  - Polyp.
❖ *Collagen vascular disease:*
  - Vasculitis
  - Polyarteritis nodosa.
❖ *Vascular:*
  - A-V malformation
  - Bladder varices.
❖ *Drugs:*
  - Cyclophosphamide
  - Analgesic
  - Anticoagulant.
❖ *Systemic disease:*
  - Scurvy
  - Vitamin K deficiency
  - Uremia
  - Thrombocytopenia.

Hemoglobinuria

It is defined by excretion of extracellular hemoglobin in urine:
It should be differentiated from myoglobinuria by:

- *Spectroscopic examination:* Myoglobin has molecular weight of 17,500.

    Hemoglobin has molecular weight of 68,000.
- *Concomitant color of plasma:* If color of plasma is red—it suggests presence of hemoglobin in plasma, not myoglobin—because myoglobin is rapidly cleared off from the blood.

Primary Causes

- Congenital—Glucose—6-phosphatase deficiency.
- *Acquired:*
  ❖ *Endocrine:*
    - Pregnancy
    - Puerperium.

- ❖ Paroxysmal nocturnal hemoglobinuria
- ❖ Immune—Autoimmune hemolytic anemia
- ❖ Infections—Malaria, yellow fever, gangrene
- ❖ Mechanical—March hemoglobinuria. Mechanical heart valves, major burns
- ❖ Vascular—microangiopathic hemolytic anemia TTP, HUS.

Myoglobinuria

Excretion of myoglobin from damaged muscles—released in urine—producing myoglobinuria.

Proteinuria: Excretion of protein in urine called proteinuria. Normal excretion of protein in urine—30–150 mg/day—in adult male.

In children and adolescent—normal urinary protein excretions twice the amount excreted by adult.

In tubular proteinuria is 2 g/day.

In glomerular proteinuria is >2 g/day to <3.5 g/day. If it is nephrotic range of proteinuria protein excretion >3.5 g/day.

In these cases, patient usually complains of frothing of urine during micturition.

Pneumaturia

Passage of air or fizzing during micturition. This is due to development of fistula tract between alimentary tract and urinary tract.

Urethral Discharge

Purulent discharge per urethra—between the times of micturition.

History is like:
- Discharge of whitish pus like secretion per urethra
- Staining of underwear with yellowish secretion
- Any pain during micturition
- Whether the discharge contains blood.

Bloody penile discharge:
- Urethritis
- Neoplasm
- Ulcerations.

Purulent discharge: Thick yellowish green:
- Gonococcal urethritis
- Chronic prostatitis.

Pain Due to Renal Cause

- Pain in loin—colicky in nature—radiating to groin, scrotum, or labia—acute urinary tract obstruction.

- In contrast—chronic urinary tract obstruction:
  - ❖ At the level of bladder—hesitancy, poor flow and terminal dribbling.
  - ❖ Above this level—asymptomatic.
- In case of acute glomerulonephritis—dull acting pain in loin.
- In case of acute pyelonephritis—pain is in renal angle and dull aching in nature.
- In case of perirenal abscess—pain in loin—radiates along the tract through which pus will pass or may patient complains of cough, chest pain due to diaphragmatic irritation.

Past medical history:
Recent renal disease may be the consequences of either past medical disease or its complication or the complication of treatment.

- Childhood recurrent urinary tract infection, late nocturnal enuresis—may be due to vesica—ureteral reflux, which may be responsible for future chronic pyelonephritis.
- Systemic lupus erythromatosus—early involvement of joint and skin—later on involve progressive renal disease.
- Gastrointestinal disease—Crohn's disease—produces AA Amyloidosis—may involve kidney.
- Oncological drugs—cyclophosphamide—produce hematuria, later on develop bladder cancer.
- *Hemoptysis:*
  - ❖ Good-pasture syndrome
  - ❖ Vasculitis.
- Gout—urate nephropathy.
- Diabetes—diabetic nephropathy.
- Deafness—alport syndrome.
- Chronic pain—analgesic use producing nephropathy.
- *Raynaud's phenomenon:*
  - ❖ Systemic sclerosis
  - ❖ SLE.
- Tonsillitis—poststreptococcal glomerulonephritis.
- Cirrhosis with ascites—may produce hepatorenal syndrome
- Infective diarrhoea may produce hemolytic uremic syndrome
- Tuberculosis may be responsible for:
  - ❖ Urogenital tuberculosis
  - ❖ Amyloidosis
  - ❖ Sterile pyuria.
- HIV injection in long course may produce HIV nephropathy.

Gynecological history:
- Patient with chronic renal disease may produce menorrhagia due to development of platelet abnormalities and coagulation abnormalities.

- Patient with chronic renal dysfunction produces infertility.
- OCP in patient may be responsible for hypertensive renal disease.
- In case of pregnant patient—pregnancy induced hypertension may produce proteinuria, edema—may precipitate renal failure.
- Recurrent thrombophlebitis, recurrent abortion—antiphospholipid syndrome.

Drug history:
- A small amount of any drug may be responsible for allergic nephritis.
- Chronic use of some drugs, e.g. analgesic—may produce interstitial nephritis—lithium—may produce progressive renal disease.
- Few antihypertensive drugs may be responsible for prerenal failure.
- Few antihypertensive drugs—angiotensin—converting enzyme inhibitor or angiotensin receptor blockers—may be harmful in patient with renal artery stenosis, because they may produce deterioration of renal function.
- Oral contraceptive pills, corticosteroids may be responsible for hypertensive renal disease in case of long-term use.
- Drugs are used in treatment of rheumatoid arthritis, e.g. Gold, penicillamine—may produce membranous nephropathy.
- A type of Chinese herb may produce nephropathy.

Dietary history:
- High protein, high K^+ containing fruits (citrus fruit) may produce cardiovascular complication or deterioration of consciousness in patient with chronic kidney disease not in hemodialysis.
- High salt and water content may produce circulatory overload and respiratory distress due to development of pulmonary edema.
- High animal protein, calcium, purine containing vegetables may be responsible for gouty nephropathy.
- Excessive alcohol intake may produce increase in blood pressure.
- High intake of fruit juice or acidic food may increase K^+ intake produces worsening of cardiovascular symptom or increase oxalate content producing urate nephropathy.
- High intake of tea or coffee, which contain methylxanthine responsible for polyuria.

Social history:
This varies according to socio-economic status.

In low socio-economic group:
- Recurrent bacteriuria—in pregnant women.
- Low cost hypotensive drugs.

In high socio-economic status:
- High protein containing diet
- Increase consumption of tobacco is associated with development of atherosclerosis, may worsen chronic kidney disease.
- Illicit drug use—may be responsible for:
  - Glomerulonephritis
  - Acute renal failure
  - Vasculitis
  - Rhabdomyolysis.

Occupational history:
- Aniline days—urothelial tumor.
- Excessive exposure to very hot climate—increase the urinary concentration—responsible for renal stone formation.
- Exposure to infection:
  - Leptospirosis—in sewage workers, farm workers
  - Hantavirus—in laboratory workers handling rodents.
- Inhaled hydrocarbon—good-pasture syndrome.

Family history:
This is responsible for identification of few family related diseases.
Few hereditary diseases are:
- Polycystic kidney disease.
- Alport syndrome.
- Metabolic disease:
  - Fabry's disease
  - Hyperoxaluria
  - Congenital urate nephropathy.
- Other inherited disorders:
  - von Hippel-Lindau disease
  - Congenital nephritic syndrome.
- Familial IgA nephropathy.
- Tubular disease:
  - Renal tubular acidosis
  - Cystinuria
  - Nephrogenic diabetes incipidus.
- Polygenic influences:
  - Diabetic nephropathy
  - Reflux nephropathy.

Geographical influences:
- In black African Caribbean:
  - In patient with diabetes hypertensive renal failure is more common.
  - End stage renal failure is three times higher than in Caucasians.
- In black, hispanic, oriental population incidence of SLE is more common than Caucasians.

- In white population IgA nephropathy is more common.
- In Indian and Russian population, incidence of tuberculosis is more common in immunosuppressive patient getting immunosuppressive therapy after transplantation.

■ Physical Examinations

Peripheral Signs

Inspection

- Kayser-Fleischer ring—brown ring at the periphery of cornea — due to deposition of copper in Descemet's membrane—Wilson's disease (Fig. 5.38).
- Perioral hyperpigmentation—Peutz-Jeghers syndrome—associated with hamartomatous polyps in jejunum (Fig. 5.39).
- Oral and tongue telangiectasias—Rendu-Osler-Weber syndrome —associated with gastrointestinal tract lesion with iron deficiency anemia (Fig. 5.40).
- Nontender enlargement of parotid—alcoholic liver disease, Alcohol misuse.
- Dupuytren contracture—thickening and shortening of palmar fascia—producing flexion deformity of fingers, occurs in more than 65 years of age—history alcohol intoxication, CLD (Fig. 5.41).

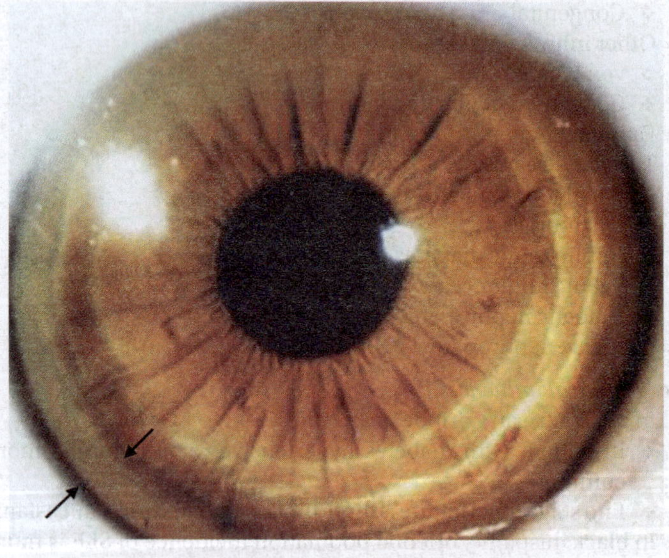

FIG. 5.38 Kayser-Fleischer ring

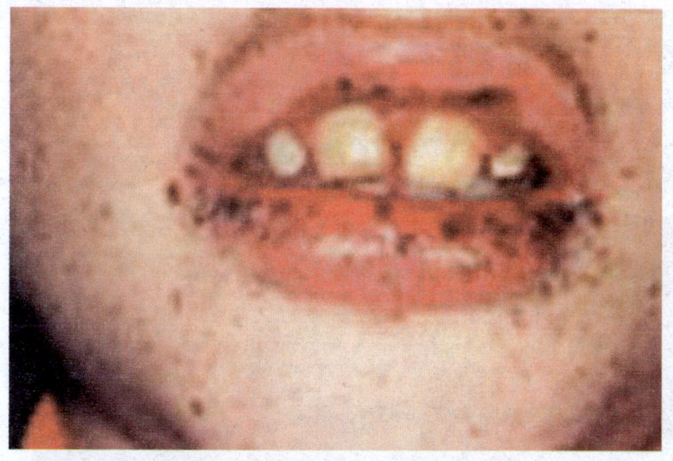

FIG. 5.39   Peutz-Jeghers syndrome

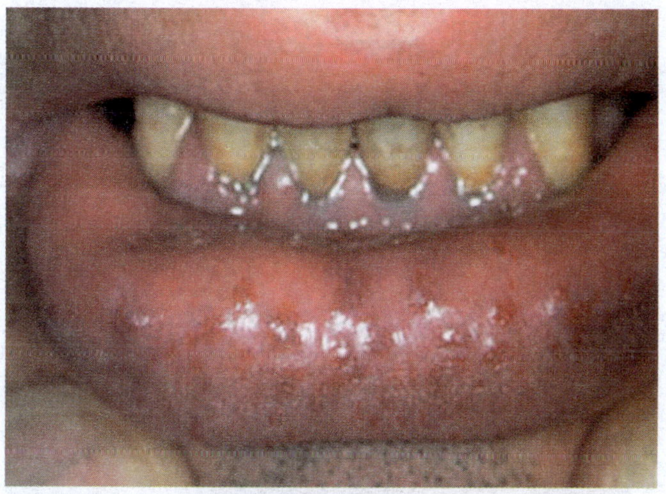

FIG. 5.40   Rendu-Osler-Weber disease

- Tattoo marks, all over the body may indicate Hepatitis infection (Fig. 5.42).
- Symmetrical yellowish plaques around eyelids—xanthelasma — primary or secondary biliary cirrhosis (Fig. 5.43).
- Wide set eyes, prominent forehead, flat nose, small chin, persistent intrahepatic cholestasis in childhood.
- Subconjunctival hemorrhages—leptospirosis—acute liver failure (Fig. 5.44).

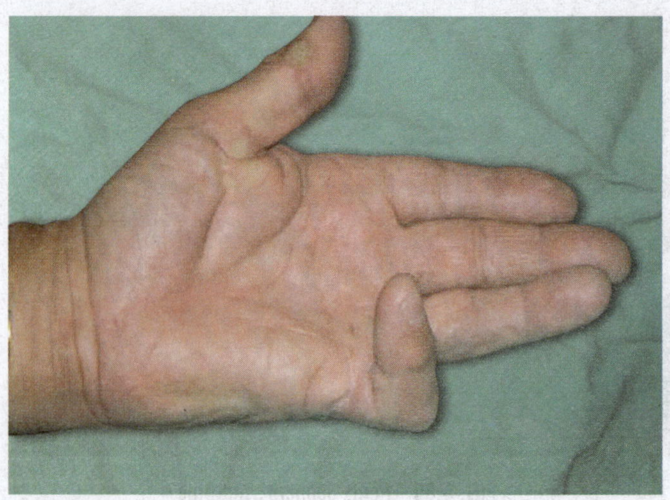

FIG. 5.41 Dupuytren contracture

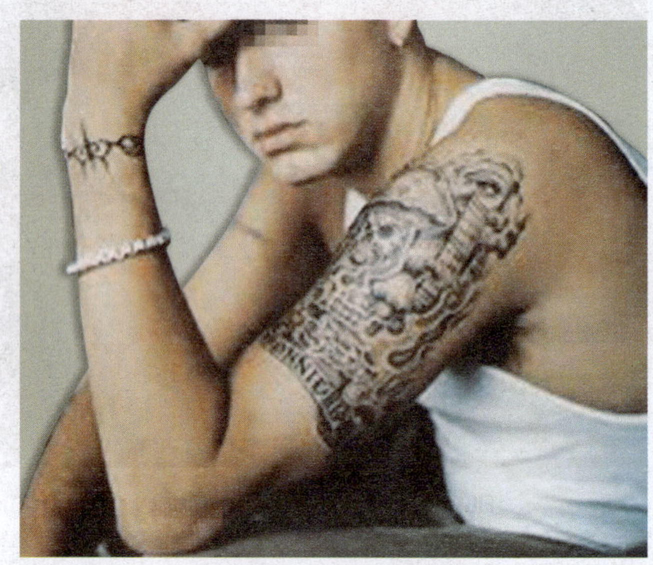

FIG. 5.42 Tattoo marks

- Periorbital skin bruises—suggestive of amyloidosis.
- Jaundice—yellowish discolorations of conjunctive and skin—any cause producing jaundice.
- Vitiligo—patchy cutaneous depigmentation—immune destruction of melanocytes—autoimmune hepatitis
  Primary biliary cirrhosis (Fig. 5.45).

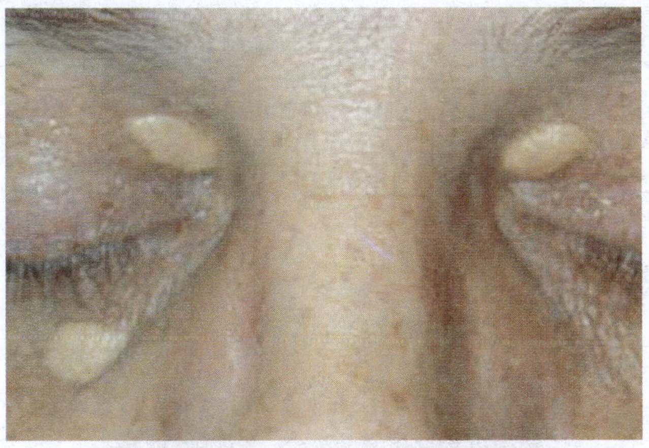

FIG. 5.43 Symmetrical yellowish plaques around eyelids

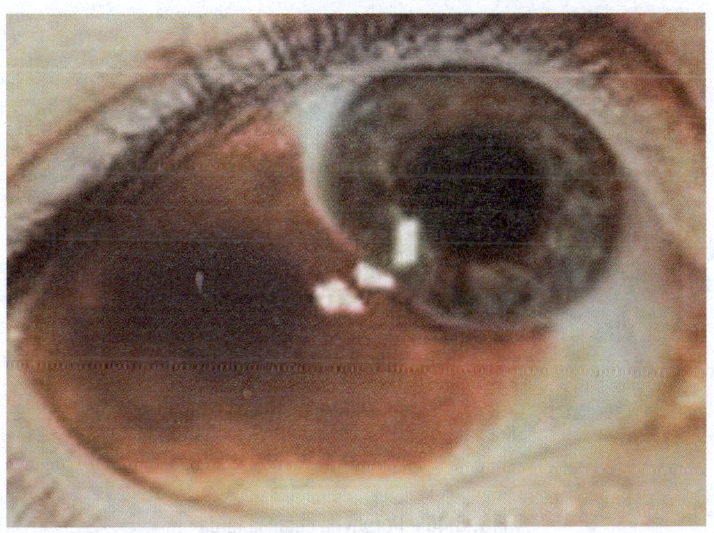

FIG. 5.44 Subconjunctival hemorrhages

- *Hyperpigmentation—bronzing of skin (Fig. 5.46):*
  - ❖ Hemochromatosis
  - ❖ Porphyria cutanea tarda
  - ❖ Cholestatic conditions.
- Glossitis, angular stomatitis—vitamin deficiency (Fig. 5.47).

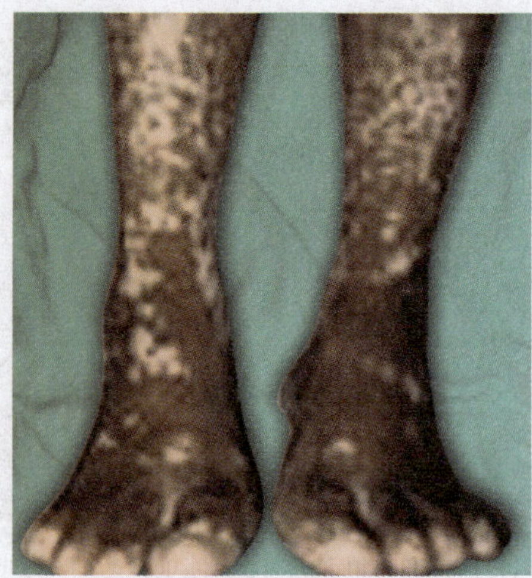

FIG. 5.45 Vitiligo

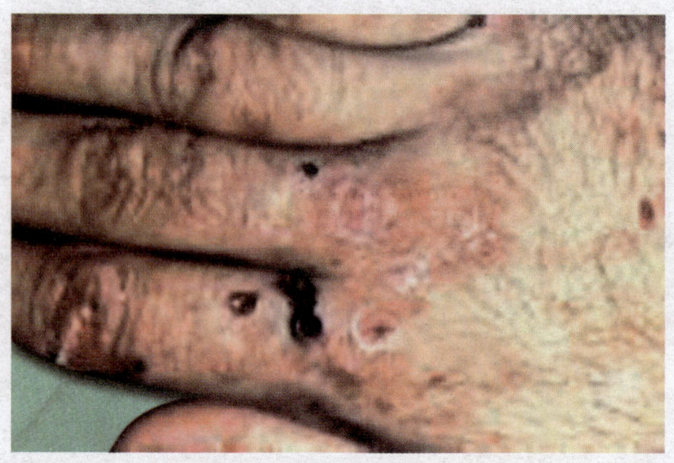

FIG. 5.46 Porphyria cutanea tarda

- Bleeding from gum, skin—due to thrombocytopenia and co-agulation abnormalities:
  - ❖ Cirrhosis decompensation
  - ❖ Acute fulminant hepatic failure.
- *Pallor due to:*
  - ❖ Anemia—blood loss, cirrhosis, coagulations abnormities (Fig. 5.48)

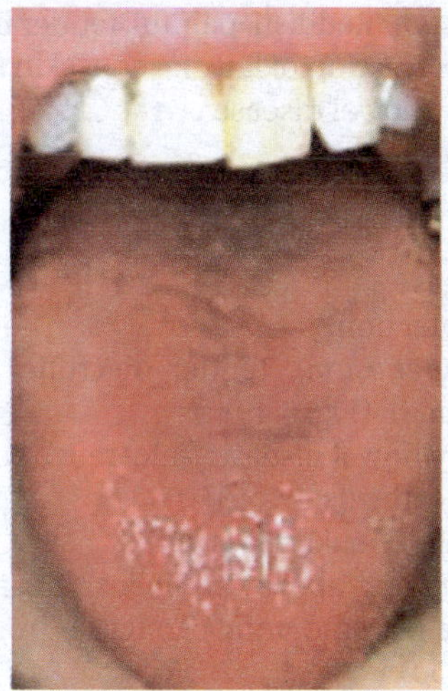

FIG. 5.47 Glossitis

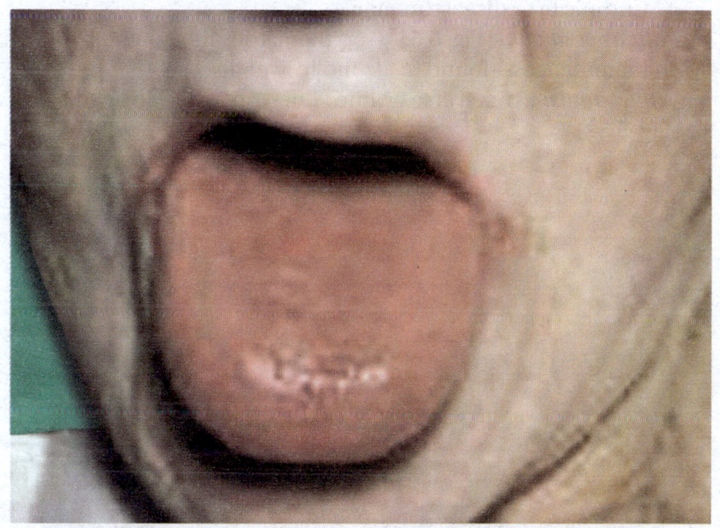

FIG. 5.48 Anemia

❖ **Without anemia—due to edema—facial puffiness**
- Myxoedema
- Hypothyroidism
- Chronic heart failure.

- *Erythema nodosum:* Reddish, painful, tender nodular lesion (1–5 cm) due to inflammation of fatty layer of skin found in lower leg.
  - ❖ Inflammatory bowel disease
  - ❖ Oral contraceptive pills
  - ❖ Pregnancy
  - ❖ Sarcoidosis
  - ❖ Behçet's disease.
  Streptococcal infection.
- *Pyoderma gangrenosum:* Tender, necrotic undermined skin ulcerations found in (Fig. 5.49):
  - ❖ Inflammatory bowel disease—ulcerative colitis
  - ❖ Rheumatoid arthritis
  - ❖ Chronic myeloid leukemia.
- *Spider nevus:* Present above umbilicus. It can be described as: Central arteriole with radiating capillaries from central arteriole found in (Fig. 5.50):
  - ❖ Alcoholic liver disease
  - ❖ Women taking oral contraceptives
  - ❖ Pregnancy
  - ❖ Chronic liver disease in men.
- *Palmar erythema* (Fig. 5.51)—erythematous thenar and hypoth-enar eminences—found in alcoholic liver disease.
- *White nails:* Transverse white lines in nail—liver disease (Fig. 5.52).

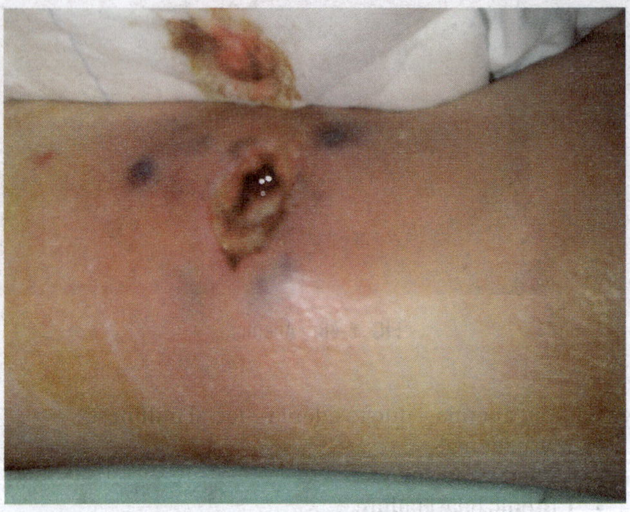

FIG. 5.49 Pyoderma gangrenosum

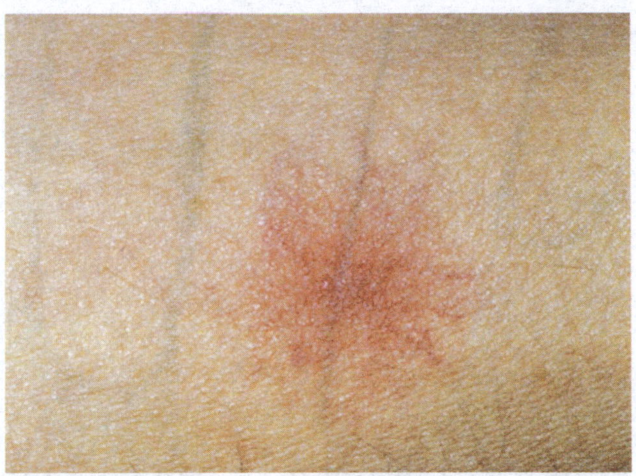

FIG. 5.50 Spider nevus

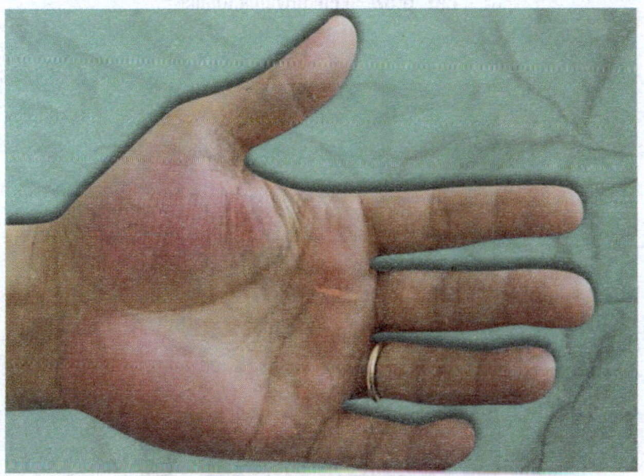

FIG. 5.51 Palmar erythema

- *Gynecomastia:* Enlarged tender palpable glandular tissues under areola seen in (Fig. 5.53):
  - ❖ Physiological adolescence, aging
  - ❖ Pathological chronic liver disease
  - ❖ Drugs spironolactone
      Here, ratio of testosterone to estradiol is less than 100:1.
  - ❖ In normal obese men—due to rapid conversion of androgen to estrogen in peripheral tissues.
- Glossitis, angular stomatitis—vitamin deficiency (Fig. 5.54).
      Cutaneous manifest.

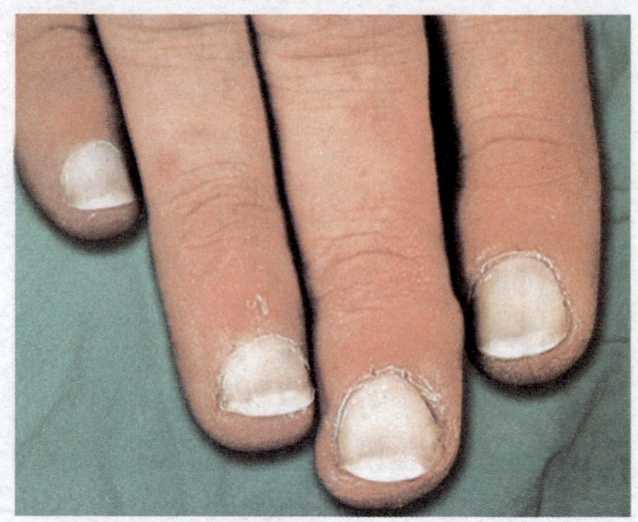

FIG. 5.52   Leukonychia totalis

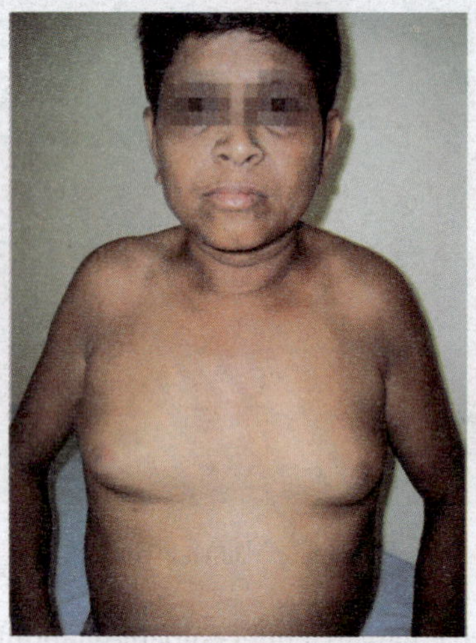

FIG. 5.53   Gynecomastia

- *Alopecia with seborrheic dermatitis*—scaly, pruritic scalp with lichenification and hair breakage (Fig. 5.55).
    Hepatic failure.
- *Livedo reticularis:* Dark pigmented skin, brown skin having hyperpigmented reticulated pattern (Fig. 5.56).

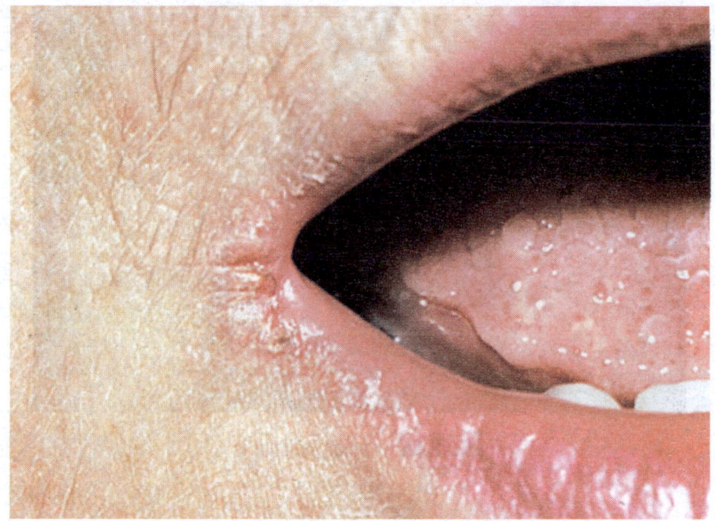

FIG. 5.54   Angular cheilitis

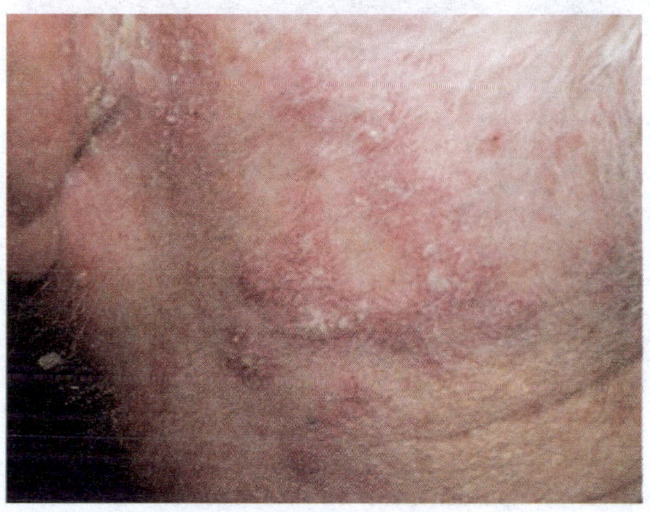

FIG. 5.55   Dermatitis seborrheic adult

- *Lichen planus:* Violaceous, flat topped pruritic red papules and plaques with overlying delicate white lines—Wickham's striae—present on flexor aspect, nails, oral and genital lesions—in hepatitis infections (Fig. 5.57).

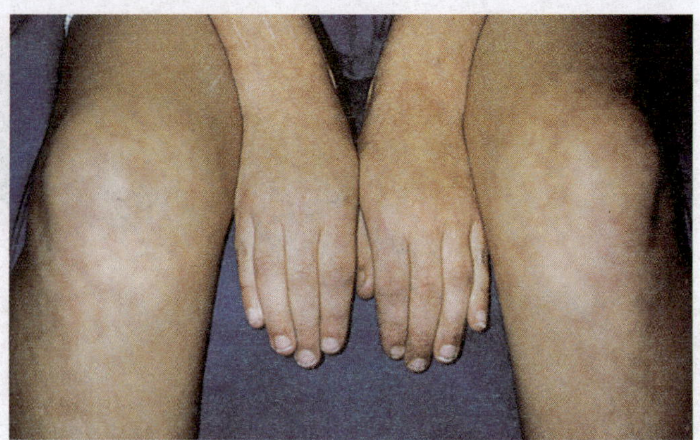

FIG. 5.56   Livedo reticularis

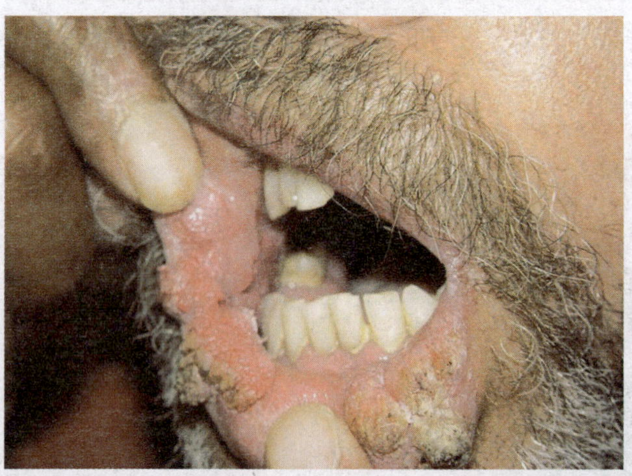

FIG. 5.57   Lichen planus

- *Palpable purpura*—if associated with arthralgia, hepatospleno-megaly, lymphadenopathy—due to mixed cryoglobulinemia—in hepatitis infection (Fig. 5.58).
- *Pruritic, acrally situated psoriasis*—like eruptions—HCV infections.
- *Blue discoloration around umbilicus due to hemoperitoneum—Cullen sign*—acute pancreatitis (Fig. 5.59).
- *Reddish-brown discoloration in the flanks—cause*—in acute pancreatitis of necrotizing variety, the retroperitoneal blood dissects along tissue plane—Grey Turner sign (Fig. 5.60).

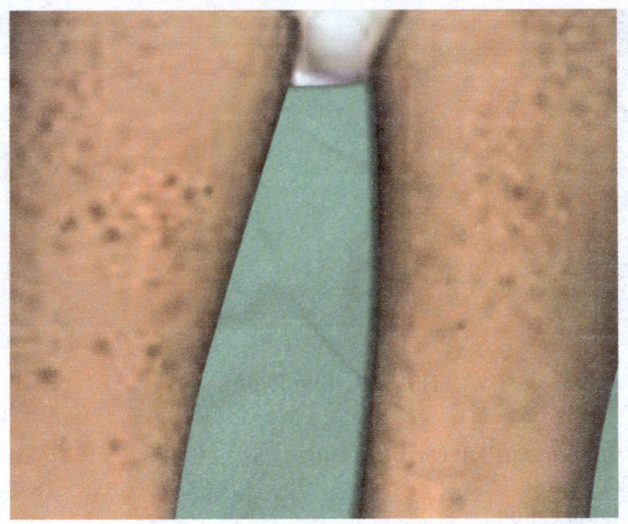

FIG. 5.58   Purpura

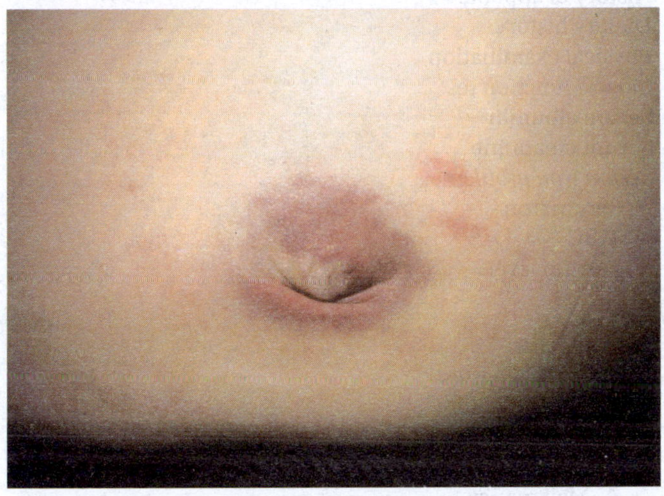

FIG. 5.59   Cullen sign

- Focal erythematous nodules due to subcutaneous fat necrosis—acute pancreatitis.
- Scratch marks all over the body associated with shining nails—signs of cholestasis.

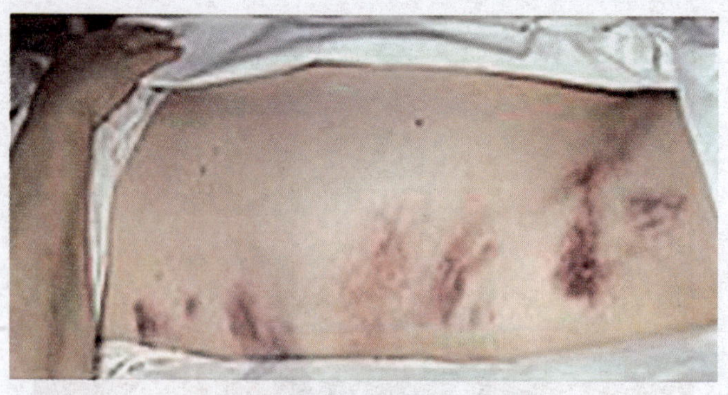

FIG. 5.60 Grey Turner sign

Nutritional status: It can be due to:
- Starvation
- Maldigestion
- Malabsorption.

To assess the nutritional status following things should be followed:
- History of appetite
- Dietary history
- Physical examination
- Muscle function test
- Serum albumin
- Serum creatinine
- *Serum iron profile:*
  - ❖ Serum iron
  - ❖ TIBC
  - ❖ Ferritin level.

History
- *Poor appetite:*
  - ❖ *Systemic illnesses:*
    - Cardiac failure
    - Renal failure
    - Viral fever
    - Malignancy
    - Mental depression
    - Drug abuse
    - Alcohol intake—patients may develop protein and vitamins malnutrition.
  - ❖ *Structural causes:*
    - Oropharyngeal
    - Esophageal—stricture, malignancy
    - Cerebrovascular disease like stroke.

- *Malabsorption:*
  - ❖ Diarrhea
  - ❖ *Steatorrhea in spite of good appetite:*
    - Celiac disease
    - Bacterial overgrowth
    - Inflammatory bowel disease.
- Diarrhea in spite of increase metabolic demand—Thyrotoxicosis.
- *Increased metabolic demands:*
  - Fever
  - Burns
  - Cancer.

Dietary History

Proper enquiry to be done regarding dietary habits, because few patients require restriction of food intake to avoid recurrence of few disease, e.g.

- Wheat product is harmful for patient with gluten sensitive enteropathy.
- Milk should be avoided by the patient proved lactase deficiency.
- High dietary fibers may be responsible for flatulence, voluminous stool, and increased bowel frequency.
- Low fiber diet is responsible for constipation.
- Strict vegetarian diet may produce vitamin B_{12} deficiency.
- High protein diet may be harmful for gouty patient.
- Vegetable or fruits containing seeds and skin may aggravate ulcerative colitis.
- High fiber diet and diet containing seeds may produce features of obstruction in patients with Crohn's disease having stricture.
- Young women, having cyclic changes in appetite, food intake; dietary fads develops in association with pathological aversion to body habitus.

Signs of malnutrition
- Temporal halo produced by gross wasting of temporalis muscles
- Loss of hair from scalp and body
- Hundreds of cracks all over the body
- Skin becomes dry and lusterless, wrinkled
- Muscles of limbs become wasted jerks are almost non-elicitable.

In protein energy malnutrition good carbohydrate intake—body becomes edematous.

The following measurements accurately estimate the nutritional status:
- *Skin fold thickness:*

Muscles: This can be measured—triceps, biceps, infrascapular, and supraspinatus regions

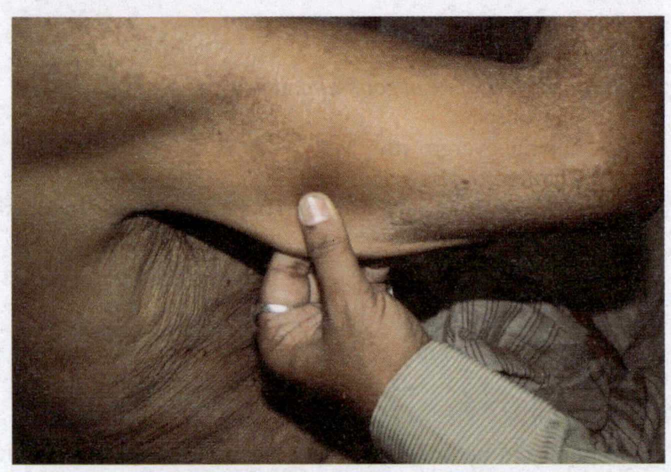

FIG. 5.61 Triceps thickness

Most commonly measured muscle is triceps—this is measured midway between tip of acromion and olecranon process (Fig. 5.61).

During measurement hand should be hanged by the side of the body.

Calipers (mm)—Schofield's calibers (in cm)

Person	Standard	80%	60%
Adult male	12.5	10.0	7.5
Adult female	16.5	13.0	10.0
Nutritional state	Normal	Moderate depletion	Severe depletion

Body composition: Body composition in 70 kg healthy man:

Substrate	Kg	Kcal/g	Kcal stored
Water	42	0	0
Protein	10	4	40,000
Fat	10	9	90,000
Glycogen			
Muscle	0.15	4	600
Liver	0.075	4	113

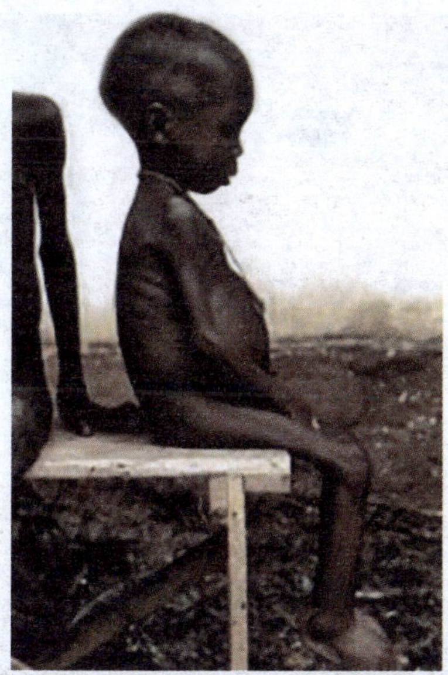

FIG. 5.62   Kwashiorkor disease from severe dietary protein deficiency

Lean body mass can be calculated from
- Measurement of total body water:

$$\text{Lean body mass} = \frac{\text{Total body water (liter)}}{0.73}$$

- Body densitometry
- Gamma nutron activation analysis of total body nitrogen.

Body mass index measured from height and weight.

In Marasmus body becomes thin, wasted, no edema, growth retarded and alert.

In Kwashiorkor body becomes edematous, child becomes miserable, sparse hair, skin changes (Fig. 5.62).

Inspection of Gastrointestinal System

Mouth

- *Lips:*
  - Cracks and fissures at the angle of the mouth—angular stomatitis—vitamin riboflavin deficiency.
  - A scar at the philtrum—(depression from nose to upper lip) nasal intonation of voice—cleft lip—may be associated with *cleft palate* (Fig. 5.63).
  - Inflammation with crustation of lips—cheilitis—in cold weather.

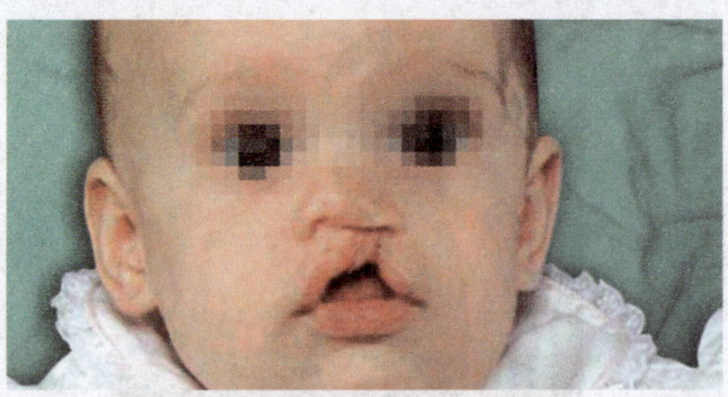

FIG. 5.63 Cleft lip

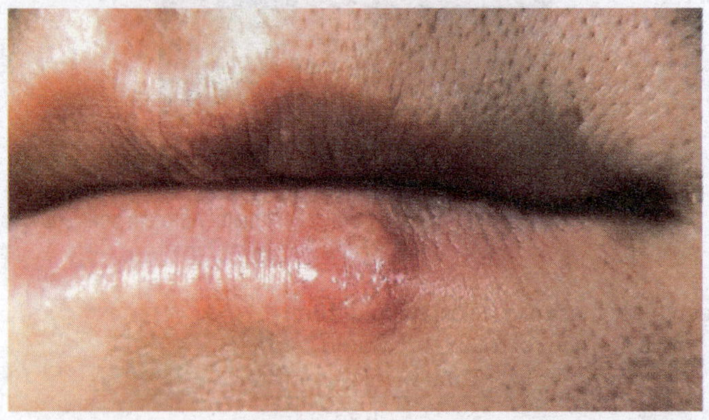

FIG. 5.64 Herpes labialis

❖ Clusters of vesicular eruption having erythematous bases (Fig. 5.64):
  - Herpes labialis
  - Common cold.
    If it is associated ulcerations and indurations—*recurrent actinic cheilitis* (Fig. 5.65).
❖ Indolent flat shallow ulcer having everted edges and indurated base in the lower lip—*epithelioma.*
❖ A firm, rounded nodular lesion occasional ulcerations due to overgrowth of stratum granulosum—in upper lip—*keratoacanthoma* (Fig. 5.66).
❖ Red raspberry-like nodule following minor trauma in upper lip—*pyogenic granuloma* (Fig. 5.67).
❖ Small rounded indurated firm lesion—in upper lip— *chancre* (Fig. 5.68).

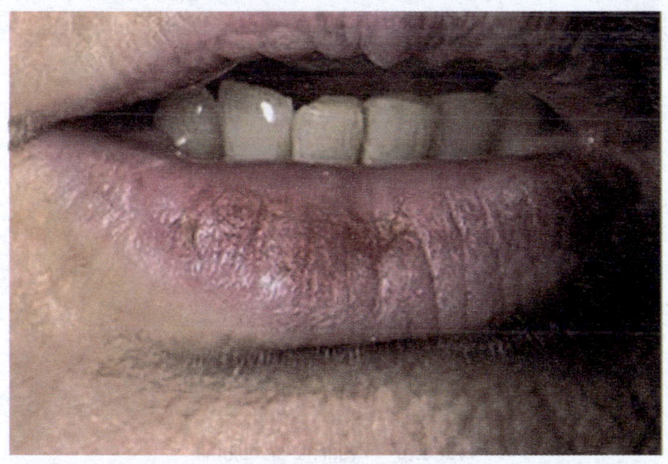

FIG. 5.65   Actinic cheilitis

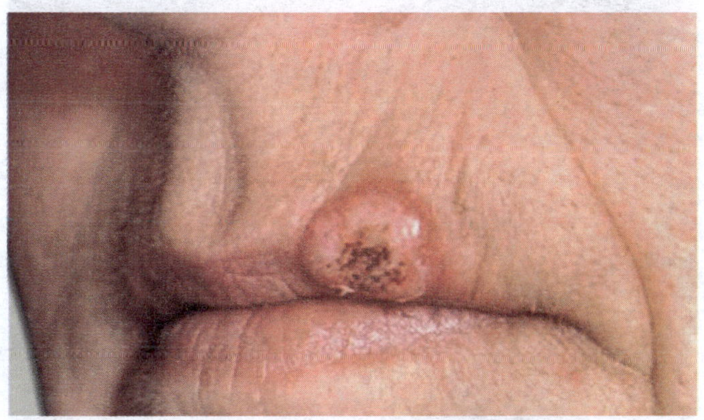

FIG. 5.66   Keratoacanthoma

- ❖ Serpiginous ulcer in upper lip—*secondary syphilis.*
- ❖ White scars extending from angle of mouth into the mouth —*Rhagades.*
- ❖ *Circumoral pigmentation:* Peutz-Jeghers syndrome.
- ❖ If pigmentation is present in inner mucous membrane of lip—*Addison's disease* (Fig. 5.69).
- ❖ In mucous membrane of lip—small superficial, painful ulcer surrounding erythematous bases—*Aphthous ulcer* (Fig. 5.70).
- ● *Teeth:*
- ❖ Impacted teeth.

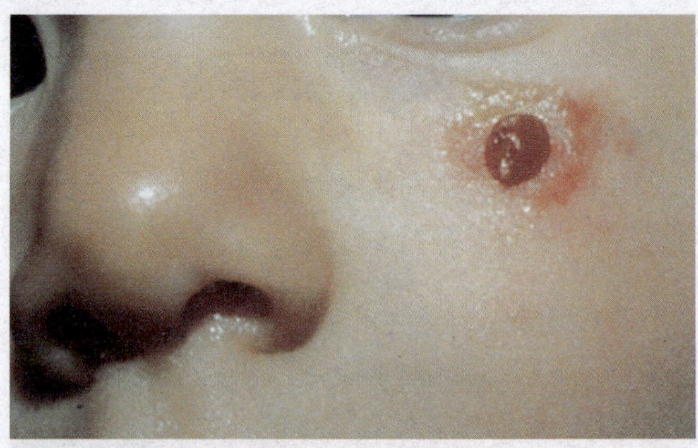

FIG. 5.67 Pyogenic granuloma

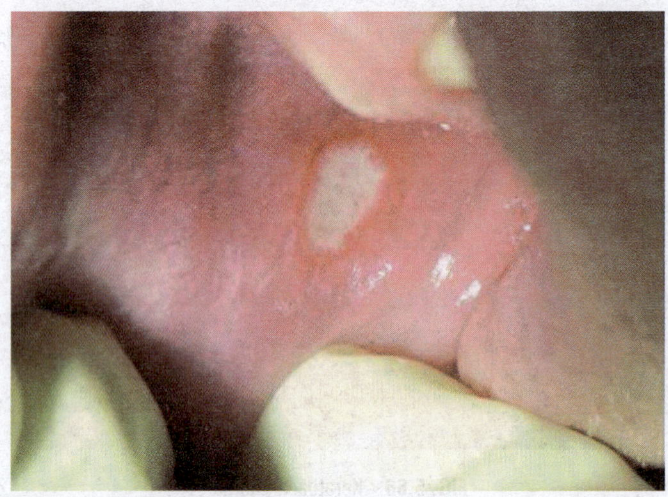

FIG. 5.68 Chancre in lip

- ❖ Unerupted teeth—third mandibular tooth—*wisdom tooth* (Fig. 5.71).
- ❖ Decay in tooth—*dental caries* (Figs 5.72A to D)
- ❖ Ridging—transverse ridging—vitamin C and D deficiency.
- ❖ *Color:*
  - Brown color—smoker (Fig. 5.73).
  - Reddish brown—chewing of betel nut.
  - Yellowish or grayish horizontal bands in deciduous or permanent teeth. Treatment with tetracycline in children at the age of 8.

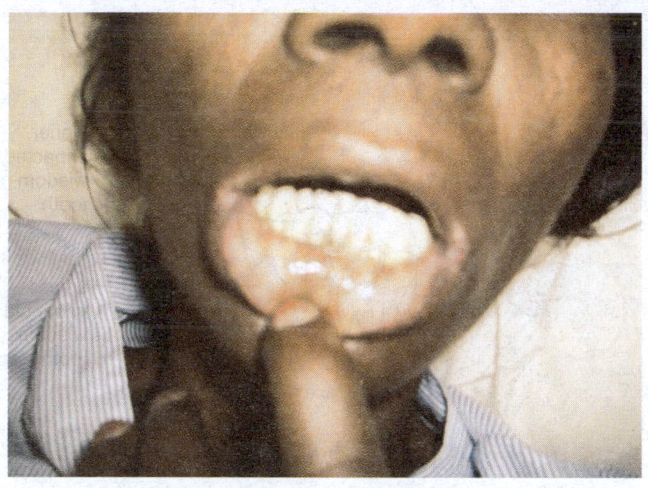

FIG. 5.69   Addison's disease

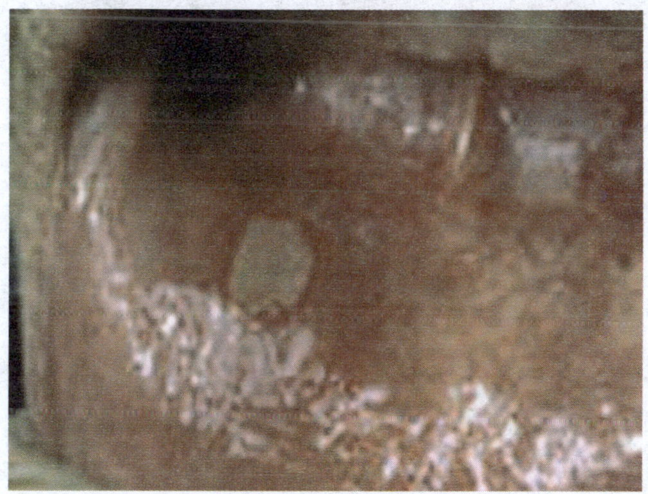

FIG. 5.70   Aphthous ulcer

- Band of hyperplasia on enamel—Exanthematous fever.
- Chalk-white patches over the teeth sometimes pitting and brown staining—*dental fluorosis* (Fig. 5.74).
- ❖ *Shape:*
  - Broad concave biting edge of incisor teeth having a notch—persons who uses to bite cotton or hold hairclips in between teeth.

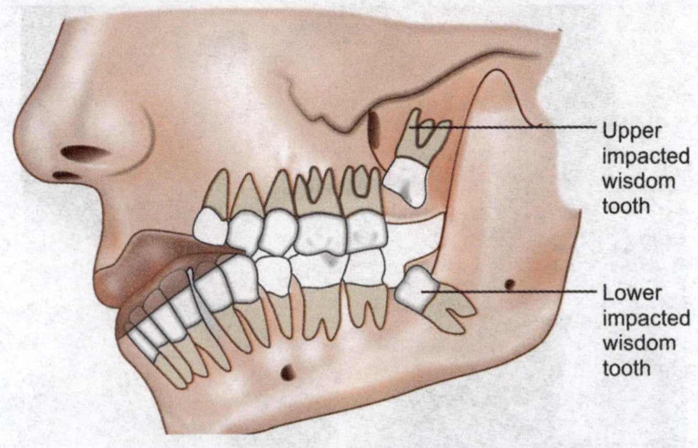

FIG. 5.71   Wisdom teeth

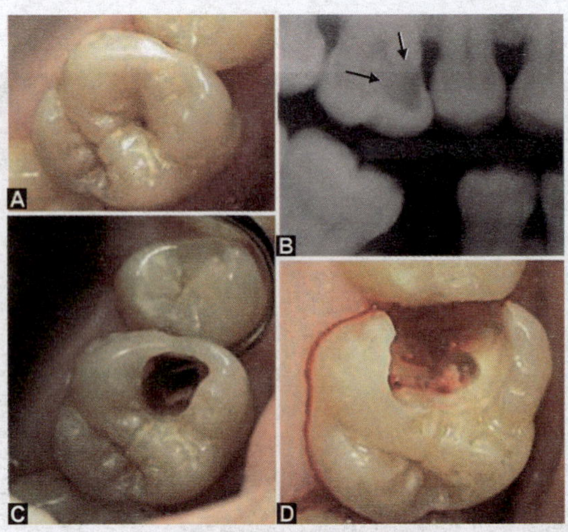

FIGS 5.72A TO D   Dental caries

- Peg-shaped teeth—upper incisors—with a notch at their biting edge and broadbase—*Hutchinson teeth* (Fig. 5.75).
- Central two upper incisors are lost—*leprosy.*
- Erosions at inner sides of incisors—due to acid in induced injury—aggravated by vomiting.

- *Gum:*
  ❖ Gradual recession of the gingival margin from the teeth producing the teeth more longer—*age related.*

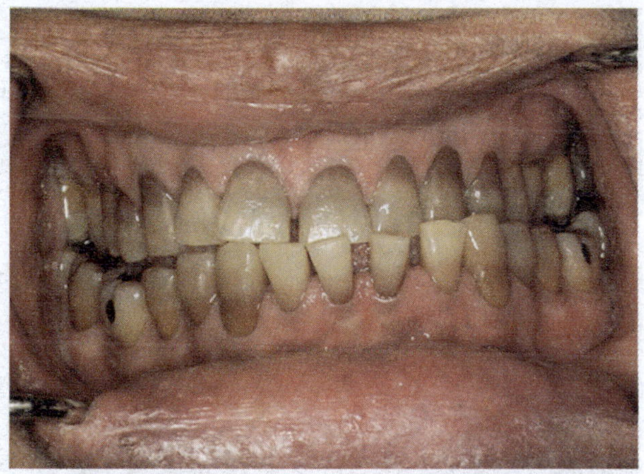

FIG. 5.73 Brown teeth

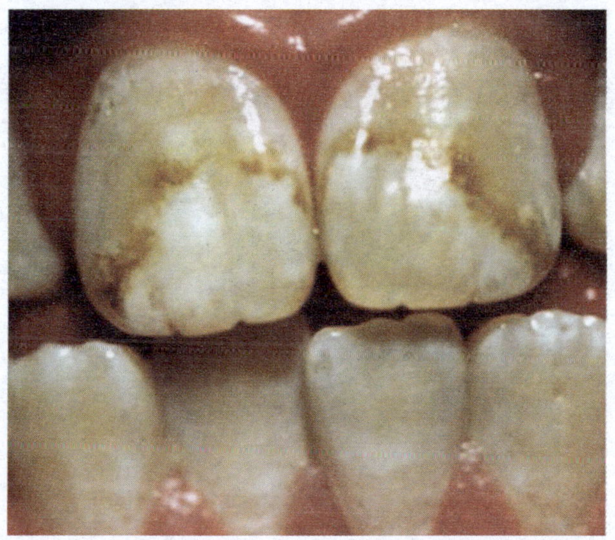

FIG. 5.74 Dental fluorosis

- ❖ *Marginal gingivitis with pyorrhea:* Gum margin is inflamed and bleeds easily, sometimes pus seen coming out from the gingival margin.
- ❖ Scattered vesicles with shallow ulcers having yellow bases after rupture of vesicles—in gum, cheeks, lips, tongue— *Herpetic gingivostomatitis*—in children, infant.

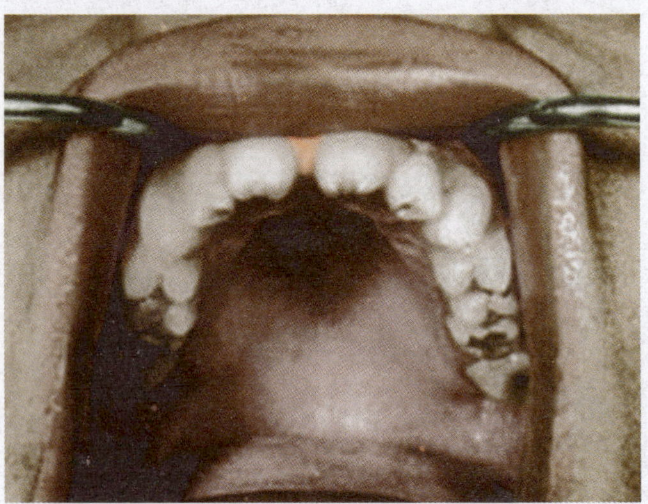

FIG. 5.75 Hutchinson teeth

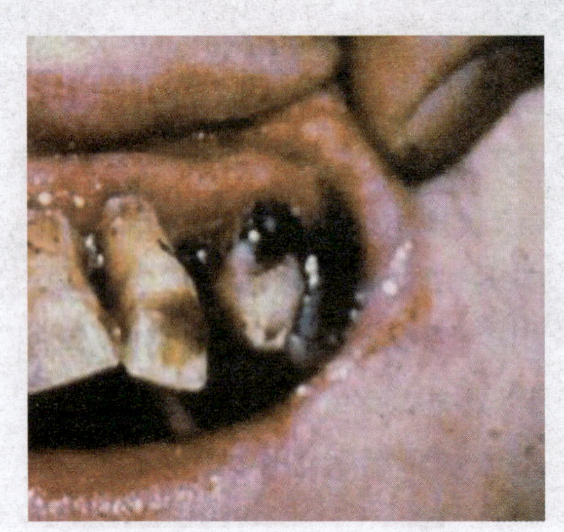

FIG. 5.76 Scurvy symptoms teeth

❖ *Blue line running transversely at the edge of gum:*
  • Bismuth, mercury poisoning, lead poisoning.
  • Opposite the teeth showing gingivitis.
❖ Thickened grayish slough—in gum *gingivostomatitis—vincent fusiform spirochates.*
❖ Spongy, fragile, red gum bleeds on touch—*scurvy* (Fig. 5.76)—vitamin deficiency.

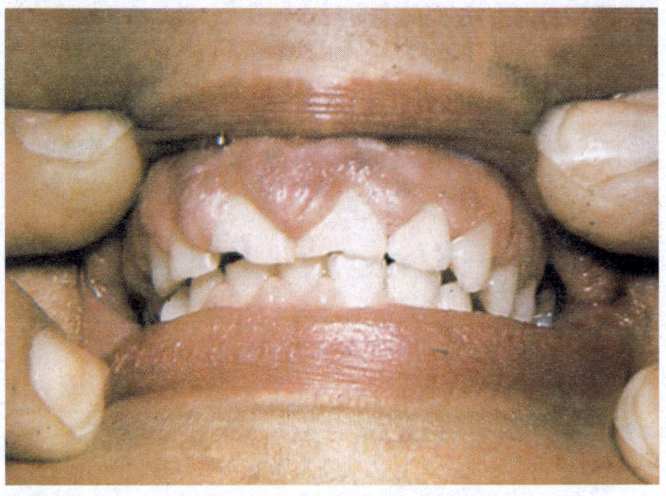

FIG. 5.77   Gingival hyperplasia from phenytoin

❖ *Hypertrophied gum:*
  • Pregnancy.
  • Long-term treatment with phenytoin (Fig. 5.77).
❖ *Bleeding gum:*
  • Thrombocytopenic purpura.
  • Leukemia.
❖ *Ulcer on the gum:*
  • Due to ill-fitted denture site where the dentures do not fit properly.
  • Malignant ulcer.
❖ *Epulis*—swelling of gum of the maxilla or mandible (Fig. 5.78).
● *Tongue:*
❖ Inability to protrude the tongue—*ankyloglossia* (Fig. 5.79).
  • In infant—tongue tie—due to small *frenulum linguul.*
  • In carcinoma of tongue—involving the floor of the mouth.
❖ *Deviation of tongue to one side:*
  • Carcinoma tongue involving sides of tongue—deviation to same side.
  • In hemiplegia—towards the paralyzed side.
  • Involvement of hypoglossal nucleus—there is fasciculation, hemiatrophy, deviation to same side.
❖ *Macroglossia:*
  • Acromegaly
  • Cretinism
  • Myxedema.

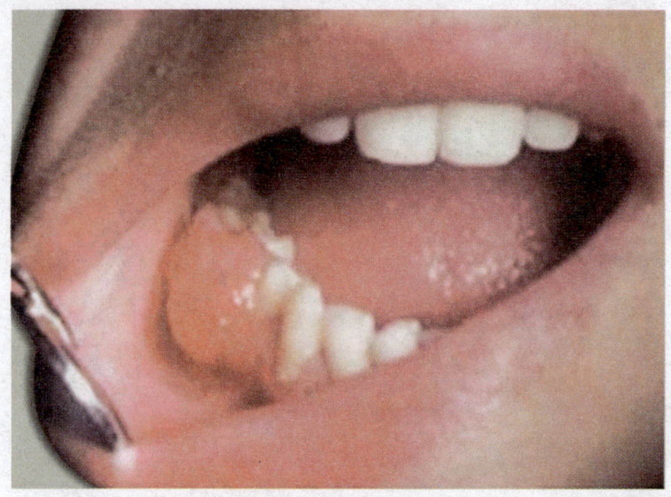

FIG. 5.78   Epulis

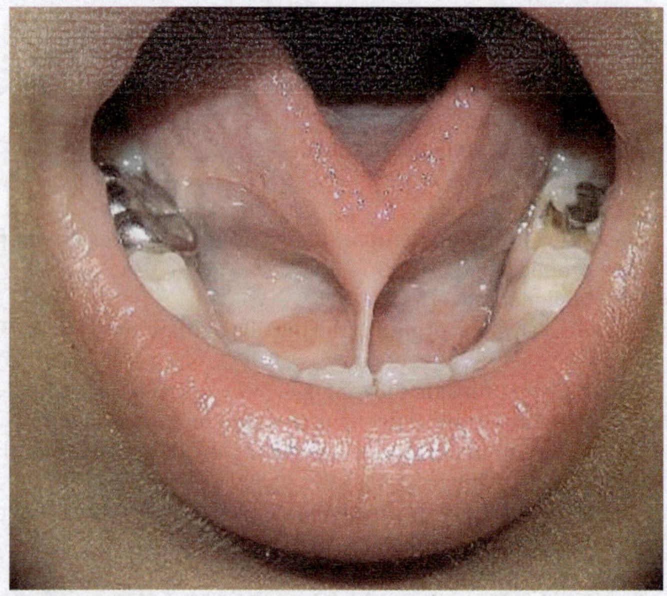

FIG. 5.79   Ankyloglossia

❖ *Tremor:*
- Thyrotoxicosis
- Depression
- Delirium tremens.

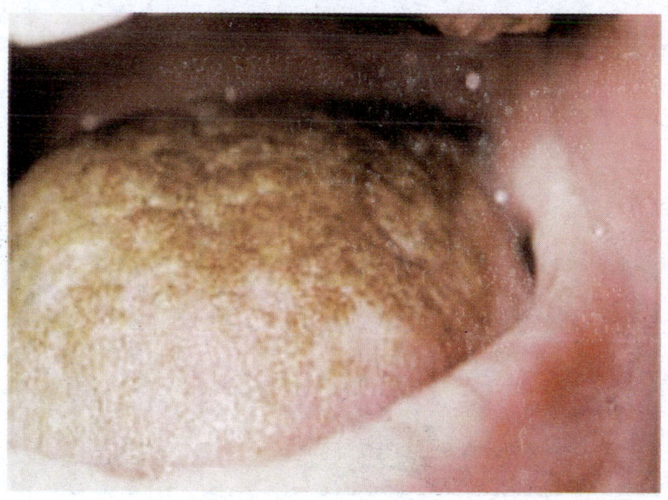

FIG. 5.80 Black hairy tongue

❖ *Surface of tongue:* Dorsal surface of tongue:
- Color—pallor—anemia
  Blue—central cyanosis
  Other colors—due to ingestion of foods.
- *Hydration*—any
  - Moderate to severe dehydration
  - Uremia
  - Acute intestinal obstruction.
- *Furring:*
  - Heavy smokers
  - *Black hairy tongue*—fungal infection (Fig. 5.80)
  - Strawberry tongue—bright red papillae standing within white fur—scarlet fever
  - Hairy leukoplakia—HIV infection.
- *Papillae:*
  - Gross atrophy of papillae—producing smoothed tongue—vitamin B_{12} deficiency, iron deficiency, niacin deficiency
  - *Scrotal tongue*: Excessive wrinkling of tongue surface—no significance
  - *Congenital fissuring of tongue*: Papillae are normal, but surface are interrupted by numerous symmetrical folds—normal (Fig. 5.81)
  - *Median rhomboid glossitis*: Lozenge—shaped area—papillae are atrophied—anterior to foramen cecum (Fig. 5.82).

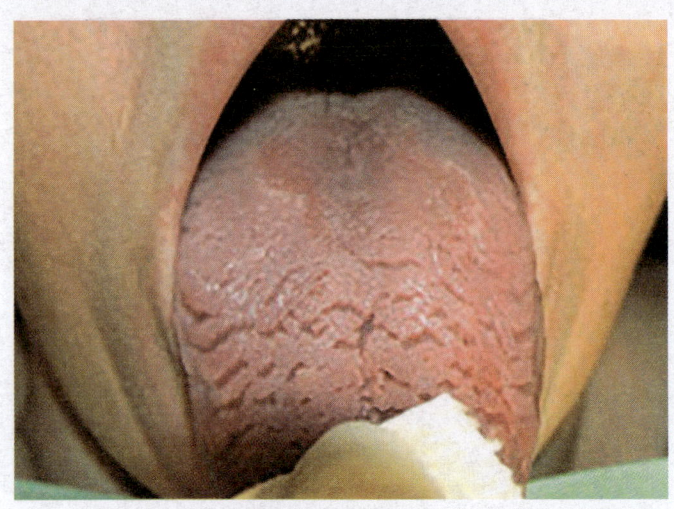

FIG. 5.81 Fissured tongue

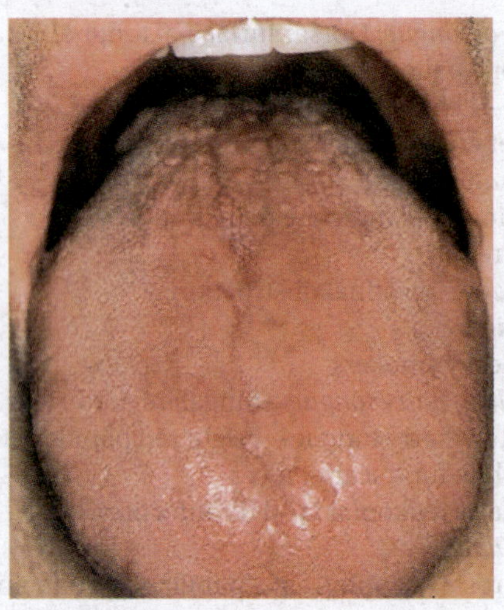

FIG. 5.82 Rhomboid glossitis

- *Lingual thyroid*: Posterior to foramen cecum
- *Geographical tongue*: Areas of desquamated epithelium and filiform papillae, surrounded by whitish yellow border (Fig. 5.83).

Sides of tongue:
- ❖ Painful, nonindurated shallow ulcers at the sides of tongue due to ill-fitting dentures

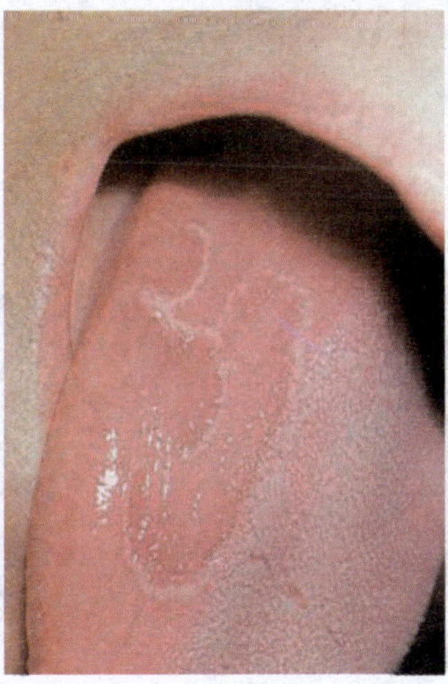

FIG. 5.83   Geographical tongue

Carries teeth
* Indurated, hard ulcer with everted margin—malignant unless—should be biopsied.

Under surface of tongue:
* Calculi—white of yellowish bleb at the site of orifice of submandibular gland
* *Yellowish discoloration*—jaundice
* A small *ulcer on the frenulum* due to long standing coughing.
* *Sublingual varicosities*
* *Ranula*—bluish white translucent swelling due to blockage of duct of mucous gland
* *Sublingual dermoid cyst.*

* *Buccal mucosa:*
* Opening of the duct of parotid gland on upper 2nd molar tooth.
* Bluish white spots opposite molar teeth—Koplik spot—*Catarrhal stage of measles* (Fig. 5.84)
* Black pigmented spot—in opposite molar teeth—*Addison's disease*
* *Ulcers on the buccal mucosa:*
  * Inflammatory bowel disease
  * Behçet's syndrome
  * Idiopathic aphthous ulcers
  * Lichen planus.
* *Thrush:* Multiple small whitish plaques surrounded by erythematous areas— *Monilial infection* (Fig. 5.85).

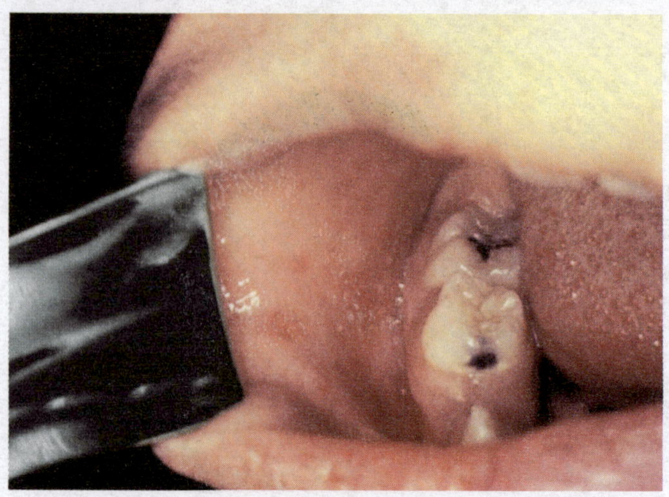

FIG. 5.84   Koplik spots, measles

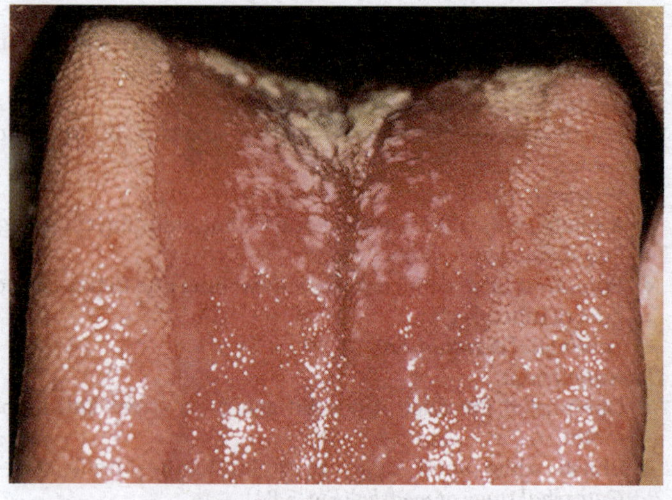

FIG. 5.85   Thrush on tongue

This can be separated from milk spots by:
❖ It can be easily detached.

Thrush cannot be easily detached. After removal, there are raw surfaces.

The causes of thrush:
- Debilitated person
- Person on immunosuppressive therapy
- Immunodeficiency states.

- *Palate, fauces, tonsils, pharynx:* There are two methods by which one can examine the above areas:
  - ❖ Ask the patient to put head back and to keep his mouth wide open.
  - ❖ To get good view of above structures—depress the base of the tongue with spatula.

The lesions
- *In herpes zoster infection:*
  - ❖ Small vesicles in the hard palate along with painful ulcers involve maxillary division of trigeminal nerve.

    Associated lesions in the areas same dermatome of the face
  - ❖ Similar vesicles and painful ulcers in pharynx involved nerve is glossopharyngeal nerve.
- *Malignant ulcers*—present on hard palate
- *Ectopic salivary gland*—most common site—hard palate.

  Malignant tissue—projects from hard palate, hard swelling having central ulceration.
- *Hole in the bone*—due to:
  - ❖ Repair of cleft palate
  - ❖ Radio necrosis following radiotherapy for localized carcinoma
  - ❖ Tertiary syphilis.
- *Petechiae—in palate:*
  - ❖ Glandular fever—associated features enlarged tonsils covered with white exudates—with edema of faces and soft palate.
  - ❖ *Streptococcal tonsillitis:* Yellow punctuate follicular exudates on tonsils
  - ❖ Rubella
  - ❖ Thrombocytopenia.
- Diphtherial membranes over tonsil—color varies from white to green spreads to pharynx.
- Small round swelling like sagu grains—in pharynx—normal
- *Herpangina*—oval, round ulcers with white slough—in oropharynx, soft palate and uvula—Coxasackie infection—common in young (Fig. 5.86).
- Erythema on buccal mucous membrane—which progress to vesicles and ulcers chickenpox.
- Mucopus seen on posterior wall of pharynx running down from nasopharyx—common cold.
- Small punctuate yellowish spots on tonsillar surface—*tonsil-abscess* (Fig. 5.87).

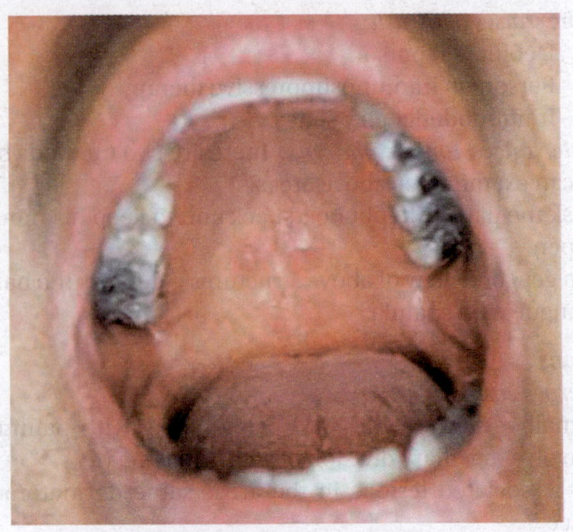

FIG. 5.86 Herpangina

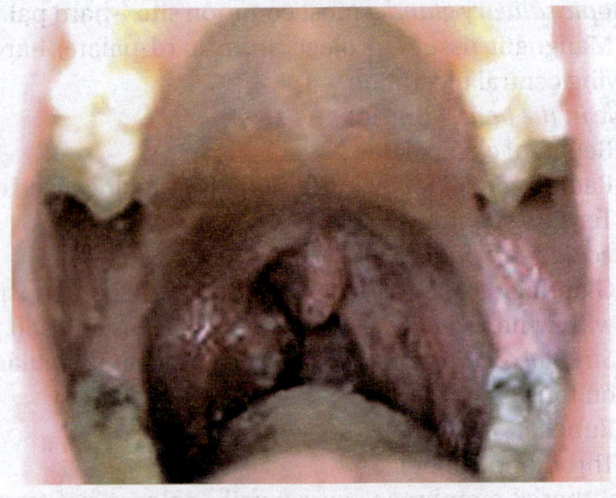

FIG. 5.87 Tonsillar abscess

Breath

- Breath of acetone—ketosis
- Breath of ammonia—uremia
- Breath of sweetish smell mousy odor—hepatic failure
- Breath of apple blossom with hint of stale feces—bronchiectasis.
- Characteristic smell of alcohol—alcoholism
- Putrid smell breath in suppurative conditions of lung.

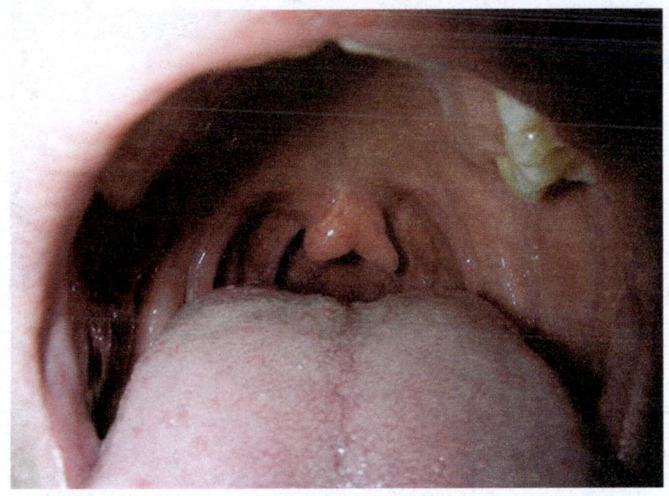

FIG. 5.88 Bifid uvula

Uvula

Midline structures are projecting from root of the posterior pharynx.

Types of uvula
- *Absent uvula:* Surgical removal for obstructive sleep apnea syndrome.
  If results in inhalation of swallowed fluids.
- *Bifid uvula:* Congenitally forked associated with occult cleft palate (Fig. 5.88).
- *Bobbing uvula:* Rhythmic pulsation of uvula associated with aortic regurgitation—Muller sign.
- Neoplastic uvula—as a result of neoplastic squamous cell degeneration (Fig. 5.89).

Localized reddening of anterior pillars
Localized crimson colored nontender reddening of anterior pillars. It is associated with chronic fatigue syndrome.
   As the disease regresses, reddening will also disappear.

Causes of exudates on posterior pharynx
- Viral
- Streptococcal
- Epstein-Barr virus
- *Mycoplasma pneumonia*
- *Chlamydia pneumonia*
- *Neisseria gonorrhoeae*
- Candidiasis
- Diphtheria.

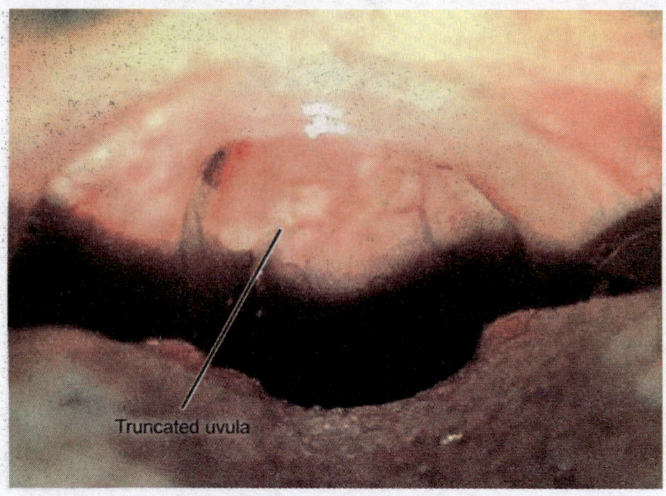

FIG. 5.89 Uvula carcinoma

Causes of nodules on posterior pharynx
- Human papilloma virus—present on tonsils, pillars, buccal mucosa—degenerates to squamous cell carcinoma
- Squamous cell carcinoma—present as papule or nodule on the posterior pharynx
- Lymphoma—most common type tonsillar cancer—presenting as submucosal mass or asymmetric tonsillar enlargement.

Causes of fleshy covered palpable lesions in the oral mucosa
- *Wharton ducts:* Two papules at the floor of the mouth—represents opening of submaxillary gland
- *Stensen's duct:* This represents opening of parotid glands
- *Ranula:* Unilateral painful dome-shaped fluctuant nodular lesion at the floor of the mouth—cause—obstruction of duct of sublingual or submandibular glands
- *Torus:* It is nontender exostosis—mucosa lined cartilage or bony spur called mandibularis.

Inspection of Abdomen

Position of the Patients and Doctors
- Patient should be in supine position with hands by the sides of the body on a comfortable mattress
- Head is supported by pillow
- Room should be properly lighted, proper room temperature
- Examiner should stand on the right side of the patient

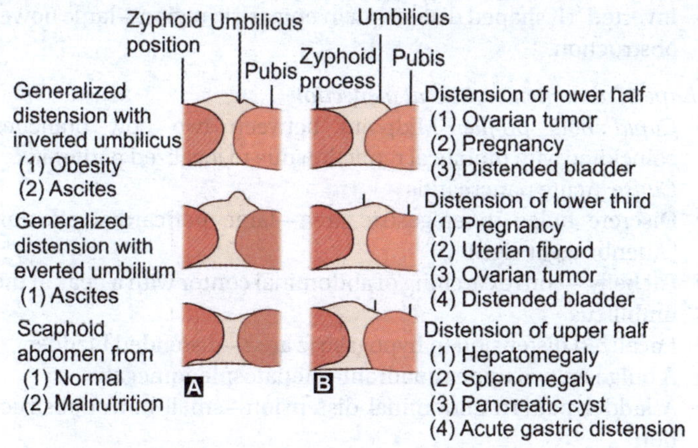

FIGS 5.90A AND B   (A) Shape of abdomen; (B) Position of umbilicus

- Patient should be properly exposed. Abdomen should be exposed from xiphisternum to symphysis pubis and if required genitalia should be exposed
- Hernia sites should be properly exposed.

Inspection

Shape of abdomen (Figs 5.90A and B)
- *Scaphoid shape:* Looking like boat:
  - ❖ Rib margins representing the stem
  - ❖ Iliac spines and symphysis pubis representing bow
  - ❖ Abdominal wall representing the hulk.
  Causes:
  - ❖ Normal
  - ❖ Cachexia
  - ❖ Starvation
  - ❖ Malignant disease—carcinoma of esophagus and stomach.
- Generalized fullness with flanks full—ascites.
- *Generalized fullness:*
  - ❖ Obesity
  - ❖ Flatus.
- *Localized distension:*
  - ❖ Symmetrical around umbilicus—small bowel obstruction
  - ❖ Asymmetrical involvement:
    - • Liver
    - • Spleen.
- Distension of lower abdomen—urinary bladder fullness.
- A ladder pattern abdominal distension—small bowel obstruction.

- Inverted 'U' shaped distension in epigastric region—large bowel obstruction.

Shape of abdomen on lateral inspection
- *Cupid bow profile:* Midpoint between two bow branches coinciding with umbilical retraction due to localized peritonitis.
  Cause: Acute pancreatitis
- Discrete bulge in epigastric area—large pericardial effusion (Auenbrugger sign)
- Fat belly—convex arching of abdominal contor with a peak at the umbilicus
- Localized distension in hypogastric area—distended bladder
- A bulge on two upper quadrant—hepatosplenomegaly
- A ladder pattern abdominal distension—small bowel obstruction
- Inverted 'U'-shaped distension in epigastria region—Large bowel obstruction.

Umbilicus

Normally umbilicus is slightly retracted and inverted—it is the center of abdomen.

Abnormalities of Umbilicus

- *Protuberances:* Most common protuberances are:
  - ❖ *Eversion:* Umbilical scar is everted and flushed with skin causes are:
    - Obesity with flushed abdomen
    - Ascites.
  - ❖ *Sister Mary Joseph's nodules:* If represents metastatic node developed due to intra-abdominal malignancy.
    It is nontender, irregular, replaces umbilicus.
  - ❖ *Ompholith:* It is umbilical nodule due to collection of sebum and keratin. It occurs in poor hygienic condition.
- *Purplish discoloration of umbilicus:* It is due to subcutaneous intraperitoneal bleed due to acute pancreatitis, may be associated with:
  - ❖ Periumbilical ecchymoses—Cullen sign
  - ❖ Bilateral reddish discoloration of the flanks—Grey Turner's sign.
- *Vertical shift of umbilicus (Figs 5.91A and B):*
  - ❖ *Downward displacement:*
    - Ascites (Fig. 5.91A)
    - Longstanding hepatosplenomegaly.

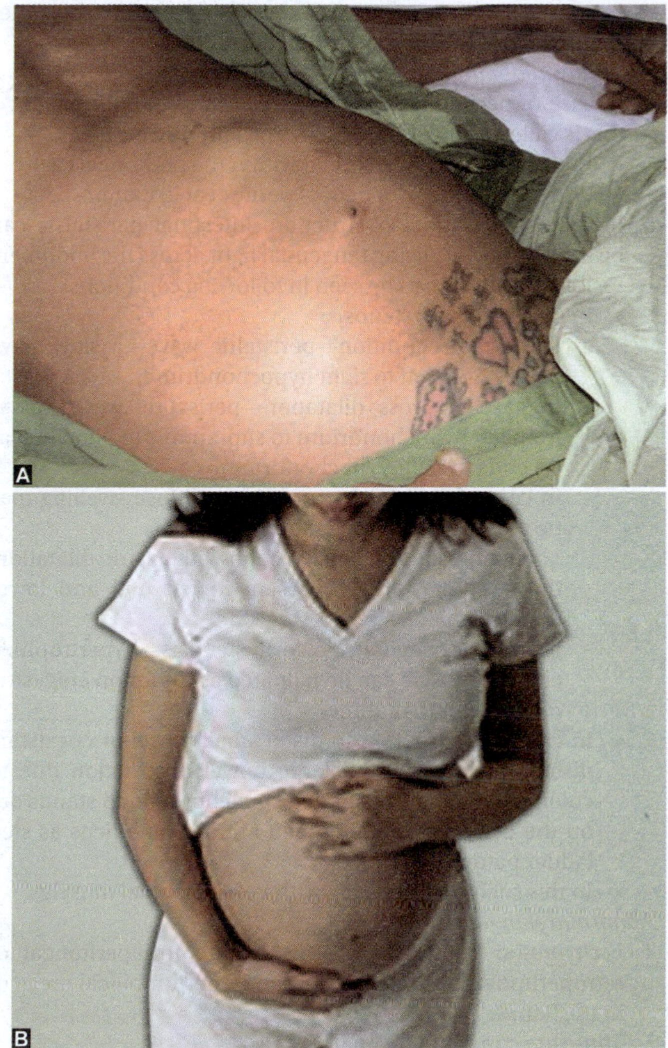

FIGS 5.91A AND B   (A) Umbilicus in ascites; (B) Umbilicus in pregnancy

◆ *Upward displacement:*
  - Pregnancy (Fig. 5.91B)
  - Pelvic tumor.

Inspection of Abdominal Wall

- *Abdominal respiratory motion:* During inspiration abdomen expands and during expiration abdominal wall retracts

In respiratory muscle weakness—respiration becomes abdominal—this is called abdominal paradox.

Normally abdominal movement is equal in both sides:

❖ In case of peritonitis, the abdominal movement is absent—this is called silent abdomen. It is usually due to:
  - Prevention infection spread within the peritoneal cavity
  - Prevention spread of pain of peritoneal irritation.
❖ In case of intestinal obstruction, intestinal peristalsis can be detected by throwing tangential light across the abdomen. Visible peristalsis can be seen in following conditions:
  - In case of pyloric stenosis:
    - In normal condition—peristaltic wave—a slow wave passes from left to right hypochondrium.
    - In case of gross dilatation—peristaltic wave passes from left hypochondrium to suprapubic region, then as ascends to right hypochondrium.
    - In case of pyloric obstruction—a diffuse swelling may be present in left upper abdomen.

      In long-standing obstruction with gastric dilatation, the swelling may be present in left mid and lower quadrants.
    - In case of congenital pyloric stenosis—hypertrophied circular muscle can be palpated as tumor on epigastric region right to midline.
  - In case of obstruction to distal small bowel or coexisting distal small bowel and large bowel obstruction due to colonic pathology, distended small bowel loop stands out on the center of the abdomen around umbilicus as step ladder pattern.
  - In this cachectic person—with lax abdominal muscles.
● *Abnormal skin markings:*
  ❖ *Ecchymoses:* These are bruises due to intraperitoneal or retroperitoneal hemorrhage—seen in periumbilical areas or in the flanks:

    These are commonly seen in:
    - Necrotizing acute pancreatitis (3%)
    - Ruptured pregnancy (1%)
  ❖ *Striae (Fig. 5.92):*
    - Location—lateral aspect of abdomen
    - They are 1–6 cm long, multiple
    - They are developed due to chronic stretching
    - They are present in abdomen, shoulder, thigh, and breasts
    - *Causes:*
      - Obesity
      - Pregnancy
      - Cushing.

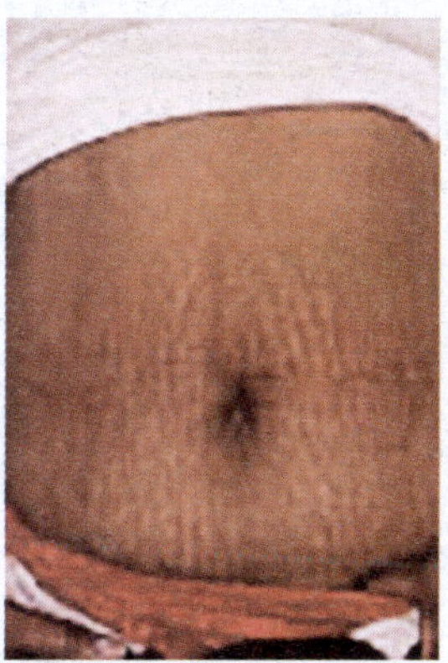

FIG. 5.92 Abdominal striae

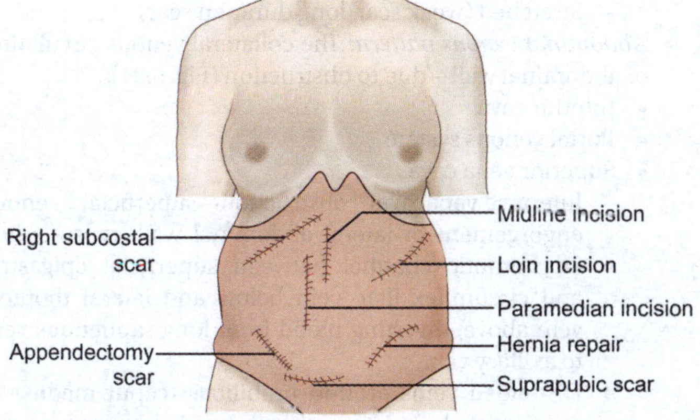

FIG. 5.93 Surgical scar in abdomen

❖ *Scars:* This scar may be the sign of previous pathology (Fig. 5.93).

The sites of scars are:
- Right subcostal scar
- Midline incision and scar
- Paramedian scar
- Suprapubic scar
- Appendectomy scar
- Hernia scar.

  Duration of scars can be identified by the following characters of scars:
- Old (white)
- Pink (recent)

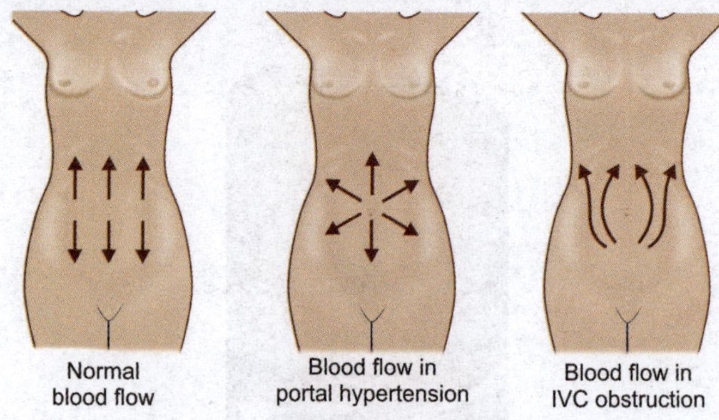

FIG. 5.94 Abdominal venous flow pattern

- Linear (recent)
- Stretched (weak scar, long duration scar).
❖ *Abdominal venous pattern:* The collateral venous circulation of abdominal wall—due to obstruction (Fig. 5.94):
  - Interior cava
  - Portal venous system
  - Superior vena cava.
    - Inferior venacaval obstruction—superficial venous engorgement of lateral abdominal wall, representing anastomotic channel between superficial epigastric and circumflex iliac vein below and lateral thoracic vein above, diverting blood from long saphenous vein to axillary vein.
    - Distended veins around umbilicus (caput medusae), representing anastomotic channel between portal veins and systemic veins. This is usually associated with splenomegaly, ascites, esophageal varices. Caput medusae present tuff of veins radiating from umbilicus as spokes of a wheel or nest of snake; draining the blood from portal veins to internal mammary rostally and inferior mammary caudally through subcutaneous veins of abdominal wall.
    - Superior vena caval obstruction—venous engorgement seen in upper abdomen.

Detection of direction of blood flow (Fig. 5.95):
By milking the abdominal wall vein:
- Place the two index fingers over the vein and give pressure to collapse it.

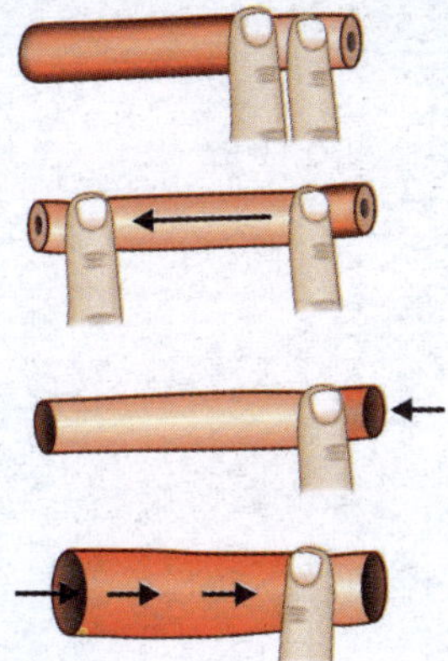

FIG. 5.95   Method of detection of venous flow direction

- Then slide the finger apart, producing 1-2 inches of gap on collapsed vein.
- Release the pressure of the caudal end of vein and then the rostral end of the vein.
- By above methods, direction of venous flow can be determined:
    - ❖ Blood flow from below upwards—inferior vena cava
    - ❖ Blood flow from above downwards—superior vena cava
    - ❖ Blood flow away from umbilicus—portal vein obstruction.

Pigmentation on the abdominal wall:
- Linear pigmentation from below the umbilicus—Linea nigra—signs of pregnancy (Fig. 5.96)
- Mottle patchy pigmentation due to placing hot water bottle, hot pad on the skin of abdominal wall—erythema ab igne. Signs of constant application of heat—commonly associated with chronic pancreatitis (Fig. 5.97).

Inspection of hernial sites: To see any obvious thing coming out—in normal position, during any type of straining (coughing, sneezing) (Fig. 5.98).

▮Palpations

Method of Palpation

- Ask the patient to lie relax and breath quietly
- Ask the patient to expose the area of examination from xiphisternal region to symphysis pubis
- Warm your hand

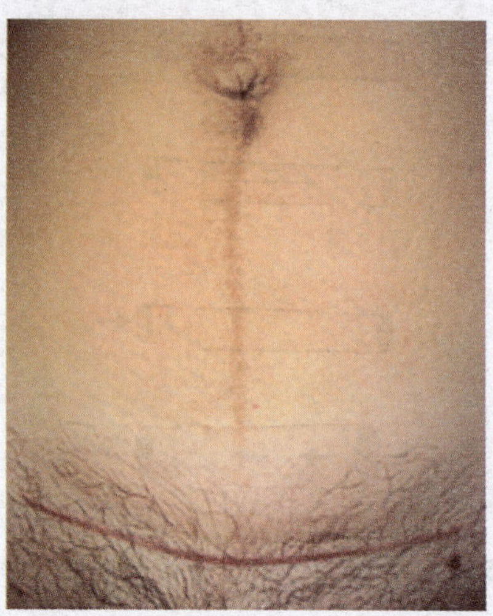

FIG. 5.96 Cesarean section scar and linea nigra

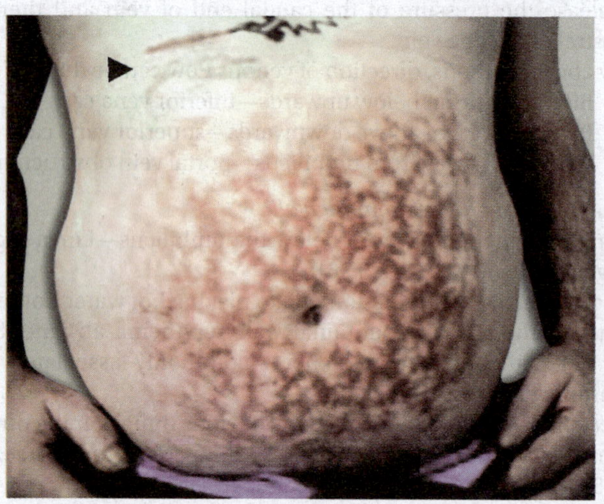

FIG. 5.97 Erythema ab igne

- Palpate the abdomen on following areas:
  Right upper quadrant to left upper quadrant, then down to left lower quadrant, then to right lower quadrant finally ending in periumbilical region.

Cross palpation (testing for pain in right lower quadrant while palpating left upper quadrant) may be more important for eliciting pain (Rovsing's sign).

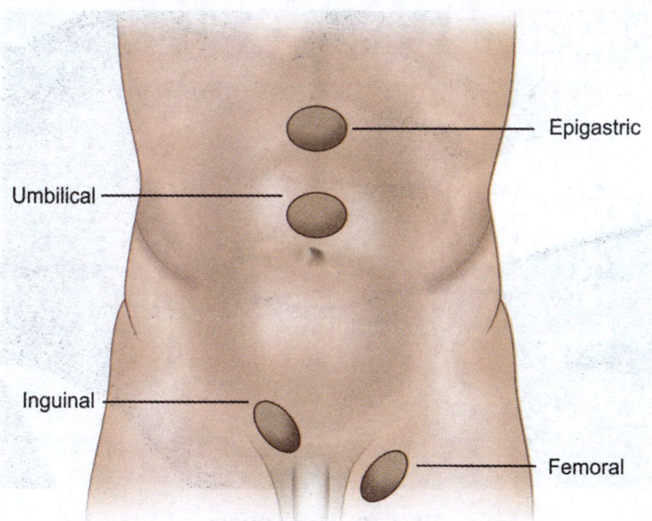

FIG. 5.98 Hernial sites

Types of Palpation

- *Superficial palpation (light palpation):* Palm of the hand rest on abdominal wall gently and fingers are pressed up to 1 cm depth in the abdomen
- *Deep palpation:* Same method of light palpation, but the depth of palpation is more than 1 cm
- *Reinforced palpation:* Pushing on the fingers of the palpating hand with the fingers of the other hand placing them above the former fingers.

Light Palpation (Fig. 5.99)

- The entire abdomen should be symmetrically palpated by ulnar border or pads of fingers of right hand not by fingertips
- Jabs to be avoided
- Fingers should be always together during palpation
- Hands should be lifted from the examination area very gently
- This palpation should be done during both phases of respiration.

Light palpation should be done to defect:

- Stiffness of rectus abdominis muscles
- To detect superficial lump tenderness
- To detect rebound tenderness.

Usually during expiration, respiratory muscles are relaxed and soften. If during expiration, muscle is rigid, this is called rigidity.

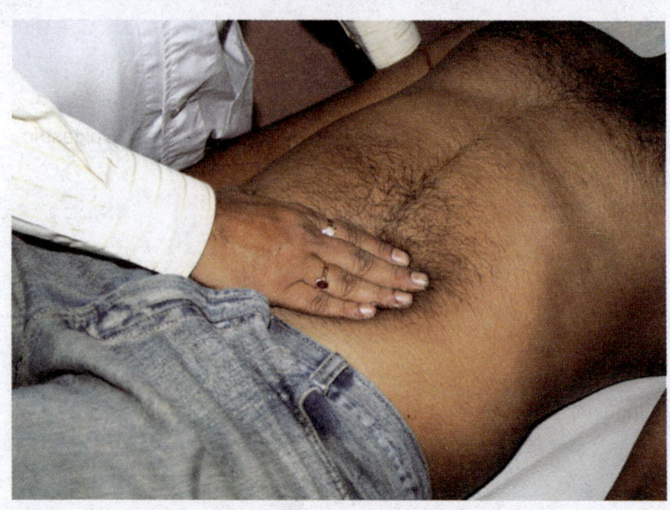

FIG. 5.99 Light palpation

It may be:
- Localized—as over inflamed appendix or gallbladder.
- Generalized—over whole abdomen—generalized peritonitis—in this case the abdomen will be board-like.

In few cases stroking the abdomen gently with pin—may produce increased sensation due to inflammation of parietal peritoneum. This is called hyperesthesia.

Differentiation between intra-abdominal masses and intramural masses (Fig. 5.100):
- Place the right hand over the abdominal mass.
- Ask the patient to elevate his head from the bed. This produces tensing of abdominal wall muscles.
- This pushes intra-abdominal mass in ward but parietal mass will be prominent.

Detection of Abdominal Aortic Aneurysm (Fig. 5.101)

- Place both the hands over the epigastria area, parallel to recti muscles, fingers pointing towards patient's head.

  This position is required, because aortic bifurcation is above umbilical region.
- As a result of expansile pulsation, your hands will be apart away from each other.
- In case of horizontal pulsation, hands will not be apart, only there is lifting—seen in normal thin built patient.

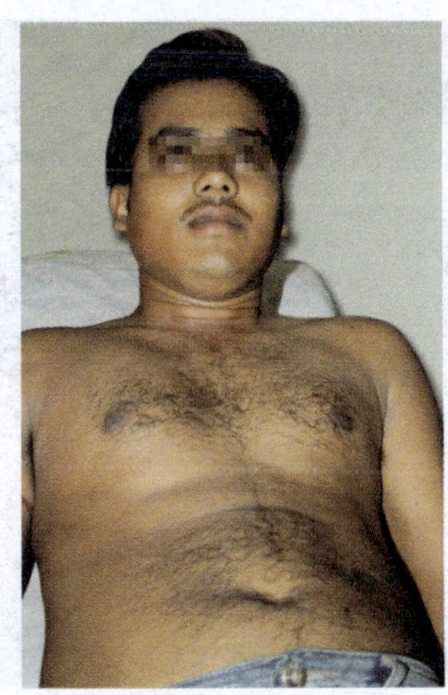

FIG. 5.100   Differentiation between intra-abdominal and intramural masses

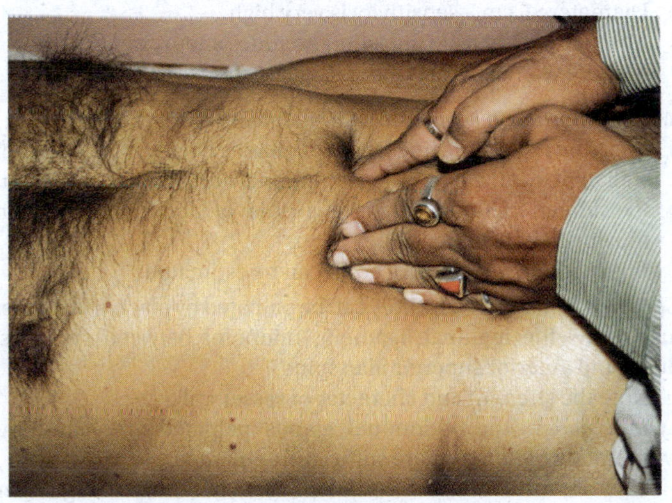

FIG. 5.101   Abdominal aorta palpation

According to Diameter of Aneurysm

- Diameter of expansile mass <3 cm—this method is positive. (Diameter of pulsation reflects the diameter of aneurysm).
- Diameter 3–5 cm—finding is very specific.
  False positive—reflects tortuous aorta.

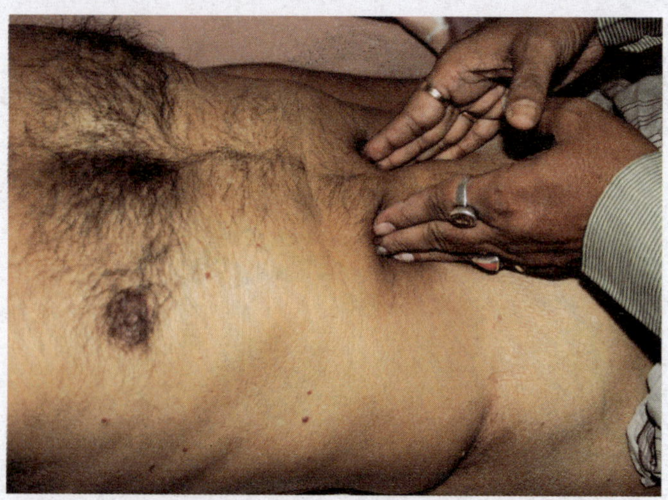

FIG. 5.102 Width of abdominal aorta detection

- Diameter >5 cm—sensitivity is very high.
  Absence of expansile pulsation excludes aneurysm.
  In these women with lumbar lordosis aorta is easily palpable.

Width of aorta can be measured by following manner (Fig. 5.102):
- Press the expanding fingers of both hands deeply into abdominal wall to detect the left wall of abdominal aorta and its pulsation.
- By similar methods detect rightside of abdominal aorta by moving fingers to right side.

By this method, pulsation of aorta can be estimated.

Common femoral vessels: They can be palpated by placing the fingers just below the inguinal ligament, midpoint between symphysis pubis and anterior superior iliac spine.

Note the strength and character of vessel wall.

Lymph nodes: The abdominal glands palpated are para-aortic lymph nodes when they are sufficiently enlarged.

They are firm, rounded, confluent, fixed in umbilical region and epigastric region along left border of aorta.

Palpation of liver: During liver palpation—following information should be sought.
- Size
- Shape
- Margin
- Surface
- Consistency
- Tenderness.

Method of palpation of liver: Only lower border of liver can be palpated, because, upper border of liver is under rib cage, thus beyond the reach of examiner's finger.

The following approaches to palpate the liver are:

- *Cephalad approach (Fig. 5.103):*
  - ❖ Place the right hand on right hypochondrium in such a position that ulnar border is parallel to rectus muscles and direction of finger towards the head
  - ❖ Left hand should be placed on patient's back to support it
  - ❖ Ask the patient to take deep breath.

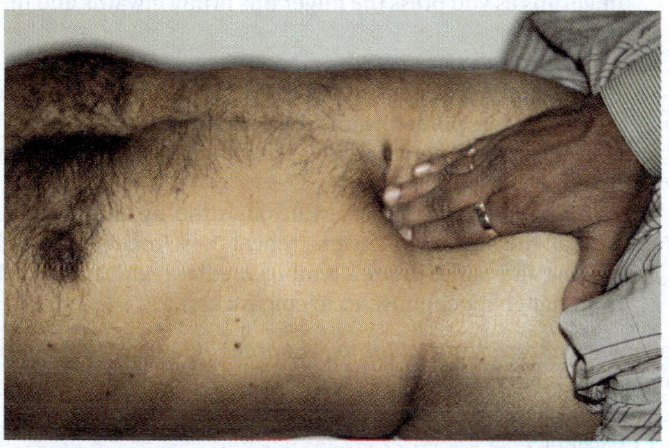

FIG. 5.103 Liver palpation with fingers towards head

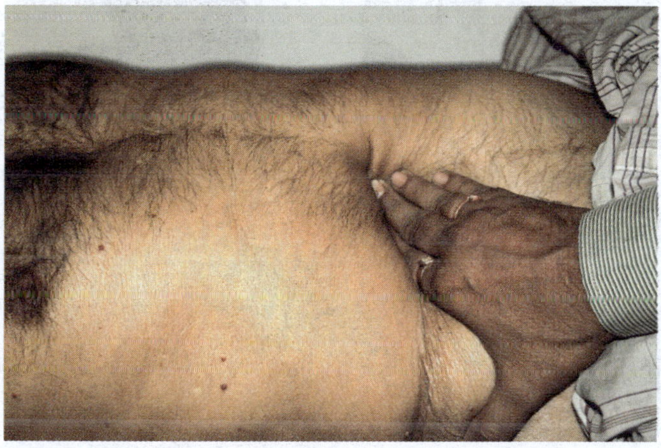

FIG. 5.104 Liver palpation with radial border of hand

- ❖ During deep inspiration, respiratory excursion of the diaphragm displaces the liver edge downward, so it will come in contact with fingertips, as you press the fingertips firmly inwards and then upwards.
- *Transverse approach (Fig. 5.104):*
  - ❖ Place your hand on right upper abdomen in such a way that its ulnar border parallels with costal margin and fingertips pointing towards flank.
  - ❖ Place the left hand on the patient's back to support it.
  - ❖ Here interior border of liver will touch hand's margin.

    Remember that Hand's margin is not as sensitive as fingertips as you press the finger tips firmly inwards and then upwards.
- *Hooking methods (Fig. 5.105):*
  - ❖ Place your both hands in such a way in right hypochondrium so that, fingers point towards the patient's feet.
  - ❖ Now try to hook gently while asking the patient to take deep breath.

    Inferior margin of liver will touch the tip of the fingers with all the above maneuvers, repeat these maneuvers while moving the hands from lateral to medial regions and cross from right hypochondrium to epigastrium.

Following characteristics of the lower border of liver can be assessed from above maneuvers:
- Sharpness
- Consistency

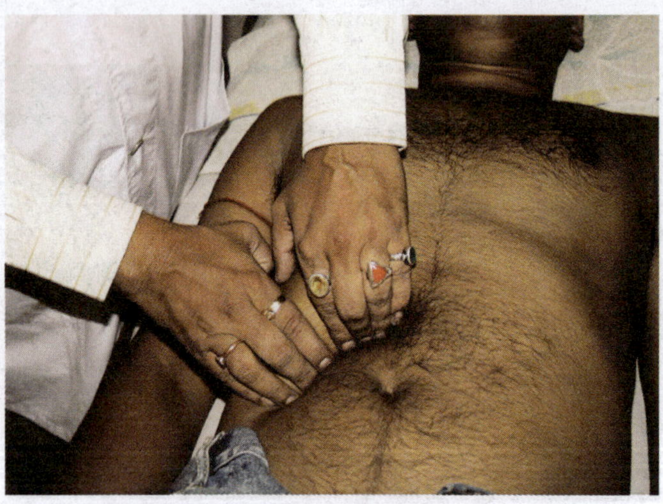

FIG. 5.105 Liver palpation by hooking method

- Tenderness
- Abnormalities of surfaces
- Presence of systolic pulsations
- Presence of friction rub and thrills.

Tenderness may occur from:
Congestion of liver—due to distension of the hepatic capsules.

Significance of firm and hard margin of liver:
- Very hard margin—tumor
- Sharp margin—cirrhosis
- Margin neither sharp nor hard—congestive
- *Nodules on the liver:*
  - ❖ Large nodules nontender—neoplasm, metastatic carcinoma
  - ❖ Small nodules—cirrhosis.

Pulsatile liver: Transmissions of aortic pulsations through the enlarged liver. The conditions responsible are:
- Tricuspid regurgitation
- Constrictive pericarditis.

Above two conditions can be distinguished by:
Inspiratory increase in systolic pulsation magnitude seen in tricuspid regurgitations (especially held in mid or late inspiration) but not in constrictive pericarditis.

In tricuspid regurgitation, hepatic movement can be felt as double movement of liver edge:
- One with jugular 'V' wave at the neck.
- Strong diastolic dip immediately after carotid pulse.

Presence of pulsation of liver in presence of hepatomegaly indicates. Constrictive pericarditis. Absence of it eventually excludes the diagnosis.

Palpability of inferior border of liver is nonspecific, because it can be palpable in following conditions in absence of hepatomegaly:
- Chronic obstructive lung disease
- Pleural effusion
- Pneumothorax.

So, to diagnose a case of hepatomegaly:
- Palpate inferior border of liver
- Detect the upper border of liver by light percussion
  But in case, where lower border cannot be palpated, only percussion method is available to detect upper and lower border of liver
- Measure the distance in cm in midclavicular line.

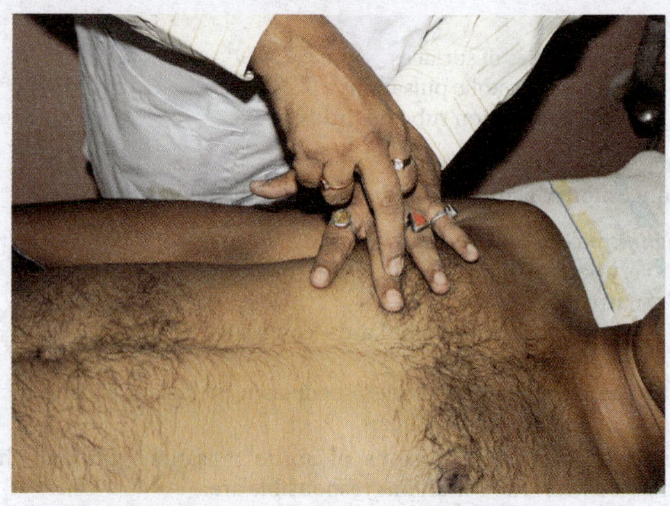

FIG. 5.106 Percussion method of liver

Percussion Method of Liver (Fig. 5.106)

- Distal interphalangeal joint of left middle finger is placed on the intercostal space in right midclavicular line.
    [To avoid damping of vibrations while finger is not placed]
- Opposite middle finger is used as plexor
- Light percussion should be done in right midclavicular line from above downwards during normal breathing
- Change percussion note from resonant (lung parenchyma) to dull (liver) indicates the upper border of liver
- Again, continuing percussion downwards, change of note from dull (liver) to tympanic note (air in intestine) indicates lower border of liver
- The normal distance between upper and lower border of liver is <12–13 cm on midclavicular line.

Problems Regarding Liver

Jaundice: It is defined as yellow to range discoloration of skin and mucous membrane and bulbar conjunctiva. Traditionally, three types of jaundice:

1. Pale yellow—hemolytic jaundice.
2. Orange yellow—hepatocellular jaundice.
3. Yellow green—obstructive jaundice.

The pseudojaundice is due to:
- *Subconjunctival fat:* This is collection of yellow fat in conjectural folds, never to pericorneal region.

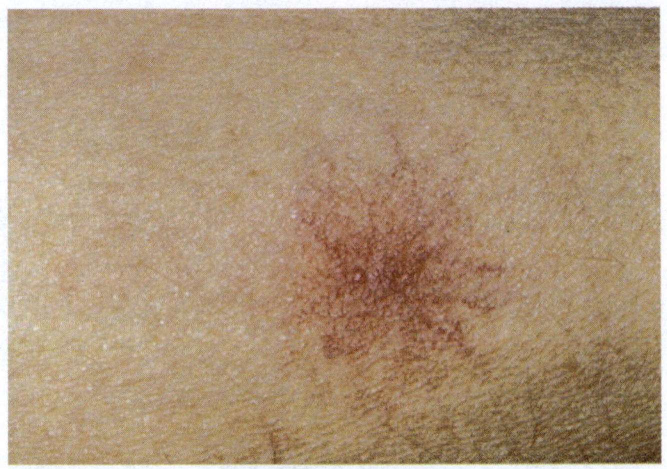

FIG. 5.107   Spider nevus

- *Hypercarotenemia:* This is due to excessive ingestion of carrots or pigmented fruits and vegetables. It involves palms, soles, nasolabial folds, but spares conjunctiva.

Spider nevi (Fig. 5.107): Intense blushing over the face, neck, shoulder, arms and torso, rare in the palms, scalp, never below umbilicus. It consists of central arteriole (body of the spider), and radiating vessels (legs of spider).

Size: Pinhead size to 0.5 cm in diameter. There can be blanched by giving pressure by the pin head to central arteriole.

They can be differentiated from:
Cherry angioma: Round venous, associated with aging.

The conditions where spider nevi are commonly found:
- Liver disease—alcoholic cirrhosis
  Combination of alcohol and hepatitis C associated
- Pregnancy—2nd to 5th months of gestation
- Thyrotoxicosis
- Malnutrition.

Mechanisms involved in cirrhosis are:
- Increased ratio of serum estradiol to testosterone.
- High levels of substance – P.

Palmar erythema (Fig. 5.108): Symmetrical reddening of thenar and hypothenar eminences, coexisting with spider nevi, waxes and wanes.

Dupuytren's contracture (Fig. 5.109):
- This is slowly progressive fibroproliferative disease
- Thickening of ulnar side of palmar fascia

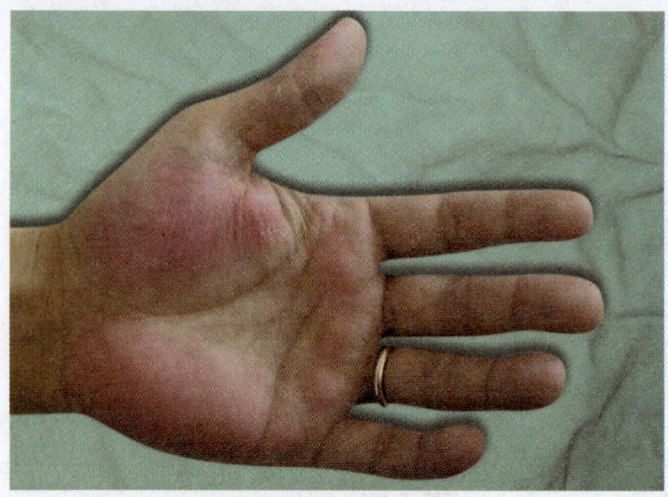

FIG. 5.108 Palmar erythema

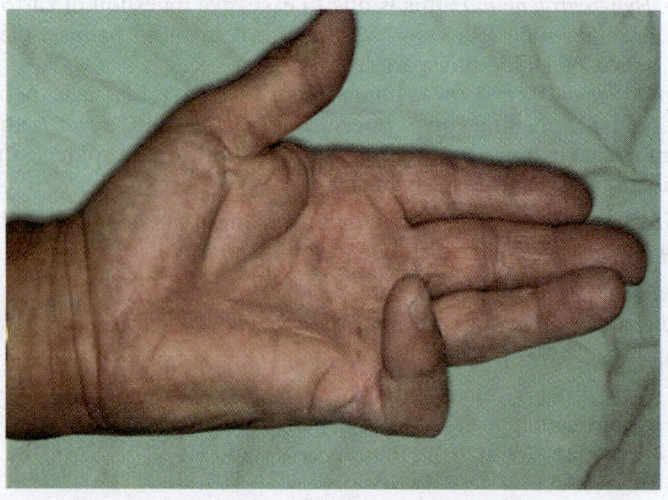

FIG. 5.109 Dupuytren's contracture

- Usually bilateral, may be unilateral, where it involves right side
- Contraction of fourth and fifth digits:
  - ❖ Flexion deformity of metacarpophalangeal joints
  - ❖ Flexion deformity of proximal interphalangeal joints
- There may be firm pulmonary nodules, palpable cords proximal to nodules

- Males are predominantly affected
- 10–15 percent of adult and young children.

Asterixis: Ask the patient to stretch the arms, at the same time holding the fingers spread apart as they are stopping traffic.

In case of asterixis, fingers and hands starts flapping in myoclonic fashion.

Brisk movement occurs at an interval of less than 1 second to more than 1 second.

Fetor hepaticus: It is a special odor coming out of the mouth in hepatocellular disease with porto-systemic shunt.

If occurs due to accumulation of dimethylsulfide in the breath—simulating rotten egg and garlic.

Auscultation of liver: This detects:

- *Hepatic friction rub:* This is rare finding. It may occur:
  - ❖ Hepatoma
  - ❖ Ten percent cases of metastasis
  - ❖ Much less common in localized or disseminated inflammatory processes.
- *Hepatic arterial murmur:* It occurs in:
  - ❖ Hepatoma
  - ❖ Hepatic secondary
  - ❖ In few cases hepatitis.

Hepatic venous hum: If indicates the presence of portal hypertension.

Difference between venous hum and arterial murmur:

- Arterial murmur is systolic
  Venous hum is both systolic and diastolic
- Venous hum originates from a communication between umbilical vein and abdominal wall veins.

Gallbladder

Normally gallbladder cannot be palpated. The gallbladder may be palpated in the following situations:

- *Mucocele of gallbladder:* When gallstone is impacted at the neck of uninfected, collapsed, empty gallbladder. Mucus is continuously secreted into the gallbladder making it distended and palpated.
- *Carcinoma head of pancreas:* This enlarged head of pancreas compresses and obstructs the common bile duct, making gallbladder passively distended.
- Carcinoma of common bile duct.
- *Carcinoma of gallbladder:* Here gallbladder becomes stony hard and irregular.

Method of palpation of position of distended gallbladder:
- Distended gallbladder can be palpated as firm, smooth, rough or globular swelling.
- Its borders just lateral to edge of rectus abdominis near the tip of right 9th costal cartilage.
- It moves with respiration.
- Its lower border is usually palpated; upper border merges with interior border of liver or disappears beneath costal cartilage.
- In case of gross hepatomegaly and hugely distended gallbladder, gallbladder may be palpated in right lumbar region or even in right iliac fossa.

Murphy's sign: There is inspiratory arrest in painful inspiration, when edge of inflamed gallbladder is being touched.

Method:
- Ask the patient to take deep breath
- You press your finger in right costal margin, along the mid-clavicular line, fingers point towards patient's head
- As soon as you touch the inflamed edge of gallbladder, there is catch of hold of patient's breath, and arrest of respiration.

Significance of Murphy's sign: It is highly accurate.

Its significance increases—when patient with acute cholecystitis present with nausea, vomiting right upper quadrant pain.

Sonographic Murphy's sign: During ultrasonography the examiner locates the gallbladder and detects whether it corresponds to the point of maximum tenderness by pressing the gallbladder directly with ultrasound transducer.

Scratch test to elicit liver edge (Fig. 5.110): The diaphragm of stethoscope is held with the left hand of the examiner—below the right costal margin over the liver.

The examiner listens through the stethoscope; right index finger scratches the abdominal wall at a semicircular distance from the stethoscope. As finger scratches over the liver edge, there is marked increase in intensity of sound.

Abnormal liver shape:

Sometimes a tongue like projection from right lobe of the liver projects towards right iliac crest—this is called Riedel's lobe—anatomical variant.

It is more common in female, palpable as mobile mass on right side of the abdomen. It moves with respiration.

Riedel's can be misdiagnosed as right kidney to be resolved by ultrasonography.

Small size of the liver: It can be detected when:
- Lower border cannot be palpable
- On percussion, liver dullness of lower margin is well above right costal margin.

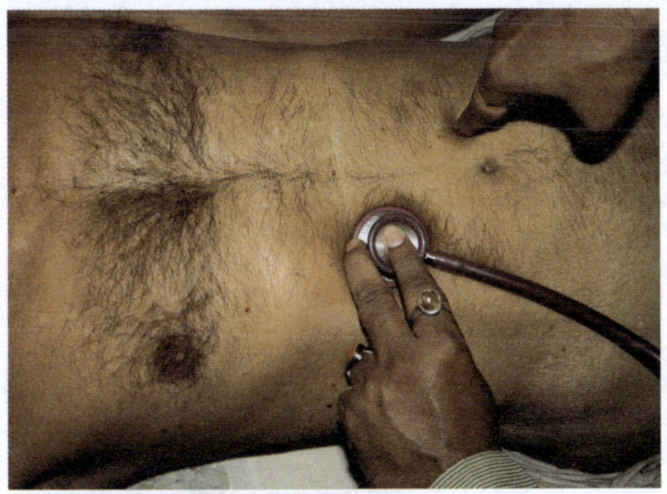

FIG. 5.110   Scratch test to detect edge of the liver

Causes of small liver:
- Micronodular postnecrotic cirrhosis
- Fulminant hepatitis
- Toxic hepatitis.

Palpation of Spleen

Normal spleen cannot be palpated unless it will be increased 2–3 times normal in size. Spleen enlarges inferior and posterior direction to become palpable subcostally.

Spleen enlarges along its axis towards right iliac fossa.

Methods of Palpation (Figs 5.111A to C)

- Patient should lie in supine position
- Expose the abdomen sufficiently to palpate abdominal organs
- Place your left hand around the back and side of the lower rib cage to:
    - ❖ Provide support of rib cage
    - ❖ Elevate spleen anteriorly.
- Start examination from umbilical region toward left anterior axillary line along splenic axis
- Place the right hand anteriorly and obliquely across the abdomen with finger tips pointing at left costal margin towards axilla
- Ask the patient to take deep breath, at the same time give moderate amount of pressure with right index and middle fingers inwards and upwards

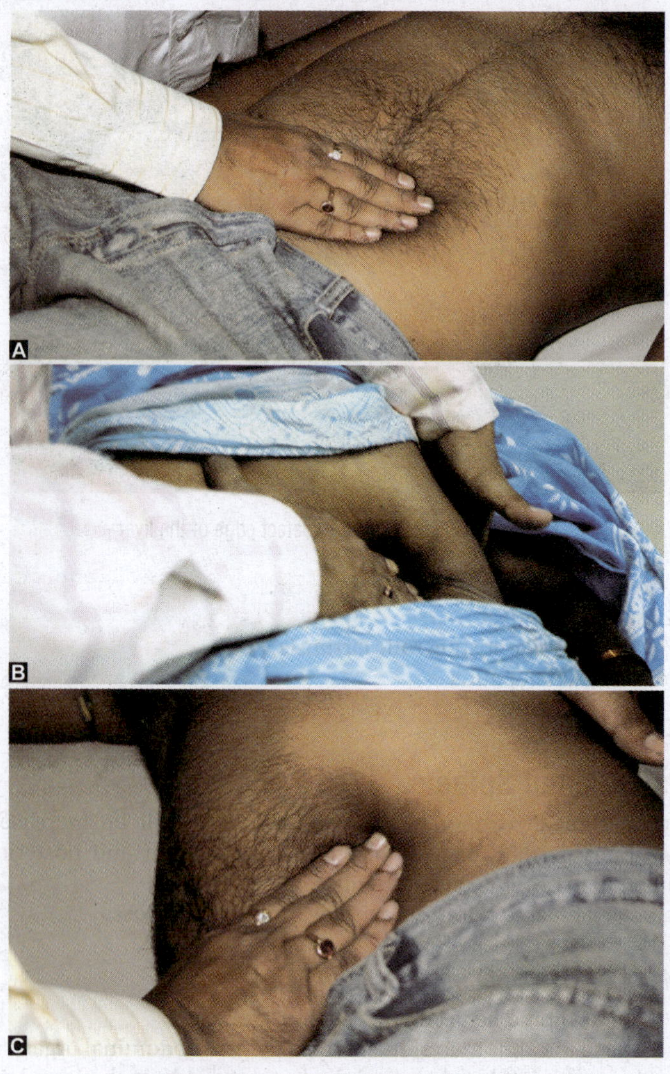

FIGS 5.111A TO C Methods of palpation of spleen

- At the midpoint of inspiratory effort, avoid or lessen inward pressure, only maintain upward pressure, allowing the fingers to drift in the direction of enlarging spleen
- The notched leading edge of spleen can be felt as passing under the fingers
- If spleen is impalpable, at the start point, move the fingers of right hands progressively closure to left lower rib cage

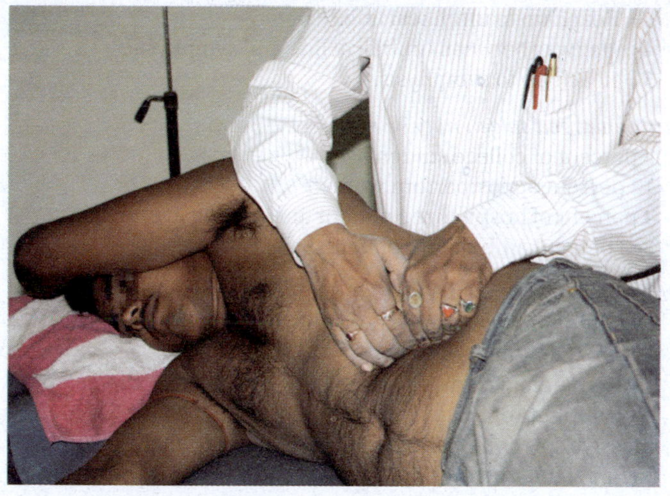

FIG. 5.112 Hooking method of palpation of spleen

- If the spleen cannot be palpated in this position, patient should be moved to lie on right lateral position with flexed knee and hip, and elevates the left hand upwards above the head to increase the area of palpation
- This maneuver helps the minor to moderately enlarged spleen to gravitate anteriorly and downwards position
- Now the examiner place his left hands on the patient's left costal margin and right hand palpates in left quadrant.

Other methods of palpation: Palpation from above (Fig. 5.112).

- Ask the patient to lie in supine position or right lateral decubitus position
- Stand on the left side of the patient
- Point all finger towards patient's feet, and try to hook the spleen gently with both hands while ask the patient to take deep breath

One Hand Hook Technique

This method should detect enlarged spleen weeks before it becomes palpable by other conventional maneuvers.

As soon as splenic tip will be palpated, this should be diagnosed as splenomegaly.

Spleen size is progressively graded according to position of spleen during palpation:

    0 = Not palpable.
    1 = Palpable only after deep inspiration.
    2 = Reaching between left costal margin and a line halfway to the umbilical line.

3 = Reach up to umbilical line.
4 = Halfway between umbilical line and symphysis.
5 = Reach up to symphysis.

Truly enlarged spleen may be normal in:
- 3 percent of college students
- 12 percent of postpartum women
- 4 percent of hospitalized patient undergoing liver scans
- 2–3 percent ambulatory patients.

Other findings help to identify the cause of splenomegaly:
- Concomitant hepatomegaly signify primary liver disease
- Lymphadenopathy signify:
  ❖ Hematological disorders
  ❖ Lymphoproliferative disorders.
- Massive splenomegaly myeloproliferative etiology.
- Kehr's sign—splenic rupture.

Causes of splenomegaly:
- Portal hypertension.
- *Infection:*
  ❖ Bacterial—tuberculosis
  Subacute bacterial endocarditis.
  ❖ Malaria.
- Chronic myeloid leukemia.
- Chronic lymphatic leukemia.
- Myelofibrosis.
- Storage disease.
- Hemolytic anemia.

Kehr's sign: There is referred pain to left shoulder due to left crus of diaphragmatic irritation—splenic rupture with intraperitoneal spillage of blood.

Percussion of Spleen

There are three techniques of percussion to get splenic dullness in case of enlargement:

1. *Nixon technique (Fig. 5.113):*
   ❖ Patient should be in right lateral decubitus position. As a result spleen will come above stomach and colon.
   ❖ Percussion will be initiated at lowest level of pulmonary resonance in posterior axillary line.
   ❖ Line of percussion will be oblique along a line perpendicular to lowest mid anterior costal margin.
   ❖ Normally, upper border of splenic dullness is 6–8 cm above left costal margin.

If it is more than 8 cm → It indicates splenic enlargement.

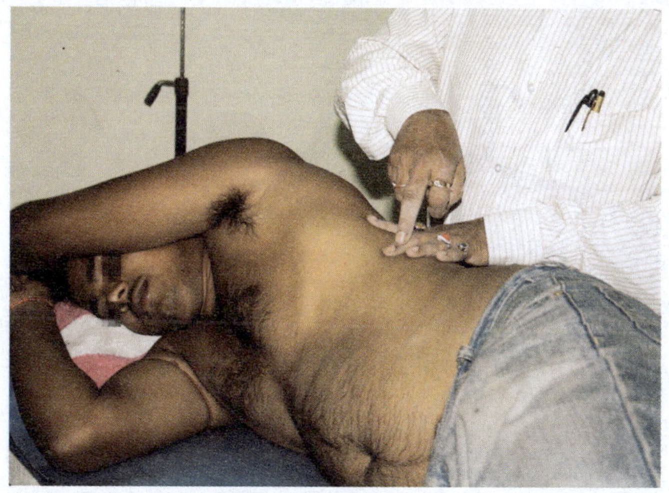

FIG. 5.113   Nixon technique

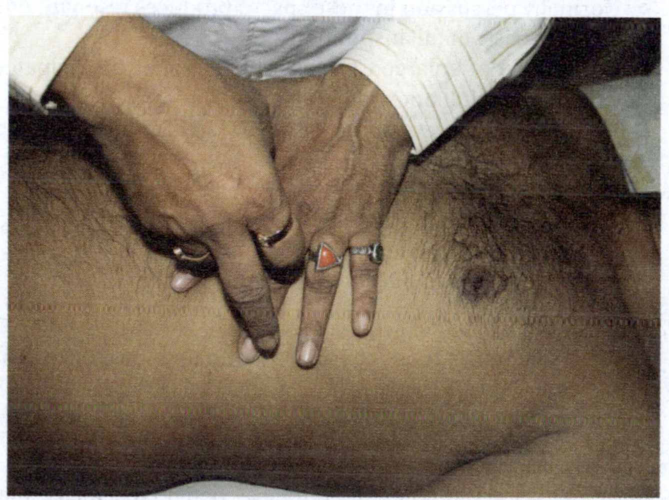

FIG. 5.114   Castell's technique

- *Castell's technique (Fig. 5.114):*
  - ❖ The patient should be in supine position
  - ❖ Ask the patient to breathe deeply
  - ❖ Percussion will be started at 8th or 9th intercostal space in anterior axillary line
  - ❖ Percussion will be carried out in both phase of respiration

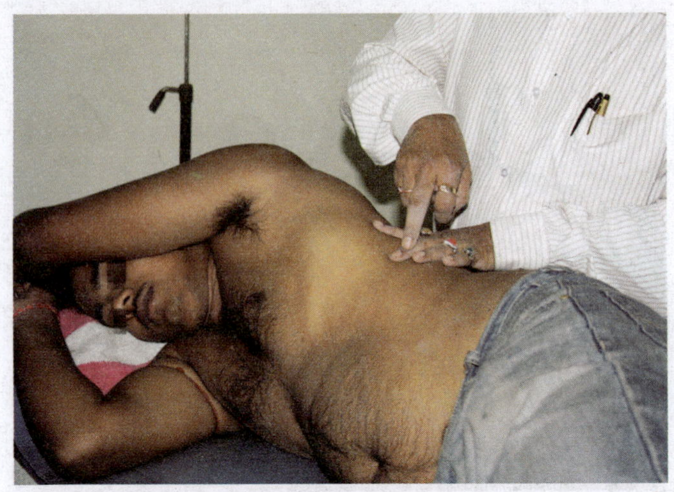

FIG. 5.115 Percussion in Traube's space

- ❖ Normally percussion in these spaces produces resonant note and it persists in full inspiration
- ❖ But in case of enlarged spleen which cannot the palpated, usually elicit dull note in this area.
- *Percussion in Traube's space (Fig. 5.115):* Traube's space is bounded by:
  - ❖ Sixth rib superiorly
  - ❖ Left mid-axillary line laterally
  - ❖ Left costal margin inferiorly.

  Percussion in this area may detect: Splenomegaly.

Values of above method of percussions:
- Castell's method is more sensitive than palpation (82% versus 71%) but less specific
- Nixon's method is more specific than palpation, but less sensitive.

Recommendation for bedside assessment of splenic size:
- Both palpation and percussion have better specificity than sensitivity
- Palpation is most accurate
- Percussion is adjunct to palpation. So both methods are complementary to each other.

Auscultation of Spleen (Fig. 5.116)

Auscultation of spleen is usually done to detect:
- Rub—in case of splenic infarct—producing irritation of visceral peritoneum.

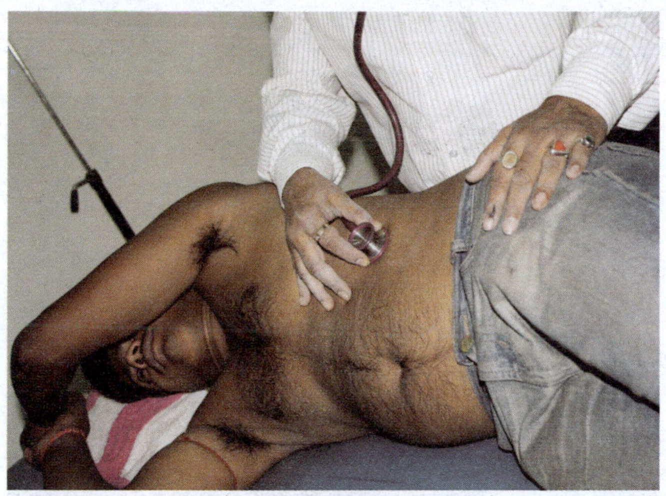

FIG. 5.116 Auscultation of spleen

- *Murmur:*
  - ❖ Massive splenomegaly
  - ❖ Carcinoma of the pancreas compressing splenic artery.

Stomach

Two methods to detect gastric retentions:

1. *Clapotage:* It is a splashing sound produced by movement of fluid within stomach cavity. It can be elicited by following method (Figs 5.117A and B):
   - ❖ Epigastric should be relaxed and properly exposed
   - ❖ Tapping should be done with two fingers apposed together
   - ❖ Tapping should be started in lower abdomen little left to midline
   - ❖ From there tapping should be progressed upwards up to xiphoid process
   - ❖ Splash only can be elicited in first few tapping. Later on it will be blunted as muscle guarding will occur.
2. *Succussion splash (Fig. 5.118):* It is also a type of splashing sound by elicited by making movement of stomach content. It can be elicitated by:
   - ❖ Place the diaphragm of stethoscope on the epigastrium little left to midline
   - ❖ Hold the patient's flank of abdomen and jerk it from right to left
   - ❖ *In empty stomach:* It is absent

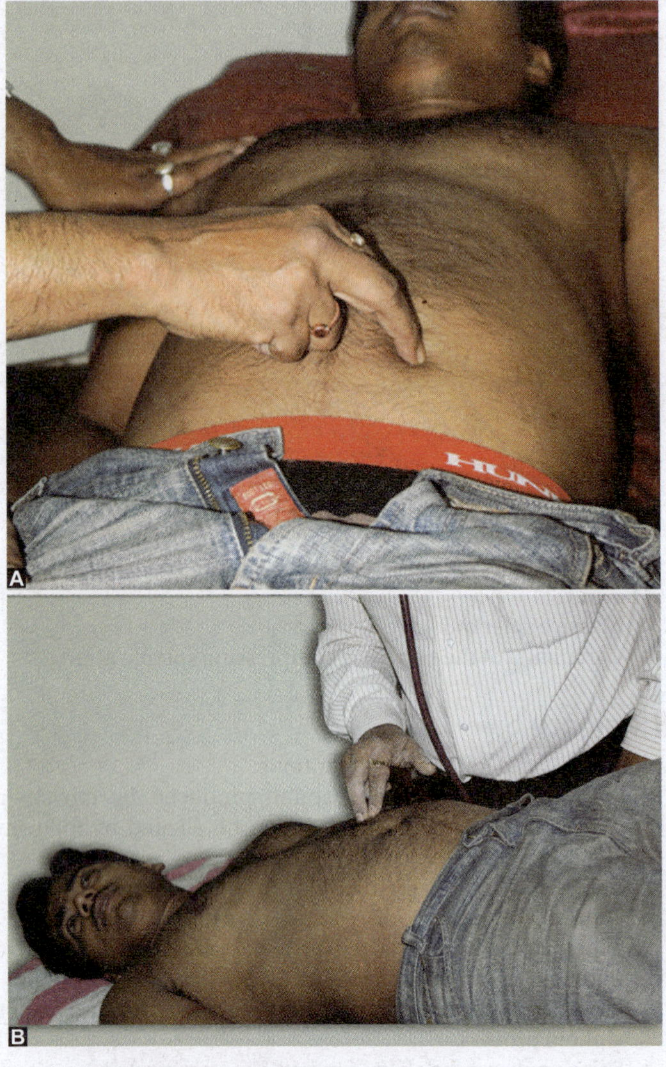

FIGS 5.117A AND B Detection of gastric retention

* It can diagnose delay in gastric emptying if:
  * It present after 5 hours of full meal
  * It present 2 hours after taking a glass of water.

It can be frequently false positive, if splashing sound can come from other visceral gurgling sound, e.g. small intestine.

So it can be confirmed, by both flat and upright film of abdomen, which can detect air fluid level.

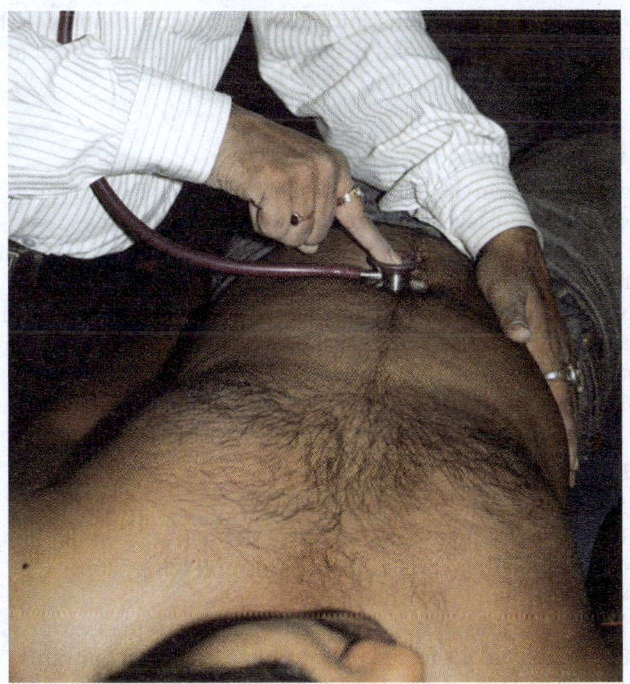

FIG. 5.118　Succussion splash

Other use of auscultation in stomach:
- After nasogastric intubation of Ryle's tube to confirm whether the tube is properly placed in stomach cavity.
- Stomach size can be detected by auscultation of stomach.

Pancreas

Usually pancreas cannot be palpated even in acute pancreatitis, diagnosis is mainly based on—history, related physical signs and laboratory and radiological investigations.

Pancreas can only be palpated in:
- Large pancreatic pseudocyst
- Pancreatic carcinoma.

Other findings of pancreatitis is:
- Cullen's sign
- Grey Turner's sign
- Arching of abdominal wall—Cupid's bow profile.

- Tenderness on percussion of thoracolumbar spine—when patient is lying in lateral decubitus position knees flexed to the chest (Mallet – Guy's sign).

Kidneys

Two kidneys can be palpated is bimanually. Two kidneys are present from the level of T_{12} to L_3 in retroperitoneal area.

Large right lobe of liver displaces the right kidney 2 cm lower than the left kidney.

Normal kidney may be palpated in lean and thin person, right is easier to palpate, because it is present slightly lower than the left kidney, palpation of both kidney requires bimanual palpation.

Examiner must stand on the right side of the patient.

Examination of Kidney (Fig. 5.119)

- Patient should lie in supine position
- Right hand of the examiner is placed anteriorly on left lumbar area and left hand is placed posteriorly on the left loin
- Ask the patient to take deep breath
- At the same time, posteriorly placed left hand is pressed forwards and right hand is pressed upwards, backwards and inwards
- When left kidney is enlarged, round firm swelling can be felt between right and left hands
- When kidney is pushed by one hand to other hand it is called balloting.

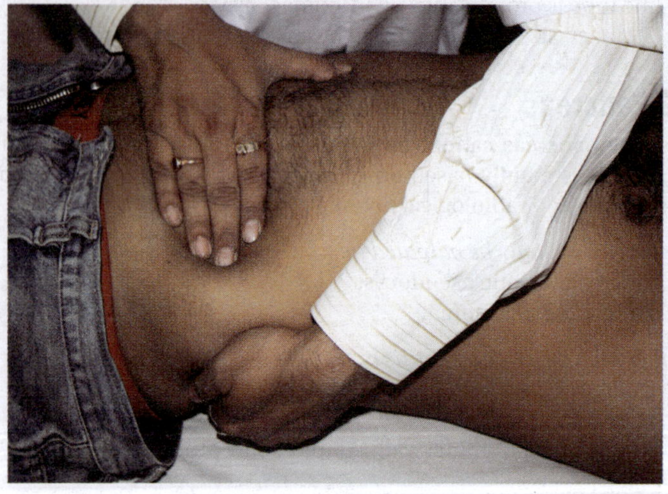

FIG. 5.119 Examination of kidney

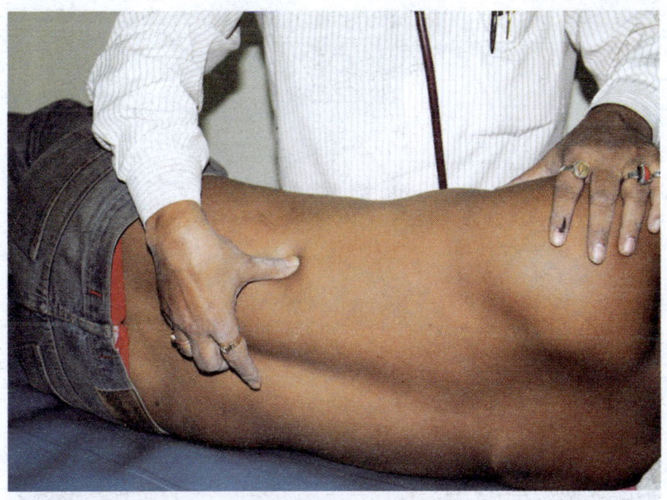

FIG. 5.120 Detection of costophrenic angle

In case of right kidney
Similar method of palpation is used. But right kidney can be palpated in thin person as smooth, round swelling, which descends on inspiration.

Method of percussion of costophrenic angle: Strike the costophrenic angle by ulnar aspect of your hand—can elicit tenderness (Fig. 5.120).

Causes of costophrenic angle tenderness:
- Acute pyelonephritis
- Any condition that distends or irritates renal capsule:
  - Perinephric abscess
  - Renal infarction
  - Hypernephroma.

Auscultation of kidneys: Auscultation is usually done to exclude renovascular disease which can be diagnosed if murmur can be heard.
- *Anterior systolic murmur:* Renal arterial bruit is heard at a point 2.5 cm above and lateral to umbilicus in:
  - Atherosclerotic disease
  - Fibromuscular hyperplasia.
  This is less specific, but more sensitive.
- *Posterior systolic murmur:* It is localized between the lumber column and costal margin. Its presence is highly specific of renovascular disease. It is highly specific, but less sensitive.

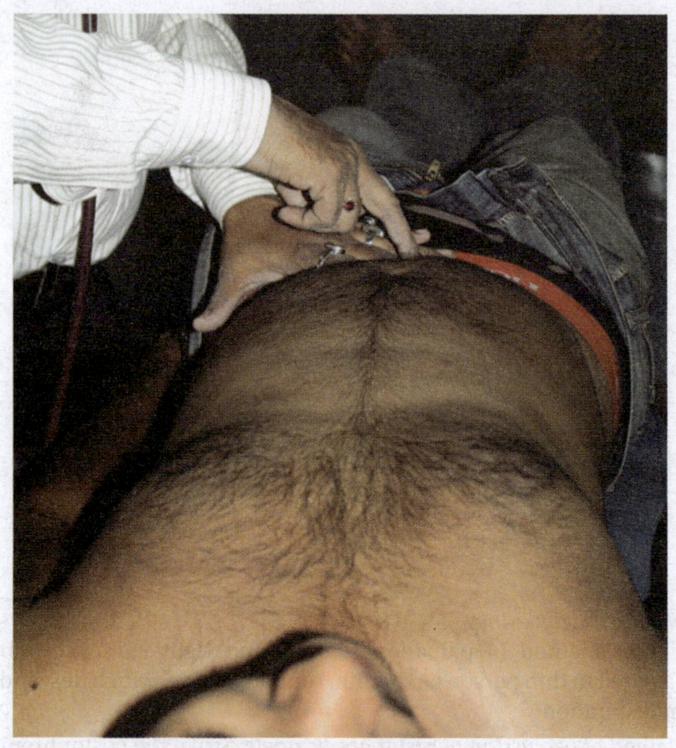

FIG. 5.121   Percussion of urinary bladder

Urinary Bladder

Normally urinary bladder cannot be palpated. But if there is any outflow obstruction the bladder will be distended above symphysis pubis in suprapubic area, then urinary bladder can be palpated.

Methods of Percussion of Urinary Bladder (Fig. 5.121)

- *Subjective palpation:*
  - ❖ Patient will lie in supine position
  - ❖ Start percussion from above downwards from umbilicus up to symphysis pubis
  - ❖ If the patient urge to urinate—it indicates the funds of the bladder has been reached.
- *Objective palpation:*
  - ❖ Patient will lie in supine position
  - ❖ Short percussion from the umbilicus along the midline towards symphysis pubis.

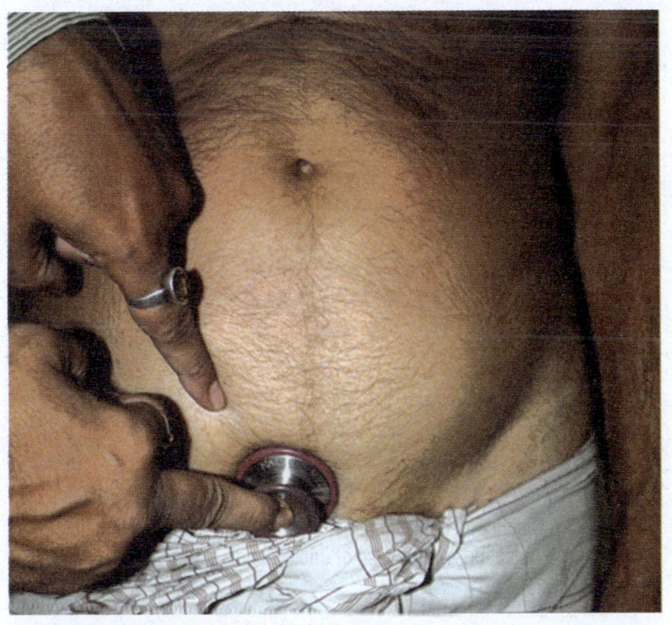

FIG. 5.122   Auscultatory percussion of the urinary bladder

❖ The area is usually tympanic, but, if the bladder is full, the area, above the symphysis pubis is dull depending upon the amount of urine accumulated in the bladder.

The full bladder can be felt as globular smooth swelling above the symphysis pubis.

- *Auscultatory percussion (Fig. 5.122):* This is a combination of auscultation and percussion to evaluate the upper border of bladder.
  - ❖ Place the diaphragm of stethoscope in the midline above the symphysis pubis
  - ❖ Start scratching from umbilicus downwards and then in radiating fashion centering umbilicus
  - ❖ The points at which scratching sound intensify—indicates the upper border of urinary bladder
  - ❖ Otherwise, if superior border of bladder is identified, rest of the globular shaped margin can be readily defined from adjacent bowel, which is resonant.

Palpation of Aorta (Fig. 5.123)

Descending aorta emerges through aortic hiatus in the diaphragm descends by the side of vertebral bodies up to L_4 where it bifurcates into common iliac arteries.

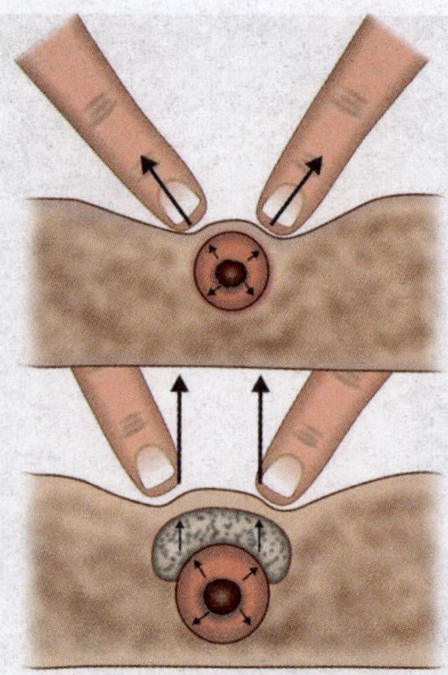

FIG. 5.123 Distinction between direction aortic pulsation and indirect aortic pulsation by presence of understanding structure

It lies adjacent to interior vena cava.

Descending aorta give rise to a number of branches to supply major abdominal organs.

Method of Palpation

- Between the thumb and index finger of one hand
- Placing the fingers of both the hands on both sides of aorta at mid-point between xiphisternum and umbilicus
- Abdominal aorta pulsation can be felt by pressing the fingers posteriorly and slightly medially
- Abdominal aorta may be abnormally prominent in elderly person because marked spinal curvature displaces the aorta anteriorly and laterally.

Ascites

Presence of free fluid in peritoneal cavity is called ascites.

The bedside maneuvers for detection of ascites:

Four maneuvers:

1. *Bulging flank:* Flanks are full due to:
   - Weight of free fluid
   - Gravity effect of the fluid.

   So, in supine position flanks are bulged outwards like a belly of a frog.

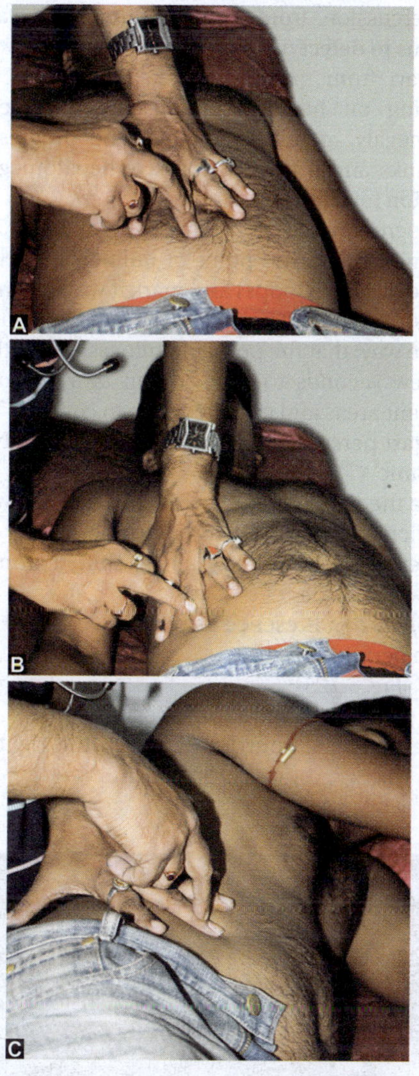

FIGS 5.124A TO C   Detection of shifting dullness

This abdomen may stimulate the abdomen of obese person. The above can be differentiated by shifting dullness maneuver.

2. *Percussion for shifting dullness (Figs 5.124A to C):* The method:
   ❖ Ask the patient to lie in supine position
   ❖ Palpate liver and spleen by above method to defect any massive hepatic or splenic enlargement.

- ❖ Start percussion from xiphisternum downwards towards umbilicus to detect maximum area of tympani
- ❖ Then start from maximum area of tympani to any flank depending on hepatosplenomegaly—if there is massive splenomegaly, percussion should be progressed towards right flanks and if there is massive hepatomegaly, progress percussion towards left side
- ❖ Now progress percussion towards right flank, if there is no hepatomegaly, till the point of dullness (junction between fluid and gas filled loops) and mark it with a pen
- ❖ Now ask the patient to rotate to left lateral decubitus position in such a way; that the point of dullness will be the summit
- ❖ Allow few seconds to fluid to run away towards gravidity dependant areas and gas filled loop to come up
- ❖ Again start percussion from the marked area. Now this area is tympanic
- ❖ Progress the percussion towards midline. You will notice the area which was tympanic, now becomes dull.

The interpretation is free fluid is shifted from left side of abdomen to right side.

Accuracy of the test: Presence of at least 500—1000 mL of fluid is required to perform this test.

3. *Fluid thrill (Fig. 5.125):*
   - ❖ Ask the patient to lie on supine position.
   - ❖ Place left palm of your left hand on the right flank of the patient.

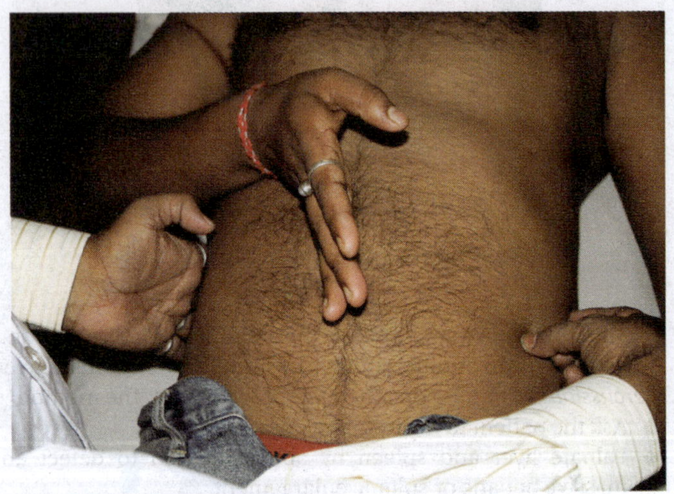

FIG. 5.125 Detection of fluid thrill

- ❖ With the finger of right hand just tap on the right flank of the patient.
- ❖ To prevent transmission of false wave, which usually occurs through abdominal wall by ripples of mesenteric fat towards contralateral side, place the ulnar sides of patient's hands on the midline at the level of umbilicus.

This test is highly specific—90 percent specificity, truly bed side method of diagnosis of ascites.

Dipping methods: This is a maneuver by which the organ may be palpated in patient with huge ascites.

- ❖ Turn the patient towards the side of the organ to be palpated— the organ is liver or spleen.
- ❖ Apply with your fingers a quick pushing motion to the organ to be palpated.
- ❖ Displace the free fluid during deep inspiration and at the same time to palpate the organ.

Puddle Sign (Fig. 5.126)

- Ask the patient to lie in prone position on his/her belly for at least 5 minutes
- Then ask the patient to raise himself by supporting the body with folded knees and elbows
- As a result middle portion of abdomen is pendulous and dependent

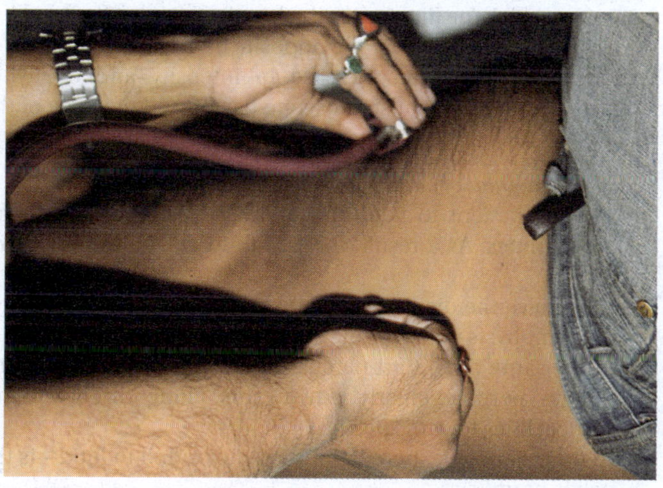

FIG. 5.126   Puddle sign

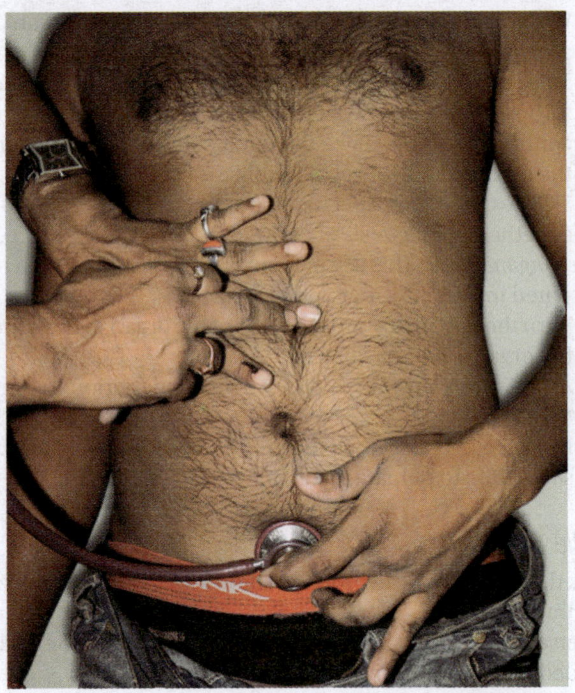

FIG. 5.127 Guarino's method of ascitic fluid detection

- Now place the diaphragm of stethoscope over this area, at the same time, flick the finger over the localized area of flank
- Move the stethoscope over the opposite flank gradually
- When there is sudden increase in intensity and clarity of sound—it indicates that stethoscope has passed the edge of the peritoneal fluid—then this test is positive.

4. *Guarino's method of ascitic fluid determination (Fig. 5.127):*
   ❖ Ask the patient to void and allow him to stand or sit for 3-5 minutes. As a result, the free fluid gravitates into pelvic cavity
   ❖ Now place the diaphragm of stethoscope midline just above the symphysis pubis (pubic crest)
   ❖ At the same time, start percussion the abdomen from costal margin perpendicularly downwards along three anterior vertical lines towards pelvis
   ❖ In normal people, percussion note turns dull to loud—is the pelvic border
   ❖ In patient with ascites this level is raised above the baseline.

Accuracy of diagnosing ascites can be done by:
- Fluid thrill—specificity—80–90 percent, sensitivity—50 percent.
- Shifting dullness—specificity—50 percent, sensitivity—83 percent.

Auscultation of intestinal sounds
- Place the diaphragm of stethoscope on the anterior abdominal wall right of umbilicus and keep it for sometime until sounds can be heard
- Normal peristaltic sound—5–8/minutes
- Keep the diaphragm for at least 1 minute.

Interpretation
- Absent bowel sound—paralytic ileus with abdominal distension.
- Rapid, metallic bowel sound—early stage of mechanical intestinal obstruction may be associated with colicky abdominal pain
- In case progressive bowel obstruction due to accumulation of large amount of gas and fluid—bowel sound will be high pitched and tingling quality—impending bowel paralysis
- In bowel obstruction with strangulation, if gangrene supervenes peristalsis gradually decreases ultimately stops
- In generalized peritonitis, bowel movement disappears; paralytic ileus ensues with gradual abdominal distension.

At the end of this period, examiner can hear the high pitched tingling sound—this indicates transfer of fluid filled loop from one segment to another.

Auscultation of abdominal aorta end its branches (Fig. 5.128)
- Place diaphragm on the abdominal wall over the aorta, above and to the left of umbilicus
- In the iliac fossa for iliac arteries
- In the groin for common femoral arteries.

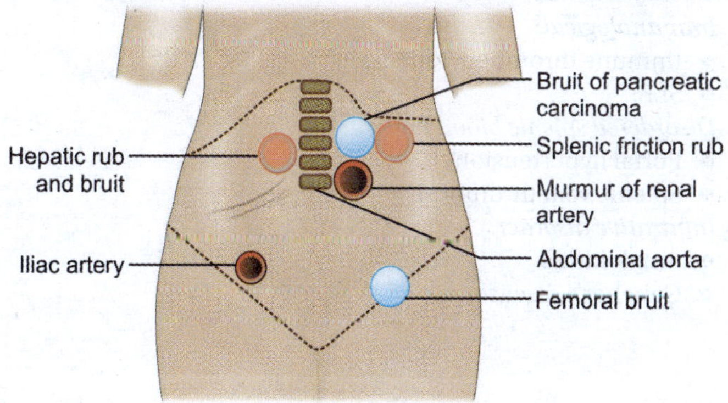

FIG. 5.128 Abdominal bruit and rub

- In the epigastrium for celiac axis or superior mesenteric artery
- On either side of midline in mid abdomen in hypertensive patient for renal artery
- Over the liver form hepatoma.
  Sound is usually murmur or bruit due to narrowing of artery.

Difference between gross ascites and ovarian cyst:
- *Ascites:*
  - ❖ Fullness in flank
  - ❖ Dull in flank
  - ❖ Umbilicus is transversely flushed with skin
  - ❖ Fluid thrill
  - ❖ Shifting dullness.
- *Ovarian cyst:*
  - ❖ No fullness in the flanks
  - ❖ Resonance in the flanks
  - ❖ Umbilicus in vertical and ascends up
  - ❖ No shifting dullness
  - ❖ No fluid thrill
  - ❖ Swelling coming from pelvis so one cannot get lower border.

Causes of splenomegaly
- *Infections:*
  - ❖ Infections mononucleosis
  - ❖ Infective endocarditis
  - ❖ Malaria
  - ❖ Leishmaniasis
  - ❖ Viral hepatitis.
- *Hematological:*
  - ❖ Myeloproliferative disorders
  - ❖ Lymphoma
  - ❖ Spherocytosis
  - ❖ Thalassemia.
- *Immunological:*
  - ❖ Immune thrombocytopenia
  - ❖ SLE.
- *Disordered splenic blood flow:*
  - ❖ Portal hypertension
  - ❖ Splenic vein thrombosis.
- *Infiltrative disorder:*
  - ❖ Amyloidosis
  - ❖ Gaucher's disease.

Differences between left kidney and spleen

Left kidney	Spleen
• Absence of notch	• Presence of notch on medial surface
• Can go upper margin of the mass	• Cannot go upper margin of the mass
• Direction of movement from above downwards	• Move along splenic axis towards right iliac fossa
• Bimanually palpable and ballotable	• Not bimanually palpable but in case of massive splenomegaly, it is ballotable
• Can insinuate finger between costal margin and kidney	• Examiner cannot insinuate finger between costal margin and mass in case of massive splenomegaly
• Lobulated or irregular mass	• Firm mass
• Little movement with respiration	• More movement with respiration

Bowel Sounds

Bowel sounds are produced in:
- Mostly in stomach
- Secondly from large intestine
- Small intestine.

No particular quadrant is necessary for hearing bowel sound because the sounds are transmitted to abdominal wall.

The bowel sounds are produced by:
- Propulsion of food through various part of intestinal segment
- Tone of the intestinal wall.

Difference between arterial bruit or murmur:
Murmur is usually systolic.

Bruit is continuous heard in both phases.

Significance of epigastric murmur:
- *Located in epigastrium:*
  - ❖ Healthy Individual
  - ❖ Pregnancy
  - ❖ Mitral regurgitation.
- *Located between xiphisternum and umbilicus:* Renal artery stenosis.

Significance of right upper quadrant bruit:
- Hepatic tumor
- Hepatic metastasis
- Hepatitis
- Cirrhosis.

- Hepatic arteriovenous fistula
- Tricuspid regurgitation.

The causes are:
- Due to neovascularization
- Due to compression by the cancer mass.

Significance of left upper quadrant bruit:
- Cancer of pancreas
- Vascular anomaly of spleen
- Aneurysmal lesions in abdominal aorta or renal, celiac or mesenteric vessels
- Renal artery stenosis.

Venus hum: It is a continuous sound of venous origin—heard over epigastric and umbilical areas—this is called Cruveilhier-Baumgarten murmur.

Mechanism: Recanalization of umbilical vein in case of portal hypertension results in reverse flow from cirrhotic liver into abdominal wall veins with final decompression into various porto-systemic shunts.

This is aggravated by:
- Forced expiratory phase.
- Valsalva maneuver.

This is softened by: Epigastric pressure.

Cruveilhier-Baumgarten syndrome: This is characterized by acquired reopening of umbilical vein or high flow in paraumbilical or anastomotic veins. This is typical of portal hypertension from cirrhosis.

Cruveilhier-Baumgarten disease: This is characterized by congenital patency of umbilical veins in absence of cirrhosis, ascites, but may have shrunken liver.

▇ Hernia

Two main hernias (Fig. 5.129):
1. More common—femoral hernias.
2. Most frequent—inguinal hernias.

Two types of inguinal hernias
1. *Indirect inguinal hernia:*
   - It occurs in both sexes, all ages, more common in children
   - It originates above inguinal ligament near mid point (in internal inguinal ring) due to defect in the abdominal ring, through which spermatic cord exits the scrotum and enters the pelvis.

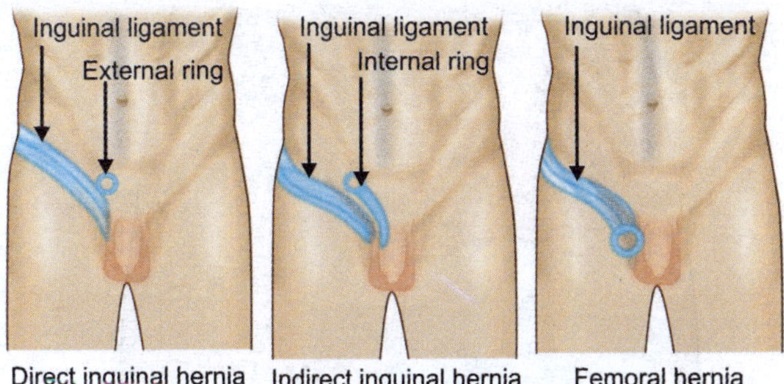

FIG. 5.129   Different types of hernia

2. *Direct inguinal hernia:*
   - ❖ It originates above inguinal ligament through a congenital defect near external inguinal ring and pubic tubercle
   - ❖ It affects persons more than 40 years of age
   - ❖ It rarely progresses to scrotum
   - ❖ It bulges anteriorly.

Method of Detection of Hernia

Inspection
- Ask the patient to stand up
- You should sit by the side of the patient on a chair
- Observe the external ring to see any localized bulging
- If not present, ask the patient to cough or strain or Valsalva maneuver and see whether any bulging is coming out.

Palpation (Fig. 5.130)
- Palpation should be started—right inguinal ring is palpated with right index finger, left inguinal ring is to be palpated with left index finger
- Insert the index finger along the spermatic cord through the invaginated scrotum to reach external inguinal ring
- When you will reach external inguinal ring, put the finger of opposite hand over the inguinal canal or over the swollen area
- Ask the patient to strain and feel whether any impulse is felt by the left hand or size of bulging is increased.
   - ❖ A strong palpable impulse—that pushes the finger outward—direct inguinal hernia.
   - ❖ A soft impulse without any bulge

     Or

     Something coming down through inguinal canal—*indirect inguinal hernia.*

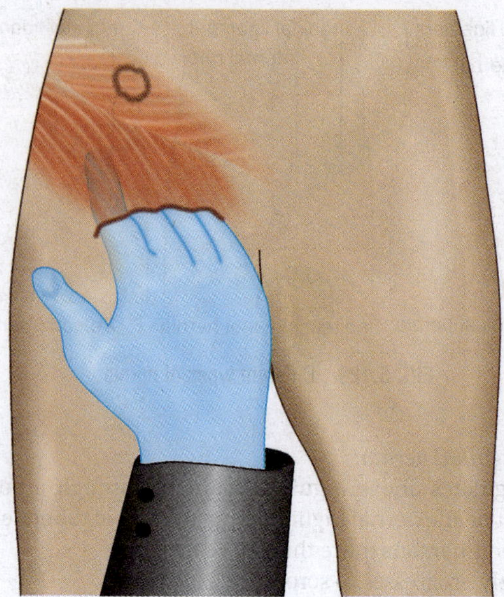

FIG. 5.130 Examination of inguinal floor by insertion of finger through invaginated upper scrotum

Palpation of femoral hernia
- Inserts the index finger and middle finger into femoral triangle lying medial to femoral artery
- A bulge is palpable
- If no bulging is palpable, ask the patient to strain—something coming out and palpable by the finger—*femoral hernia.*

During auscultation over inguinal hernia
If intestine is coming out, bowel sounds can be heard. Since direct inguinal hernia develops through the weakness of the posterior wall of inguinal canal, its reappearance cannot be controlled by pressure over the internal ring.

Inguinal hernia can be differentiated from femoral hernia
- Inguinal hernia lies above and medical to pubic tubercle
- Femoral hernia lies below and lateral to pubic tubercle.

Zieman's tridigital examination for hernia
By this procedure both inguinal (direct + indirect) and femoral hernia can be palpated at the same time.
- You should stand by the right side of the patient
- Patient is also in standing position
- Place the palm of right hand over the right lower abdomen.

- *Place the fingers in the following manner:*
  - ❖ Finger tips on right inguinal ligament.
  - ❖ Tip of the long finger in the external inguinal ring.
  - ❖ Tip of the index finger in the internal inguinal ring.
  - ❖ Ring finger tip is placed in femoral triangle.
- Ask the patient to cough or do Valsalva maneuver. There is increase in intra-abdominal pressure, as a result hernia in any of the above places manifests itself as gliding motion of the walls of hernial sac or as impulse produced by protrusion of virus into the sac.

■ Rectum and Anal Canal

- Rectum is curved segment of bowel, 12 cm long.
- Anterior 2/3rd of rectal surface covered with peritoneum which is reflected to the bladder base in men.
- Peritoneum is reflected to uterine wall to form rectouterine pouch of Douglas (in women) which contains loops of bowel.
- Anterior to lower 1/3rd of rectum lies:
  - ❖ Prostate
  - ❖ Bladder base
  - ❖ Seminal vesicle in men and vagina in women:
    - Anus is 3–4 cm long
    - It joins rectum to perineum
    - Anal wall is supported by voluntary external sphincter muscles and involuntary internal sphincter muscles.

These muscles are responsible for:
- Continence
- Tone.
  Rectal mucosa can be visualized through sigmoidoscope.

Value of digital rectal examination
- Palpation of prostate
- Palpation of genital organs
- Assessment of gastrointestinal infections
- Evaluation of malignancy.

Methods of digital examination of rectum
- Ask the patient to lie in left lateral position with hips and knee flexed
- Buttock should be positioned at the edge of the bed
- Put on the gloves and gently spread the buttock of the patient
- Look for perianal area, any skin abnormalities, any ulcer, any fungal infection is present or not
- Then adequately lubricate your finger with xylocaine jelly
- Tell details of the method of insertion to the patient

- Ask the patient to take deep breath
- Place the finger against the anus and ask the patient to bear down as if he was having bowel movement
- As a result anal sphincter muscles are relaxed and you will slowly enter the finger into anal canal
- During insertion you must estimate the sphincter tone
- Palpate prostate (posterior and lateral wall) by the pad of index finger. Anterior wall is not accessible
- Push the inserted finger upwards towards umbilicus and try to palpate seminal vesicles—if it is enlarged due to any disease—then only it is palpable
- Then you rotate the finger posteriorly to search for the rectal lesions or mass
- Then rotate the finger again 180° to palpate female genital organ—retroverted uterus, cervix
- Lastly withdraw the finger and see—the soiling present on the wall of the gloves—stool, blood, mucus or any other things—color of stool—if black—it indicates the bleeding from above the ligament of Treitz
- Then you can test the stool for occult blood
- Then take a cotton or napkin to clean the anal area.

The following findings can be diagnosed from rectal examination:
- *Skin lesions—sexually transmitted diseases:*
  - ❖ Papilloma
  - ❖ Herpes.
- *Parasitic infestations:* Pinworm.
- *Fungal infection: Candida.*
- *Anal mucosal lesion:*
  - ❖ Anal fissure
  - ❖ Anal fistula
  - ❖ Solitary rectal ulcer
  - ❖ Hemorrhoids.
- *Assessment of sphincter tone:* Ask the patient to contract his anal sphincter by trying to "hold on" your finger.

Reduced tone reflects central or peripheral nervous system compromisation—may produce rectal incontinence—may be due to neoplastic conditions of cord producing compression of sacral roots or spinal cord.

Anal examination should not be deferred in case of myocardial ischemia or it introduces arrhythmia, but no such study proves it.

▊ Prostate Gland

- Normal prostate gland measures 3.5 cm from side to side
- It protrudes 1 cm into rectum.

Palpation of Prostate—Assess

- Size
- Consistency
- Nodularity
- Tenderness
- Symmetry
- Fixation:
  - ❖ Normal gland is smooth surfaced, rubbery, symmetrical, nontender and has a well demarcated median cleft.
  - ❖ Firm nodular gland—fixed to pelvic structure—malignancy
  - ❖ Firm gland—chronic prostatitis.

Causes of Prostatic Nodules

- Benign prostatic hyperplasia—most common cause (>60 years of age)
- Various inflammatory processes–prostatitis, prostatic abscess
- Malignancy.

Tender nodules in prostate:
- Chronic prostatitis
- Prostatic abscess.

If prostatic infection is suspected, massage the organ from within the rectum to squeeze the prostatic fluid through urethral meatus for microscopy and culture.

Acute Abdomen

Peritoneal signs

Importance of bedside diagnosis of peritonitis: In spite of valuable accurate diagnostic methods like MRI, CT Scan, Clinical diagnosis of peritonitis is still valuable for urgent diagnosis and proper interventions.

Most commonly used maneuvers to diagnose peritonitis are:
- Muscle guard/muscles rigidity
- Abdominal wall tenderness
- Rebound tenderness.

Muscle guarding: It means tensing of abdominal wall muscles. It may be:
- Diffuse or localized
- Involuntary.

But voluntary muscle guarding does not indicates peritoneal inflammation, because it may occur from:
- Examiner's cold hand's touch
- Anxiety of the patient
- Abnormal sensation of abdominal wall which may be from birth.

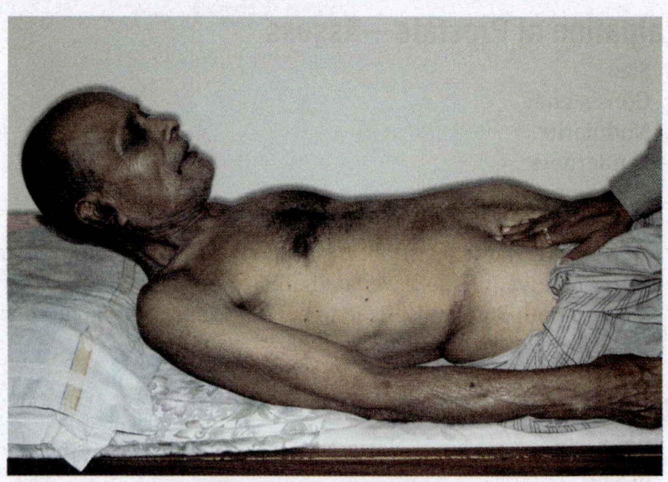

FIG. 5.131 Method of induced guarding

Localized rigidity: It may arise from localized involvement of peritoneum overlying inflamed viscous. It can be evidenced by localized freezing of abdominal wall motion during respiration.

Induced guarding: It is called induced tension of abdominal wall muscles.

Method (Fig. 5.131):

- Ask the patient to raise his head above the pillow and to touch his chin against the anterior chest
- This makes anterior abdominal wall muscles taught to prevent the examiner's finger to touch the inflamed viscous present under the muscles
- Throughout the above procedure examiner must maintain same pressure on the inflamed viscous.
- If during induced tensing of abdominal wall muscles:
  - ❖ The pain is maintained with pressure by examiner's finger—positive Carnett's sign
  - ❖ The pain disappears with maintained pressure on abdominal wall—negative Carnett's sign.

Abdominal tenderness: This is nothing but modified muscles guarding.

- Ask to patient to lie in flat and relaxed position
- Identify the wall of maximum tenderness
- Place the examining finger on the site of maximum tenderness and keep it throughout the procedure
- Ask the patient to cross arms and sit forward
- When the patient is in midway between sitting and recumbent position—anterior abdominal wall muscles become tensed

- Now, after giving pressure with fingers on the same site:
  - ❖ If pain is increased—positive abdominal wall tenderness
  - ❖ If pain is reduced—negative abdominal wall tenderness.

Causes of abdominal wall tenderness:
- Diabetic neuropathy of lower thoracic segments associated with hyperesthesia and weakness
- Viral myositis
- Fibrositis
- Nerve entrapment
- Trauma.

Limitations of elicitation of abdominal wall tenderness:
- In case children and elderly patient because of risk of misinterpretation
- It is useless in patient with diffuse abdominal tenderness or rigidity
- It is dangerous to perform this test in patient with intra-abdominal abscess because there is chance of rupture.

Accuracy of abdominal wall tenderness maneuvers:
Different studies show that it is clinically useful in evaluation of acute or chronic abdominal pain.

In few studies it has been shown that there are false positive test, inspite of no intra-abdominal pathology.

Again few studies shown false negative test in spite of presence of intra-abdominal pathology.

In spite of above controversies, anterior abdominal wall tenderness maneuvers are very useful differentiating intra-abdominal pathology from abdominal wall pathology.

Rebound tenderness: This can be defined as severe abdominal pain arising from sudden release of hand pressure from abdominal wall underlying in flamed peritoneum.

This is called Blumberg's sign: This can be elicited by following methods:
- Ask the patient to lie in supine position
- Palpate the area of tenderness gently but deeply, then sudden release the pressure
- As a result there is recoil back of abdominal wall muscles to baseline position and thus produce exquisite tenderness in localized area

  Alternative method is indirect percussion on the localized area.

Referred rebound tenderness test:
Examiner compresses the quadrant contralateral to the quadrant having pain.

The test is positive when pressure elicits pain at the site of original pain.

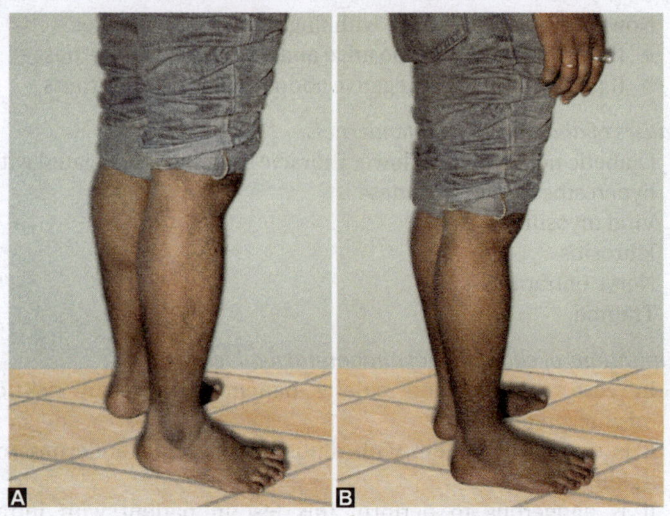

FIGS 5.132A AND B Jar tenderness detection

This test is negative when this pressure elicits pain at the site of applied pressure.

Cough test: Cough increases sudden increase in intra-abdominal pressure, which in turn increases abdominal pain.

This test is indicative of peritonitis.

This test is more valuable when absent than present.

Jar tenderness (Figs 5.132A and B): In this maneuver:

- Ask the patient to stand on out stretched toes, then tell him to fall on his heels with his body weight.
- Sudden jerk produces abdominal wall into motion, which automatically elicits pain on a localized area.

Role of valsalva maneuver in acute abdominal pain:
This maneuver suddenly distends the abdominal wall which increases the intensity of abdominal pain and identify the area of tenderness.

Stethoscope tenderness: First you palpate the abdomen twice—first by your hands then with your stethoscope. In this method:

- First, you distract the patient from the maneuver you are doing
- Then slowly and gently give pressure on the anterior abdominal wall
- In case of unreal pain, the patient does not show any facial expression of pain.

In this method, you always look towards the facial expression of the patient. Any grimacing or other reaction is the clue to the diagnosis.

Closed—eyes sign: This is peculiar face of nonspecific abdominal pain because patient with false abdominal pain often closes his eyes with beautiful smile during abdominal palpation.

But patient with true intra-abdominal pain, always keeps his eyes open and monitor what you are doing.

The following points are responsible for closed eyes:
- These patients will not monitor the physician's activity to avoid unnecessary pain
- They must be aware that this palpation will not produce severe pain.

Hyperesthesia: It is hypersensitivity to light touch in the areas overlying inflamed viscous. This can be elicited by drawing lightly by a cotton, or pin or fingernail.

It may be due to—inflamed viscera or herpes zoster.

Boas' sign: This is hyperesthesia applied to gallbladder in case of acute cholecystitis. The hyperesthetic area is right costophrenic angle even light touch will produce exquisite tenderness.

Acute appendicitis
Following signs can be used to detect acute appendicitis:
- *McBurney's sign:* This sign can be elicited by giving pressure by one finger on McBurney's point (Fig. 5.133).

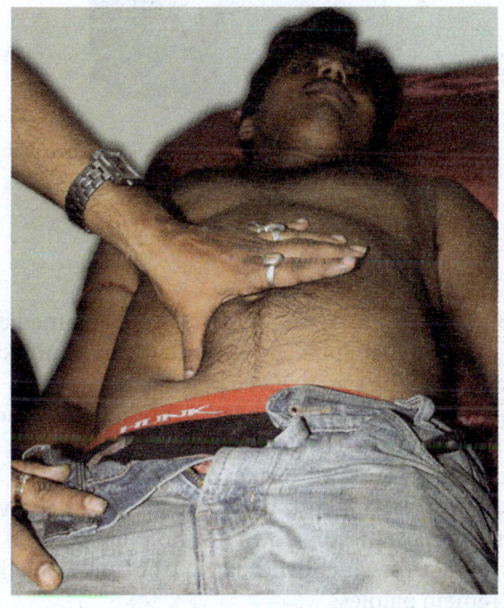

FIG. 5.133 McBurney's sign

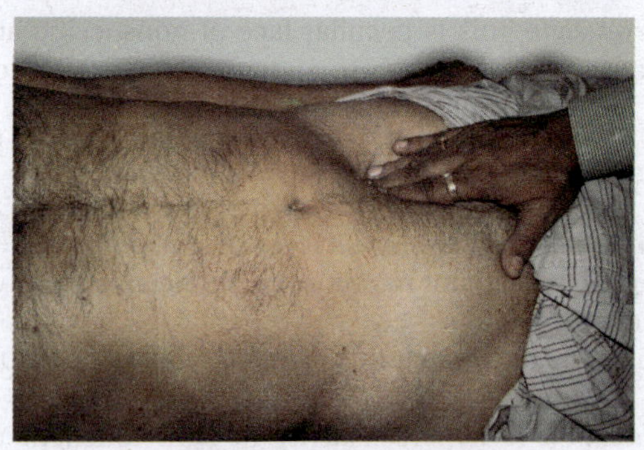

FIG. 5.134 Rovsing's sign

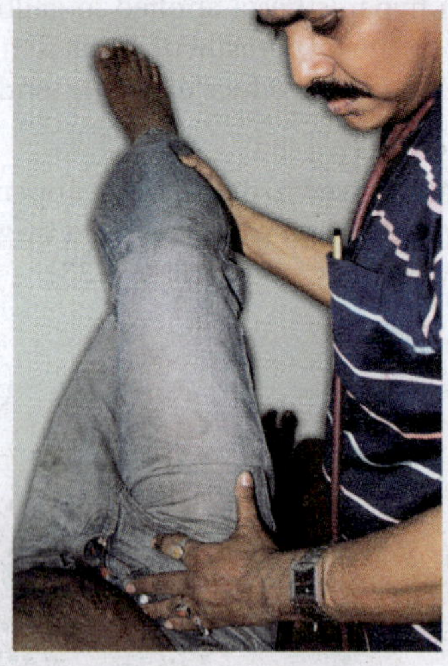

FIG. 5.135 Obturator test

McBurney's point is situated 1.5–2 inches medial to right antero-superior iliac spine, on a line that joins umbilicus.

Specificity of the sign is 75–85 percent.

- *Rovsing's sign (Fig. 5.134):* This sign is nothing but tenderness in right iliac fossa elicited by giving pressure on left lower quadrant.

  Specificity of sign is 75–85 percent.

- *Obturator test:* In this test, ask the patient to flex the hip and rotate it internally in lying down position (Fig. 5.135).

  This maneuver should be carried out on both thighs and should remain painless.

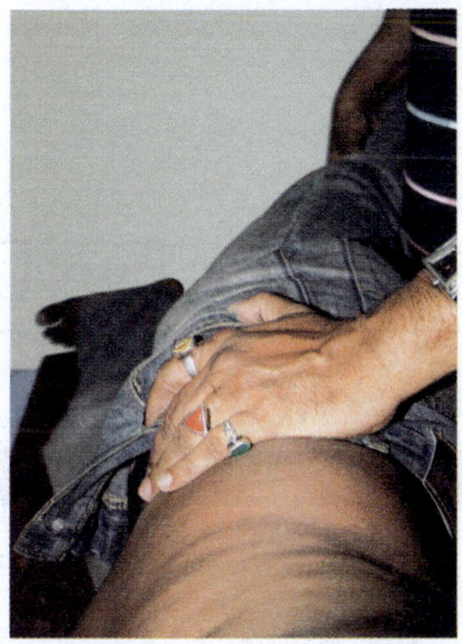

FIG. 5.136   Reverse psoas maneuvers

Pain indicates inflammation in any organ surrounding obturator internus muscles.

This test is positive in:

* *Retrocecal appendicitis:* Positive in right leg
* Intrapelvic pus—Positive in both legs.

● *Reverse psoas maneuvers (Fig. 5.136):* Ask the patient to roll towards left side and hyperextend the hip. The test is positive if his maneuver elicits tenderness.

This test is positive in:

* Retrocecal appendicitis
* Any collection of pus of blood on psoas muscle.

● *Rectal tenderness:* There is tenderness during rectal examination in case of rectal appendicitis.

Eye Disease

Orbit (Fig. 6.1)

It is a pair of bony cavities contain:
- Eyeball
- Orbital muscles
- Nerves
- Vessels
- Fat
- Lacrimal apparatus.
  Orbital opening is guarded by eyelids.

Eyelids: Two eyelids—upper eyelid and lower eyelid:
- Upper eyelid is larger, more movable
- Lower eyelid is smaller
- Both eyelids meet each other at medial and lateral angles
- Palpebral fissure is the area between the eyelids
- *During close position:* Upper eyelid covers full eye
- *During opened eye:*
  - ❖ Upper eyelid covers upper margin of cornea
  - ❖ Lower eyelid covers lower margin of cornea.
- Inner surface of eyelid is covered by palpebral part conjunctiva
- Eyelashes—short, curved hairs on free edge of eyelids
- Ciliary glands—open in between adjacent lashes
- Tarsal glands—sebaceous glands pouring their secretion on the margin of lid
- Median angle is separated from eyeball, by a space—called *lacus lacrimalis* at the center of it there is reddish brown elevation *caruncula lacrimalis*
- Near median angle—there is an elevation lacrimal papilla at the top of it there is an opening—called lacrimal punctum which leads to lacrimal canaliculi

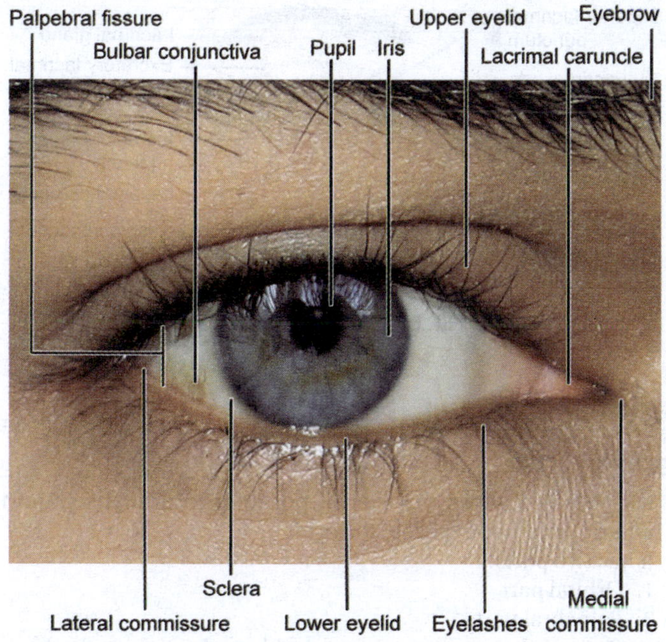

FIG. 6.1   External features of eye

- Palpebral conjunctiva is continuous with bulbar conjunctiva through superior and interior fornices
- Superior fornix is pierced by lacrimal gland
- Framework of eyelids is formed by fibrous sheet orbital septum
- *Thickened orbital margin form superior and interior tarsal plates:*
  - ❖ Lateral ends of tarsal plats is attached with lateral palpebral ligaments
  - ❖ Medical end of plates is attached to medial palpebral ligaments.
- *Two muscles are attached with eyelids:*
  1. Levator palpebrae superioris—responsible for upward movement of upper eyelids
  2. Orbicularis oculi—its tone and contraction are responsible for closing of eyelids, when levator palpebrae superior is relaxed.

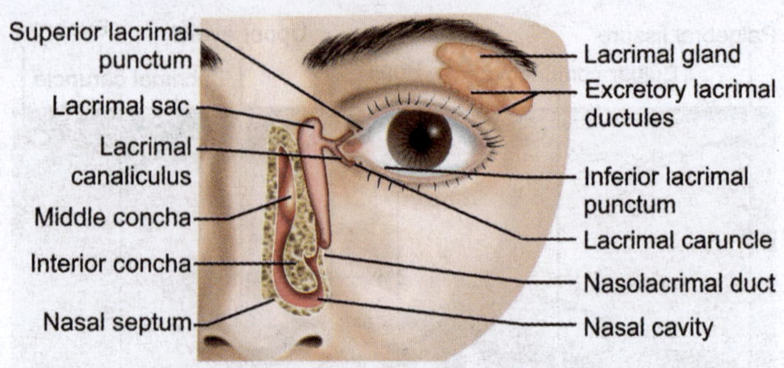

FIG. 6.2   Lacrimal apparatus

Lacrimal Apparatus (Fig. 6.2)

Lacrimal Gland

- It is situated above the eyeball posterior to orbital septum in anterior and upper part of the orbit
- It has two parts:
  1. Orbital part
  2. Palpebral part.
  Both of them are continuous with each other at the lateral edge of aponeurosis of levator palpebrae superioris.
- Glands open into lateral part of superior fornix by twelve ducts
- *Nerve supply:*
  - ❖ *Parasympathetic secretomotor nerve supply:*
    Lacrimal nucleus of facial nerve
    ↓
    Preganglionic fibers reach pterygopalatine ganglion via nervus intermedius, and greater petrosal nerve
    ↓
    Postganglionic fibers join maxillary nerve
    ↓
    Zygomatic branch of zygomaticotemporal nerve
    ↓
    Lacrimal nerve
    ↓
    Lacrimal gland
  - ❖ *Sympathetic postganglionic nerve supply:*
    From nerves round internal carotid plexus
    ↓
    Deep petrosal nerve
    ↓
    Nerve of pterygoid canal
    ↓
    Maxillary nerve

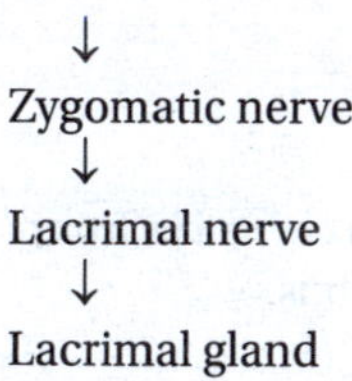

$$\downarrow$$

Zygomatic nerve

$$\downarrow$$

Lacrimal nerve

$$\downarrow$$

Lacrimal gland

Lacrimal Duct

Tear circulates across cornea to lacus lacrimalis

$$\downarrow$$

Tear enters into lacrimal canaliculi through lacrimal punctum

$$\downarrow$$

Canaliculi open into lacrimal sac

Lacrimal sac lies behind medial palpebral ligament and upper blind end of nasolacrimal duct (1.3 cm long).

Nasolacrimal duct opens into interior meatus of nose. This opening is guarded by a fold—lacrimal fold.

This lacrimal fold prevents air from entering into nasolacrimal duct and reaching lacrimal sac.

Structures of Eye (Fig. 6.3)

Coatings of Eyeball

- *Fibrous coat:* It consists of two parts:
  1. *Sclera:*
     - Opaque posterior fibrous white part
     - It is pierced by optic nerve area is called lamina cribrosa. Sclera is fused with optic nerve sheath

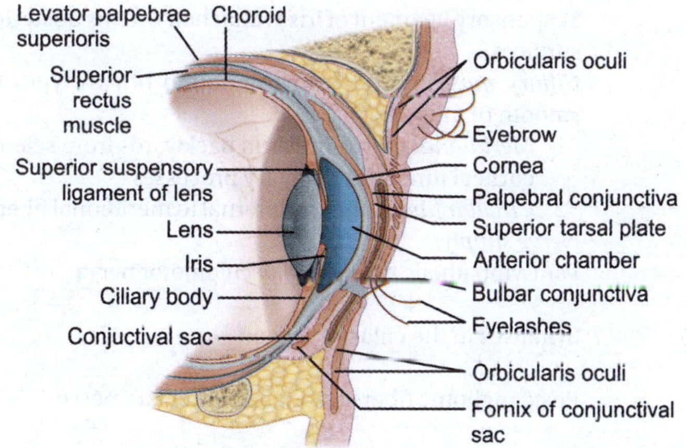

FIG. 6.3 Sagittal section of eye

- It is also pierced by:
  - Ciliary arteries
  - Ciliary veins—venae varicose
- Anteriorly sclera is continuous with cornea in front
- Sclerocorneal junction is called limbus.

2. *Cornea:*
  - It is the continuation of sclera—inferiorly
  - It is in contact with aqueous humor posteriorly
  - Blood supply—avascular, no lymphatic drainage—nourishment occurs through diffusion from:
    - Aqueous humor
    - Capillaries at its edge.
  - Nerve supply:
    - Long ciliary nerves
    - Ophthalmic division of trigeminal nerve.
  - Functions:
    - Most important refractory medium of the eye. Refractive index—1.38
    - Tear is responsible for survival of corneal cells.

- *Vascular pigmented coat:* It consists of—from behind forward.
  - ❖ *Choroid:* It consists of:
    - Outer pigmented layer
    - Inner highly vascular layer.
  - ❖ *Ciliary body:*
    - Posteriorly it is continuous with choroid layer
    - Anteriorly it lies behind the peripheral margin of iris.
    - It is composed of:
      - *Ciliary ring:* It is the posterior part of the body, has shallow grooves—called ciliary striae
      - *Ciliary process:* These are radially arranged folds. Suspensory ligament of iris is attached with its posterior surfaces
      - *Ciliary muscles:* They run compound of two types of smooth of muscles:
        1. *Meridional fibers:* They run backwards from sclerocorneal junctions to ciliary processes
        2. *Circular fibers:* They lie internal to meridional fibers.
      - *Nerve supply:*
        Parasympathetic fibers from occulomotor nerve
        ↓
        Synapses in the ciliary ganglion
        ↓
        Postganglionic fibers through short ciliary nerve

- *Action:*

Contraction of meridional fibers
↓
Pulls the ciliary body forward
↓
Increased tension of suspensory ligament
↓
Elastic lens becomes more convex
↓
Increases refractive power of lens

- ❖ *Iris and pupil (Fig. 6.4):*
  - Iris is a contractile diaphragm present in between cornea anteriorly and lens posteriorly, suspended in aqueous humor
  - It forms the aperture of the pupil
  - It is attached with ciliary body at its periphery
  - It divides the space between cornea and lens into anterior chamber and posterior chamber
  - *Muscles of iris consist of:*
    - Circular fibers—involuntary, arranged around the margin of iris—forms sphincter pupillae
    - Radial fibers—involuntary, radially arranged close to its posterior surface—forms dilator pupillae.

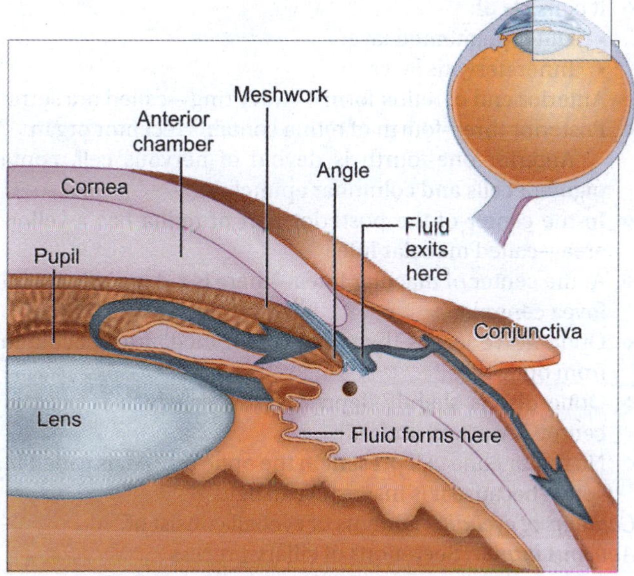

FIG. 6.4   Anterior chamber

- *Nerve supply:*
  - Parasympathetic fibers
    ↓
    Oculomotor nerve—preganglionic fibers
    ↓
    Synapse with ciliary ganglion
    ↓
    Postganglionic fibers (short ciliary nerves)
    ↓
    Sphincter pupillae
  - Sympathetic fibers
    ↓
    Dilator pupillae
    ↓
    Dilatation of pupil
- *Actions:* Sphincter pupillae.
  Constricts the pupil:
  - In relation to accommodation
  - In presence of bright light.
  Dilator pupillae dilates the pupil in presence of:
  - Light of intensity
  - Fright due to excessive sympathetic activity.

- *Nervous coat—retina (Figs 6.5A and B):*
  - ❖ This layer is in contact with vitreous body at its inner surface and at its outer surface in contact with choroid layer
  - ❖ It consists of:
    - Outer pigmented layer
    - Inner nervous layer
  - ❖ Anterior end of retina forms—wavy ring—called ora serrata
  - ❖ Posterior three-fourth of retina contains receptor organ
    Anterior one-fourth is devoid of nervous cell, contains pigment cells and columnar epithelium.
  - ❖ In the center of the posterior part of retina has a yellowish area—called macular lutea
  - ❖ At the center of macular lutea—there is a depression—called fovea centralis
  - ❖ Optic nerve leaves the retina 3 mm medial to macula lutea from optic disc
  - ❖ Optic disc is slightly depressed center which is pierced by central are artery and vein
  - ❖ No rod or cone cell present in the optic disc—it is called blind spot—because it is insensitive to light.
- *Contents of eyeball:* Contents of eyeball consist of:
  Aqueous humor: Secretions of ciliary process
    ↓

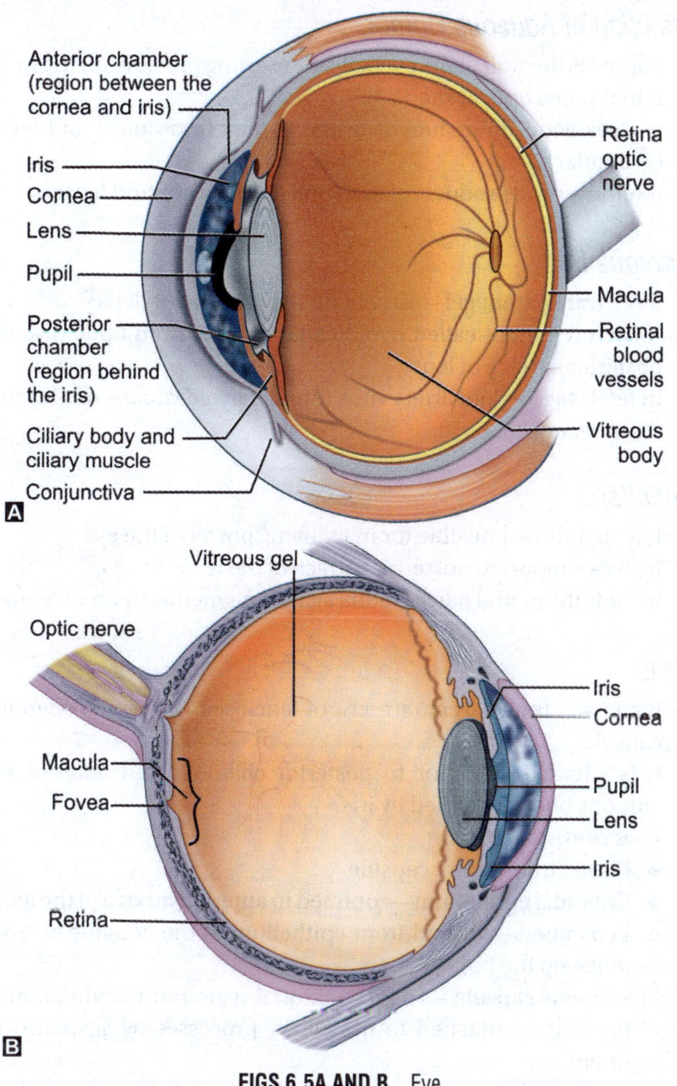

FIGS 6.5A AND B   Eye

It enters the posterior chamber

It flows through anterior chamber through pupil

It is then drained away through spaces at the irido-corneal angle—called canal of Schlemm.

Obstruction to drainage of aqueous humor—it is a condition called glaucoma.

Function of Aqueous Humor

- Supports the wall of the eyeball—by exerting pressure on the wall
- It maintains optical shape
- It gives good nourishment to the cornea (avascular) and lens (avascular)
- It removes the products of metabolism of cornea and lens.

Vitreous Body

- It is a transparent gel—present on the posterior to lens
- A narrow canal—called hyoid canal extends from optic disc to posterior surface of lens
- In fetal stage hyloid artery runs through hyoid canal—this artery disappears after birth.

Function

- It is slightly responsible for magnifying power of the eye
- It gives support to posterior surface of the lens
- It holds the neural part of retina against pigmentary part of retina.

Lens

- Biconvex transparent structure—enclosed in a transparent capsule
- It is situated posterior to posterior chamber and anterior to vitreous body, encircled by iris
- *Lens consists of:*
  - Elastic transparent capsule
  - Cuboidal epithelium—confined to anterior surface of the lens
  - Lens fibers—formed from epithelium at the equator of lens make up the bulk of fibers.
- Elastic lens capsule—on its equatorial region or circumference of the lens is attached to the ciliary processes by suspensory ligament.

The pull of this ligament makes the elastic lens flattened—so that eye can be focused on the object.

Accommodation of Eye

Objects close to eye

↓

Ciliary body are pulled forward and inward by contraction of ciliary muscles

↓

Radiating fibers of suspensory ligaments are relaxed

↓

Elastic lens areas globular in shape.

Extrinsic Muscles of Eyeball (Fig. 6.6)

- Superior rectus
- Inferior rectus
- Medial rectus
- Lateral rectus
- Superior oblique
- Inferior oblique.
    - ❖ Oculomotor nerve supplies:
        - Superior rectus
        - Inferior rectus
        - Medial rectus
        - Inferior oblique.
    - ❖ Trochlear nerve supplies—superior oblique
    - ❖ Abducent nerve supplies—lateral rectus.

Movement	Primary Muscle	Secondary Muscle
Abduction	Lateral rectus	Superior oblique Inferior oblique
Adduction	Medial rectus	Superior rectus Inferior rectus
Elevation	Superior rectus	Inferior oblique
Depression	Inferior rectus	Superior oblique
Extortion	Inferior oblique	Inferior rectus
Intorsion	Superior oblique	Superior rectus

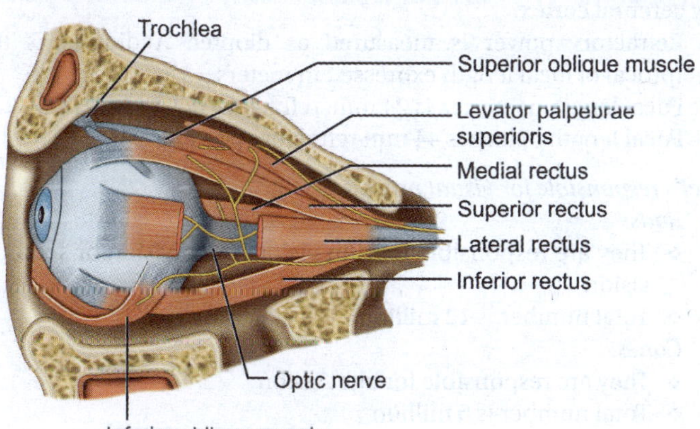

FIG. 6.6 Extraocular muscles of eyeball

Simultaneous movement of both eyeballs
- *Conjugate movement:* Movement of both eyeballs in same direction.
  - ❖ Visual axes of both eyeballs remain parallel
  - ❖ Simultaneous contraction of medial rectus of one eye and lateral rectus of other eye.
- *Disconjugate movement:* Movement of both eyeballs in opposite direction. Two types of movement:
  1. *Convergence:* Movement of both eyeball towards nose. It is mainly due to:
     - Contraction of both medial recti
     - Simultaneous relaxation of both lateral recti
     - Visual axes are close together.

     It occurs during accommodation.
  2. *Divergence:* Movement of two eyeballs towards temporal side—visual axes of both eyes move away from each other. It is mainly due to:
     - Contraction of both lateral recti
     - Relaxation of both medial recti.
- *Pursuit movement:* Movement of eyeballs along the objects when eyes are fixed on a moving object
- *Saccadic movement:* Jerky movement of both eyeballs when fixation of eyes is shifted from one object to another object.

Visual process

During looking to an object

↓

Light rays from the object is refracted and brought to the focus on retina.

The image formed is in inverted position, which is made upright by cerebral cortex.

Refractory power is measured as diopter. A diopter is the reciprocal of focal length expressed in meters.
- Focal length of cornea is 24 mm, refractory power is 42D.
- Focal length of lens is 44 mm refractory power is 23D.

Cells responsible for visual process
- *Rods:*
  - ❖ They are responsible for dim vision, night vision or scotopic vision
  - ❖ Total number is 12 million.
- *Cones:*
  - ❖ They are responsible for light vision
  - ❖ Total number is 6 million.

Distribution of Cells in Retina

- Fovea has only cones, no rods
- *From fovea to periphery:* Rods increase and cones decrease in number
- *At the periphery of retina:* All are rods, no cone cell.

Function of rods
- Responsible for dim vision, night vision or scotopic vision
- Do not resolve details or boundaries of the object (visual acuity)
- Do not resolve the color of the object (color vision)
- Vision of rod is black, white or combination of black and white, i.e. gray.

Function of cones
- They are responsible for light vision, photic vision or day light vision
- Responsible for acuity of vision
- Responsible for color vision.

Dark Adaptation

It is the process by which the person is able to see the object in dim light.

A person enters from highly lighted room to dim lighted room

↓

At first he cannot see the object

↓

Pigment is transformed to rhodopsin, necessary for rod cell function

↓

As a result patient starts seeing in dim vision.

Cause of dark adaptation

Increased sensitivity of rods as a result of increased resynthesis of rhodopsin.

Dilatation of pupil—it allows more and more light to enter in the eye.

Field of Vision

Part of external world seen by one eye when it in fixed in one direction

Types of Field

- Temporal field extends up to 100°
- Nasal field extends up to 60°—restricted by nose
- Upper field extends up to 60°
- Lower field extends up to 75°.

Binocular vision: In this vision, both eyes are used same portion of external world together.

Monocular vision: In this vision each eye is used separately for vision of particular object, e.g. dogs, horse.

Blind spot: It is the small area of retina where visual receptors are absent. For example—optic disc of retina does not have visual receptors.

- Mapping of visual field is done by Goldmann perimeter. This technique is called perimetry
- Bjerrum's screen
- Confrontation perimetry
- Humphrey field analyzer.
  - *Visual pathway* and site of lesions to be delt during discussion of 2nd cranial nerve—optic nerve
  - *Pupillary reflexes* to be delt during discussion of 3rd cranial nerve; optic nerve.

Color vision: Human eye identifies 150 different colors in visible spectrum.

The series of colored light produced by prism is called visible spectrum. Spectrum of colors is—according to wavelengths from maximum to minimum:

- Red
- Orange
- Yellow
- Green
- Blue
- Indigo
- Violet.

Red color—maximum wave length—8000 Å. Light rays longer than this color is called infrared rays.

Violet color—minimum wave length—3000 Å. Light rays shorter than minimal wave length is called ultraviolet rays.

Extraspectral colors: These colors are not present in spectrum, e.g. purple color—combination of red and violet colors.

Primary colors: Red, blue and green—there are combined to produce while color.

Complementary color: These are pair of two colors which when combined produce white color.

- Red and greenish blue
- Orange and cyan blue
- Yellow and indigo blue
- Violet and greenish yellow.

Color sensitive areas of retina

- Peripheral part of retina is devoid of cones—so this area is insensitive to color, sensitive to black, white and gray only

- Central part of retina—fovea centralis—mostly cones—sensitive to color
- Retinal sensitivity to blue is highest—next green then yellow.

For measurement of visual acuity: Following things are used:
- Snellen chart
- Pinhole occluder
- Pocket size near vision test card
- Rosenbaun card—in case of bed ridden patients.

Method of measurement of vision who cannot read any letter on the chart.
- Reducing the distance between patient and the chart—it should be recorded as numerator of new visual acuity measurement
- If the patient cannot read largest letters on snellen chart at 3 feet, vision can be measured in terms of counting numbers—during this examination, examiner should record the distance between eye and finger
- If patient cannot count the finger—followings are required:
  ❖ Hand movement
  ❖ Flash light perception
  ❖ No light perception.
- *In case illiterate patient or children:* 'E' chart and asking the patient to designate stroke's direction.

Causes of reduced visual acuity
- *Refractive errors:*
  ❖ Hypermetropia—in which axial length of the eye is too short
  ❖ Myopia—in which axial length is too long
  ❖ *Astigmatism:* Here refractive error of eye is different—from one meridian than another.
- Treatable and reversible blindness—cataract, uveitis.
- *Systemic disorders:*
  ❖ Diabetes
  ❖ Hypertension.
- Central nervous system disease—multiple sclerosis, glioma
- *Congenital disorders:*
  ❖ Rubella
  ❖ Toxoplasmosis.
- *Infectious diseases:*
  ❖ Cytomegaly virus
  ❖ Retinitis
  ❖ Toxoplasmosis.

Confirmation of cause of reduced visual acuity
- Vision improves with a pinhole occluder—uncorrected refractive errors

- Simple ophthalmoscopy or examining red reflex—opaque media
- *Neurological or retinal disorders:* Ophthalmoscopy, visual field testing, swinging flash light test
- *Amblyopia:* History of reduced visual acuity often by strabismus.

SYMPTOMS OF EYE DISEASE

■ Presenting Problems

Red Eye

- *Foreign body sensation in the eye:* Conjunctivitis.
- *Pain during movement of the eyes:*
  - ❖ Bacterial conjunctivitis
  - ❖ Glaucoma
  - ❖ Scleritis.
- *Foreign body sensation with itchy sensation:*
  - ❖ Allergic conjunctivitis
  - ❖ Winter conjunctivitis.
- *Redness of eye:*
  - ❖ Trauma
  - ❖ Infection
  - ❖ Allergy
  - ❖ Increased pressure in the eyes
  - ❖ Occasionally coughing or recurrent vomiting
  - ❖ Use of contact lens producing irritation.

The main causes are:
- Acute conjunctivitis
- Acute iritis
- Narrow angle glaucoma
- Corneal abrasion.

History

- Sudden onset, contact with patient having conductivities
- Fairly sudden onset, recurrence
- Rapid onset, history of previous attack
- Pain, history of trauma.

Vision

- Normal
- Gradually lost if untreated
- Rapidly lost if untreated.

Pain

- Gritty sensation
- Photophobia
- Severe
- Severest.

Bilateral Involvement

- Frequent
- Occasional
- Unilateral.

Ocular Discharge

- Watery or mucopurulent
- Watery
- Mucopurulent.

Systemic Effects

- Absent
- May be present
- Many
- None.

Cornea Examination

- Clear
- Clear or cloudy
- Steamy
- Irregular light reflex.

Pupil

- Normally reactive
- Shape irregular, sluggishly reactive
- Shape—dilated, oval, reactive
- Shape—normal, reactive.

Iris

- Normal
- Anterior chamber may show cells
- May be invisible due to corneal edema
- May be shadow of corneal defect.

The following questions to be asked in case of red eye

- History of injury to eye
- History of injury to eye in his family
- History of coughing or any other straining
- History of any associated pain
- History of any associated discharge
- Any effect of light
- History of wearing contact lens.

Discharge

- *Watery discharge:*
  - ❖ Conjunctivitis
  - ❖ Glaucoma
  - ❖ Iritis.
- *Purulent discharge:*
  - ❖ Bacterial conjunctivitis
  - ❖ Corneal abrasion with infection.
- *Sticky discharge:*
  - ❖ Winter conjunctivitis
  - ❖ Allergic conductivitis.
- *Mucopurulent discharge: Chlamydia* infection unilateral involvement.

Involvement of One or Both Eyes

- *Superficial structure (conjunctiva)—involvement may be unilateral:*
  - ❖ Conjunctivitis (except *Chlamydia*)
  - ❖ Blepharitis.
- *Involvement of deeper structures:*
  - ❖ Iritis
  - ❖ Uveitis
  - ❖ Glaucoma—acute angle
  - ❖ Chlamydial conjunctivitis.

History of Photophobia

- Iritis
- Anterior uveitis
- Corneal ulcer
- Corneal trauma.

Disturbance in Vision

- *Loss of vision:*
  - ❖ Optic neuritis
  - ❖ Detachment of retina
  - ❖ Retinal hemorrhage
  - ❖ Central nervous system disease.
- *Spot.* May precede retinal detachment
- *Flashes of light:*
  - ❖ Aura of migraine
  - ❖ Retinal hemorrhage
  - ❖ Posterior vitreous detachment.

- *Loss of visual field:*
  - ❖ Retinal detachment
  - ❖ Retinal hemorrhage.
- *Distortion of vision:*
  - ❖ Retinal detachment
  - ❖ Macular edema.
- *Difficulty in seeing in dim light:*
  - ❖ Retinal degeneration
  - ❖ Vitamin A deficiency
  - ❖ Myopia.
- *Colored spots around light:*
  - ❖ Lenticular opacities
  - ❖ Corneal opacity
  - ❖ Narrow angle glaucoma.
- *Distorted color vision:*
  - ❖ Cataract
  - ❖ Drugs—digitalis increases yellow vision.
- *Loss of vision:*
  - ❖ *Sudden loss:* Due to vascular cause:
    - Ischemia—involving—retina, optic nerve or brain
    - *Hemorrhage:*
      - – Anterior chamber
      - – Posterior chamber
      - – Vitreous body
      - – Age related macular degeneration.
  - ❖ *Gradual loss:* Due to slowly progressive:
    - Degeneration or deposition
    - Cataract
    - Open angle glaucoma.
  - ❖ *Painful loss of vision:*
    - Uveitis—anterior
    - Keratitis
    - Optic neuritis
    - Giant cell arteritis
    - Disease of orbit.
  - ❖ *Painless loss of vision:*
    - Cataract
    - Diabetic neuropathy
    - Optic neuropathy
    - Retinal vein occlusion, retinal artery occlusion
    - Open angle glaucoma.
  - ❖ *Transient loss of vision:* Due to transient ischemia:
    - Giant cell arteritis
    - Amaurosis fugax
    - Vertebra basilar insufficiency.

- ❖ *Persistent loss of vision:*
  - Hemorrhages in eye
  - Retinal artery occlusion
  - Cataract
  - Optic nerve damage.
- ❖ Unilateral—glaucoma
- ❖ Bilateral—systemic disease
- ❖ *Central loss of vision:*
  - Macular disease
  - Optic nerve head disease
  - Patient complained of scotoma.
- ❖ *Peripheral loss of vision:* Superior or inferior hemianopia—superior or inferior vascular event involving retina or optic disc
  - Retinitis pigmentosa
  - Retinal detachment
  - Bitemporal hemianopia—due to strokes, tumor, vascular cause.
- **Floaters:**
  - ❖ *If it is of gradual onset:* Vitreous degeneration with increasing age and myopia
  - ❖ *If it is of sudden onset with normal vision:* Posterior vitreous detachment with increasing age and myopia
  - ❖ *If it is of sudden onset with diminished vision:* Vitreous hemorrhage with involvement of macula
- **History double vision:**
  - ❖ If it is monocular—due to ocular problem
  - ❖ If it is bilateral—due to nervous system damage from brainstem to ocular muscle.
  - ❖ *Horizontal double vision:*
    - Sixth nerve palsy
    - Raised intracranial pressure
  - ❖ *Diagonal separation of object:* 3rd or 4th nerve palsy.
- **History of proptosis:**
  - ❖ Thyroid disease
  - ❖ Retro-orbital cause.
- **Ptosis (Drooping of eyelids):** 3rd cranial nerve palsy.
- **History of headache:**
  - ❖ Meningitis
  - ❖ Refraction error
  - ❖ Sinusitis
  - ❖ Migraine.
- **Eye heaviness:**
  - ❖ Eyelid edema
  - ❖ Stye
  - ❖ Fatigue.

- *Excessive blinking:*
  - ❖ Corneal irritation
  - ❖ Facial tic.
- *Excessive tearing:*
  - ❖ Conjunctivitis
  - ❖ Blockage of lacrimal duct.

Past History

Local

- Trauma
- Surgery
- Refractive error
- Previous recurrent history of eye disease—anterior uveitis. Recent history of eye operation—postoperative endophthalmitis.

Systemic

- Hypertension
- Diabetes
- Hyperlipidemia
- Arthritis
- Ulcer in penis
- Recurrent headache
- Recurrent vertigo
- Other systemic events of vasculitis.

Family History

It may disclose the hereditary conditions—like:
- Retinitis pigmentosa
- Corneal dystrophies
- Early onset cataract.
  Or, acquired disease like—conjunctivitis.

Social History

History of smoking or alcohol intake—it may disclose—traumatic, vascular or hypertensive cause as precipitating factor.

▪ Drug

History of intake of digitalis—in case disturbed color vision. History of allergy to any drugs.

Examination

Eyelids

Note the position of eyelids:

- Normally in opened eye condition, upper eyelid covers upper margin of iris
- In closed eye condition—upper lid and lower lid approximate each other completely.

  The gap between upper and lower eyelid is called palpebral fissure.

  ❖ *Droping of eyelid*—called ptosis—produce narrowing of palpebral fissure—when bilateral, it is due to myasthenia gravis or any other muscle wasting disease

  ❖ *Kearns-Sayre syndrome*—bilateral ptosis—symmetrical progressive, symmetrical external ophthalmophegia, retinal pigmentary degeneration and cardiac conduction defect; short stature, may be deaf.

  Lagophthalmos: Inability to close the eyes completely. The causes are:
  - Thyroid disease
  - Consequence of the surgery.

  ❖ *Ectropion (Fig. 6.7):* Eversion of lower eyelid—as a result tarsal conjunctiva is exposed to external stimuli—producing irritation and keranization

  ❖ *Entropion (Fig. 6.8):* Inversion of eyelids producing mechanical irritation of conjunctiva by eyelashes—causes may be:

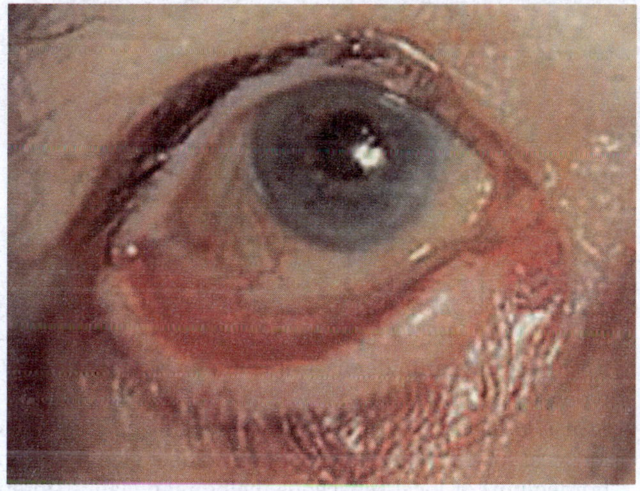

FIG. 6.7   Ectropion

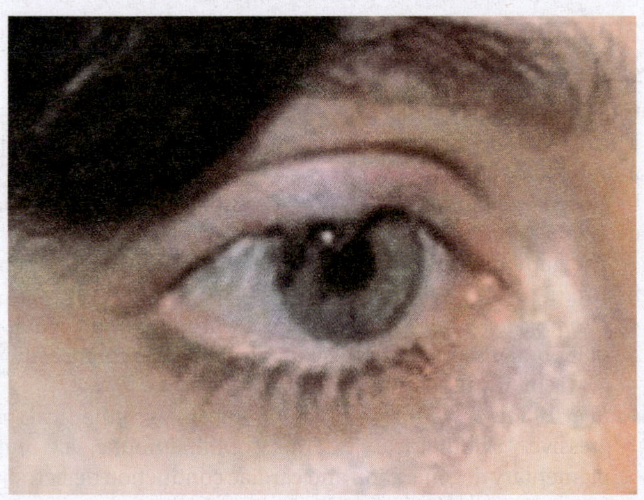

FIG. 6.8 Entropion

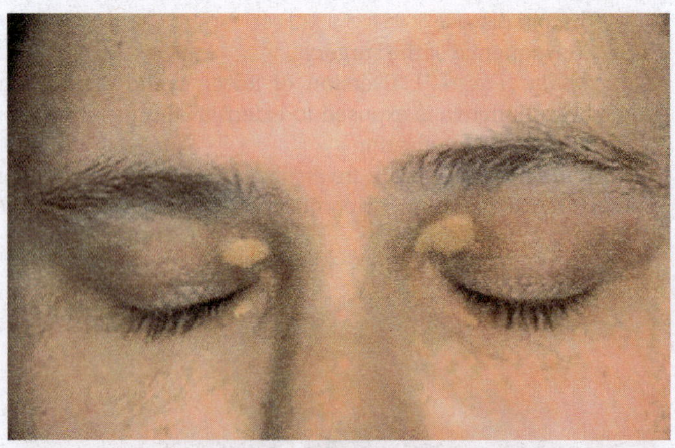

FIG. 6.9 Xanthelasma palpebrarum

- Trachoma
- Aging.

❖ *Xanthelasma palpebrarum (Fig. 6.9):* Yellowish deposits over the eyelids—it may occur with or without hyperlipidemia—if it is due to hyperlipidemias—it is due to type III; type IV or type V

❖ *Stye (Hordeolum) (Fig. 6.10):* It is mainly due to staphy-lococcal local inflammation of hair follicle glands (external hordeolum) or local sebaceous meibomian glands (internal hordeolum)

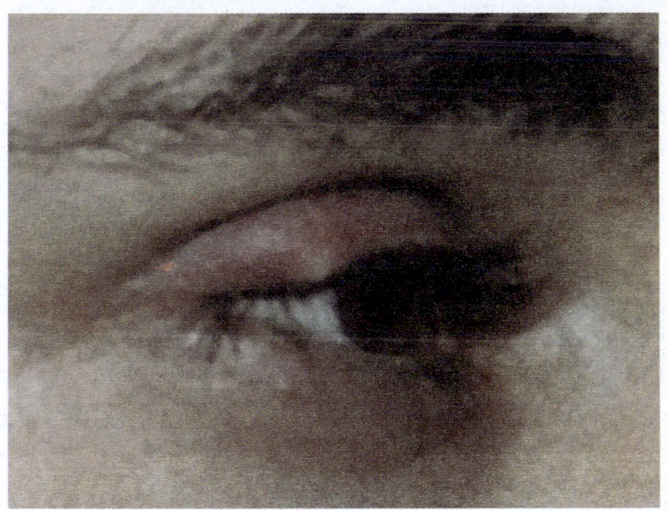

FIG. 6.10   Stye (Hordeolum)

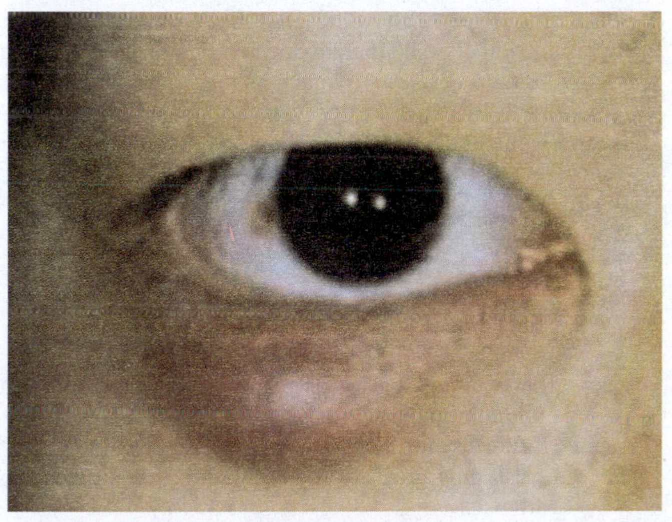

FIG. 6.11   Chalazion

This may present with—local redness, swelling and tenderness.

❖ *Chalazion (Fig. 6.11):* It is subacute painless slowly emerging inflammation of meibomian glands—producing nodules. It may be a consequence of blepharitis

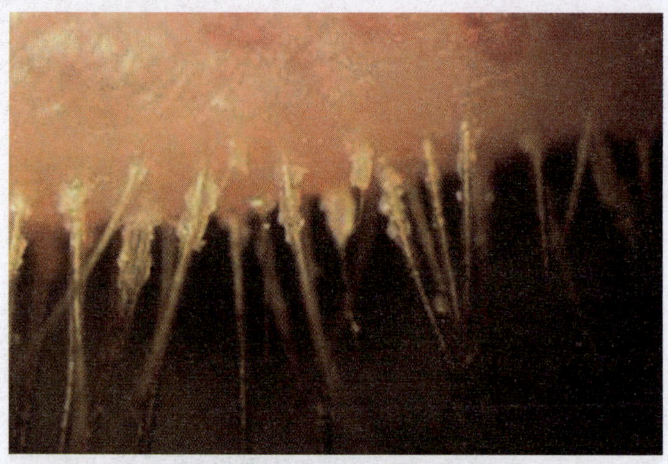

FIG. 6.12 Blepharitis

Difference between blepharitis and chalazion is:
Blepharitis is painful, chalazion.

* *Blepharitis (Fig. 6.12):* It is diffuse, swollen crusted erythematous inflammation of eyelid margin due to *Staphylococcus aureus or Staphylococcus epidermidis* infection, may hire hypersensitivity component. There may be dry eye sensation and ciliary cuffing

* *Ptosis:* Unilateral or bilateral drooping of eyelids—the causes are:
  * Myogenic
    - Aging
    - Trauma
    - Surgery
    - Congenital.
  * Neurogenic
    - Third nerve palsy—associated with diplopia and ophthalmoplegia
    - Horner's syndrome—associated with myosis
    - Myasthenia gravis—progressive increase in weakness with use.

* *Proptosis (Fig. 6.13):* Unilateral or bilateral protrusion of eyeball.
  Causes of unilateral proptosis:
  * Orbital cellulitis
  * Space occupying lesion in orbit
  * Rhabdomyosarcoma in children.
  Causes of bilateral proptosis:
  Graves' disease.

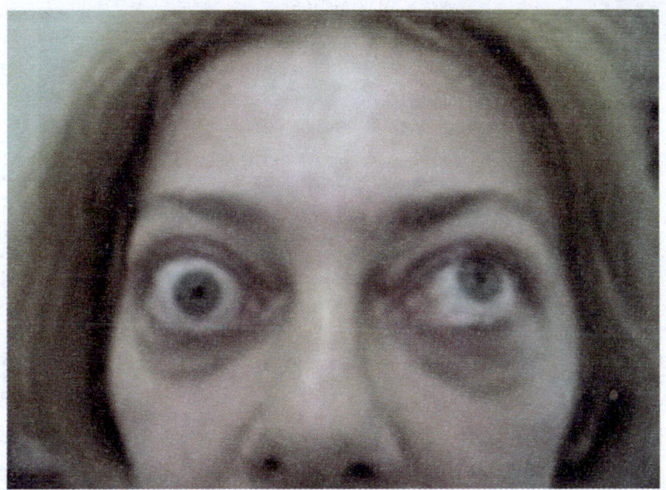

FIG. 6.13 Graves' disease

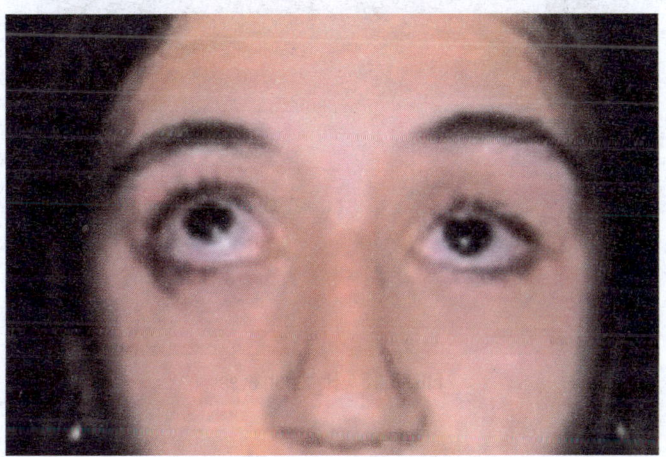

FIG. 6.14 Enophthalmos

* *Enophthalmos (Fig. 6.14):* Inward displacement of eyeball into tho orbit
* *Herniation of orbital pad of fat:* Due to weakening of orbital septum
* *Port-wine stain:* In lower eyelid—it may be associated with Sturage-Weber syndrome—staining on one side of the face following the distribution of one or more divisions of trigeminal nerve

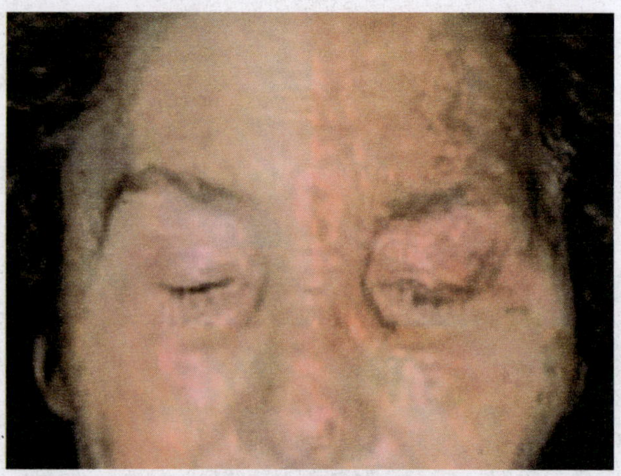

FIG. 6.15   Herpes zoster ophthalmicus

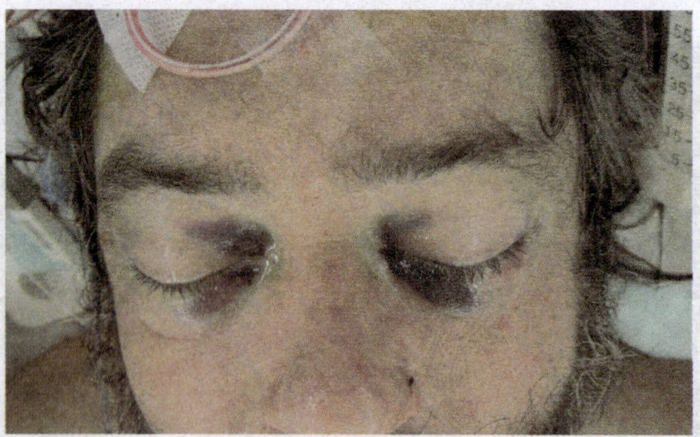

FIG. 6.16   Raccoon eyes

- *Hemangioma on episclera, ciliary body and choroid* may be associated with unilateral glaucoma—when uveal hemangioma.
- *Herpes zoster ophthalmicus (Fig. 6.15):* Painful, rows of vesicles, ulcers and crusted scads—distributed along one or more branches of ophthalmic division of trigeminal nerve
- *Raccoon eyes (Fig. 6.16):* In basilar skull fracture, extravasated blood produces discoloration of orbit—diagnostic sign in unconscious patient without any history
- *Carcinoma of eyelids (Fig. 6.17):* Malignant ocular tumor occurs at 50–60 years age, males are mostly affected.

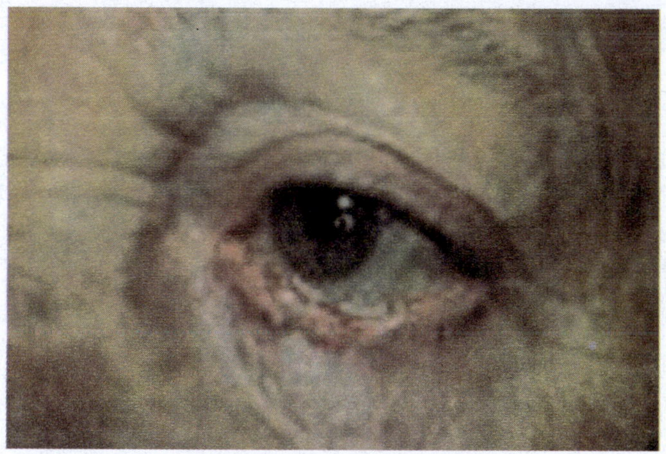

FIG. 6.17   Carcinoma of eyelids

Types of carcinoma:
- Basal cell carcinoma of lower eyelid
- Squamous cell carcinoma—upper eyelid, faster growing
- Meibomian gland carcinomas
- Kaposi's sarcoma—in patient will AIDS.

Inspection of lacrimal apparatus
- *Epiphora:* Some obstruction to flow through punctum. Whether there is blockage of nasolacrimal duct—can be tested by pressing the lacrimal sac.

  If blockage is present—materials may be expressed through punctum sluggishly.
- *Massive enlargement of lacrimal gland:* Sarcoidosis
- *Dacryocystitis (Fig. 6.18):* Chronic inflammation of lower lacrimal passage—present in children or elderly individuals.
  Causes:
  - ❖ Congenital
  - ❖ Infection
  - ❖ Stenosis of lacrimal duct.

Inspection of conjunctiva
Conjunctive should be examined for:
- Inflammation (congestion or dilatation of blood vessels)
- Pallor
- Unusual pigmentation
- Swelling
- Masses
- Hemorrhage.

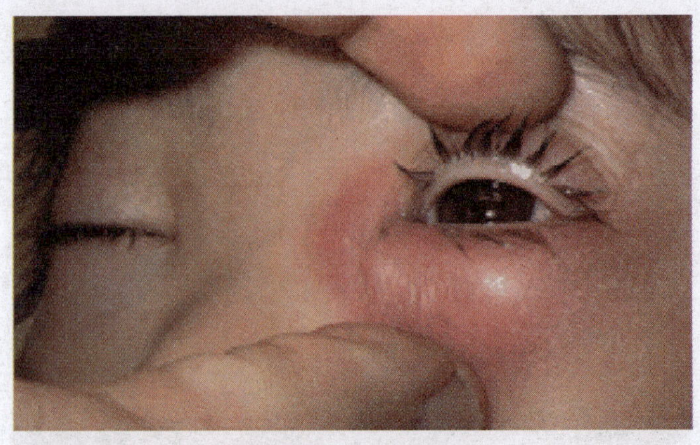

FIG. 6.18 Dacryocystitis

Method of conjunctival examination
- Tarsal conjunctive can be examined by everting eyelid
- Keep the eyes open and look downward
- Grasp the eyelashes of upper eyelid and make it everted.

Normal conjunctiva
- ❖ Color-pink
- ❖ Small number of blood vessels is usually seen
- ❖ Compare vascularity of two eyes.

Conjunctivitis
Inflammation of conjunctiva—causes are:
- Bacterial
- Viral
- Fungal
- Parasitic
- Allergic
- Traumatic
- Chemical
- Idiopathic.

Bacterial conjunctivitis (Fig. 6.19)
- *Mostly due to:* Pneumococci, *Haemophilus influenzae*
- It is usually bilateral, diffusely red
- Discharge—watery or mucopurulent
- Vision—normal, may be blurred—clears on blinking
- Preauricular lymph node—enlarged
- In few cases—upper respiratory tract infection.

Allergic conjunctivitis (Fig. 6.20)
- Usually bilateral
- Watery or sticky discharge

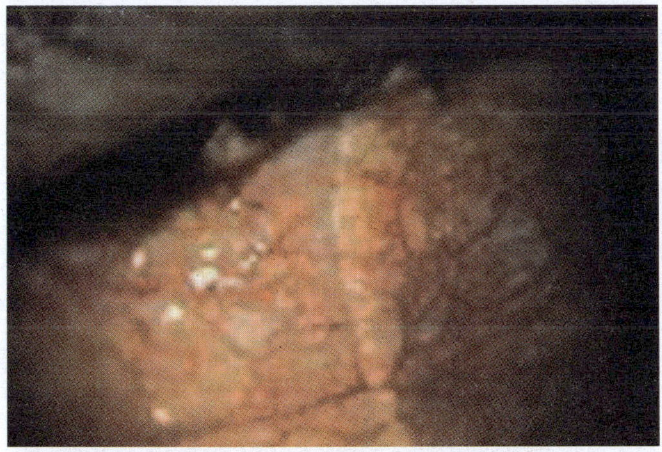

FIG. 6.19 Bacterial conjunctivitis

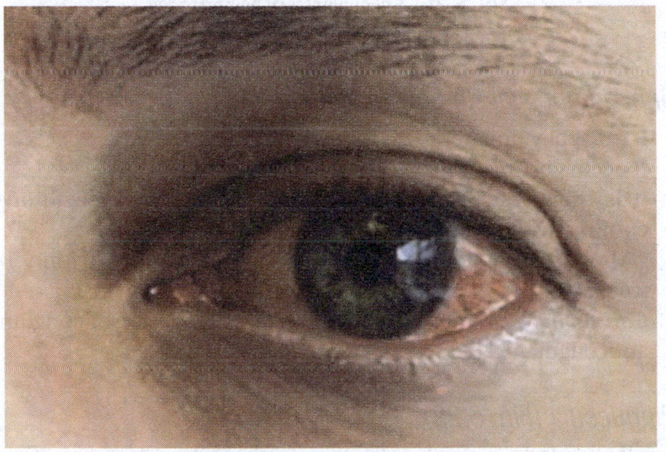

FIG. 6.20 Allergic conjunctivitis

- Itchy
- Mild to moderate redness
- Vision normal.

Giant Papillary Conjunctivitis

Excessive secretion of conjunctival mucus, itchy, development of giant papillae on the tarsal conjunctiva. May be seen in:

- Patient with contact lenses
- Patient with occular prosthesis
- Foreign body in eye.

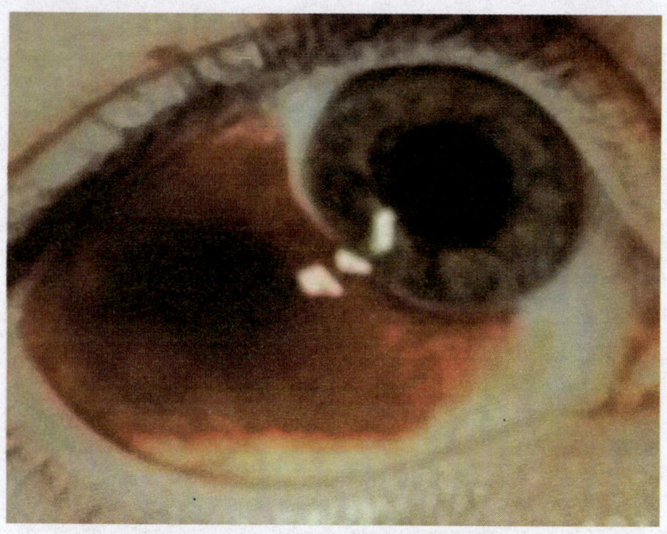

FIG. 6.21 Subconjunctival hemorrhages

Subconjunctival Hemorrhages (Fig. 6.21)

- It is usually unilateral, may be bilateral
- It occurs in any age
- It is bright red in color—due to diffusion of oxygen through conjunctival epithelium.

  It becomes yellow in color, eventually resolve within 1–2 weeks.
- *Causes may be:* Traumatic, precipitated by sneezing or coughing, anticoagulant.

Pinguecula (Fig. 6.22)

Small rounded yellowish collection on nasal canthus secondary to sunlight (actinic) exposure.

Pterygium (Fig. 6.23)

It is excessive conjunctival vascular growth starting from nasal or temporal canthus of bulbar conjunctiva.

As it approaches over cornea and involve visual axes, vision may be impaired.

The cause may be sunlight exposure—may produce irritation, dryness.

Significance of palpebral preauricular lymph node: Tender—viral conjunctivitis.

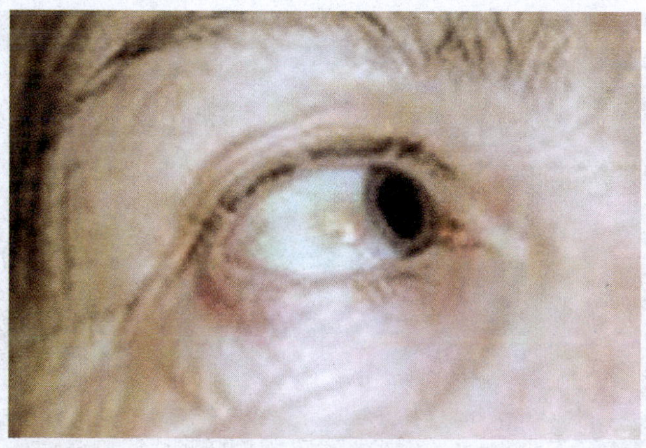

FIG. 6.22   Pinguecula

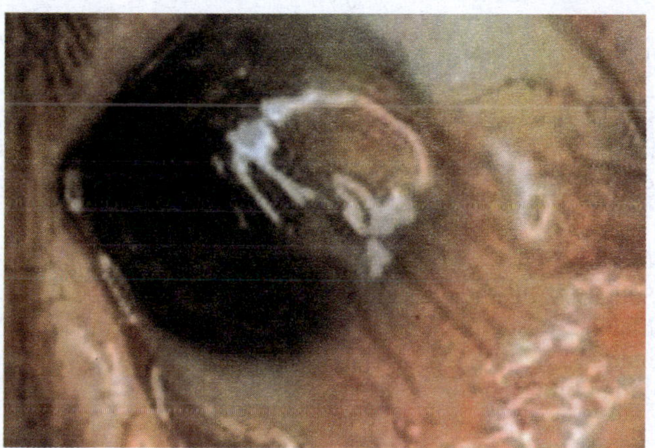

FIG. 6.23   Pterygium

Difference of vascular distribution in case of uveitis and conjunctivitis:
In uveitis—pericorneal vessels are congested.

In conjunctivitis—whole conjunctival vessels are congested diffusely.

Chemosis of Bulbar Conjunctiva (Fig. 6.24)

- Edema of bulbar conjunctiva
- If edema is very severe, it may protrude anteriorly.
- It may be due to allergic conjunctivitis, trauma, proptosis in hyperthyroidism, neurological deficit
- It may occur in melanoma, hemorrhage.

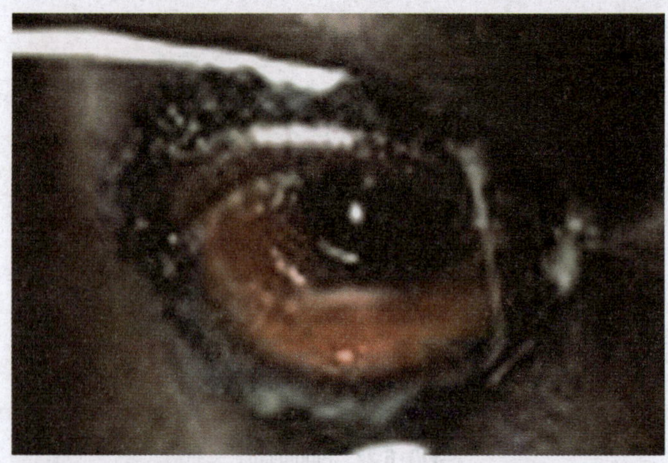

FIG. 6.24 Chemosis of bulbar conjunctiva

Primary Acquired Melanosis

- Unilateral
- Melanotic pigment at develops in conjunctival or corneal epithelium
- Starts at middle age.

Conjunctival Nevus (Fig. 6.25)

- Solitary, well defined, slightly elevated lesion
- May be present in limbus, plica semilunaris, caruncle and lid margin
- Tan or brown in color.

Papilloma (Fig. 6.26)

Congenital, bilateral tumor, present on superotemporal quadrant of conjunctiva near lateral canthus.

Often fine hairs protrude from its surface.

Examination of Sclera

Sclera should be examined for

- Color
- Nodules
- Hyperemia

Normal sclera is

- White
- Muddy in dark-skin individuals.

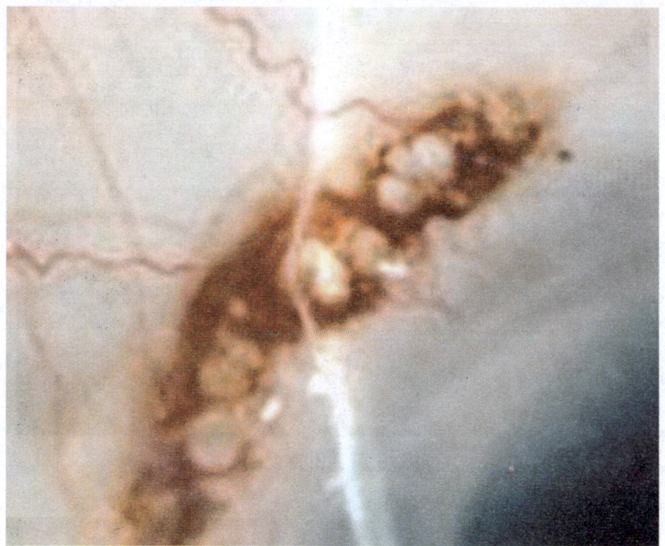

FIG. 6.25 Conjunctival nevus

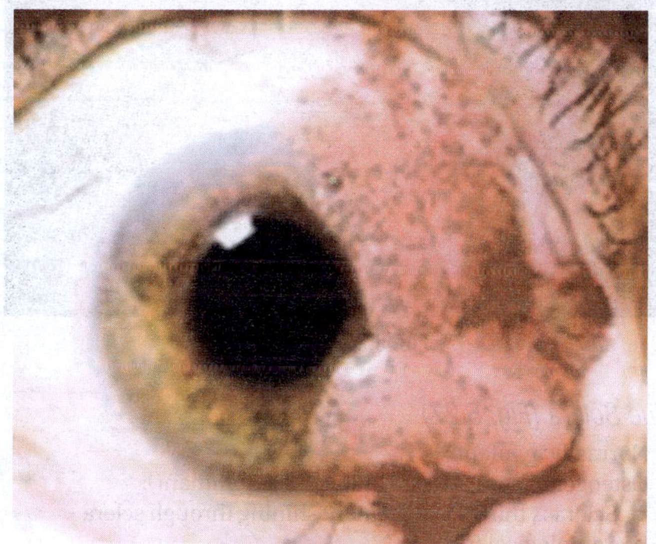

FIG. 6.26 Papilloma

Jaundice

Yellowish discoloration of sclera, skin and mucous membrane due to retention of bilirubin or its product of metabolism.

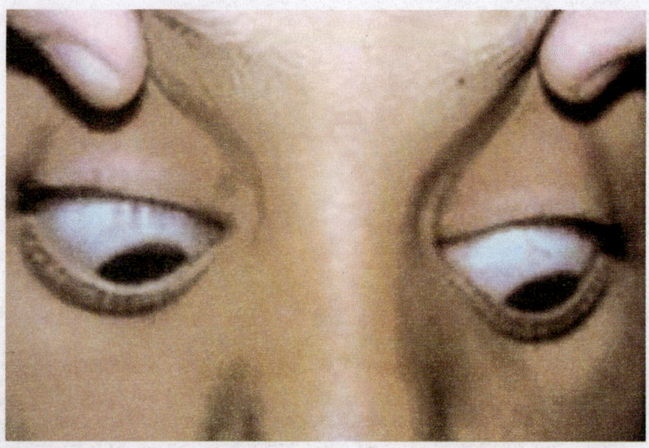

FIG. 6.27   Blue sclera

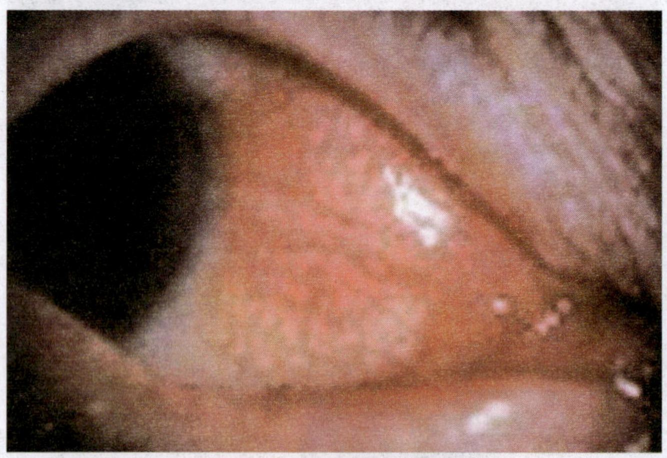

FIG. 6.28   Episcleritis

Blue Sclera (Fig. 6.27)

- Normally in infant
- Osteogenesis imperfecta (autosomal dominant):
  - ❖ Sclera is thin, uveal pigment shining through sclera
  - ❖ Pathological fracture
  - ❖ Deafness.

Episcleritis (Fig. 6.28)

- Recurrent painless benign flat, diffuse or localized and nodular noninfectious inflammation present in sclera
- Frequently bilateral

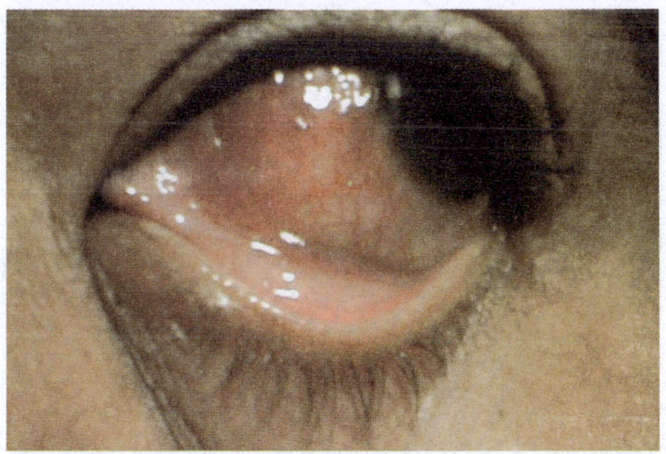

FIG. 6.29 Scleritis

- The causes are:
  - ❖ Inflammatory bowel disease
  - ❖ Herpes zoster
  - ❖ Collagen vascular disease
  - ❖ Syphilis
  - ❖ Rheumatoid arthritis.

Scleritis (Fig. 6.29)

- It is painful recurrent diffuse or localized nodular bilateral inflammatory lesion in sclera associated involvement of cornea, uveal tract or retina
- Photophobia
- Causes—connective tissue orders
- Condition may resolve spontaneously.

Scleromalacia Perforans

Uncommon painless condition characterized by appearance of dehiscence in the sclera in absence of inflammatory changes. As a result:

- Uveal tissue may bulge through dehiscence
- Anterior synechia is present.

Corneal tissue should be inspected for:

- Color
- Cloudiness
- Ulceration
- Opacities.

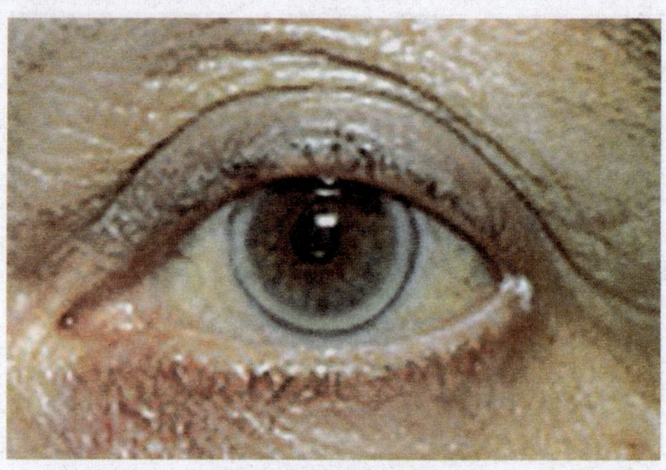

FIG. 6.30 Arcus senilis

Arcus Senilis (Fig. 6.30)

Whitish ring seen at the periphery of cornea in person older thin, aged ≥ 70 years.

It may occur in less than 40 years of age in hypercholesterolemia.

Kayser-Fleischer's Ring (Fig. 6.31)

Greenish yellow ring present in limbus mainly superiorly and inferiorly—due to deposition of copper in Descemet's membrane of the peripheral cornea.

This occurs in Wilson's disease—a disorder of hepatolenticular degeneration due to disorder of copper metabolism.

Corneal Ulcers (Fig. 6.32)

This is painful progressive erosion and loss of necrotic tissue of cornea—caused by:

Bacterial
- Pneumococcal—most common
- *Pseudomonas*—less common, but if affected, produces rapid spread and perforation of cornea
- Herpes simplex—most common virus related infection produces corneal pathology related blindness—dendritic ulcer in cornea
- Patient may present with photophobia, lacrimation, pain in eye, conjunctival hyperemia
- Later stage, corneal ulcer may be painless—due to corneal anesthesia.

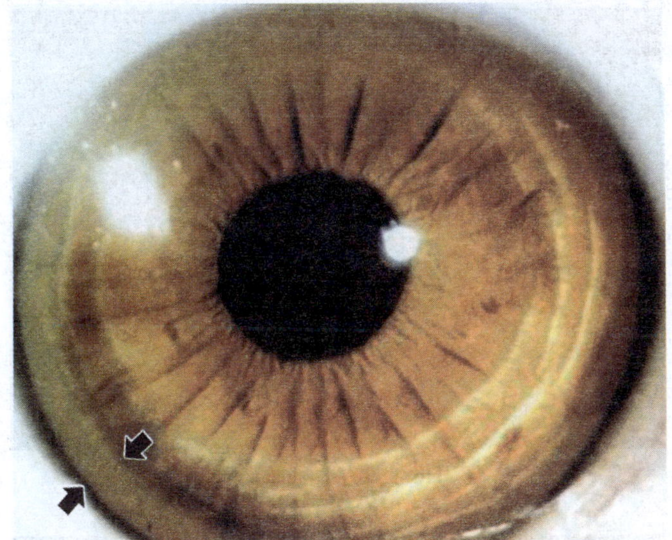

FIG. 6.31   Kayser-Fleischer's ring

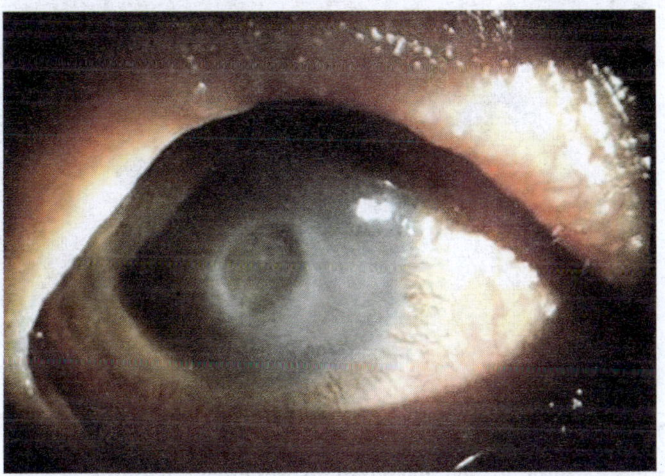

FIG. 6.32   Corneal ulcers

Keratoconus (Fig. 6.33)

- In this condition, cornea protrudes like cone, apex being scarred.
- It is bilateral but asymmetrical
- When the patient is asked to look downwards, keratoconus will be obvious.

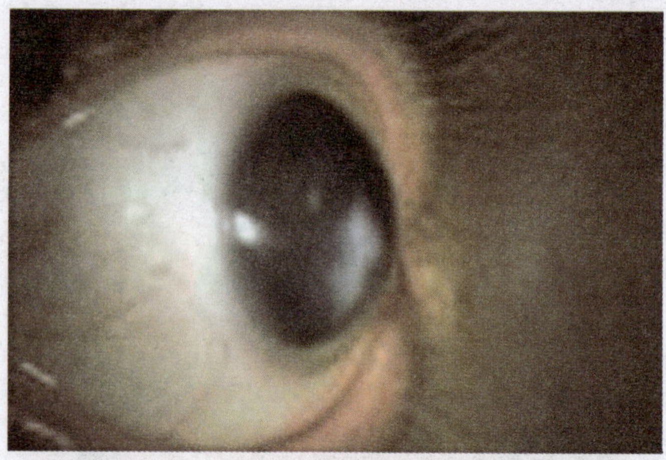

FIG. 6.33 Keratoconus

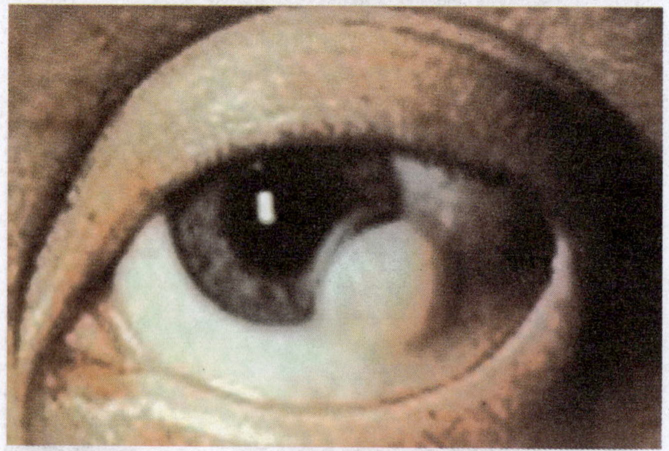

FIG. 6.34 Dermoid

Dermoid (Fig. 6.34)

Smooth, rounded, yellowish benign growth at the limbus.

Iris

Iris should be checked for:
- Shape
- Color
- Nodules
- Vascularity.

Normally blood vessels of iris cannot be seen in naked eye.

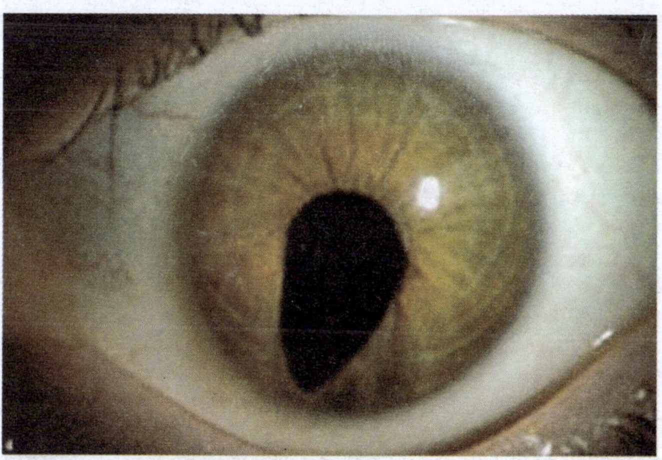

FIG. 6.35   Coloboma of iris

Coloboma of Iris (Fig. 6.35)

- This is a notch or gaping in iris due to failure of fusion of embryonic tissue
- It is usually unilateral, but may be bilateral
- It is usually located in inferior quadrant
- Associated structures involved are—choroids, retina
- It is autosomal dominant
- Visual acuity is normal—if macula is spared.

Iritis or Iridocyclitis (Fig. 6.36)

This is characterized by:
- Congestion of deep episcleral vessels—ciliary flush
- Transudation of protein into anterior chamber and deposition of inflammatory cells on corneal epithelium—keratic precipitates

$$\downarrow$$

Iris will be blurred—called muddy iris.
- *Causes are*
  - ❖ *Infection:*
    - Exogenous from cornea, iris, sclera, retina
    - Endogenous—Tuberculosis, syphilis, gonorrhea, viral infection, mycotic infection.
  - ❖ *Systemic disease—autoimmune diseases:*
    - Rheumatoid arthritis
    - SLE
    - Reiter's disease
    - Behçet's syndrome
    - Relapsing polychondritis.

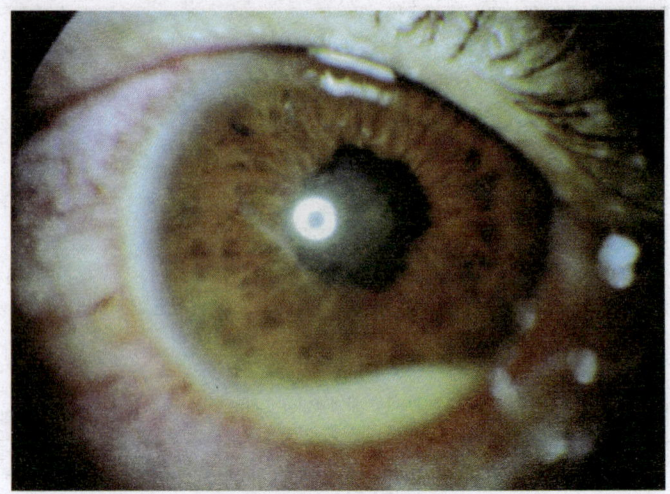

FIG. 6.36 Iridocyclitis

FIG. 6.37 Iris heterochromia

- *Complications:*
  - ❖ Adhesion with cornea—anterior synechiae
  - ❖ Adhesion with retina—posterior synechiae
  - ❖ Glaucoma.

Iris Heterochromia (Fig. 6.37)

Different pigmentation in two iris. It is rare but may occur in:
- Iritis
- Iris melanoma
- Normal variant
- Horner's syndrome—congenital—in this case one iris is lighter than the other.

Uveitis (Fig. 6.38)

Inflammation of middle coat is called uveitis.

Causes: Autoimmune diseases or systemic manifestation of rheumatoid arthritis.

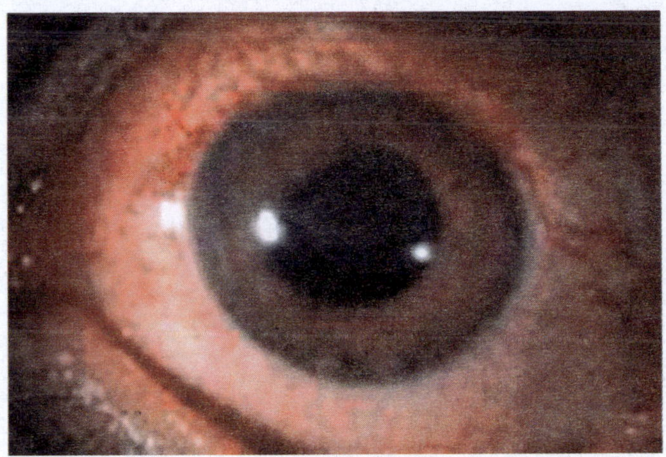

FIG. 6.38   Uveitis

Classification of Uveitis

- *Anterior:* It is also called iritis or iridocyclitis
- *Intermediate:* It is called pars planitis
- *Posterior:* It is also called choroiditis.

Symptoms
- Aching pain
- Photophobia
- Smaller pupil.

In case of intermediate and posterior uveitis:
- No pain or acting sensation
- Blurred vision
- Floaters (Fig. 6.39).

It differs from conjunctivitis: It has no discharge.

It differs from keratitis: Pain is unrelieved by topical anesthetics.

It differs from glaucoma: Intraocular pressure is normal.

Anterior Chamber

- *Hypopion (Fig. 6.40):* A layer of white cells at the bottom of anterior chamber
  Cause:
  - ❖ Infections—sequelae of endophthalmitis
  - ❖ Noninfections—Behçet's disease.
- *Hyphema (Fig. 6.41):* Blood in anterior chamber—if it is small in amount. It is seen at the bottom of the chamber.

  If it is large in amount, it occupies whole of the chamber. Hyphema can be seen by penlight as dark red layer.

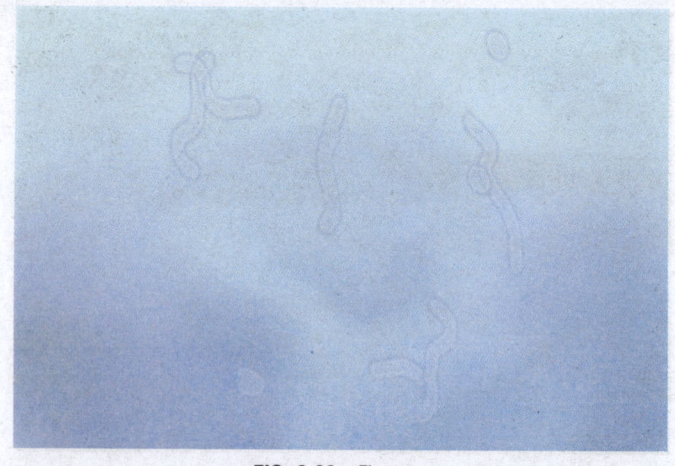

FIG. 6.39 Floaters

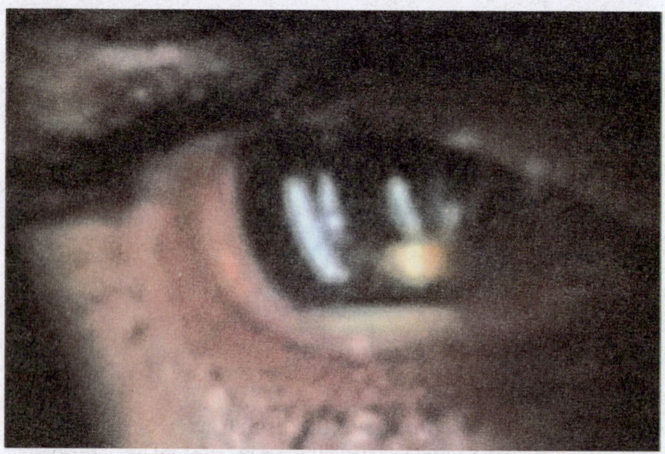

FIG. 6.40 Hypopion

- *Eight-ball hyphema:* If blood occupies whole of anterior chamber—eyes looks black like eight ball
Hyphema may occur from hematological disorders.
  - ❖ *Corneal light reflex:* When the light is thrown into the cornea:
    - In case of normal corneal surface—reflex will be clear, white spot, smooth and round border
    - In case of scarring or drying of cornea—reflex will be irregular and broken up.
  - ❖ *Strabismus (Fig. 6.42):* Misalignment of eyes—it may be:
    - Congenital

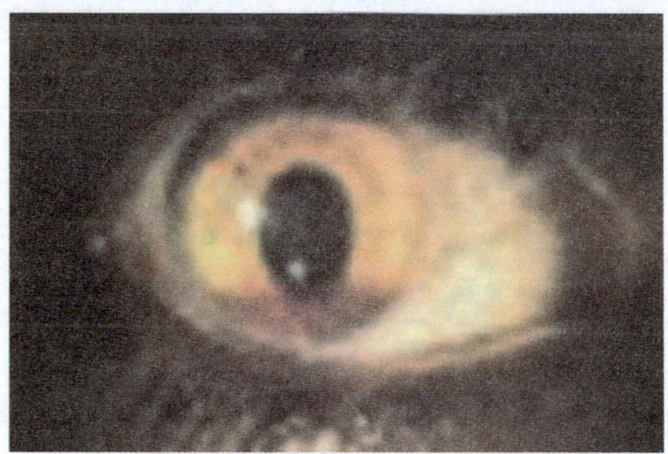

FIG. 6.41 Hyphema

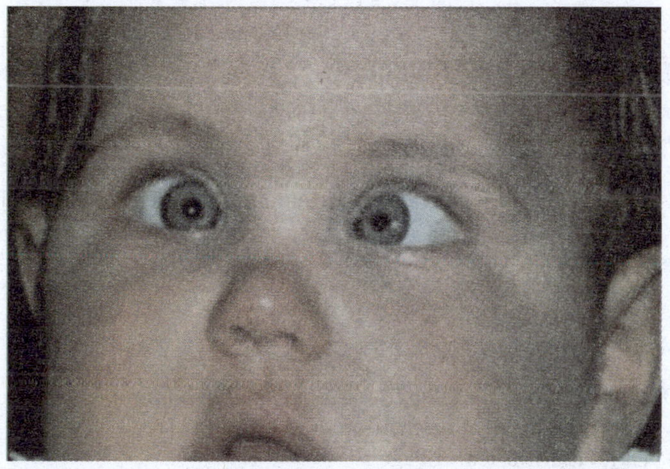

FIG. 6.42 Strabismus

- Acquired
  - Neurogenic
  - Neuromuscular
  - Myogenic

❖ *Pseudostrabismus (Fig. 6.43):* Apparent misalignment of eyes. *Cause:* Children with prominent epicanthic folds—obscuring nasal side of sclera.

Differentiation between strabismus and pseudostrabismus:
Corneal reflex test of both eyes: If the reflexion is centered in both the eyes—diagnosis is pseudostrabismus.

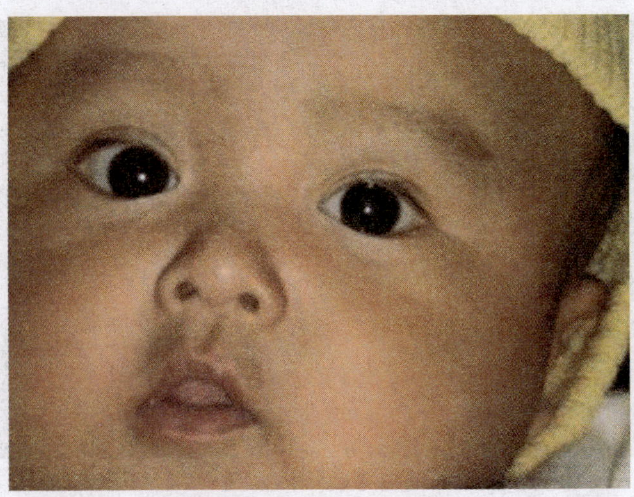

FIG. 6.43 Pseudostrabismus

Value of Ophthalmoscopy

Following structures can be viewed by ophthalmoscopy:

- Anterior end of optic nerve—optic disc
- Retina and its blood supply
- *Red eye reflex:* It provides information of all clear media of the eye:
  - ❖ Cornea
  - ❖ Lens
  - ❖ Anterior chamber
  - ❖ Vitreous.

Ophthalmoscopy should be done all following conditions:

- Complaining of altered vision
- Older than 40 years of age
- Neurological disorders responsible for increase intracranial pressure
- Patient with diabetes and hypertension.

Dilatation of pupil can be done by:

- Tropicamide—0.5 or 1 percent
- 2.5 percent phenylephrine.

Red Reflex

It is the light reflected by the retina—because of its rich vascular supply. This reflects the transparency of light-reflecting media.

Red eye reflex can be viewed through ophthalmoscope, observing the pupil from a distance of 1–2 feet.

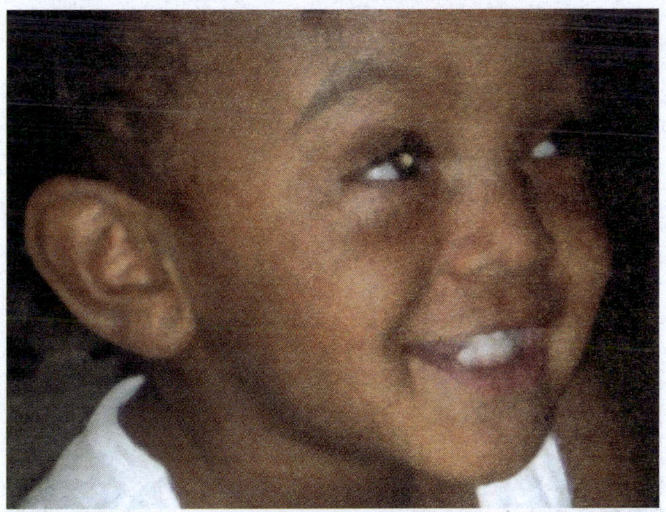

FIG. 6.44   Leukocoria

Leukocoria (Fig. 6.44)

While pupil or opaque pupil—occurs in following conditions:
- In children—retinoblastoma
- Cataract
- Severe intraocular inflammation
- Retinopathy
- Retinal detachment.

Causes of abnormal red eye reflex:
All, those are responsible for opacity of light transmitting media, produce abnormal red eye reflex:
- *Anterior eye structures:*
  - ❖ Lens—cataract
  - ❖ Cornea—scars, abrasion, ulcers.
- *Posterior eye structures:*
  - ❖ *Vitreous:* A clear gel like fluid—fills the area between lens and retina. Vitreous opacities can result from:
  - ❖ Vitreous hemorrhage:
    - Proliferative retinopathy:
      - Diabetes
      - Hypertension
      - Sickle cell disease
      - Blood dyscrasia
      - Thrombocytopenia.
    - Tearing of retinal vessels due to retinal detachment.
  - ❖ *White blood cells may be present in vitreous chamber due to:*
    - Choroiditis
    - Retinitis.

The following structures should be visualized by ophthalmoscopy.

Optic disc (Fig. 6.45A)

Optic disc—can be identified by following the vessels path:

- Seeing its caliber—as it is increasing its caliber
- Arrow head appearance at the bifurcation of retinal vessels.

Normal optic disc (Fig. 6.45B) is:

- Oval
- Yellowish margin
- Sharp margin.

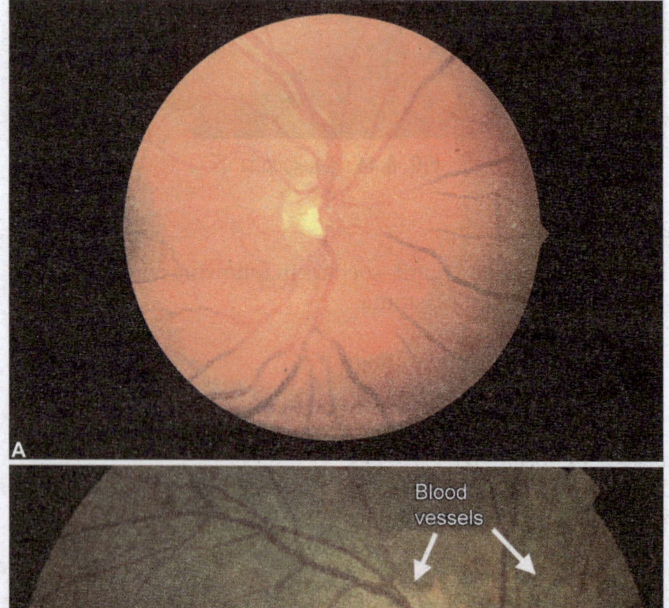

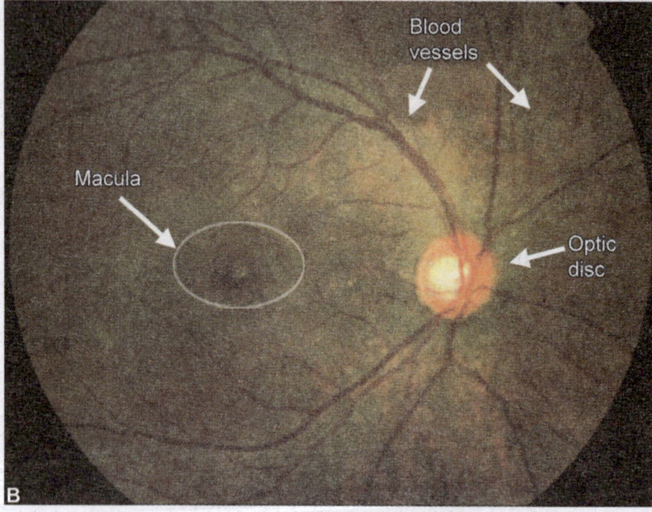

FIGS 6.45A AND B Normal fundus

Variant of optic disc:
- *Hypopigmented crescent surrounding optic disc:* Due to failure of pigmented layers to extend to optic disc margin
- Hyperpigmented area surround optic disc.

Optic cup:
- It is central excavation in optic disc—where retinal vessels exit or enter the optic up
- It is not greater than 50 percent of optic disc.

Pathologic changes in optic disc

Redness of disc:
- Retinal vessel occlusion
- Papilledema
- Polycythemia
- Neovascularization of the disc.

Pale optic disc:
- Normal variant
- Myopic eye
- Optic atrophy—due to death of axon cells.

Causes of optic atrophy (Figs 6.46 and 6.47)
- Optic neuritis—in multiple sclerosis
- Ischemic optic neuropathy (Fig. 6.48) Vasculitis (temporal arteritis)
- Compression of optic nerve, optic chiasma, optic tract—tumor, aneurysm, meningioma.
- Toxin
  - ❖ Ethylene glycol
  - ❖ Methanol.

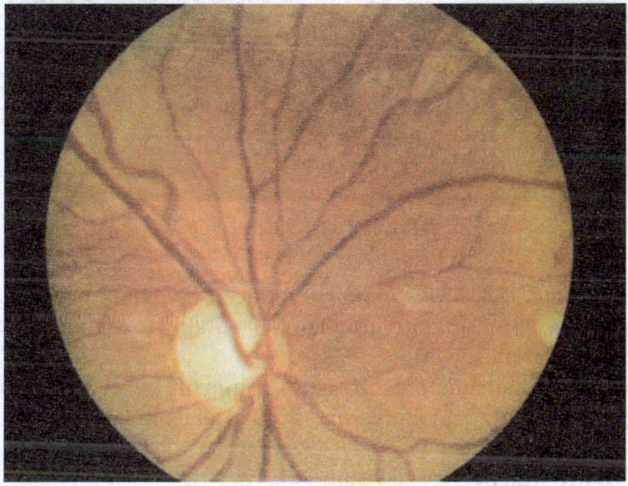

FIG. 6.46 Optic atrophy (primary)

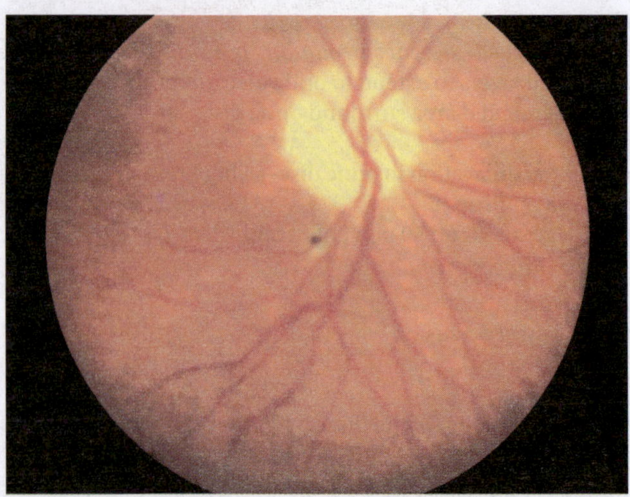

FIG. 6.47   Optic atrophy (secondary)

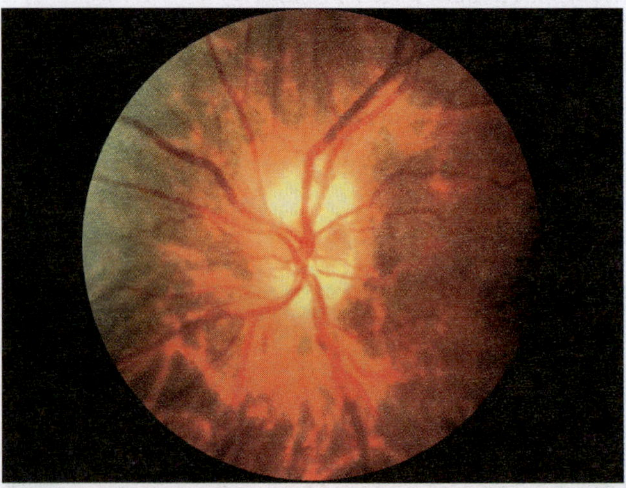

FIG. 6.48   Ischemic optic neuropathy

Normal flow of aqueous humor: Produced by ciliary body, flows through the pupil to anterior chamber—drains to venous system via trabecular meshwork.

Normal intraocular pressure is 10–21 mm of Hg.

Increased intraocular pressure is called glaucoma.

Eye findings in glaucoma (Figs 6.49 and 6.50)

- Red eye with decreased vision
- Cloudy cornea

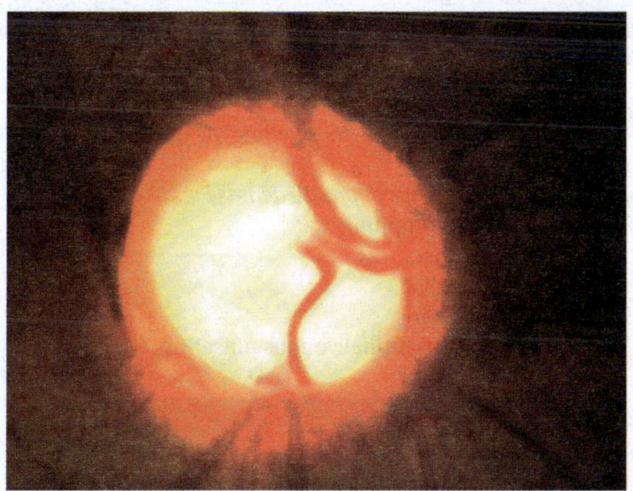

FIG. 6.49   Glaucomatous cupping

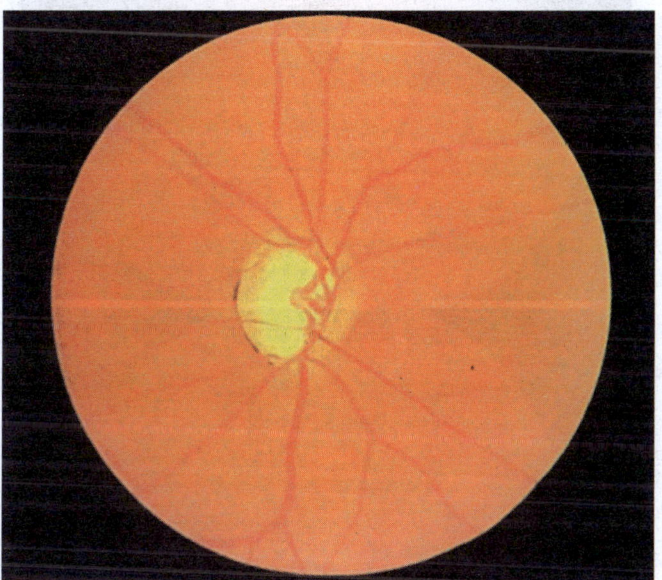

FIG. 6.50   Glaucomatous fundus

- Irregular light reflex
- *Ciliary flush:* All these finding are due to high intraocular pressure.

Optic disc of glaucoma: >50 percent of size of optic disc—occupied by optic cup—pathological cupping—its vertical diameter or oblique diameter is increased —oval cup.

Symptoms of acute glaucoma: Pain, nausea, abnormal visual acuity, lacrimation, seeing halos around light.

Disc size
Swelling of optic disc—due to swelling of optic nerve head—is called papilledema.
Ophthalmoscopic findings in papilledema (Figs 6.51A and B)
- Loss of physiologic cupping
- Blurring of optic disc
- Hyperemia of the disc
- Engorged retinal veins
- Loss of spontaneous retinal venous pulsation.

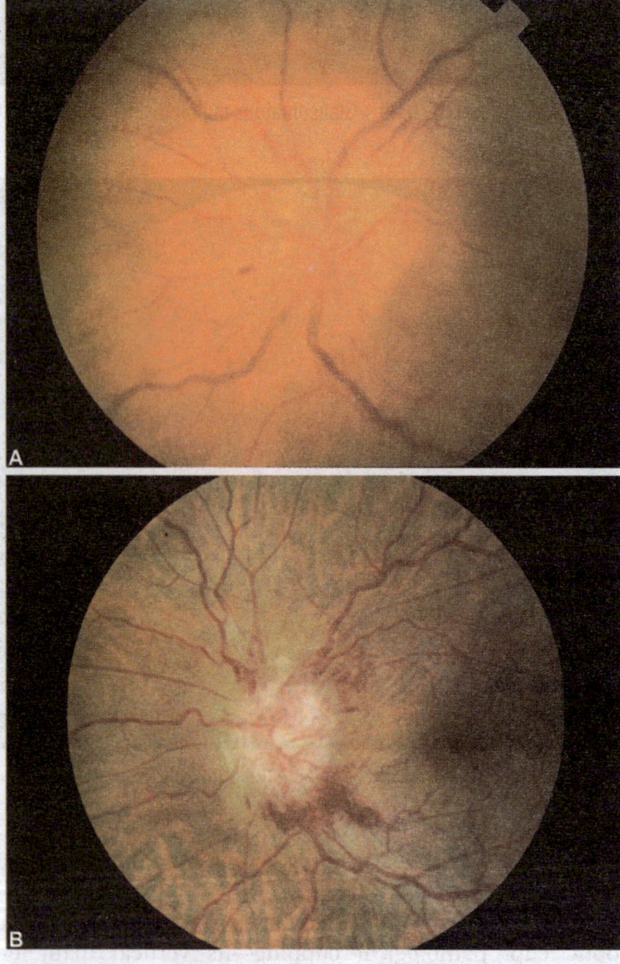

FIGS 6.51A AND B   Papilledema

- Cotton-wool spots
- Peripapillary hemorrhage.

Retinal venous pulsations are visible, collapse and refilling of largest branches of central retinal vein—seen as they emerge from the cup and cross the disc.

When intracranial pressure increases—retinal veins become much engorged.

In papilledema—visual acuity will be lost.

Cause of papilledema:

- Congenital
- Central retinal vein occlusion
- Ischemic optic neuropathy
- Infiltrative—lymphoma
- Inflammatory
- Metabolic—thyroid ophthalmopathy
- Increased intracranial pressure.

Optic neuritis: Inflammation of optic serve—called optic neuritis. Two forms of optic neuritis:

1. *Papillophlebitis:* Visible swelling of optic disc (Fig. 6.52) Complaining of:
   - Acute unilateral loss of vision
   - Eye pain
   - Afferent pupillary defect
   - Impairment of color vision.
2. *Retrobulbar neuritis:* Inflammation of optic nerve behind optic nerve head—produces:
   - Visible scotoma
   - No optic disc swelling

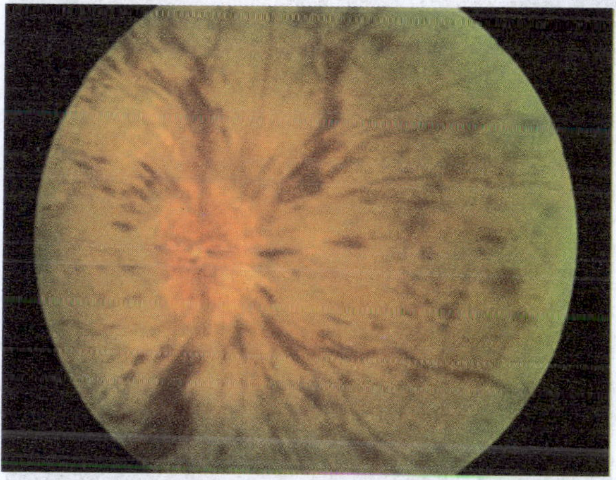

FIG. 6.52   Papillophlebitis

- ❖ Afferent papillary defect
- ❖ Impairment of color vision.

Acute ischemic optic neuropathy (Fig. 6.53): Infarction of optic nerve head. Causes of AION:

- *Nonarteritic:*
  - ❖ Hypertension
  - ❖ Diabetes
  - ❖ Myocardial infarction.
- *Arteritic:* Giant cell arteritis—inflammation of medium size arteries. Triad of scalp tenderness, headache and jaw claudication.

Retinal circulation: This circulation includes (Fig. 6.54).

- Central retinal artery
- Central retinal vein.

Artery branches originates at optic disc

↓

Distributed centrifugally toward retinal quadrants

↓

Distributed in superficial nerve fiber layer

Venous branches—arranged similarly in opposite direction centripetally towards optic disc.

Differentiation of retinal vein from retinal artery:

- Retinal vein is darker than arteries.
- Arteries are more glistening.

Arterial light reflex increases with progressive hypertension

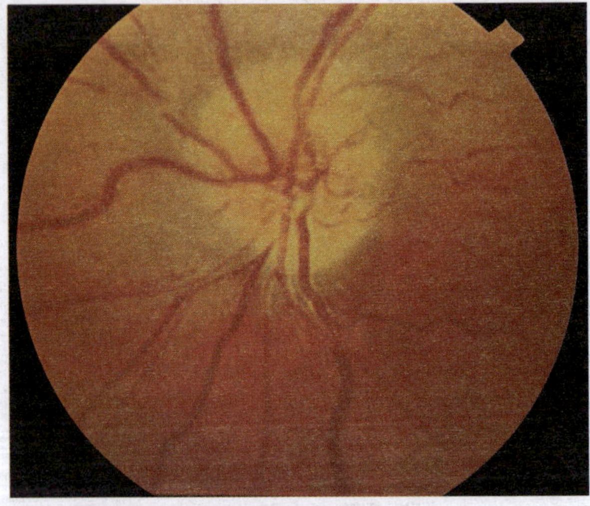

FIG. 6.53 Acute ischemic optic neuropathy (AION)

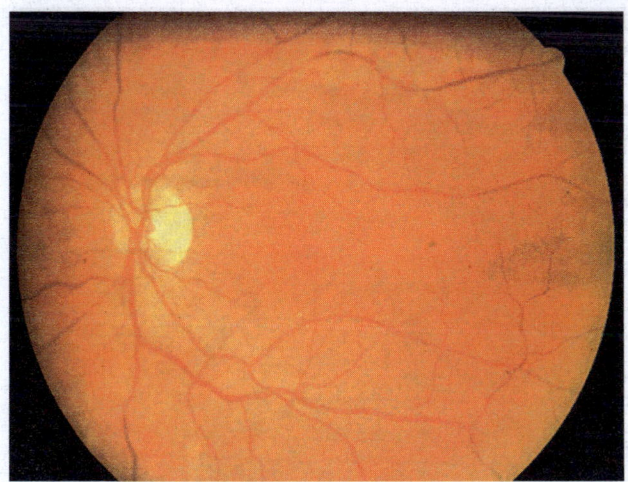

FIG. 6.54 Normal retina

Arteriolar wall progressively thickness
↓
Resembling copper wire at first due to increased light reflex
↓
Silver wire appearances

Eye pictures of hypertensive retinopathy (Figs 6.55 and 6.56)
- Leaking of serum—hard exudates
- Leaking of blood—dot, blot or flame shaped hemorrhage
- *Late stage of hypertension:* Retinal infarct (cotton-wool spots) (Fig. 6.57)
- *In hypertensive crisis:* Papilledema
- *In chronic hypertension:* Arterial wall thickening—producing copper wire followed by silver wire appearance
- *When more thickening of arteriolar wall:* Arteriovenous nicking.

Central retinal artery occlusion: Painless loss of vision in one eye.
- Retina is pale swelled
- Macula is cherry red—due to visualization of choroidal circulation through fovea
- Afferent pupillary defect.
  Cause is—embolus from carotid artery.

Manifestation of central retinal vein occlusion (CRVO):
- Dilated and engorged vein
- Retinal hemorrhages in all quadrants
- Microaneurysm close to retinal vein
- Multiple cotton-wool spots
- Optic disc edema.

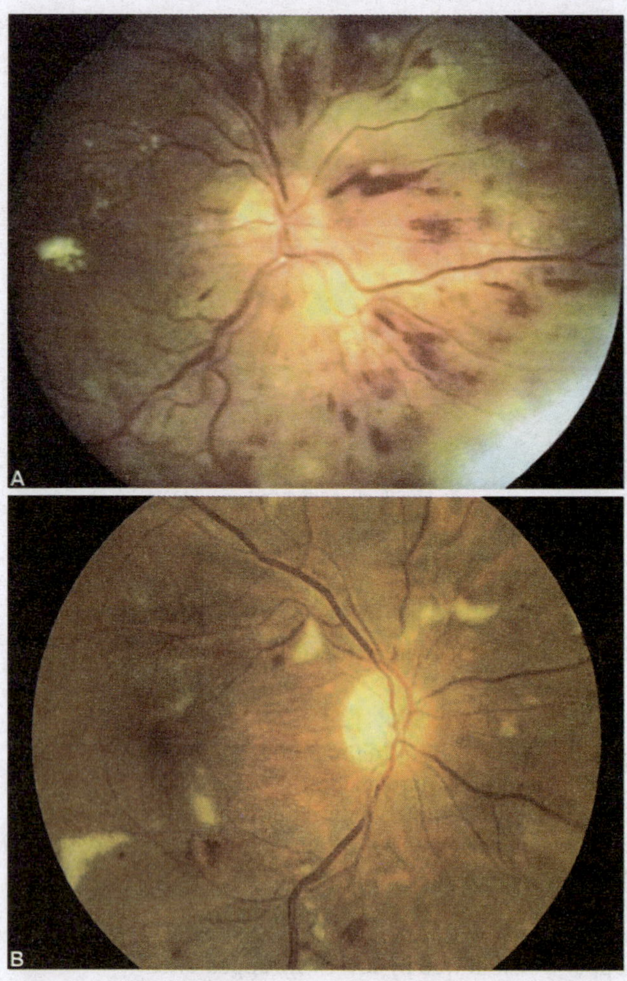

FIGS 6.55A AND B   Hypertensive retinopathy

Fundoscopic findings in branched retinal vein occlusion (BRVO) (Fig. 6.58):
- Cotton-wool spots
- Flame shaped hemorrhages in the affected retinal quadrant
- Dilated and tortuous vein distal to occlusion
- It occurs in superotemporal quadrant.

Causes of BRVO: Arterial compression of vein—in case of following pre-existing disease:
- Atherosclerotic diseases
- Inflammatory disease
- Thromboembolic disease.

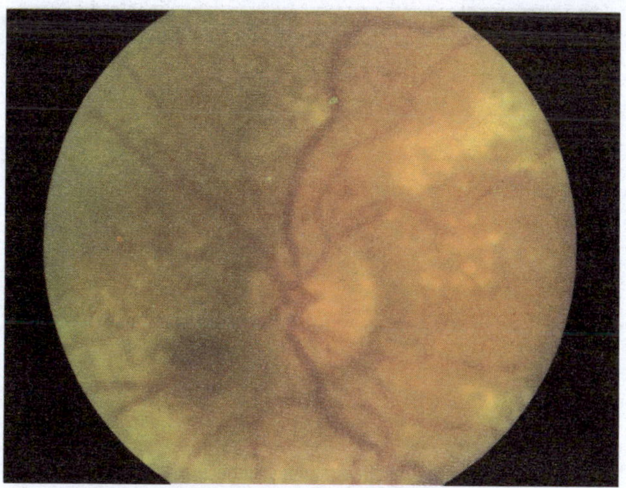

FIG. 6.56   Hypertensive arteriosclerotic retinopathy

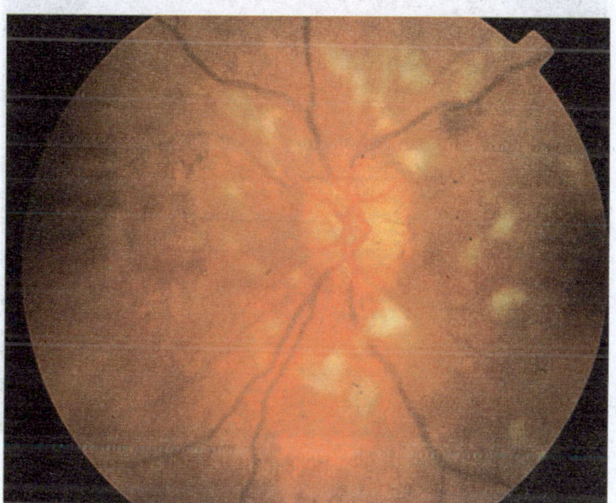

FIG. 6.57   Cotton-wool spots

Hollenhorst plaque (Fig 6.59): Yellowish bright arteriolar wedge shaped deposits at the bifurcation of retinal artery, larger than the artery where they sit.

It is due to arterial cholesterol embolus—originating from ulceration of atheromatous plaque in proximal artery.

Clinical significance: It indicates severe atherosclerotic disease, patient may suffer from myocardial infarction or stroke in future.

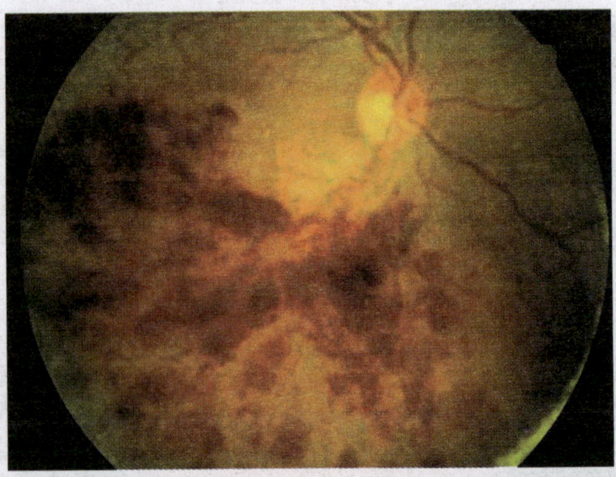

FIG. 6.58 Branched retinal vein occlusion (BRVO)

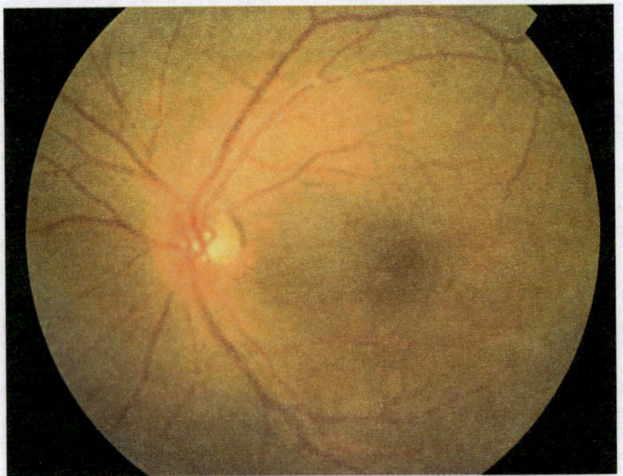

FIG. 6.59 Hollenhorst plaque

Neovascularization of retina (Fig. 6.60)
- Formation of new vessels—in retina, may begin in retina. Ultimately clusters around optic disc
- Cause:
  - ❖ Diabetes
  - ❖ Retinal ischemia due to hemoglobinopathies.

Background retinopathy (Fig. 6.61)
- *Yellow-white retinal spots:* Following are yellow-white retinal spots:

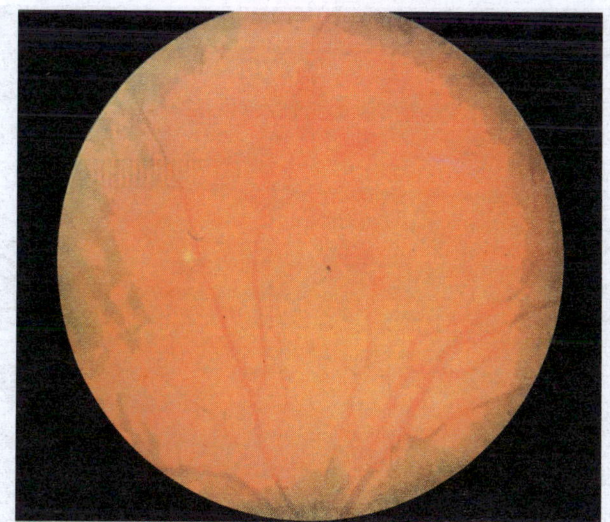

FIG. 6.60   Neovascularization of retina

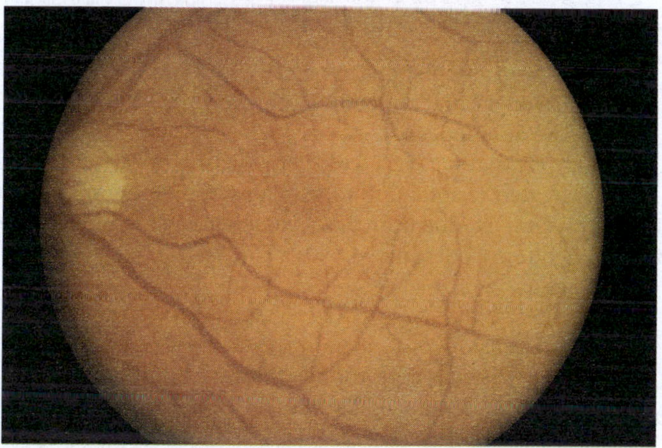

FIG. 6.61   Background retinopathy

❖ *Cotton-wool spots:* These are oval, white, superficial ill-defined borders—obscuring retinal vessels. Cause—retinal infarct due to microvascular disease.
  - Diabetes
  - Hypertension
  - Leukemia
  - Lymphoma
  - Infection subacute bacterial endocarditis

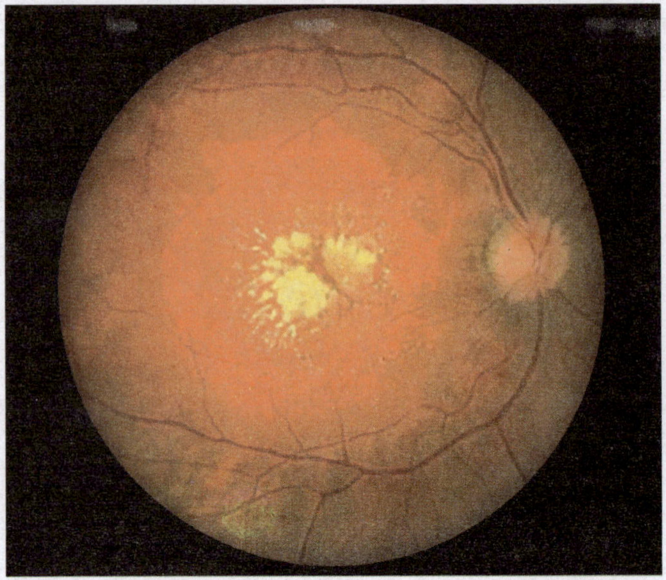

FIG. 6.62 Hard exudates

- Collagen vascular disease
- Increased intracranial pressure
- Serve anemia.

❖ *Hard exudates (Fig. 6.62):* Yellowish or whitish, well demarcated lesions due to exudates containing cholesterol and serum residue from leaky vessels. They are more deeper than cotton-wool spots.

Causes are:

- Diabetes
- Hypertension.

❖ *Drusen bodies:* Discrete, round, yellowish lipoprotein deposits in retinal pigmentary epithelium, near macular region, rarely causing visual disturbances.

Causes: Age related macular degeneration.

Optic disc drusen (Fig. 6.63): There are globular deposits located near optic nerve head. It is made up of:

- Mucoproteins
- Mucopolysaccharides
- Calcification.

Cause: Retinitis pigmentosa.

Chorioretinal scar: Lesions are present in retina and choroids—may be sequelae of inflammation, trauma, surgery or toxoplasmosis.

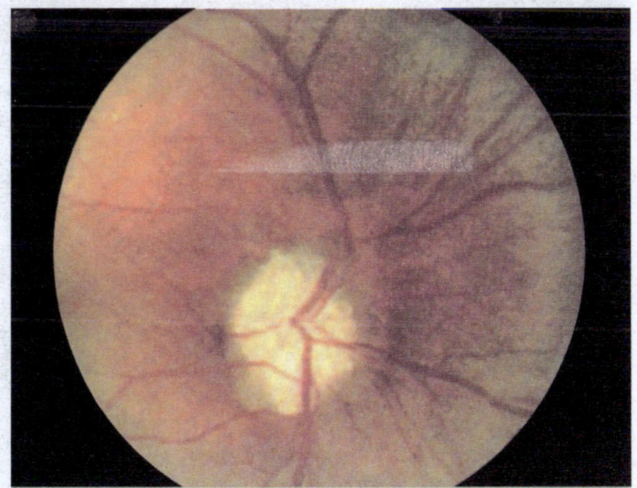

FIG. 6.63 Optic disc drusen

- ❖ *Myelinated nerve fibers:* They are congenital myelinated nerve fiber—bright while color, varying size, superficial, obscuring blood vessels.
- *Red spots:* Following red spots can be seen in ophthalmoscopy.
  - ❖ *Retinal hemorrhage:*
    - They are released from leaky vessels
    - They are of different shapes:
      - Flame shaped—arranged superficially along the orientation of nerve fiber layer. These are more common in hypertension
      - Dot shaped—arranged vertically in middle retinal layer, circular shape, well demarcated. These are common in diabetes.
  - ❖ *Microaneurysm:* These are secular out pouching of retinal capillaries—looking like well demarcated red dot
  - ❖ *White centered hemorrhage:* These are red spot with white centers—called Roth's spot.
    Causes:
    - Subacute bacterial endocarditis
    - Diabetes
    - Intracranial hemorrhage
    - Anemia
    - Thrombocytopenia.
- *Brown-black spots:*
  - ❖ *Retinitis pigmentosa (Figs 6.64A and B):* These are aggregation of pigment in retina arranged like bony specule. These are degenerative condition.

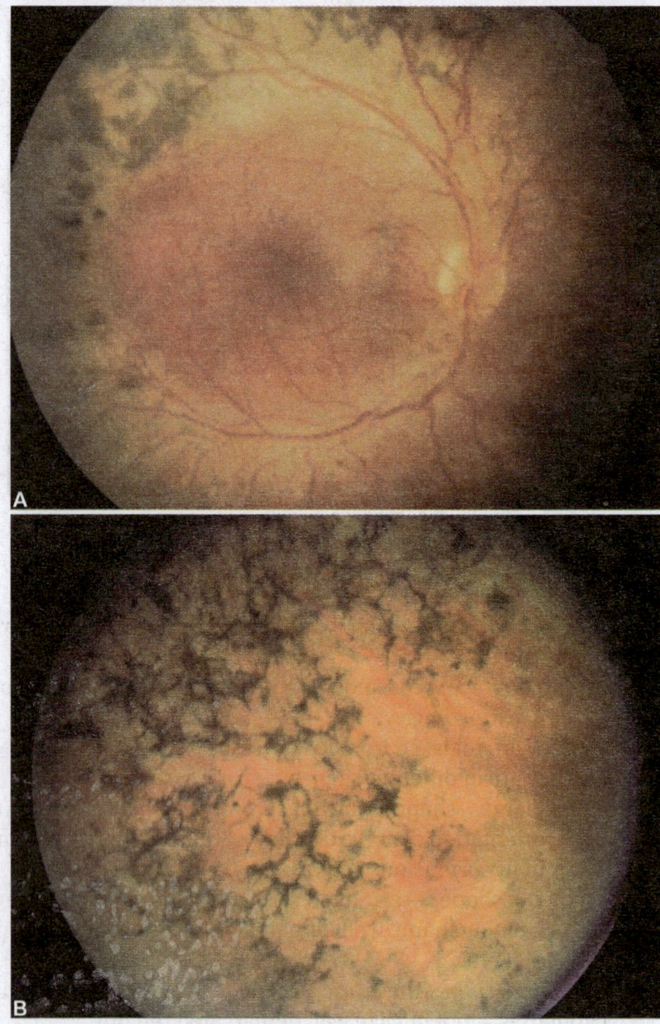

FIGS 6.64A AND B Retinitis pigmentosa

Case:

- Congenital
- Vitamin A deficiency.

❖ *Retinal pigment epithelium hypertrophy:* They are >4 in number, different sizes, never larger than optic disc, do not compromise vision
❖ Normally they are <4
❖ *Melanoma (Fig. 6.65):* Most common malignancy of eye. They are raised highly pigmented and symptomatic
❖ *Benign nevi.*

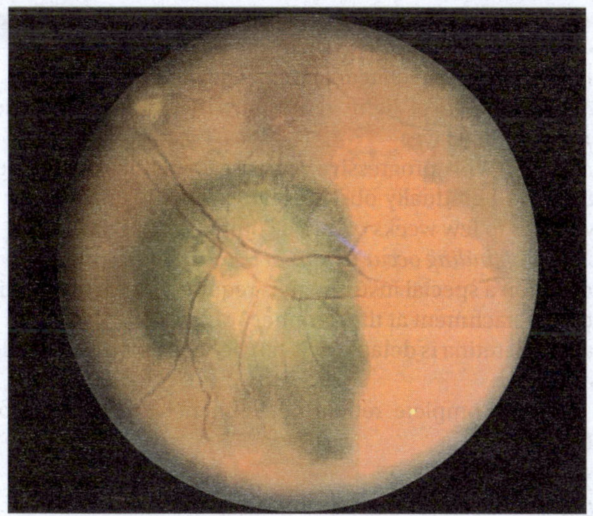

FIG. 6.65 Melanoma

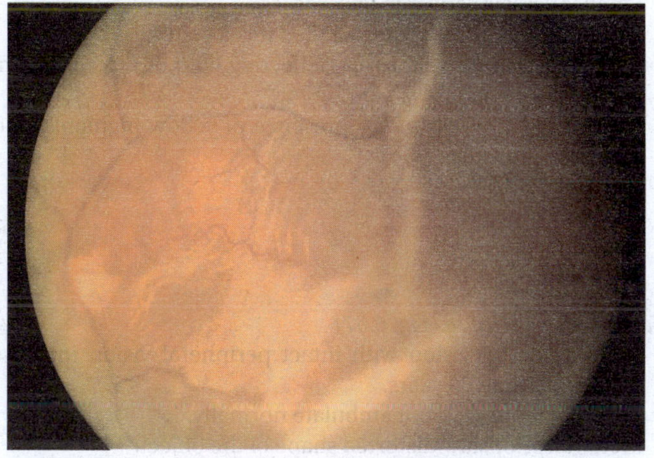

FIG. 6.66 Retinal detachment

Retinal detachment (Fig. 6.66): The shearing of retina into two layers:

1. Outer one—pigment epithelial layer.
2. Inner one—sensory neural part of retina.

Causes of retinal detachment:

- Degenerative tear of sensory retina—allows vitreous fluid enters in between the layers of retina—producing detachment
- In diabetic—proliferative retinopathy, neovascular membrane contracts and pulls the retina from retinal pigmentary epithelium.

Presentation in patient with retinal detachment: Three 'F's:

- *Floaters:* Sudden appearance of floaters—clusters of cells released at the time of tear and float in vitreous body
- *Flashes:* 'Shown of light' represents mechanical activation of sensory retinal layer
- *Field loss:* With progressive increase in retinal detachment, a curtain will gradually obscure the vision. This may occur from few hours to few weeks of initial complaints.

Three types of finding occur in retinal detachment:

1. Most often a special instrument is required for early detection of retinal detachment at the periphery of retina.
2. If a part of retina is detached, it can be seen as white fine folds on its surface.
3. In case of complete retinal detachment—there is loss of red reflex.

Macula

- It is temporal to optic disc, one-forth of its size
- It is darker than surrounding retina
- Smaller vessels converge towards it
- Little dipping in the center—called fovea centralis.
  It acts as concave mirror—reflecting light of the ophthalmoscope.
- It is yellow in color due to presence of yellow pigment abnormalities in macula.
  - ❖ Edema
  - ❖ Hemorrhage
  - ❖ Exudates
  - ❖ Drusen.

Macular degeneration (Fig. 6.67)

- Loss of central vision with intact peripheral vision in person aged more than 50 years.
- Patient cannot read but ambulate normally.
- Metamorphopsia—distorted shape of the object.
- Micropsia—small size of object.

Findings of diabetic retinopathy: It is divided into:

- *Background diabetic retinopathy* (Figs 6.68A and B):
  - ❖ Microaneurysm—earliest sign
  - ❖ Intraretinal hemorrhages—dot-shaped
  - ❖ With progression of retinopathy:
    - Dot and blot shaped hemorrhages
    - Hard exudates
    - Soft exudates
    - Venous beading
    - Intraretinal microvascular abnormalities.

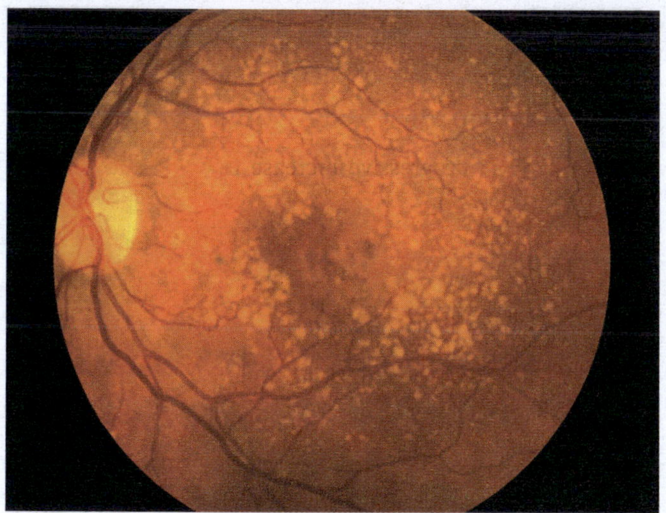

FIG. 6.67   Age-related macular degeneration

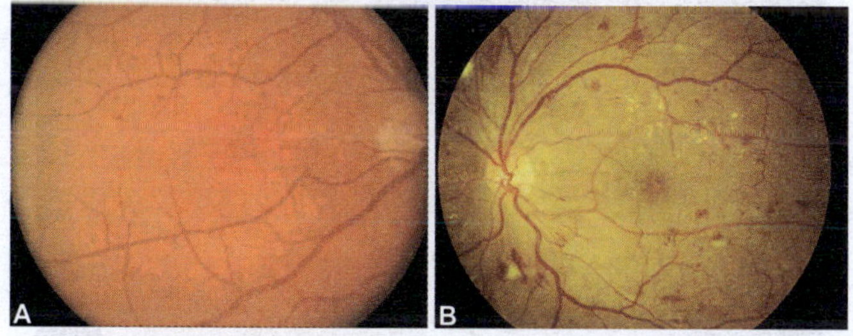

FIGS 6.68A AND B   Background diabetic retinopathy

- *Proliferative diabetic retinopathy* (Figs 6.69A and B)
  - ❖ Neovascularization in the inner surface of retina, vitreous, optic disc
  - ❖ Vitreous hemorrhage
  - ❖ Retinal detachment
  - ❖ Late manifestation—new vessels may extend into drainage system of the anterior chamber—producing neovascular glaucoma
  - ❖ Macular edema—due to break down of blood-brain barrier with leakage of plasma into central portion of retina—(Macula)—producing swelling.

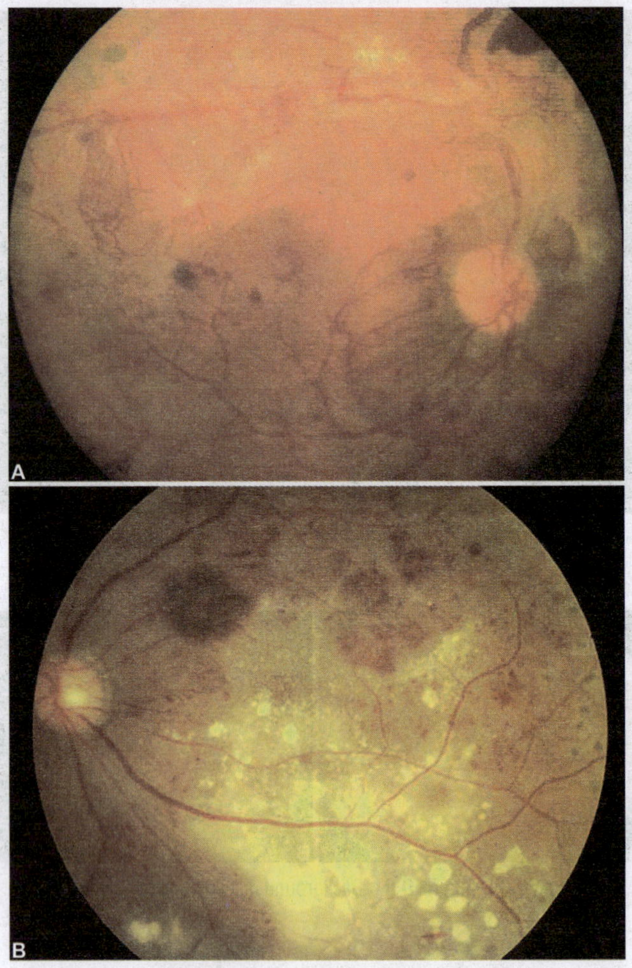

FIGS 6.69A AND B Proliferative diabetic retinopathy

Optic Disc Abnormalities

Disc swelling

- Disc swelling is a sign not a diagnosis
- *Test for optic nerve function:*
  - ❖ Visual acuity
  - ❖ *Pupillary response*
    - Direct reflex
    - Indirect reflex
  - ❖ Visual field
  - ❖ Color vision

Causes of optic disc swelling:
- Optic neuritis
- Papilledema.

Differences	Papilledema	Optic neuritis
Definition	Passive swelling of optic disc secondary to increased intracranial pressure	Inflammations optic nerve head two types: 1. Papillitis 2. Retrobulbar neuritis
Visual acuity	Transiently obscured	Reduced
Pupil reaction	Normal, no RAPD	Positive RAPD in unilateral cases
Visual field	Enlarged blind spot	Central or centrocecal scotoma
Color vision	Normal	Red desaturation

Causes of disc swelling

Unilateral
- Vascular—AION, CRV, diabetes
- Inflammatory—papillitis—uveitis, sarcoidosis, viral, SLE
- Hereditary—optic neuropathy
- Infiltrative—tumor—retinoblastoma, lymphoma
- Infective—toxoplasmosis, herpes, Lime's disease.

Bilateral
- Raised intracranial pressure—BIH, SOL
- Malignant hypertension
- Diabetic papillopathy
- Infiltrative papilledema
- Toxic—ethambutol.
  Chloramphenicol, uremia.

Findings in glaucomatous optic neuropathy
- Increased cup/disc ratio—(normal 0.1–0.3) (Abnormal—>0.4)
- Nasalization of vessels in optic disc—displacement of retinal vessels from center to nasal aspect of cup in optic disc
- Bayoneting of vessels in optic disc—double angulations of vessels as they climb up the optic disc
- Very deep cup.

Optic disc revascularization
- Disorganized vessels archimedes seen in optic disc
- Shape—Fronds with thin and fragile vessels
- Revascularization—may involve periphery—assume the shape of 'seafan'.

Nose

■ External Nose (Fig. 7.1)

The normal structures in external nose are
- *Bridge:* It represents bony upper third of the nose
- *Alae:* Cartilage, that makes inferior, medial and lateral two-thirds of the nose
- *Nares:* The paired orifices
- Tips and columella.

Rhinophyma (Fig. 7.2)

Rhino (nose), phyma (tumor). It is also called brandy nose, Topper's nose, run nose. It is described as-thickened, erythematous, non-tender areas covered with multiple telangiectasias. The cause of rhinophyma—is exposure to alcohol.

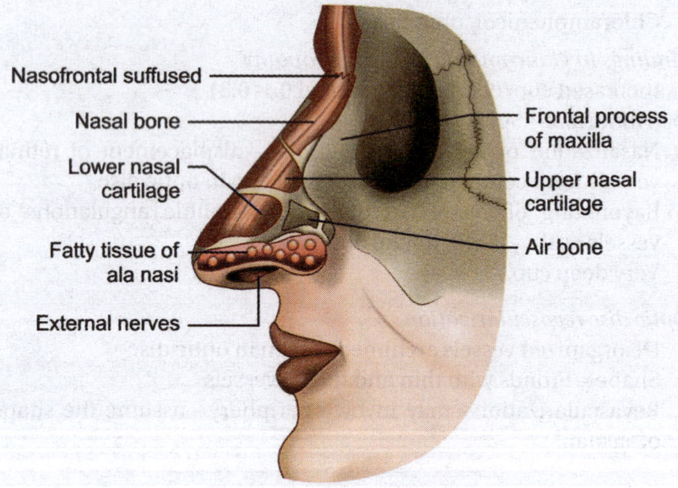

FIG. 7.1 External nose

Saddle Nose

- *True saddle nose (Fig. 7.3):* Due to destruction of bony portion of nose—causes are:
  - ❖ Congenital lues
  - ❖ Wegener's granulomatosis.
- *Pseudo saddle nose:* Due to destruction of cartilaginous portion of nose—due to relapsing poly chondritis.

Nasal Fracture

This is due to trauma. Patient present with:
- Severe pain.
- Anterior epistaxis.
- Periorbital ecchymosis develops 24 hours later after trauma.

Septal Hematoma

It is a painful nodule in the nasal septum easily spottable through nostrils.

Deviation of nasal septum is difficult to be visible in early post-traumatic phase due to edema obscuring the visibility.

Lupus Pernio (Fig. 7.4)

- Chronic
- Nonblanching
- Diffuse
- Purple discoloration of external nose.

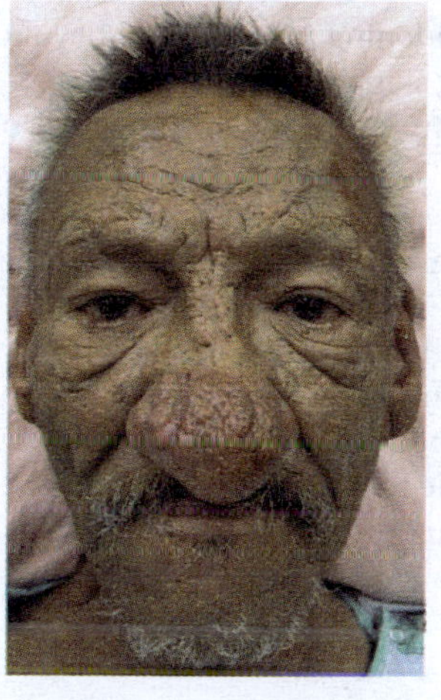

FIG. 7.2   Rhinophyma

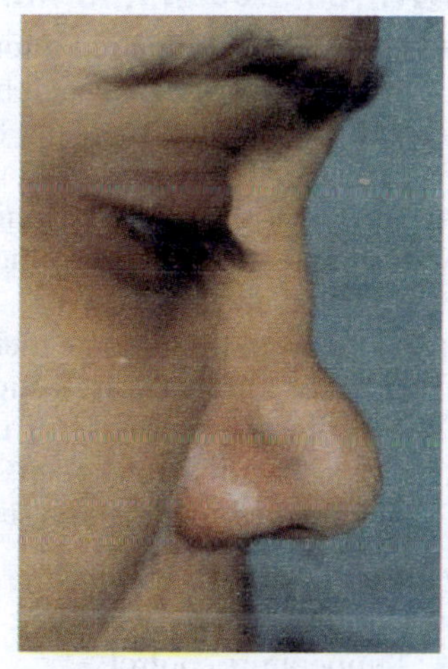

FIG. 7.3   True saddle nose

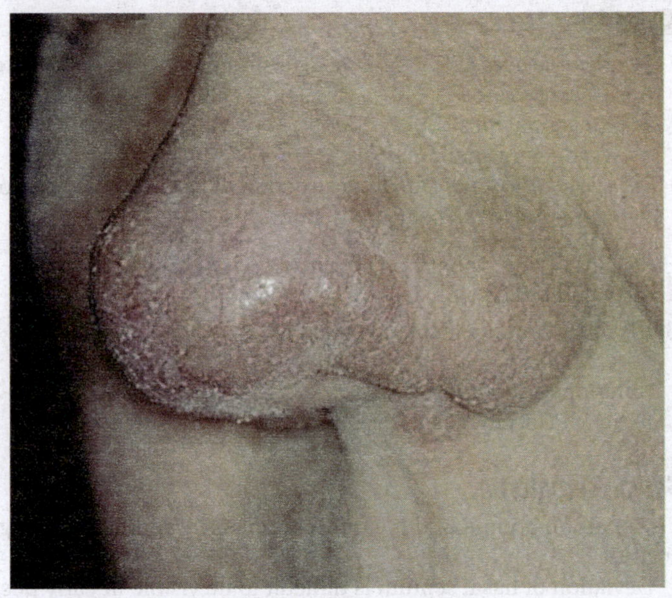

FIG. 7.4 Lupus pernio

In active sarcoidosis (Figs 7.5A and B), it may occur with:
- Uveitis
- Erythema nodosum
- Pulmonary involvement
  Coexisting lesions may occur in ears, checks, fingers and hands.

Structures of Internal Nose (Figs 7.6 and 7.7)

- *Vestibule:* It is a paired internal widening immediately beyond the nares. It is lined by hair bearing skin, not the mucosa
  It is bounded medially by septum and laterally by wall of cartilage.
- *Turbinates:* Deeply beyond the vestibules there are three turbinates—covered by highly vascular mucous membrane, protrude into nasal cavity.
  - ❖ Below each turbinate there is a groove, called meatus
  - ❖ Three turbinates are—superior, middle and inferior
  - ❖ Name of the meatus is given according to the turbinate above it
  - ❖ Nasolacrimal duct opens into the inferior meatus
  - ❖ Openings of paranasal sinuses are present in middle meatus.

Functions of the turbinates are:
- Humidification
- Temperature control
- Filtering of inhaled air.

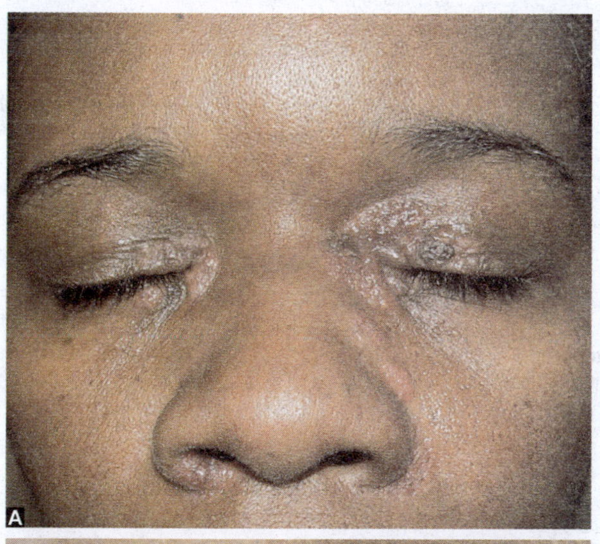

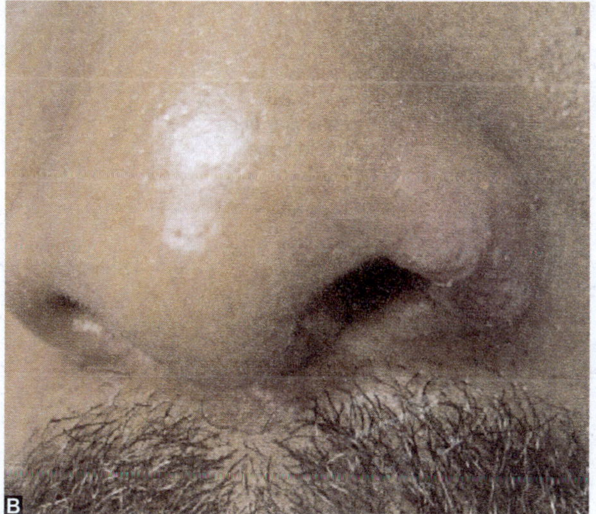

FIGS 7.5A AND B Nasal cutaneous sarcoidosis

Paranasal Sinuses

- These are the airfilled cavities within the bones of skull
- They are lined by mucous membranes
- All the sinuses open into meatus—middle meatus
- The sinuses are:
  - ❖ Paired frontal sinuses
  - ❖ Paired maxillary sinuses

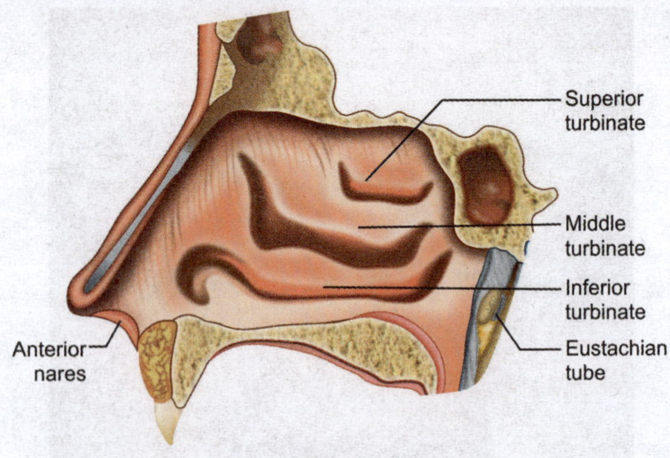

FIG. 7.6 Lateral wall of nasal cavity

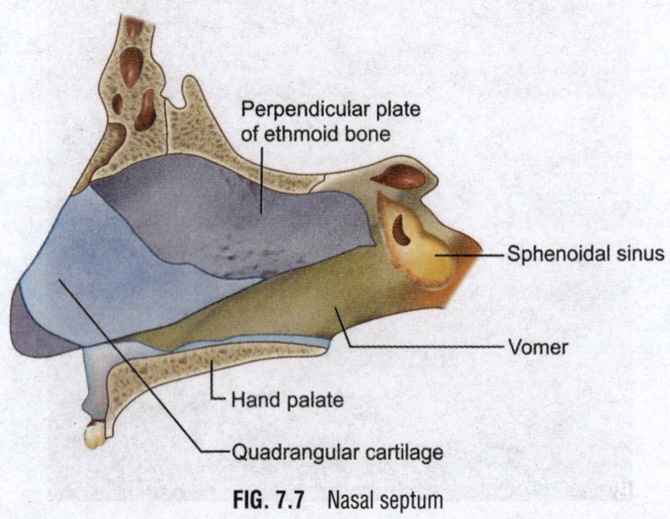

FIG. 7.7 Nasal septum

- ❖ Paired ethmoidal sinuses
- ❖ Sphenoidal sinus.

Significance of Flaring of Nostrils

It is the finding of distress, like:

- Increased work of breathing, i.e. impending respiratory failure
- Respiratory alternans

- Abdominal paradox
- Peritonitis result of impaired and painful excursion of diaphragm.

Best Tools for Inspecting Nares and Internal Nose
- Otoscope
- Handled Vienna Nasal Speculum.

Causes of Airflow Obstruction in One or Both Nares
- Septal hematoma
- Septal abscess
- Nasal polyp
- Papilloma
- Tumor
- Nasal mucosa edema
- Septal deviation
- Foreign bodies.

Nasal Manifestations of Basilar Skill Fracture
The following manifestations of basilar skill fracture:
- Facial trauma
- Nasal bone fracture
- Periorbital ecchymosis
- Swelling and tenderness of nasal bridge
- Cerebrospinal fluid rhinorrhea.

Difference between CSF rhinorrhea and allergic rhinorrhea
- Put a drop or nasal secretions over a paper of tissue
  ↓
  Show a halo around nasal secretions (CSF rhinorrhea).
- Glucose control of secretions may be measured at the bedside by using chemostrip (CSF rhinorrhea).

Causes of swelling of nasal mucosa:
- *Viral cause:* Nasal and oropharyngeal infection by rhinovirus and adenoviruses
- *Atopic:* Pollen and dander exposure causing nasal congestion, allergic rhinitis
- *Vasomotor:* Response to respiratory inhalant causing boggy edema of the mucosa and tearing.

Diagnosis of GI bleeding by peeping into the patient's nose
- Epistaxis—swallowed blood results in guaiac—positive stool
- Osler-Weber-Rendu disease—multiple telangiectasias in gut, mouth, face. Extremities and chest. It is autosomal disorder

Anosmia

Absence of smell. It may be congenital or acquired.

Congenital Anosmia

Kallmann's syndrome

- Sex-linked recessive trait or autosomal trait
- Familial hypogonadotropic hypogonadism
- Anosmia.

Acquired

- *Central nervous system:*
    - ❖ Parkinson's disease
    - ❖ Diabetes
    - ❖ Pernicious anemia
    - ❖ Cirrhosis
    - ❖ Chronic renal insufficiency
    - ❖ Cushing syndrome
    - ❖ Cystic fibrosis
    - ❖ Sarcoidosis.
- *Nasal:*
    - ❖ Allergic rhinitis
    - ❖ Nasal polyp.

Palpation for Sinuses

- Press frontal sinuses under the bony brows
- Press maxillary area for maxillary sinuses.
  Local tenderness with fever, nasal discharge—due to sinusitis.

Oral Cavity and Pharynx

Two main structures of posterior pharynx (Figs 8.1 and 8.2).
1. Hard palate.
2. Soft palate supported by anterior and posterior pillars.

Cleft Palate (Fig. 8.3)

It is a congenital deformity which is usually corrected in childhood, but may persist in adult. It is common in native Americans. Of 100 percent cases—30 percent are isolated cleft palate, 20 percent isolated cleft lip, and 50 percent combined, cleft lip and cleft palate.

Uvula

It is a grape-like midline structure hanging from the roof of the posterior pharynx.

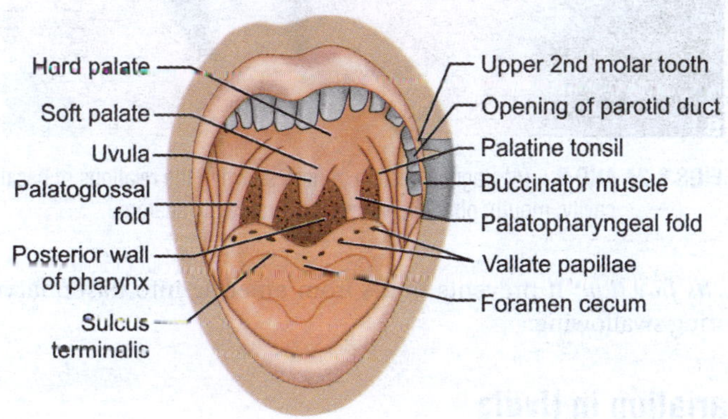

FIG. 8.1 Cavity of the mouth

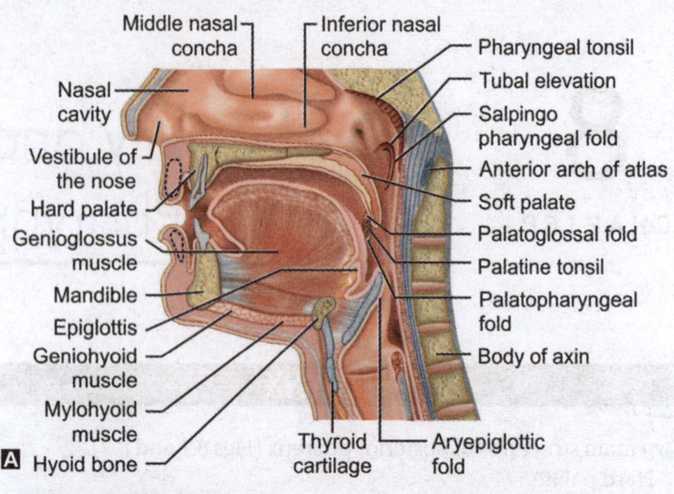

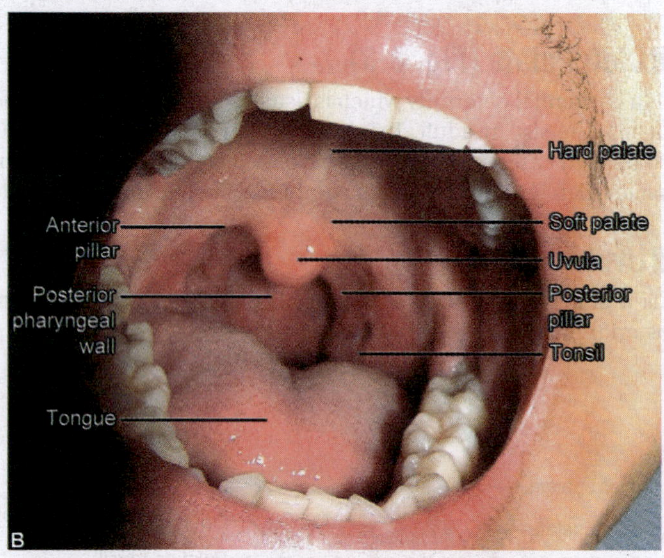

FIGS 8.2A AND B (A) Sagittal section of neck showing the relations of nasal cavity, mouth, pharynx, larynx; (B) Oral cavity anatomy

Its function: It prevents fluids from entering into nasopharynx during swallowing.

Variation in Uvula

- *Absent uvula:* Surgical removal during uvulopalatopharyngoplasty. It results in inhalation of swallowing liquid.

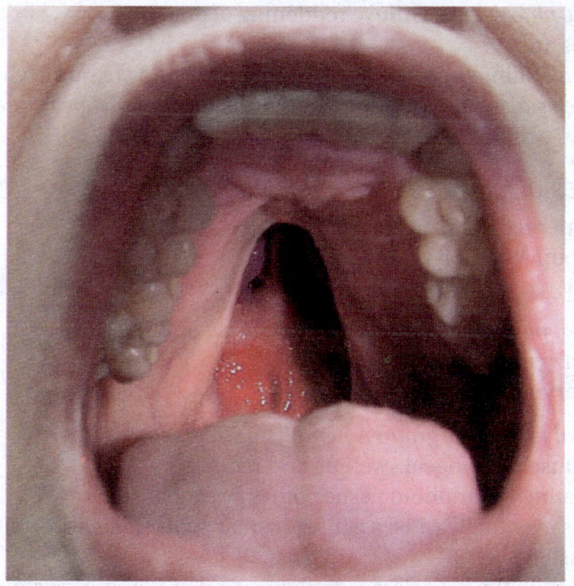

FIG. 8.3 Cleft palate

- *Bifid uvula:* Uvula is usually forked. It may be associated with cleft palate. It is entirely benign.
- *Bobbing uvula:* Patient with aortic insufficiency may have rhythmic pulsatile movement of uvula (Müller's sign). This is equivalent to DeMusset's sign.
- *Neoplastic uvula*
- *Uvulomegaly:* Swollen and elongated uvula. Causes are:
  - ❖ Pharyngitis
  - ❖ Gamma heavy chain diseases—extremely rare.

  Uvulomegaly of pharyngitis is associated with oral manifestations. But uvulomegaly of gamma heavy chain disease is associated with pancytopenia and β-symptoms of lymphoproliterative disorders.

  Uvulomegaly is associated with coughing, snoring and gagging when uvula is large enough.

Localized reddening of anterior pharyngeal pillars
It may be present in patient with chronic fatigue syndrome (FS). In this disease, peculiar purplish discoloration of the anterior pillars present bilaterally, it is brisky demarcated from rest of the pharynx. It gradually fades with remission of the disease. During exacerbation, it reappears. There is no tenderness, no sore throat, no pain and no other feature of pharyngitis.

Diffuse pharyngitis: Diffuse reddening of pharynx.
Causes are:
- *Viral:* Rhinovirus, adenovirus, HIV, CMV and coxsackie virus.
- *Bacterial:* Group A streptococci, Neisseria *gonorrhoeae*, previous days—diphtheria.

Causes of Exudates on the Posterior Pharynx
- Upper respiratory tract viruses
- Group A hemolytic streptococci
- EPV.

Clinical pictures of upper respiratory tract infections
- Pharyngeal vesicles
- Pharyngeal ulcers.

Clinical features of group A hemolytic Streptococcus
- Diffuse pharyngeal swelling and redness
- Coating of lymphoid tissue with gray exudates
- This eventually causes white tonsillar spots (follicles)—follicular tonsillitis
- There is the associated erythema and swelling of surrounding structures—faucial pillar, uvula and base of the tongue
- Associated symptoms—fever chill and rigor, mild nausea
- Enlarged jugulodigastric nodes, anterior cervical nodes, mainly submandibular gland
- Pain may present during swallowing—often radiating to ear.
- *Complications:*
  - ❖ *Local:*
    - Retropharyngeal abscess (<1% patients treated with antibiotics)
    - Suppurative cervical lymphadenitis
    - Otitis media
    - Sinusitis
    - Mastoiditis.
  - ❖ *Systemic:*
    - Meningitis
    - Pneumonia
    - Septicemia
    - Rheumatic fever.

■ Scarlatina (Scarlet Fever) (Fig. 8.4)
- Scarletiniform rash—fine scarlet like papules—starts on the trunk, spreads to the extremities, spares palms and soles.
- Tongue is usually coated, but later becomes denuded.
- Circumoral pallor, rash accentuation in anticubital fossa (Pastia's sign).

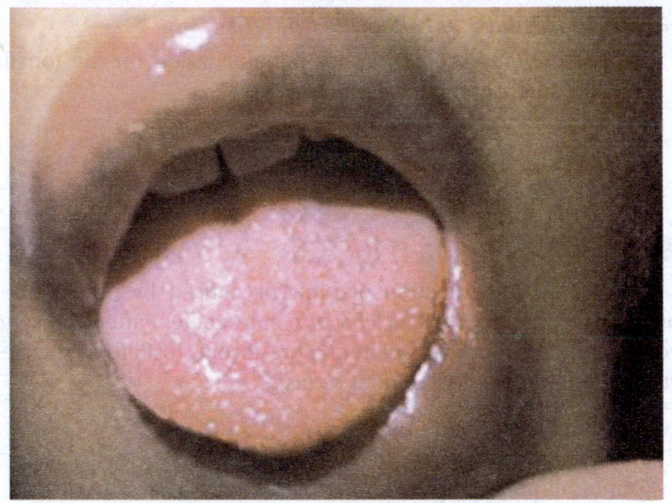

FIG. 8.4 Scarlatina (Scarlet fever)

- Rash typically blanches on pressure, sandpaper like feeling, eventually subsides in 6–9 days.

Gonococcal Pharyngitis
- Exudative and ulcerative pharyngitis
- Enquire about sexual activities.

Infectious Mononucleosis

Caused by EB virus:
- Exudative severe pharyngitis, tonsillar swelling, sore throat and often dysphagia
- Often hepatomegaly and splenomegaly
- Prominent anterior bilateral cervical lymphadenopathy
- Severe constitutional symptoms like fatigue, arthralgia
- Hemolytic anemia may occur.

Causes of Glandular Fever-like Syndrome

- HIV (at the time of seroconversion)—viremia present. HIV antibody is negative
- CMV—comparing with infectious mononucleosis—lymphadenopathy is less prominent and pharyngitis is severe
- Toxoplasmosis.

Causes of Nodules in Posterior Pharynx

- *Human papilloma virus:* Warty papular lesion on the tonsils, tonsillar pillars and buccal mucosa
- Squamous cell carcinoma
- Lymphoma
- Peritonsilar abscess.

Vincent's Angina (Fig. 8.5)

It is a necrotizing infection of pharynx caused by organisms—fusiform bacilli and *Borrelia vincentii* spirochete. Patient presents with rapidly developing unilateral sore throat, ipsilateral referred lymphadenopathy and bad odor or taste.

Examination reveals:
- Ulcerated tonsil
- Submandibular lymphadenopathy.

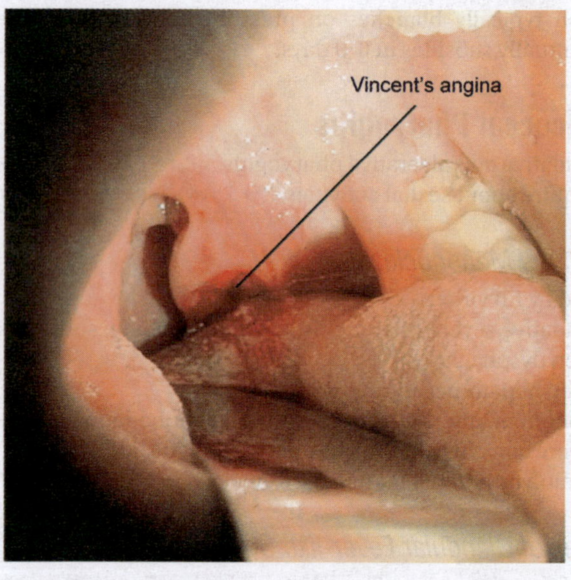

FIG. 8.5   Vincent's angina

ORAL MUCOSA

Significance of examining the oral mucosa by saying 'Ahhh':
- *It elevates soft palate, thus allows visualization of:*
  - ❖ Uvula
  - ❖ Tonsillar pillars
  - ❖ Base of the tongue
  - ❖ Hypopharynx.
- *It helps to assess the motor division of IX (glossopharyngeal) and X (vagus) nerve:*
  - ❖ *In case of bilateral damage of these nerves:* This 'Ahhh' fails to elevate soft palate
  - ❖ *In case of unilateral damage of these nerves:* The uvula is deviated towards the intact side. It will fail to elevate soft palate from paralyzed side.

Oral Mucosa

Palpable Lesions

- *Most common normal anatomic structures:*
  - ❖ *Wharton's duct:* Two tiny papules seen on the floor of the mouth—just under the tongue and 5 mm lateral to frenulum—it indicates opening of submandibular gland
  - ❖ *Stensen's duct:* This ductal opening present on both sides of buccal mucosa, directly opposite to 2nd upper molar tooth near the bite line. It indicates the opening of parotid gland.
- *Abnormal structures:*
  - ❖ *Ranula (Fig. 8.6):*
    - Small, painful, dome shaped, fluctuant, nodule on the floor of the mouth
    - It indicates salivary duct obstruction of submandibular or sublingual gland resulting mucus retention.
  - ❖ *Torus:* Nontender exostosis cartilage capped, mucosa lined bony spurs—arising either from:
    - Mandible
    - Palate.
      - *Mandible:* It is called exostosis mandibularis (Fig. 8.7). It in smaller, arising from lingual surface of mandible. It is benign
      - *Palate:* It is called exostosis palatinus (Fig. 8.8). It is larger, arising from midline of the palate. It is benign.
    - *Buccal exostosis (Fig. 8.9):* It is painless bony spur, arising on the facial surface of either upper or less commonly lower jaw. No neoplastic transformation occurs.

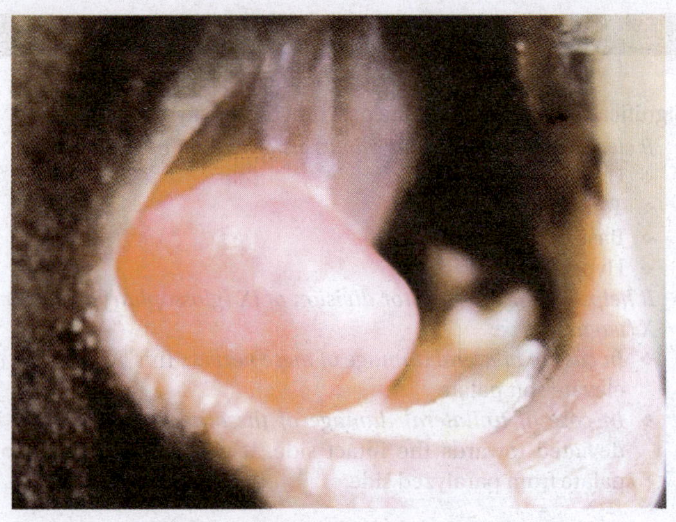

FIG. 8.6 Ranula

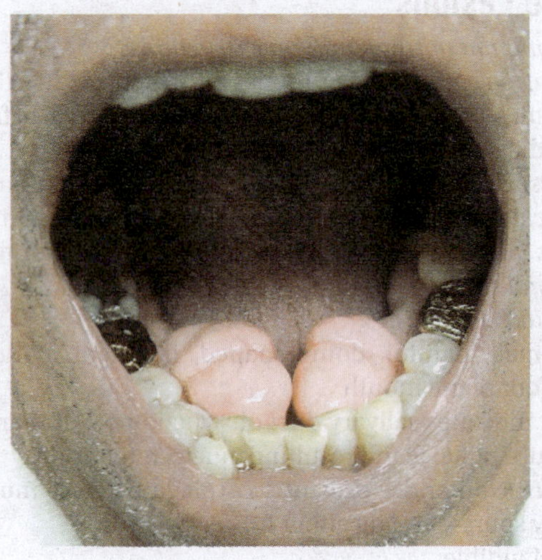

FIG. 8.7 Torus mandibularis

White Lesions

- *Thickening of oral mucosa:*
  - ❖ It is caused by biting the sides of the mouth
  - ❖ It is horizontal white line present on the buccal mucosa extending from opening of Stensen's duct to the angle of mouth
  - ❖ It is created by juxtaposition of upper and lower teeth. It is also called occlusal bite.

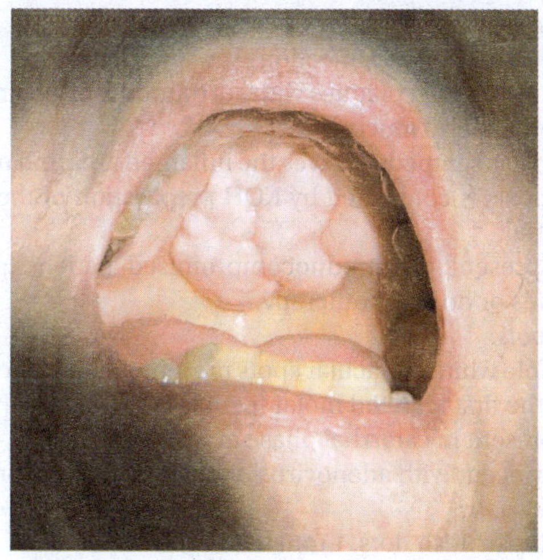

FIG. 8.8   Torus palatinus

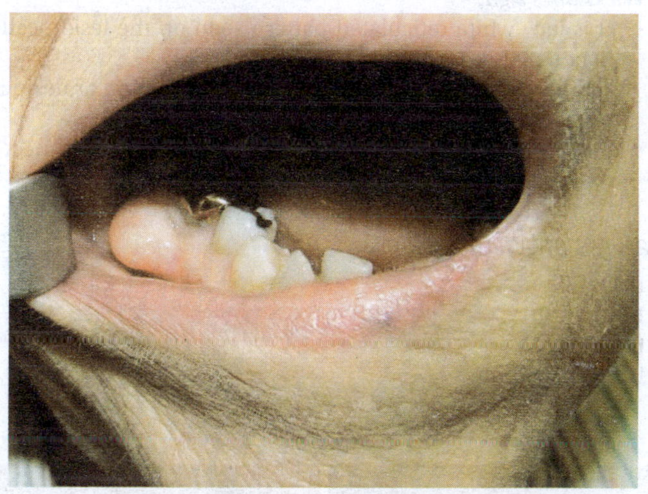

FIG. 8.9   Buccal exostosis

- *Squamous cell carcinoma:* It is most common cause of whitish spots.

Less Common Causes

- *Hairy leukoplakia:* White lesions on the:
  - ❖ Lateral aspect of the tongue
  - ❖ Buccal mucosa of cheeks.

- *Oral thrush:*
  - It is due to *Candida* infection
  - Multiple whitish plaques with surrounding erythematous rim present on oral mucosa
  - When it is scraped, it leaves the inflamed area and often bleed
  - Diagnosis is confirmed by KOH preparation of the scrapped material
  - It is present in immunocompromised patient, patient on steroids or on chemotherapy.
- *Koplik spots:*
  - Multiple whitish macular spots present on the buccal mucosa near the first and 2nd molar teeth (Figs 8.10A and B)
  - It is present in catarrhal phase of measles
  - It may occur with adenovirus or echovirus infection.
- *Fordyce's spots:*
  - It is tiny whitish dots, 1 mm in size
  - It is present in check, lips and tongue
  - It represents mucosal sebaceous cysts.
- *Wickham's sign:*
  - It is lacy white reticulated pattern seen on the lesion called lichen planus (Fig. 8.11).
    This lesion is flat topped violaceous papular lesion—pruritic, shiny, whitish, or grayish in color.
  - This lesion is present in buccal mucosa and flexor aspect of male genitalia.

Features of White Lesion

- Palpability
- Induration
- Bleeding
- Ulcer formation.

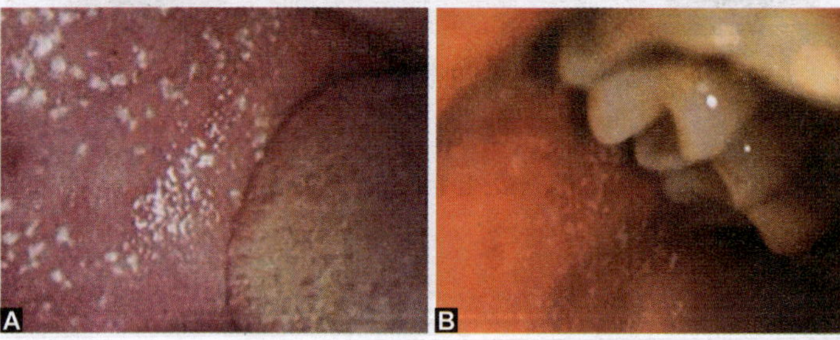

FIGS 8.10A AND B   Koplik spots

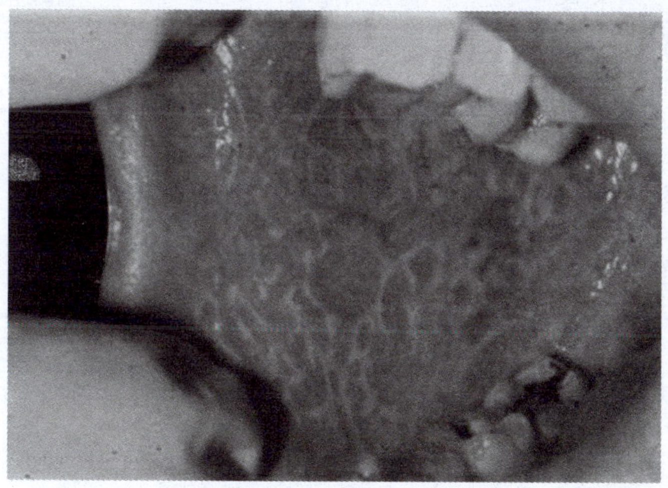

FIG. 8.11   Wickham's striae

- Concomitant risk factors responsible for malignant transformation:
  - ❖ Alcohol ingestion
  - ❖ Tobacco smoking or chewing.

Pigmented Spots

- *Amalgam tattoo:*
  - ❖ It is blackish or grayish stain in buccal mucosa adjacent to the area of tooth restoration
  - ❖ It is caused by mucosal exposure to dental amalgam.
- *Peutz-Jeghers syndrome:*
  - ❖ It is multiple melanin deposits on the mucocutaneous junction of mouth, anus (Fig. 8.12)
  - ❖ They are also present in lips, buccal mucosa, dorsal aspects of fingers and toes 1–5 mm in diameter
  - ❖ They are present at birth or early childhood
  - ❖ The pigmented mucosal lesions fade with increasing age, but lesions in fingers and toes become more prominent
  - ❖ Associated multiple pigmented and hamartomatous intestinal polyps
  - ❖ Risk of gastrointestinal malignancies.
- *Smoker's melanosis:*
  - ❖ It is focal flat, <1 cm multiple, irregular shaped brownish macular lesions
  - ❖ It is present in maxillary, labial gum, buccal mucosa, floor of the mouth

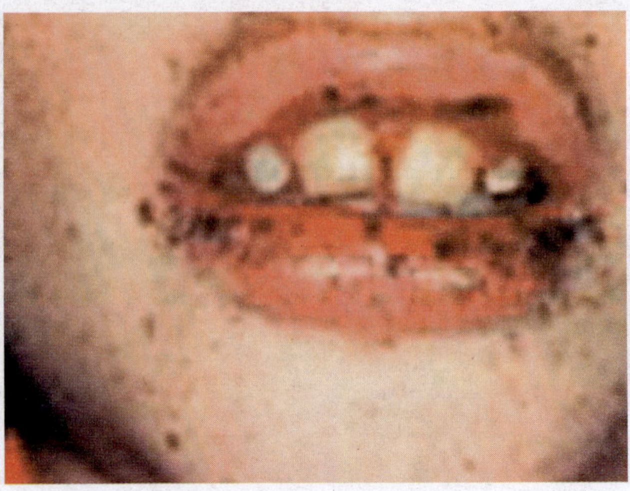

FIG. 8.12   Peutz-Jeghers syndrome

- ❖ If occurs due to chronic cigarette smoking, occurs in 3rd decade of life
- ❖ It is due to deposition of melanin pigment. Since melanocytes are stimulated by estrogen and progesterone, it is more common in females
- ❖ It is associated with yellowish staining of teeth and fingernails.
- ❖ There is increased risk of carcinoma.
- *Addison's disease:* Skin and buccal mucosa (inner side of lips, tongue and gingiva) are hyperpigmented.
- *Hemochromatosis:* Bluish-gray pigmentation of hard palate and to a lesser degree, gums.
- *Malignant melanoma:* Pigment lesions, ulcerated, palpable irregular margin.
- *Melanoplakia:* One or more pigmented patches in buccal mucosa of dark skinned individual. It is of little clinical significance.

Common Causes of Red Spots

- *Pyogenic granuloma:*
  - ❖ Well demarcated red, small nodular lesion
  - ❖ Composed of highly vascular granulation tissue
  - ❖ It projects from buccal mucosa
  - ❖ It frequently ulcerates.
- *Erythema migrans:*
  - ❖ Multiple red irregular patches with raised white rims
  - ❖ It is usually present in buccal mucosa and ventral surface of tongue and gums

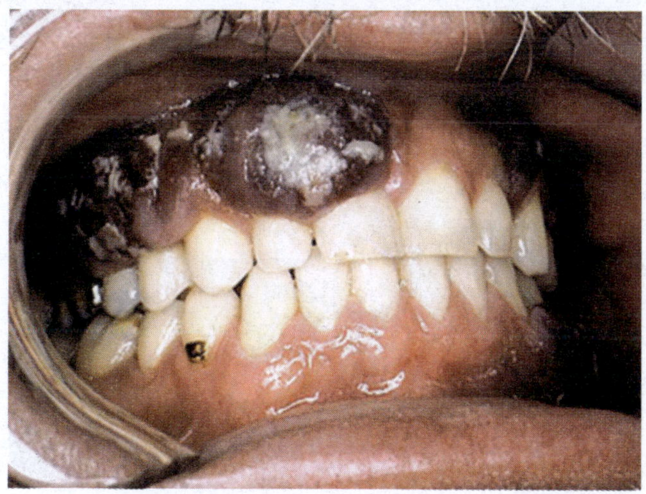

FIG. 8.13 Kaposi's sarcoma

- ❖ It is associated with geographical tongue, which is also referred as erythema migrant lingualis.
- *Palatal petechiae:*
  - ❖ Red scattered lesions present on the border of hard and soft palate
  - ❖ It is associated often with infectious mononucleosis.
- *Oral lesion of Kaposi's sarcoma (Fig. 8.13):*
  - ❖ Raised or flat purplish lesion.
  - ❖ May be associated with AIDs.
  - ❖ Occasionally may be associated with nonimmunocompromised patient of Mediterranean origin.

Ulcers or Erosions in Oral Mucosa

- *Thermal injuries:* By any hot liquid or solid food.
- *Aphthous ulcers (Fig. 8.14):*
  - ❖ *Minor aphthous ulcers:*
    - • Shallow, <1 cm in diameter, yellowish or grayish bases with surrounding erythematous rim
    - • They are isolated or multiple
    - • They are present in labial, buccal mucosa, palate, tongue and floor of the mouth.
  - ❖ *Major aphthous ulcer:* Large, deep, often heel with scarring
  - ❖ *Herpetiform ulcer:* More numerous, vesicular in morphology
    Associated symptoms: If fever, adenopathy, gastrointestinal symptoms and arthritis or mucous membrane involvement

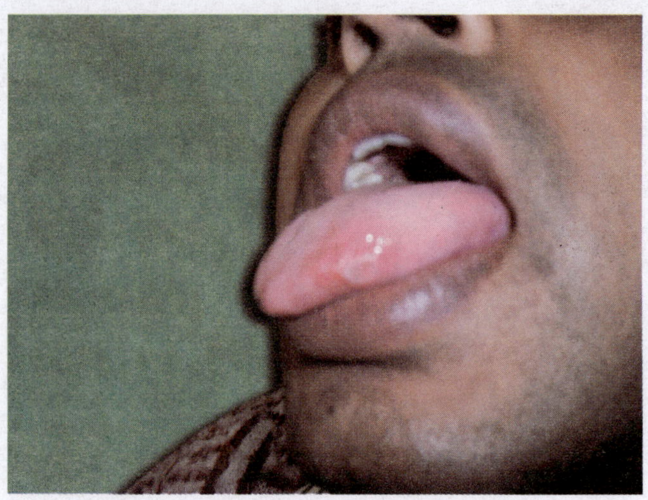

FIG. 8.14 Aphthous ulcer

(uveitis, conjunctivitis, and genital ulcerations) present—indicates systemic disease.

- *Autoimmune gingivostomatitis:* Pemphigus, pemphigoid and Stevens-Johnson syndrome painful tender, inflammatory sloughing of mucosa preceded by vesicles and bulla
- *Chancre:* Painless ulcer of primary syphilis, it is solitary.

Importance of vermilion border of the lip in identifying the cause of oral ulcers and vesicles

- Lesion, that cross the vermilion border of the lip and involve the skin are due to herpes simplex
- Lesion that do not cross the vermilion border of the lip are due to autoimmune diseases or Coxsackie virus infection.

TONGUE

Anatomy of the Tongue (Figs 8.15A and B)

- *It consists of skeletal muscles covered with mucosa—Dorsum of the tongue contains:*
  - ❖ Covered with exophytic structures (papillae)—increases the surface area
  - ❖ Taste buds for gustatory sensation.
- *Papillae are of:*
  - ❖ Filiform papillae both cover the entire dorsal surface of the organ
  - ❖ Fungi form papillae, they are small
  - ❖ *Circumvallate papillae:* Larger, located on the posterior dorsum in semicircular arrangement.
- Undersurface of tongue has no papillae.
- Midline structure, lingual frenulum connects tongue to the floor of the mouth
- Duct of submandibular gland (Wharton's duct) passes forward and medially at the base of the tongue. This duct opens on the papillae on each side of lingual frenulum.

Dysgeusia

Altered perception of taste—it may be:
- Local (involving tongue)
- Central (involving CNS).

Method of Inspection of Tongue

- *Ask the patient to do 'AHHH':* See the dorsum of the tongue
- *At the same time ask the patient to protrude and curl the tongue upward:* See the undersurface of the tongue
- *Place gauze on the tip of the tongue, gently grasping it and pull it out:*
  - ❖ See the lateral surfaces of the tongue
  - ❖ Any deviation of tongue to one side—indicating paralysis of ipsilateral hypoglossal nerve.

Tongue Abnormalities

Macroglossia (Fig. 8.16)

- Large size of tongue
- Presence of indentations caused by patient's teeth.

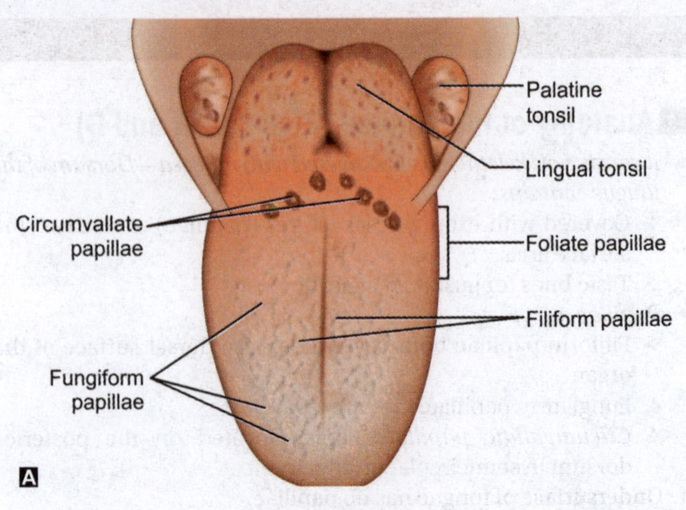

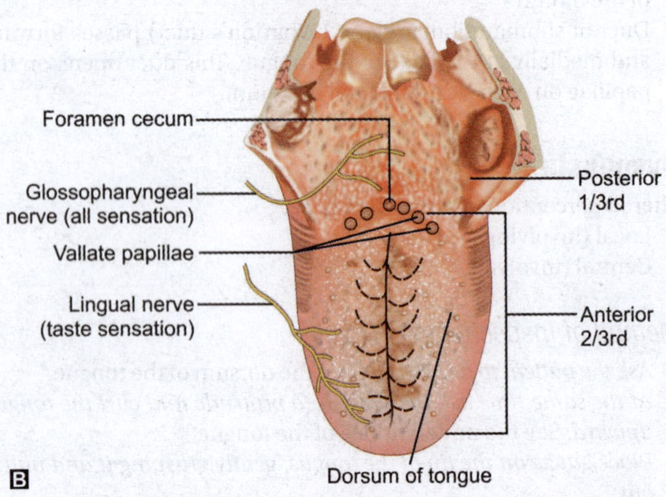

FIGS 8.15A AND B (A) Human anatomy of tongue; (B) Dorsum of tongue

Patient may present with:
- ❖ Thickened speech
- ❖ Snoring
- ❖ Sleep apnea.

The causes of enlargement
- Hypothyroidism
- Acromegaly.

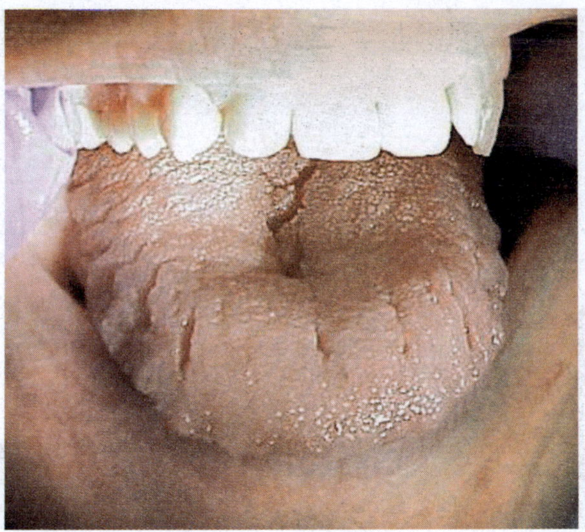

FIG. 8.16   Macroglossia

- Amyloidosis
- Down's syndrome.

Pathogenesis behind enlargement
- Proteinaceous infiltrations
- Hypertrophy of muscles.

Exception
Normal tongue with lateral indentation:
- Politicians (tongue in cheek)
- Some normal people.

Scrotal Tongue (Fig. 8.17)
- Occurs in elderly
- Ugly looking fissures on the dorsum of the tongue
- It is of no clinical significance.

Hairy Tongue (Fig. 8.18)
Abnormal desquamation of the filiform papillae, as a result 1 mm long filiform papillae become 15 mm in length producing hairy looking appearance. The color of hairy tongue may be:
- Black (black hairy tongue)
- Brownish
- Green
- Pinkish.

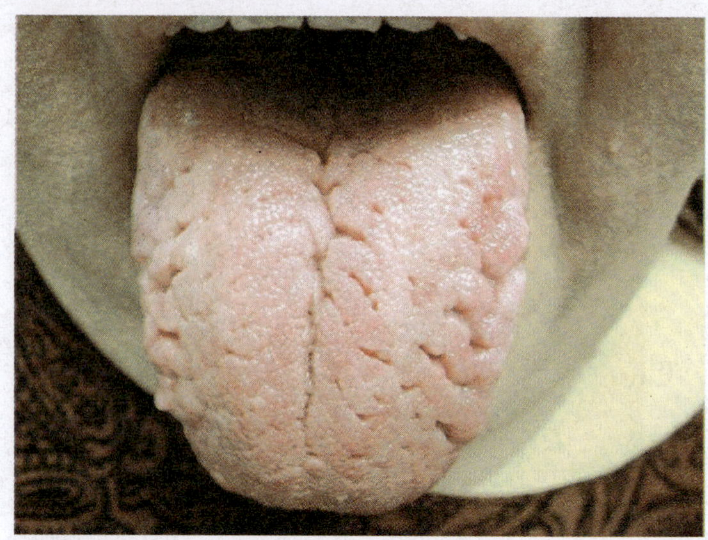

FIG. 8.17   Scrotal tongue

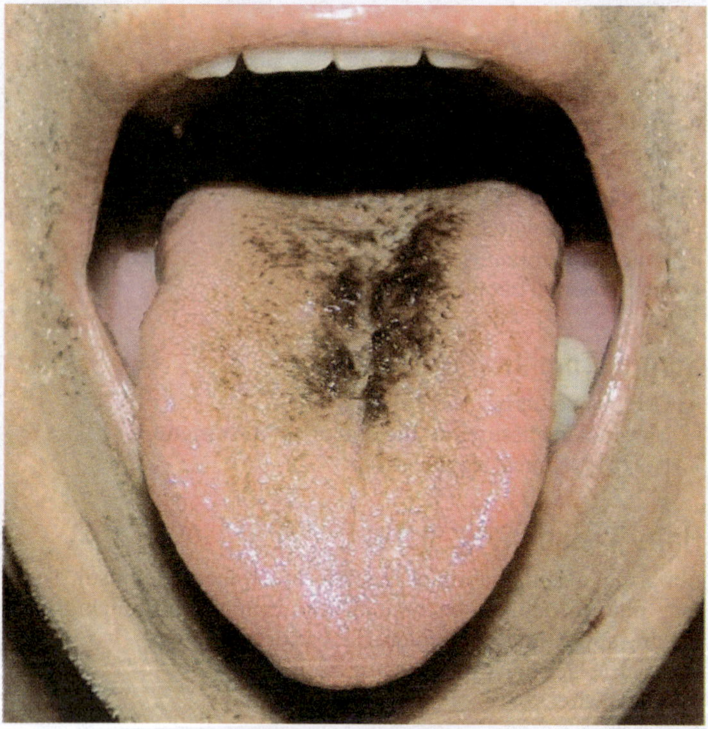

FIG. 8.18   Black hairy tongue

Common causes are:
- Idiopathic
- Broadspectrum antibiotics
- Radiation therapy
- Inadequate toothbrushing
- Diet too little roughage to mechanically debride the dorsum of tongue.

Prevalence is higher with age and more prevalent in:
- Males
- Smokers
- Tea/coffee drinkers
- HIV patients.

Symptoms
- Asymptomatic
- Overgrowth of *Candida* result is burning feeling (glossopyrosis)
- Retention of food debris between the elongated papillae secondary bacterial and fungal infection producing halitosis.

Treatment
Removal of elongated papillae with tongue scraper.

Geographic Tongue
- Multiple smooth red glossy patches of glossitis, each is surrounded by whitish hyperkeratotic patches
- Primarily affects dorsum of the tongue, occasionally extends to the lateral wall
- Histologically—there is atrophy of filiform papillae
- It waxes and wanes with time, resolves spontaneously, and may reappear with time in different mucosa (if lesions occur in family, it terms erythema migrans).
  - ❖ It runs in families
  - ❖ It is more common in adult than in children
  - ❖ It is more common in women
  - ❖ It is idiopathic
  - ❖ It is four times more common in psoriatic patient.

Median Rhomboid Glossitis (Fig. 8.19)
- It occurs on the dorsum of the tongue just anterior to the 'V' region of circumvallate papillae
- It is rhomboidal, sharply demarcated, flat or raised firm texture

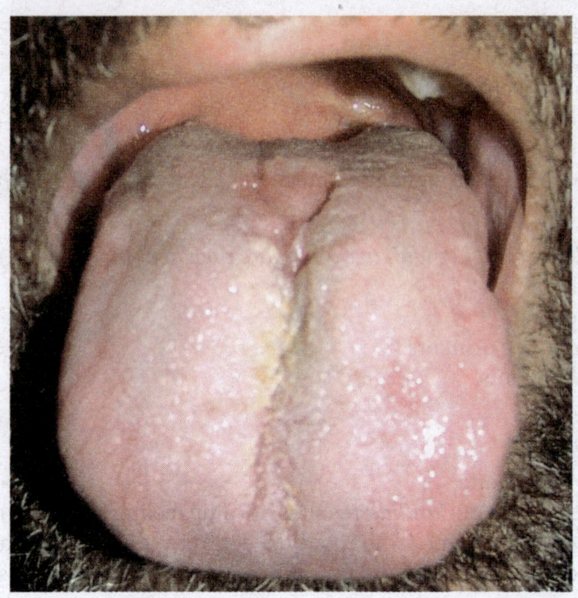

FIG. 8.19 Median rhomboid glossitis

- It is either asymptomatic or present with burning sensation after spicy food
- It may be inflammatory, or infectious in nature.

Tongue-tie (Fig. 8.20)

- It is a congenital condition characterized by short lingual frenulum
- This prevents protrusion of tongue
- It may interfere with breastfeeding
- It usually requires surgery.

White Hairy Tongue

- Multiple white, warty, corrugated, painless plaques, full of hairy projections of keratin overgrowth
- It is present on the lateral margin of the tongue, occasionally involves buccal mucosa of cheek.
- It may be caused by:
  - ❖ HIV infection—in this case, it is of worst prognosis
  - ❖ It may occur in immunocompromized patient, infected with Epstein-Barr virus.
- Unlike thrush it cannot be scrapped off.

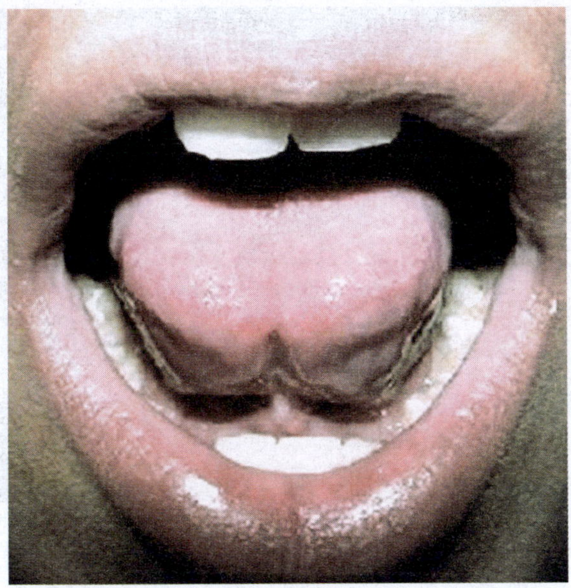

FIG. 8.20   Tongue tie

Smooth Red Tongues (Atrophic Glossitis) (Fig. 8.21)

- Initially hypertrophy of papillae
  ↓
  Then flattening of papillae
  ↓
  Atrophy of all except circumvallate papillae.
- It is at first shiny red color (beefy tongue).
  Later on smooth and sore on tongue (because of atrophy).

Palpable Lingual Nodules

- *Circumvallates papillae:* Sometimes it may be prominent. It is usually normal.
- *Lingual thyroid (Fig. 8.22):*
  ❖ It is a vestigial remnant of thyroid, present in thyroid embryologic site, before being migrated in front of the neck during 1st trimester of pregnancy
  ❖ It is smooth, round, red midline nodule at the base of the tongue
  ❖ It is more common in females
  ❖ It is usually >1 cm diameter. Lesion may interface with swallowing or respiration

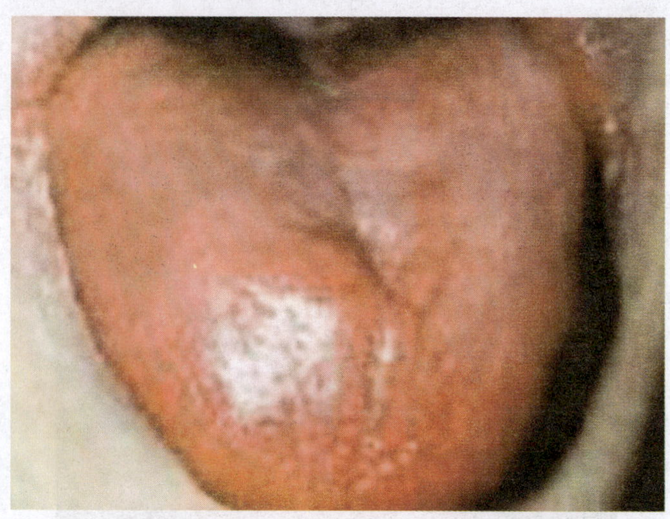

FIG. 8.21 Atrophic glossitis

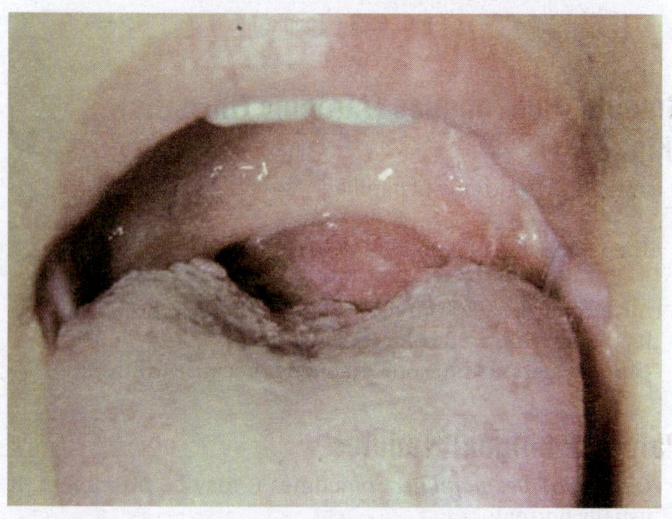

FIG. 8.22 Lingual thyroid

- ❖ 70 percent patients present with hypothyroidism, 10 percent cretinism
- ❖ Confirmed by iodine uptake and radionuclide scan.
- ● *Lingual tonsils:*
  - ❖ Smooth round nodule/papule present on the posterior lateral border of the tongue in the foliate papilla
  - ❖ It is hypertrophic lymphoid tissue.

- *Papilloma (Fig. 8.23):*
  - ❖ Soft pedunculated well circumscribed nodule present on lingual mucosa
  - ❖ It is caused by papilloma virus.
- *Carcinoma (Fig. 8.24)*
  - ❖ Nontender, firm, whitish papule and nodule
  - ❖ It is on the lateral aspect of the tongue.

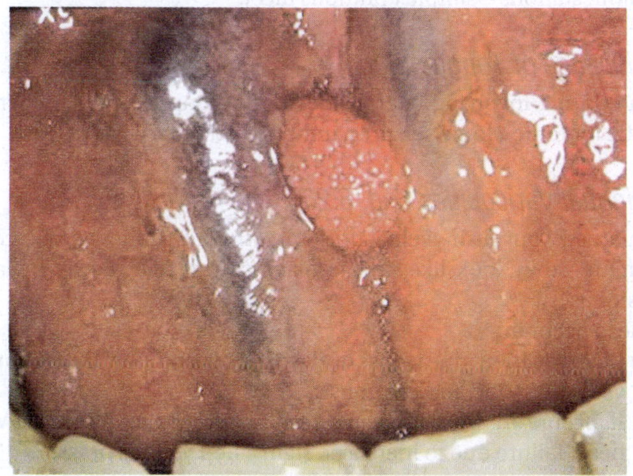

FIG. 8.23 Tongue papilloma

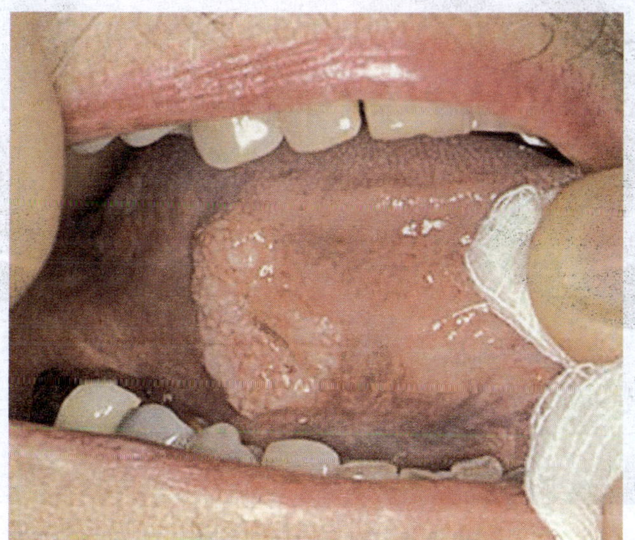

FIG. 8.24 Cancer of the tongue

Tongue Ulcer

- Indurated midline ulcer—on the dorsum of the tongue—suggest granulomatous disorder—tuberculosis or histoplasmosis
- Ulcer—indurated, located on the lateral or inferior surface of the tongue—diagnosis of Behçet syndrome
- Nonindurated peripheral ulcer—unassociated with systemic manifestations—simple aphthous ulcer.

Significance of Tongue Biting

Tongue biting involving lateral sides of the tongue is 100 percent specific for tonic-clonic seizures, until proved otherwise.

Sublingual Varicosities (Fig. 8.25)

- Enlarged purplish vein—present on the undersurface of tongue—they look like purple-black caviar, referred as caviar lesion.
- These occur in:
  - ❖ Elderly patient due to loss of elasticity of venous wall, resulting venodilatation and tortuousity
  - ❖ If occurs in superior vena cava syndrome and congestive heart failure due to increased right sided venous pressure.

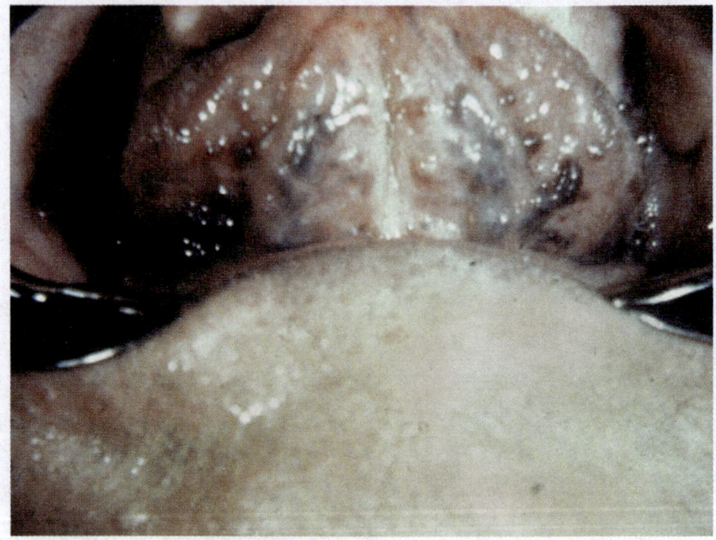

FIG. 8.25 Sublingual varicosities

Observe the color, moisture, lump, ulcers, cracking, or scaling of the lips. Difference between cheilosis and cheilitis is given below:

Cheilosis (Fig. 8.26)

It is reddening and cracking of one or both angles of mouth—it is called angular stomatisis.

- *In edentulous patient:* With ill-fitting dentures:
  - ❖ There is recurrent dribbling of saliva
  - ❖ Maceration of surrounding tissue
  - ❖ Secondary superimposed infection by bacteria—endogenous—including *Candida* for dentures and *Staphylococcus* for dentate individuals.
- Concurrent vitamin deficiencies including vitamin B_{12} Folates riboflavin, pyridoxine.
- HIV infection.
- Iron deficiency anemia.
- Plummer-Vinson syndrome.

Cheilitis (Fig. 8.27)

- It is dry scale of the lips with vertical fissures, painful, perpendicular to the vermilon border of lip—mainly lower lip.
- It is caused by exposure to wind, sunlight; nutritional deficiency, vitamin deficiencies, ultraviolet radiation.
- It can be prevented by sun blockers—lipstick, bam.

Causes of Ulcer or Erosions on Lips

- *Squamous cell carcinoma:* Solitary, nontender, firm ulcer.
- Herpes labialis—multiple tender, vesicles or erosions.

Angioedema (Fig. 8.28)

- It is nonpruritic, nonpitting, well-circumscribed edema due to vascular permeability.
- It involves head, neck, face, floor of the mouth, lip, tongue, and larynx.
- In some cases, it may produce laryngeal edema stridor, upper respiratory tract infection, respiratory failure.
- In some cases, gastrointestinal involvement producing intestinal wall edema resulting colicky abdominal pain, nausea, vomiting, diarrhea.

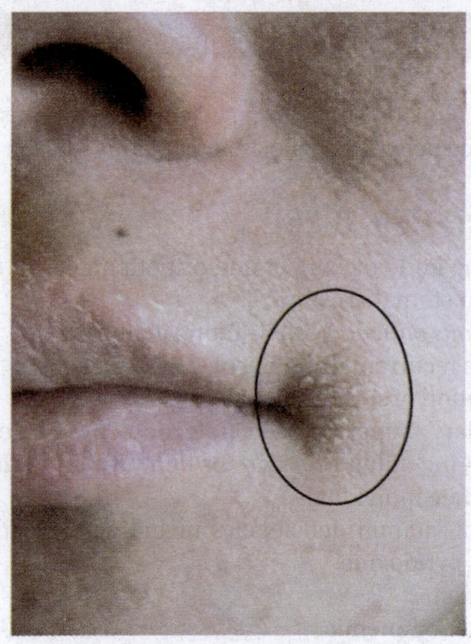

FIG. 8.26 Angular cheilosis

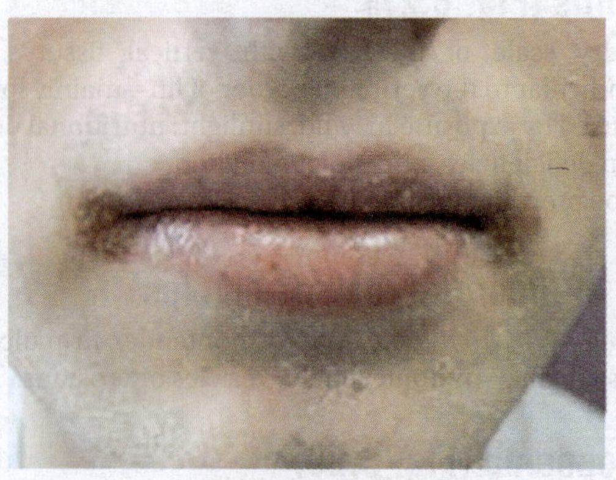

FIG. 8.27 Cheilitis

Causes

- ❖ Medications
- ❖ Foods (berries, fish, shellfish, eggs, nuts)
- ❖ Environmental (sunlight, cold, heat)
- ❖ Insect bite
- ❖ Pollen
- ❖ Animal dander
- ❖ Associated with autoimmune disorder.

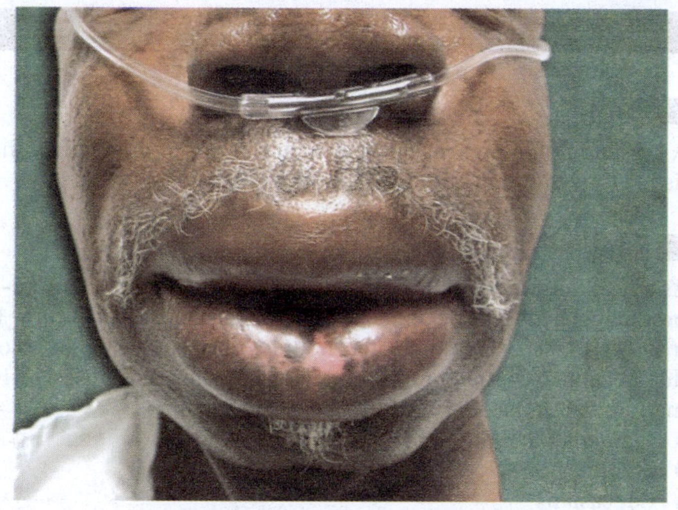

FIG. 8.28 Angioedema of lips and face

Pigmented Areas of Lip

- Peutz-Jeghers syndrome.
- *Simple ephelides:* Pigmented macules, 2-3 mm in diameter solitary or multiple, benign.

GUM AND TEETH

Parulia

A sessile nodule present on gingiva at the site of drainage of the fistula tract draining from tooth infection.

Epulis Fissuratum

As a result of exuberant response to trauma by ill-fitting denture—producing hyperplastic folds of mucosa around the denture. It may be sessile or pedunculated nodule, purplish brown in color due to capillary proliferation producing bleeding. It is observed in mandibular or maxillary area. It usually present in:

- Women than men
- Elder person
- Caucasians
- Asymptomatic person.

Causes of Thickening of Gum

- Gingivitis vulgaris
- Scurvy
- Leukemic infiltration—most ominous cause—Acute monocytic leukemia
- Medications—Phenytoin, cyclosporine.

In Gingivitis vulgaris: There is association with:

- Periodontal disease
- Coronary artery disease.

Coronary artery disease occurs in gingivitis vulgaris because:

- Increased plasma level of inflammatory mediators—fibrinogen, C-reactive protein, several cytokines
- Periodontal pathogen enters the bloodstream—producing atherosclerosis.

Scurvy

Gum is thickened, swollen, friable, having bleeding.

There may be concurrent petechiae in perifollicular areas. Dysmorphic and cork-screw hair.

This occurs due to vitamin C deficiency.

Complications of Gingivitis Vulgaris

- Tooth loss.
- Recurrent aspiration pneumonia due to anaerobic infection and lung abscess.

- Severe gingival infection and even, pain, gum swelling and gum erosions, halitosis maligna.

Long of Teeth

'Long of teeth' does not mean elongation of teeth, rather there is regression of gum (due to gingivitis). So patient with 'long of teeth' may become short of teeth within few years.

Causes of Tooth Loss

- *Tooth abrasion (Fig. 8.29):* Causes are:
  - ❖ Localized grinding
  - ❖ Recurrent trauma due to tooth picks, pipes.
- *Tooth attrition (Fig. 8.30):* As a result of disorders of mastication teeth become yellow brown surrounded by worm-down enamel.
- *Tooth erosion (Fig. 8.31):* This occurs due to:
  - ❖ Corrosive chemicals
  - ❖ Persons who regularly consume large quantities of squeezed citrus fruits
  - ❖ Persons consume regularly sweetened carbonated beverages
  - ❖ Bulimic patient—teeth mainly posterior surface of incisor are exposed to gastric acids
  - ❖ In nonbulimic patient—due to acid reflex disease.

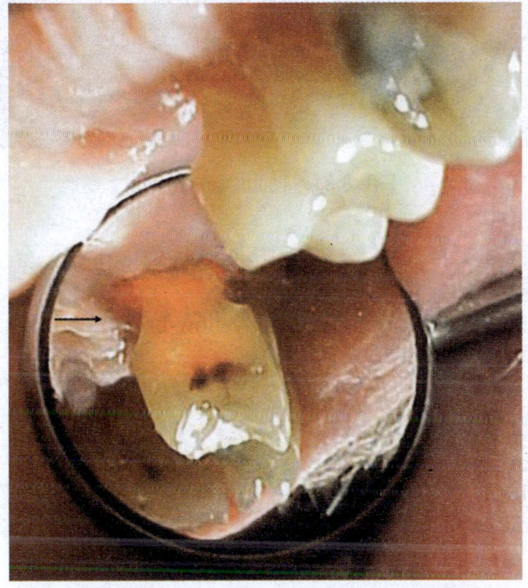

FIG. 8.29 Toothbrush abrasion and abfraction

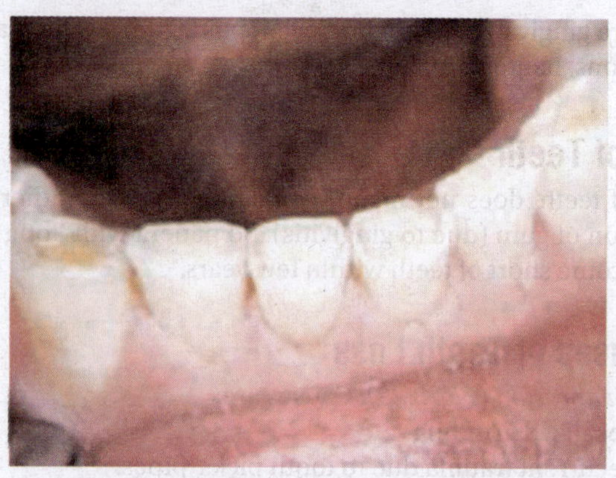

FIG. 8.30 Attrition

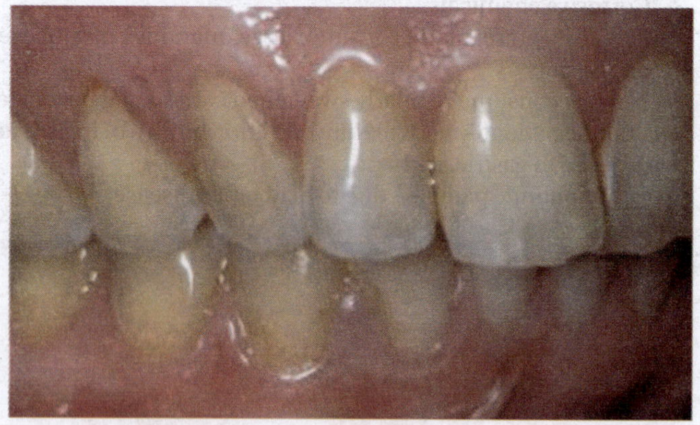

FIG. 8.31 Tooth acid erosion

Condition of Teeth

Enamel becomes eroded exposing yellow-brown dentin, yellowish discoloration and cavity formation.

Blue Line in the Gum

This occurs in:

- Plumbism
- Chronic exposure to bismuth.

In plumbism:
The blue lines are produced by conglomeration of multiple dots present at the point of tooth insertion in the gum. They are produced by tartar bacteria synthesizing lead sulfide (bluish black).

Other signs of plumbism are renal insufficiency, peripheral neuropathy, saturnine gout (monoarticular arthritis), cognitive delay.

Hutchinson's Teeth

- It is one of the manifestations of congenital syphilis (triad are interstitial keratitis, labyrinthine deafness, Hutchinson's teeth)
- Upper incisor is shorter than normal and notched.

Halitosis

It is bad breath. The factors are:
- *Nonpathological:*
  - Age related changes
  - Hunger breath
  - Menstrual breath
  - Tobacco breath
  - Various other breath—onion, garlic, fish, metronidazole.
- *Pathologic:*
  - *Local causes:*
    - Disorder of oral cavity—stomatitis, gingivitis, glossitis, periodontal abscess
    - *Disorder of nose and sinuses:* Sinusitis, chronic atrophic rhinitis, nasal septal perforation, ozena (atrophic disease of nose and turbinates), retained foreign bodies
    - Disorders of tonsils, pharynx—chronic tonsilitis, pharyngitis, Zenker's diverticulum, adenoiditis
    - *Disorders of digestive systems:* Achalasia, gastroesophageal reflux
    - *Disorders of lung:* Bronchiectasis, lung abscess, pneumonia, empyema.
  - *Systemic causes:*
    - Smell of acetone in DKA
    - Ammoniacal odor in uremia
    - Sweet odor of hepatitis (fetor hepaticus).

Ear

EXAMINATION OF EARS

■ Components of Ear (Fig. 9.1)

- External ear
- Middle ear
- Inner ear.

External Auditory Canal

1 cm long; opens outside through auricle and limited inside by eardrum.

It is made up of bony part its inner 2/3rd and cartilage its outer 1/3rd.

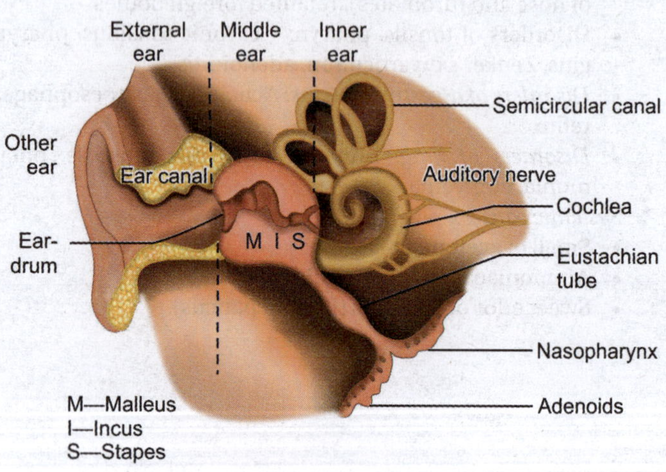

FIG. 9.1 Diagrammatic representation of ear

Nerve supply—outer thirds by trigeminal nerve—highly sensitive. Inner parts by vagus nerve, its stimulation cause vagal response, produces dry cough.

Lesions in External Ear

- *Keloid:*
  - ❖ Firm nodular, hypertrophic mass of scar tissue extends beyond the area of injury
  - ❖ It is most common in shoulder and upper chest, it is also present on the earlobe, it has cosmetic effect.
- *Tophi:*
  - ❖ Deposits of uric acid crystals, characteristics of chronic tophaceous gout
  - ❖ It is hard nodule present in helix and antihelix of ear
  - ❖ It may discharge chalky substances through skin
  - ❖ It is also present in the joints of hands, feet and other areas
  - ❖ It occurs after chronic sustained high blood levels of uric acid.
- *Cutaneous cyst:*
  - ❖ A dome shaped benign closed firm sac having blackhead at the top
  - ❖ Histologically it may be epidermoid cyst—common in face and neck or it may be pillar cyst commonly in the scalp.
- *Chondrodermatitis nodularis chronica helicis:*
  - ❖ Chronic inflammatory painful tender papule present on helix or antihelix
  - ❖ Later stage—it becomes ulcerated and crusted
  - ❖ Biopsy to rule out carcinoma.
- *Basal cell carcinoma:*
  - ❖ Raised nodule having lustrous surface and telangiectatic vessels
  - ❖ Slowly growing malignant tumor, rarely metastasize.
- *Rheumatoid nodules:*
  - ❖ In chronic rheumatoid arthritis small lumps on the helix and antihelix
  - ❖ Additional nodules may be present on the hands, along surface of ulna, distal to elbow, on the knees and heels.
- *Darwin's tubercle:*
  - ❖ Benign and congenital tubercle near auricular apex (on the helix at the junction of upper and mid third).
  - ❖ Nontender and rarely bilateral.
- *Congenital creases:* Present in newborn with Beckwith syndrome (gigantism, macroglossia, umbilical abnormalities, hepatosplenomegaly, renal hyperplasia, microcephaly)
- Earlobe transverse crease in adult is acquired, associated with coronary artery disease.

- *Auricular red spot:*
  - ❖ Trauma results in ecchymoses, even hematomas
  - ❖ Port-wine stain—congenital, only cosmetic importance
  - ❖ Sturge-Weber disease—Port-wine nevus on the upper part of scalp associated with intracranial vascular abnormalities, that may be responsible for seizures, cerebellar calcifications.

Causes of Tender Swollen Auricle

- Trauma
- Malignant otitis externa
- Relapsing polychondritis palpation of temporal artery anterior to tragus:

     Temporal artery is a branch if external carotid—it supplies lateral areas of scalp.

This artery may be compromised in:
- Polymyalgia rheumatica
- Temporal arteritis
- Patient with proximal muscle weakness and jaw claudication. In this case temporal artery may be tender.

Finding during inspection in the postauricular space:
In mastoiditis
- Exquisite tenderness in the 1 cm crescent shaped depression immediately behind the external auditory canal and also mastoid tip
- Palpable posterior auricular node in the mastoid process
- Positive Battle sign—ecchymoses over the mastoid mostly due to traumatic basilar skull fracture. It occurs 48 hours after traumatic event.

Auscultation over the Auricle

- A bruit can be heard over the auricle consistent with arterio-venous malformation of the carotid artery. This patient may present with tinnitus (without vertigo, nausea, nystagmus, abnormal audiogram or MRI of posterior fossa)
- Crepitus—due to temporomandibular disease.

Functions of Middle Ear (Fig. 9.2)

- To accommodate three auditory ossicles—those are responsible for transmission of sound from eardrum to cochlea
- To connect mastoid antrum and rhinopharynx.

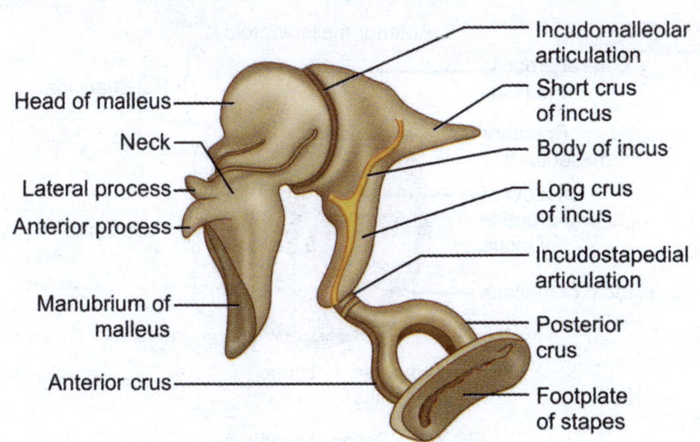

FIG. 9.2 Ossicles of middle ear

Functions of Eustachian Tube

To equalize the pressure on both side of eardrum. Though it is closed, but it reopens during yawning, swallowing and during valsalva maneuver.

Two muscles are in middle ear:
1. *Stapedius:* It attaches to the neck of the stepes, it is supplied by VII nerve
2. *Tensor tympani:* It is attached to malleus, supplied by V nerve (trigeminal nerve).

Factors preventing proper visualization of tympanic membrane:
- Cerumen
- Otitis externa
- Exostosis
- Furuncle.

Findings of tympanic membrane by otoscope (Fig. 9.3):
- Pale, gray translucent, surrounded by ring—this is the site of perforation
- Umbo of the malteus—which coincides with head of hammer
- Reflective triangular cone of light located inferiorly and anteriorly to umbo.
- Flaccid portion of tympanic membrane (pars flaccida).
- Pars tensa—located posteriorly to manubrium.

Otoscopic features of eardrum in purulent otitis media:
- Redress
- Prominent vessel dilatation
- Outward building of eardrum

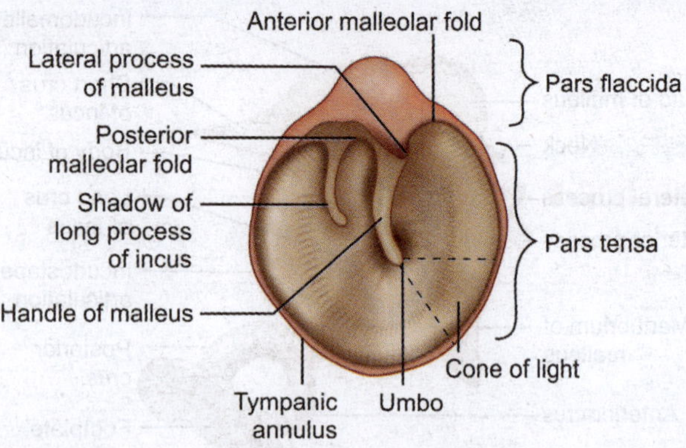

FIG. 9.3 Bones of middle ear

- Loss of markings for the umbo
- Loss of light reflex
- Loss of mobility of eardrum on pneumatic endoscopy.

Distinguishing Features of Serous Otitis Media

- Air-fluid level and bubbles behind the eardrum
- Loss of cone of light reflex
- Retraction of tympanic membrane
- Malleus becomes prominent and white
- Eardrum acquires yellowish hue.

Retraction of eardrum is due to:
Drop of pressure in tympanic cavity due to obstruction of eustachian tube.

Ramsay Hunt syndrome: It is herpes zoster infection of the geniculate ganglion with

- Fascial paresis
- Hyperacusis
- Unilateral loss of taste
- Reduced salivation and tear formation
- Earache
- Vesicles in ear canal.

Cholesteatoma:

- Chole (biliary like mass), steat (tallow), toma (tumor). This is benign, tumor like mass of cholesterol and keratinized squamous epithelium, located in middle ear and result of chronic otitis media
- Histologically it is squamous metaplasia linings the expanding cystic cavity

- Cholesteatoma sometimes present adjacent to the postero-superior perforation of tympanic membrane
- It can grow into external canal or mastoid.

Horseshoe-shaped Eardrum Plaque

- It occurs due to presence of tympanosclerosis—it is hyalinization and calcification of eardrum
- It may occur due to insertion of ventilatory tubes.

Test for Inner Ear

Functions of inner ear:
- Acts as receptor for hearing
- Acts as receptor for balance.

Two methods of testing
Whisper voice test → if it is normal → Patient's hearing is normal
↓
If it is abnormal
↓
Tuning fork test

Method of Whisper Voice Test

- Stand behind the patient at 2ft distance
- Occlude one ear by rubbing in circular fashion or putting finger in external auditory canal and continuous irrigating it
- Exhale completely, then whisper three letters
- Ask the patient to repeat if entire sequence
- *Interpretation:*
    - If patient can repeat complete sequence—hearing is normal (negative test)
    - If patient can repeat only 2 of three items, the other is wrong—repeat a new sequence in same technique
    - If patient repeat two or more items wrong—then hearing of the patient is abnormal (positive test)—do the tuning fork test
- Repeat this method on the other ear also.

Accuracy of whisper voice test
It is highly specific, sensitive test:
- Positive test rules if significant hearing loss
- Negative test rules out hearing loss

Tuning Fork Test

This test differentiates between—conductive deafness and sensori-neural deafness.

- Conductive deafness involves defect in transmission of sound involving external and middle ear. In this case speech is softer than normal
- Sensorineural deafness involves perception of sound due to problem in inner ear (cochlea), neural connections and center of auditory area

  In this case speech is louder than normal.

  Most sensorineural loss is due to presbycusis (age related degenerative loss of ear receptor/auditory nerve).

Weber Test

- Place the base of vibrating tuning fork over the midline of the skull, or on forehead or on nasal bridge equidistant from both ears
- Ask the patient in which ear the buzzing of tuning fork is best heard
- *Interpretation:*
  - ❖ In normal subject the sound should be in midline
  - ❖ In conductive deafness—the sound should be best heard in diseased ear
  - ❖ In sensorineural deafness the sound is best heard in normal ear.
- In 40 percent of normal people, sound is lateralized. So only when screening test (when per voice test) is abnormal, Tuning fork test should be performed.

Rinne's Test

- Place the vibrating tuning fork base on the mastoid process of one ear and keep it there until no sound will be heard by the patient
- At that point place the vibrating limb of tuning fork in front of ipsilateral ear.

  This method will test bone conduction (BC) and air conduction (AC).
- *Interpretation:*
  - ❖ Normally AC is greater than BC (AC > BC) due to amplifying effects of eardrum and middle ear
  - ❖ Patient with conductive deafness cerumen and middle ear disease has normal bone conduction but impaired air conduction due to impaired air transmission. So in this case BC is greater than AC (BC > AC) or Rinne's test negative
  - ❖ In the case of a patient with sensorineural deafness, due to impaired perception of sound, there is equal reduction of BC and AC. So in this case AC is greater than BC (Rinne's test positive)
- This test will be performed in other ear also.

Interpretation on the bases of Weber test and Rinne's test
- *In conductive deafness:*
  - Rinne's test is negative
  - Weber test is lateralized to diseased ear.
- *In sensorineural deafness:*
  - Rinne's test is positive
  - Weber test is lateralized to normal ear.

Limitations of tuning fork test
- *Weber test:*
  - It is less sensitive, because many patients with unilateral hearing loss does not exibit lateralization
  - It cannot identify bilateral symmetrical hearing loss
  - It cannot differentiate pure conductive deafness from mixed conductive and sensorineural hearing loss.
- *Rinne's test:* Quite accurate in detecting conductive hearing loss.

Frequencies of tuning fork used for tests
- 512 Hz has better sensitivity for detecting conductive hearing loss
- 512 Hz has better specificity than 256 Hz

Tuning fork should be strucked against soft surface, because, strucked against hard surface generate multiple overtones.

Discharge in the ear—called otorrhea. Discharge may be:
- *Bloody discharge:* Traumatic, cancer
- *Serous discharge:* Infection, CSF leakage in case of trauma to head
- *Purulent discharges:*
  - Infection in middle ear following perforation in eardrum—otitis interna
  - Infection of external ear—otitis externa.

Method of examination of ear canal and drum:
- Use otoscope with the largest ear speculum that the canal can accommodate
- Hold the ear in such a way to straighten the ear canal, grasp the auricle and pull it gently upward, backward and slightly away from the head
- Hold the otoscope with thumb, press the hand against the patient's face
- Insert the speculum gently to ear canal, directing it some what down and forward through the ear.

Findings:
- Movement of auricle and tragus is painful in acute otitis externa (inflammation of ear canal)

But not painful in acute otitis media (inflammation of the middle ear). In otitis media there is tenderness behind the ear.

- Nontender nodular swellings covering the normal skin deep in the ear canal suggest exostoses—this is nontender, nonmalignant, it may obscure drum
- *Otitis externa:*
  - ❖ Simple otitis externa is due to psoriasis, eczema, dermatitis or narrow ear canal. It may be so swollen, so that it may produce temporary deafness. It may be very painful and impede sleep
  - ❖ Malignant otitis externa. It may occur due to poor neutrophillic function due to qualitative and quantitative disorders (leukemia, diabetes, chemotherapy, corticosteroid therapy). This may be due to pseudomonas infection, may spill into blood stream producing sepsis.
- *Otalgia:* It may be due to—referred pain from pharynx, teeth and spine. It may occur when any process affecting the territory of the distribution of:
  - ❖ Trigeminal nerve
  - ❖ Facial nerve
  - ❖ Glossopharyngeal nerve
  - ❖ Vagus nerve
  - ❖ $C_2 - C_3$ cervical nerve.
- *Vesicles in the external ear:* It may be due to:
  - ❖ Contact dermatitis—due to poison Ivy
  - ❖ Varicella zoster
  - ❖ Ramsay-Hunt syndrome—vesicular rash in the inferior portion of auricle due to herpetic infection of geniculate ganglion.
    Producing:
    - Ipsilateral facial paresis
    - Hyperacusis
    - Ipsilateral loss of taste.

10

CHAPTER

■ Anatomy (Fig. 10.1)

- It is the largest organ of the body.
- *Its thickness varies in different areas of the body:*
  - ❖ Average thickness is 1-2 mm
  - ❖ Thickest in palm, sole, interscapular region—5 mm
  - ❖ Thinnest over eyelids and penis—0.5 mm.
- *It has two layers:*
  1. *Epidermis:* It is outermost layer of skin, composed of stratified epithelium. It consists of five layers:
     i. *Stratum corneum:* Outermost layers—consists of dead cells—called corneocytes—it is horny layer. Cytoplasm of dead cells is flattened with fibrous protein called keratin.
     ii. *Stratum lucidum:* Consists of flattened epithelial cells containing either degenerated nucleus or no nucleus.

     This layer looks like translucent zone hence called stratum lucidum.

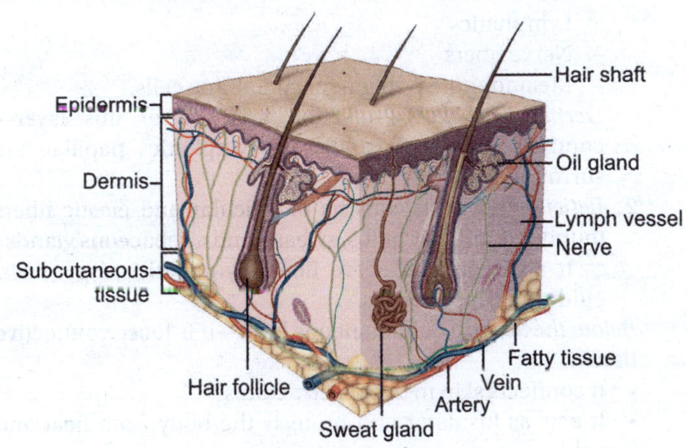

FIG. 10.1 Skin layers

iii. *Stratum granulosum:* Two to three layers of flattened rhomboid cells having granular cytoplasm and kerato hyaline protein, precursor of keratin.

iv. *Stratum spinosum:* This is called prickle cell layer having spine like projection in the cells by which cells of this layer are connected with each other.

v. *Stratum germinativum:* This layer has two sublayers of cells:
1. Polygonal cells superficially.
2. Columnar or cuboidal cells deeply.
   Newly formed cells move towards stratum corneum.
   The stem cells, which give rise to new cells called keratinocytes.
   - Melanocytes scalloped between keratinocytes.
     Melanocyte secretes melanin, which is responsible for color of skin.
     From this layer, projection, called rete ridges projects down the dermis. This rete ridges responsible for:
     - Anchoring
     - Nutrition.

2. *Dermis:* Inner layer of skin. It is made up of:
   - Dense and stout collagen fibers
   - Fibroblast
   - Histiocytes.

   Collagen fibers contain collogenase, which is responsible for wound healing.

   Dermis made up of two layers:
   1. *Superficial papillary layer:* It projects into epidermis. It contains:
      - Blood vessels
      - Lymphatics
      - Nerve fibers
      - Melanophores—pigment containing cells.

      Dermal papillae: Projection arises from this layer— contains plexus of capillaries, lymphatics papillae are surrounded by rete ridges.
   2. *Reticular layer:* It consists of reticular and elastic fibers found around hair bulbs, sweat glands, sebaceous glands.
      It also contains nerve fibers, lymphatics, mast cells, epidermal appendages.

   Below the dermis: Subcutaneous layer—it is loose connective tissue.
   - It connects skin to deeper structures
   - It acts as insulator and protects the body from heat and cold.

Appendages of Skin

- Hair follicles with hairs, nail, sweat gland.
- Sebaceous gland.
- Mammary gland.

Color of Skin

- *Pigmentation of skin—color of skin:* It is due to amount of melanin pigment in the skin produced by melanocytes.
  Melanocytes are present in:
  - Stratum germinativum
  - Stratum spinosum.
  Darkening of skin depends upon amount of melanin.
- *Amount of hemoglobin in the blood control color of skin in following ways:*
  - When hemoglobin content decreases—skin is pale
  - When blood rushes into skin and normally oxygenated—skin is pink
  - When hemoglobin becomes desaturated—skin color— cyanosed.

Functions of the Skin

- *Protection:* Skin covers whole body except few body orifices thus protects the organs from following factors:
  - *Protection from bacterial and toxic substances:* Keratinized stratum corneum is responsible for protective function of the skin—protect the skin from acid, alkali and bacterial toxins. Invasion occurs only when skin is traumatized or abraded. During this time keratinocytes secrete:
    - Antibacterial peptides—like β-defensin—it prevents invasion of microbes.
    - Cytokines like interleukins, tumor necrosis factor, gamma interferon have important role on:
      - Inflammation
      - Immunological reaction
      - Wound healing
      - Repair.
  - *Protection against mechanical blow:* Since skin is not tightly adhered to the underlying organ, hence any mechanical blow, unless very severe, do not damage underlying organ.
  - *Protection against ultraviolet rays:* Skin protects the body from ultraviolet rays or sunlight.
    - Melanin absorbs sunlight and ultraviolet rays.
    - Thickness of stratum corneum increases the above function.

- *Sensory function:* Skin has afferent cutaneous receptors, which respond to pain, touch, temperature and pressure, send these signals to brain via afferent nerves and perception of sensation occurs.
- *Storage function:* It can store:
  - ❖ Sugar
  - ❖ Water
  - ❖ Chloride
  - ❖ Fat
  - ❖ Blood by dilatation of cutaneous blood vessels.
- *Synthetic functions:* By action of ultraviolet rays from sunlight on cholesterol.
- *Body temperature regulation:* Heat is lost from body by:
  - ❖ Conduction
  - ❖ Convection
  - ❖ Radiation
  - ❖ Evaporation.

  Lipid content of sebum prevents loss of heat from the body in cold environment.
- *Regulation of water and electrolyte balance:* It excretes water and salts through sweat.
- *Excretory function:* Skin excretes urea, salt and fat.
- *Secretory function:*
  - ❖ Sebum through sebaceous gland
  - ❖ Sweat through sweat gland.

Diagnosis of Skin Disease

Nondermatologist has difficulty in diagnosing skin disease because:

- There are literally hundreds of skin diseases.
- A single skin disease has varying appearance, e.g. seborrheic keratosis has smooth, rough or eroded surface, uniform or irregular border like that of melanoma.
- Dynamicity of skin disease—regular changes in morphology.
- Few diseases have different stages of evaluation, e.g. herpes simplex presents as red papule → blister → to erosion or ulcer → scarring.

So to diagnose a skin disease following methods are very helpful:

History

- *Brief history:*
  - ❖ Duration
  - ❖ Onset of symptoms
  - ❖ Location
  - ❖ Area of spread

- ❖ Family history of similar episode
- ❖ Allergies
- ❖ Occupation
- ❖ Previous treatment.
- *Distribution:* Extent of eruption. Distribution of primary lesion and appearance of secondary lesion.

Anatomic Distribution of Skin Lesion

- *Head and neck:*
  - ❖ *Acne:*
    - Face
    - Neck
    - Shoulder
  - ❖ *Actinic keratosis:* Face
  - ❖ *Amyloidosis:* Eyelids
  - ❖ *Atopic dermatitis:*
    - Face
    - Neck
  - ❖ *Contact dermatitis:*
    - Eyelids
    - Face
  - ❖ *Cancer:*
    - Face
    - Lips
    - Nose
    - Ears
  - ❖ *Discoid lupus erythematosus:*
    - Cheek
    - Nose
  - ❖ *Herpes zoster:* Trigeminal distribution in the face.
  - ❖ *Psoriasis:* Scalp
  - ❖ *Rosacea:* Face
  - ❖ *Seborrhea:*
    - Face
    - Eyelids
    - Eye brows
    - Nasal alae
  - ❖ *Secondary syphilis:* Face
  - ❖ *Spider angioma:* Cheek, neck
  - ❖ *Tinea capitis:* Scalp
  - ❖ *Xanthelasma:* Eyelids
  - ❖ *Vareola:* Face and head → Extremities.
- *Trunk:*
  - ❖ *Candidiasis:*
    - Under breast

- Axillae
- Sacrum
❖ *Dermatitis herpetiformis:*
  - Scapulae
  - Buttock
  - Sacrum
❖ *Drug eruption:* Thorax, abdomen any site
❖ *Petechiae:* Abdomen
❖ *Pityriasis rosea:* Front and back of trunk
❖ *Secondary syphilis:* Front and back of abdomen, thorax
❖ *Spider angioma:* Chest, shoulder, abdomen
❖ *Varicella:* Trunk → extremities → face.
- *Extremities:*
  ❖ *Actinic keratosis and cancer:* Back of the hands
  ❖ *Atopic dermatitis:* Antecubital fossa
  ❖ *Contact dermatitis:* Arm, hands, legs
  ❖ *Erythema nodosum:* Skin, legs
  ❖ *Granuloma annulare:* Back of hands and fingers
  ❖ *Onycholysis:* Fingernails, toenails
  ❖ *Petechiae:* Forearm, hands, feet
  ❖ *Pityriasis rosea:* Upper arm, upper legs
  ❖ *Plantar wart:* Sole
  ❖ *Psoriasis:* Elbows, hands, fingernails.

Pattern of Lesion

- *Annular or arciform:* Arranged in circles, arcs:
  ❖ Tinea infection
  ❖ Drug eruption
  ❖ Urticaria
  ❖ Psoriasis
  ❖ Erythema multiforme.
- *Serpeginous pattern:* Occurs in wavy outline:
  ❖ Granuloma annulare
  ❖ Larva migrans
  ❖ Late syphilis.
- *Iris pattern:* As an encircled round spot, more than one may be present—erythema multiforme.
- *Irregular pattern:* No regular shape, but collection of irregular patterns:
  ❖ Urticaria
  ❖ Insect bite.
- *Dermatomal pattern:* Lesions occur in dermatomal distribution—along spinal root with sensory abnormalities—Herpes zoster.

- *Linear lesion:* Lesions arranged along cutaneous or subcutaneous structures like, nerve, blood vessels, lymphatic:
    - ❖ Lymphangitis
    - ❖ Vasculitis
    - ❖ Contact dermatitis
    - ❖ Jellyfish envenomation.
- *Reticular pattern:* Lesion produces a network pattern consistent with arterial or venous anatomy:
    - ❖ Venous pattern—Erythema ab igne, livedo reticularis
    - ❖ Arterial pattern—Necrotizing vasculitis.
- *Extrinsic pattern:* Lesion follows no anatomic pattern, has a relatively straight border:
    - ❖ Radiation injury
    - ❖ X-ray dermatitis
    - ❖ Contact dermatitis.

Morphology of Lesion

Primary lesions

When the lesions have not been changed or triggered by several factors—like scratching, trauma, and medicines. The following are the primary lesions:

- *Macules:* Flat nonpalpable, discolored skin <0.5 cm in diameter. *Example:*
    - ❖ Freckles
    - ❖ Drug eruptions
    - ❖ Measles
    - ❖ Flat nevi.
- *Patches:* Circumscribed flat discolored skin >0.5 cm in diameter. *Example:*
    - ❖ Vitiligo
    - ❖ Senile freckles
    - ❖ Melasma.
- *Papules:* Circumscribed, raised palpable lesion. Size <0.5 cm in diameter. *Example:*
    - ❖ Lichen planus
    - ❖ Elevated nevi
    - ❖ Wart.
- *Wheal.* Large papule, edomatous, transitory present for less than 24 hours. *Example:*
    - ❖ Drug allergy
    - ❖ Food allergy
    - ❖ Insect bite.

- *Plaques:* Raised palpable, superficial, circumscribed solid lesion >0.5 cm in diameter.
  Examples:
  - Psoriasis
  - Mycosis fungoides
  - Lichen chronicus.
- *Nodule:* Raised, palpable solid lesion >0.5 cm in diameter, penetrated deeper into dermis. Overlying cutis is mobile.
  Example:
  - Neurofibromatosis
  - Erythema nodosum
  - Basal cell cancer
  - Xanthoma.
- *Tumor:* Nodules larger than 2 cm in diameter with depth, poorly demarcated margin.
  Example:
  - Basal cell carcinoma
  - Mycosis fungoides.
- *Bulla:* Circumscribed, raised serous fluid filled >1 cm in diameter.
  Examples:
  - Pemphigus
  - Bullous pemphigoid
  - Burn.
- *Cyst:* Raised, encapsulated lesion containing fluid or semisolid material.
  Examples: Cysts of acne.
- *Pustules:* Purulent fluid containing raised, circumscribed lesions of skin.
  Examples:
  - Impetigo
  - Acne
  - Infected cyst.
- *Petechiae:* Reddish to purple discolorations due to deposition of blood or blood pigment. Size >0.5 cm in diameter.
  Examples:
  - Thrombocytopenia
  - Vasculitis
  - Drug eruption
  - Typhus.
- *Purpura:* Deposition of red blood cells or blood pigment >1 cm in diameter.
  If purpura is palpable: Vasculitis—due to antigen—antibody complex—localized to lower extremities—Henoch-Schönlein purpura.

- *Ecchymoses:* Reddish to purple discoloration, larger than petechiae—resembling plaque or patches.
- *Spider angioma:* This is arterial telangiectasia, fills from center, blanch whenever this is compressed.
- *Venous spider:* This venous telangiectasia—they fill from periphery, they empty with pressure.

Secondary lesion

This lesion may be altered by medical treatment, outside manipulation, or own natural course.

- *Scales:*
  - ❖ Represent the thickening of stratum corneum
  - ❖ Color may be white, tan, or gray
  - ❖ They may be small or large
  - ❖ They provide squamous component to papulosquamous disease
  - ❖ They are present in scalp.
  - *Example:*
  - ❖ Seborrheic dermatitis
  - ❖ Tinea capitis
  - ❖ Dandruff
  - ❖ Psoriasis.
- *Excoriation:* Linear erosions produced as a result of scratching on normal skin or on the primary lesion.
  Example: Eczema.
- *Lichenification:*
  - ❖ Due to recurrent scratching in chronic pruritus.
  - ❖ Due to recurrent trauma in patient's palms and soles.
  - ❖ Skin is hardened, leather like with prominent markings, occasional scaling.
  Example: Eczematous skin disease.
- *Crust:* It is a colored mass of blood, serum, pus, or combination of these on the skin.
  Example:
  - ❖ Impetigo
  - ❖ Infected dermatitis.
- *Erosion:*
  - ❖ Depressed lesions whenever epidermis is either removed or sloughed
  - ❖ Color is red, shallow, circumscribed.
  Example: Chickenpox after rupture of vesicle.
- *Ulcer:*
  - ❖ Depressed circumscribed lesion
  - ❖ Epidermis and part of dermis is abraded
  - ❖ Concave, sharp margin, red clear base or clot at base
  - ❖ It is healed with scarring.

Examples:
- ❖ Venous ulcers
- ❖ Pyoderma gangrenosum
- ❖ Tertiary syphilis.
- *Fissures:*
  - ❖ Depressed, linear, vertical cracks
  - ❖ It involves epidermis and part of dermis.
  Examples: Athlete's foot.
- *Atrophy:*
  - ❖ It is pale, shiny area, loss of cutaneous marking
  - ❖ It involves full thickness skin.
  Example:
  - ❖ Third degree burns
  - ❖ Discoid lupus erythematosus
- *Sinus:* It is a channel connecting deeper tissue to exterior of skin.
- *Keloid:*
  - ❖ Hypertrophied scar beyond the border of original injury
  - ❖ Elevated, progressive
  - ❖ Triggered by trauma
  - ❖ They can be numb or painful.
  Example:
  - ❖ Full thickness trauma healed with scar
  - ❖ Earlobe after trauma.

Special lesions
- *Burrows:*
  - ❖ It may be short and small—scabies
  - ❖ Long and tortuous—creeping eruption.
  These are tunnels in the epidermis.
- *Blackhead comedones:* These are plug of whitish or blackish sebaceous or keratinous material—deposited in pilosebaceous follicles. Plural number of comedo is comedones.
  Site—Face, chest, back, upper part of arms.
  Examples:
  - ❖ Acne
  - ❖ Favre-Racouchot on sun damaged skin on temporal areas (Fig. 10.2).
- *Cutaneous horn:* This is spike shaped cutaneous deposits stuck above the skin, half inch or more 0.5–1 cm width.
  Example: It is overlying above:
  - ❖ Actinic keratosis
  - ❖ Seborrheic dermatitis
  - ❖ Wart
  - ❖ Parakeratosis
  - ❖ Hyperkeratotic basal cell cancer.

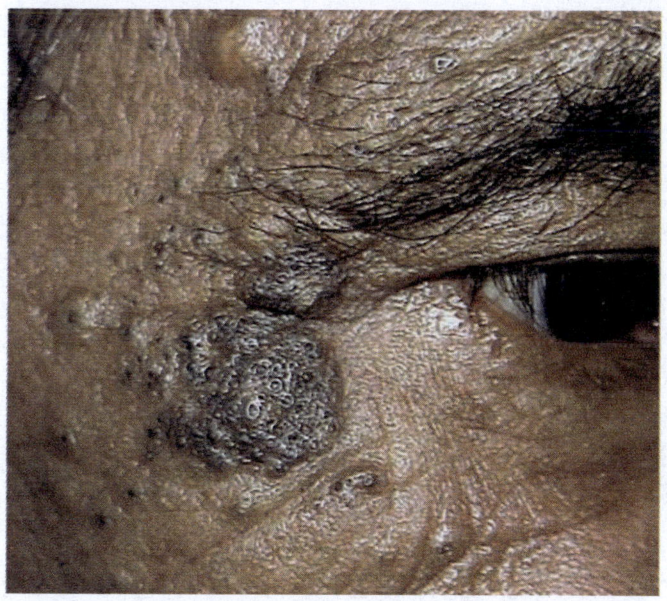

FIG. 10.2 Blackhead comedones

- *Keratin plug:* This is 1–3 mm in size present in the hair follicle.
  Example:
  - Systemic lupus erythematosus (SLE)
  - Lichen planus.
- *Ulcer malum perforans (Fig. 10.3):* Since it is associated neuropathy hence, it is painless, deep and destructive.
  Cause:
  - Diabetes
  - Leprosy.
- *Milia (Fig. 10.4):* Whitish papule—1–2 mm in diameter haring no opening at the top. Site—face in adult and wider spread in newborn.
  Example:
  - Healed burn or superficial traumatic sites
  - Healed bullous disease sites.
- *Cutaneous striae distensae (Fig. 10.5):*
  - Red, while resolved turns white
  - Linear areas of atrophy may be indentation
  - Sites—buttocks, lower abdomen, breast in case of:
    - Rapid weight loss
    - Prolonged use of corticosteroids—topical or systemic
    - Pregnancy.

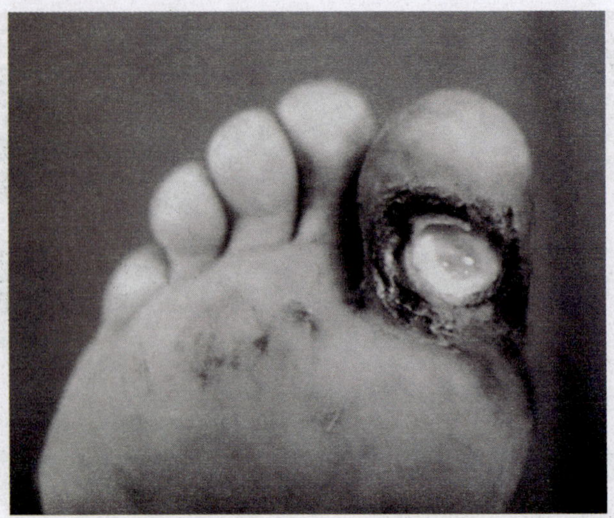

FIG. 10.3 Ulcer malum perforans

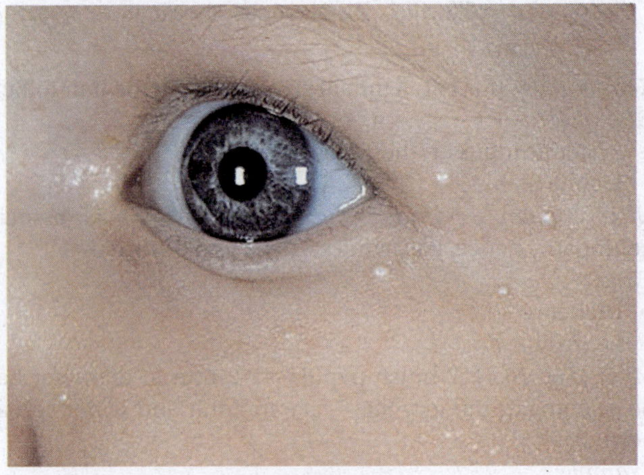

FIG. 10.4 Milia

- *Telangiectasias:* Dilated superficial tortuous blood vessels.
  Example:
  - Spider angioma
  - Chronic radiation exposure
  - Basal cell cancer
  - Sebaceous hyperplasia
  - Rosacea.

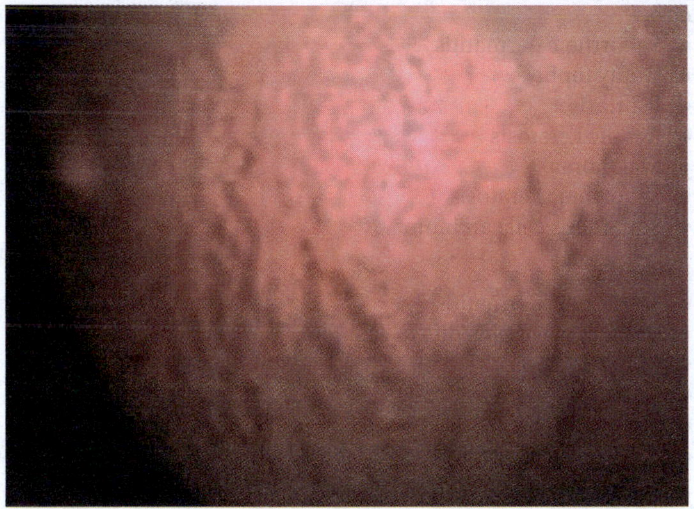

FIG. 10.5   Cutaneous striae distensae

Diagnosis by Location

Head and scalp

- Male or female pattern of hair distribution
- Alopecia areata
- Discoid lupus erythematosus
- Tinea capitis
- Seborrheic dermatitis
- Contact dermatitis
- Vitiligo
- Psoriasis
- Trichotillomania
- Postpregnancy alopecia.

Face

- Seborrheic dermatitis
- Contact dermatitis
- Acne rosacea
- Psoriasis
- Atopic eczema
- Impetigo
- Systemic lupus erythematosus
- Dermatomyositis
- Based cell cancer
- Actinic keratosis
- Acne
- Squamous cell cancer
- Seborrheic keratosis.

Ears
- Seborrheic dermatitis
- Gouty tophi
- Psoriasis
- Actinic keratosis
- Melanoma
- Seborrheic keratosis
- Squamous cell carcinoma.

Eyelid
- Seborrheic dermatitis
- Contact dermatitis due to cosmetics
- Atopic eczema
- Skin tags
- Syringoma
- Basal cell cancer.

Posterior neck
- Lichen simplex chronicus
- Seborrheic dermatitis
- Seborrheic keratosis
- Psoriasis
- Contact dermatitis
- Acne keloidalis in dark-skinned people
- Folliculitis.

Mouth
- Vitiligo
- Herpes labialis
- Aphthous ulcer
- Geographic tongue
- Syphilis
- Glossitis
- Oral hairy leukoplakia
- Candidiasis
- Pemphigus
- Stevens-Johnson syndrome
- Squamous cell cancer.

Axillae
- Seborrheic dermatitis
- Contact dermatitis
- Erythrasma (Fig. 10.6)
- Acanthosis nigricans
- Fordyce disease
- Hidradenitis suppurativa.

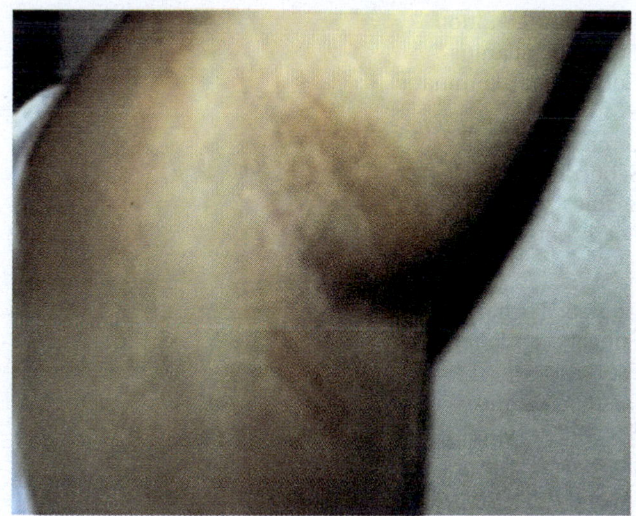

FIG. 10.6 Erythrasma

Chest and back
- Tinea versicolor
- Fixed drug rash
- Erythroderma
- Psoriasis
- Seborrheic dermatitis
- Acne
- Sebaceous cyst
- Seborrheic keratosis
- Spider angioma
- Vitiligo
- Epidermoid cyst
- Melanomas.

Groin and crural areas
- Tinea infection
- *Candida* infection
- Impetigo
- Wart
- Granuloma inguinale
- Pediculosis
- Seborrhea
- Folliculitis.

Penis
- Primary and secondary chancre
- Contact dermatitis

- Fixed drug eruption
- Candidal balanitis
- Condyloma acuminata
- Psoriasis
- Circinate balanitis
- Seborrhea
- Scabies
- Pearly penile papules.

Hand
- Contact dermatitis
- Fungal eruption
- Psoriasis
- Pustular psoriasis
- Secondary syphilis
- Eczema
- Squamous cell carcinoma
- Atopic eczema
- Warts.

Cubital fossa and popliteal fossa
- Eczema
- Contact dermatitis
- Prickly heat.

Elbow and knee
- Psoriasis
- Eczema
- Granuloma annulare
- Xanthomas
- Dermatomyositis.

Feet
- Contact dermatitis
- Atopic eczema
- Verrucae
- Primary and secondary bacterial infection
- Psoriasis
- Erythema multiforme
- Dyshidrotic eczema (Fig. 10.7).

Seasonal disease
Few skin diseases are prevalent in certain seasons.
- *Winter seasons:*
    - ❖ Atopic eczema
    - ❖ Psoriasis
    - ❖ Contact dermatitis
    - ❖ Seborrheic dermatitis

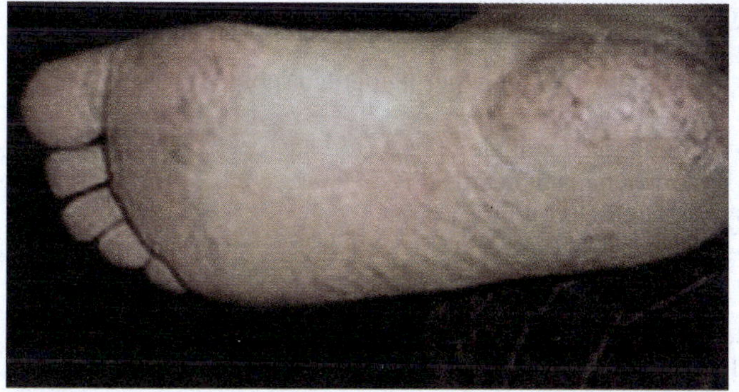

FIG. 10.7 Dyshidrotic eczema

- ❖ Nummular eczema
- ❖ Ichthyosis.
- *Summer seasons:*
  - ❖ *Candida* infection
  - ❖ Fungal infection of feet and groin
  - ❖ Contact dermatitis due to poison ivy
  - ❖ Miliaria or prickly heat
  - ❖ Insect bite
  - ❖ Tinea versicolor
  - ❖ Polymorphous reaction.
- *Spring seasons:*
  - ❖ Acne
  - ❖ Pityriasis rosea
  - ❖ Erythema multiforme
  - ❖ Viral exanthems.
- *Fall:*
  - ❖ Acne
  - ❖ Senile pruritus
  - ❖ Pityriasis rosea
  - ❖ Contact dermatitis
  - ❖ Tinea of scalp
  - ❖ Contact dermatitis due to ragweed
  - ❖ Viral exanthems.

Certain dermatosis may occur or may be aggravated due to:
- Poor hygiene
- Inadequate food
- Overcrowding

The following dermatoses are:
- Scabies
- Pediculosis
- Pyoderma
- Miliaria.

Following dermatosis are common in dark skinned people:

- Keloid
- Hypopigmented or hyperpigmented spot
- Pyoderma in legs
- Granuloma inguinale
- Ingrown hairs of beard
- Acral lentiginous melanoma
- Tinea capitis
- Seborrheic dermatitis.

Acne vulgaris (Figs 10.8A and B)
This is a disorder of pilosebaceous unit due to:

- Excessive sebum production
- Comedone formation
- Propionibacterium acne.

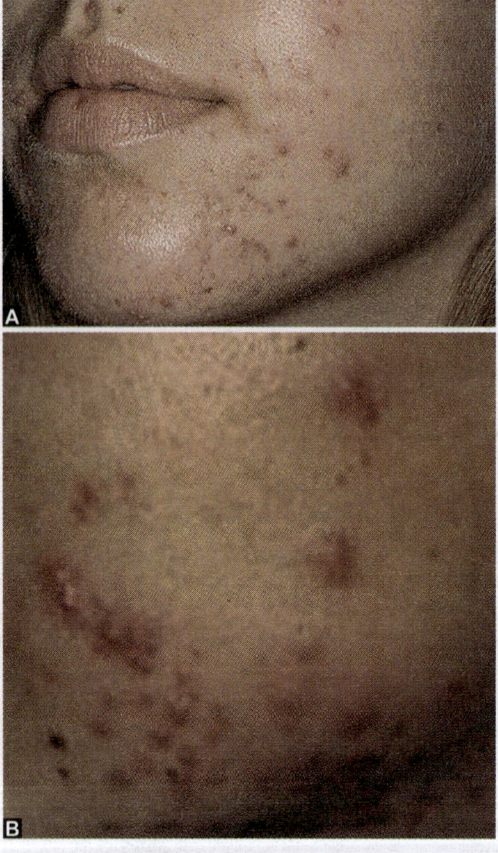

FIGS 10.8A AND B Acne vulgaris

If occurs in:

- Pubertal girls or boys.
- Perimenstrual women.
- Iatrogenic-steroid.

The following are the types:

Acne may be noninflammatory or inflammatory.

Noninflammatory lesion may be: (No proliferation of P acne)

- Closed comedo (Fig. 10.9) dome shaped papule, 1–2 mm in size
- Open comedo 1–2 mm papule with blackened keratinous plug closing the orifice of sebaceous follicles.

Inflammatory lesions may be due to proliferation of P acne:

- *Mild inflammatory acne:* Mild papular or pustular inflammatory <20 in number
- *Moderate-to-severe inflammatory acne:* Number of papules >20 in number, inflammatory, patient may have disfigured face. This may be gradually worsening or virulent at onset due to psychological stress.
- *Nodular cystic acne:* It includes:
  - ❖ Localized cystic acne—(Fig. 10.10) face, chest and back
  - ❖ Diffuse cystic acne—wide areas of face, chest and back
  - ❖ Pyoderma faciale—inflamed cyst on face in female predominantly in central portion of cheek. After drainage of purulent material, there may be scarring (Fig. 10.11)
  - ❖ *Acne fulminans:* In adolescent boys, ulcerative necrotic lesion with systemic symptoms—arthralgia, fever, weight loss.

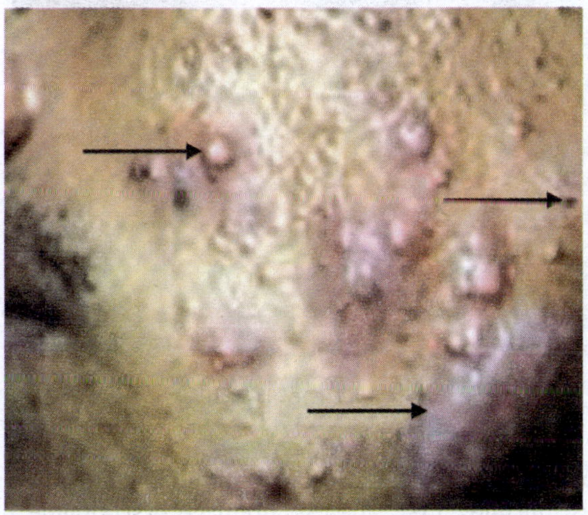

FIG. 10.9   Comedones

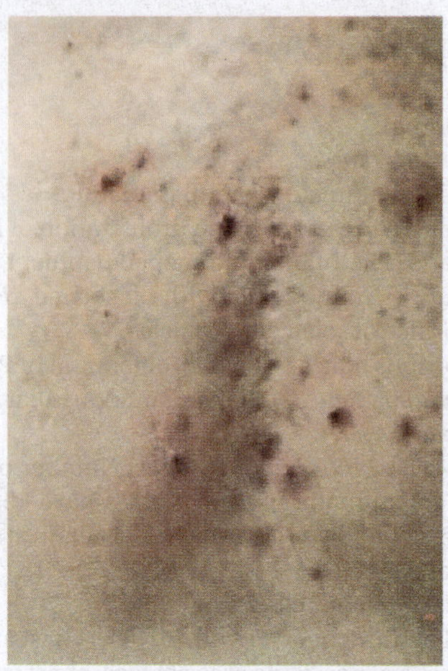

FIG. 10.10 Acne cystic

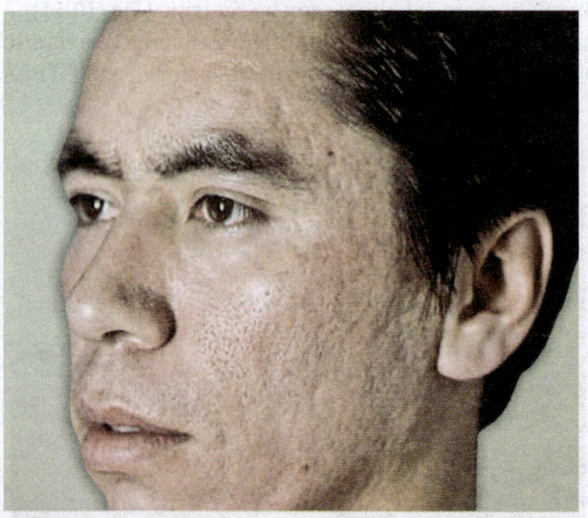

FIG. 10.11 Acne scarring

❖ *Acne conglobata (Fig. 10.12):* Chronic inflammatory, papules, pustules, cyst, abscess, drainage cyst, double headed comedones. No fever or weight loss is associated with it

❖ *Acne rosacea (Fig. 10.13):* In early childhood or early teen, facial flushing is triggered by:
  - Alcohol
  - Emotional stress
  - Spicy foods
  - Temperature changes.

In third to fifth decade rosacea may present with, telangiectasia, acne like papulopustular eruptions affecting forehead, nose, cheeks, and chins.

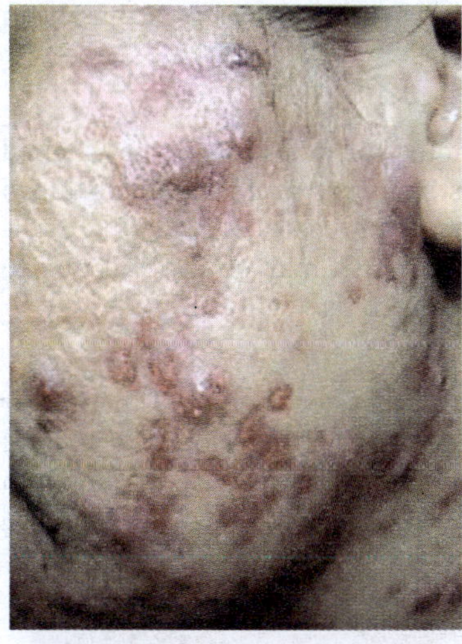

FIG. 10.12 Acne conglobata

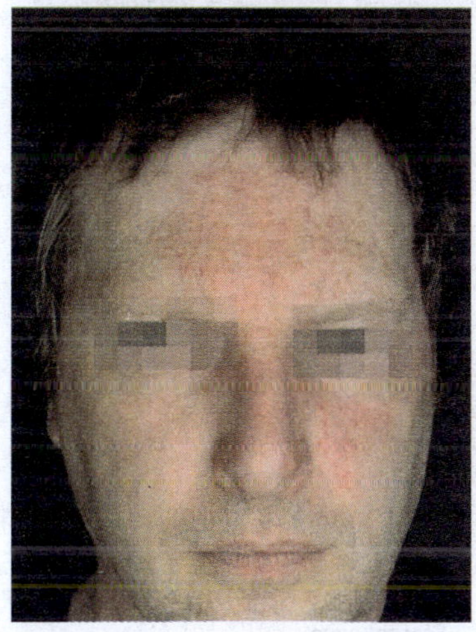

FIG. 10.13 Acne rosacea

The differences with acne vulgaris are:
- Absence of scarring.
- Lack of comedones.

Ocular rosacea may present with episcleritis, chalazion, and blepharitis. Extra facial involvement may include neck and upper chest.

The symptoms may be intermittent to start with, but in later stages there is permanent flushing of skin of cheeks, nose with lymph edema.

In chronic acne rosacea, there is hyperplasia of sebaceous glands leading to thickened and disfigured nose called rhinophyma.

Acne rosacea is more frequent in celtic ancestry, it has been described in dark skin individual.

Steroid acne (Fig. 10.14)
- Acne-like rash monomorphous (pustules or dome shaped papules) involving upper chest, upper arm and shoulders due to >2 weeks continuous used of systemic corticosteroids
- Perioral dermatitis—rosacea like rash may be evolved due to prolonged use of topical corticosteroids (Fig. 10.15).

Herpes simplex (Fig. 10.16)
Description of lesion: This lesion starts as erythematous papule or plaques of uniform size and shapes which develop into painful umbilicated vesicles on an erythematous base—these develop into pustules—finally ulcerate and develop crust.

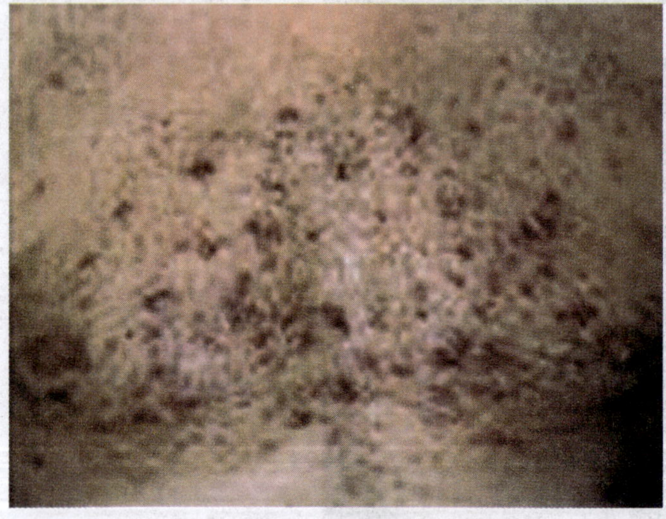

FIG. 10.14   Steroid acne

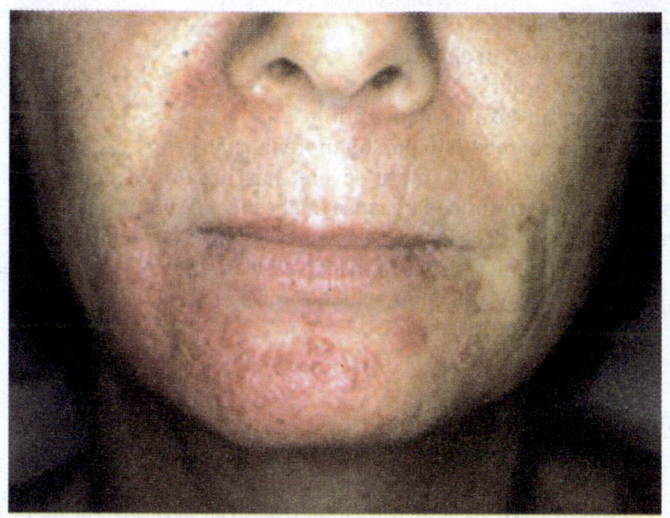

FIG. 10.15 Steroid cream induced acne

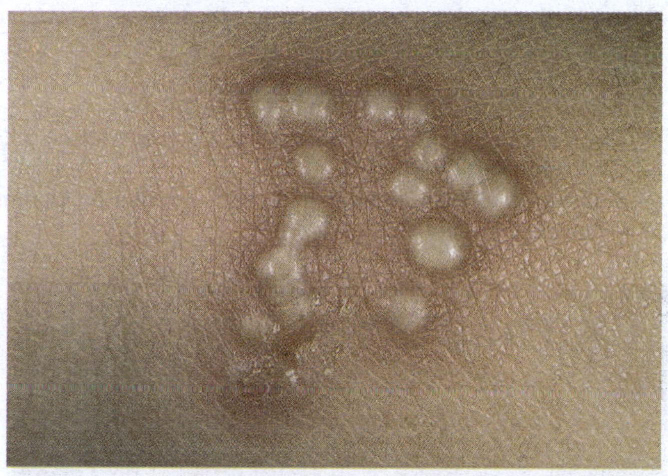

FIG. 10.16 Herpes simplex

Site:
- Vermilion border of the lip
- Genital areas
- Eye
- Presacrum.

Age: Specific site:
- Perioral region in children
- Labialis in adult
- Genitalias in sexually active adult
- Lumbosacral region in person more than 40 years.

Primary lesion: This is more severe, has prolonged course, few lesions may go unnoticed because of absence of symptoms.

Secondary lesion: This lesion is less severe, have short course.

The main characteristics of this disease are the presence of virus in dorsal ganglia as dormant, which is the source of recurrence.

Recurrences occur in case of:
- Genital lesion
- Labial lesion.

Other herpes simplex lesions:
- *Herpetic gingivostomatitis (Fig. 10.17):*
  - ❖ It occurs in children and young adult
  - ❖ Patient may present with malaise, fever, sore throat, painful vesicles, erosions in tongue, lips, buccal mucosa, gingiva, palate
- *Herpetic Whitlow:* This lesion occurs in digits of medical or dental professionals as vesicles surrounding edema associated with lymphangitis, lymphadenopathy.

Diagnosed by:
- ❖ Tzanck preparation
- ❖ Direct immunofluorescent antibody staining of infected cells
- ❖ Viral culture
- ❖ Biopsy of the lesion demonstrates reticular and ballooning degeneration of epidermis.

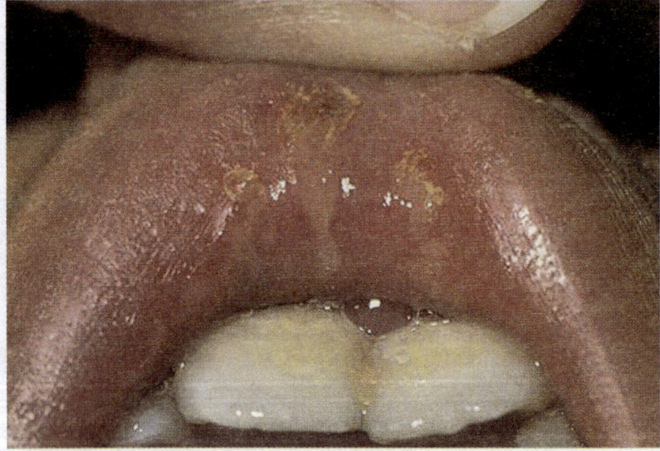

FIG. 10.17 Herpetic gingivostomatitis

Varicella (Fig. 10.18)
Incubation period: Two weeks.
Infections period: Highly contagious for 2–4 weeks (1–2 days prior to exanthems to the development of crust).
Description of lesion: 2–3 mm elliptical vesicles surrounded by erythema as dew drop in rose petal appearance.

It starts in face and scalp then to trunk, lastly to arms and legs —so thesis centrifugal lesion.

This vesicles will be converted into pustules and umbilication — lastly to crust and scab formation. The scab falls off in 1–3 weeks.

As a result there is pink depression followed by scarring.
Age: Mainly children less than 10 years old.
Severity:

- More severe in adult with high constitutional symptoms
- In case of pregnancy, it can be transmitted to fetus, responsible for developmental congenital abnormalities
- In immunocompromised patient, it may be so virulent that it may produce hemorrhagic manifestations.

Herpes zoster (Fig. 10.19)
In this case prodormal discomfort starts as paresthesia and pain in the involved dermatome (Saint Anthony's fire) with no historical or physical explanation.

This is followed by appearances of erythematous plaques, which is transformed into—Vesicles → Pustules → Umbilication → Development of crust.
Site of lesion

- This lesion affects a single dermatome, never cross the midline
- Trigeminal nerve distribution or T_3 to L_2 distribution.

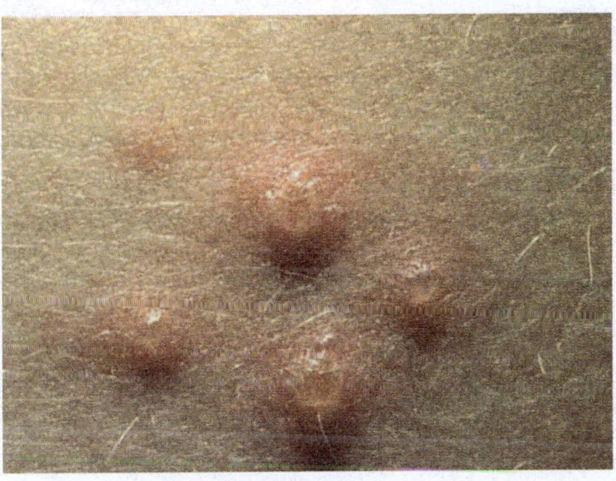

FIG. 10.18 Chickenpox primary lesions

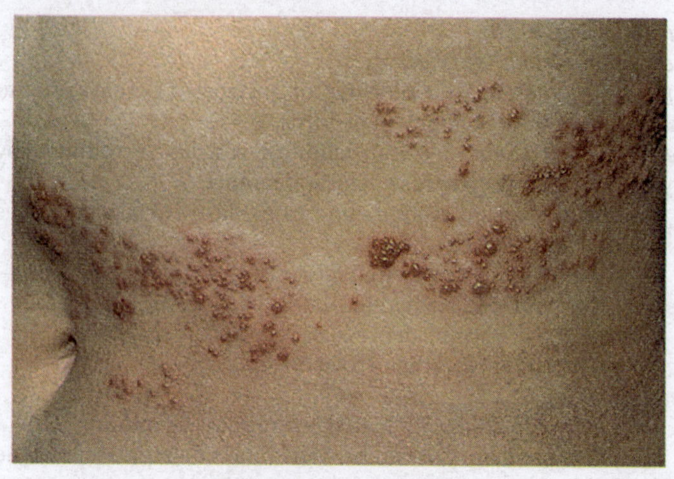

FIG. 10.19 Herpes zoster

Affected persons are:
- Ages more than 50 years (90% cases).
- Immunocompromised patient.
- Pregnant women.

Fate of lesion
- The crust will be developed in 1 week and resolved in several weeks
- In few cases, postherpetic neuralgia (15% of cases)—more common in older persons.

Other sites of involvement
- Involvement of nasociliary nerve—lesions appears at the tip of the nose
- *Ramsay-Hunt syndrome:* Involvement of geniculate ganglion.

With facial paralysis—lesion on external auditory canal or tympanic membrane—produces vertigo, tinnitus, deafness unilateral loss of taste, decreased tear formation and salivation.

Dermatitis herpetiformis (Fig. 10.20)
It is immune mediated blistering disease may occur in gluten enteropathy.

Description of lesion: Flesh-colored herpetiform popular lesion-pruritic, inflammatory may progress into erosions and crusts.

Site of involvement: It is usually present on extensor surface of elbow, knee, shoulder and buttocks, never in buccal mucosa palms and soles.

Course: It usually waxes and wanes—responds to dapsone and gluten free diet.

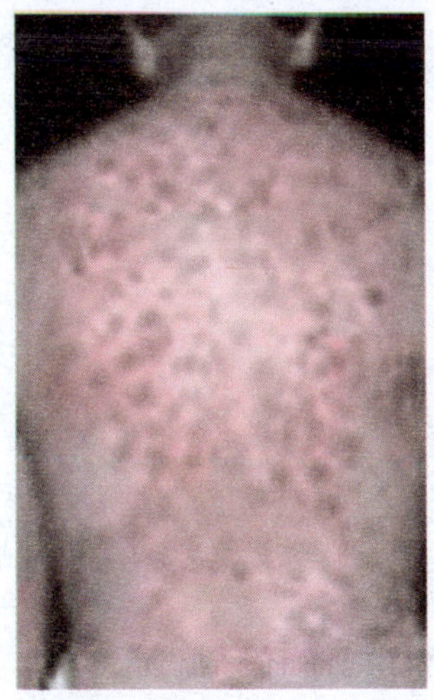

FIG. 10.20 Dermatitis herpetiformis

Pemphigus
It is a group of disorders—characterized by:
- Intradermal blisters.
- IgG antibodies against keratinocytes.

The group of disorders are:
- Pemphigus vulgaris
- Pemphigus foliaceus (Fig. 10.21)
- Paraneoplastic pemphigus.

Pemphigus vulgaris (Fig. 10.22)
Oral lesions (Fig. 10.23) precede the cutaneous involvement by several months. Since, bullae are rare in mouth—main lesions are large shallow irregular shaped erosions present in gingival, buccal mucosa, and palatine mucosa slow to heal, interferes with drinking, swallowing and eating.

Other mucosal involvements are conjunctiva, larynx, esophagus, labia, vagina, penis, cervix, urethra, and anus.

Cutaneous involvement: Primary lesion is usually blister containing clear fluid, but they usually rupture easily and produce shallow superficial painful ulcers, slow to heal. Bullae are usually intraepidermal.

It affects all races, more in Jews in 5th to 8th decade.

Drug-induced pemphigus:
- Penicillamine
- Captopril
- Rifampin
- Thiol-containing compound.

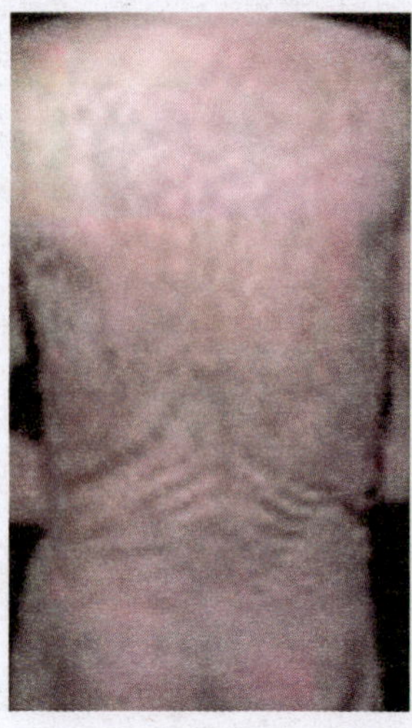

FIG. 10.21 Pemphigus foliaceus

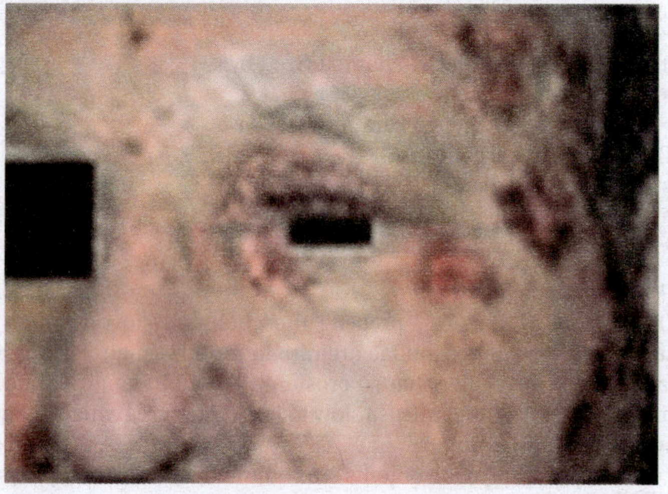

FIG. 10.22 Pemphigus vulgaris

Pemphigus in autoimmune diseases:
- Myasthenia gravis
- Thymoma.

Bullous pemphigoid (Fig. 10.24)
- Bullous pemphigoid involves mainly skin, rarely oral or conjunctival mucous membrane
- The onset is acute or subacute or chronic, age 65 years
- In contrast to pemphigus vulgaris, pemphigoid blisters are subepidermal having thick base, hence rarely rupture, they are pruritic.

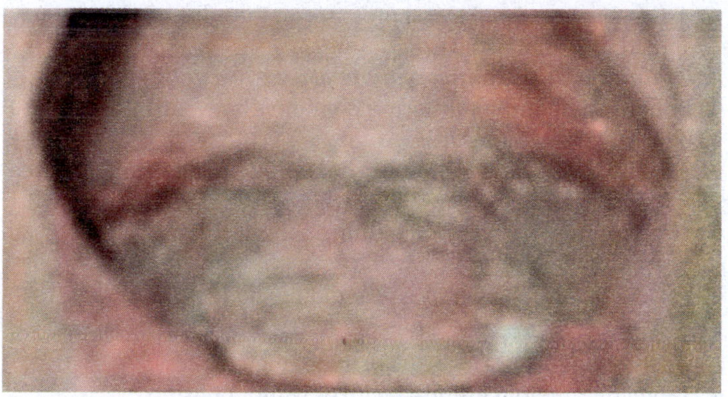

FIG. 10.23 Pemphigus vulgaris oral lesions

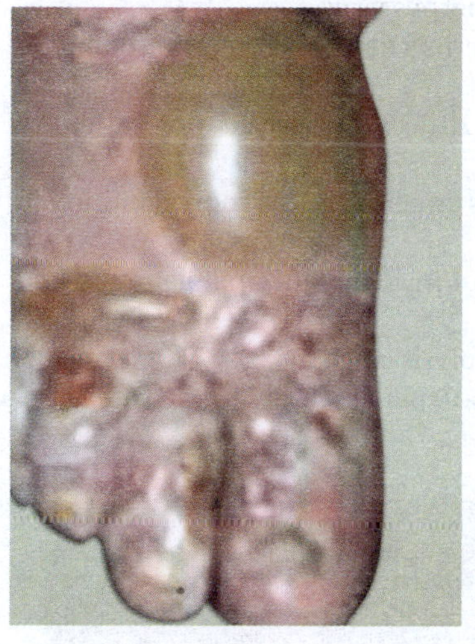

FIG. 10.24 Bullous pemphigoid

- When rupture, they produce painful disabling erosions mainly involving palms and roles
- The pathogenesis is IgG antibodies to skin mucous membrane.
- If it involves oral mucosa, it may produce dysphagia.

Pemphigus vulgaris and bullous pemphigoid can be separated by:

- *Nikolsky's sign:* There is separation of epidermal cells due to shearing stress produced by sliding finger, due to poor adhesion of epidermal cells (acantholysis).

  It occurs in pemphigus vulgaris, not in pemphigoid.

  It may occur in scalded skin syndrome.

- *Asboe-Hansen sign:* Lateral pressure on the edge of a blister may spread into unaffected skin.

Important cutaneous manifestations of drug reactions:

- Bullous erythema multiforme denuding body surface area <10 percent target lesions
- Stevens-Johnson syndrome, denuding body surface area <10 percent
- Overlapping SJS/TEN, denuding body surface area 10–30 percent
- Toxic epidermal necrolysis denuding body surface area >30 percent.

Erythema multiforme (Fig. 10.25): It is benign process:

- Target or targetoid lesions—with or without blisters
- Symmetrical acral distribution involving palms, soles, dorsum of hands, extensor aspect of extremities
- If it involves mucosal surface, it affects only one surface
- If may be caused by drugs or herpes virus
- If may be associated with epidermal detachment having denuded body surface area <10 percent.

Stevens-Johnson syndrome (Fig. 10.26): If is dermatological emergency.

- Widespread purpuric macules targetoid lesion more common in face and torso
- More than two mucosal site of involvement oral, genitalia and eyes
- Full thickness epidermal necrolysis occurs
- If may involve denudation of >10 percent body surface area.

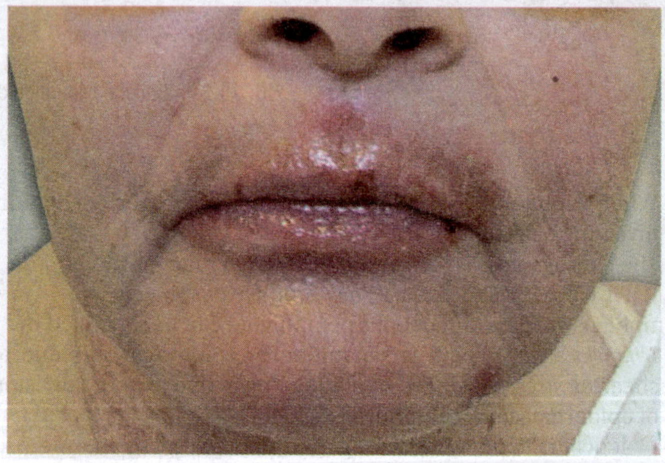

FIG. 10.25 Erythema multiforme

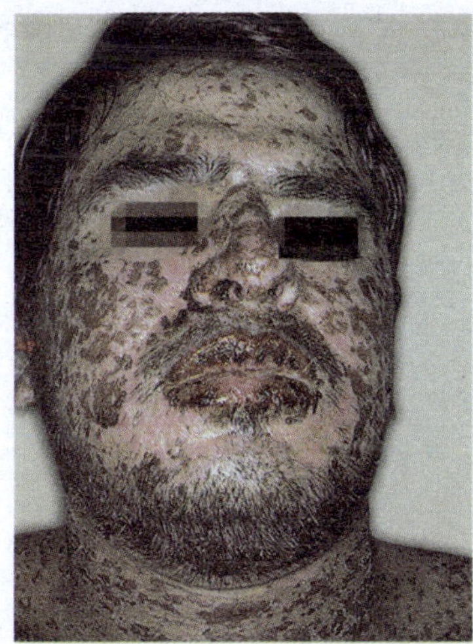

FIG. 10.26 Stevens-Johnson syndrome

Toxic epidermal necrolysis (Fig. 10.27): Also called Lyell's syndrome. If involves:

- *Cutanaous lesion:* Erythematous and target like macules.
- Full thickness epidermal necrosis, involving >30 percent body surface area.
- It may be fatal and produces respiratory distress.
- It also involves mucosal lesions.
- Lesions may involve sun-exposed areas also affect entire epidermis, including nail bed.
- Palms and soles develop painful edematous erythema, flaccid blisters with full thickness epidermal necrosis.
- Nikolsky's sign demonstrated in the lesions present in shoulder, sacrum or buttock.

Stevens-Johnson syndrome (SJS)/Toxic epidermal neurolysis (TEN)

- Constitutional symptoms—fever, cough, sore throat.
- Photophobia appears—followed by diffuse cayenne symmetrically distributed in face and upper torso. This is macular lesion with pepper eruptions purpuric center → coalesce to form blister and ulcerate.

Difference between targetoid lesions of SJS/TEN and target of EM:
Targetoid lesion of SJS/TEN have two zones of color:

1. Central dusky purpura or central bulla
2. Surrounding macular erythema.

Target lesion of erythema multiforme have three zones of color:

1. Central dusky purpura or central bulla
2. Surrounding pale edematous zone
3. Surrounded by macular erythema.

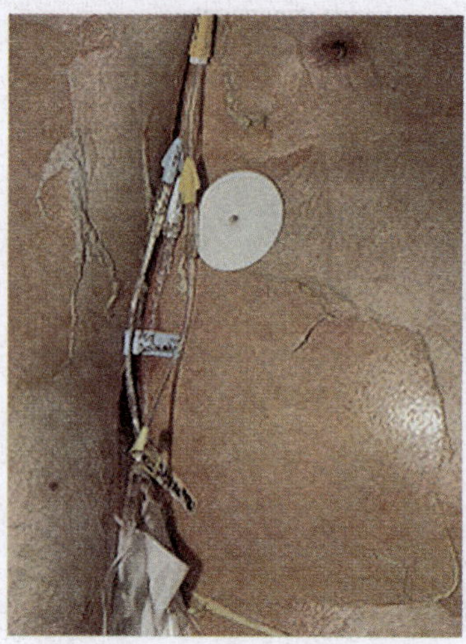

FIG. 10.27 Toxic epidermal necrolysis

Sequelae of SJS/TEN
- Some patients loose large surface areas, some patients develop rapid re-epithelization of denuded areas.

  Re-epithelization is completed within 3 weeks, but pressure and mucosal areas remain eroded and crusted for 2 weeks or more.
- *Long-term sequelae:*
  - ❖ Eye—blindness, sicca syndrome
  - ❖ Skin—mottling of hyperpigmentation and hypopigmentation
  - ❖ Genital lesion—phimosis, vaginal synechiae
  - ❖ Nail—fingernail and toenails—abnormally regrow.

Causes of SJS/TEN
- *Antibiotics:*
  - ❖ Trimethoprim-co-trimoxazole
  - ❖ Sulfonamide
  - ❖ Cephalosporins
  - ❖ Quinolone.
- *Anticonvulsant:*
  - ❖ Phenobarbitone
  - ❖ Phenytoin
  - ❖ Carbamazepine
  - ❖ Valproic acid.
- NSAIDs.
- Corticosteroid.
- Allopurinol.

Other cutaneous lesions due to drugs:
- Urticaria—hives.
- Bullous lesion.
- Pigmentary changes.
- Vasculitis.
- Lichenoid eruptions.
- Photosensitivity.
- Erythema nodosum.
- Fixed drug eruptions.

Photosensitizing drugs:
- Diuretics.
- Antibiotics.
- Retinoid.
- Diltiazem, amiodarone, enalapril.

Urticaria (Fig. 10.28)
- Flat-topped balanced well-demarcated edematous papule or plaque.
- This lesion is surrounded by pale or erythematous pruritic annular, linear, round, oval, arcate halo.
- They may arise anywhere in the body size few millimeters to 10 cm.
- It may resolve spontaneously without any residual sign.
- If it persists for more than 24 hours, biopsy should be taken to exclude vasculitis.

Causes of urticaria:
- *Acute urticaria:* Persists for 4 to 6 weeks. The causes are:
  - ❖ Drugs—Sulfonamides, Penicillin
  - ❖ Food allergens—shellfish, eggs, chocolates, cheese, nuts, butter, strawberries

FIG. 10.28 Urticaria

- ❖ Pets
- ❖ Infection (respiratory infection)
- ❖ Pregnancy—it may be aggravating factors.
- *Chronic urticaria (Figs 10.29A and B):* It lasts for more than 6 weeks. Causes are all the above. The other causes are:
  - ❖ Virus
  - ❖ Parasites
  - ❖ Neoplasm
  - ❖ Stress
  - ❖ *Physical factors:*
    - Cold water
    - Pressure
    - Vibrations
    - Stroke (dermographism).

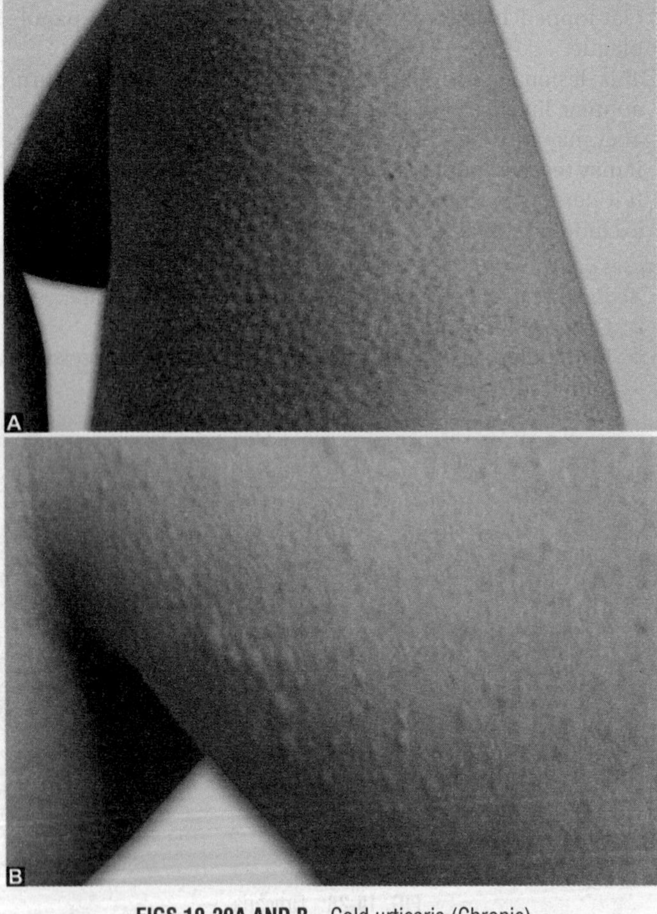

FIGS 10.29A AND B   Cold urticaria (Chronic)

Angioedema (Fig. 10.30)
It is a variant of urticaria—as evidenced by swelling of tissues of eyelids, oral mucosa, lips and tongue—may be responsible for respiratory distress.

Warts
- This benign, rough-surfaced mucocutaneous proliferation due to human papillomaviruses
- It occurs in 10–20 percent of school children, immunocompromised patients, meat handler (Butcher's wart)
- It can be spreaded by direct or indirect contact, when normal epithelial barrier will be interrupted.

Types of wart
- *Common wart (verruca vulgaris) (Fig. 10.31):* Rough surfaced, often tender scaly, circumscribed papule, 1 mm to 0.5 cm in diameter, often black headed due to thrombosed capillaries present on hands, knees, or other areas of the body
- *Filiform wart (Fig. 10.32):* Long slender growth-present usually on lips, eyelids, or nares
- *Condyloma (Fig. 10.33):* Flat-topped rough surfaced pink to brown papule present on labia, glans, vulva, or anus
- *Palmoplantar wart (Fig. 10.34):* White, irregular surfaced papule with or without black dot when present on sole may be painful and impair ambulation. These lesions may progress into sharply defined nodular, round keratotic surfaced lesions and smooth collar of thickened horn.

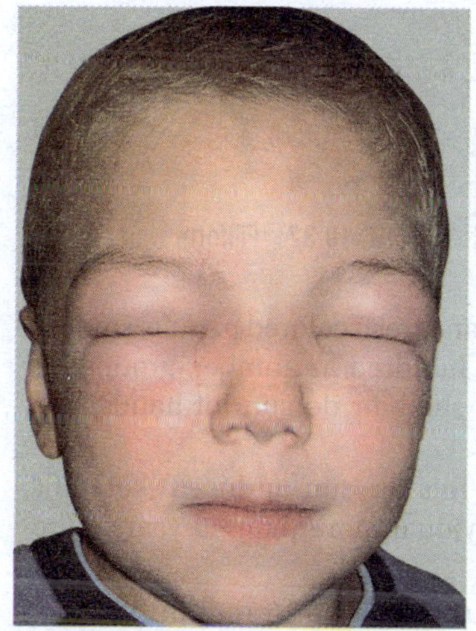

FIG. 10.30 Angioedema

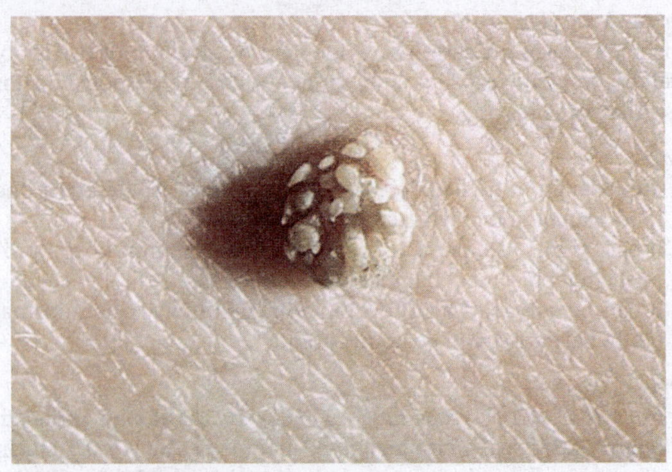

FIG. 10.31 Common wart (verruca vulgaris)

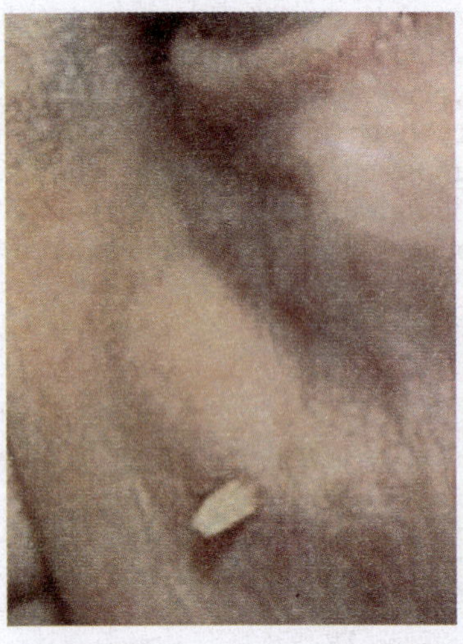

FIG. 10.32 Filiform wart

- *Flat wart (verruca plana):* Flat and fresh colored papule, smooth, slightly hyperkeratotic, few to hundred in number, grouped or confluent, present on face or shins or dorsum of hands, may regress spontaneously.

Actinic keratosis (Fig. 10.35): This is sun induced keratotic, premalignant lesion, affects individual more than 40 years, blue-eyed persons.

Lesion: Single small erythematous papule, 3–10 mm in diameter, located over exposed surfaces—nose, forehead, temples, cheeks, ears, bald scalp, forearm, and dorsum of the hand.

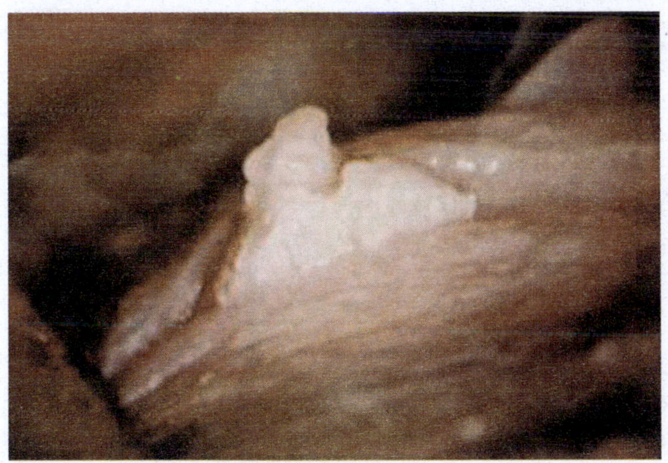

FIG. 10.33 Condyloma

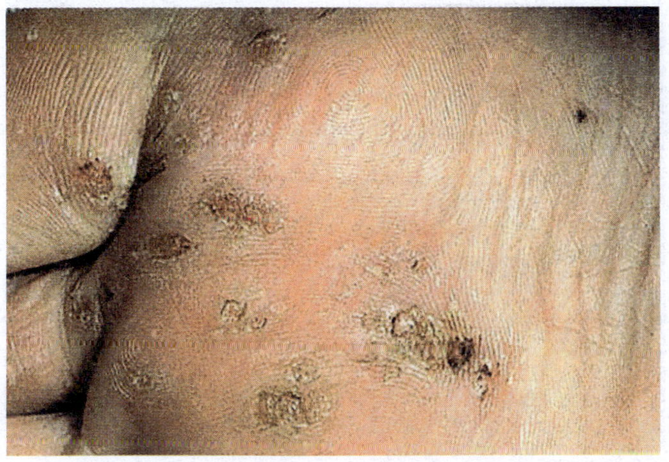

FIG. 10.34 Plantar wart

Lesions are scaly on background of solar damaged skin with telangiectasias, elastosis, multiple erythematous keratoses.

All mainly affects older individual, but may affect the person of 20–30 years especially fair skinned red-headed/blond-headed individual.

Squamous cell carcinoma (Fig. 10.36) (SSC)
Areas most commonly affected: Lower lip, external ear, preauricular region, forehead, scalp.

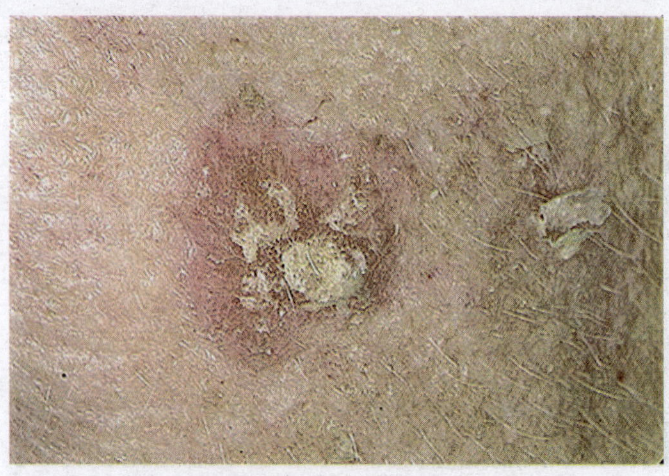

FIG. 10.35 Actinic keratosis

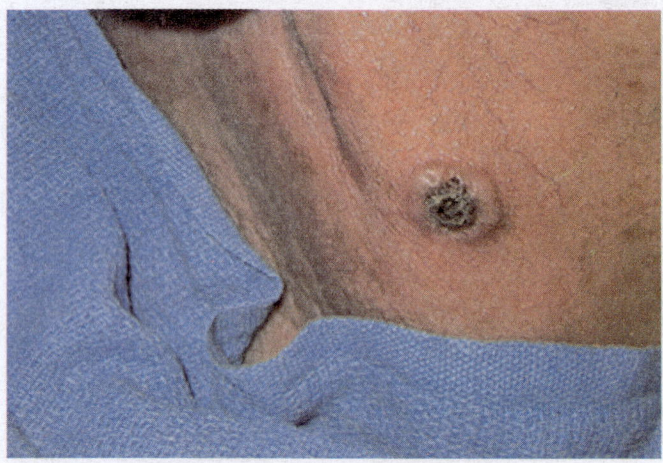

FIG. 10.36 Squamous cell carcinoma

Evolution of lesion: It starts as actinic keratosis. As atypical cells fill the entire epidermis, but do not breach the basal layer—produce carcinoma *in situ* (Bowen's disease).

Later on atypical cells invade dermis—producing invasive squamous cell carcinoma.

Spread of SCC depends upon following factors:
- Depth of invasion
- Degrees of cellular differentiation
- Origin in mucous membrane.

Bowen's disease (Fig. 10.37): This is squamous cell carcinoma *in situ*.
Causes:
- Human papillomavirus (HPV)
- Arsenic
- Solar damage.

It more commonly affects older people, head, neck, hands, limb, glans of penis. (Erythroplasia of Queyrat).

Lesion: Slowly enlarging erythematous plaque, scaly hyperkeratotic, crusted, fissured, eventually ulcerated.

Basal cell carcinoma:
- Parlcy nonkeratotic papule, occasionally central necrosis due to decreased vascularity, rolled out everted margin
- Present in face or ears
- Locally metastatic, rarely metastasize.

Skin tags (Fig. 10.38)
- Soft benign, nonkeratotic, occasionally variegated, pedunculated neoplasm 2–5 mm in diameter
- Present in face, neck, axilla, grains, eyelids, trunk, abdomen, and back
- Size increases with age
- Causes—HPV, obesity, paraneoplastic, hormone imbalance.

Vitiligo (Figs 10.39A and B)
- Milky white macular patches, symmetrical in distribution, involving the areas of trauma elbows, ventral wrist, knees, axilla, dorsal hands and feet, circumorificial areas (nose, lips, eyes, ears, genitals, nipples).

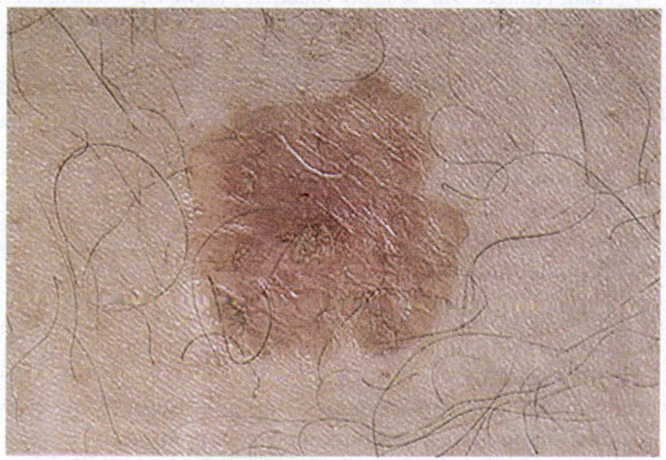

FIG. 10.37 Bowen's disease

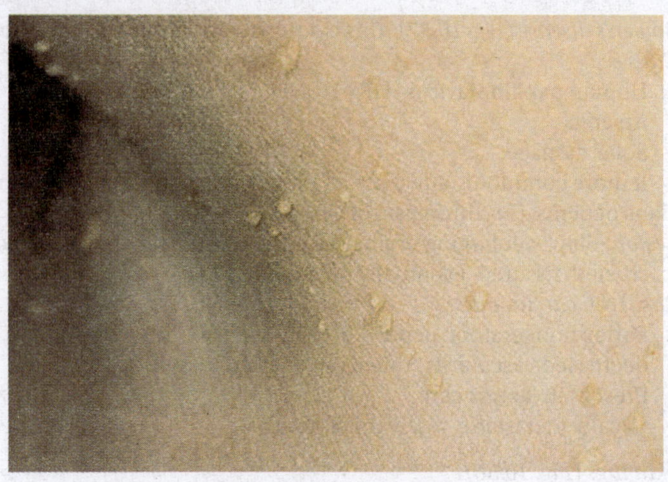

FIG. 10.38 Skin tags

- Number and size of the patches gradually increase, confluent.
- *Other cutaneous findings are:*
  - Premature graying of hair
  - Alopecia areata
  - Piebaldism
  - Halo nevi
  - Retinal pigmentary abnormalities.
- It occurs at any age, but mainly in 1st two decades of life.
- Course is unpredictable; it may be stable or slowly progresses.
- *Types of vitiligo:*
  - *Focal vitiligo:* One or more macular patches in a single area
  - *Segmental vitiligo:* Unilateral depigmented macules in a dermatomal or quasi-dermatomal distribution
  - *Universal vitiligo (Fig. 10.40):* Whole body becomes affected.
- *Diseases associated with vitiligo:*
  - Alopecia areata
  - Addison's disease
  - Diabetes
  - Hypothyroidism
  - Pernicious anemia.

Tinea versicolor (Fig. 10.41)

- Common benign fungal superficial infection caused by *Malassezia furfur*
- Predisposition factors—genetics, immune suppression, malnutrition, Cushing's disease, humid environment
- Numerous well-demarcated hypopigmented macules, occasionally scaly—present in chest and trunk

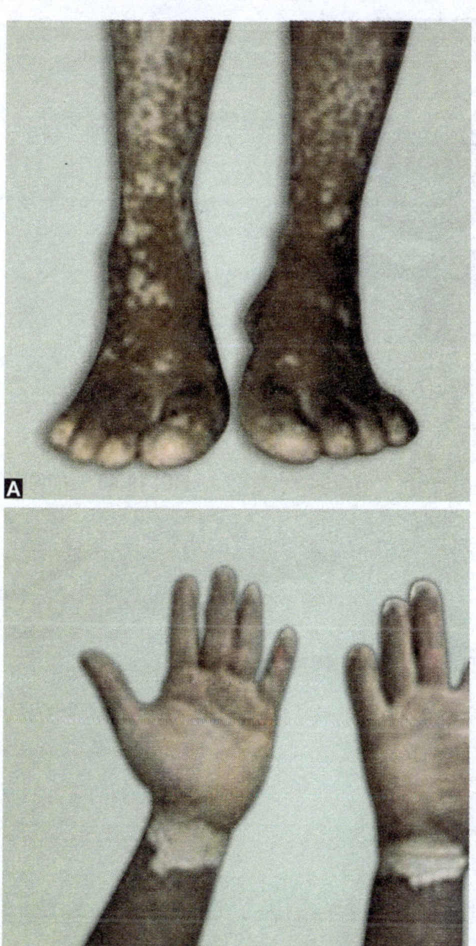

FIGS 10.39A AND B Vitiligo

- Color reddish brown to white macules
- Diagnosed by KOH preparation—cigar-buff mycelial hyphae and round thick walled spores.

Acanthosis nigricans (Fig. 10.42)
- Brown to black, poorly defined velvety plaques occurs anywhere in the body, but usual sites are:
  - ❖ Intertriginous areas, e.g. axilla, groin
  - ❖ Umbilicus
  - ❖ Posterior and lateral folds of the neck

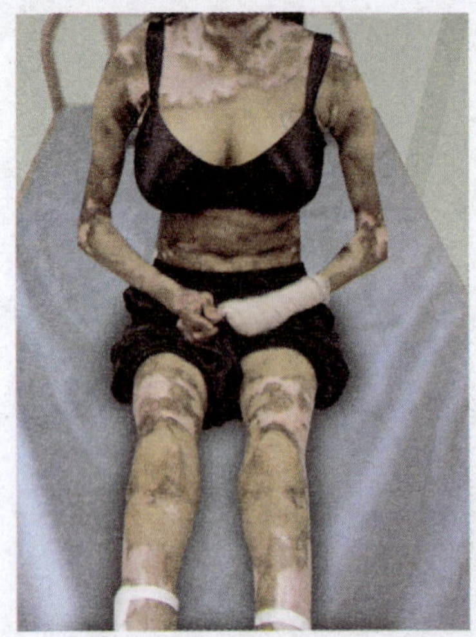

FIG. 10.40 Universal vitiligo

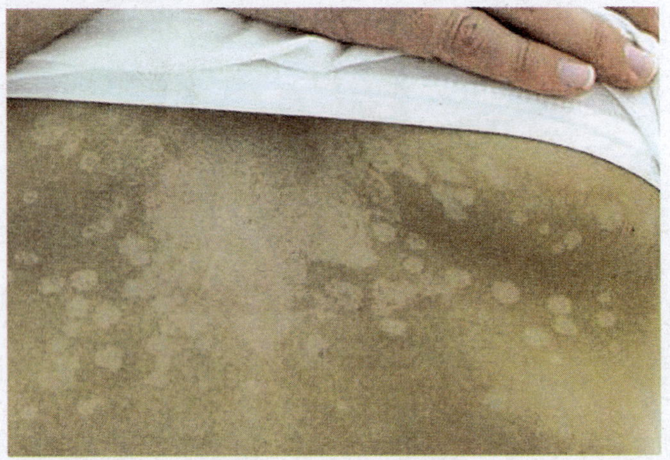

FIG. 10.41 Tinea versicolor

- ❖ Mucous membranes are:
  - Oral cavity
  - Esophagus
  - Nasopharyngeal mucosa
  - Nipples.
- Causes:
- ❖ Obesity
- ❖ Insulin resistance
- ❖ Congenital syndrome—Type A and Type B syndrome.

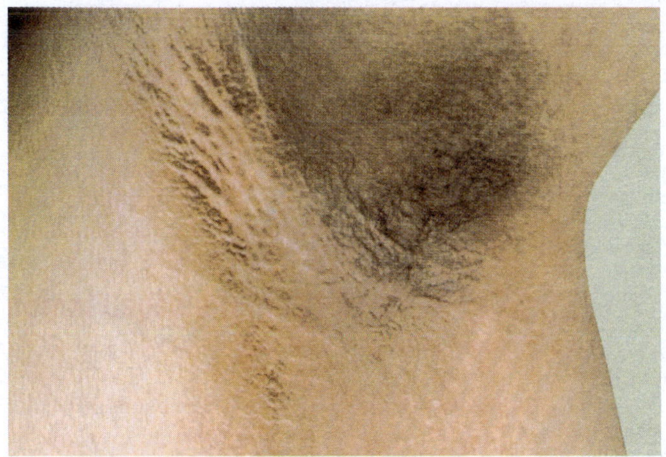

FIG. 10.42   Acanthosis nigricans

Type A syndrome—HAIR-AN syndrome (Hyperandrogenemia insulin resistance, AN syndrome).

Type B syndrome—occurs in women with uncontrolled diabetes, ovarian hyperandrogenism, other autoimmune diseases (SLE, scleroderma, Hashimoto thyroiditis).

❖ Drug reaction—pituitary extract, nicotinic acid, systemic corticosteroids
❖ Internal malignancy.

Common nevi: These are benign neoplasm composed of melanocytes can be described as part of skin.

Different types of nevi: Histological classification:

- *Junctional nevus (Fig. 10.43):* Macules to thin papule, brown to black pigment, well circumscribed. Cells are located at dermoepidermal junction
- *Compound nevus (Fig. 10.44):* Raised papules—brown to tan, often lighter pigmentation at dermoepidermal/upper dermis
- *Dermal nevus (Fig. 10.45):* Brown, fleshy dome shaped pedunculated lesion present in dermis.

Features of melanotic nevi

- Stability—size, height, outline
- Color—tattoo, brown
- Lack of symptoms—painful, irritation, bleeding
- Size—<1 cm.

Dysplastic nevi: Acquired, typically runs in families.

Characteristics:

- Larger than common (5–15 mm) moles
- Color—dark brown to pink
- Occurs in sun exposed to sun protected areas

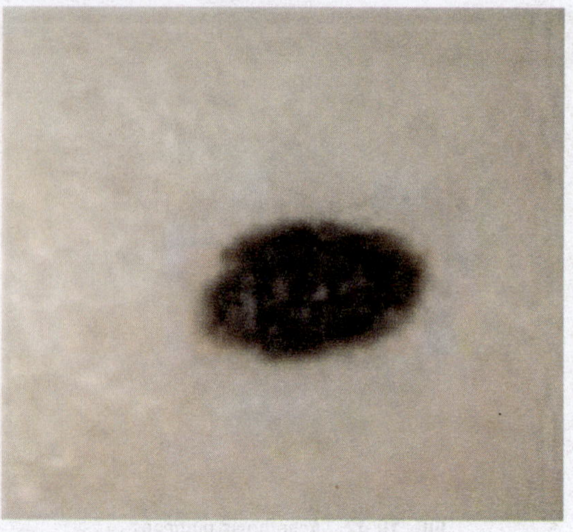

FIG. 10.43 Junctional nevus

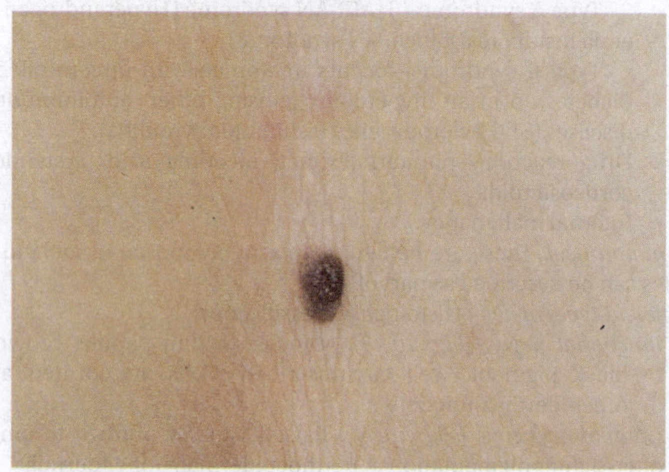

FIG. 10.44 Compound nevus

- Occurs in back, chest, buttock, breast, scalp
- Central papule with surrounding macular areas of different pigmentation.

Seborrheic keratosis (Fig. 10.46)

- It is a benign tumor of old age due to proliferation of epidermal cells. These are sometimes called benign senile verrucae
- These are round or oval, <1 cm to start with, grow thicker and larger, soft and greasy, grow along skin-folds more common in exposed areas.

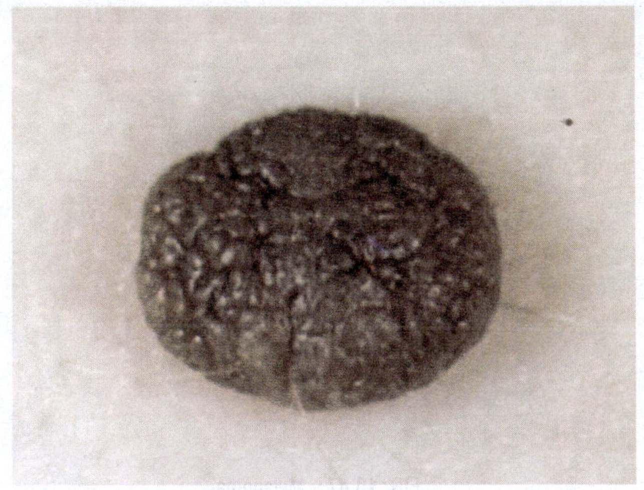

FIG. 10.45   Dermal nevi

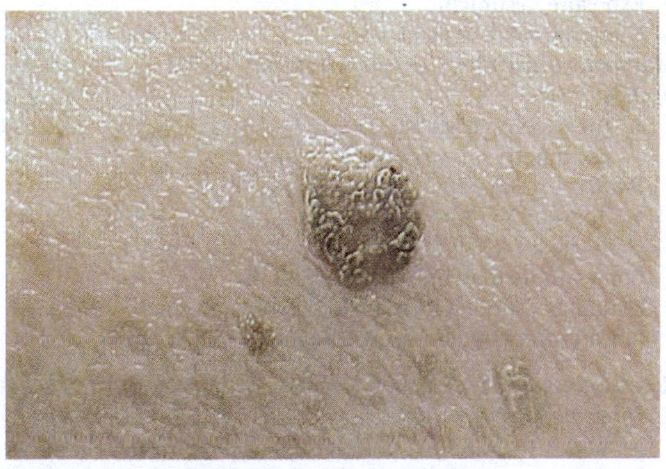

FIG. 10.46   Seborrheic keratosis

Dermatosis papulosa nigra
- Seborrheic keratosis variant
- It affects upper cheeks, lateral orbits in dark skinned individual
- This lesion is small pedunculated, pigmented.

Melanoma (Fig. 10.47)
Age of onset:
- Median age of onset of superficial spreading melanoma is 44.
- Most common ages during 2nd to 3rd decades.

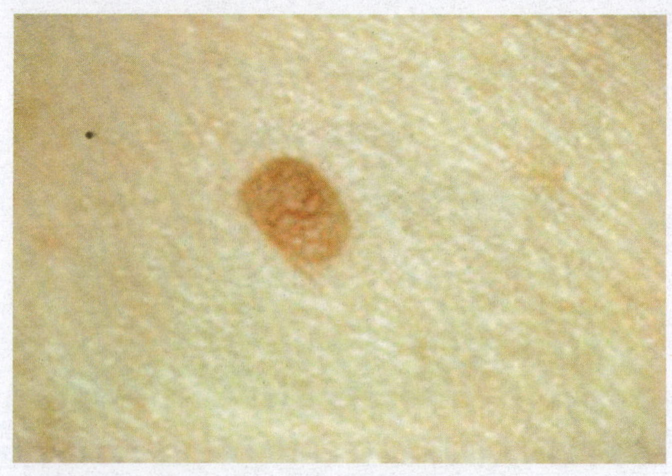

FIG. 10.47 Melanoma

- Exposure to sunlight.
- Numerous and atypical nevi.

Morphologic warning signs of melanoma: ABCD (E)
- *Asymmetry:*
  - ❖ The lesion is bisected
  - ❖ Asymmetry on two sides of lesion.
- *Border–irregularity:*
  - ❖ Uneven
  - ❖ Ragged.
- **C**olor—more than one shade of color.
- **D**iameter—sudden increase in diameter >6 cm.
- **E**levation/enlargement/evolvement.

Reverse glasgow 7 points checklist
- *Three major criteria:*
  1. Size
  2. Shape
  3. Color.
- *Four minor criteria:*
  1. Inflammation
  2. Crusting or bleeding
  3. Sensory changes
  4. Diameter >7 mm is size.

Types of melanoma
- *Superficial spreading melanoma:*
  - ❖ Occurs in 3rd to 5th decade
  - ❖ Present on back of men, legs of women, trunk of both sexes

- ❖ Flat, slightly raised, brown, variegated, >6 mm diameter, irregular borders.
- *Nodular melanoma (Fig. 10.48):*
  - ❖ Present on legs or trunk
  - ❖ Papule or nodular lesion, black or brown in color, rapidly growing, sometimes ulcerates and bleeds.
- *Lentigo melanoma:*
  - ❖ Intraepithelial precursor of lentigo maligna melanoma
  - ❖ Present on sun exposed areas—head, neck and arms
  - ❖ >3 cm, hyperpigmented, variegated, irregular bordered lesion.
- *Lentigo maligna melanoma (Fig. 10.49):* Large >3 cm, slowly grown, more variegated in color.
- *Acrolentiginous melanoma (Fig. 10.50):*
  - ❖ Present in palms and soles, beneath the nail plate
  - ❖ One or more dark papule, pigmented, uneven surface
  - ❖ Nail bed melanoma presents as longitudinal pigmented melanoma within nail plate.

Freckles (Fig. 10.51)
- It appears early in life
- 1–2 mm in diameter
- It may disappear with time
- It has no malignant potential.

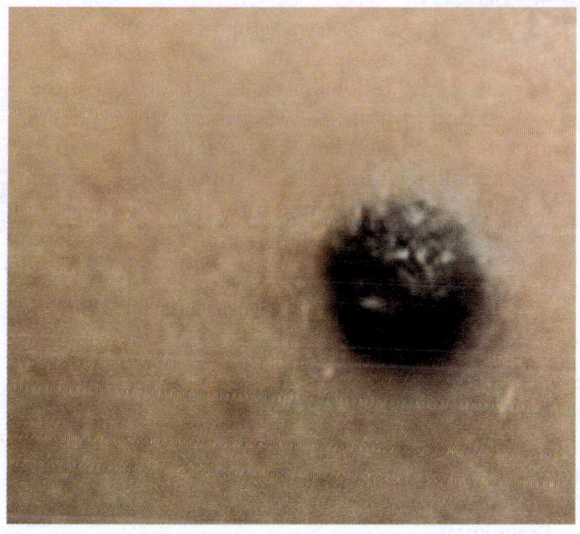

FIG. 10.48 Nodular melanoma

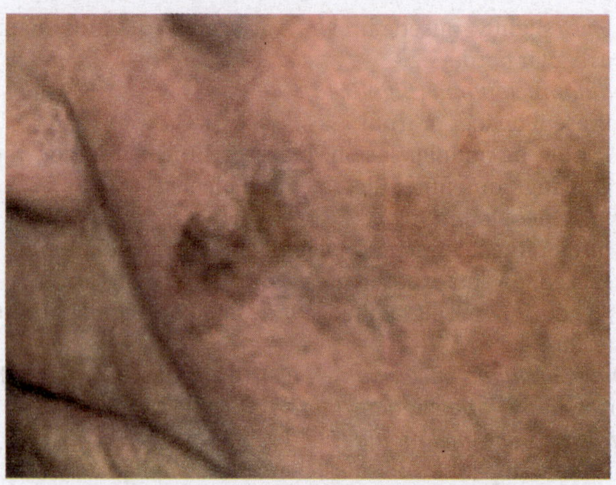

FIG. 10.49 Lentigo maligna melanoma

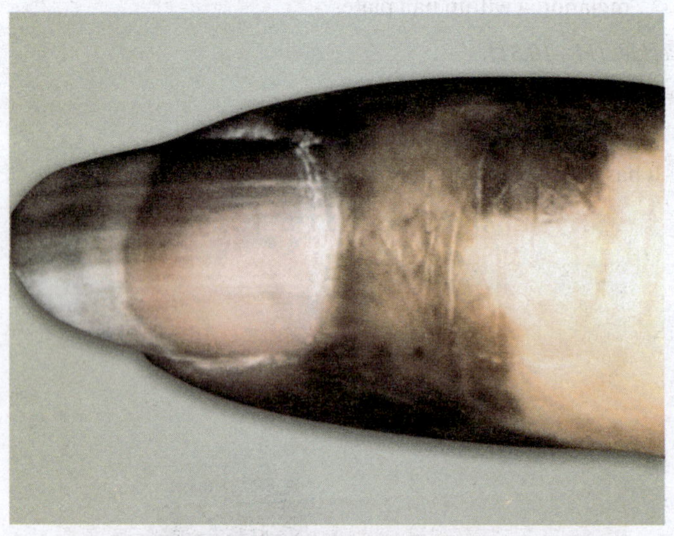

FIG. 10.50 Acrolentiginous melanoma

Cutaneous xanthoma
Causes
- Primary idiopathic
- *Secondary:*
  - ❖ *Hypercholesterolemia:*
    - Pregnancy
    - Hypothyroidism
    - Cholestasis.

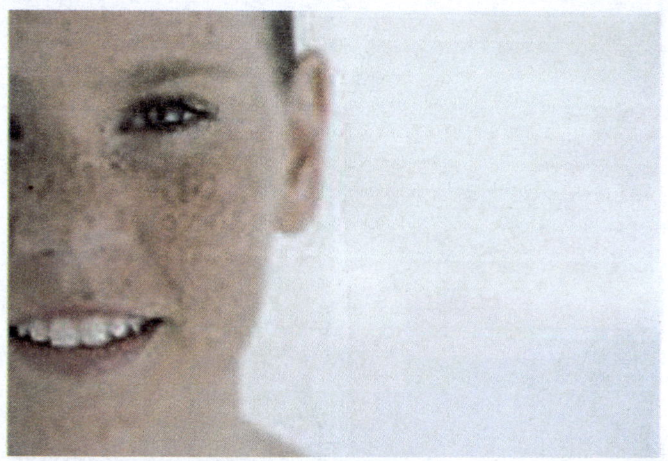

FIG. 10.51 Freckle

- ❖ *Hypertriglyceridemia:*
  - Diabetes
  - Alcoholism
  - Pancreatitis
  - Gout
  - Oral contraceptives.

Types of xanthoma
- *Tuberous xanthoma (Figs 10.52A and B):* Firm yellowish painless nodules present on pressure areas of body, e.g. buttock, extensor surface of knees and elbows, eyelids. It indicates hypercholesterolemia, increased LDL.
- *Tendinous xanthoma (Fig. 10.53):* These are subcutaneous nodules present over tendons (Achilles), extensor surface of feet and hands.

  It indicates hypercholesterolemia, high LDL.
- *Eruptive xanthoma (Fig. 10.54):* These are red-yellow papules on erythematous bases seen on buttock, shoulders, and extensor surfaces of extremities.

  It is associated with hypertriglyceridemia—type I, IV and V, high level of VLDL, chylomicrons.
- *Plane xanthoma (Fig. 10.55):* Macular yellowish lesions seen in face, neck, thorax and flexural areas.

Psoriasis
- *Psoriasis vulgaris (Fig. 10.56):* Sharply demarcated erythematous papules circular or oval in shapes present on extensor aspects of the body.

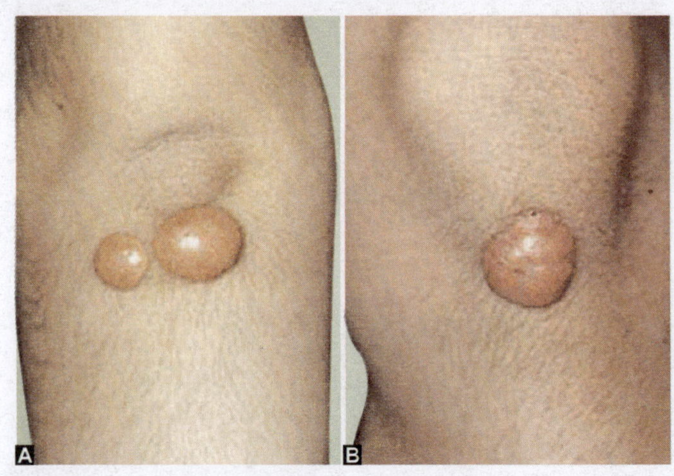

FIGS 10.52A AND B Tuberous xanthoma

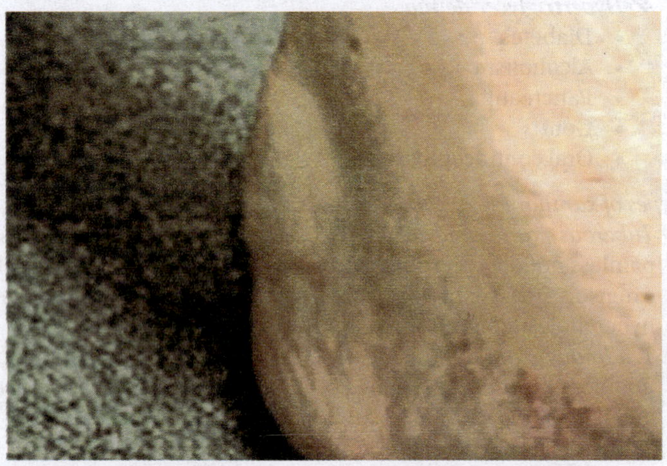

FIG. 10.53 Tendinous xanthoma

The lesion is usually covered by silver white scale.

On removal of scale, there is usually an area of bleeding spots (Auspitz sign).

Areas of predilection:

- ❖ Scalp
- ❖ Knees
- ❖ Elbows
- ❖ Genitalia
- ❖ Extensor surface of extremities
- ❖ Lumbosacral region.

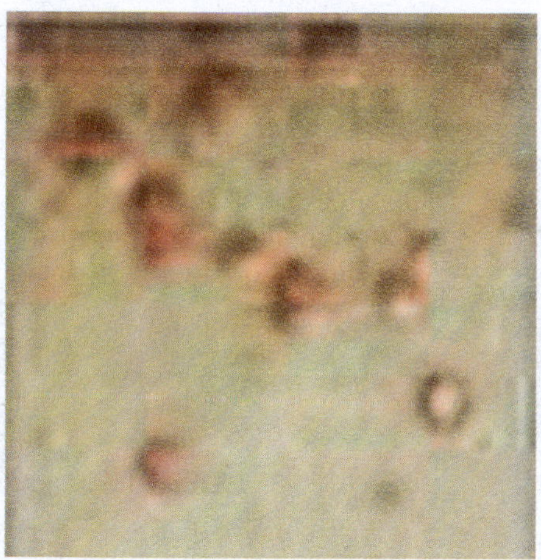

FIG. 10.54   Eruptive xanthoma

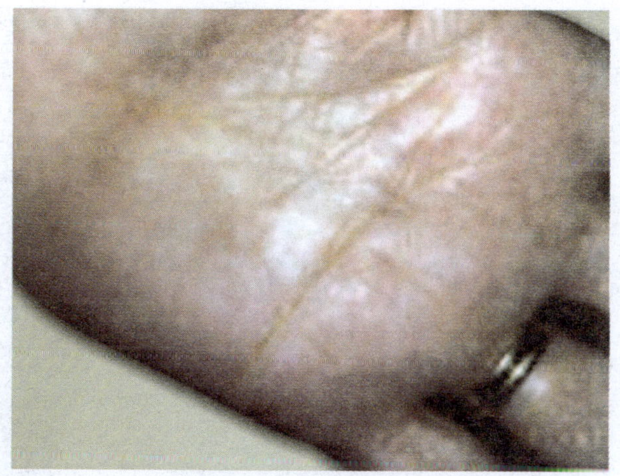

FIG. 10.55   Plane xanthoma

Presence of Koebner's phenomenon: After 7–14 days of direct trauma, the lesion appears.
- *Intertriginous psoriasis (Fig. 10.57):* Areas involved:
  - ❖ Axilla
  - ❖ Inguinal region
  - ❖ Perianal region
  - ❖ Inframammary region.
- *Guttate psoriasis (Fig. 10.58):* Sudden appearance of crops of nonconfluent papules—widely distributed, not very scaly.

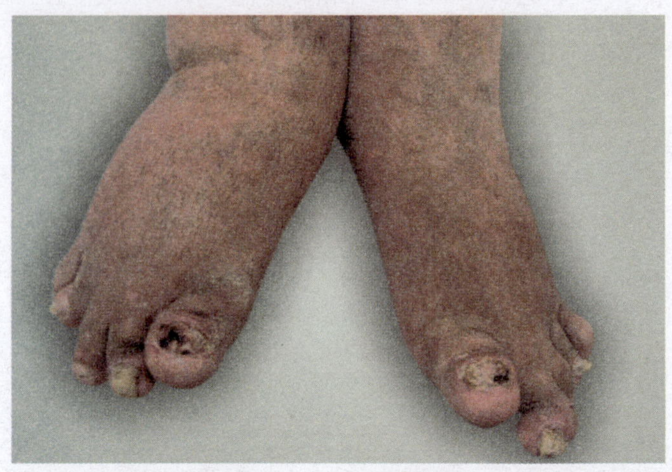

FIG. 10.56 Psoriasis vulgaris

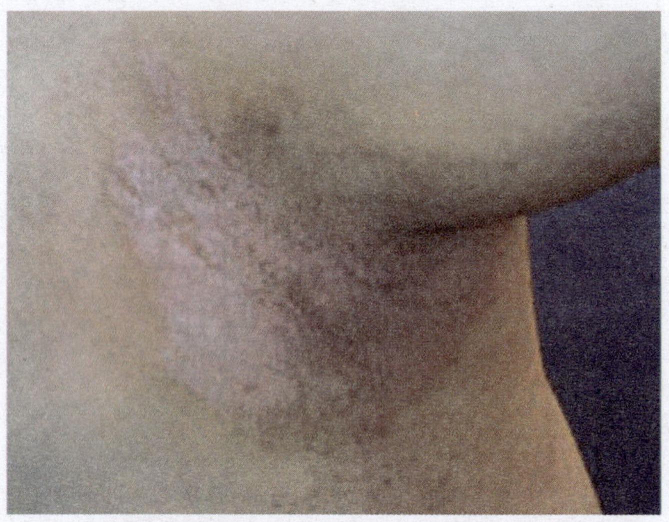

FIG. 10.57 Intertriginous psoriasis

This lesion can be triggered by *Streptococcus* infection, viral respiratory infection.

This lesion can be exacerbated by respiratory infection by streptococci and staphylococci.

Erythroderma (Fig. 10.59): It includes—total body erythema with scaling.

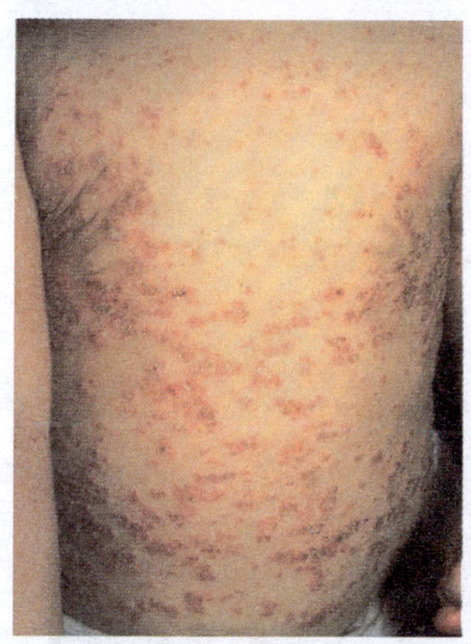

FIG. 10.58   Guttate psoriasis

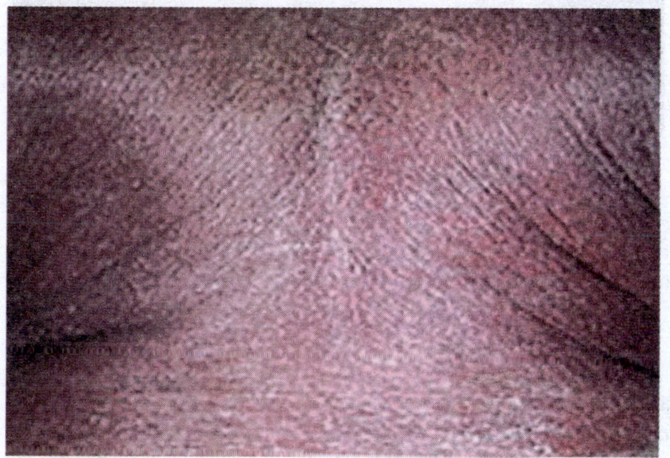

FIG. 10.59   Erythrodermic psoriasis

Pustular psoriasis: There are two types of pustular psoriasis (Fig. 10.60):

1. *Zumbusch type:*
   - ❖ Systemic symptoms—fever, anemia, leukocytosis
   - ❖ Psoriasis with surrounding erythema.
2. *Barber type:*
   - ❖ No systemic involvement
   - ❖ Localized psoriasis involving palms and soles.

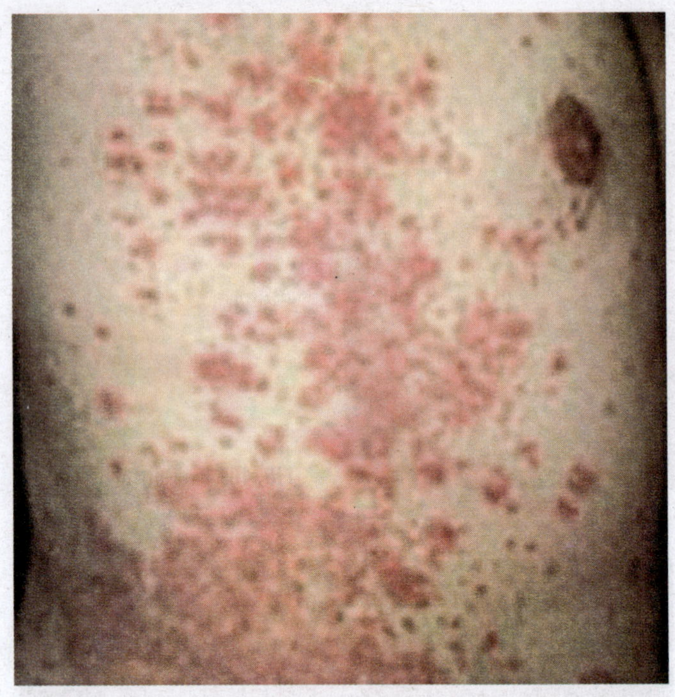

FIG. 10.60 Pustular psoriasis

Dermatophytosis

Hallmark is invasions of dead keratin:

- Skin
- Hair
- Nail.

Causative organism—ring worm.

Hallmark of lesion

- Pruritic erythematous scaly plaques, having active border, and central clearing
- Papules
- Vesicles
- Bullae.

Age of frequency

- Tinea corporis—in any age group
- Tinea capitis—disease of children
- Tinea cruris—in adult population
- Tinea pedis—in adult population.

Tinea cruris and pedis are common in people using common pools.

Tinea capitis (Fig. 10.61): Infection of scalp hair.
- Scaly erythematous patches, broken hair
- *Kerion celsi:* Tender abscess with purulent discharge followed by development of scarring alopecia
- *Favus:* Severe form, yellow cup shaped crust around infected hair follicles.

Tinea corporis (Fig. 10.62)
Body:
- Circular lesion, erythematous raised borders, central clearing evolving into annular scaly plaques
- Papules, vesicles.

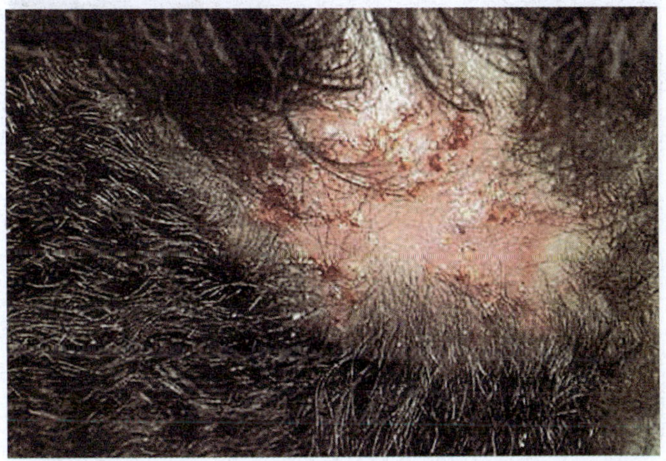

FIG. 10.61 Tinea capitis

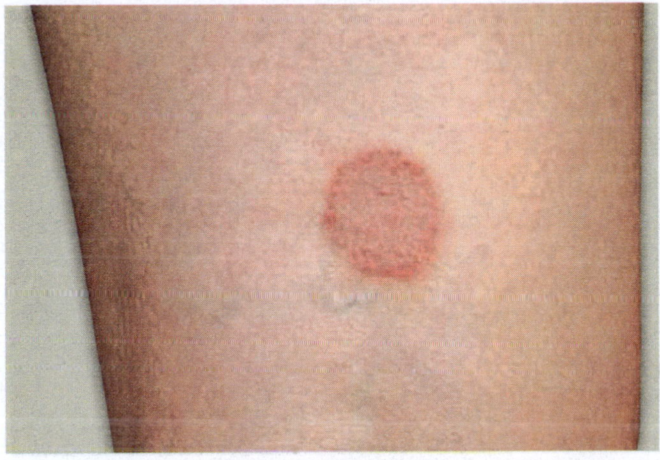

FIG. 10.62 Tinea corporis

Tinea faciale (Fig. 10.63)
Face: Red scaly plaques, having raised erythematous border and no central clearing.
Tinea barbae (Fig. 10.64)
Beard: Erythematous papules, pustules, scaling—in beard area and neck.
Tinea cruris (Fig. 10.65)
Groin:

- Erythematous plaque with central clearing and erythematous raised border
- Site—inguinal folds and adjacent skin, not scrotum.

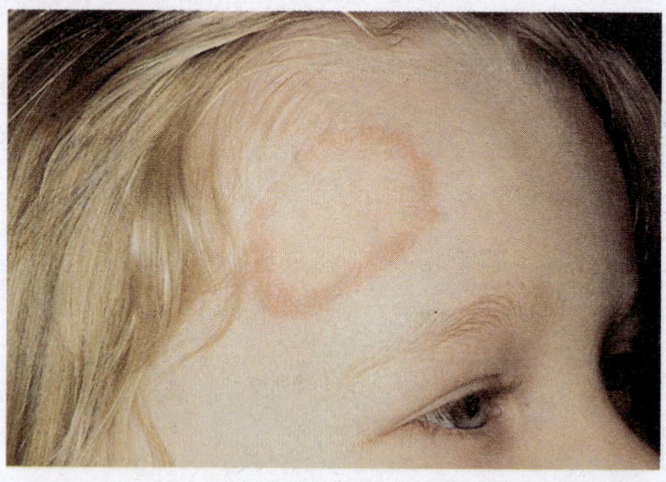

FIG. 10.63   Tinea faciale

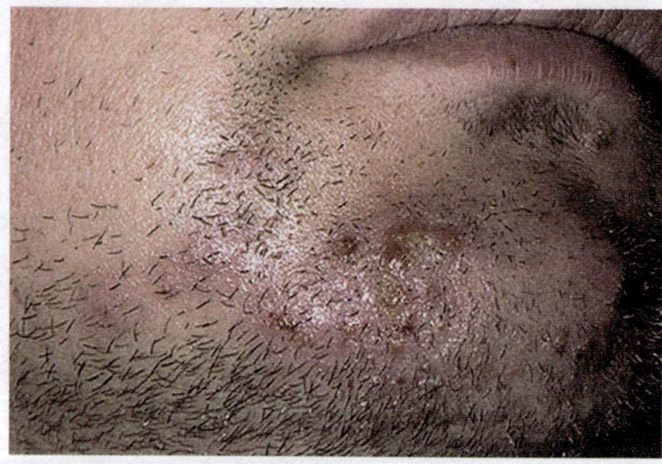

FIG. 10.64   Tinea barbae

Tinea manus (Fig. 10.66)
Hand:

- Annular plaques on dorsum of hand with hyperkeratosis of palms
- Scaling and erythema
- Palms, finger webs—in association with tinea pedis.

Tinea pedis (Fig. 10.67)

- Erythematous scaly plaques, fissuring and maceration (Athlete's foot)
- Third and fourth interdigital webs are usually involved.

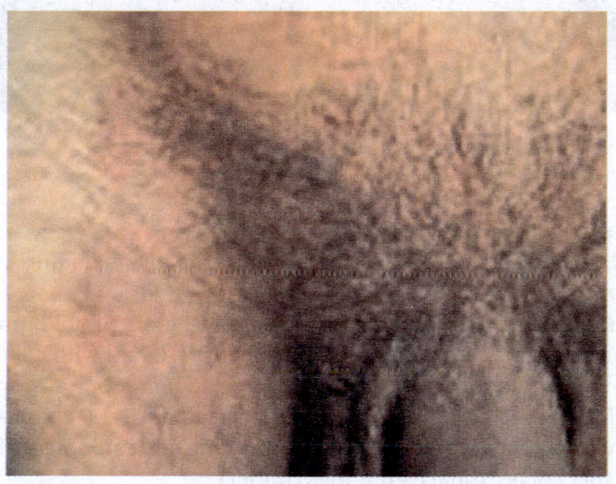

FIG. 10.65   Tinea cruris

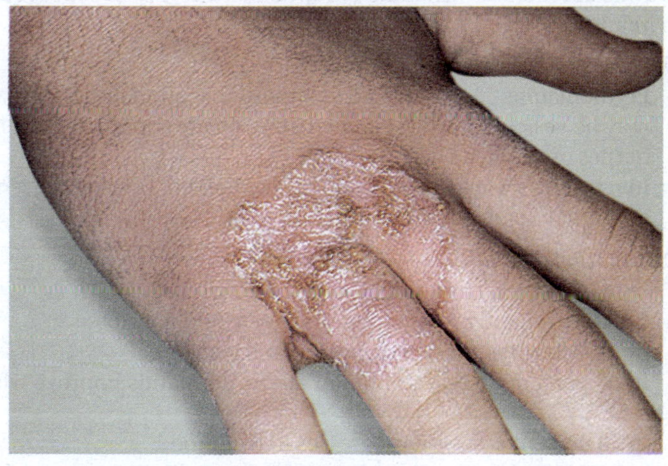

FIG. 10.66   Tinea manus

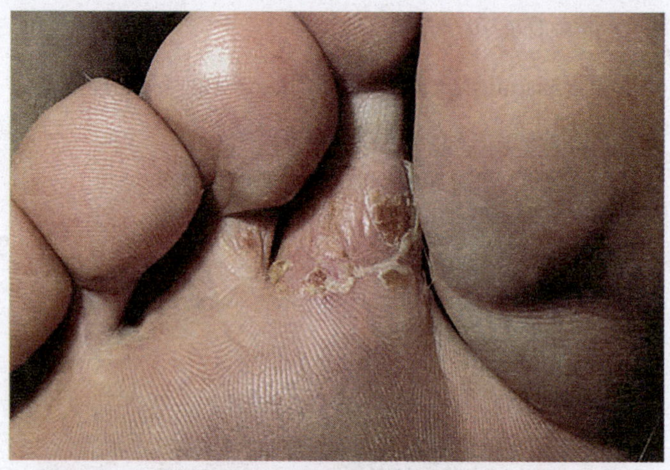

FIG. 10.67 Tinea pedis

Tinea unguium (Fig. 10.68)
Nail: Yellowish brown macule with subungual hyperkeratosis.
Pityriasis rosea (Fig. 10.69)
- *Herald patch:* Round or oval macules, salmon colored, present on the trunk. It enlarges into large patch (10 cm) with collarette of scale (pityron) having well demarcated border.
- Herald patch is followed by 50–100 isolated 0.5–1.0 cm bilateral symmetrical less scaly macules present on trunk, neck, inner aspect of proximal extremities (upper).

Atopic dermatitis (Fig. 10.70)
Pruritic eczematous lichenified eruption and xerosis of skin occurs in infancy.

The sessions are:
- Erythematous papules and plaques, occasionally follicular, may be vesicles, pustules and crusting due to super infection by herpes or staphylococci
- In chronic case—lesion may be lichenified (thickening and accentuation of skin creases).

Distribution of lesion
- In infant—face, mainly cheeks, extensor surfaces.
- Children—hands, feet, anticubital fossa, popliteal fossa
- Adult—flexures, face, neck, hands and feet.
  In 50 percent cases—childhood atopic dermatitis improve with age.
  In 50 percent cases—it progresses to adulthood.

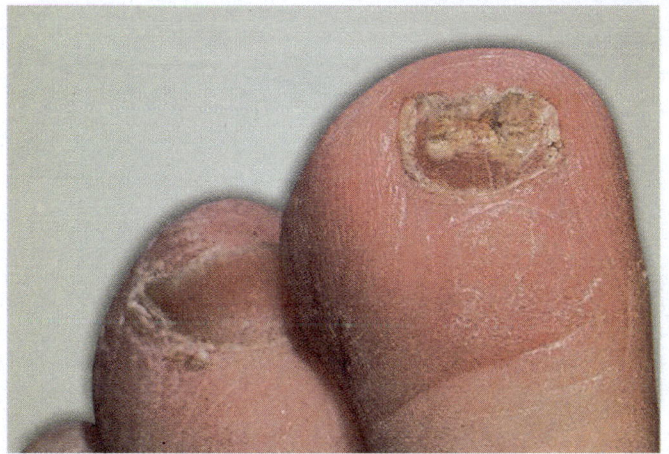

FIG. 10.68 Tinea unguium

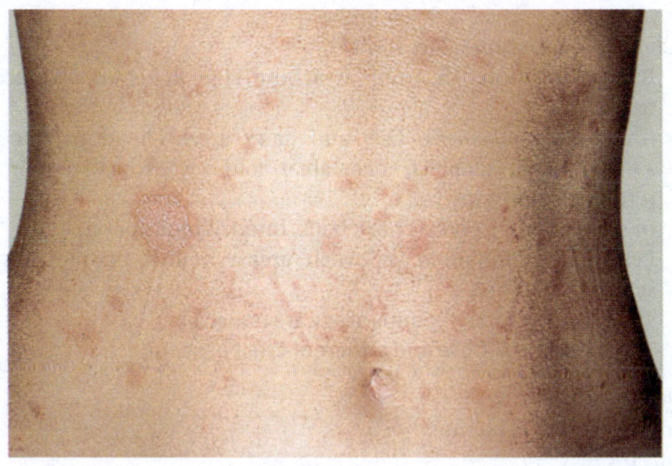

FIG. 10.69 Pityriasis rosea torso

The risk factor
- Family history
- Severe cutaneous lesion
- Early disease of childhood.

Associated skin disease are:
- Secondary infection by *Staphylococcus aureus*.
- Warts.
- *Molluscum contagiosum*.
- Dermatophytosis.
- Herpes simplex.

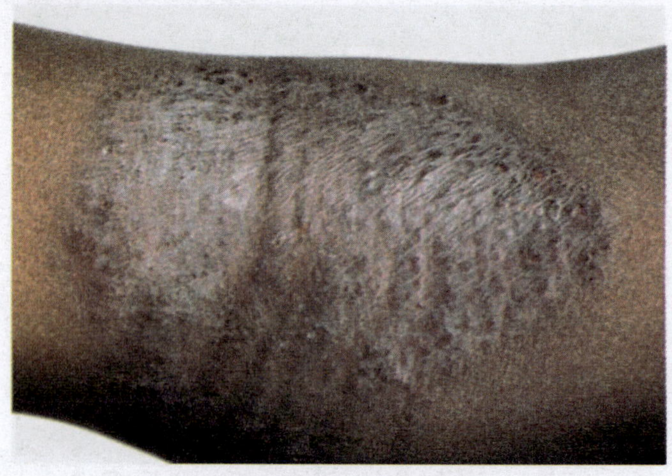

FIG. 10.70 Atopic dermatitis

Seborrheic dermatitis (Fig. 10.71)
- Papulosquamous disorder in sebum rich areas—scalp, face, trunk
- *Areas of involvement:* Oily and hairy areas—head and neck → Forehead, glabella, nasolabial fold, eyebrow, lash line, retroauricular skin
  In serves cases: Central chest, back, intertriginous areas.
- *Lesion:* Erythematous yellowish greasy yellow papules with scaling and crusts
  The lesion in intertriginous areas are nonscaly
  There may be diffuse and adherent crust in scalp.

Lichen planus (Fig. 10.72)
Primary lesion is papule:

Five Ps:
1. Pruritus
2. Planar
3. Purple
4. Polygonal
5. Papular.

Description of lesion: Shiny 1–4 mm, violaceous flat-topped pruritic papules, occasionally with scaling, may be verrucoid.
Site of involvement:
- Trunk (including sacral areas).
- Extremities (tibial areas, flexor surfaces of wrist).
- Orally—Wickham striae (Fig. 10.73)—reticular pattern of white streaks on violaceous background.

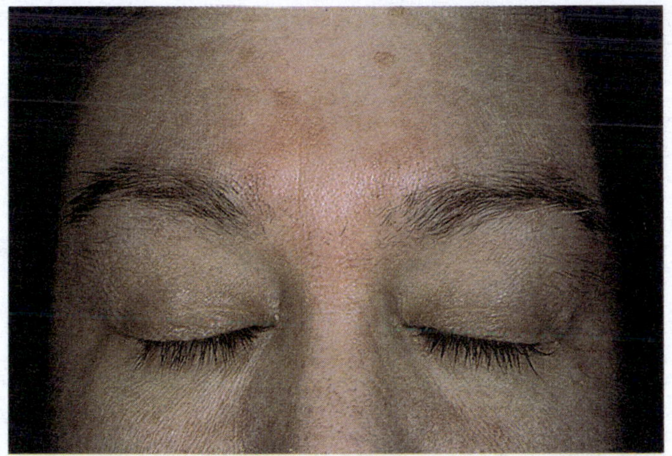

FIG. 10.71 Seborrheic dermatitis

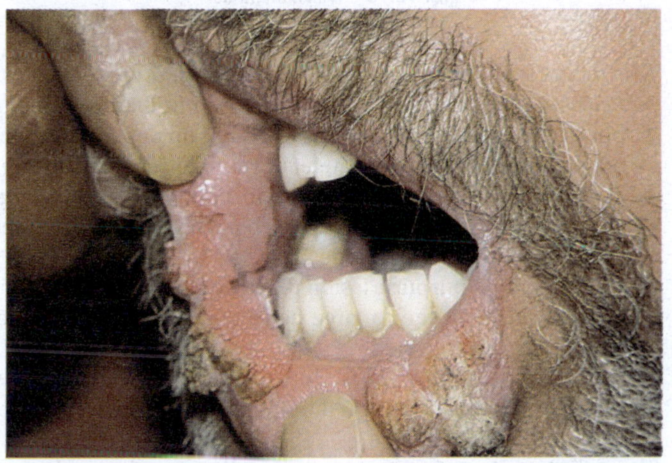

FIG. 10.72 Lichen planus

- Glans—papules—annular configuration.
- Vulval involvement—reticulates papules to severe erosions—producing dyspareunia, vulval stenosis.

Purpura: There are two types of purpura:

1. *Noninflammatory purpura:* Extravasation blood into skin and mucous membrane. It may be due to:
   ❖ Thrombocytopenia
   ❖ Thrombocythemia
   ❖ Vascular disorder.

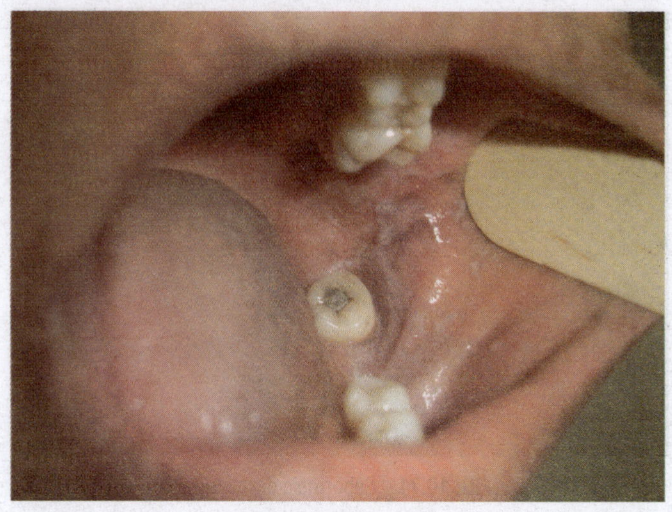

FIG. 10.73 Wickham striae

Extravasations of blood can be divided into 4 subtypes:
* *Petechiae (Fig. 10.74):* Superficial <3 mm in diameter, red or purple, nonblanching macules—present on dependent areas of body may be due to—platelet or vascular related disorder
* *Ecchymoses (Fig. 10.75):* >3 mm in diameter, due to large amount of extravasations, purple color to start with followed by yellow and ultimately fades out
* *Vibices:* Linear purpuric lesion due to scratching
* *Hematoma:* It is due to large collection of blood in deeper tissue.

2. *Inflammatory purpura:* It is due to small vessel vasculitis. Producing extravasations of red blood cells, leukocytes—hence it is indurated and palpable.

These lesions is 1–3 mm in size, coalesce to form plaques, palpable; mainly occur in legs.

If it is due to large vessel vasculitis, it usually ulcerates.

Causes of cutaneous vasculitis
* *In children:*
  * Henoch-Schönlein purpura
  * Leukoclastic vasculitis.
* *In adult:*
  * Immune mediated
  * *Drugs:*
    * Beta lactum
    * Nonsteroidal anti-inflammatory drug (NSAID)
    * Diuretics.

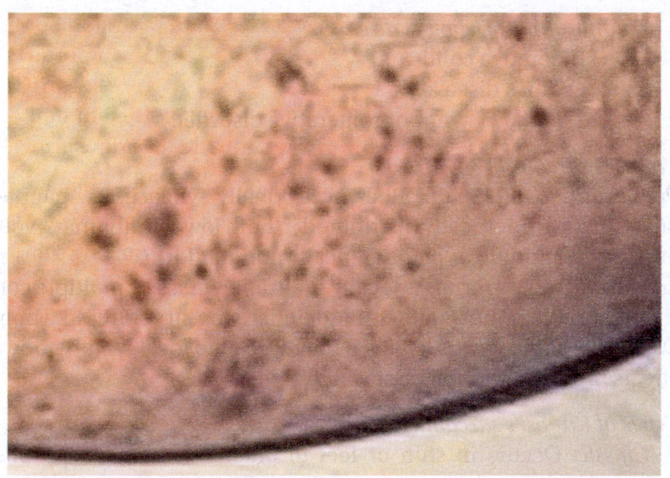

FIG. 10.74 Petechiae

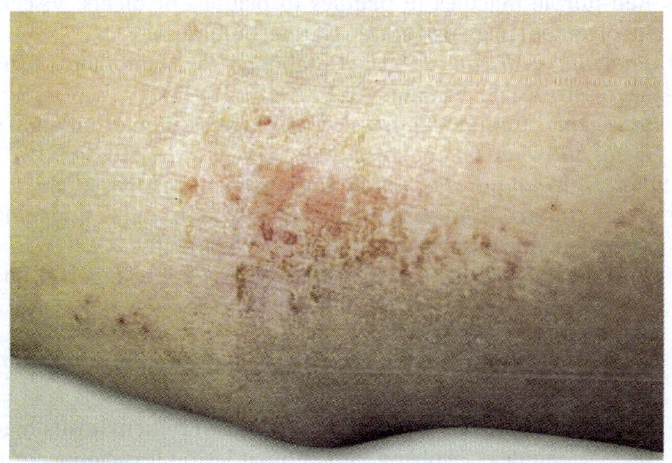

FIG. 10.75 Ecchymoses

- ❖ *Infection:*
  - Respiratory tract infection by Streptococci
  - Viral hepatitis (Hepatitis C virus)
  - HIV
  - Endocarditis.
- ❖ *Collagen vascular disease:*
  - SLE
  - Rheumatoid arthritis
  - Sjögren syndrome
  - Rarely polyarteritis nodosa, Wegener's granulomatosis.

- ❖ *Inflammatory bowel disease:*
  - Ulcerative colitis
  - Crohn's disease.
- ❖ *Malignancy:* Lymphoproliferative disorder.

Kaposi's sarcoma (Fig. 10.76)
Presentation of lesion: Red occasionally violaceous papules, bilaterally symmetrically distributed in both lower limbs may evolve into spongy nodule or plaques locally nodular form.
Locally aggressive form: As locally infiltrating mass or multiple cone shaped friable tumor—adherent to underlying structures like bone.
Distal spreading form: Distally it may spread to local lymph node or affects multiple internal organs.

Types of Kaposi's sarcoma
- *Classic:* Occurs in shin or feet of older men. Lesion purplish papules progresses to plaques. Rarely fatal
- *Epidemic (AIDS associated):* More wide spread than classic form. Red-purple-macules to papules to plaques or ulcers. Visceral involvement in glans, mouth, GI tract or lung
- *Endemic (African form):* Cutaneous or lymphatic form, aggressive, Male: Female—15:1
- *Iatrogenic:* Immunosuppression may regress after termination of drugs and often GI tract bleeding.

Lupus erythematosus (Fig. 10.77): The cutaneous manifestations:
- *Acute cutaneous lupus erythematosus:* Butterfly maculopapular rash involving nasal bridge and cheeks bilaterally.

  It may be pruritic and distributed over forehead, peri-orbital areas, chin, ears and neck. Theses may be associated with sun exposure.

  It can be protracted or resolves spontaneously with post-inflammatory hyperpigmentation.
- *Subacute cutaneous lupus erythomatosus:* Erythematosus macules or papules—evolving into annular lesion (erythema annulare) or papulosquamous scaly lesion.
  - ❖ If may be asymptomatic or mildly pruritic
  - ❖ Wax and wane with scaling and atrophy, may be hypo-pigmented.
- *Discoid lupus erythematosus (Fig. 10.78):* Sharply demarcated erythematosus macules or papules, asymptomatic or pruritic or painful, arise over sun exposed areas in cheeks, nose, ears, face and scalp, evolve into chest, back and arms.

  The lesions may evolve into adherent scales with areas of hyperpigmentation or hypopigmentation.

  There are also areas of telangiectasias.

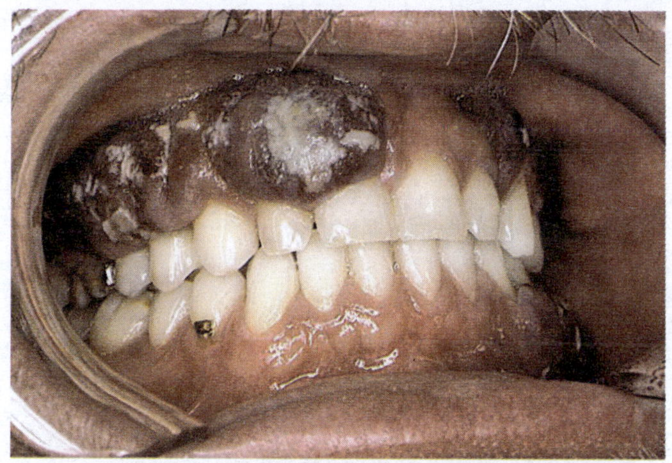

FIG. 10.76 Kaposi's sarcoma

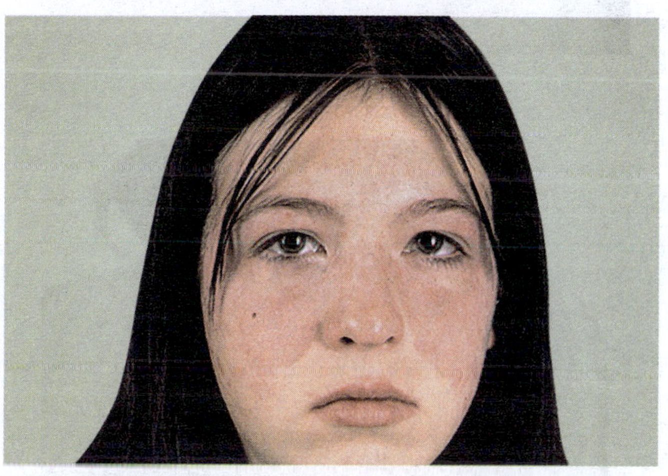

FIG. 10.77 Acute systemic lupus erythematosus

Lesion of scalp first appears as pink lesion, evolve into white depressed scar and alopecia.

- *Lupus profundus (Fig. 10.79):* Lupus involvement of adipose tissue. Multiple subcutaneous nodules with overlying discoid lesion of face, breast, buttocks, trunks or proximal arms and legs. The nodules ulcerate subcutaneous atrophy.

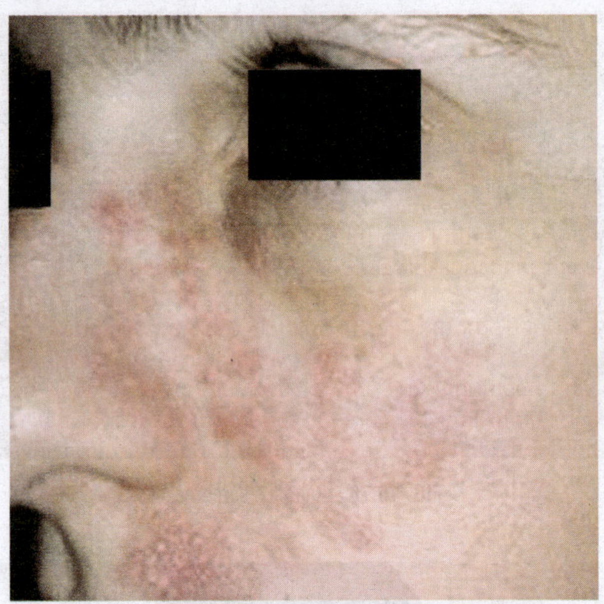

FIG. 10.78 Discoid rash

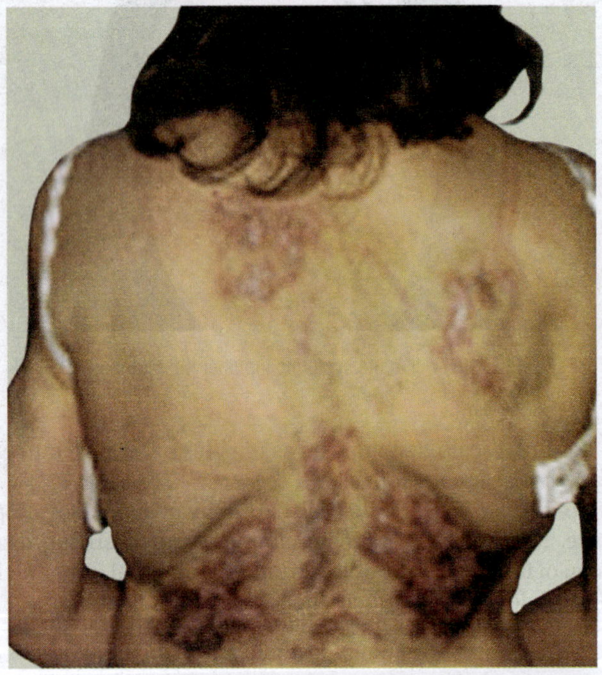

FIG. 10.79 Lupus profundus

The following drugs are responsible for development of lupus:
- Hydralazine
- Procainamide
- Methyldopa
- Sulfonamides
- Phenytoin
- Penicillamine.

Necrobiosis lipoidica (Fig. 10.80)

1–3 mm papular or nodular circumscribed slowly enlarging shiny lesions appear on pretibial areas, in few cases these may appear on trunk, scalp, face, and upper extremities.

Lesions eventually form red to brown atrophic round patches may progress into depressed atrophic, yellowish plaques scaly, violaceous border producing underlying vasculature more visible.

These plaques may ulcerate and infected. There may be surrounding telangiectasias.

The disease responsible—diabetes mellitus, microangiopathy.

Porphyria cutanea tarda (Fig. 10.81)
- Most common cutaneous manifestation of porphyria due to increased excretion of uroporphyrin in urine
- It is associated:
  - HIV infection
  - Liver dysfunction—hepatitis, alcoholism, iron overload. Hemochromatosis, liver malignancy—hepatocellular carcinoma

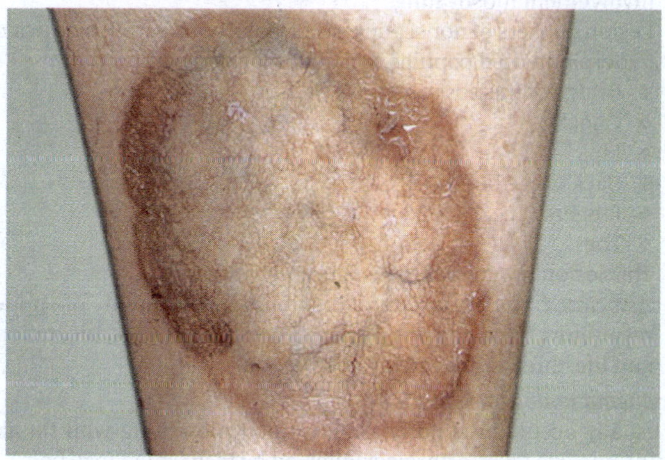

FIG. 10.80 Necrobiosis lipoidica diabeticorum

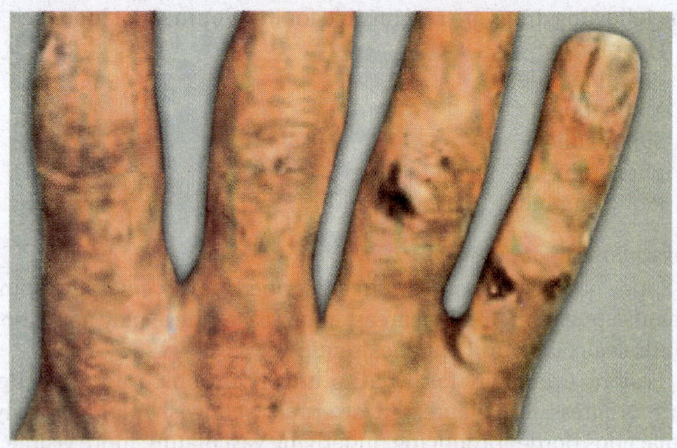

FIG. 10.81 Porphyria cutanea tarda

- Lesion full thickness epidermal erosion and blistering followed by crusting and secondary infection, evolving into hyperpigmentation and scarring.

Sarcoidosis

There are two types of lesion (Fig. 10.82).

Specific lesion

Lupus pernio (Fig. 10.83)

- It occurs in African-American women with chronic systemic involvement mostly lung.
- Lesion clusters of nonscaling small violaceous, reddish brown or hyperpigmented papules or plaques located over:
  - Bridge of the nose
  - Cheeks
  - Lips
  - Back of the hands
  - Fingers
  - Toes.

  This lesion progresses to disfigurement of face.
- *Associated features:* Granulomatous involvement of upper respiratory tract, and nasal mucosa resulting masses, ulcerations and life-threatening airway obstruction.

Erythema nodosum (Fig. 10.84)

It usually occurs in child bearing women presenting with flu like syndrome like fever, arthralgia followed by rash which may be:

- Tender, nonscaling erythematous nodule or papule present on pretibial region in 1st week it is bright red, hard, tense, painful

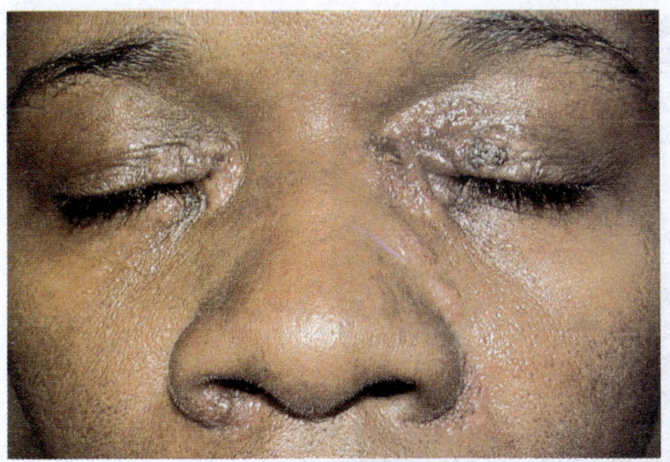

FIG. 10.82 Sarcoidosis

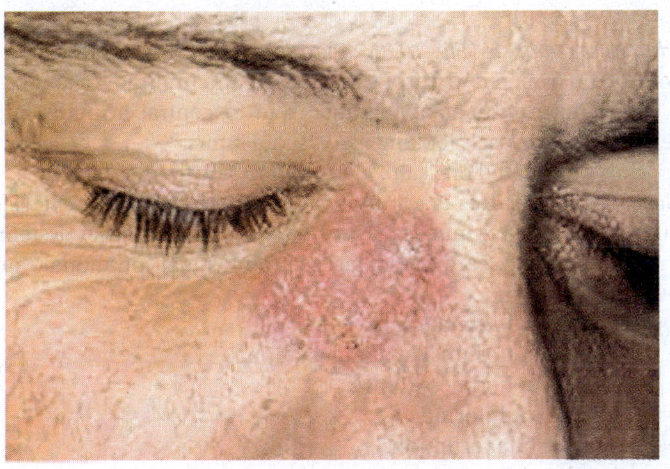

FIG. 10.83 Lupus pernio

- In 2nd week it becomes bluish to livid and occasionally fluctuant
- Eventually it fades to a yellowish hue often leaving with hyperpigmentation and desquamation of overlying skin.

Lofgren's syndrome
Characteristic and febrile form of acute sarcoid include:
- Erythema nodusum.
- Anterior uveitis
- Hilar adenopathy
- Polyarthritis.

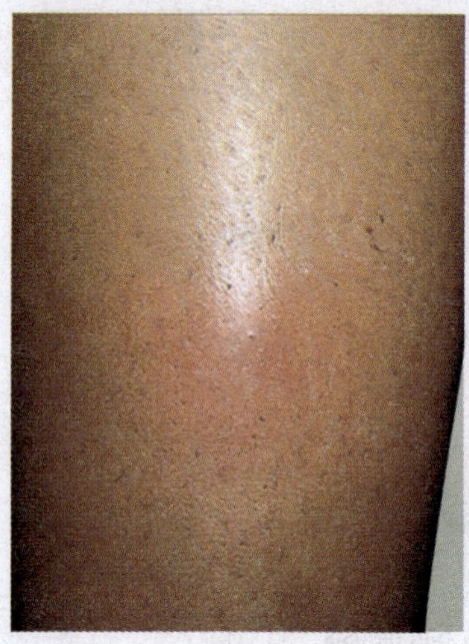

FIG. 10.84   Erythema nodosum

Plaque sarcoidosis (Fig. 10.85): Plaque results from coalescence of round and oval, red to purple, flat topped and infiltrated papules.

They have annular appearance due to central atrophy, large telangiectatic vessels looking like discoid lupus.

They are located on scalp, back, button, extremities, and face.

Behçet's disease: This is a multisystem disease involving eye (Figs 10.86A to D), skin, mucosa (Fig. 10.87), joints and other systemic involvement, e.g. cardiovascular, gastrointestinal, pulmonary and neurological.

Dermatological manifestation

- Erythema nodosum like manifestation.
- Actinic form nodules
- Erythema multiforme
- Papulopustular eruption.

Associated manifestations may be:

- Posterior uveitis (eye)
- Aphthous ulcerations in scrotum, penis and groin (male), and vulva, vagina, groin (female)
- Arthritis.
- GI involvement
- Neurological involvement
- Glomerular involvement
- Myocarditis.

Dermatomyositis

- Skin involvement occurs in half of patient dermatomyositis.

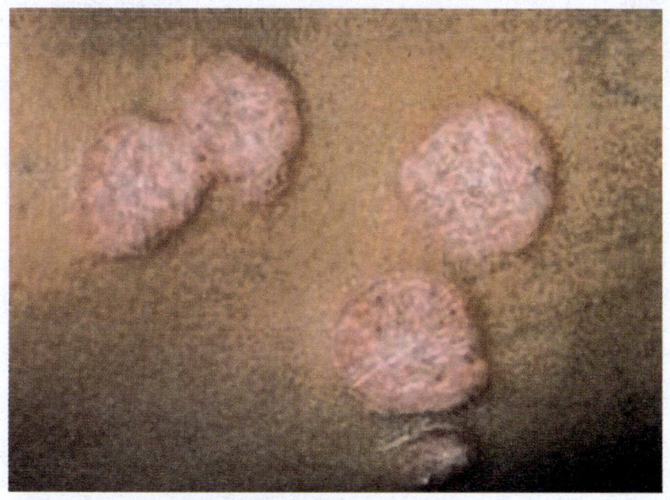

FIG. 10.85 Plaque sarcoidosis

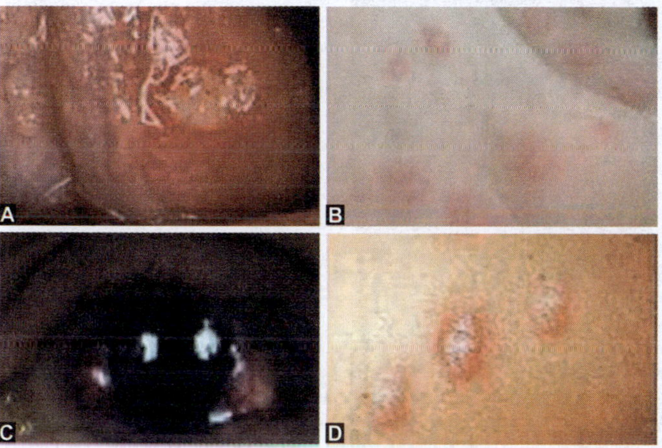

FIGS 10.86A TO D Eye in Behçet's disease

- Two characteristic and pathognomonic of this disease are:
  1. *Heliotrope rash (Fig. 10.88):* Violaceous to dusky, erythematous rash in periorbital area with or without edema and mild discoloration of eyelid margin
  2. *Gottron's papules (Figs 10.89A and B):* Slightly elevated violet-to-red papules and plaques found in bony prominences, distal surfaces of knuckles metacarpophalangeal, proximal and distal interphalangeal, knee, elbow joints, feet. Sometime they are scaly and thickened.

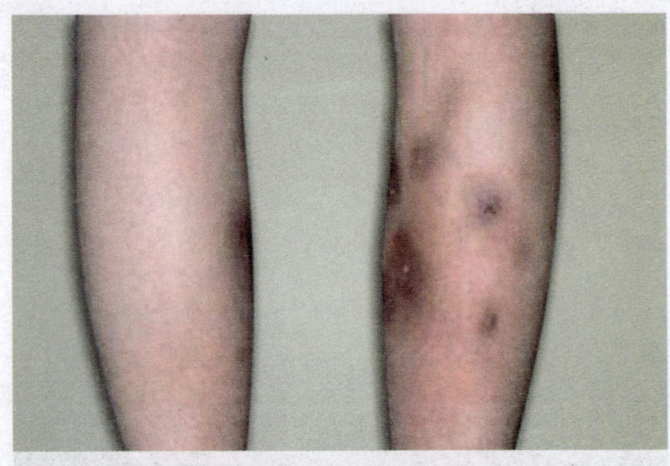

FIG. 10.87 Skin in Behçet's disease

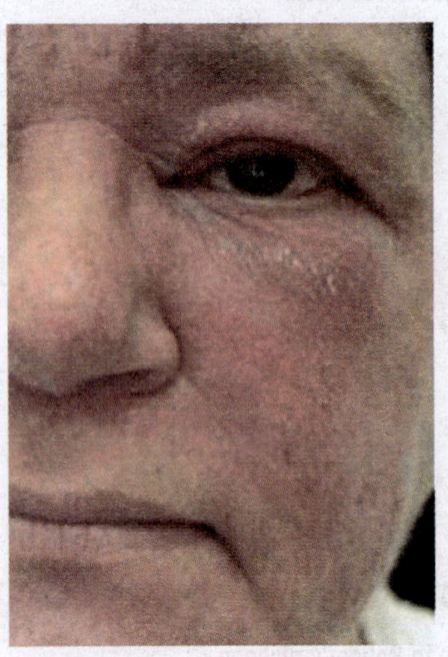

FIG. 10.88 Heliotrope rash

Poikiloderma (Fig. 10.90): Hypo or hyperpigmented, erythematous telangiectatic atrophic lesion present on:

Cheek, lateral sides of neck of middle aged women other sun exposed areas, extensor surfaces of arms, upper part of back (Shawl sign).

Scleroderma
- *Two major cutaneous manifestations of scleroderma:*
  1. *Sclerodactyly:* Thickening, tightening, and induration of fingers (Fig. 10.91).

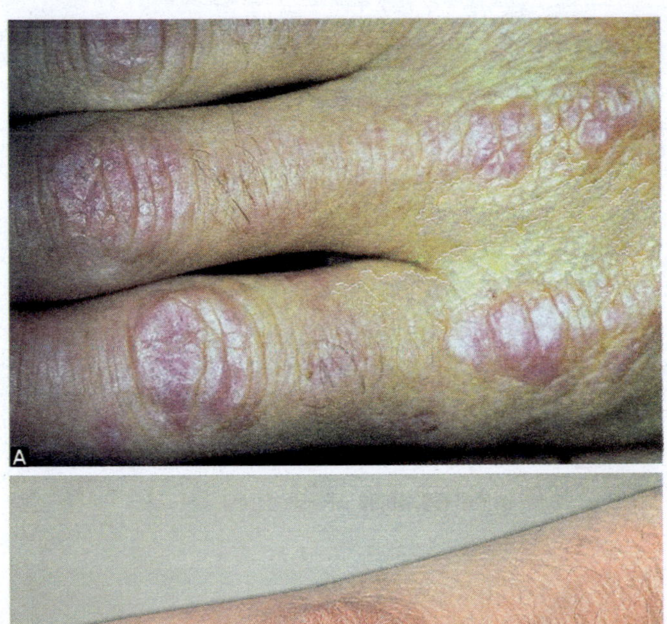

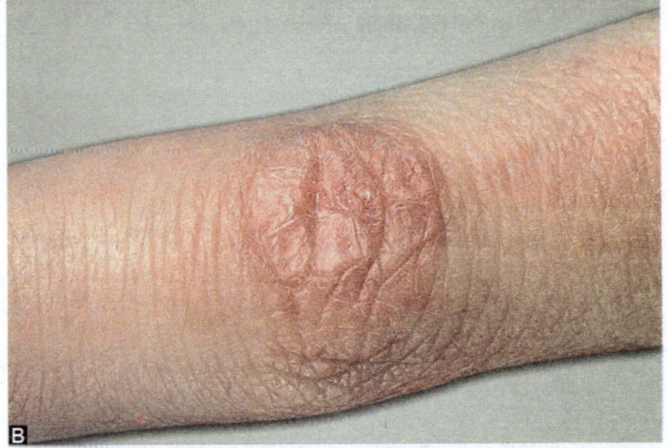

FIGS 10.89A AND B   Gottron papules

Proximal scleroderma: Induration of skin proximal to metacarpophalangeal and metatarsophalangeal joints, face, neck, thorax, and abdomen (Fig. 10.92).

- *Minor cutaneous manifestations of scleroderma:*
  - ❖ Due to ischemia, fingertips are pitted, tapered and loss of digital pad.
  - ❖ *Raynaud's phenomenon:* Seventy percent patients develop in early phase, 95 percent patients develop during the course of disease.

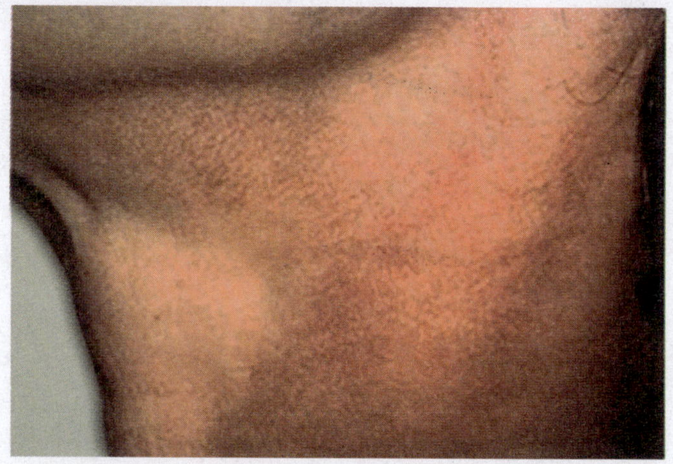

FIG. 10.90 Poikiloderma

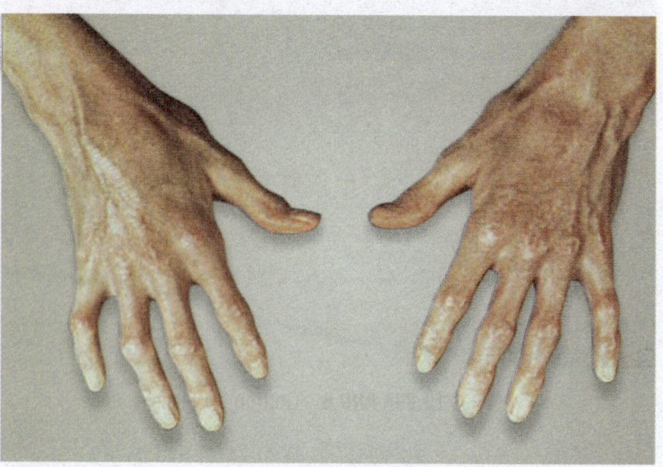

FIG. 10.91 Sclerodactyly

❖ *Pigmentary changes:*
  • There may be salt and paper appearance
  • Alternate areas of hyperpigmentation and hypopig-
    mentation
  • Overall hyper or hypopigmentation
❖ *Telangiectasias:* Dilatation of blood vessel under the dermis of
  face, periorbital areas an neck.
Limited cutaneous scleroderma: Thickening of skin distal to elbows
or knees, also involve face.

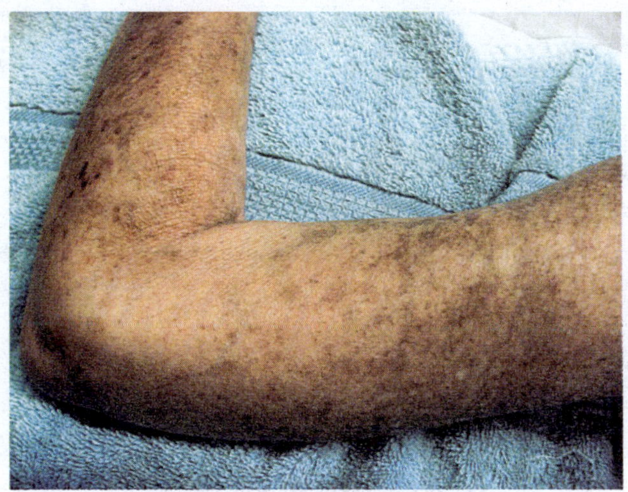

FIG. 10.92 Proximal scleroderma

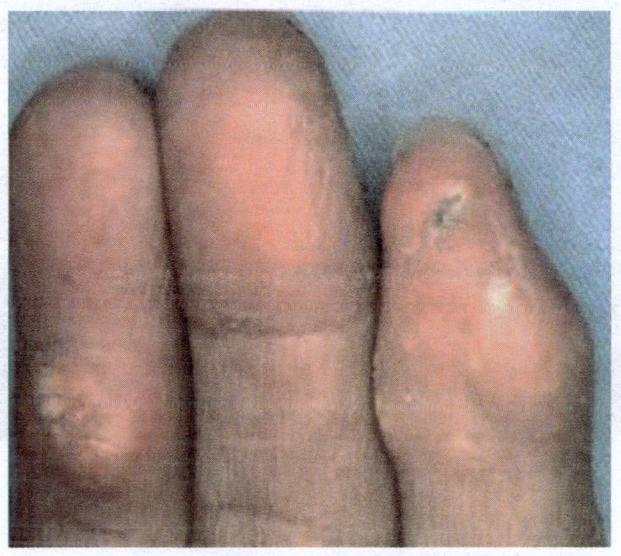

FIG. 10.93 Calcinosis

CREST syndrome is a term of cutaneous scleroderma:
C—Calcinosis (Fig. 10.93)
R—Raynaud's phenomenon
E—Esophageal dysphagia

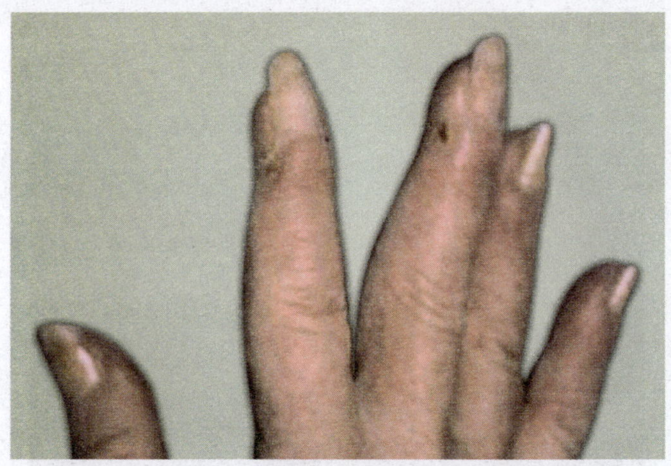

FIG. 10.94 Sclerodactyly (closer view)

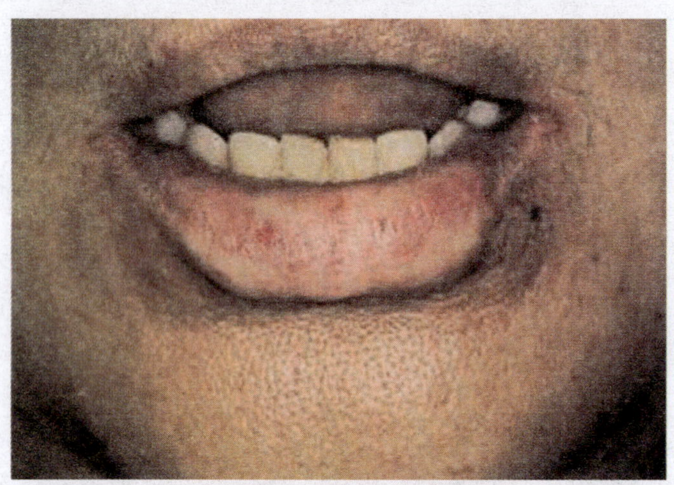

FIG. 10.95 Telangiectasia

S—Sclerodactyly (Fig. 10.94)

T—Telangiectasias (Fig. 10.95).

Diffuse cutaneous scleroderma: Thickening of skin of proximal extremities, trunk, and face.

Fish mouth appearance due to thickening and contracture of skin (Fig. 10.96).

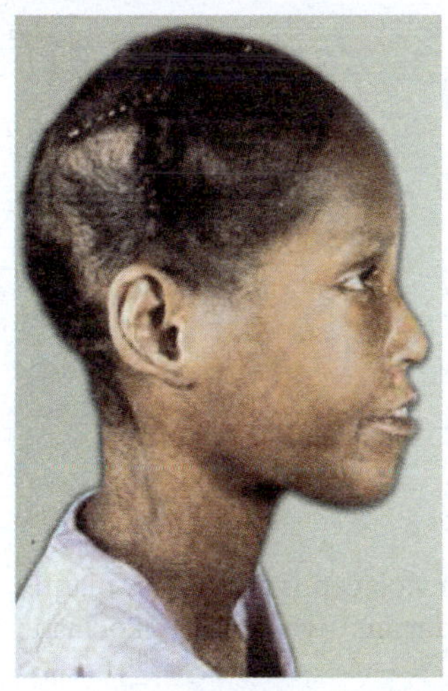

FIG. 10.96 Face in scleroderma

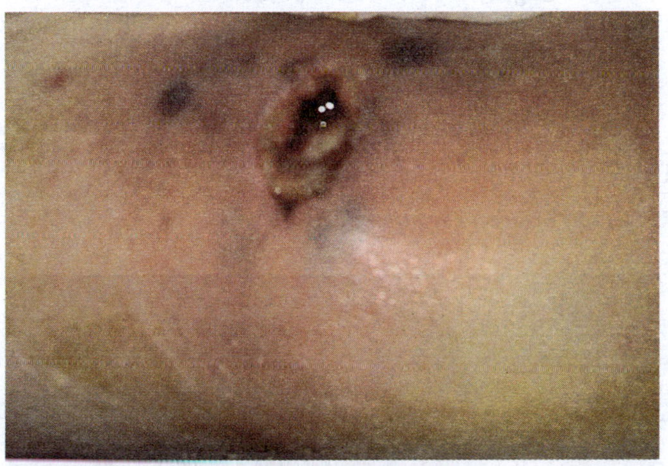

FIG. 10.97 Pyoderma gangrenosum

Pyoderma gangrenosum (Fig. 10.97): This starts as erythematous tender nodules or pustules, which undergo necrosis to form ulcers having raised margins, extending into dermis

The lesion may be solitary or multiple. If multiple, they coalesce into single ulcer—it is painful, dusky margin.

Site of lesion:
- Mainly in lower extremities.
- May appear on the trunk, abdomen.
- Rarely appear on head and neck.

Causes of lesion:
- Ulcerative colitis.
- Crohn's disease.
- Arthritis.
- Neoplastic disorders.
- Myelodysplastic syndrome:
    - ❖ Polycythemia
    - ❖ Myelofibrosis
    - ❖ Essential thrombocythemia.

Sweet's Syndrome

Criteria:
- *Major criteria:*
    - ❖ Abrupt onset of erythematous or violaceous nodules or plaque
    - ❖ Eosinophilic infiltration of dermis without leukoclastic vasculitis.
- *Minor criteria:*
    - ❖ Preceding history of fever or infection
    - ❖ Accompanying fever, arthralgia, and conjunctivitis or underlying malignancy.
    - ❖ Leukocytosis, increased ESR
    - ❖ Good response to corticosteroid, not to antibiotics.

Both major and any two minor criteria are necessary for diagnosis of Sweet's syndrome.

Skin lesions in Sweet's syndrome (Fig. 10.98)

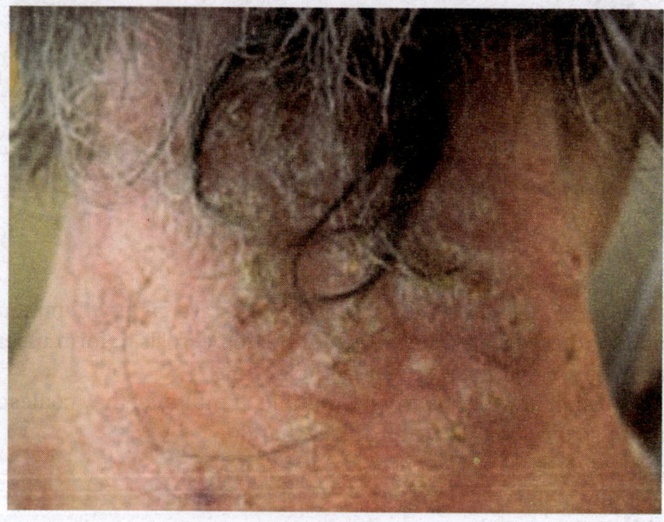

FIG. 10.98   Sweet's syndrome

Lesion: Erythematous, beefy-red or violaceous nodules or plaques often have purulent base with central clearing ultimately develop into ulceration.

Lesion may be papular, vesicular, pustular or bullous.

Associated systemic signs include—fever, leukocytosis, elevated erythrocyte sedimentation rate, arthralgia, myalgia, conjunctivitis.

There may be pulmonary, hepatic, or renal involvement.

Sites: Sudden eruption on face, neck and extremities.

Malignancies associated are—hematological malignancy in 90 percent of cases—most common is acute myelogenous leukemia, followed by lymphoma, multiple myeloma, Myelodysplastic syndrome.

Neurology

ANATOMY OF NERVOUS SYSTEM

▮ Diencephalon

It is a part of cerebrum. It includes:
- Thalamus
- Geniculate bodies
- Hypothalamus
- Subthalamus
- Epithalamus.

Third ventricle lies between the half of diencephalon.

Thalamic nuclei: Five groups of thalamic nuclei (Fig. 11.1):

1. *Anterior nuclei group:* It receives fibers from mammillary bodies via Mammillothalamic tract and projects to cingulate cortex of cerebrum.
2. *Nuclei of midline:* They connect with:
   - ❖ Hypothalamus
   - ❖ Periaqueductal gray matter.

   Centromedian nucleus connects with:
   - ❖ Cerebellum
   - ❖ Corpus striatum.
3. *Medial nuclei:* They include:
   - ❖ Intralaminar nuclei
   - ❖ *Dorsomedial nucleus:* It projects into cerebral cortex.
4. *Lateral nuclear mass*
   - ❖ Reticular nucleus
   - ❖ *Anteroventral nucleus:* It connects with corpus striatum
   - ❖ *Lateroventral nucleus:* It connects with cerebral cortex
   - ❖ *Posteroventral nuclei:* These are subdivided into:
     - Posterolateral nucleus
     - Posteromedial nucleus
   - ❖ *Dorsolateral nucleus:* It connects with parietal lobe of cortex.

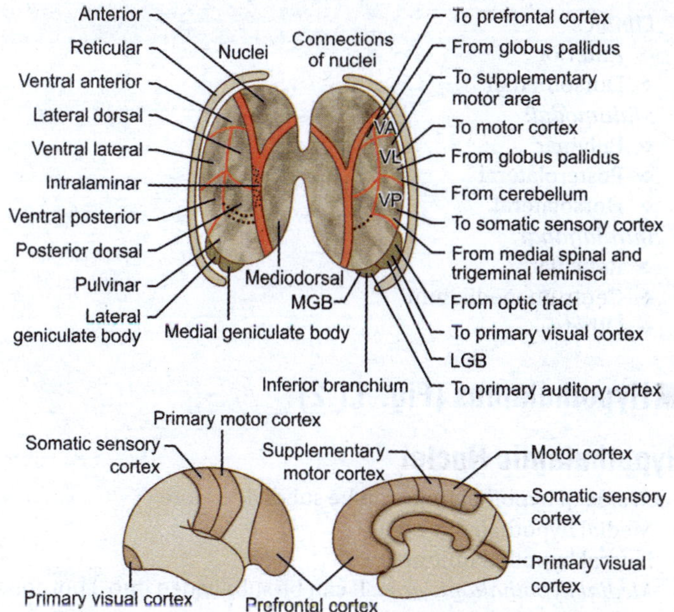

FIG. 11.1 Thalamic nuclei and connection with specific nuclei

5. *Posterior nuclei:* They include:
   ❖ *Pulvinar nucleus*: It connects with parietal and temporal cortex
   ❖ *Medial geniculate nucleus*: It receives aquastic fibers from:
      • Lateral leminiscus
      • Inferior colliculus.
         It project fibers to—temporal lobe cortex via acoustic radiation.
   ❖ *Lateral geniculate nucleus*: It receives fibers from optic tract.
   It projects fibers via geniculocalcarine radiation to visual cortex around calcarine fissure.

Functional Division of Thalamic Nuclei

● *Sensory:*
   ❖ Lateral geniculate nucleus
   ❖ Medial geniculate nucleus
   ❖ Posteroventral:
      – Posterolateral
      – Posteromedial.
● *Motor:*
   ❖ Anteroventral
   ❖ Lateroventral.

- *Limbic:*
  - ❖ Anterior
  - ❖ Dorsomedial.
- *Multimodal:*
  - ❖ Pulvinar
  - ❖ Posterolateral
  - ❖ Dorsolateral.
- *Intralaminar:*
  - ❖ Reticular
  - ❖ Centrum medianum
  - ❖ Others.

◼ Hypothalamus (Fig. 11.2)

Hypothalamic Nuclei

Each side of hypothalamus can be subdivided into:
- Medial hypothalamic area
- Lateral hypothalamic area
- *Medial hypothalamic area:* It can be subdivided into 3 portions:
  1. *Supraoptic portion:*
     - Supraoptic nuclei
     - Suprachiasmatic nuclei
     - Paraventricular nuclei.
  2. *Tuberal portion:*
     - Ventromedial nuclei
     - Dorsomedial nuclei
     - Arcuate nuclei
     - Medial eminence.

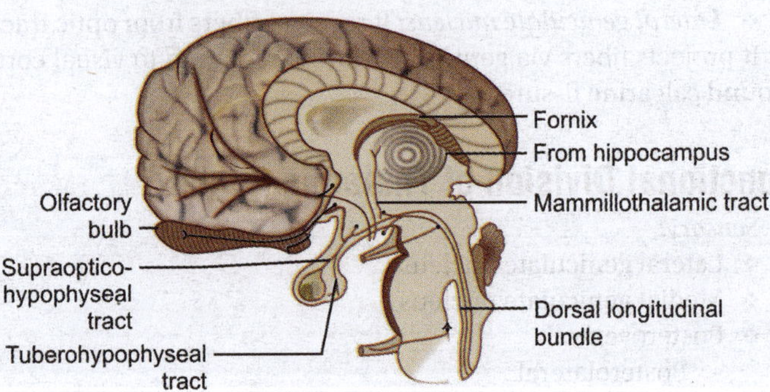

FIG. 11.2 Afferent and efferent connections of hypothalamus

3. *Mammillary portion*:
   - Premammillary nuclei
   - Medial mammillary nucleus
   - Lateral mammillary nucleus
   - Posterior hypothalamic nucleus.

- *Lateral hypothalamic area:* It contains fiber systems.
  - ❖ *Afferent connections:* To the hypothalamus:
    - *Part of medial forebrain bundle*
      - – From nuclei of par olfactory area
      - – From corpus striatum
  - ❖ Thalamohypothalamic fibers from medial and midline thalamic nuclei
  - ❖ *Fornix:* It brings fibers from hippocampus and mammillary bodies
    - *Stria terminalis:* it brings fibers from amygdala
    - *Inferior mammillary peduncle:* It brings fibers from tegmentum of midbrain
    - *Pallidohypothalamic fibers:* It brings fibers from lenticular nucleus to ventro-medial hypothalamic nucleus
    - *Ventral noradrenergic bundle:* It brings fibers from nucleus of tractus solitarius and other hind brain nuclei to paraventricular nuclei
    - *Dorsal noradrenergic bundle:* It brings noradrenergic fibers from locus ceruleus to dorsal hypothalamus
    - *Serotonergic neurons:* It brings serotonergic fibers from medulla
    - *Adrenergic neurons:* It brings adrenergic fibers from medulla
    - *Retinohypothalamic fibers:* Optic nerve fibers from optic chiasma to supraoptic nuclei.

- *Efferent connections:* From the hypothalamus:
  - ❖ Supraopticohypophyseal tract and paraventricular hypophyseal tract
  - ❖ Mammillothalamic tract (tract of Vicq d'Azyr) connects mammillary body to thalamic nuclei
  - ❖ *Mamillotegmental tract:* It connects mammillary body to tegmentum of midbrain
  - ❖ *Periventricular system (including dorsal longitudinal fasciculus):* It connects hypothalamus to midbrain, efferent projections to spinal cord
  - ❖ *Tuberohypophyseal tract:* It projects fibers from tuberal portion of hypothalamus to posterior pituitary
  - ❖ Fibers from septal region through fornix to hippocampus.

"Temperature Regulating Mechanism" (Table 11.1)

- *Mechanisms activated by cold*
  - ❖ Shivering   } Increased
  - ❖ Hunger   } Heat
  - ❖ Increased voluntary activity } Production
  - ❖ Increased secretion of nor epinephrine and epinephrine.
  - ❖ Curling up   } Decreased
  - ❖ Cutaneous vasoconstriction } Heat
  - ❖ Horripilation } Loss
- *Mechanisms activated by heat*
  - ❖ Cutaneous vasodilatation } Increased
  - ❖ Increased sweating } Heat
  - ❖ Increased respiration } Loss
  - ❖ Anorexia } Decreased
  - ❖ Apathy } Heat Production

Subthalamus

Subthalamic nucleus or body of Luys medial to internal capsule. Fibers from globus pallidus—as afferent connection.

Anterior to Red Nucleus

There is an area—field of Forel. It has three parts:
1. Ventromedial portion—Field H
2. Dorsomedial portion—Field H_1
3. Ventrolateral portion—Field H_2

Epithalamus

It consist of:
- *Habenular trigone:* It contains:
  - ❖ *Habenular nuclei:* It receives fibers from stria medullaris thalami
  - ❖ *Habenulopeduncular tract:* It extends from habenular nuclei to interpeduncular nucleus in midbrain.
- *Pineal body*
  - ❖ Tumor of pineal body—obstructs cerebral aqueduct, or inability to move eyes in vertical plane—Parinaud syndrome
  - ❖ *Other tumor—Germinoma:* It produces precocious sexual development.
- *Posterior commissure:* This band lies at the boundaries between diencephalon and midbrain.

  Interruption of posterior commeasure—It abolishes consensual light reflex.

Table 11.1 Principle of hypothalamic regulatory mechanism

Function	Afferent from	Integrating areas
1. Temperature regulation	Cutaneous cold receptors, temperature sensitive cells in hypothalamus	Ant hyp: Response to heat Post hyp: Response to cold
2. Neuroendocrine control		
a. Catecholamine	Emotional stimuli via limbic system	Dorsomedial and posterior hypothalamus
b. Vasopressin	Osmoreceptors – volume receptors	Supraoptic and paraventricular nuclei
c. Oxytocin	Touch receptors in breast, uterus, genitalia	Supraoptic and paraventricular nuclei
d. TSH via TRH	Temperature receptors	Dorsomedial nuclei
e. ACTH and Beta to LPH via CRH	i. Limbic system (emotional stimuli) ii. Reticular formation (systemic stimuli) iii. Suprachiasmatic nuclei (diurnal rhythm)	Paraventricular nuclei
f. FSH and LH via LHRH	Hypothalamic cells sensitive to estrogen	Preoptic areas
g. Prolactin via PRH and PIH	Touch receptors in breast, other unknown receptors	Arcuate nucleus, other areas (hypothalamus inhibits secretion)
h. Growth hormone via GRH and somatostain	Unknown receptors	Arcuate nucleus, periventricular nucleus
i. Hunger	"Glucostat" cells sensitive to glucose utilization	Ventromedial satiety center, lateral hunger center
j. Sexual behavior	Cells sensitive to circulating estrogen and androgen	Anterior and ventral hypothalamus in male, piriform cortex
k. Thirst	Osmoreceptors	Supraoptic hypothalamic nuclei

Cerebral Hemisphere (Figs 11.3 and 11.4)

Surfaces of hemispheres contain many fissures and sulci that separate the frontal, parietal, temporal and occipital lobes from each other.

The portions of brain lying between sulci are called convulations or gyri.

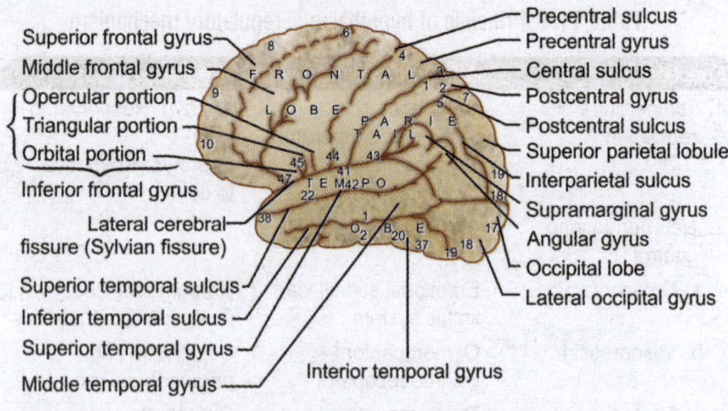

FIG. 11.3   Lateral surface of cerebral hemisphere

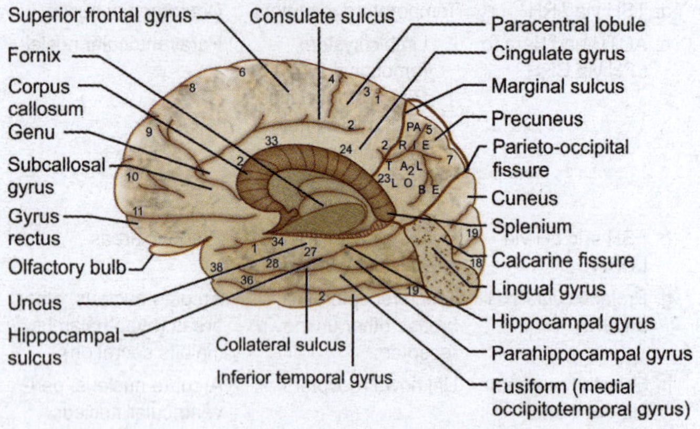

FIG. 11.4   Medial surface of cerebral hemisphere

Fissures

- *Lateral cerebral fissure:* It separates temporal lobe from frontal lobe.
- *Longitudinal cerebral fissure:* Hemispheres are being separated.
- *Parieto-occipital fissure:* It passes along the medial surface of the posterior portion of cerebral hemisphere, separates parietal lobe from occipital lobe.
- *Calcarine fissure:* It presents on the medial surface of the hemisphere near occipital pole.
- *Circuminsular fissure:* It surrounds insula and separates it from frontal, parietal and temporal lobes.

Carpus Callosum

Large myelinated bundle of fibers: It crosses longitudinal cerebral fissures and interconnects large portions of cerebral hemispheres.

Frontal Lobe

Gyri
- Superior frontal gyrus
- Middle frontal gyrus
- *Interior frontal gyrus:* It is divided into 3 parts from anterior:
  1. Orbital portion—rostral to anterior horizontal ramus
  2. Triangle-shaped portion—between anterior horizontal ramus and ascending ramus
  3. Opercular portion
- Precentral gyrus parallel to central sulcus
- Orbital gyrus
- Straight gyrus
- Cingulate gyrus
- Paracentral lobule—quadrilateral gyrus—around the end of central sulcus on medial surface of cerebral hemisphere.

Sulcus
- Precentral sulcus
- Central sulcus.

Parietal Lobe

Gyri
- Postcentral gyrus
- Superior parietal lobule
- Inferior parietal lobule
- *Supramarginal gyrus:* It arches above the ascending end of the posterior ramus of lateral fissure
- *Angular gyrus:* It arches above the end of superior temporal sulcus
- *Precuneus:* It is present on the posterior portion of medial surface.

Sulcus
- Postcentral sulcus
- Interparietal sulcus dividing superior and inferior parietal lobule.

Occipital Lobe

- Lateral occipital sulcus extends transversely and divides occipital lobe into:
  - ❖ Superior gyrus
  - ❖ Inferior gyrus.
- Calcarine fissure divides medial surface of occipital lobe into:
  - ❖ Wedge-shaped cuneus
  - ❖ Lingual gyrus.
- Posterior part of fusiform gyrus—on the basal surface of occipital lobe.

Temporal Lobe

- *Superior temporal gyrus* and middle temporal gyrus are divided by superior temporal sulcus
- *Middle temporal gyrus* and inferior temporal gyrus are divided by middle temporal sulcus
- Inferior temporal gyrus
- *Transverse temporal gyrus:* It occupies on the posterior part of superior temporal surface
- *Fusiform gyrus:* It is medial and interior temporal gyrus lateral to interior temporal sulcus on basal aspect of temporal lobe
- Parahippocampal gyrus—between hippocampal fissure and anterior part of collateral fissure
- *Uncus:* Most medial part of temporal lobe.

Insula

Shrunken portion of cerebral cortex. It lies deep in cerebral fissure
- *Short gyri:* It lies on anterior portion of insula
- *Long gyri:* It lies on posterior portion of insula.

White Matter in Cerebrum

White matter contains myelinated nerve fibers of many sizes. White center of cerebrum is called centrum semiovale. It contains three types of fibers:
1. *Transverse commissural fibers:* It connects two cerebral hemispheres.
   a. *Corpus callosum:* It connects homologous neocortex of cerebral hemisphere.
   b. *Anterior commissure:* It connects two olfactory bulbs and temporal lobe structures.
   c. *Hippocampal commissural fibers:* It connects two hippocampi.
2. *Projection fibers:* These fibers connect cerebral cortex with lower portions of brain and spinal cord.
   - *Afferent fibers (corticopetal fibers):*
     - Geniculocalcarine radiation—from lateral geniculate body to calcarine cortex
     - Auditory radiation—from medial geniculate body to auditory cortex
     - Thalamic radiation—from thalamic nuclei to specific cerebrocortical areas.
   - *Efferent fibers (corticofugal fibers):* From cerebral cortex to:
     - Thalamus
     - Brainstem
     - Spinal cord.

3. *Association fibers:* These fibers connect various portion of cerebral hemisphere. Two main types of association fibers:
   - ❖ *Short association fibers (U fibers):* These connects adjacent gyri:
     - • *Intracortical fibers:* It is located in deeper portion of cerebral cortex
     - • *Subcortical fibers:* It is located just beneath the cortex.
   - ❖ *Long association fibers:* It connects widely separated areas
     - • *Uncinate fasciculus:* It connects the interior frontal lobe gyri with anterior temporal lobe
     - • *Cingulum:* White band lying within cingulate gyrus, connects anterior perforated substance with parahippocampal gyrus
     - • *Arcuate fasciculus:* It connects superior and middle frontal gyri to temporal lobe and frontal pole
     - • *Superior longitudinal fasciculus:* It connects portions of frontal lobe with occipital and temporal areas
     - • *Inferior longitudinal fasciculus:* It connects temporal and occipital poles
     - • *Occipitofrontal fasciculus:* It connects frontal lobe with temporal and occipital lobes.

Areas of Cortex

- *Frontal lobe:*
  - ❖ Area 4 (precentral gyrus)—primary motor area
  - ❖ Area 6 (premotor area)
  - ❖ Area 8—Frontal eye field
  - ❖ Area 9, 10, 11—Frontal association areas
  - ❖ Area 44—Motor areas (Broca's area).
- *Parietal lobe:*
  - ❖ Area 3, 1, 2—Primary sensory areas
  - ❖ Area 5, 7—Sensory association areas
  - ❖ Area 39, 40—Association areas.
- *Temporal lobe:*
  - ❖ Area 41—Primary auditory areas
  - ❖ Area 42—Auditory association areas
  - ❖ Remaining areas—Association areas.
- *Occipital lobe:*
  - ❖ Area 17—Primary visual cortex
  - ❖ Area 18 and 19—Visual association areas.

■ Basal Ganglia (Figs 11.5 and 11.6)

Basal ganglia includes:

- Caudate nucleus
- Lentiform nucleus—external medullary lamina divides lentiform nucleus into 2 parts:
  1. Putamen
  2. Globus pallidus.

      A medullary lamina divides the globus pallidus into two portions.

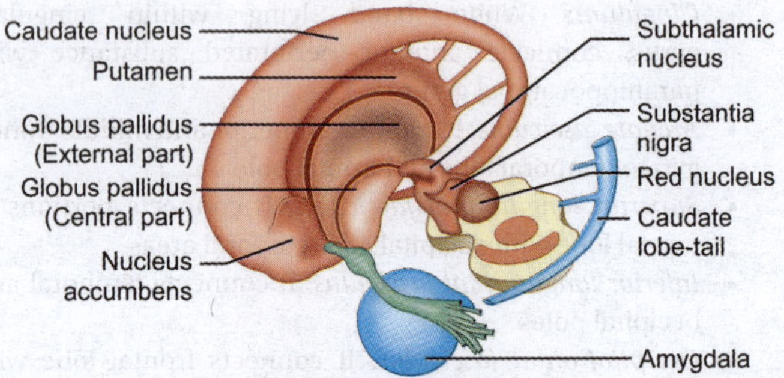

FIG. 11.5   Basal ganglia

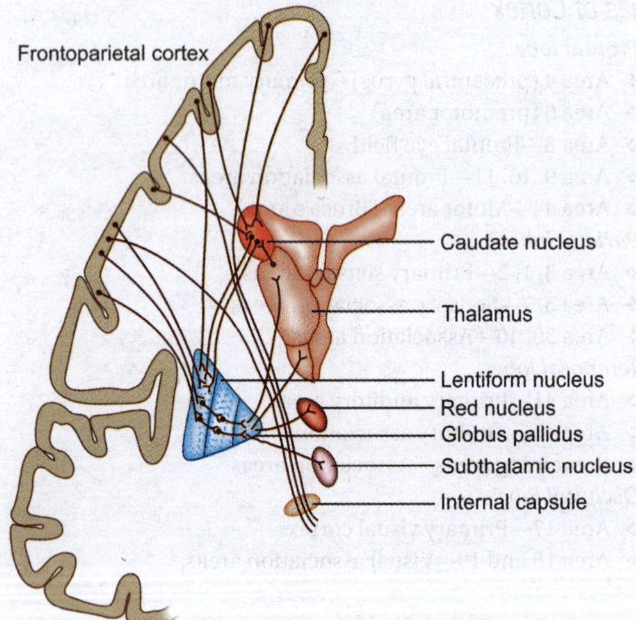

FIG. 11.6   Connections between basal ganglia, thalamus and cortex

Efferent tract
- Pallido—rubral tract
- Pallido—subthalamic tract
- Pallido—thalamic tract.

Afferent tract
- Putamen and globus pallidus receives some fibers from substantia nigra
- Thalamus sends fibers to caudate nucleus.

Internal Capsule (Fig. 11.7)

- It lies between lentiform nucleus and caudate nucleus and thalamus
- It is 'V' shaped in two appearances. It has two limbs:
  1. *Anterior limb*: It contains:
     - Thalamocortical and corticothalamic fibers join lateral thalamic nucleus and frontal lobe cortex
     - Frontopontine tract connecting frontal lobe to pontine nuclei
     - Fibers from caudate nucleus to putamen.
  2. *Posterior limbs is divided into 3 parts*:
     i. *Central part:*
        - Corticobulbar tract
        - Corticospinal tract
        - Corticorubral tract from frontal lobe cortex to red nucleus.
     ii. *Retrolenticular part:*
        Thalamocortical tract—from posterolateral nucleus of thalamus to postcentral gyrus.

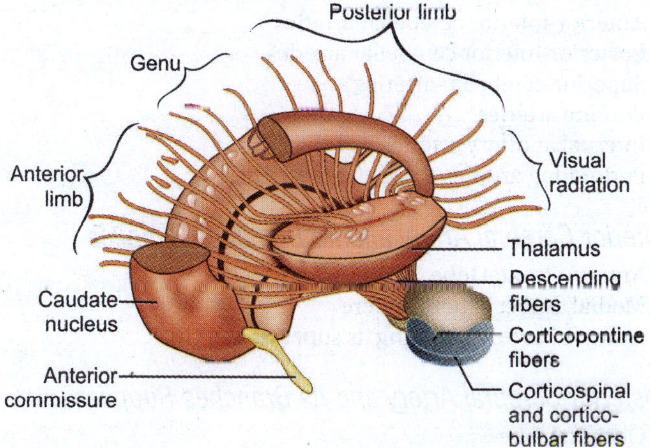

FIG. 11.7 Internal capsule and nucleus

iiii. *Sublenticular part:*
- *Parietotemporopontine tract:* It is connecting parietal lobe, temporal lobe cortex to pontine nuclei
- *Auditory radiations:* Fibers from medial geniculate body to transverse temporal gyrus
- *Optic radiations:* Fibers from lateral geniculate body to visual cortex.

Arterial Supply (Figs 11.8 to 11.10)

Arterial blood for brain enters the cranial cavity by 2 pairs of large vessels:
1. *Internal carotid*—branch of common carotid arteries
2. *Vertebral arteries*—branch of subclavian arteries.

Vertebral Arterial System Supplies

- Cerebellum
- Brainstem
- Occipital lobe
- Part of thalamus.

Two vertebral arteries are joined to form a basilar artery—it ends by forming two posterior cerebral arteries.

Internal carotid arteries—end dividing in into:
1. Anterior cerebral artery
2. Middle cerebral artery.

Anterior cerebral artery of one hemisphere is joined with the same of opposite side by anterior communicating arteries.

Ist branch of internal carotid artery is ophthalmic artery.

Vertebral arteries and basilar arteries give several branches:
- Anterior-inferior cerebellar arteries
- Posterior-inferior cerebellar arteries
- Superior-cerebellar arteries
- Pontine arteries
- Internal auditory arteries
- Perforating arteries.

Anterior Cerebral Artery and Its Branches Supplies

- Anterior frontal lobe
- Medial aspect of hemisphere
- A strip of cortex spanning its superior margin.

Posterior Cerebral Artery and Its Branches Supplies

- Occipital lobe
- Choroid plexus of IIIrd and IVth ventricle
- Lower surface of temporal lobe

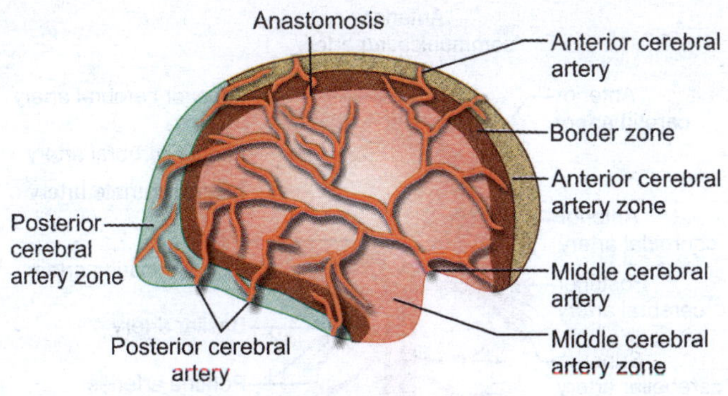

FIG. 11.8   Vascular supply of cerebral cortex

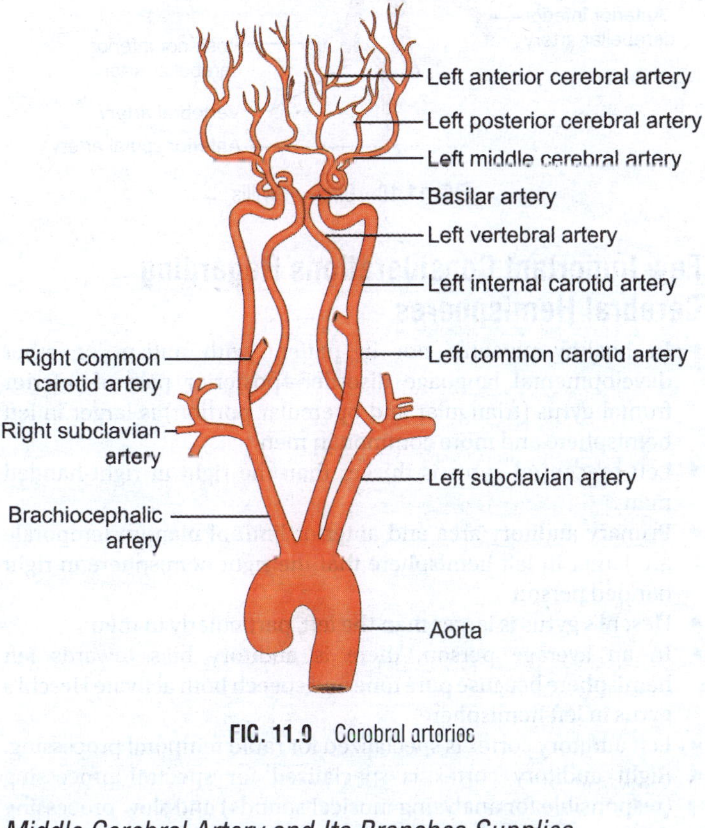

FIG. 11.9   Cerebral arteries

Middle Cerebral Artery and Its Branches Supplies

Much of lateral aspect of the cerebrum.

Normal cerebral blood flow—55 mL/100 gm/mb—it is 15 percent of cardiac output.

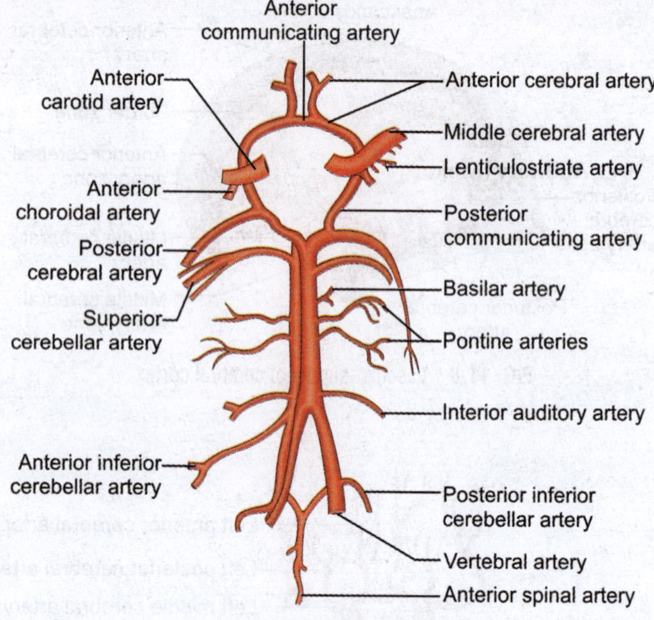

FIG. 11.10 Circle of Willis

Few Important Considerations Regarding Cerebral Hemispheres

- In healthy persons—not in patient with autism or other developmental language disorder—posterior part of inferior frontal gyrus (triangular and opercular portion) is larger in left hemisphere and more common in men
- Left precentral gyrus is thicker than the right in right-handed man
- Primary auditory area and anterior limit of planum temporale are larger in left hemisphere that the right hemisphere in right handed person
- Heschl's gyrus is larger than the left, particularly in men
- In an average person, there is auditory bias towards left hemisphere because pure tone and speech both activate Heschl's gyrus in left hemisphere
- Left auditory cortex is specialized for rapid temporal processing.
- Right auditory cortex is specialized for spectral processing (responsible for analyzing musical sounds) and slow processing mode
- Right frontal lobe is larger than the left frontal lobe. Left occipital lobe is larger than the right occipital lobe

- Right hemisphere is dominant for:
  - ❖ Skillful task
  - ❖ Constructional skills
  - ❖ Nonvisuospatial perception
    - Somesthetic
    - Auditory (Melody and tone discrimination)
    - Emotional functions—comprehension of emotional tone, voice and body gestures.
- Retrorolandic potion of cerebral hemisphere (postcentral gyrus) is involved in processing sensory information of outside world and about the motor act performed by individual.

  The latter action requires integration of different modalities of sensations (visual, somatosensory, auditory).

  Lesions in primary sensory area cause loss of specific modality of sensation.
- *Cortex—adjacent to primary sensory area* is called secondary sensory cortex—process unimodal sensory information
- *Cortex—lying between different secondary sensory areas* are called tertiary sensory cortex—responsible for processing multimodal sensory information.

  Example:

  Somatosensory information reaches somatotopically to postcentral gyrus, which projects somatotopically upwards to superior parietal lobule (arm and leg) and downwards to interior parietal lobule (head).

  Somatosensory information is integrated with auditory and visual information in angular gyrus.

  With visual in vegetative information in precuneus (posteromedial portion of parietal lobe).
- *Lesion in primary sensory area*—results in sensory loss.

  Lesion in multimodal association areas shown lack in multimodal sensations. For example, bilateral lesions in posterior portion of superior parietal lobule result in impairment of hand movement under visual guidance.
- *Activation of primary, secondary and multimodal sensory areas* are stimulus specific and touch specific.

  For example,
  - ❖ Activation of left posterosuperior temporal gyrus is activated by acoustic changes in speech and nonspeech sounds
  - ❖ Activation of left supramarginal gyrus is engaged in detection of changes in phonological units.
- Activation of sensory areas are modulated by prefrontal cortex, cingulate cortex, insular cortex
- *Prerolandic portion* of cortex is responsible for planning, initiation and execution of movements in a meaningful way,

getting information from the area of mesial frontal cortex (cingulate gyrus and supplementary motor areas) linked with reticular activating system and limbic lobe.

Lesion in these areas produces akinetic mutism.

From limbic system—information reaches frontal lobe—here it is integrated with sensory information from thalamus and multimodal association areas of hemisphere.

- *Precentral gyrus* is responsible for fine distal movements whereas subcortical structures are responsible for axial movements.

Cerebellum, brainstem and vestibular complexes are responsible for essential feedback information.

Regarding Lesions in Cerebral Hemisphere

- Lesions involving cerebral hemisphere is less pronounced than similar volumes of lesion involving brainstem because of:
  ❖ Redundancy of pathways
  ❖ Plasticity of hemisphere
  ❖ Large number of cortical neurons.
- Neurological deficit caused by cerebral hemisphere lesions is inconsistent than deficit involving lower brainstem
- Patient may be unaware of extent and quality of deficit especially when it involves multimodal behavior (apraxias, aphasia).
  For example,
  ❖ Patient with right hemisphere lesion is unaware of his deficits than patient with left hemisphere lesion—Anton syndrome—patient may be unaware of blindness related to parieto-occipital lesion
  ❖ Patient peripheral ulnar neuropathy may delineate the area accurately, but patient with lesion in primary sensory area cannot definitely delineate the exact area of sensory loss.
- For adequate localization, multimodal deficits must be analyzed.
  For example, Alexia—unable to understand written material.

In right parietooccipital lesion—saccades to left side is incomplete, hence he will miss beginning of words.

In left occipital lesion—patient cannot understand the meaning of array, used for making up written words.

- Same function is represented in different areas of cortex and contralateral hemisphere in different patients
- Hemispheric functions are subserved by:
  ❖ Extensive networks
  Hence, single lesion may be silent and becomes symptomatic when additional areas will be involved impairing network functions.

- A similar amount of tissue may be responsible for global aphasia in acute state, but, becomes responsible for motor aphasia few weeks later—it may be due to:
  - Perilesional edema
  - Metabolic abnormalities
  - Dysfunctions of the areas of brain away from the damaged area of brain.
- Lesions affecting same portions of cerebral hemisphere present with variable clinical pictures depending upon nature and tempo of lesion.

  For example, Infarcts—small infarct in brain produces aphasia in acute presentation.

  Tumor involving the brain—will be gradually, progressively increased in size before producing aphasia so it is slowly progressive.
- Cortical plasticity results is more or less complete recovery from elemental motor and sensory deficit, although more complex motor or sensory deficits remain—this occurs as a result of functional reorganization of cortex—so that sound cortical area take over the functions of lesioned cortical area.

  In case of subcortical lesions, the newly organized area, when firstly developed, become larger than the lesioned area. But as the time progresses, the area of activation gradually shrinks.
- *Cortical plasticity is mediated by multicentric arrays* which are susceptible to metabolic insult—as a result, processing and elaboration of neurotransmitters will be hampered. The newly organized area is more susceptible to toxic insult.
- *Lesions involving cortex (hypoxic laminar necrosis)*—giving rise to clinical picture—that differs from clinical picture produced as a result of lesions involving white matters (multiple sclerosis).

  Characteristics of cortical lesions
  - Seizures
  - Multimodal motor and sensory deficits.

  Characteristics of white matter lesion
  - Weakness
  - Spasticity
  - Pure motor syndromes
  - Urinary incontinence
  - Visual field deficit.
- Localization of the lesion can be diagnosed by following neuroimaging study:
  - Computed tomography (CT) scan
  - Magnetic resonance imaging (MRI) brain
  - Positron emission tomography (PET)
  - Single photon emission computerized tomography.

Brain infarct or cortical lesion may be passed unnoticed by CT scan if:

- It is restricted to cortex
- If there is coagulative necrosis.

Diffusion-weighed MRI can depict—them earlier and provides the timing of the lesion.

Tumor can be depicted by CT scan, but structural and metabolic changes of Alzheimer's disease are so subtle, that they cannot be imaged by CT scan.

Main output of brain is motor output; the physician becomes aware of it by observing patient's motor performances. This motor performance depends on:

- Level of alertness, mediated by ascending reticular activating system
- Cortical attention
- Perception of sensory stimuli and their relation with past experiences
- The ability to carry out sequence of events—those make up motor act itself.

HISTORY TAKING AND SYMPTOMS

◼ Neurological Examination

Neurologist—It deals with two types of diagnoses:
1. Site and severity of lesion—Anatomical diagnosis
2. Etiology or pathophysiology of diagnosis—Etiological diagnosis.

The following clinical features are helpful in neurological diagnosis:
- *Distribution of weakness*
  - ❖ Unilateral or bilateral
  - ❖ Symmetrical or asymmetrical
  - ❖ Primary proximal or primary distal.
- *Presence or absence of sensory symptom*
  - ❖ Type of distribution
  - ❖ Unilateral or bilateral.
- Presence or absence of pain
- Presence or absence of cranial nerve abnormalities
- Presence or absence or exaggeration of reflexes
- Presence or absence of pathological reflexes
- Involvement of bladder and bowel disturbances
- Presence or absence of symptoms relating to cortical involvement.

The level of lesion may be in:
- Muscle
- Neuromuscular junction
- Peripheral nervous system
- Nerve roots
- Spinal cord
- Brainstem
- Hemisphere.

Cranial Nerve

- Optic neuropathy or optic neuritis
- Third cranial nerve palsy—it is producing ptosis or diplopia, squint
- Seventh cranial nerve palsy—Bell's palsy.

Cerebellar Disease

- Signs of cerebellar disease—Tremor, in co-ordination, ataxia, vertigo, dysarthria, difficulty in walking and nystagmus
- No muscle weakness
- No sensory loss

- Normal reflexes
- No pathological reflexes
- No sphincter dysfunction
- No cortical dysfunction.

Basal Ganglia Disease

- No motor weakness
- No sensory loss
- Hypokinetic reflex—in Parkinsonism
- Hyperkinetic reflex—in Chorea
- Muscle rigidity
- Abnormal movements—Huntington's chorea
- Tremor.

Cortical and Subcortical Involvement

- Unilateral cortical involvement usually produces hemideficit in the form of:
  - ❖ hemiparesis
  - ❖ hemisensory deficit
  - ❖ hemianopsia
  - ❖ hemiseizures.
- Hyper-reflexia
- Pathological reflexes—Babinski response
- No bladder—bowel involvement—till bilateral cortical involvement will occur
- If thalamus is involved—pain will be a feature
- *If dominant hemisphere is involved*: Language disturbances like—agraphia, alexia, and aphasia will occur
- If nondominant hemisphere is involved—agraphia
- *If any cortical hemisphere is involved*: Astereognosis, impaired two points discrimination, memory defect, cognitive defect
- *If subcortical structures are involved*: Hemidistribution of dysfunction other than agraphia, language disturbance, cognitive defect, seizures.

Common causes of muscle disease
- Muscular dystrophies
- Inflammatory
- Toxic
- Metabolic
- Congenital.

Common causes of neuromuscular junction disorders
- Myasthenia gravis
- Eaton-Lambert syndrome

- Botulism
- Hypermagnesemia.

Common causes of peripheral neuropathy
- Guillain-Barré syndrome
- Alcoholism
- Diabetes mellitus.

Common causes of plexus diseases
- Trauma
- Neuralgic amyotrophy:
  - ❖ Parsonage—Turner syndrome
  - ❖ Plexitis.

Common causes of nerve root disease
- Disc prolapse
- Spondylosis.

Common causes of spinal cord disease
- Transverse myelitis
- Trauma
- Infective—tuberculosis.

Common causes of cranial nerve disease
- Optic neuritis—multiple sclerosis
- More than one cranial nerves involvement:
  - ❖ Lyme's disease
  - ❖ Sarcoidosis
  - ❖ Cavernous sinus thrombosis.

Some disorders may involve more than one locations
- *Devic disease*
  - ❖ Involvement of optic nerve
  - ❖ Involvement of spinal cord.
- *Amyotrophic lateral sclerosis:* Involve spinal cord to cerebral cortex—spares sensory function and cortical function.

History Taking

- *Presenting complaint—followed by history of present illness:*
  - ❖ History taking should be started with presenting complaint—to avoid unnecessary time consumption—you can ask
    - What problem makes you ill and for which you are brought to this hospital?
    - What is wrong with you?
    - Is there any immediately previous problem—after which you are attached by presenting problem—it may discover few following very necessary incidences:

- Immunization may lead to neuralgic amyotrophy
- Watery diarrhea may be followed by Guillain-Barré syndrome.

❖ Next step is to elaborate the presenting complaint. This can be done by a series of questions to the patients:
- Onset of illness
- Duration of illness
- Character of illness
- Constant or intermittent type
- Frequency of symptoms
- Severity of illness
- Any provocating of relieving factors
- Progression or regression of symptoms
- Localization.

During above type of questioning—you may have to do few leading questions—like:
- Pricking type pain or knife like pain
- Throbbing or bursting type of headache
- Associated blurring of vision, nasal congestion, etc.
- Relived by sleep or medication or after taking spectacle.

Time and Course of Symptoms

- Abrupt onset followed by progressions of symptoms—vascular, trauma
- Abrupt onset followed by gradual regression of symptoms—trauma, vascular
- Gradual onset of symptoms followed by variable rate of progression—degenerative diseases
- Gradual onset of symptoms—followed by progression, which may vary according to type of tumor

  If there is sudden hemorrhage in the tumor there will be sudden worsening of symptoms.

  ❖ Exaggeration and remission of symptoms with progressive increase in severity of symptoms in each exacerbation—Multiple sclerosis. In few cases the symptoms may be stationary or intermittent.

- Comparatively sudden with or without fever, gradual deterioration followed by progressive recovery if patient will get proper treatment. But if time of commencement of treatment is delayed, complete recovery may not occur.

Recent previous history may be important in some cases to get light in the present illness, e.g.
- Trauma
- Hypertension

- Vascular events
- Demyelinating diseases—like episodes of visual loss—within 3–5 years—may strengthen the recent symptoms.

Past Medical Relevant History

Following history may be relevant:
- History of trauma
- Operation
- Chronic illness
- Hospitalization
- Accidents
- Infectious diseases
- Venereal diseases
- Over the counter drugs.

For example:
- Radical gastric surgery, ileal bypass, ileal surgery—it may produce symptoms of vitamin B_{12} deficiency—subacute combined degeneration
- Few comorbid disease like—diabetes, thyroid disease, connective tissue diseases, sarcoidosis may produce neurological complications of systemic diseases
- History of mitral stenosis—with or without obvious appearances of thrombus in left atrium may produce cerebrovascular events
- History of hypertension—it may be responsible for vascular events
- Systemic neurological complication of cancer—it may start from Eaton-Lambert syndrome to cerebrovascular events or cerebral metastasis
- History of birth trauma, complications during pregnancy, labor, delivery, neonatal periods, age of schooling, performance in school
- *Drug history*
  ❖ Confusion from β blocker ophthalmic solution
  ❖ Aseptic meningitis from NSAID
  ❖ BIH—from thiamine infusion
  ❖ Headache from proton pump inhibitors.

Relevant Family History

There may be a linkage of family history with patient's disease:
- *Family history of:*
  ❖ Cancer
  ❖ Diabetes
  ❖ Hypertension
  ❖ Cardiovascular disease

Level	Weakness of muscle	Sensory loss	Deep tendon reflexes	Pathological reflexes	Bladder or bowel disturbances	Cortical function	Other symptoms
1. Muscle disease	Symmetrical proximal	Absent	Intact but in severe cases absent	Nil	Normal	Normal	May or may not have muscle tenderness
2. Neuro-muscular junction	Symmetric and proximal may be bulbar involvement (1) Eye movement weakness—producing double vision or ptosis, (2) Dysphagia, (3) Nasal regurgitation of fluid	Absent	Normal in Myasthenia gravis Depressed in Eaton-Lambert syndrome	Nil	Normal	Normal	Nil
3. Peripheral neuropathy	Symmetric and predominantly distal type may be proximal	Present	Depressed or absent	Nil	Normal	Normal	Pain may be present

Contd...

Contd...

Level	Weakness of muscle	Sensory loss	Deep tendon reflexes	Pathological reflexes	Bladder or bowel disturbances	Cortical function	Other symptoms
4. Plexus disease	Weakness of involved muscle	Sensory loss	Depressed or absent	Nil	Normal	Normal	
5. Nerve root disease	Motor weakness	Sensory loss	Depressed in the distribution of root	Nil	Normal	Normal	i. Pain along the distribution of root—aggravated by movement of neck or low back ii. Signs of irritability—positive straight leg rising test iii. Presence of pathological reflexes

Contd...

Contd...

Level	Weakness of muscle	Sensory loss	Deep tendon reflexes	Pathological reflexes	Bladder or bowel disturbances	Cortical function	Other symptoms
6. Spinal cord disease	Bilateral weakness below the level of lesion—paraparesis or quadriparesis	Sensory loss below the level, tingling and paresthesia at the level	Exaggerated below the level Lost at the level	Babinski sign	Difficulty in sphincter control and bladder dysfunction	Normal	
7. Brainstem disease	Crossed cranial nerve on the side of lesion and weakness of limb on opposite side	May or may not be present	Hyperactive	Babinski sign	Present in case of bilateral involvement	If RAS not involved— normal	If posterior fossa structure is involved – vertigo, ataxia, dysphagia, nausea, vomiting, abnormal eye movements

- ❖ Alcoholism
- ❖ Abuse of drugs.
- *If patient is suffering from*
  - ❖ CVA
  - ❖ Peripheral neuropathy
  - ❖ Myopathy
  - ❖ Movement disorder
  - ❖ Cerebellar disease—family history questionnaires may be important.
- In few cases, pes cavus, stork-leg deformities may have a family relation but in this case, the history taking is being neglected since these diseases are very common among people. In this case the apparently negative family history is not really negative.
- History of consanguinity among parents is also very important. Because some neuralgic disease common in one ethnic group. It may transmit to another ethnic group through sexual relationship.

Relevant Social History

Social history includes:
- *Marital status*
  - ❖ Number of marriages
  - ❖ Duration of present marriage
  - ❖ Any disturbance in marital adjustment
  - ❖ Health of the wife and children.
- *Occupational status*
  - ❖ Present occupation
  - ❖ Working environment
  - ❖ Any personal protection during working time
  - ❖ Level of exertion
  - ❖ If the patient is no longer working—when and why he stopped.
- *Hobbies:* Enquiry regarding hobbies or avocations
- *Personal habits*
  - ❖ Use of alcohol, tobacco, street drugs, coffee, tea or soft drinks
  - ❖ Any abstinence
  - ❖ Cause of abstinence.

Regarding Alcohol Abuse

CAGE Question

- Have you ever felt the need to *cut down* on your drinking?
- Have people *annoyed* you by criticizing your drinking?
- Have you ever felt *guilty* about your drinking?
- Have you ever had a morning *eye-opener* to steady your nerves or get rid of a hangover?

HALT Questions

- Do you usually drink to get *high*?
- Do you drink *alone*?
- Do you ever find yourself *looking* forward to drinking?
- Have you noticed that you are becoming to tolerant to alcohol?
- Abuse of inhaling less refined substances—spray paints, paint thinner, gasoline, airplane glue.

Enquiring about following Symptoms in a Suspected Neurologic Patient

- *Headache*
- *Loss of consciousness:* It may be mainly due to:
  a. Cardiological causes
  b. Neurological causes.

  If cardiological causes can be excluded, neurological causes may be excluded by following questionnaires:
- Can you describe each attack—till you will become unconscious?
- During onset of attack is anyone present in front of you?
- Have you describe any premonitory symptoms preceding attack?
- Is there any body movement during the period of unconsciousness?
- After the period of unconsciousness, were you ever confused?
- What was the length of period of unconsciousness?
- Any history of bowel and bladder movements during the period of unconsciousness.

Black out: Black out may be described as acute transient loss of consciousness, dimming of vision.

Epilepsies: It is described in involuntary movement.

Dizziness

It may be described as light headedness, vertigo or ataxia. So, it is necessary to differentiate ataxia from vertigo by following questions:

- Do you feel dizziness as spinning sensation of head?
- Do you spin or your surroundings spins?
- Have you any unsteadiness during walking?

Vertigo—It means sensation that objects are moving around or spinning. In this case following questions should be asked:

- Do you feel nausea and vomiting?
- Have you noticed any disturbance in hearing or any ringing in ears?
- Have you any history of intake of aminoglycosides?

  If vertigo us associated with tinnitus or deafness, patient becomes unsteady, having horizontal nystagmus directed away from affected ear.

Ataxia

Any patient having dizziness—must be evaluated for abnormal functions of vestibular, ocular, cerebellar and proprioceptive systems—equilibrium requires the integration of sensory input and motor output to maintain balance. The following questions to be asked to enquire about ataxia:

- Are you unsteady during walking?
- Are you unsteady when your eyes become closed?
- What about your diet?
- Have you ever had syphilis?

The causes of ataxia

- Abnormal proprioceptive sensation from lower limbs
- Posterior column damage from—syphilis, vitamin B$_{12}$ deficiency, multiple sclerosis—producing sensory ataxia—high stepping gait
- Motor ataxia from:
  - ❖ Abnormalities in cerebellum
  - ❖ Central vestibular pathways.

It is characterized by—wide based, irregular, occasionally poorly placing limbs and poor placement of center of gravity.

Change in Consciousness

This may be described as changes in attention, perception, arousal or combination.

In confusional states—Reception is normal, but processing is disturbed.

In delirium—perception of information is abnormal.

If any patient has history of change in consciousness—the following questions should be asked:

- Whether this change occur suddenly or slowly?
- Is there any associated symptom with change in consciousness?
- Is there any history of medication—depressants, insulin, alcohol abuse?
- Is there any history of liver disease, thyroid disease, renal disease?
- Is there any history of injury of head?
- Is there any history of psychiatric illness?

Any level of lesion may produce change in consciousness

- History of hemiparesis, hemisensory defect, paresthesia, garbled speech, hemianopia—due to supratentorial lesion
- Brainstem lesion—It may produce nausea, vomiting, nystagmus, doubled vision, yawning
- Toxic metabolic changes
- Psychiatric illness
- Any type of drug

Visual Disturbances

This is common neurological symptom. It consists of:

- *Acute visual loss*
  - ❖ Painless—vascular accident, retinal detachment
  - ❖ Painful—acute narrow angle glaucoma.
- *Chronic visual loss*
  - ❖ Painless—compression on optic nerve, tract or radiation, glaucoma—open angle.
    - Migraine—it may be associated with transient loss of vision.
    - Amaurosis fugax—it may be associated with internal carotid artery disease—it usually lasts for 3 minutes.
- *Diplopia:* Double vision. It may occur in the following conditions:
  - Ocular muscle palsies
  - Myasthenia gravis
  - Brainstem lesions
  - Thyroid disease.

Regarding visual loss, you have to ask following questions:
- Duration of visual loss.
- Whether visual loss is sudden, or slowly progressive.
- Any history of diabetes, thyroid disease, hypertension.
- Any previous history of glaucoma.

Regarding double vision following questions should be asked:
- In which gaze, patient complains of double vision?
- Whether it occurs suddenly or gradually?
- Any history of diabetes, hypertension, thyroid disease.
- Is there any associated pain?
- Any history of trauma to head or eye.
- Is double vision get worse with tiredness?

Dysphasia—Described

Following questions should be asked in case of dysphasia:
- Did you recognize any change in your speech pattern recently?
- Do you understand the words said to you?
- Do you find any difficulty in using proper words during expression?
- Have your hand writing changed recently?

Dementia

Progressive impairment of memory, orientation judgement and other aspects of neurological function. The causes are:
- Alzheimer's disease
- Parkinson's disease
- Vascular disorder

- Metabolic disorder
- Tumor
- Drugs
- Vitamin B_{12} deficiency
- Normal pressure hydrocephalus.

The following questions are to be asked for enquiry of dementia:
- Have you noticed any change in memory?
- Have you any difficulty in reading or understanding?
- How many years—during which the patient is abnormal?
- Any change in personality of the patient.

Gail Disturbances

It may occur due to:
- Pain in foot
- Pain in joint
- Claudication of the hip or leg
- Bone disease
- Cerebellum
- Vestibular problem
- Corticospinal tract involvement
- Extrapyramidal disorder.
  So, enquiries should be done—pointing above problem.
  History of hypertension, diabetes, sexually transmitted disease should be taken.

Gait

Stance: This is the position assumed in standing position.
Gait: This is patient's ambulating style.

Phases of Normal Gait Cycle

- *Stance:* Stance begins when one heel strikes the floor and it last for the entire period during which the foot is grounded
- *Swing:* This phase starts when the toes are off the ground and the time when heel of the same foot on the ground again.

Co-ordination of Gait

The gait is highly precised display of different structures:
- *Sensory input* (visual, vestibular and proprioception)
- *Motor output* (muscles and joints)
- *Good integration:* The different structures of CNS:
  - ❖ *Basal ganglia*—for automatic movement and swinging of arm
  - ❖ *Locomotor region* in midbrain for initiation of motion

- *Cerebellum:* For maintaining posture and balance, major characteristics of movement—trajectory, acceleration and velocity
- *Spinal cord:* For sending proprioceptive signals from joints and muscles to brain for feedback autoregulation.
- Vision.

Common Causes of Gait Disturbances

1. Pain
2. Immobile joints
3. Muscle weakness
4. Abnormal neurological control.

Information to be taken to evaluate gait disturbances:
- Acute onset or chronic onset
- Presence or absence of muscle weakness
- Limb stiffness or not
- Difficulty in initiation or termination of movement
- Associated bladder or bowel disturbances
- Associated vertigo or light headedness
- Associated alteration of pain, touch or temperature sensation
- Difficulty worsens at night or not.

Watch the following movements of patients:
- How does the patient climb up from chair (limb girdle muscle dystrophy, Parkinson's disease)?
- How does the patient climb upstairs?
- How does the patient start walking (Parkinson's disease)?
- Pace of walk—slow or fast.
- How does the patient turn?
- Whether patient walks on toes (Parkinson's disease, spastic paraplegia, sensory ataxia)?
- Whether patient walks on heels (sensory ataxia, spastic paraplegia)?
- Whether the patient walks on straight line?
- How does the patient walk with eyes open first followed by closed eyes?
- How does the patient stand with closed eyes?

Abnormal Gait due to Pain

Antalgic gait: This is due to pain and associated stiffness of weight-bearing joint, e.g. hip, knee, ankle or heel—it is more common by the age of 75—These can present with following fashion:
- *Gonarthrosis:* This is associated with knee stiffness; inability to extend or flex during gait

- *Coxarthrosis:* There is difficulty in hip extension and adduction. Patient shifts his upper body towards the affected limb, which effectively relocates his center of gravity, thus decreasing weight load—the other name of this gait is coxalgic gait.

Gait Disturbances due to Immobile Joints

- Osteoarthritis
- Plantar flexor contracture following prolonged immobilization. Patient fails to clear the foot off the grounds with compensatory dragging of stiff foot during walking.

Gait Disturbances due to Muscle Weakness

Muscles involved in abduction of hip:

- Gluteus medius
- Gluteus minimus.

Function of above muscles

- Abduction of ipsilateral hip with internal rotation
- Internal rotation of ipsilateral hip.

Abnormal gait

- *Trendelenburg gait:* Normally during walking pelvis of nonweight bearing side drops few degrees. But contraction of abductors of weight bearing side prevents this fall.

  In case of weakness of abductions of hip, there is sagging of pelvis on nonweight bearing side, hence, swinging limb is too low to clear the ground.
- *Waddling gait:* This occurs due to weakness of iliopsoas muscle. In this gait, patient utilizes gluteus medius and minimus muscles (abductors of hip) to lift and rotate the pelvis to compensate the inability of iliopsoas muscle of the same side to flex the knee joint.

  The patient can utilize his trunk muscles in this gait. The diseases involved:
- Limb girdle muscle dystrophy
- Progressive muscle dystrophy (Duchenne type)
- Congenital dislocation of hip.

Gait Disturbances due to Neurological Abnormality

- *Spastic gait:* Patient stands with hips adducted and intensely rotated, legs slightly flexed at knees and hip. The arm is flexed at elbow and wrist.

  Patient cannot lift the leg high enough to clear the foot off the ground, so there is compensatory abduction of hip to elevate the pelvis upwards and circumduct in a form arc. So this is also called circumduction gait. Arm is flexed across the body.

Lesion responsible: Unilateral upper motor tract lesion.

- *Scissor's gait:* Here both the legs are adducted and internally rotated, the legs are stiff and do not clear the floor during walking.

  So patient during walking leans forward, steps are small. The ankles are plantar flexed, so the patient walks on toes, feet scrapping the floor, bilaterally adducted limb—*(Scissor's gait).*

  To compensate stiff legs of both sides, patient may move trunk from side to side.

  Lesion responsible—bilateral upper motor neuron lesion (brainstem stroke or injury).

- *High stepping gait:* Patient flexes the hip and knee to raise the affected foot from the floor. Since the toes of lifted food look downwards, during grounding toes first touch the floor followed by heel. During this process, toes may scrape still on the floor, stumbling and fall.

  Cause:
  - ❖ *Unilateral*—peroneal nerve palsy—lesion at L4–L5 level
  - ❖ *Bilateral:*
    - Hereditary sensory motor neuropathies (loss of all muscles below the knee)
    - Cauda equina lesion
    - Distal myopathies
    - Anterior compartment atrophy
    - Autoimmune neuropathies (Guillain-Barré syndrome).

- *Stamping gait or thumping gait:* When patient is unware of his position sense and joint sense, foot may flail side to side, base is wide, patient is unware of his position of knee, so foot may strike the ground with much force, heels strike the ground first followed by the toes.

  Patient may not be able to walk in dark as visual compensation is lost in dark (sensory ataxia).

  Lesion: Posterior column lesion in tabes dorsalis.

- *Cerebellar gait—Reeling gait*
  - ❖ *In lateral cerebellar hemispheric lesion:* Patient is unstable, sway and fall to ipsilateral side, base is wide, legs moves irregularly, when flexed and extended
  - ❖ *In bilateral cerebellar hemispheric lesion:* Patient may sway from side to side, base in broad
  - ❖ *If vermis is involved:* Loss of tone of extensor paraspinal muscles—leads to sway and reeling in all direction titubation of head. While walking, patient may fall in any direction, and has to hold anything to prevent falling.

When arm is outstretched, the drift is upwards.
Lesions responsible
Vermain lesion caused by:
- Cerebellar hemorrhge
- Tumor
- Demyelinating disease
- Compression from tonsillar decent into foramen magnum.

❖ *Martionette gait:* Patient's leg becomes stiff in extensor posture, tends to lean backwards.
Lesion: Lesion in anterior vermis—caused by severe alcoholism.

- *Festinant gait:* Patient is flexed forward, carrying angles are increased in flexed position. There is difficulty in initiation of motion, suddenly there is increased in steps (festination), suddenly patient become freeze. Steps are short shuffling with bends forward as if patient is trying to catch his center of gravity. There is lack in associated movement.

Lesion
❖ Basal ganglia disease—severe Parkinsonism
❖ Normal pressure hydrocephalus.

   In normal pressure hydrocephalus: Patient may be at gait ignition failure (foot grasp on the floor).

   Patient may lift the leg with feet and again lower the leg and feet in same place (egg-walking)—patient may frequently fall backwards.

- *Lurching gait*
  ❖ *In Huntington's chorea*—wide-based, reeling from heel to heel, steps irregularly, associated with vigorous grimace and movements of hands and wrists and choreatic eye movements
  ❖ *Sydenham's chorea*—in it, gait is less involved, but involvement of arm, neck and face is prominent
  ❖ *Dystonic movement due to dopaminergic drugs*—shoulder, face and extremities are affected more than gait
  ❖ *In central dystonia*—patient walks on everted foot, but posture of foot will be normal in recumbency
  ❖ *In peripheral dystonia*—patient walks on sole, in recumbency foot is inverted and dropped.

- *Hysterical gait:* This gait becomes bizarre, do not show any specific pattern of movement, differs from examination to examination

- *Apraxic gait (frontal gait):* Wide base gait, hesitation in start, short shuffling steps, feet rarely off the floor—magnetic as if feet are glued to floor.

   Trunk is stooped forward, lack of reflexes.

Lesion: Disconnection of prefrontal and frontal regions with other parts of motor control system (involvement of frontopontocerebellar fibers at their origin in frontal lobe).

Causes of apraxic gait:
- ❖ Subcortical strokes in white matter in frontal region
- ❖ Frontal lobe tumors
- ❖ Normal pressure hydrocephalus.

Aparaxic gait is associated with urgency, urinary incontinence, dementia, CSF pressure <180 mm Hg.

Response to removal of 40–50 mL of CSF is diagnostic.

- *Tremor:* Rhythmic oscillation of distal parts of the limbs and head—it may be physiological—10–12 cycles/second or pathologic tremor. Simple tremor involves a single muscle groups, whereas complex tremor involves several muscle groups. Tremor can be classified in various ways by:
  - Location
  - Rate
  - Amplitude
  - Rhythmicity
  - Relationship to rest and movement
  - Etiology
  - Underlying pathology
  - Relationship to fatigue, emotion, head, cold, medication, alcohol, street drugs.

Parkinson tremor: At rest, diminished during movement.

Ataxic tremor: Increased during movement, worsens during anxiety.

Intention tremor: It may occur in multiple sclerosis.

Liver failure, renal failure, withdrawal of alcohol: It may precipitate tremor.

So, following questions should be asked to delineate tremor:
- History of thyroid disease, liver, kidney disease
- History of alcohol abuse
- Increase or decrease during movement
- Any history of large amount of intake of coffee or chocolate.

Tremors

It is defined as symmetric movement of body parts.

Central generation of discharge—results from cerebellum and thalamus.

Peripheral feedback from proprioceptive fibers through peripheral nerve.

Fine tremor: It is difficult to see. It can be amplified by placing a piece of paper on the outstretched fingers.

Coarse tremor: It is slower, can be seen.

Nonspecific trigger factors are:
- *Postural kinetic tremor:* When patient tries to maintain a fixed prosture
- *Orthostatic tremor:* It occurs only when the patient is in up right posture
- *Tremor at rest:* It occurs with lesion in basal ganglia.

Types of Tremor

Nervousness
- It is most common tremor
- It is physiologic, universal tremor
- It affects hands predominantly, in severe cases—voice, body and extremities may be involved
- It is present at rest, increased during voluntary movement, not increased by automatic movements
- It is due to β-adrenergic stimulation of segmental stretch reflex
- Oscillation in between 10–15 Hz.

Anxiety State
- It is similar to nervousness tremor
- *It is associated with:*
  - ❖ Dilated pupil
  - ❖ Tachycardia
  - ❖ Hyperhidrosis
  - ❖ Cold and calmy extremities.
- It is caused by excessive circulation of noradrenaline from the adrenal gland or discharge from the sympathetic neurons in the lateral column of spinal cord.

Thyrotoxicosis
- This is fine tremor—It can be evidenced by placing a paper on the patient's outstretched hands
- This is associated with:
  - ❖ Pathologic lid retraction (Collier's sign)
  - ❖ Tachycardia
  - ❖ Warm extremities
  - ❖ Hyperhydrosis

- Circulation is hyperdynamic, venous pulsation is observed in optic disc
- This tremor can be treated by β adrenergic blocker.

Alcoholism

- Tremor is postural, between 6–11 Hz
- This is exacerbated by voluntary movements or emotions
- The associated gait is ataxic gait—*"Martinette gait"*
- The associated sign is *Quinquaud's sign*—The examiner when presses his or her palm against patient's outstretched finger tips—there is extension of interphalangeal joints and flexion of metacarpophalangeal joints
- The causative lesion is cerebellar dysfunction which regulates agonist and antagonist muscles of proximal and distal joints
- Tremor of alcohol withdrawal may be close to 8–10 Hz.

Toxic Tremor

- Withdrawal from opiate produces physiologic tremor due to excessive sympathetic nervous system stimulation
- Lithium produces—myoclonus, postural kinetic tremor and coarse tremor of outstretched extremities
- Lithium and nicotine can mimic alcohol—type tremor
- Toluene abuse produces intention tremor.

Essential Tremor

- This is characterized by rapid side to side head tremor or coarse side to side head tremor with slow intention tremor
- This tremor is constant, worsened by emotional upset and decreased by—intake of alcohol or during execution of fine movements (picking up a pencil)
- There are two varieties:
  a. Autosomal dominant
  b. Autosomal recessive with incomplete penetrance and intrafamilial and interfamilial variance.
- Normal frequency is 8 Hz.

Intention Tremor

- This is characterized by tremor of side to side oscillation in last 1/3rd voluntary movement as the target is approached
- The frequency range is 4–6 Hz
- In milder form it can be tested by finger nose test and in severe form, it is present during voluntary movement
- This tremor is absent at rest.

- The causative lesions are:
  - ❖ Cerebellar infarction due to involvement of anterior, inferior cerebellar artery
  - ❖ Multiple sclerosis
  - ❖ Spinocerebellar atrophy
  - ❖ Genetic cerebellar disease
  - ❖ Postanoxic states.

Pill Rolling Tremor

- Hand flexed at metacarpophalangeal joint, extension and flexion of thumb
- As tremor progresses—the thumb rubs against forefinger—this initiates flexion tremor at 1st interphalangeal joint
- Further progression—all the fingers are flexed together.
  - ❖ It is exacerbated by emotion
  - ❖ It is present at rest
  - ❖ It is absent in sleep and just after awakening
  - ❖ It is suppressed by voluntary movements.
- It is associated flexed posture and other manifestations of Parkinson's disease—cog-wheel rigidity, up and down tremor of head
- Tremor is not a feature of drug-induced Parkinsonism or a kinetic states.

Tremor of Collagen Disease

- Side to side irregular movement of finger
- Exacerbated by emotion and postural maintenance
- Disappears by total relaxation.

Red Nucleus Tremor

- It is unilateral, coarse and rhythmic (Claude's syndrome)
- It is present at rest and during all times of voluntary movement
- It is due to embolic occlusion of thalamoperforate branches of posterior cerebral or paramedian division of top of the basilar artery
- Frequency 2.5–4 Hz—it increases as hand reaches its target
- Sometimes it is accompanied by contralateral third nerve palsy and contralateral choreathetoid movement (Benedict syndrome).

Tremor of Wilson's Disease

- Vertical, asymmetric, flapping irregular tremor—of wrist and shoulder girdle.

- It is increased by voluntary movements and decreased at repose
- It has chorea and intention component
  Kayser-Fleischer ring—Golden brown crescent in the superior part of iris in blue-eyed person—is pathognomonic.
- Patient is hypotonic, dysarthric, demented.

Asterixis

- Patient is asked to hold his arms outstretched with wrist dorsiflexed.
  There is sudden loss of tone, so there is wrist drop
  ↓
  There is compensatory jerk to reposition his wrist in former position
  ↓
  So there is flapping tremor.
- It occurs in:
  ❖ Hepatic failure
  ❖ Renal failure
  ❖ Pulmonary failure
  ❖ Hyperosmotic states.

Pseudoathetosis

- Patient holds the arms outstretched or placing the extremity on the surface
  ↓
  Sinuous movements of the fingers with wrist flexion at metacarpophalangeal joints
  ↓
  This elevates extremity from the surface
  Fingers closed, wrist further flexed and arms internally rooted.
- It is suppressed when patient watches his hands
- There is associated loss of joint and position sense
- In Tabes dorsalis, there is damage of posterior root ganglia and posterior column lesion—producing tabetic athetosis
- Severe degeneration of dorsal column occurs in:
  ❖ Degenerative disease
  ❖ HIV
  ❖ Vitamin B_{12} deficiency
  ❖ Autoimmune diseases
  ❖ Myelopathy
  ❖ Carcinomatous large fiber destruction.

Parietal lesion—updrift of extremity—contralateral to the side of lesion with or without sinuous movement of the fingers.

Lesion in thalamus—it produces updrift of extremity with sinuous movement of finger and flexion of wrist, adduction of thumb into the palm.

Weakness

It is a symptom of motor system. Weakness may be proximal or distal.

Patient with proximal muscle weakness—have a difficulty in combing hair, shaving, washing his head.

Patient with distal muscle weakness has history of difficulty in putting a button through a button-hole, using pen, keys or pencil.

Patient with proximal lower limb weakness has history of climbing upstairs, getting into bed or bathtub.

Patient with distal lower limb weakness has history of foot drop.

Pain

It is an infrequent symptom—it may be facial type:
Facial pain may be due to:
- Trigeminal neuralgia
- Herpes Zoster infection
- Trauma.

Low back pain may be due to:
Sciatica—intense pain shooting down the leg in the distribution of sciatic nerve—it may be due to arthritis of lumbosacral joint.

Pain around the neck may be due to—primarily
- Cervical spondylosis
- Meningitis
- Subarachnoid hemorrhage.

So, we can deduce organ specific symptoms in following process:
Head
- *Headache:*
  - Migraine
  - CVA
  - Brain tumor
  - Benign intracranial hypertension
  - Meningitis
  - Brain abscess
- *Trauma:* Subdural hematomas.

Headache (Figs 11.11A to G)
- *Location:*
  - Unilateral in 70 percent, bifrontal or global in 30 percent—*Migraine*
  - Usually bilateral, may be generalized, or localized to back of the head, upper neck or to frontotemporal area—*Tension*

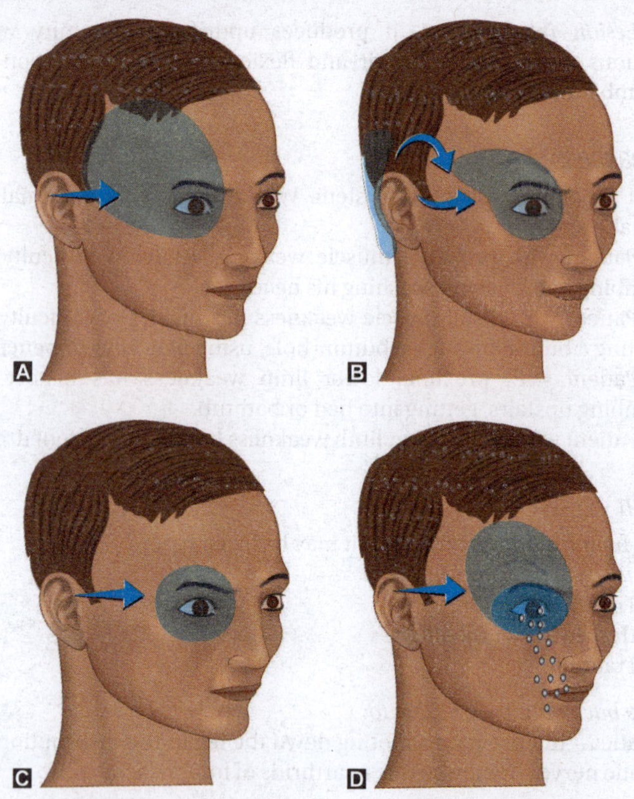

FIGS 11.11A TO D (A) Classic migraine—Starts in the temple on one side, then spreads to whole side of head; (B) Occipito-orbital migraine—Less dramatic, dull ache, in occipital area, then extends forwards in around the temple, or dull bursting pain behind the eye; (C) Oribital migraine—Less painful, predominantly nagging pain behind the eye. Photophobia, light and sudden movement provoke pain; (D) Clauster headache—Middle-aged male, without prior history of migraine, pain around eye with lacrimation, nasal congestion

- ❖ Unilateral, behind or around the eye—*Clauster*
- ❖ Around and over the eyes, may radiate to occipital area—*Errors of refraction* (farsightedness, astigmatism but not nearsightedness)
- ❖ Above the eyes—*Frontal sinus*, maxillary area—*Maxillary sinus*, center of head—*Sphenoidal sinus*
- ❖ Generalized—*Meningitis, Subarachnoid hemorrhage*
- ❖ Varies with location of tumor—*Brain tumor*

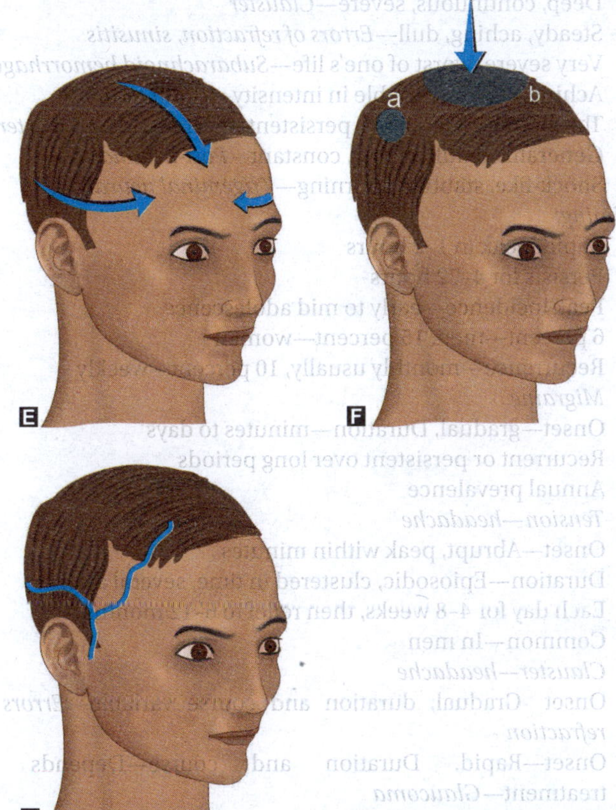

FIGS 11.11E TO G (E) Tension headache; (F) Psychogenic headache—(a) Specific spot-complaint bone is going bad, worms crawing under the skin, lumpish feeling, (b) Relentless pressure feeling over the vertex-depressive headache; (G) Temporal arteritis—Swelling, redness and tenderness of the temporal artery and headache in the distribution of temporal artery

- ❖ Localized near involved artery:
  - Temporal region—temporal artery *Gaint cell arteritis*
  - Occipital region—Occipital artery
- ❖ It may be localized to involved traumatic area—*Post-traumatic*
- ❖ Around cheeks, jaws, lips, gums—*Trigeminal neuralgia involving nerve division 2, 3 >1.*
- ● *Quality and severity:*
  - ❖ Throbbing, aching, variable in severity—*Migraine*
  - ❖ Tightening pain, mild to moderate intensity—*Tension*

- ❖ Deep, continuous, severe—*Clauster*
- ❖ Steady, aching, dull—*Errors of refraction, sinusitis*
- ❖ Very severe, worst of one's life—*Subarachnoid hemorrhage*
- ❖ Aching, steady, variable in intensity—*Brain tumor*
- ❖ Throbbing, generalized, persistent, severe—*Gaint cell arteritis*
- ❖ Generalized dull aching, constant—*Post-traumatic*
- ❖ Shock-like, stabbing, burning—*Trigeminal neuralgia.*

- *Timing:*
  - ❖ Rapid, peak in 1–2 hours
    Persists for 4–72 hours
    Peak incidence—early to mid adolescence
    6 percent—men, 15 percent—women
    Recurrence—monthly usually, 10 percent—weekly
    Migraine
  - ❖ Onset—gradual, Duration—minutes to days
    Recurrent or persistent over long periods
    Annual prevalence
    Tension—headache
  - ❖ Onset—Abrupt, peak within minutes
    Duration—Epiosodic, clustered in time, several attacks
    Each day for 4–8 weeks, then relief to 6–12 months
    Common—In men
    Clauster—headache
  - ❖ Onset—Gradual, duration and course variable—*Errors of refraction*
  - ❖ Onset—Rapid. Duration and course—Depends on treatment—*Glaucoma*
  - ❖ Onset—Variable
    Duration—Several hours at a time, recurring over days
    Course—Recurrent in repetitive daily pattern
    Sinusitis
  - ❖ Onset fairly rapid, Duration—Variable
    Course—Persistent, in acute illness
    Meningitis
  - ❖ Onset—Abrupt, severe, prodromal symptoms may occur.
    Duration—Variable
    Course—Persistent, in acute illness
    Subarachnoid hemorrhage
  - ❖ Onset—Variable, Course—Intermittent but progressive
    Brain cell tumor
  - ❖ Onset—Gradual or rapid
    Course—Recurrent or persistent over weeks to months
    Giant cell arteritis
  - ❖ Onset—Within 1–2 hours of injury, persist for weeks, months to years

Tends to diminish overtime
Post-traumatic headache
  ❖ Onset—Abrupt, paroxysmal
    Each jab lasts for seconds to minutes, recurs at intervals of seconds to minutes last for months, reappears after month.
    Trigeminal neuralgia
- *Associated factors:*
  ❖ Nausea, vomiting.
    Photophobia, visual auras (flickering zigzagging lines), motor auras (affecting hand or arm), sensory aura (numbness, tingling preceding attack)
    —*Migraine*
  ❖ Sometimes photophobia
    Nausea—Absent
    —*Tension*
  ❖ Lacrimation, rhinorrhea, miosis, ptosis, eyelid edema, congestive conjunctiva
    —*Clauster*
  ❖ Eye fatigue, sandy sensation in eyes, redness in conjunctiva
    —*Errors of refraction*
  ❖ Diminished vision, sometimes nausea vomiting
    —*Glaucoma*
  ❖ Local tenderness, nasal congestion, discharge, fever
    —*Sinusitis*
  ❖ Fever, stiff neck—Meningitis
  ❖ Nausea, vomiting, neck pain, loss of consciousness
    —*Subarachnoid hemorrhage*
  ❖ Aggravated by coughing, sneezing, sudden movements
    —*Brain tumor*
  ❖ Tenderness of adjacent scalp, fatigue, weight loss, jaw claudication (50%), visual loss (15–20%), polymyalgia rheumatica (50%).
    —*Giant cell arteritis*
  ❖ Poor concentration, memory problem, vertigo, irritability, fatigue, restlessness
    —*Post-traumatic*
  ❖ Exhaustion from recurrent pain—*Trigeminal neuralgia.*

Aggravating Factors

- Alcohol, certain foods or tension—provoke, common—premenstrually
  Aggravated by noise, bright light —*Migraine*
- Sustained muscle tension, as in driving or typing —*Tension*

- During an attack, alcohol may increase sensitivity —*Clauster*
- Prolonged use of eyes, for close work—*Errors of refraction*
- Provoked by mydriatic drop—*Acute glaucoma*
- Aggravated by coughing, sneezing or movement of head —*Sinusitis*
- Movement of neck and shoulder—*Giant cell arteritis*
- Mental and physical straining, stooping, emotional excitement, alcohol—*Post-traumatic*
- Touching certain areas of lower face, lips, mouth, chewing, brushing, talking—*Trigeminal neuralgia.*

Relieving Factors

- Quite darkroom, sleep. Early in course
  Transient relief from pressure on involved artery—*Migraine*
- Massage, relaxant—*Tension*
- Rest on eyes—*Errors of refraction*
- Nasal decongestants, antibiotics—*Sinusitis*
- Rest—*Post-traumatic.*

Dizziness and Vertigo

Dizziness: It is a nonspecific term, used by patient that encompassing several disorders.

Vertigo: It is spinning sensation accompanied by nystagmus, ataxia.

- *Peripheral vertigo:*
  - ❖ Benign positional vertigo
  - ❖ Vestibular neuronitis
  - ❖ Meniere's disease
  - ❖ Drug toxicity
  - ❖ Acoustic neurinoma
- *Central vertigo:*
  - ❖ Atherosclerosis
  - ❖ Multiple sclerosis
  - ❖ Vertebrobasilar migraine
  - ❖ Transient ischemic attack

Vertigo

- *Onset:*
  - ❖ Sudden, rolling onto affected side or fitting head up— *Benign, positional vertigo*
  - ❖ Sudden—*vestibular neuronitis, Meniere's disease*

- ❖ Acute or indious, linked to loop diuretics, aminoglycoside, alcohol, salicylates—*Drug toxicity*
- ❖ Insidious from cranial nerve VIII compression Vestibular branch—*Acoustic*
- • *Duration and course:*
  - ❖ Onset—few seconds to <1 minutes Last for few weeks, may recur—*Benign positional vertigo*
  - ❖ Onset—hours up to 2 weeks May recur over 12–18 months—*Vestibular neuronitis*
  - ❖ Onset—several hours to <1 days Recurrent—*Meniere's disease*
  - ❖ May or may not reverse Parital adaption occurs—*Drug toxicity*
  - ❖ Variable— *Acoustic neurinoma*
  - ❖ Variable, but rarely continuous—*Central vertigo*
- • *Hearing:*
  - ❖ Not affected—*Benign positional vertigo, vestibular neuronitis, central vertigo*
  - ❖ Progressive sensorinural deafness—*Meniere's disease*
  - ❖ May be impaired—*Drug toxicity*
  - ❖ Impaired on one side—*Acoustic neurinoma*
- • *Tinnitus:*
  - ❖ Absent—*Benign positional vertigo, vestibular neuronitis, central vertigo*
  - ❖ Present:
    - • Fluctuation—*Meniere's disease*
    - • May be present—*Drug toxicity*
  - ❖ Present—*Acoustic neurinoma*
- • *Additional features:*
  - ❖ Nausea, vomiting, nystagmus—*Benign, positional vertigo, vestibular neuronitis drug toxicity*
  - ❖ Nausea, vomiting, nystagmus, pressure or fullness in affected ear—*Meniere's disease*
  - ❖ May involve V and VII cranial nerve—*Acoustic neurinoma*
  - ❖ Other brainstem deficit dysarthria, ataxia, crossed motor or sensory deficit—*Central vertigo.*

Eye

- • *Episodic blindness:* Multiple sclerosis
- • *Painful loss of vision:*
  - ❖ Acute closes angle glaucoma
  - ❖ Retrobulbar neuritis.

- *Painless loss of vision:*
  - ❖ Open angle glaucoma
  - ❖ Optic neuropathy
  - ❖ Compression of optic nerve, optic tract, optic radiation
  - ❖ Retinal detachment
  - ❖ Vascular.
- *Diplopia*
  - ❖ 3rd, 4th or 6th cranial nerve palsy
    Without levator palpebrae superior is paralysis
  - ❖ Ophthalmoplegic migraine.
- *Ptosis*
  - ❖ Myasthenia gravis
  - ❖ Eaton-Lambert syndrome
  - ❖ Paralysis of levator palpabrae superioris.
- *Dry eyes:* Sjögren syndrome
- *Photophobia:* Migraine
- *Pain in eye:* Optic neuritis.

Ear

- *Deafness:* Acoustic neurinoma
- *Tinnitus*
  - ❖ Acoustic neurinoma
  - ❖ Meniere's disease
  - ❖ Middle ear disease
  - ❖ Eustachian tube blockage.
- *Vertigo*
  - ❖ Cerebellar cause
  - ❖ Vestibular cause.
- *Discharge:* Cholesteatoma

Nose

- *Anosmia:* Olfactory groove meningioma
- *Parosmia:* Trauma to base of brain
- *Discharge through nose:* If glucose content of discharge is high—CSF rhinorrhea:
  - ❖ Trauma
  - ❖ Tumor.

Mouth

- Sore tongue—Vitamin deficiency
- *Tremor on tongue*
  - ❖ Cranial nerve palsy (if associated with atrophy and fasciculation)

- ❖ ALS
- ❖ Bulbar involvement, when associated other cranial nerves (X, XI, XII) are involved.
- *Deviation of tongue:* Same side XII cranial nerve involvement.

Neck

- *Pain*
  - ❖ *Cervical spondylosis:* It may be associated vertigo or radiation of pain
  - ❖ Radiculopathy.
- *Stiffness*
  - ❖ Meningitis
  - ❖ SAH
  - ❖ Gross cervical spondylosis.

Cardiovascular

- *Valvular heart disease:* Cerebral embolism
- *SBE:* Cerebral embolism—It may turn into cerebral abscess
- *Hypertension:* CVA
- *Cardiac arrhythmia:* Cerebral embolism.

Respiratory

- *Dyspnea*
  - ❖ Any neurological disease with bulbar involvement
  - ❖ Guillain-Barré syndrome
  - ❖ Myasthenia gravis
  - ❖ Sedative poisoning.
- *Tuberculosis:* Meningitis
- *Asthma:* Systemic vasculitis.

Gastrointestinal

- *Change of appetite:* Hypothalamic lesion
- *Excessive thirst*
  - ❖ Diabetes insipidus
  - ❖ Diabetes mellitus.
- *Dysphagia*
  - ❖ Pharyngeal
  - ❖ Myasthenia gravis.
- *Constipation*
  - ❖ Any neurological disease involve nerve supply to bowel
  - ❖ Dysautonomia.
- *Vomiting:* Increased intracranial pressure

- *Hepatitis*
  - ❖ Cryoglobulinemia
  - ❖ Vasculitis.

Genitourinary

- *Urinary frequency:* Diabetes
- *Urinary retention:* Neurogenic bladder
- *Polyuria:*
  - ❖ Diabetes mellitus
  - ❖ Diabetes insipidus.
- *Spontaneous abortion:* Anticardiolipin syndrome
- *Pus in urine or at glans:* Syphilis
- *Red urine:* Myoglobinuria—Polymyositis, Rhabdomyolysis.

Menstrual History

- *Use of oral contraceptive:* Hypertensive stroke
- *Hormone replacement:* Migraine.

Blood

- Anemia—Vitamin B_{12}—subacute combined degeneration
- VT—Anticardiolipin syndrome.

Musculoskeletal

- *Arthritis:* Connective tissue diseases
- *Muscle*
  - ❖ Myositis
  - ❖ ALS
- *Myalgia:* Myositis.

Skin

- *Rash*
  - ❖ Drug reaction
  - ❖ Lyme disease
- *Infection:* Tick paralysis
- *Birth mark:* Phakomatosis.

Endocrine

- *Galactorrhea:* Chromophobe tumor—in Pituitary fossa
- *Amenorrhea:* Pituitary insufficiency
- *Club-shaped hand:* Acromegaly
- *Thyroid:*
  - ❖ Carpal Tunnel syndrome
  - ❖ Thyrotoxic myopathy.

Relevant History Regarding Pain in Neck and Arm
- Onset—time of onset—acute subacute or chronic
- Duration of pain
- Radiation to arm, shoulder, pectoral girdle, periscapular region
- History of birth injury, trauma to neck, infection, immunization
- Any history of disc prolapse.
- *Aggravation*
  - ❖ Neck movement
  - ❖ Movement of arm and shoulder
  - ❖ Coughing
  - ❖ Sneezing
  - ❖ Straining during defecation.
- Any history of weakness of arm or hand
- Any site of anesthesia or peresthesia in arm or hand
- Any history of bladder or bowel involvement or sexual dysfunction—It indicates spinal cord compression.

Relevant History of Low Back Pain
- Onset—time of onset—acute, subacute or chronic
- Duration of pain
- *Location of pain*
  - ❖ Back
  - ❖ Buttock
  - ❖ Thigh
  - ❖ Leg.
- *Radiation to*
  - ❖ Buttock
  - ❖ Back of thigh
  - ❖ Knee
  - ❖ Foot.
- *Any history of*
  - ❖ Trauma to back
  - ❖ Disc herniation
  - ❖ Disc surgery.
- Any history of weakness of lower limb muscle
- Any anesthesia or hyperesthesia of lower limb.
- *Aggravating factors*
  - ❖ Movement at low back—bending, stooping, leg motion
  - ❖ Coughing
  - ❖ Sneezing
  - ❖ Straining at stool.
- Any involvement of bladder, bowel involvement—it indicates cauda equina syndrome.

- *Any history of systemic involvement:*
  - ❖ Fever
  - ❖ Weight loss
  - ❖ Morning stiffness.

Relevant History to Differentiate Radiculopathy from Others

- Symptom—continuous or intermittent
- If intermittent—relation with time of the day, tetany for nocturnal symptoms
- Duration of each episode
- Frequency, i.e. the gap between two episodes
- Pain in hand/arm
- Relation with activities—driving
- Pain is neck, arm or wrist
- Old history of wrist or neck
- Weakness of muscles of arm or hand
- Any associated involvement of speech, vision
- Any numbness of hand
- Any involvement of opposite hand.

Symptoms in Differential Diagnosis of Peripheral Neuropathy

- Onset—acute or insidious
- Frequency—intermittent or constant
- History of injury to low back, disc herniation, disc surgery
- Associated pain in lower limb muscle
- Bilateral symmetrical or asymmetrical
- Any associated bladder, bowel or sexual dysfunction
- Any sensory symptom—like paresthesia, numbness
- Drinking of alcohol
- History of systemic disease—Diabetes, vitamin deficiency
- History of smoking
- Any associated weight loss
- Family history of similar episode.

Symptoms of Transient Ischemic Attack–Related to Vertebrobasilar Insufficiency

- Date of 1st attack, number of attacks
- Duration of each attack—from the party
- Frequency between two attacks
- Any history of premonitory symptoms

- Which part of the body is involved—whether any variation of distribution of involvement in any attack
- Any associated symptoms—like difficulty in swallowing, disturbances in vision, speech disturbances
- Any history of chest pain, shortness of breath
- Any history of systemic disease—diabetes mellitus, hypertension, coronary artery disease, hyperlipidemia
  History of drug abuse, peripheral vascular disease
- Any residual weakness of any side of the body
- Medications like oral contraceptives antihypertensive.

Symptoms Related to Alzheimer's disease—which may be Helpful to Differentiate other Conditions

- Duration of the problem
- Progress—whether it is static or getting worse or improves
- Forgetfulness—of minor one-like—date of anniversary
- Patient can control checkbook
- Any tendency to get lost
- Drug history—OCP drugs
- History of immunization, alcohol abuse
- History of headache, recent trauma to head
- History of systemic disease—thyroid disease, anemia, vitamin B_{12} deficiency, sexually transmitted disease
- History of depression
- History of involvement of bladder and bowel
- Any history of disturbances in smell or taste
- Any imbalance in walking
- Any family history of Alzheimer's disease.

PHYSICAL EXAMINATION

Physical examination: It includes:
- General examination
- Neurological examination.

■ General Examination

Vital Signs

- *Blood pressure:* It should be examined in supine, sitting and standing position
  - ❖ High—in case of CVA
  - ❖ Orthostatic hypotension—syncopal attack
  - ❖ Low pressure—syncope, septicemia in case of CVA.
- *Pulse:*
  - ❖ Bound in anemia, thyroid disease, aortic regurgitation
  - ❖ Low volume—aortic stenosis.
- *Temperature:*
  - ❖ High, in meningitis, septicemia, brain abscess
  - ❖ Low temperature—thyroid disease, septicemia.

General Appearance

- *Evidence of acute or chronic illness:* Pain, fever or distress
- *Abnormal posture*—of head, trunk and extremities
- *Motor activities:* Bizarre activity, unusual mannerism, irritability, restlessness, no movement
- *Weight loss with evidence of malnutrition:* Hyperthyroidism, Whipple's disease, celiac disease, Amyloidosis, Alzheimer's disease
- *Body fat and hair distribution and secondary sexual development:* Endocrine disorder, hypothalamic disorder
- *Abnormal development:* Gigantism, acromegaly, dwarfism, Cushing's syndrome, gross contracture, deformities, amputation, cretinism
- *Specific abnormal posture*
  - ❖ *Spastic hemiplegia:*
    - *In affected upper limb:* Flexion and adduction at shoulder. Flexion at elbow and at wrist
      Flexion and adduction of fingers.
    - *In affected lower extremity:* Extension at hip, knee and ankle.
      Equinus deformity of foot.
  - ❖ *Parkinson disease and Parkinson plus disease:*
    - Flexion of neck, shoulder, trunk, elbow and knee with rigidity and stooping

- Masked face
- Slowness of movement
- Pill-rolling tremor.
- ❖ *Myopathies:*
  - Protrusion of abdomen
  - Lordosis of back
  - Calf muscle hypertrophy
  - Waddling gait.
- ❖ *Peripheral neuropathy:*
  - Foot drop
  - Wrist drop
  - Claw hand.

These neurological deformities can be confused with following deformities.

- Pes cavus
- Changes due to trauma, arthritis
- Developmental abnormalities
- Abnormal habitual posture.

Head

Inspection

Size, shape, contour, symmetry of head, scar, suture, dilated veins, telangiectatic areas should be observed.

- Premature closure of skull may produce deformity
- Shape—hydrocephaly, microcephaly, macrocephaly
- Scar—it indicates previous trauma, surgery
- Port-wine Angioma—in scalp, face—in trigeminal nerve distribution or overlie cerebral hemangioma.

Palpation

If may disclose:

- Craniotomy
- Burr-hole
- Tenderness
- Scar.
  - ❖ *In children:* Bulging of fontanels and separation of suture—it occurs due to increased intracranial pressure.
  - ❖ *Palpable skull defect occurs in:*
    - Meningocele
    - Encephalocele.
  - ❖ *Palpable masses:* In scalp and skull:
    - Lymphoma
    - Leukemia
    - Multiple myeloma

- Dermoid
- Metastatic carcinoma.
- ❖ *Localized masses in the scalp*—Osteomyelitis
- ❖ *Exostoses*—Underlying meningioma
- ❖ *Before closure of suture massive enlargement of skull and frontal bossing-sunset appearance*-Hydrocephalus
- ❖ *Tenderness of superficial temporal arteries*-Giant cell arteritis.
- ❖ *Transillumination test*—positive in:
  - Hydrocephalus.

Percussion

It may disclose:
- *Dullness*
  - ❖ Side of the tumor
  - ❖ Sides of subdural hematoma.
- *Tympany*
  - ❖ Hydrocephalus
  - ❖ Increased intracranial pressure.

Auscultatory Percussion

Percussion in midfrontal area and auscultation over the various parts of the head discloses:
- Sides of tumor
- Subdural hematomas.

Auscultation

Bruit can be heard in following areas:
- **Cephalic bruit:** It can disclose:
  - ❖ Arteriovenous malformation
  - ❖ Aneurysm
  - ❖ Angioma
  - ❖ Neoplasm compressing over large arteries
  - ❖ Presence of atherosclerotic plaques occluding partially cerebral or carotid arteries
  - ❖ In absence of any disease.
- *Ocular bruit*
  - ❖ Intracranial arteriovenous malformation
  - ❖ Intracranial arteriovenous aneurysm.
    Bruit can be disappeared by compressing carotid arteries.
- *Carotid bruit:* Over carotid arteries due to carotid artery stenosis in presence of atherosclerotic plaque—carotid bruit can be transmitted to mastoid
- *Murmur:* It can be transmitted to cranium from heart and great vessels.

Facial Expressions

- *Gross facial deformities:*
  - ❖ Cretinism
  - ❖ Myxedema
  - ❖ Acromegaly
  - ❖ Gigantism
  - ❖ Down's syndrome.
- *Special facial expression*—characteristic of few diseases:
  - ❖ Masked face—Parkinsonism
  - ❖ Masked face with precipitated laughter and crying—pseudobulbar palsy.
  - ❖ *Grimacing:*
    - Athetosis
    - Dystonia
  - ❖ *Ptosis and weakness of facial muscles:*
    - Myasthenia gravis
    - Myopathies.

Eye Examination

Ophthalmologic examination may reveal:
- Etiology of neurological disease
- Presence of systemic disease.
  - ❖ Bilateral exophthalmoses—Grave's disease
  - ❖ *Unilateral proptosis:*
    - Carotid—cavernous fistula
    - Encephalocele
    - Meningocele
    - Histiocytosis x.
  - ❖ *Brushfield spots:* Down's syndrome
  - ❖ *Corneal clouding:* Mucopolysaccharidosis
  - ❖ *Lisch nodules:* Neurofibromatosis
  - ❖ *Tortuous conjunctival vessels:* Ataxia telangiectasia
  - ❖ *Keratoconjunctivitis sicca:* Sjögren syndrome
  - ❖ *Kayser-Fleischer ring:* Wilson's disease
  - ❖ *Scleritis:* Wegener's granulomatosis
  - ❖ *Unilateral arcus senilis:* Unilateral carotid stenosis
  - ❖ *Interstitial keratitis:* Cogan syndrome
  - ❖ *Pigmented pingueculae:* Gaucher disease

Ear examination is necessary in patient with hearing loss or vertigo.
Following informations can be found:
- Perforation of tympanic membrane
- *Glomus tumor:* Jugular foramen syndrome
- *Vesicles in external ear:* Herpes Zoster
- *CSF otorrhea:* Trauma–fluid may be scrous or bloody

- *In comatose patient:* Calorie test to be done—but it must be cleared that:
  - ❖ Tympanic membrane must be intact
  - ❖ Canal must be clear.

Nose

- Perforation of nasal septum—cocaine abuse
- Saddle-shaped nose—congenital syphilis
- Bacterial infection—cavernous sinus thrombosis
- Watery discharge—CSF rhinorrhea.

Mouth

Tongue

- Smooth translucent tongue with atrophy of filiform and fungiform papillae, reddened: Pernicious anemia
- *Smooth reddened, atrophic tongue:* Thiamine deficiency
- *Triple furrowed tongue:* Myasthenia gravis
- *Lingua plicata:* Melkersson-Rosenthal syndrome
- Macroglossia:
  - ❖ Amyloidosis
  - ❖ Myxedema
  - ❖ Acromegaly
  - ❖ Down's syndrome.
- *Xerostomia:* Sjögren syndrome
- *Lead line (blue) in the gum:* Lead poisoning
- *Trismus:* Tetanus, polymyositis
- *Mucosal ulcer:* Behçet disease
- *Notched teeth:* Congenital syphilis.

Neck

Neck should be examined for:

Adenopathy, thyroid enlargement, tenderness, masses, rigidity, pain during movement, posture abnormalities.

Normal Movement of Neck

- Chin rest on the chest.
- Rotary movement from side to side.
  - ❖ Nuchal rigidity, neck retraction, opisthotonus:
    - Meningeal irritation
    - Cervical spondylosis
    - Cervical radiculopathy
    - Dystonia.

- ❖ Neck short, broad, movement limited, low hair line:
  - Klippel-Feil syndrome
  - Syringomyelia
  - Platybasia.
- ❖ Carotid artery auscultation—for bruit.

Respiratory system
Respiratory rate, rhythm, depth, movement of chest during respiration should be examined.

Breathlessness, orthopnea dyspnea—it may occur in case of neuromuscular inco-ordination, myasthenia gravis.

Cardiovascular system
Neurological diseases may be linked with:
- Hypertension
- Valvular heart disease
- Subacute bacterial endocarditis
- Ischemic heart disease
- Arrhythmia
- Atherosclerosis.

Abdomen
Examination of abdomen should be done for.
Abdominal masses, enlarged viseras, fluid, abnormal pulsation.
The following findings may be found:
- *Hepatomegaly*
  - ❖ Hepatitis
  - ❖ Cirrhosis
  - ❖ Hepatocellular carcinoma
  - ❖ Amyloidosis
  - ❖ Carbohydrate storage diseases.
- *Splenomegaly*
  - ❖ Lymphoma
  - ❖ Leukemia
  - ❖ Cirrhosis
  - ❖ Infectious mononucleosis
  - ❖ Amyloidosis.
- *Ecchymosis:* Retroperitoneal hematoma
- *Ascites:* It is due to hepatic encephalopathy.

Genitalia and Rectal Examination

Following findings may be a due to neurological disease.
- Chancre in penis—Syphilis
- Ulceration in penis—Behçet disease
- Angioma in scrotum—Fabry's disease

- Rectal examination is necessary—in:
  - ❖ Myelopathy
  - ❖ Cauda-equina syndrome
  - ❖ Conus medullaris syndrome.

Spine

Here mobility, deformity, abnormality of posture, tenderness should be examined.

- *Marked kyphosis (gibbus):*
  - ❖ Tuberculosis
  - ❖ Neoplasm
- *Marked lumbar lordosis*—Muscular dystrophy
- *Marked scoliosis*
  - ❖ Friedreich ataxia
  - ❖ Syringomyelia.
- Localized rigidity + slight scoliosis + absence of lumbar lordosis—Lumbosacral radiculopathy
- Dimpling of skin and unusual hair growth over sacrum—spina bifida.

Extremities

Here limb deformities, contracture, edema, size and shape of hands to be examined.

Wasting, ulceration, localized tenderness can be visualized.

Following findings may be found

- Edema—congestive cardiac failure, cardiomyopathy
- *Arthritis*
  - ❖ Connective tissue disease
  - ❖ Whipple's disease
  - ❖ Sarcoidosis.
- Painless arthropathy—Sarcoidosis
- *Decreased peripheral pulses*
  - ❖ Takayasu disease
  - ❖ Atherosclerosis.
- *Acrocyanosis:* Ergotism
- *Palmar erythema:* Alcoholic liver disease.

Hair and Nails

- *Premature graying of hair*
  - ❖ No obvious cause
  - ❖ Pernicious anemia
  - ❖ Hypothalamic disorder.
- Transverse lines on the nails (Mees lines)—Arsenic poisoning

- *Clubbing of fingers*
  - ❖ Bronchogenic carcinoma
  - ❖ Heart disease.
- Abnormal capillary loop in nail bed—Dermatomyositis.

Nodes

Lymphadenopathy—it may occur in:
- Lymphoma
- Leukemia
- HIV
- Mononucleosis
- Niemann-Pick disease
- Gaucher disease
- Sarcoidosis.

Skin

- Spider angioma—Alcoholic liver disease
- Erythema chronicum migrans—Lyme disease
- *Purpura*
  - ❖ Meningococcemia
  - ❖ Rocky mountain spotted fever
  - ❖ TTP.
- *Livedo reticularis*
  - ❖ Antiphospholipid syndrome
  - ❖ Cryoglobulinemia.
- *Hyperpigmentation*
  - ❖ Addison's disease
  - ❖ Nelson syndrome
  - ❖ Carotenemia.
- *Trophic ulcers*
  - ❖ Syringomyelia
  - ❖ Tabes dorsalis
  - ❖ Syphilis.
- Heliotropic erythema in the face—Dermatomyositis
- Needle mark, scar mark—IV drug user
- Skin nevi—Hemangioma of spinal cord
- Greasy and seborrheic skin—Parkinsonism
- Vesicular eruption along the spinal root—Herpes Zoster
- Signs of vitamin deficiency—Subacute combined degeneration of spinal cord.

■Outline of Neurological Clinical Examination

Major sections in neurological examination and short screening to elicit abnormalities:

- *Mental status:* It can be elicited during conversation of examiner. It is barometer of mental status.
  - ❖ If patient is logical, coherent alert and gives sensible to the point answer—he is mentally alert
  - ❖ If patient is incoherent, gives incomplete, disjointed, scattered history—he is mentally impaired.
- **Cranial nerves**
  - ❖ *Using penlight:*
    - Pupillary light reaction—direct and indirect (III and II cranial nerve)
    - Visual field—(II cranial nerve)
    - Extraocular movement—(III, IV, VI cranial nerve)
      If the patient does not give the history of diplopia—there may not be any necessity to examine III, IV and VI cranial nerve.
  - ❖ Fundoscopic examination of retina.
  - ❖ *Motor function of V cranial nerve:*
    - If unilateral—jaw moves towards affected side during history taking
    - If bilateral—patient's jaw drops—during conversation.
  - ❖ *XII cranial nerve:* While opening the mouth:
    - If unilateral—tongue moves towards affected side
    - If bilateral—tongue becomes atrophic
      In both cases—fasciculation is present.
  - ❖ *VIII cranial nerve:* If patient does not give any history of tinnitus or deafness—one need not examine this cranial nerve
  - ❖ *IX and X cranial nerve:* If patient does not give the history of dysphagia, dysphonia, nasal regurgitation of fluid there is unnecessary to examine these cranial nerves
  - ❖ *VII cranial nerve:*
    - During history taking—history of saliva dribbling, lacrimation, difficulty in answering questions examination of VII cranial nerve is essential
    - Checking of nasolabial furrow
    - During grimacing—Following things should be seen:
      - Deviation of angle of mouth
      - Number of teeth of both sides
    - Tight closure of eye
    - Relective amplitude and velocity of lower facial contraction and symmetry of upper facial contraction.
- *Screening examination of motor function, sensory function and co-ordination of upper and lower extremities:* Cortico-spinal tract (CST) innervates the following muscle groups of upper and lower extremities:
  - ❖ *In upper extremities:*
    - Finger extensors

- Wrist extensors
- Forearm supinators
- External rotation of shoulder
- Triceps
- Deltoid.
  ❖ *In lower extremities:*
  - Hip flexors
  - Hamstring
  - Dorsiflexors of feet and toes
❖ Fine motor control to distal muscles
  - *In upper extremity the best muscles to examine are:*
    - Deltoid
    - Triceps
    - Wrist extensors
    - Finger extensors
    - Small muscles of hand—mainly interossei.
  - *In CST lesion:* Finger flexors and wrist flexors are not innervated
  - Pronator drift—It should be examined with eyes closed
  - Upper extremity stereognosis
  - Upper and lower extremity simultaneous stimulation, while waiting for drift
  - Finger-nose test, eyes closed
  - Examination of finger and arm roll
  - Examination of lower extremity strength, heel-knee test
  - Sensory assessment
  - Deep tendon reflexes of upper and lower extremities
  - Plantar response—bilateral
  - Romberg test.

Mental Status

Orientation

Normally all the people are orientated in:

- Time
- Place
- Person.
  ❖ Most people of modern world are oriented to time within 15 minutes. Ask the patient to know, what is the time now?
  ❖ Ask the patient, "Where you are staying now?" "Where is your residence?"
  ❖ Patient with right parietal lobe lesion is usually disoriented to place, sometimes have bizarre ideas of place orientation.
  ❖ "Who is he?"—patient cannot recognize him is acute state or chronically with severe dementia.

Memory

Insight

The patient may have insight into his illness and implication of any functional impairment.

Patient with nondominant parietal lobe illness has lack of insight.

Judgment

Ask the patient that what he will do if he finds a sealed addressed, stamped envelope on the sidewalk in a theater. The patient will answer properly normally. But if there is lesion in orbitofrontal region, the patient behaves inappropriately and impulsively.

Abstract thinking

Ask the patient few common proverbs to interpret, e.g.

- A rolling stone gathers no moss
- A stitch in time saves time.

Patient sometimes cannot interpret if:

- He does not know the proverb
- Patient has psychiatric disease.

So it may be useful to ask mixed and confused proverb, "The hand that rocks the cradle, should not throw stones". It can test patient's abstraction ability and sense of humor.

The abstraction ability is impaired in frontal lobe lesion.

Frontal lobe function

- *Formal test* requires the patient to sort the cards by color, shape and number and then recognize the change in scheme.

  Patient with lesion in dominant prefrontal cortex cannot recognize the scheme.
- *Trail making test*
  - ❖ Patient is asked to connect the letter or number in sequence
  - ❖ Patient is asked to connect the letter and number in alternate manner, e.g. A-1-B-2-C-3 ....
- *Luria fist edge-palm test:* The patient is asked to repetitively place his hand in a series of motion—fist—followed by edge followed by palm over and over
- *Copy of task:* It involves drawing simple figures with extra-multiple loops within already drawn loops
- *Little-big test:* The words "little" and "big" are written in separate cards in upper case and lower case letters.

  The patient is required to respond "big" if the written word is in upper case even if the letter is print "little" or vice versa.

  The patient with frontal lobe lesion, all above tests are abnormal.

Calculation

Calculation depends upon
- Native intelligence
- Mathematical ability
- Educational level
- Number sense.

Following types of calculation can be tried:
- To perform mental calculation of two digit
- To perform calculation of moderate level of difficulty
- Addition or subtraction of a column of two or three digit number.
- Subtraction of serial 7 from 100.
- Counting backward from 30.

Impaired calculation ability may occur from posterior dominant hemisphere lesion.

Attention

Disturbances in attention

Attention can be defined as awakening state in which sensory stimulation can be perceived from peripheral organ system to cerebral cortex through thalamic nuclei, basal ganglia and mesencephalic formation.

Alertness is always associated with attention, but reverse is not true, e.g., Akinetic mutism in which patient is alert, although his eyes dirt towards the stimulus, but he is immobile and mute.

Alertness preceding attention may be specific for a stimulus or nonspecific.

Alertness for specific stimulus is called attention. This attention may be passive—involuntarily triggered by external stimuli, or may be active—where external stimuli triggers attention directly.

Active attention is mediated by
- Superior parietal lobule
- Superior portion of dorsal prefrontal cortex.

    Both hemispheres participate in active attention. Systems activated by external stimuli are lateralized to right hemisphere in right handed person—It involves:
    - Inferior parietal lobule
    - Posterior portion of superior temporal gyrus
    - Inferior portion of prefrontal cortex.

Cortical alerting mechanism—activated by brainstem structures
- Mesenchymal reticular formation—sends sensory stimuli—responsible for arousal
- MRF—facilitates the relay of sensory information to cortex by inhibiting—nucleus reticularis thalami, which projects to and inhibits thalamic relay nuclei

- ❖ Lesion in unilateral MRF—It produces contralateral neglect or contralateral inattention—because thalamic sensory nuclei are being inhibited by nucleus reticularis thalami
- ❖ Bilateral lesion of MRF—It produces coma
- ❖ Dorsal mesencephalic lesion produces contralateral visual inattention due interruption of uncrossed pathways from superior colliculus to dorsolateral prefrontal cortex

Primary sensory cortical area for vision (Brodmann area 17)

↓

Projects to visual association area (Brodmann area 18) (unimodal specific area)

↓

Projects to multimodal sensory association area—in parieto-occipital lobe.

This area combines information from vision, hearing and somatosensory stimuli

↓

Corticofugal pathways—It inhibits nucleus reticularis thalami and potentiates thalamic relay nuclei

↓

Provides further arousal of cortex.

Unimodal sensory areas of cortex inhibit a specific area of nucleus, reticularis thalami, where as multimodal areas inhibit nucleus reticularis thalami in general fashion.

Basal ganglia sends sensory input to cortex through thalamus.

Pulvinar sends impulse through thalamus to parietal and frontal attention areas.

- ❖ Lesions of any component of network or their interconnections including white fiber bundle—results in neglect.
- ❖ Lesions—in unilateral posterior parietal areas—It produces sensory extinction associated with neglect.
- ❖ Lesion in frontal or basal ganglionic areas—It produces neglect which includes disruption of orientation towards neglected hemisphere (Fig. 11.12).

Unilateral inattention or neglect is characterized by:

- *Hemi in attention or hemi neglect:* Lack of orientating response to unilateral visual or tactile stimuli—in the absence of primary sensory or motor deficit.
- Extinction to double simultaneous stimulation—patient perceives on the affected side to single stimulation, not on simultaneous stimulation to both sides.
- *Hemiakinesia or motor neglect:* Patient directs all his activities on one hemisphere.
- *Allesthesia:* All contralateral stimuli are attributed to ipsilateral stimuli.

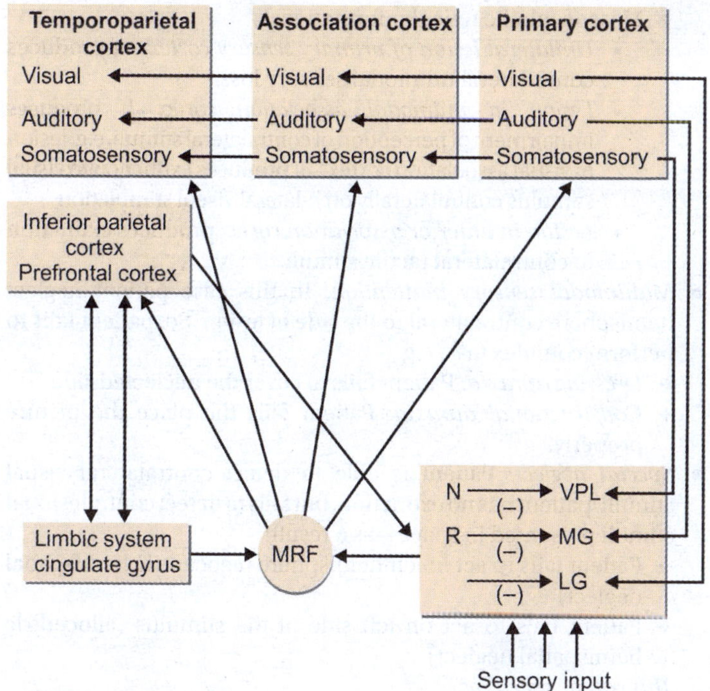

FIG. 11.12 Pathways of attention, arousal and neglect

Neglect may be:
- *Primary sensory (sensory inattention):* This sensory neglect is unilateral (e.g. visual inattention), so that specific sensory modality is less well perceived on one side.

  There is also sensory extinction to double simultaneous stimulation, patient fails to detect the stimulus contralateral to the side of lesion.

  This can be explained by following fact:

  Stimuli from one side compete with the stimuli from other side for cortical activation. So, in case of unilateral lesion, cortical activation of the affected hemisphere will be present, even if patient does not see the visual stimulus on the affected side.

  Contralateral inattention can be seen with the lesion of:
  - Inferior parietal lobule
  - Lesion in temporoparieto-occipital junction
  - Dorsolateral frontal lobe
  - Cingulate gyrus
  - Insular cortex
  - Thalamus

- ❖ Mesencephalic reticular formation
  - *Unilateral lesion of primary sensory cortex*—it produces contralateral unimodal sensory loss
  - *Lesion in unimodal association cortex*—It produces impairment of perception of contralateral stimuli, e.g. lesion of visual association cortex—It produces extinction to visual stimulus contralaterally on bilateral visual stimulation
  - *Lesion in anterior association cortex* produces extinction to contralateral tactile stimuli.
- *Multimodal sensory inattention:* In this case patient neglect hemisphere contralateral to the side of lesion. So, patient fails to perform complex task, e.g.
  - ❖ *Dressing apraxia:* Patient fails to cover the neglected side
  - ❖ *Constructional apraxia:* Patient fails the place the picture properly.
- *Special neglect:* Patient is able to detect contralateral visual stimuli, patient has no extinction, but fails to detect contralesional stimuli presented in space—as a result:
  - ❖ Patient fails to act in left hemisphere (egocentric hemispatial neglect)
  - ❖ Patient fails to act on left side of the stimulus (allocentric hemispatial neglect)
- *This can be tested by:*
  - ❖ *Line bisection test*
  - ❖ *Cancellation task* (whether patient can cross out all the lines presented on the paper).
- *This spatial neglect may be:*
  - ❖ Horizontal neglect
  - ❖ Vertical neglect
  - ❖ Radial neglect.

Involved lesion producing special neglect
- Inferior parietal lobule
- Insula
- Caudate nucleus
- Lenticular nucleus
- Striatum
- Internal capsule
- White matter tract (cortico-strito-nigral tract).

Severity of neglect is determined by
- Size of lesion
- Degree of prior diffuse cortical damage.

Lesion in right nondominant hemisphere
- Responsible for inattention to both hemisphere
- Inattentive to their bodies
- Distracted by right sided extracorporeal stimuli.

Hemiakinesia

It is an unilateral motor neglect—as a result:

- Patient may not look towards one side of the space, but readily react when stimulus will come from that space
- Patient cannot move limbs contralateral to the side of lesion—unless he is asked to do so.

The areas involved and responsible for hemiakinesia: Hemiakinesia may be developed as a result of lesion of either hemisphere—affecting dorsal, goal directed attentional network.

- Hemiakinesia occurs contralateral to the side of lesion
- Ipsilateral hemiakinesia may occur with lesion of ipsilateral basal ganglia and frontal lesions
- In few cases unilateral neglect and extinction are associated with hemiakinesia—lesion involving area and of the medial and lateral premotor area of frontal lobe—mainly right hemisphere—may be responsible for this syndrome
- Akinesia may also result from lesion of:
    - ❖ Basal ganglia
    - ❖ Ventral thalamic
    - ❖ Frontal lobe
    - ❖ Limbic system.

Nonspatial inattention: Inattention to non spatial behavior, e.g. inability to concentrate on a task, with consequent motor or verbal impersistance.

Motor impersistence: Inability to keep closed eyelids—it occurs in right sided hemispheric lesion—right central and frontal lesions are mainly responsible—Patient are more distractible.

Lesions in left caudate and frontal lobe: It produces impairment in ability to divide attention between two sources and to focus the attention to one source.

Verbal impersistence: Patient may be laconic and tends to repeat sentences spoken to them or near them—Echolalia.

Patient may try to imitate gesture (echopraxia).

The lesions responsible are:

- Advanced Alzheimer's disease
- Metabolic encephalopathies—impairing subcortical mechanism
    - ❖ When focal lesion—responsible—it affects mesial aspect of frontal lobe
    - ❖ When large lesion responsible—it produces akinetic mutism—patient becomes mute and motionless with normal sleep-wall cycles
    - ❖ Medial diencephalon—mesencephalic lesion
    - ❖ Unilateral or bilateral caudate nuclear lesion—It produces apathy, disinhibition, effective disturbances

❖ Unilateral or bilateral basal ganglia lesion—It produces in apathy, failure to thrive, stereotyped behavior, compulsive and obsessive behavior.

Perseveration behavior can be divided into three categories:

1. *Recurrent perseveration*: Repetition of previous response to subsequent stimulus—lesion of left temporoparietal cortex.
2. *Stuck-in-set perseveration*: Inappropriate maintenance of activity. Lesion—frontosubcortical and mesolimbic lesion.
3. *Continuous perseveration*: Abnormal prolongation of a current activity. Lesion—right hemisphere damage.

Intrusion

Abnormal verbal utterances. Cholinergic deficiency is responsible for intrusion in Alzheimer's disease.

- *Intrusion during free recall*—It is due to impaired activation of right superior prefrontal cortex
- *Intrusion during cued recall*—It is due to impaired activation of left anterior medial temporal cortex
- *Verbal intrusion*—It occurs in delirium
- *Motor intrusion*—It occurs in Parkinson's disease.

Emotional Disturbance

Emotions and their expressions depend upon several factors

- *State of arousal are mediated by:*
  - ❖ Reticular activating system
  - ❖ Thalamic nuclei
  - ❖ Medial frontal cortex.
- *Vegetative functions are governed by:*
  - ❖ Periaqueductal structures
  - ❖ Brainstem regions
  - ❖ Limbic system
  - ❖ Dopaminergic structures
  - ❖ Striatum
- *Memory is mediated by:*
  - ❖ Hippocampus
  - ❖ Limbic system.
- *Ability to perceive the affective component of various stimuli* such as verbal threat, angry face, threatening utterance. This is controlled by various structures of cerebral and subcortical structures
  - ❖ *Patient with bilateral damage of amygdala nucleus*—It can recognize the expression of fear when directed to look at the eyes

- ❖ *Aphasic patient with lesion in the inferior parietal lobule and superior temporal gyrus* is unimpressed by verbal threat, but react to threatening speech or feared face
- ❖ *Patient with lesion in right parietotemporal region,* can understand the meaning of verbal threat, but perception to emotional tone is impaired (sensory aprosodia)
- ❖ *Patient with right parieto-occipital lesion* has impairment of ability to perceive facial expression
- ❖ *Patient with right fronto-parieto-occipital lesion and orbitofrontal cortex* has reduced ability to identify and describe one's own feelings.
- *Ability to evaluate properly the importance of internal and external stimuli* for survival and well-being of the patient
    - ❖ *Patients with bilateral orbitofrontal destructive lesion* are social nonsense and trivial, they may go into rage when basic instinctive desire is not fulfilled
    - ❖ *Patient with bilateral cingulate gyrus lesion* becomes unconcerned in presence of painful stimuli
    - ❖ *Patient with bilateral anterior temporal lesions* has bland effect
    - ❖ *Patient with lesions in septal regions*—has irritability and rage reactions
    - ❖ *Patient's right orbitofrontal penetrating wounds* have edginess, anxiety, depression
    - ❖ *Patient with left dorsofrontal penetrating wounds* has anger and hospitality
    - ❖ *Patient with left temporal lobe epileptogenic focus* has paranoid, antisocial behavior
    - ❖ *Patient with right temporal lobe epilepsy* has emotional extremes (elation, sadness)
    - ❖ *Patient with medial temporo-occipital lesions* (parahippocampal fusiform and lingual gyri) are disorientated, agitated, abusive
    - ❖ *Patient with lesion in brainstem and thalamic reticular activating system* has delirium, confusional state
- *To express emotion, it requires intact motor system:*
    - ❖ *Lesion in right frontal hemisphere*: There is impairment of voluntary emotional intonation of speech
    - ❖ *Pathological crying or laughing result from:*
        - Bilateral lesion in internal capsule
        - Lesion in basal ganglia
        - Lesion in substantia nigra
        - Cerebral peduncle
        - Hypothalamus
        - Corticobulbar fibers.

- ❖ *Pathological laughing may rarely occur from:*
  - Acute basal ganglia lesion
  - Brainstem stroke
  - Left carotid infarction.

Dominant hemisphere subserves positive feelings and non-dominant hemisphere subserves negative feeling because:

- Left hemisphere lesions induce pathological crying. Right hemisphere lesion induces pathological laughing
- Left hemisphere lesion tends to produce more depression than the right hemisphere lesion
- Patient with left hemisphere damage are anxious, tearful and abusive where as patient with right hemisphere damage are indifferent and jocular
- Patient with single stroke involving left anterior cortical or subcortical lesion have severe depression than the lesion involving other areas
- Patient with single stroke involving right hemisphere shows no sign of depression
- Mood is depressed by endogenous depression and mania. Few anatomic sites are involved in mood control.

  Stimulation or disruption of circulatory near subthalamic nucleus—It results in depression or mania.

- Temporal lobe contains limbic system that is involved in modulation of emotional behavior:
  - ❖ *Patient herpes simplex encephalitis has:*
    - Emotional disturbances
    - Hypermetamorphosis
    - Agnosias
    - Eating and drinking problems
    - Improper sexual display
    - Irritability
    - Aggressiveness
    - Emotional blunting.
  - ❖ *Patient with complex partial seizures involving temporal lobe has:*
    - Altered sexual behavior
    - Hyper religiosity (sudden religious conversion, excessive bible reading, attachment with unorthodox religious group)
    - Hypergraphia
    - Aggressive behavior.

Memory

It is a type of information which is stored in different parts of brain. Types of memory along with storage area in brain:

- *Episodic memory:* Events in life of an individual or data base type of information. Areas involved are—Amygdala and hippocampal region of medial temporal region and other portion of Papez circuit
- *Procedural memory:* Memory of skill based learning (how to use tools)
  Area involved: Prefrontal cortex and basal ganglia
- *Immediate memory:* Retaining memory of short periods of life. *This is of three types:*
  1. Immediate memory for verbal material—*Dominant presylvian cortex.*
  2. *Prosopagnosia*—Immediate memory for faces—*Both lingual gyri.*
  3. *Immediate tactile memory:* Somatosensory area.
- *Focal lesion in the above area:* It produces loss of above immediate memory
- *Antegrade amnesia:* Loss of ability to create new memories after the event caused by amnesia.
- *Retrograde amnesia:* Loss of ability of recall of memories of some duration. As these memories relate to older material, they are gradually better and the patient can remember the materials that occurred 11–30 years before the event.

How far back the memories are lost depends upon:
- Degree of mesial temporal damage
- Additional frontal or temporal damage
- Type of memories.

Cortical amnesic syndrome is characterized by:
- Episodic memory will be lost but procedural memory is unaffected
- Immediate memory will be lost if focal areas responsible for immediate memory is affected
- Multimodal impairment
- Variable deficit of recall of memories, acquired within certain interval (1–2 years).

The areas involved in amnesic syndrome:
- Medial temporal lobes (hippocampal gyrus, amygdala)
- Anterior and dorsomedial nucleus of thalamus
- Connection structures.
  The above circuit determines which memory requires saving and which do not.

According to new most widely accepted view:
Hippocampus—works with neocortex → allow memories to be encoded and then accessible.

Co-ordinated works of hippocampus and neocortex—gradually strengthens the neocortico—neocortical connections. Ultimately neocortical memory can be accessed without the help of hippocampus.

Then these remote memories are stored in distributed cortical frame works—associated with other modalities—visual, auditory, tactile.

Many patients with memory loss do not have typical amnesic syndrome, they have attentional difficulties, typical of frontal lobe dysfunction.

Working Memory

This is a temporarily stored memory in frontal cortex which can be used for cognitive function. It is composed of two components:
1. *Short term storage* (on order of seconds)
2. *Executive process*—that operates on contents of storage.

Storage Areas

- **Storage of verbal material:** Broca's area, left hemisphere supplementary and premotor areas.
- **Storage of spatial material:** Right hemisphere, premotor cortex.
- **Storage of object information:** Right prefrontal cortex.

Two types of executive process:
1. Selective attention
2. Task management.

Both the processes activate anterior cingulated gyrus and dorsolateral prefrontal cortex (Fig. 11.13).

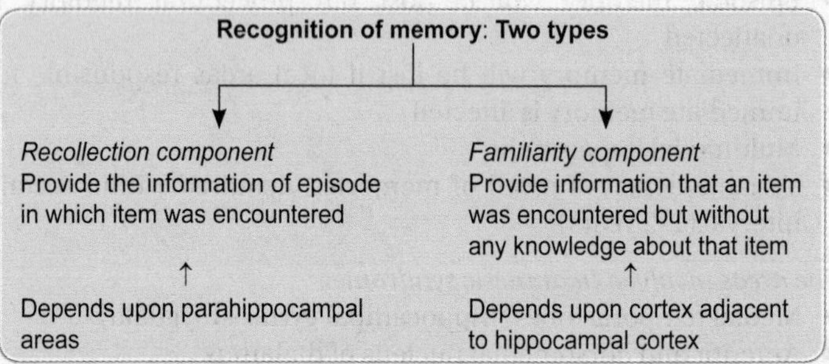

Difference between medial temporal and thalamic lesion producing amnesic syndrome:
Patient with lesion in anteromedial thalamic nucleus—confabulate—i.e. patient gives factitious responses to "fill-in" memory gaps (results from impaired activation of orbitofrontal and medial prefrontal structures).

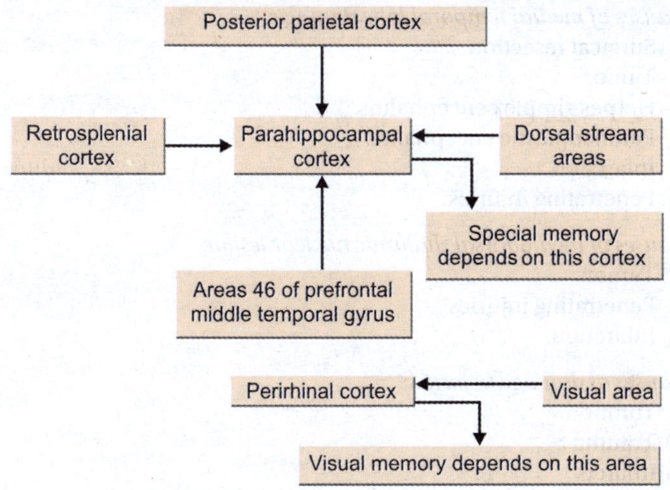

FIG. 11.13 Pathways of memories

But patient with bilateral lesions in medial temporal areas—is aware of deficit.

Patient with left temporal lobe lesion—impairs the storage of language related information.

Patient with right temporal lobe lesion—impairs the storage of visual related information.

In acute lesion—even in case of unilateral lesion—both verbal and nonverbal materials are equally affected. But with time, in left hemisphere lesion only verbal information are affected than nonverbal materials.

Because verbal tasks are used often to test memory, impairment of verbal memory usually involves left hemisphere.

Papez Circuit

- Hippocampus
- Fornix
- Mammillary body
- Mammillothalamic tract
- Anterior and dorsomedial thalamic nuclei
- Cingulate gyrus
- Cingulum.

    Lesion bilaterally and involvement of any of above structure producing amnesic syndrome.

- Retrosplenial cortex connecting anterior thalamus with medial temporal structures → it is an alternative route between hippocampus and thalamus.

Causes of medial temporal lobe damage:
- Surgical resection
- Tumor
- Herpes simplex encephalitis
- Paraneoplastic encephalitis
- Infarction
- Penetrating injuries.

Causes of mediodorsal thalamic nuclear lesion:
- Tumor
- Penetrating injuries
- Infarction.

Causes of damage to fornix:
- Tumor
- Trauma
- Infarcts
- Surgery (removal of colloidal cyst).

Unilateral amnesic stroke involves territories of:
- Posterior cerebral arteries
- Choroidal arteries
- Thalamic penetrating arteries.

Hallucination

Smell hallucination

Epileptogenic foci in temporal lobe—it produces hallucination of smell accompanied by mouthing and chewing movements.

Gustatory hallucination

If occurs in parietal, temporal or temporo parietal seizures.

Visions

Visual hallucination: It is caused by:
- Psychiatric, disorder
- Medical
- Neurological
- Ocular disorder
- Drug-induced states
  - *Vitreous detachment:* Brief vertical flash of light (Moore's lightening streaks) in the temporal field of vision, predominantly with eye movements—best seen in eye closed or in the dark—it indicates mechanical stimulation of retina
  - *Optic neuritis:* It is associated bright flashes of light with eye movements or in responds to sudden loud sounds
  - *Amaurosis fugax:* Patient experiences bright light flashes or scintillations.

Mainly two types of hallucinations:
1. *Simple visual hallucination:* It consists of:
   - ❖ Flashes of light (photopsia)
   - ❖ Different colored lines in zigzag, circle or fortification pattern with defective field of vision.

   Diseases associated are:
   - ❖ Inferomedial occipital epileptic focus—Multi-colored circular or spherical pattern of light
   - ❖ In migraine involving inferomedial occipital region, it produces black and white zigzag lines
   - ❖ In occipital brain, tumor produces unformed visual hallucination in one hemifield (icteral in nature)
   - ❖ In heavy exercise produces unformed visual hallucination in one hemisphere.
2. *Complex visual hallucinations:*
   - ❖ *Temporal lobe seizure:*
     - Hallucination of landscape or animal
     - Autoscopic phenomenon (hallucination of the self)
     - Illusory phenomenon (micropsia, metamorphopsia).
   - ❖ Hippocampal stimulation
   - ❖ Structural brain lesion—Lewy body disease, tumor
   - ❖ Lesions in upper midbrain and also involve thalamus often bilaterally

     Visual hallucinations—Oneiroid (dream like) quality hypnagogic, unreal, pleasant to patient—Peduncular hallucinosis.
   - ❖ Isolated bilateral medial substantia nigral infarct—It produces visual hallucination—when it also destroys pars reticulata—produces peduncular hallucinations
   - ❖ Left cerebral peduncle infarction and right paramedian thalamic infarction—without midbrain involvement—peduncular hallucinosis occurs
   - ❖ Bilateral medial occipital region lesion and right lateral thalamic lesion—visual hallucination with preceding complete loss of dream

     Damage of ARAS
     ↓

     Rostral projections from midbrain to intralaminar thalamic nuclei affection
     ↓

     Peduncular hallucination.
   - ❖ Visual complex hallucination with impaired vision occurs in elderly *(Charles Bonnet syndrome)* with presence of normal cognition, associated visual deprivation.

This hallucination usually occurs in the evening, made up of small bright colored object or people, or cartoon like appearance. Patient is aware of this unreality and change in color and size when touched.

This occurs as a result of release phenomenon in ventral temporo-occipital cortex—an area poorly activated by visual area in these patients.

- Hallucination of colors—*It is due to activation of fusiform cortex*—area corresponding to color center.
- Hallucination of black and white color—*Activation of regions outside this area.*
- Hallucination of unfamiliar face—*Activation of left middle fusiform gyrus.*
- Hallucination of brick work fences—*Activation of collateral sulcus.*

Other types of visual phenomenon associated with visual loss:
- *Tessellopsia*—regular, repeating phenomenon
- *Dendropsia*—branching pattern
- *Hyperchromatopsia*—hyperintense bright colors.

Simple and complex hallucinations may be classified into three groups:
1. Irritable lesion in cerebral cortex—typically stereotyped, associated with other seizure manifestations.
2. Nonepileptogenic foci—Lewy body disease.
3. Those with impaired visions—with visual acuity 20/50 or less. Release hallucination—it may occur due to:
   ❖ Liberation of endogenous cerebral visual activity from control of visual inhibitory centers
   ❖ Lesion anywhere from retina to visual cortex pathways.

Cerebral Polyopia

- It occurs with lesion in occipital or parieto-occipital cortex
- It occurs with mono-ocular diplopia—both images are with equal clarity, does not resolve with a pinhole, is unchanged with viewing mono-ocularly with either eye or binocularly.

Palinopsia

Image recurs immediately after diverting the gaze from the object or the object removed from visual filed.

It recurs with each blinking, not affected by eye closure.

The image moves in the direction of head movements.

It occurs in:
- Focal nondominant parieto-occipital or occipitotemporal lesion
- Recovering from cortical blindness in the recovering area of visual filed
- Creutzfeldt-Jakob disease

- Multiple sclerosis
- Cerebral vasculitis
- Drug-induced—interleukin-2
  The above causes are due to: Ischemia, trauma, tumors, abscess, AV malformation.
- Migraine
- Cerebral abscess
- Carbon dioxide poisoning.

■ Language

Language involves:
- Speech (verbal language)
- Comprehension
- Reading
- Writing.

Speech impairment means:
- Dysphonia
- Dysarthria
- Apasia.

Dysphonia

Difficulty in phonation. Voice may be hoarse, in severe cases there is complete loss of phonation, e.g. mutism, aphonia.

The causes are:
- Laryngitis (common cold)
- Hypothyroidism (thickening of vocal cord due to myxomatous tissue deposits)
- Unilateral laryngeal nerve paralysis
- Lesion in vagus nerve.

Dysarthria

Normal articulation of speech requires:
- Tongue movements against the teeth (glottal)
- Precise movement of lips and mouth (labial)
- Closure of nasopharynx (tensor veli palatini)
- Co-ordinated movements of tongue, lips, palate, larynx, respiration is responsible for normal phonation.

Examination of Dysarthria

Ask the patient to enunciate British Artillery Brigade. This can distinguish—whether there is problem with labial (British), glottal (Artillery).

Watch the loudness, rhythm, modulation and tone of speech (Weakness of tensor veli palatini).

Types of Dysarthria

- *Spastic dysarthria:* In this type of dysarthria:
    - ❖ Tongue is small
    - ❖ Speech is spastic
    - ❖ Limited movement of lips and mouth
    - ❖ Particular difficulty with letters b, p, d, r.

    Speech becomes slow, harsh, strained, grunts at the end of phrase.

    Lesions responsible:
    - ❖ Bilateral upper motor neuron lesion disease
    - ❖ Corticospinal tract lesion
    - ❖ Brain tumor
    - ❖ All causes of pseudobulbar palsy.
- *Extrapyramidal dysarthria:*
    - ❖ *Parkinsonism:* Slow monotonous speech, loss of modulation, words run into one another, sentence starts and stops suddenly
    - ❖ *Hyperkinetic dysarthria:*
        - Inability to sustain phonation due to laryngeal articulatory interruptions
        - Prolonged interval between words
        - Inappropriate silences
        - Sometimes ends of sentence may be spoken explosively.
- *Ataxic dysarthria:* There is difficulty in co-ordination of muscles of speech and breathing.

    Speech becomes slurred, scanned (due to unco-ordination of speech and breathing). Changes from loud to soft, arrhythmic.

    The causes are: Hereditary cerebellar disease, multiple sclerosis, drug intoxication, superior cerebellar artery stroke, tumor.
- *Dysarthria from lesion of lower motor neuron and muscles:*
    - ❖ Facial paralysis (VII nerve) pronounces the following consonants—"b", "p", "m", "w", with difficulty
    - ❖ Tongue weakness and paralysis (XII nerve)—It produces severe dysarthria and pronunciation of words with "l", "d", "n", "s", "t", "x" and "7" will be difficult
    - ❖ Palatal paralysis producing weakness of tensor veli palatini, and produces nasal intonation of speech

        The letter   "b" and "d" sounds like "m"
                 "n" and "g" distorted like "rh"
                 "k" sounds like "na"
- *Myasthenic dysarthria:* Voice may be normal at the beginning of each sentence or while started after taking some rest.

As the sentence progresses—hoarseness will occur, tone becomes low—due to palatal weakness
Alternate motions of lips, tongue and mandible—(diadochokinesia).

This can be tested by—asking the patient to repeat:
Put (labial), tuh (lingual), key (posterior aspect of tongue).

Aphasia (Figs 11.14A and B)

Aphasia: Loss or impairment of language function caused by—structural and functional damage of brain.

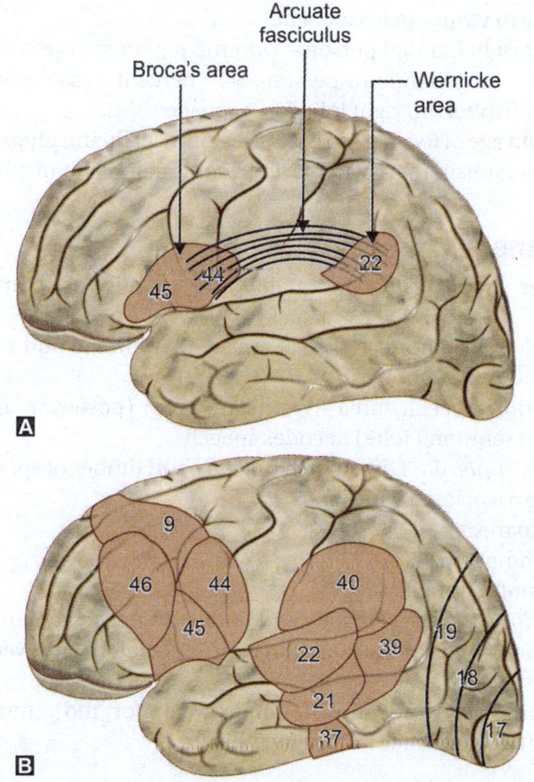

FIGS 11.14A AND B   (A) Language area; (B) Neuroanatomy of reading

Aphasia means combinations of following deficit:
- Prosody—Rhythm of speech
- Timber—Modulation of speech
- Naming—Small parts of common objects
- Ability to follow command of the midline
- Color naming
- Reading and writing
- Repetition of words or sentence.

Preliminary Information

Examiner should know:
- Native language
- Educational level
- Ability to read
- Ability to write, spell, calculate
  - ❖ For right handed person—Dominant hemisphere is left lobe
  - ❖ For left handed person—90 percent case dominant hemisphere in right lobe for language
  - ❖ Upto age of 6 years—in case of lesion in left hemisphere speech mechanism may switch over to contralateral hemisphere.

Spontaneous Speech

Examiner should listen the quality and quantity of spontaneous speech.

Anterior speech areas (Broca area, SMA) initiate and maintain spontaneous speech.

Posterior speech area—Wernicke area (posterior third of dominant temporal lobe) decodes speech

In anterior aphasia: Difficulty in prosody and timber of speech.

It may be associated with:
- Hemiparesis
- Agrammatism
- Ideomotor apraxias.

In posterior aphasia—Prosody and timber of speech are normal but comprehension is abnormal. It may be associated with Neologism (nonsense word).

Paraphasias, word substitutions (green for red), translitoral aphasia (two consonants used together).

Comprehension of Speech

Patient can utilize both hemispheres to perform midline commands, e.g.
- Stick your tongue out

- Get up
- Close your eyes.

Comprehension should be tested by avoiding midline commends. So patient should be asked:
- To point up and down with thumb
- To point to an object in the room
- To place an object in a specific places.

Naming the Object

Aphasic patient has some degree of nominal aphasia. Patient is asked to name a small part of common object, e.g. pen or watch.

Notes the speed of response, paraphasias, neologism, perseveration. Patient can be asked to pick up the object by name.

Repetition of Words

Patient is asked to repeat simple sentence of complex words.
This test evaluates:
- Wernicke area which decodes speech
- Arcuate fasciculus that connects the Wernicke area with Broca area In conduction aphasia (arcuate fasciculus) patient cannot properly repeat simple sentence, but enunciate complex words, e.g. The simple sentence "Today is Sunny day" can be repeated as "Today Sunny" but properly enunciate "Presidential address".

Reading

Patient is asked to read words or sentences and to perform specific actions.

Posterior parietal area (39, 40, 41) and Wernicke area are important for decoding language.

Writing

Patient is asked to write his or her name and address and take dictations or to write few sentences about weather.

Anterior aphasia is associated with agrammatism, *posterior aphasia* is associated with writing disabilities.

Exner's area, anterior to Broca area is responsible for writing.
Damage to this area produces difficulty in writing.

Calculation

Ask the patient to calculate small problem.

This is a component of posterior aphasia. So posterior parietal deficit produces dyscalculia.

Anatomic Points Regarding Aphasia

- Major speech areas are pre and postsylvian fissure
- If the lesion is in pre and postsylvian fissure, repetition is abnormal
- If patient is aphasic and repetition is normal, no perisylvian fissure pathology

  This type of a aphasia is transcortical aphasia. It may be:
  - Transcortical motor aphasia—present superior to Broca area
  - Transcortical sensory aphasia—present posterior and inferior to sensory area

    These aphasias occur in the water shed distribution of Anterior cerebral artery/Middle cerebral artery/(ACA/MCA) or Middle cerebral artery/Posterior cerebral artery posteriorly.

Types of Aphasias (Figs 11.15A to D)

- *Broca aphasia:*
  - Difficulty in initiation or articulation of speech
  - Difficulty in prosody or timber of speech
  - Speech is nonfluent
  - Reading comprehension is abnormal because lack of comprehension of grammatically sensory words
  - Writing difficulties
  - Comprehension is intact
  - Repetitions of simple word is abnormal.
- *Wernicke's aphasia:*
  - Difficulty in comprehension of spoken words
  - Repetition is difficult in spoken language
  - Normal prosody or timber of speech
  - There is presence of paraphasias (verbal or literal), neologism, consonants, errors, circumlocution, word substitutions
  - Patient may be word—deaf (can understand other sounds)
  - Patient may be word—blind (cannot read words)
  - Patient may have associated superior quadrantic field defect.
- *Conduction aphasia:*
  - Speech is fluent, but repetition is abnormal
  - Naming is abnormal
  - Comprehension is preserved
  - Writing is impaired
  - No dysarthria
  - Lesion is in arcuate fasciculus or supramarginal gyrus.

Aphasia classification

According to severities:

	Fluency	Auditory comprehension	Repetition	Naming	Reading	Writing
Broca	–	+	–	–	–	–
Global	–	–	–	–	–	–
Wernicke	+	–	–	–	–	–
Conduction	+	+	–	+/–	+	+
Anomic	+	+	+	–	+	–
Transcortical motor	–	+	+	–	–	–
Transcortical sensory	+	–	+	–	–	–
Verbal aphasia	–	+	–	–	–	+
Transcortical mixed	–	–	+	–	–	–

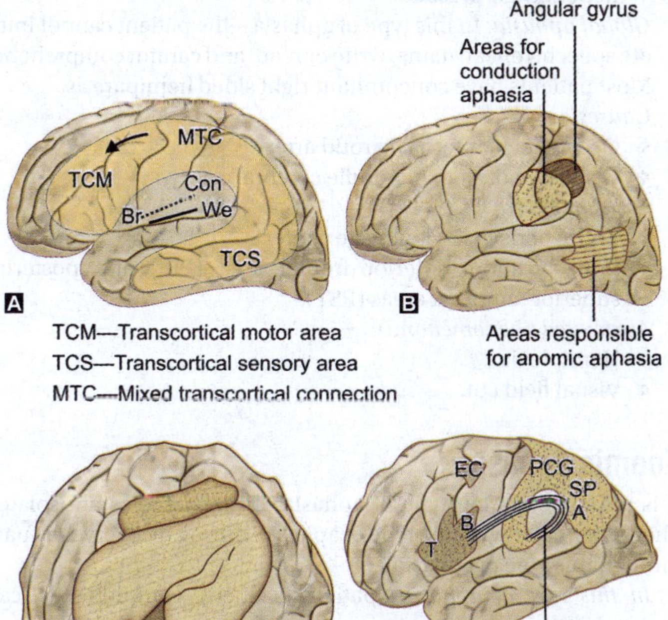

A
TCM—Transcortical motor area
TCS—Transcortical sensory area
MTC—Mixed transcortical connection

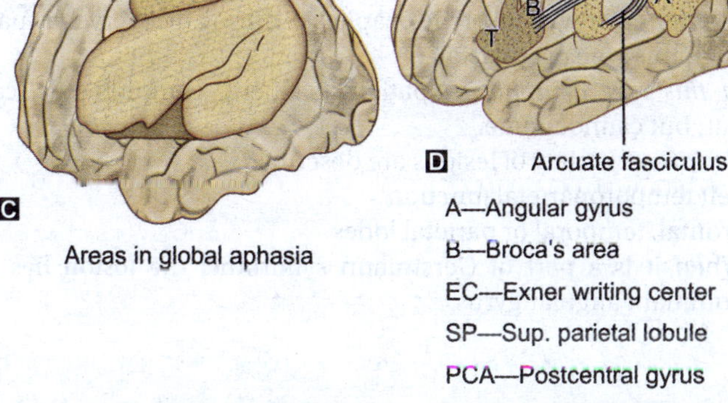

Areas in global aphasia

A—Angular gyrus
B—Broca's area
EC—Exner writing center
SP—Sup. parietal lobule
PCA—Postcentral gyrus

FIGS 11.15A TO D   Different areas of speech center in cerebrum

- *Transcortical aphasia:* This is a syndrome in which the presylvian language area is preserved but disconnected from the rest of the brain. The cause is usually water shed infarction.

  In this type of aphasia, repetition is so much intact that patient may display echolalia.

  In transcortical mixed aphasia—Repetition is intact, but comprehension or fluency of speech will be disturbed.

  In transcortical motor aphasia—anterior isolation syndrome:
  - Fluency is absent
  - Comprehension is intact
  - Repetition is present
  - Difficulty in naming.

  In transcortical sensory aphasia—(posterior isolation syndrome):
  - Fluency in present
  - Comprehension is absent
  - Repetition is present.

- *Global aphasia:* In this type of aphasia—the patient cannot initiate speech, repeat, name, write or read, and cannot comprehend. Most patients have concomitant right sided hemiparesis.
  Causes:
  - Occlusion of internal carotid artery
  - Occlusion of stem of middle cerebral artery.

  Areas involved:
  - Entire perisylvian language center
  - Both posterior inferior frontal area (PIF) and posterior superior temporal areas (PST).

  Associated phenomenon:
  - Hemiplegia
  - Visual field cut.

Anomic Aphasia

It is a most common type of aphasia. It may arise as an isolated phenomenon or with any type of aphasia, during recovery may pass through this type of aphasia.

In this type of aphasia—patient is fluent, comprehends, can repeat; but cannot name.

The lesion—A variety of lesions are described:
- Left temporoparietal junction
- Frontal, temporal or parietal lobes
- When it is a part of Gerstmann syndrome, the lesion lies in dominant angular gyrus.

Subcortical Aphasia

- In acute onset—there is initial mutism followed by aphasia of Broca type
- Verbal output is slow and poorly disarticulated, spastic, dysarthric
- Reduplicative speech, where patient can repeat the last part of the ward or sentence
- Naming and reading are unimpaired
- *The structures involved*
  - ❖ AV and DM nuclei of thalamus
  - ❖ Red nucleus
  - ❖ Putamen
  - ❖ Nuclei of basal ganglia.

All the above structures must be of the language dominant hemisphere.

Language disturbance due to nondominant hemispheres lesion:
In case of nonright-handed person—there may be some speech-controlling cells present in nondominant hemisphere. In these cases, patient may recover somewhat from aphasia but emotional and automatic speech may be present.

So, nondominant hemispheric lesion may affect non-linguistic form of speech element—like emotional and rhythm element:
Prosody is:
- Melodic form of speech
- Volume of speech
- Modulation of speech
- Intonation of speech
- Inflection.

So, *hyperprosody* means exaggeration.
Hypoprosody means diminished prosody
Aprosody means absence of prosody.

Aphemia

It is most severe form of dysarthria—*lesion is in frontal operculum—which is the cortical motor innervations of VII, X and XII cranial nerves.*

In this lesion, the patient is mute at onset followed by severe dysrhythmic—syntax and word choice normal.

Unilateral lesion may be in Broca's area or undercuts of white matter of left frontal operculum.

Echolalia

Patient can repeat the words or phrases just heard without knowing fully the meaning the same.

Lesion

Dominant temporoparietal cortex.

Pure Word Deafness

In this type of lesion, the patient can read, write, fluent, but cannot comprehend spoken words or repeat it.

Patient can recognize nonverbal sound.

Lesion:
- Damage of *Heschl's gyrus* and destruction of *radiation from medial geniculate body* and *callosal fibers* from contralateral superior temporal gyrus.

   Above lesion separates the auditory association area of left dominant hemisphere from auditory input.
- Bilateral damage of mid portion of superior temporal gyrus.

Nonverbal Auditory Agnosia

Patient cannot comprehend non-verbal sound.

Lesion in Nondominant Hemisphere
Cortical deafness: Patient cannot comprehend spoken words or nonverbal sounds—but aware of words or sound.
Lesion:
Bilateral damage to Heschl's gyrus and its connections.

Alexia

Loss of ability to read the written language in absence of any loss of vision—is called alexia. These patient can recognize the spelled word, or when written on the palm or palpate the word and recognize.

The region of angular gyrus of dominant hemisphere connect the visual cortex through some association fibers. So any *lesion in angular gyrus or its connection with visual cortex produces alexia.*
The etiology—Occlusion of posterior communicating artery producing infact to left occipital lobe and splenium of corpus callosum.
Alexia with agraphia is more common than isolated alexia.
Alexia may be accompanied by:
- Acalculia
- Nominal aphasia
- Hemianopia
- Some degree of visual agnosia.

Agraphia

This can be defined as inability to write in absence of any weakness, inco-ordination or other neurological dysfunction related to muscles of arm and hand.

Three types of agraphia:
1. *Aphasia:* All types of aphasia are usually accompanied by agraphia except—pure word blindness or pure word mutism.
2. *Constructional:* This type of apraxia is associated with agraphia.
3. *Apraxia:* This is due to inability to proper use of hand of writing—in absence of other neurological deficit.

Agraphia is usually contraction of words, transposition of words or symbols, omission of letters or symbols or syllables or mirror writing.

Lesion
Anterior frontal (Exner's area 45) or posterior parietotemporal syndromes.

Acalculia
Inability to calculate is called acalculia. It is of following types:
- *Aphasic acalculia:* Patient cannot comprehend well enough to write number correctly or substitute one number with another
  Lesion: It is in posterior parietal cortex of speech dominant hemisphere.
- *Visuospatial acalculia:* Patient is unable to place the number in correct position or place
  Lesion: Parieto-occipital junction of nondominant hemisphere.

von Gerstmann's Syndrome
The following constellation of symptoms are present:
- Agnosia
- Acalculia
- Inability to cross the midline
- Right to left confusion.

Occasionally following may be present:
- Agraphia
- Constructional apraxia
- Conduction aphasia.

If angular gyrus is extensively involved:
- Alexia
- Agraphia
- Nominal aphasia.

Apraxia
Inability to carry out purposeful, familiar acts on request in absence of any weakness, sensory loss or other neurodeficit involving affected part. There are many types of apraxia. These are the following:

- *Limb kinetic apraxia:* In this lesion, due to very mild involvement of corticospinal tract lesion, patient may not be paretic, but severe enough to produce inco-ordination and dexterity—so patient's fine motor control is impaired
- *Ideomotor apraxia*
  - ❖ Patient is unable to carry out complex commands (salute, wavy good bye, snapping fingers) with one or both extremities
  - ❖ Patient may be unable to pantomime how to use the common implements (comb, hammer, tooth brush)
  - ❖ They may substitute finger or hands for imaginary objects (finger for comb) and show how to use it without actually using it
  - ❖ Patient in few cases unable to carry out some functions imaginally, but can perform when actual object will be given.
    Lesion: Disconnection between visual center or language center that understand the command and motor areas—those responsible for carrying out such activities.
- *Sympathetic apraxia:* Inability of a patient to perform complex motor acts with nonparetic limb in presence of dominant hemispheric lesion.

  For example, patient with left hemispheric lesions causing Broca's aphasia may be unable to perform wavy good bye with his left hand.

  Lesion: Fibers connecting language areas of dominant hemisphere with motor areas of nondominant hemisphere are usually disrupted.

  Patient can understand the command, no weakness of the performing hand, but unable to carry out command because right hemisphere cannot receive any command.
- *Ideational apraxia:* In this apraxia, when a patient is asked to perform a sequences of movement, he may omit or forget some steps of that composite movement. For example:
  - ❖ When asked to derive a car he may try to put the car in before starting the enzene
  - ❖ Patient may mail a letter without putting the letter into an envelope or without affixing stamp.

  Lesion:
  - ❖ Lesion in left posterior temporoparietal junction
  - ❖ Cognitive impairment.
- *Buccofacial apraxia:* The patient is unable to execute the complex act involving muscles of mouth, lip and face without any paresis of these muscles. For example:

  Whistling, blowing horn, coughing, pursing lips.

  Patient may spontaneously perform these acts, e.g. licks his lips—but cannot perform on command.

Lesion: Degeneration of frontal operculum, which is the cortical region of all activities requiring cranial nerves for swallowing, facial muscle movement, tongue movements.

- *Constructional apraxia:* Patient is unable to construct geometric complex forms because of impaired visuospatial skills, for example:
  - ❖ Patient may copy geometric form, but three-dimensional cube cannot
  - ❖ Patient can draw individual shapes, but cannot perform or make complex figures with above shapes
  - ❖ Patient with hemineglect may fail to put the numbers on one side of the clock
  - ❖ Patient with frontal lobe involvement or confusion, may be disorganized in his work
  - ❖ Patient with cognitive impairment, may not be able to arrange the number in sequence
  - ❖ Rey-Osterrieth figure—It can bring out subtle constructional apraxia.

    Constructional apraxia can differentiate patient with neural impairment from patient with psychological impairment, in latter case there will no evidence of constructional apraxia.

    Lesion: Frontal lobe lesion.

- *Dressing apraxia:* Patient has difficulty in dressing and undressing themselves. This can be tested by following manners.

    Turn one sleeve of hospital gown inside out and ask the patient to put it on. Patient with dressing apraxia faces immense difficulty to perform this act.

    Lesion: Right occipitoparietal or bilateral occipitoparietal lesion.

    Patient with hemineglect may fail to dress one side of the body.

- *Visual apraxia:* These patients are unable to copy of one act and perform it in similar manner.

    For example, ask the patient to follow the examiner's hand. Then examiner withdraw his hand.

    Normally, patient should see the position of hand, understand and hear the task to be performed, and then he has to position his hand in exactly similar position. Patient with visual apraxia cannot perform this position.

    Lesion: "Engram" of desired movement first should be copied in the brain (in premotor cortex and supplementary motor cortex)—then it will be relayed to primary motor cortex.

    So, lesion in prefrontal cortex and supplementary motor cortex—It prevents the patient to make the "engram", and the patient cannot make proper position of his hand.

- *Gait apraxia:* There are two types of gait apraxia:
  1. *Magnetic gait:* Here the patient's foot gets stuck to the floor. He can move the foot for few inches, then it becomes stick again.
  2. *Egg-walking:* Here the patient can lift his feet up as if he is walking on eggs. Here there is no advance.

  Lesion:
  - ❖ Failing to activate various brainstem center, mainly nucleus cuneiformis of the midbrain
  - ❖ Normal pressure hydrocephalus—here descending motor fibers of corticospinal tract is compressed by expanded lateral ventricle
  - ❖ Lacunar stroke—affecting descending corticospinal fibers
  - ❖ Basal ganglia disease.

- *Callosal apraxia:* Patient is unable to perform even simple task with left hand.

  To execute the simple task following neural pathways must be considered:
  - ❖ The method and command of the task must be understood and heard by Wernicke's area (left hemisphere)
  - ❖ This information must cross the midline anteriorly along corpus callosum to reach right (nondominant) primary motor cortex for execution. So, the lesion and the causes are:
    - In patient with lesion in prefrontal cortices or corpus callosum—signals will be interrupted
    - Occlusion of prefrontal branch of superior division of middle cerebral artery
    - Strokes in anterior cerebral artery
    - Callosotomy for epilepsy
    - Frontal lobe glioma.

- *Apraxia of eyelid opening:* Here patients is unable to open their eyes on command, they think that they are blind they occasionally press their eyelids with glasses.

  One painful stimulus or startle responses open their eyes.

  Lesion: Second frontal convolution of frontal eye fields.

  Conceptual apraxia: Frontal lobe degeneration responsible for this apraxia.

Visual Agnosia (Fig. 11.16)

Impairment in ability to recognize an object visually in absence of loss of visual acuity or loss of intellectual function account for it.

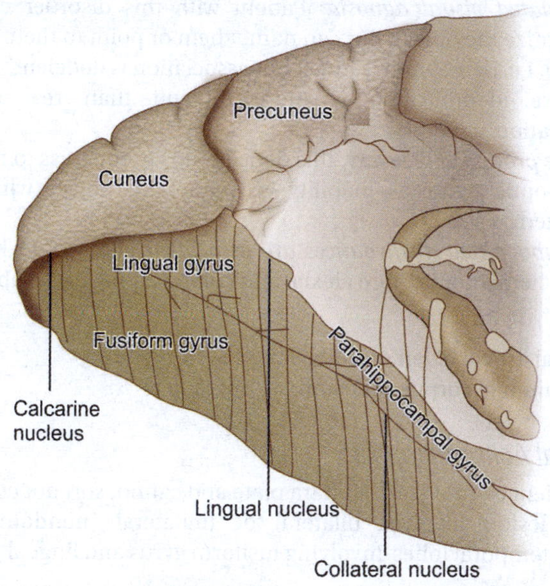

FIG. 11.16 Medial aspect of occipital lobe

Two factors are responsible for visual recognition:
1. Perception of an object
2. Correlating the newly percepted object with previously encoded percept—association.

So two types of visual agnosia occur:
1. *Appreciative visual agnosia:* These patients avoid obstacles during walking, but cannot name the item, draw the item or match the item, presented to them.

     Their visual aquity and visual fields are normal.

     Defect lies on the impairment of visual pattern recognition.
     Lesions: Bilateral ischemic lesions in calcarine cortex or occipito-temporal region in patient recovering from cortical blindness. They can distinguish change in intensity and hue of minute source of light.

     The extrastriatal pathway including pulvinar, superior colliculus, and parietal lobe may play a role in recognition of light.

2. *Associated visual agnosia:* Patient with this disorder cannot recognize the object, but can name them or point to them when asked, i.e. perception is intact but association is deficient.

Picture identification is more difficult than real object identification.

In the process of recovery, this deficit tends to progress to milder deficit—optic agnosia—inability to name the object which is recognized.

The above two disturbances are associated with—right homonymous hemianopia, pure alexia, and color-naming of the object.

Lesions
- Mesial aspect of left occipital lobe
- Splenium of corpus callosum.

Cerebral Achromatopsia

This patient cannot read ishihara plate and cannot sort out colors.

The lesion involves bilateral or unilateral (nondominant) occipitotemporal lobes-involving fusiform gyrus and lingual gyrus.
↓

Thin lesions are associated with infracalcarine lesion that damages the middle third of lingual gyrus and white matter on the posterior third of lateral ventricle.

Common causes:
- Vertebrobasilar disease
- Herpes simplex encephalitis
- Metastatic lesions
- Focal seizures
- Transient phenomenon in migraine.

The vascular lesions involves inferior branch of posterior cerebral artery sparing calcarine branch supplying visual cortex.

Color perception area involves lateral aspect of collateral sulcus involving fusiform gyrus. It mediates color perception of both upper and lower hemifields:
- Superior hemifield represented by fusiform gyrus more medially
- Inferior hemifield represented by fusiform gyrus more laterally.

Patient with achromatopsia often associated with superior quadrantanopia because inferior optic radiation is affected.

Color Agnosia

This patient can read ishihara chart or can sort out the color according to hue, but:

- It cannot name the color or spot the color directed by the examiner.
- It can perform verbal to verbal task (name the color of sky).

The lesion involves inferomedial aspect of the occipito-temporal lobe of dominant hemisphere.

Patient with color agnosia often associated with right homonymous hemianopia, alexia.

Homonymous hemianopia occurs due to involvement of:

- Optic radiation
- Lateral geniculate body
- Calcarine cortex.

Prosopagnosia

This patient:

- Fails to identify faces or objects that are visually similar (fail to identify car in car parking area)
- Fails to tell the number of members in families
- Fails to identify the picture of well-known personalities and fails to identify himself (e.g. fail to identify himself in front of mirror).

Lesion involves—fusiform gyrus—structure which functions as visual association area for recognition of specific faces.

Patient with prosopagnosia can better recognize face than object and vice versa:

- Object recognition can be represented in left temporo-occipital cortex and do not involve right hemisphere.
- Face recognition can be represented in fusiform or occipito-temporal gyrus of right hemisphere or bilaterally.

The causes are:

- Bilateral posterior cerebral artery occlusion
- Encephalitis
- Hypoxia
- Tumor
- Trauma
- Hematomas

- Alzheimer's disease
- Parkinson's disease
- Developmental defect.

Prosopagnosia may be associated with:
Strange paradoxical knowledge:
- When confronted with picture of Mona Lisa, patient usually says—it cannot be a picture of Mona Lisa
- Nonanatomical views (patient is unable to identify the eye glasses when folded, but can when unfolded).

Landmark Agnosia

Patient is unable to recognize familiar landmark.
Lesion involves: Discrete regions in the depth of right lingual sulcus straddling the lingual and parahippocampal gyrus.
- *Prosopagnosia and other visual agnosia* results from temporo-occipital lesions (vertical hatching).
- *Visual simultanagnosia*—It results from occipitoparietal lesion bilaterally (stippling).
- Unilateral lesion in either hemisphere may cause *contralateral field defect with hemiachromatopsia.*
- *Unilateral left hemisphere lesion* (occipitotemporal area) and splenium of corpus callosum—It results in alexia with agraphia.

Visual Simultanagnosia

Inability to appreciate the meaning of a whole, though the elemental parts can be recognized.

For example, patient is unable to recognize complex figure made up of multiple subunits, but can recognize the subunits separately.

Visual simultanagnosia is associated with unilateral or bilateral inferior quadrantic defect but formal testing is difficult because patient fails to keep the eyes stationary on target.

Some patients with visual simultangnosia "can look but not see" with apparent "disappearance of stationary objects from the direct view"—this occurs due to lesion in superior occipital lobe lesion.

Attentional mechanism: This is required for sustained awareness of visual target—it depends on superior vision association cortex which is being destroyed during lesion of superior occipital lobe.

CRANIAL NERVES

◼ Functional Components of Cranial Nerves (Figs 11.17A and B)

- *Olfactory nerve:* Special sensory nerve
- *Optic nerve:* Special sensory nerve
- *Oculomotor nerve:*
  - ❖ Somatic efferent
  - ❖ Visceral efferent.
- *Trochlear nerve:* Somatic efferent
- *Trigeminal nerve:*
  - ❖ Somatic afferent
  - ❖ Brachial efferent.
- *Abducens nerve:* Somatic efferent
- *Facial nerve:*
  - ❖ Brachial efferent
  - ❖ Visceral efferent
  - ❖ Visceral afferent
  - ❖ Somatic afferent.
- *Vestibulocochlear nerve:* Special nerve
- *Glossopharyngeal nerve:*
  - ❖ Brachial efferent
  - ❖ Visceral efferent
  - ❖ Visceral afferent
  - ❖ Somatic afferent.
- *Vagus nerve:*
  - ❖ Brachial efferent
  - ❖ Visceral efferent
  - ❖ Visceral afferent
  - ❖ Somatic afferent.
- *Accessory nerve:* Brachial efferent
- *Hypoglossal nerve:* Somatic efferent.

Foramina for Cranial Nerve in the Base of the Skull

- *Inferior fossa*
  Olfactory nerve: Perforation through cribriform plate.
- *Middle fossa*
  Optic nerve: Optic foramen
  III, IV, VI and ophthalmic division of trigeminal nerve: Superior orbital fissure.
  Maxillary division of trigeminal nerve: Foramen rotundum.
  Mandibular division of trigeminal nerve: Foramen ovale.

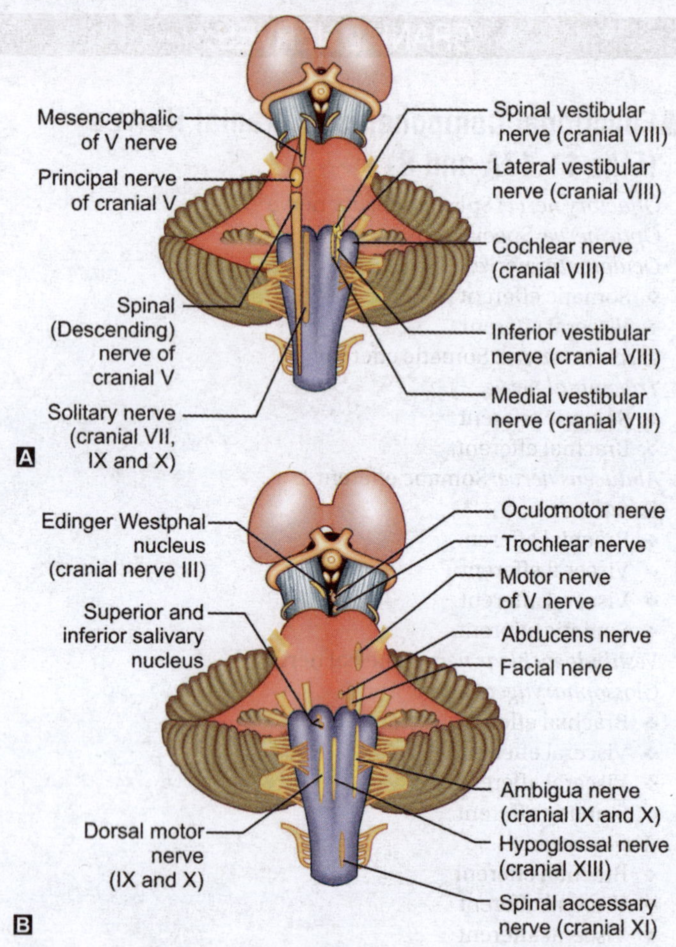

FIGS 11.17A AND B (A) Cranial nerve nuclei—sensory; (B) Cranial nerve nuclei—motor

- *Posterior fossa*
  VII and VIII nerve: Internal auditory meatus.
  IX, X and XI nerve: Jugular foramen.
  XII nerve: Hypoglossal foramen.

Somatic Efferent Fibers

Innervated striated muscles those are derived from somites:

- Involved in eye movements—III, IV and VI nerve
- Involved in tongue movements—XII cranial nerve.

TABLE 11.2 Relation of cranial nerve names to anatomy or functions

Number	Name	Functions or anatomic significance of name
I	Olfactory	It smells
II	Optic nerve	It sees
III	Oculomotor nerve	It's muscles move the eyeball
IV	Trochlear nerve	It's muscle moves the eyeball after running through the trochlea
V	Trigeminal nerve	It has three large sensory branches to the face
VI	Abducens nerve	It abducts the eyeball
VII	Facial nerve	It moves the muscles of all facial orifice
VIII	Glossopharyngeal nerve	It supplies the taste fibers to the tongue and activates the pharynx during swell owing
IX	Vagus nerve	It is vagrant, wandering from the pharynx to the splenic flexures of the colon
X	Spinal accessary nerve	It arises from neuronal bodies in cervical spinal cord, runs into the skull, out again and conveys accessary fibers to the vagus
XI	Hypoglossal nerve	It runs under the tongue

Brachial Efferent Fibers

These fibers supply the muscles those are derived from brachial arches:

- Involved in chewing movements—V cranial nerve
- Involved in facial expression—VII cranial nerve
- Swallowing movements IX and X cranial nerve
- Producing vocal sounds—X cranial nerve
- Turning the head—XI cranial nerve.

Visceral Efferent Fibers

Preganglionic parasympathetic components of cranial division:

- Courses through III nerve (smooth muscles of eye)
- Courses through VII nerve (lacrimal and salivary gland)
- Courses through IX nerve (parotid gland)
- Courses through X nerve (lung, heart and bowel muscles).

Visceral Afferent

- Convey sensations from lung, heart, great vessels, alimentary tract—IX and X nerve
- Gustatory sensation conveyed by VII, IX and X nerve.

Somatic Afferent

- Convey sensation from skin of head and face—V nerve
- Small number of efferent fibers passes through VII, IX and X nerves.

Special Sensory Fibers

- For smell—olfactory nerve
- For vision—optic nerve
- For hearing—vestibulocochlear nerve.

Difference between Cranial Nerve and Spinal Nerve

- Cranial nerves are not found at regular interval:
  - ❖ Some cranial nerve have motor component
  - ❖ Some cranial nerves have sensory component
  - ❖ Some cranial nerves are mixed—sensory and motor component
  - ❖ Some cranial nerves contain large visceral component
- Spinal nerve has no brachial and special sensory component
- In case of mixed cranial nerve, exit and entry are at the same point of brainstem.
  This point is ventral or ventrolateral.
  IV cranial nerve is dorsal.

◼ Olfactory Cranial Nerve (Figs 11.18A and B) (Flow Chart 11.1)

Method of Examination

Aim:
- Perception of smell, it is of more value.
- Identification of smell.
  - ❖ Ask the patient to sniff various nonirritating substance in each nostril separately.
  - ❖ Irritating substance has to be avoided, because it stimulates trigeminal nerve fibers in nasal mucosa and olfactory fibers simultaneously.

Abnormalities of Smell

- Anosmia—absence of smell
- Hyposmia—diminished sense of smell
- Parosmia—perversion of smell.

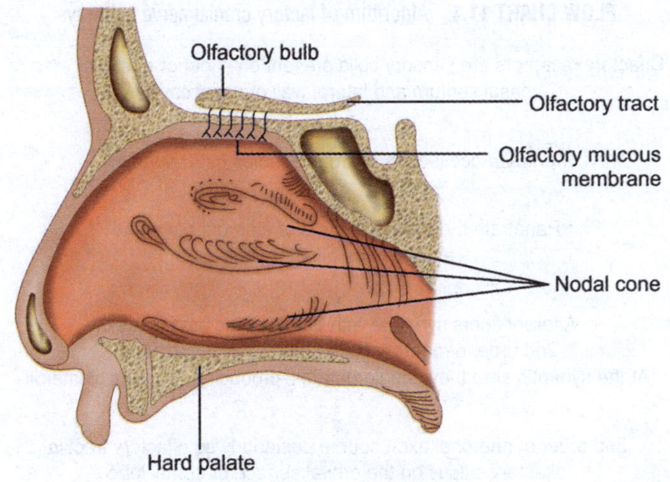

FIG. 11.18A   Olfactory nerve

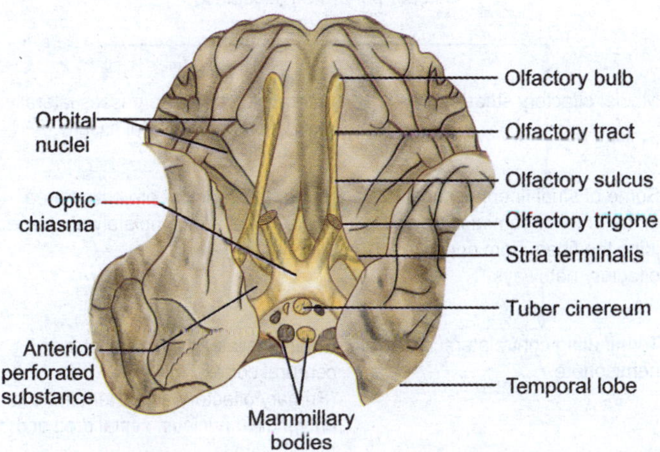

FIG. 11.18B   Olfactory nerve (inferior view)

Causes of Anosmia and Hyposmia

- *Congenital:*
  - ❖ Cleft palate in men
  - ❖ Absence or hypoplastic olfactory bulb or tracts
  - ❖ Familial dysautonomia
  - ❖ Turner's syndrome

FLOW CHART 11.1 Algorithm of factory cranial nerve pathways

Olfactory receptors are sensory cells present on superior-posterior area of nasal septum and lateral wall of nasal cavity

↓

Central processes form small bundles ($\simeq$ 20 number)

↓

Penetrate the cribriform plate of ethmoid bone and enters in the olfactory bulb

↓

Afferent fibers synapse with the dendritic processes of 2nd order of neuron, called mitral and tufted cells. At the synaptic area they conglomerate—producing olfactory glomeruli

↓

2nd order of neuronal axon course posteriorly as olfactory tract in olfactory sulcus on the orbital surface of frontal lobe

↓

Olfactory tract divides into two branches on either side of anterior perforated substance

Medial olfactory striae

↓

Some of strial fibers decussate in the anterior commissure and joins the fibers from opposite olfactory pathways

↓

Terminating contralateral cerebral hemisphere

Lateral olfactory stria passes laterally along the floor of lateral fissure

↓

Enters the olfactory projection area. There fibers are completely uncrossed

↓

Enters ipsilateral pyriform lobe of cerebral cortex (Primary olfactory area), terminate in amygdaloid nucleus, septal area and hypothalamus

❖ Kallmann's syndrome:
  • Permanent anosmia
  • Hypogonadrotropic hypogonadism
  • Cerebellar ataxia
  • Mirror movements of hands.
● *Local nasal disease:*
  ❖ Allergic rhinitis
  ❖ Nasal obstruction
  ❖ Nasal polyposis
  ❖ Sjögren's syndrome
  ❖ Tumors.

- *Neurologic:*
  - Head injury—most common cause of disruption of olfactory fibers prior to decussation.
  - Fracture involving cribriform plate of ethmoid bone tears the olfactory nerve fiber (olfactory filaments).
  - Closed head injury can impair olfactory recognition and preserve olfactory perception.
      Trauma to orbitofrontal and temporal lobes—impair olfactory naming and recognition—degree of disturbances related to severity of injury.
  - Korsakoff's syndrome
  - Lewy body disease
  - Huntington's chorea
  - Parkinson's disease
  - Spinocerebellar ataxia
  - Refsum's disease
  - Meningioma
  - Migraine
  - Seizure.
- *Endocrinologic:*
  - Adrenal insufficiency
  - Hypothyroidism
  - Diabetes mellitus
  - Pseudohypothyroidism.
- *Iatrogenic:*
  - Rhinoplasty
  - Ethmoidectomy
  - Orbitofrontal lobectomy
  - Temporal lobectomy
  - Submucous resection of nasal septum.
      After temporal lobectomy, olfactory discrimination is impaired in one nostril.
      After frontal lobe lesion (right) with involvement of orbital cortex, olfactory sensation in both nostrils are impaired. So, orbitofrontal cortex is important for olfactory discrimination.
- *Infections:*
  - Herpes simplex encephalitis
  - URTI
  - HIV
- *Liver disease:*
  - Acute hepatitis
  - Cirrhosis.
- *Psychiatric:*
  - Hypochondriasis
  - Major depression
  - Schizophrenia.

- *Miscellaneous:*
  - ❖ Cystic fibrosis
  - ❖ Giant cell arteritis
  - ❖ Occupational exposure
  - ❖ Sarcoidosis.

Tumors

- Olfactory bulb and tract are frequently affected by—tumor of olfactory groove
- Tumor of sphenoid bone and frontal bone—(glioma or abscess)
- Pituitary tumor with suprasellar extension
- Nasopharyngeal carcinoma
- Saccular aneurysm of anterior portion of circle of Willis.

Mass lesion in frontal lobe produces anosmia as earliest manifestation before clear cut frontal lobe signs and symptoms become evident.

Esthesioneuroblastoma: Tumors present in upper nasal cavity and superior and lateral wall near to ethmoid sinus—it produces:

- Nasal obstruction
- Epistaxis
- Anosmia.

If it involves orbit, it produces:

- Periorbital swelling
- Proptosis
- Diplopia
- Visual loss.

Foster-Kennedy syndrome: The causes are:

- Tumor in olfactory groove or sphenoidal masses (meningioma)
- SOL in frontal lobe.

The syndrome consists of:

- Ipsilateral anosmia—it is due to direct pressure on olfactory bulb or tract.
- Ipsilateral optic atrophy—it is due to direct injury to ipsilateral optic nerve.
- Contralateral papilledema—it is due to raised intracranial pressure secondary to mass lesion.

Pseudo-Foster-Kennedy syndrome: It occurs—when ICT is increased due to any cause, who has previous optic atrophy. It occurs:

- It is due to segmental anterior ischemic optic neuropathy.
- Optic neuritis—in which optic disc edema of one side with optic atrophy of other side.

Parosmia: Perversion of smell

Cacosmia: Perception of unpleasant odor

Hyperosmia: Increased sensitivity to smell
Phantosmia: Perception of odor which is not usually present
Hypersomnia: Present in:

- Migraine
- Hyperemesis gravidarum.

Parosmia and cacosmia occurs in:

- Head injury
- Psychiatric disorder (depression)
  Unilateral parosmia—Olfactory hallucination—it occurs with:
  - ❖ Partial seizures
  - ❖ Migraine.

▌Optic Nerve (Figs 11.19 and 11.20)

Retina extends anteroposteriorly from ora serrata to optic disc, which correspond to attachment of optic nerve, slightly nasal to posterior pole. Macula, yellow colored when viewed through ophthalmoscope. Algorithms of visual pathway shown in Flow chart 11.2.

Each retina can be divided into four quadrants by two meridian:

1. Horizontal meridian—it divides retina into superior and interior portions.
2. Vertical meridian—it divides retina into nasal and temporal portions.

First order of neuron (Fig. 11.19): Photoreceptors starts deep in the retina. Photoreceptors are rods and cones—react to visible light—generate electrical signals—which pass to ganglion cells through bipolar cells and horizontally disposed to amacrine cells.

Rod cells: It responds to dim vision—contains pigment rhodopsin—reacts with light of wave length between 400–800 mm. Hundred millions of rods cells are evenly distributed throughout the retina, tightly packed in fundus, absent in optic disc and macula.

Cones: Three different types: Sensitive to red, green and blue light.

Total 7 millions of cone cells of which 100,000 cells are concentrate in the macula in a small region—called foveola—this area is devoid of vessels and neural elements.

Ganglion cells: 1.2 million of ganglion cells—populate inner aspect of retina. These cells are more populated on the posterior pole where there is one to one connection of cone cell with ganglion cell. On the contrary, there is overlap of vision in the periphery. So, there is relative sparing of vision with lesions that affects the ganglion cells preferentially.

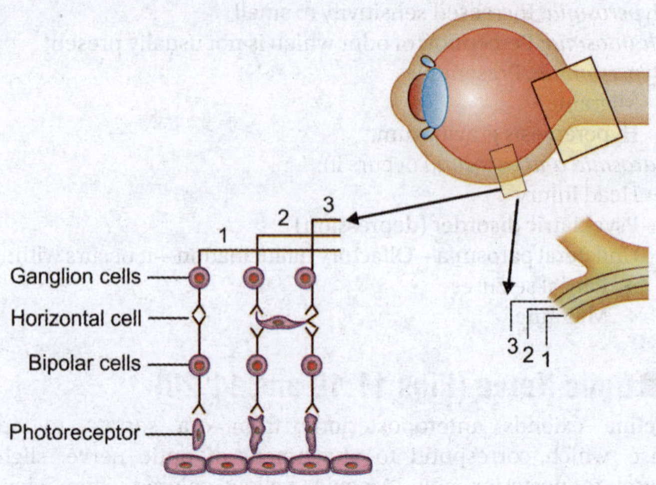

FIG. 11.19 Retinal pigment epithelium—first order of neuron

Two types of retinal ganglion cells

1. *M cells:* Ten percent of retinal ganglion cells—they are concerned with:
   - ❖ Depth of perception
   - ❖ Color ignorance
   - ❖ Low spatial resolution
   - ❖ High contrast sensitivity.

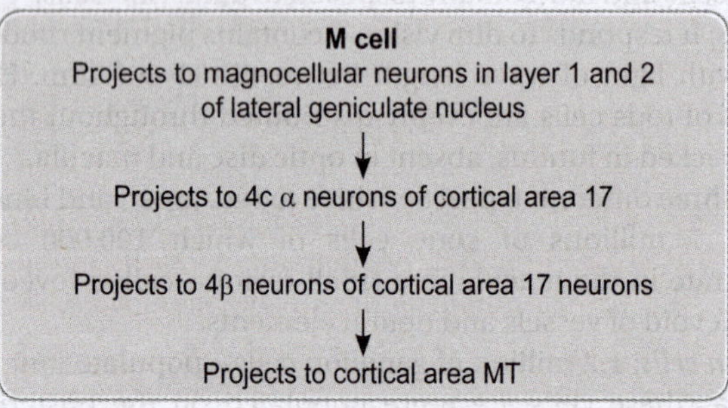

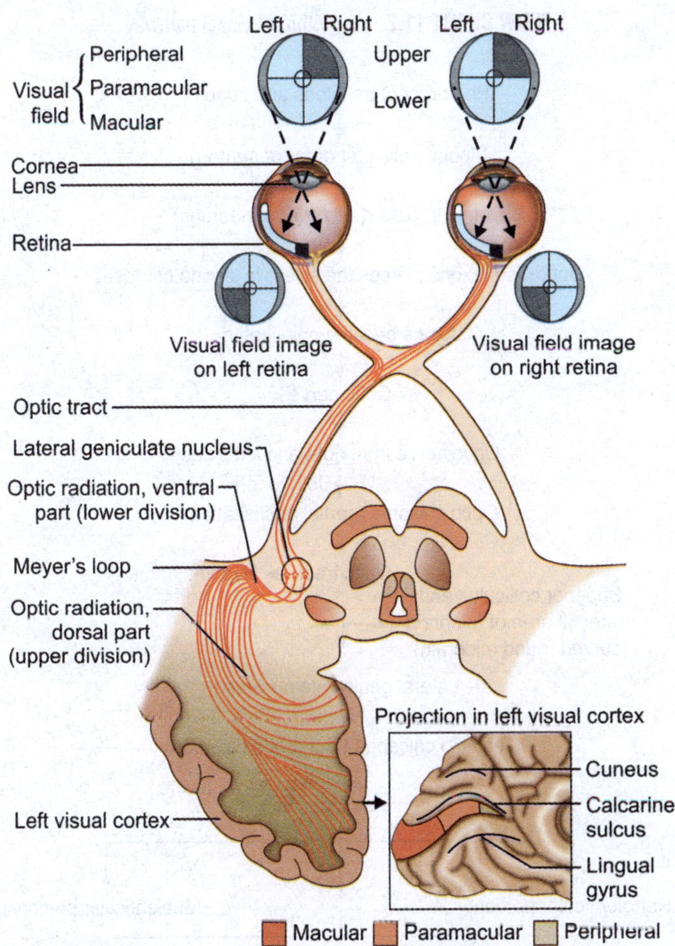

FIG. 11.20   Visual pathway and its representation in cortex

2. *P cells:* It is 90 percent of total ganglion cells. They are concerned with:
   ❖ High contrast sensitivity
   ❖ High spatial resolution
   ❖ Has color opponency.

FLOW CHART 11.2 Algorithm of visual pathway

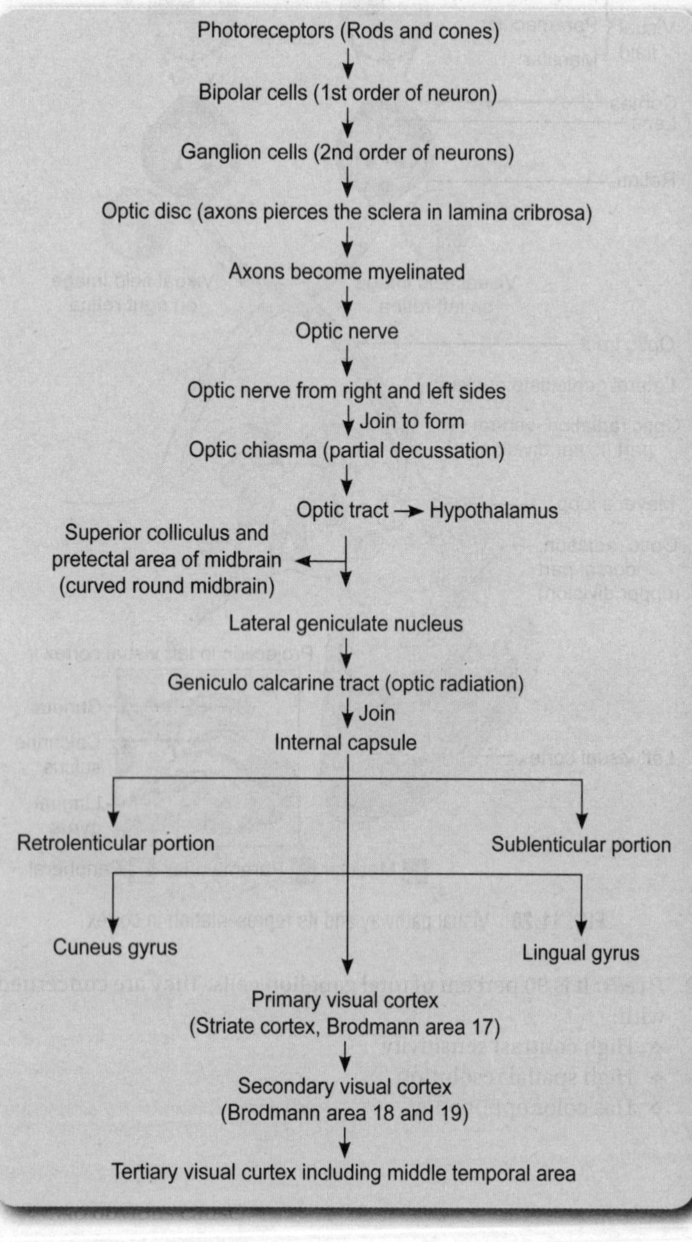

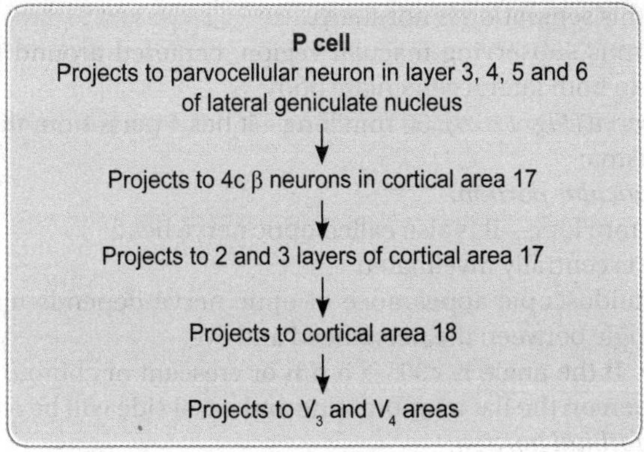

In Alzheimer's disease: There is loss of M cells—in retina. As a result:
- Difficulty in determining motions and depth
- Inaccurate fast eye movements (saccades)
- Preservation of color and acuity of vision.

In optic neuritis: There is loss of P cells in retina. As a result:
- Central scotoma
- Impairment of color vision
- Contrast sensitivity abnormalities.

Axons of ganglion cells constitute the inner layer of retina, separated from vitreous by thin basement membrane. Positions of axons in the nerve fiber layer depends on their origin from retina, so ganglion cells close to optic disc involves whole thickness of nerve fiber layer and more peripherally generated axons present in the center of the nerve fiber layer.

- Fibers from nasal side of optic disc and nasal side of macula produce a straight course—known as pillomacular bundle.
- The remaining fibers arche around the pillomacular bundle. It produces a disposition that has a bearing on visual field defect.
- Fibers form superior half of temporal aspect of retina arches superiorly and then down towards the disc.
- Fibers from inferior half of tempore aspect of retina aches inferiorly, then above towards the disc. Between the nerve fibers from superior aspect of retina and inferior aspect of retina, a raphe is formed near the horizontal meridian.
- Axon of ganglion cells on temporal side of vertical line drawn through fovea projects to ipsilateral geniculate nucleus.
- Fibers from nasal side of retina, nasal to vertical line cross in optic chiasma.

But this separation is not sharp.

Neurons subserving macular region, centered around fovea—project to both lateral geniculate body.

Optic nerve (Fig. 11.20): 50 mm long—it has 4 parts from the globe to charisma:

- *Intraocular portion:*
    - ❖ 1 mm long—it is also called optic nerve head
    - ❖ It is centrally myelinated
    - ❖ Fundoscopic appearance of optic nerve depends upon the angle between the nerve head and eye.

        If the angle is <90° → a rim or crescent of choroid will be seen on the flat temporal side and nasal side will be elevated.
- *Intraorbital portion:*
    - ❖ It is 25 mm long
    - ❖ It is 'S'-shaped to allow its mobility within the orbit.
    - ❖ It is surrounded by fat contained in cone—the apex of the cone is open to optic foramen and superior orbital fissure superomedially.
    - ❖ *Here there is relation with*
        - Ophthalmic artery
        - Nerve to extraocular muscles
        - Ciliary nerve and ganglion.
- *Intracanalicular portion*
    - ❖ This part traverses through optic canal
    - ❖ This part is 9 mm long
    - ❖ This canal is orientated posteromedially at 45°
    - ❖ *This optic canal contains:*
        - Optic nerve
        - Ophthalmic artery
        - Sympathetic carotid plexus.
- *Intracranial portion*
    - ❖ This 4–16 mm long depending upon the position of optic charisma.
    - ❖ *Optic nerve lies above the*
        - Ipsilateral internal carotid artery as the vessel exits from cavernous sinus and gives off ophthalmic branch
        - Sphenoidal sinus bony roof
        - Contents of sella turcica.
    - ❖ *Superior to optic nerve*
        - Horizontal portion of anterior cerebral artery
        - Olfactory tract
        - Anterior perforated substance
        - Anterior communicating artery lies above optic nerve or optic chiasma
        - Gyrus rectus of frontal lobe.

Arrangement of Nerve Fibers in Optic Nerve (Fig. 11.21)

- Superior retinal fibers run superiorly
- Interior retinal fibers run interiorly
- Nasal and temporal portion of fibers—it corresponds to same portion in optic nerve.
- *Macular fibers*
  - ❖ Near the globe—macular fibers occupy the wedge-shaped area temporal to central vessels.
  - ❖ More distally it occupies core of the nerve.

Chiasmal Fiber Arrangement

- More than half (53:47 → Crossed: Uncrossed) of nasal fibers cross in optic chiasma to contralateral optic tract.
  Among the nasal retinal fibers:
  - ❖ Fibers from inferior part nasal retina are ventral in chiasma and form a loop (Wilbrand's knee) in the distal part of contralateral optic nerve and reach the lateral aspect of optic tract (Fig. 11.22).
  - ❖ Fibers from superior part of nasal retina lie dorsal in chiasma and lies medial aspect of optic tract.
- Fibers from temporal retina are uncrossed and maintain their ventral and dorsal position in chiasma.
- Macular fibers—some are crossed and some are uncrossed. Both uncrossed and crossed fibers originate from nasal and temporal part of macula.
  These fibers maintain dorsal position in optic tract.

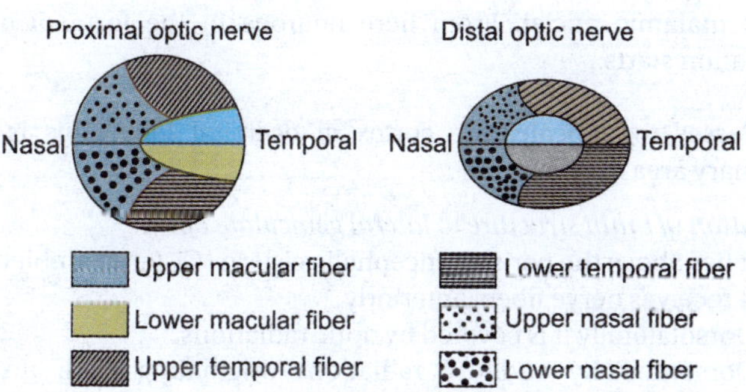

FIG. 11.21   Arrangement of fibers in optic nerve

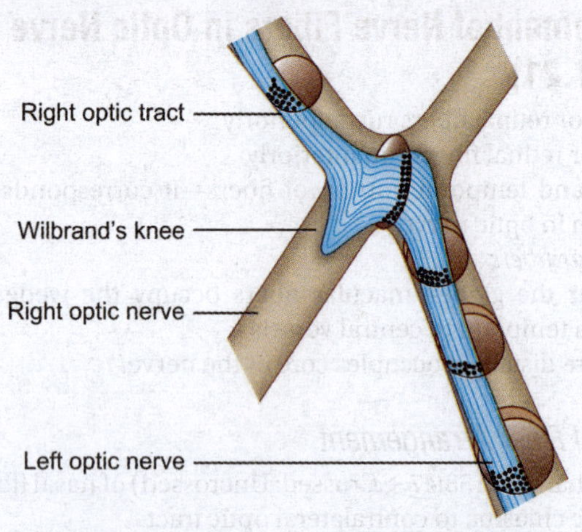

FIG. 11.22 Fiber arrangement in chiasma

Optic Tract

It extends from posterolateral aspect of optic chiasma—it extends posterolaterally, limiting hypothalamus in a triangular space

↓

Then it sweeps round the cerebral peduncles

↓

Reaches the lateral geniculate body

Several vessels lie below the optic tract. They are:
- Posterior communicating artery
- Posterior cerebral artery
- Perimesencephalic system
- Basilar cistern of Rosenthal.

Lateral geniculate body

It is thalamic nuclei. From here neurons in the form of optic radiation starts.

↓

Passes to pericalcarine cortex of occipital lobe. This is the primary area of vision.

Relation of brain structure to lateral geniculate body:
- It lies above the perimesencephalic cistern (Cisterna ambiens)
- It receives nerve fibers anteriorly
- Dorsolaterally it is covered by optic radiations
- Dorsomedially auditory radiations originating from medial geniculate body and end in primary auditory cortex in temporal gyrus of Heschl's.

Neurons in lateral geniculate body are disposed into 6 Lamina:
- Lamina I, IV and VI—from contralateral eye
- Lamina II, III and V—from ipsilateral eye.

Arrangement of fibers in optic tract (Fig. 11.23):
- Superior retinal fibers present superomedially
- Inferior retinal fibers present inferolaterally.

Optic Radiations

It runs posteriorly around the lateral aspect of posterior portion of lateral ventricles forming external sagittal striatum.

↓

It is being separated from ventricles by internal sagittal striatum, occipitio-mesencephalic fibers.

Optic radiations consist of three bundles (Fig. 11.24):
1. *Upper bundle*:
   - ❖ It occurs from media part of lateral geniculate body
   - ❖ It corresponds to the fibers from superior retina
   - ❖ It passes through deep parietal white matter and passes to upper lip of calcarine fissure.
2. *Central bundle*:
   - ❖ It corresponds to fiber of macula
   - ❖ It occurs from medial part lateral geniculate body
   - ❖ It passes through posterotemporal and occipital white matter and end in both superior and interior lips of calcarine fissure.
3. *Lower bundle*:
   - ❖ It corresponds to fiber of lower retina
   - ❖ It occurs from lateral part of lateral geniculate nucleus
   - ❖ It passes first anteriorly, then posteriorly around the temporal horn of lateral ventricle (Meyer's loop).
   - ❖ It terminates in lower lip of calcarine fissure.

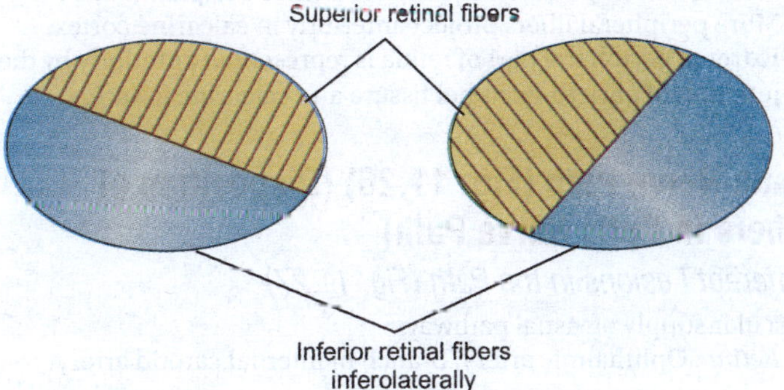

FIG. 11.23   Arrangement of fibers in optic tract

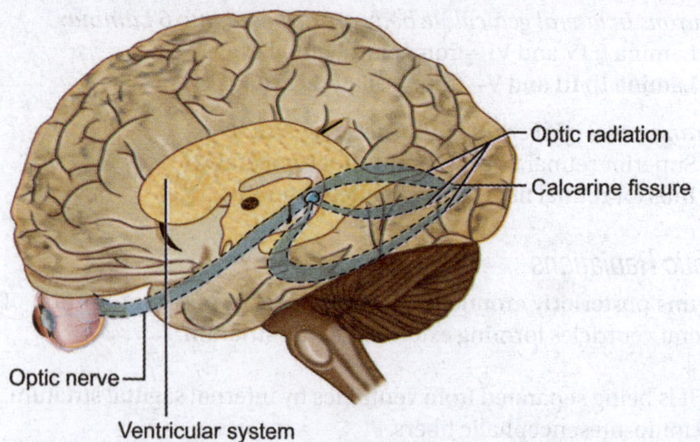

FIG. 11.24   Arrangement of optic radiation in parietal, temporal lobes, lateral to ventricular system

Visual Cortex

- Cortical area 17 of Brodmann, is located along the superior and interior lip of calcarine fissure on the medial surface of occipital lobe.
- This area also extends beyond the posterior extent of calcarine fissure and extends up to 1 cm around posterolateral aspect of occipital pole.

  This is the primary visual area—the other name of area 17 is striate cortex—this is very rich in granular cells.

Disposition of fibers in visual cortex (Figs 11.25A and B):
- Each occipital pole receives fibers from ipsilateral temporal half of retina and contralateral fibers from nasal half of retina.
- Superior lip receiver the fibers from superior retinal projection and inferior retinal projections are received by inferior lip.
- Macular fibers projects to posterior pale of occipital cortex.
- More peripheral fibers project anteriorly in calcarine cortex.
- Extreme peripheral part of retina is represented anteriorly by the junction of parieto-occipital fissure and calcarine fissure.

Optic Nerve Path (Fig. 11.26) (Disposition of Fibers in Optic Nerve Path)

Different Lesions in the Path (Fig. 11.27)

Vascular supply of visual pathways

A. *Retina*: Ophthalmic artery, branch of internal carotid artery

↓

Passes through optic canal with optic nerve

↓

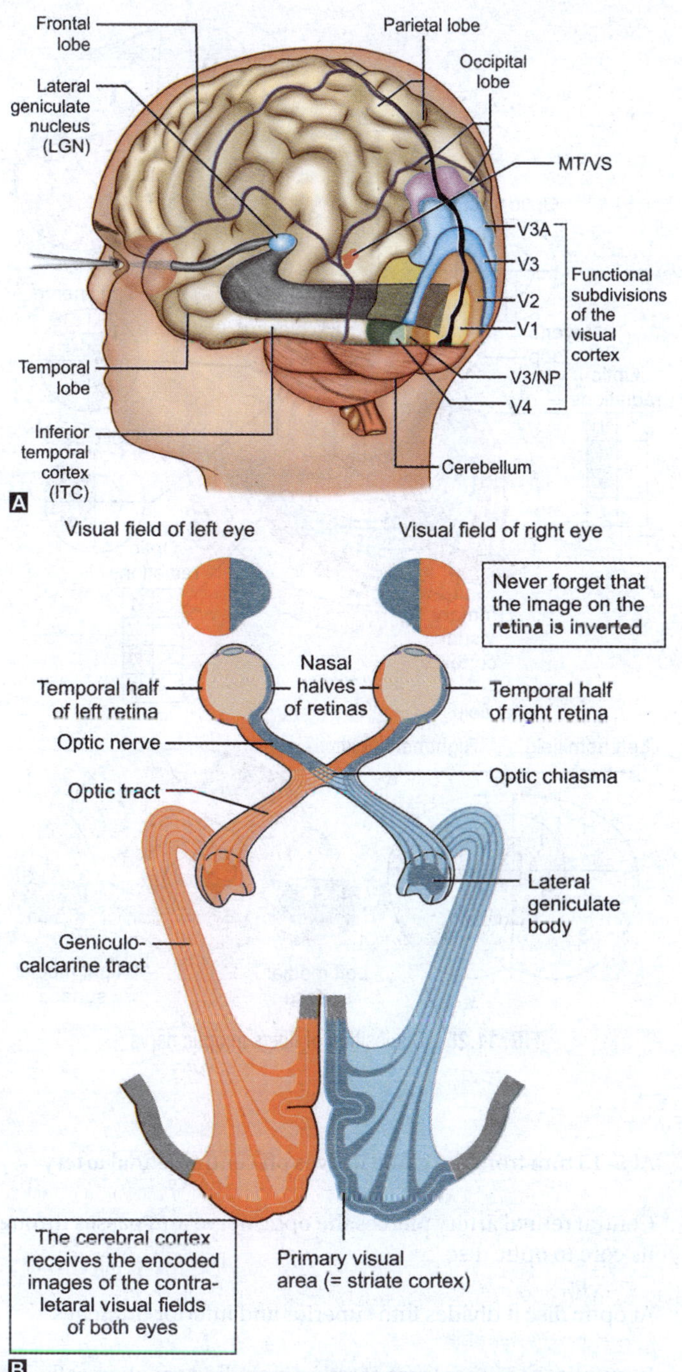

FIGS 11.25A AND B Visual cortex

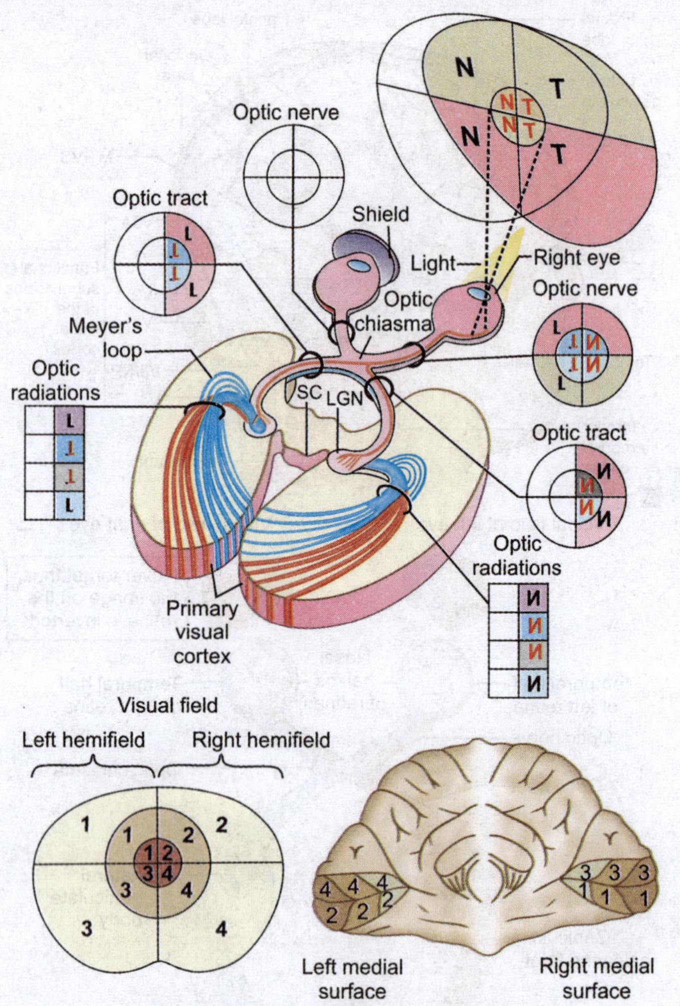

FIG. 11.26   Disposition of fibers in optic nerve

At 5–15 mm from the globe it gives off central retinal artery
↓
Central retinal artery pierces the optic nerve and passes through its core to optic disc
↓
At optic disc it divides into superior and inferior branches
↓
It supplies the inner layer of retina including ganglion cells

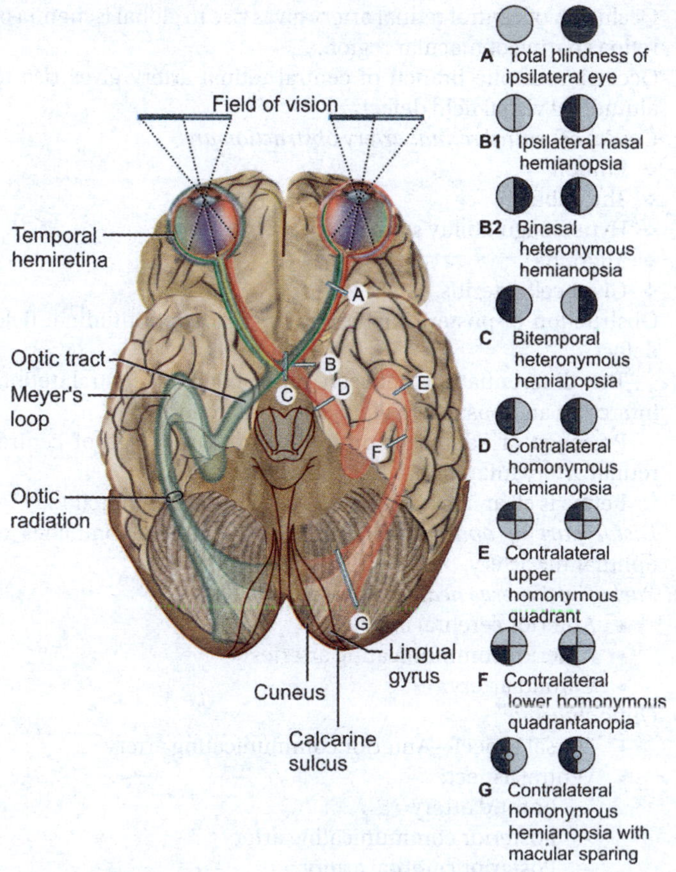

FIG. 11.27 Different sites of lesions in optic pathway

Ophthalmic artery gives other branches:

- Dural branches
- Orbital branches
- Several posterior ciliary arteries.

Posterior ciliary arteries—supply—by forming vascular arcades around globe:

- Outer layer of retina including photoreceptor
- Choroid.

Posterior ciliary artery gives:

One or more ciliospinal arteries—they supply macular region and papillomacular bundle.

- Occlusion of central retinal artery gives rise to global ischemia of retina sparing of macular region.
- Occlusion of one branch of central retinal artery gives rise to altitudinal visual field defect.
  Causes of central retinal artery obstruction are:
  ❖ Emboli
  ❖ Thrombus
  ❖ Hypercoagulability state
  ❖ Migraine
  ❖ Giant cell arteritis.
- Obstruction of posterior ciliary artery leads to altitudinal field defect.

  The differentiation between obstruction of central retinal infarction and posterior ciliary artery infarction:

  Presence of edema in optic disc in acute stage of central retinal artery infarction.

  Retina is clear in case of posterior ciliary artery infarction.

B. *Distal part of optic nerve near globe*—by small branches of ophthalmic artery.

C. *Part of optic nerve near to chiasma by*:
  - Anterior cerebral artery
  - Anterior communicating arteries
  - Carotid artery.

D. *Optic chiasma*:
  - Dorsal aspect—Anterior communicating artery
  - Ventral aspect:
    - Carotid artery
    - Posterior communicating artery
    - Posterior cerebral artery.

E. *Optic tract*:
  - Posterior communicating arteries
  - Posterior cerebral artery.

F *Lateral geniculate body*:
  - *Laterally:* Anterior choroidal artery
  - *Medially:* Posterior choroidal artery.

G. *Optic radiation*:
  - *Upper part:* Middle cerebral artery
  - *Lower part:* Posterior cerebral artery.

H. *Calcarine cortex*: Calcarine branch of posterior cerebral artery.

Location of lesions in visual pathways
Detailed qualitative testing allows:
- Detection of subtle defect, which can be escaped during bedside testing
- Exact shape of visual field defect
- Quantification of extent intensity of defect.

Lesion in visual pathways produces:
- Defect in visual acuity
- Impaired colored perception
- Contrast discrimination—Impaired discrimination of objects having little contrast with the background
- Visual field defect.

Changes in visual perception

Visual acuity: It is the discrimination of the details of high contrast, e.g. small black letter against white paper.

This reflects the lesion in macular region. Subnormal value reflects:
- Fault in visual system (optic faults, retinal lesions, visual pathways lesion)
- Faulty foveation (defect in eye motility)
- Poor co-operation.

Most common cause of impaired visual acuity is—refractory changes in eye—Patient with refractory changes can be tested with pin hole (*Pin hole test*)—this maneuver restricts the vision to central beam of light.

This is undisturbed by abnormal ocular distances.

Bed side of visual acuity test: By Snellen optotypes—this card should be well-illuminated and the distance between chart and eye should by 14 inches.

Lesions responsible are:
- Compressive and noncompressive lesions of optic nerve—it produces drop in visual acuity before visual field defect will be detected.
- Medial chiasmal lesion
- Lateral chiasmal lesion—it produces impairment of visual acuity in ipsilateral eye only.
- If crossed and uncrossed fibers from fovea will be affected by medial chiasmal lesion.

   Visual acuity is unaffected if lateral geniculate body, optic tract, optic radiation and visual cortex are affected.

Contrast sensitivity: Contrast sensitivity testing detects subtle visual field defect in macula, optic nerve and optic chiasma, even when visual acuity testing is normal.

Perception color: Color perception is impaired in the areas of visual field which corresponds to partial visual field defect.

Color vision can be tested by following methods:
- Ask the patient to identify which one of the identically bright red objects is more red.
  - ❖ In case of healthy person—there will be no difference.
  - ❖ In case of lesion in visual pathways—the red object becomes orange to yellow even colorless—according to the severity of the disease.

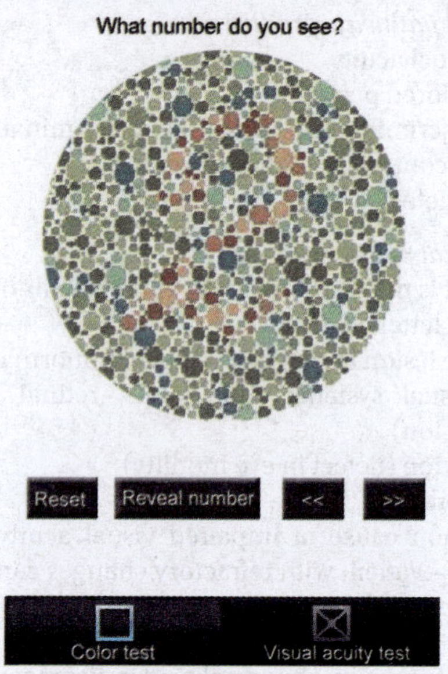

FIG. 11.28 Ishihara chart

The above test should be done by each eye, blocking the other eye at a time.

- *By using ishihara chart (Fig. 11.28):* Ask the patient to read the number made up of different colored dots against the background of different color dots.

  The number started from 1–15. If patient can identify 13 or more plates the color vision is said to be normal.

  The chart must be 75 cm distances from the eyes.

- ❖ The defects in color vision involve macular fibers.

  Since optic nerve and optic chiasma lesion involved macular fibers—so color vision may be defective on the side of lesion—when mono-ocular reading of ishihara chart is being done.

- ❖ Patient with simultanagnosia—it is due to lesion in bilateral parieto-occipital areas (in case of posterior form of Alzheimer's disease)—may have difficulty in identifying the image but their color naming and visual acuity are intact.

  Usually color vision defect runs parallel to visual acuity loss in ischemic optic neuropathy.

  But exceptions:

  - *In optic neuropathy:* Color vision is more impaired than visual acuity.
  - *In patient with nystagmus and anisometropia:* Normal color vision, but with impaired visual acuity.

- *In cerebral lesion:* Bilateral lesion in inferomedial occipital region—normal visual acuity but color blindness will be present.

  Congenital color vision defect:
- More common in men
- Defect mainly in red and green hues

  Acquired color vision defect:
- Patient optic nerve damage there is tendency for difficulty in discrimination between red and green.
- Patient with choroidal-retinal disorder—there is difficulty in discrimination between blue and yellow hues. (Kollner's rules).

  Kollner's rule's exception: Patient with open angle glaucoma—is an optic nerve disease—produces blue-yellow deficit.
- *Flight of colors perception phenomenon:* Succession of color impression that follows shining a bright light into the eye. This phenomenon is reduced in duration in acquired dyschromatopsia. Visual field and their representation in retina (Fig. 11.29).

Visual Field Defect

Lesion in optic pathways can be localized by:
- Shape
- Distribution of visual field.

The unco-operative patient may be:
- Inattentive
- Disturbances in alertness
- Disturbances in mentation.

Visual field can be tested by:
- Bedside confrontation perimetry
- Tangent (Bjerrum) screen
- Static or kinetic perimetry.

Testing of central 20°–30° is most important, because very few lesions are accompanied by peripheral visual field disturbances alone. The lesions are:
- Retinal detachment
- Tapetoretinal disorder
- Anterior visual cortex lesion.

During visual field testing, following disorders should be taken into account:
- *Shadowing facial contours:*
  - ❖ Eyebrows
  - ❖ Nose.
- Ptosis

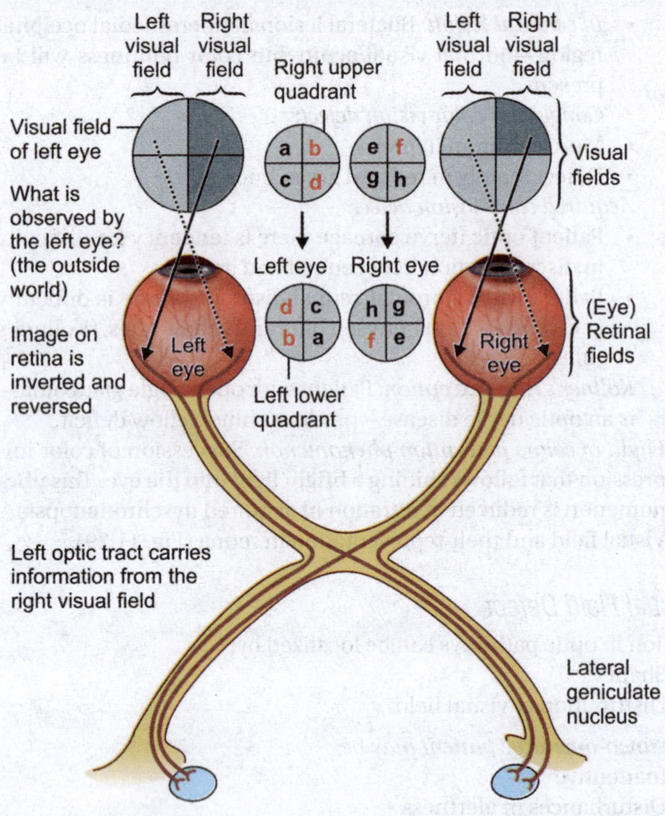

FIG. 11.29   Visual field representation in retina

- Disorders in eye motility
- Pupillary size
- Eyelashes
- Blinks
- Spectacle rim.
- *Error of refraction:*
  - ❖ Ametropia
  - ❖ Presbyopia
  - ❖ Both ametropia and presbyopia
  - ❖ Uncorrected astigmatism—it may cause temporal depression
  - ❖ Spherical ametropia—it may cause generalized visual field depression, occasional temporal depression, which may run under blind spot.

Scotoma

Localized area of poor vision surrounded by normal vision—it is called scotoma.

Physiological scotoma

- *Blind spot:* Image of optic nerve over the visual field is called blind spot—it cannot be perceived because it lacks in representation in brain.
- Image of retinal vessel—superficial on underlying retina—called angioscotoma—it can be noted in certain circumstances.
- *Contraction:* Absolute defect in outer limit of visual field.
- *Depression:* Smooth tapering in visual field.

Confrontation perimetry (Fig. 11.30).

- Patient and examiner; both sit at approximately 1 meter distance.
- For testing left visual field, patient must cover his right eye and examiner must cover his left eye.
- Ensure that patient's left eye must be fixed at examiner's right eye throughout the examination procedure.
- Limits of peripheral field can be defected by bringing the moving finger of examiner's right hand in all four quadrants of patient's visual field from just outside the limits of his or her visual field.
- A red object is better for this aspect of visual filed testing, as red color desaturation is a marker of lesion in visual pathways.
- Graying of vision or color desaturation may be noted prior to quantify the visual field defect.
- Central vision can be detected by utilizing 5 mm white disc attached to rod or long pin.

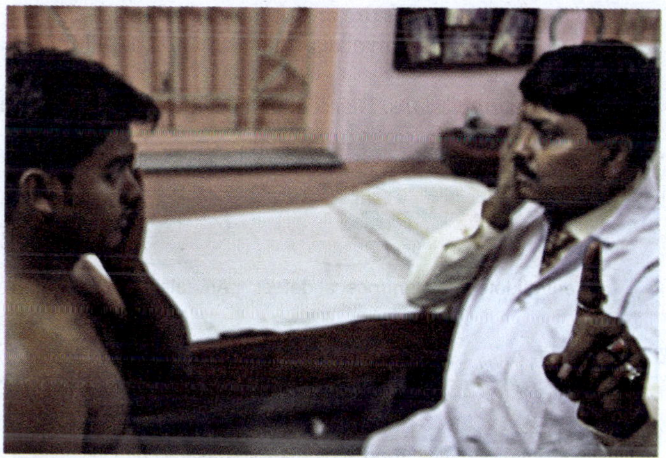

FIG. 11.30 Examination of visual field

- Move the long pin in the temporal field along the horizontal meridian.

  Explain the patient that the object will disappear briefly then reappear and that the patient should indicate when this happens.
- Once you have found the position of blind spot, its shape can be mapped.
- Both eyes should be tested simultaneously. Examiner asks the patient to fix his vision between examiner's eyes. Examiner moves his finger simultaneously in each quadrant.

  If there is visual inattention in one field and fingers are moved simultaneously, patient will not perceive the finger subserving the damaged component in visual pathway.

  This method is called double simultaneous stimulation.
- In rare occasion, patient may not perceive a stationary object in one visual filed, but may perceive the moving object in that same visual field (Riddoch's phenomenon).
- Quantitative perimetry is essential for arcuate field of vision.
- If objects of different sizes are used—patient can detect larger object in same sector of visual field where smaller object cannot be seen in that sector of visual filed—this defect is partially caused by edema or pressure phenomena.
- Constricted visual field can be detected by testing the visual field by small objects (2 mm). This can be hidden if larger objects (10 mm) are taken.
- Bjerrum screen (Tangent screen) enlarges central meridian to 30°— this can be helpful for measuring central scotoma and blind spot.

Field Defect (Fig. 11.31)

- *Central defect:* It occupies the position of macula.
- *Centrocecal defect:* It involves macula and papillomacular bundle.
- *Small deep retinal lesions:* Discrete defects localized to the point of lesion, nerve fiber layer is unaltered.

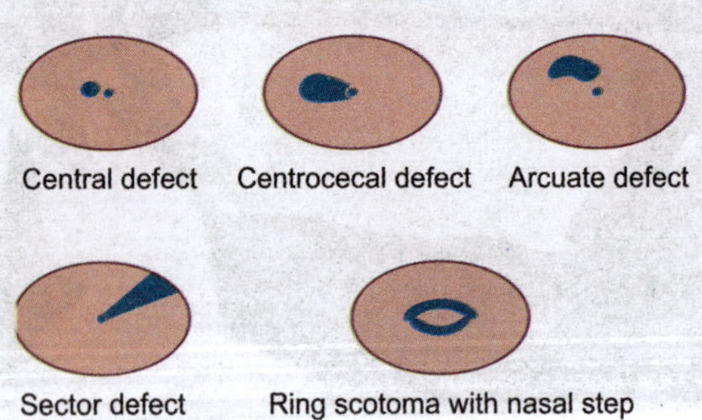

FIG. 11.31   Visual field defect

- *Large retinal lesion:* Here superficial fiber layer is involved. It gives rise to fan-shaped arcuate defect—with its tip pointing toward the lesion and base fanning peripherally towards the nasal horizontal meridian.
- *In nerve fiber defect:*
  - ❖ If nasal field is affected the defect is in arcuate shape. Arcuate shape defect is due to disposition of nerve fiber layer of temporal side is arcuate in course.
  - ❖ If temporal field is affected the defect appears as sector shape, because neither blood supply nor fiber disposition of nasal retina is along horizontal meridian. Straight course of nasal fibers towards nerve head are responsible for sector defect.
    - *Arcuate defect may occur in:*
      - Glaucoma
      - Nonarteritis anterior ischemic optic neuropathy
      - Congenital optic pit
      - Drusen of the disc.
- *Enlargements of blind spot:* It occurs in:
  - ❖ Increased optic disc swelling—increased intracranial pressure
  - ❖ *Papillary retinal disorder*: Peripapillary cons seen in:
    - Aging
    - Myopia
    - Glaucoma
    - Congenital optic nerve pit.
- *Ring scotoma:* In case of ring scotoma, vision is preserved central and peripheral to scotoma. Central vision coincides with fovea.
    - *Ring scotoma causes*:
  - ❖ Optic neuropathies
  - ❖ Retinopathies
  - ❖ Cancer associated retinopathy—it associated fundoscopic appearance—arteriolar narrowing, optic atrophy
  - ❖ Retinitis pigmentosa—it is large mid peripheral ring.
  - ❖ Chloroquine associated retinopathy—"Bull's eye" appearance
  - ❖ Retinitis
  - ❖ Choroiditis
  - ❖ Migraine
  - ❖ Myopia.
- Fusion of superior and inferior arcuate scotoma—it gives rise to central scotoma—this type of scotoma has characteristic horizontal or nasal step.
- *Physiologic ring scotoma*—caused by:
  - ❖ Corrective lenses
  - ❖ Prismatic effect of strongly curved corrective lenses.
- Shallow ring scotoma around blind spot.

Funnel vision: Central vision is intact and peripheral visual field is narrowed:

The causes of constricted visual field:

- Glaucoma
- Retinitis pigmentosa
- CAR
- Hyaline bodies in the disc
- Bilateral occipital infarct with macular sparing
- Papilledema with optic atrophy
- Feigned visual loss.

Monocular visual field loss: It may be due to defect in retina or optic nerve lesion.

Binocular visual field loss: It may be due to lesion in chiasma or beyond chiasmal lesion.

Lesion in retina and optic nerve can be differentiated by Ophthalmoscopic examination—in both cases, visual acuity will be lost.

Sparing of visual acuity—it can raise the suspicion of:

Preretinal and retrochiasmal disease.

Monocular visual field loss is due to:

- Disease of choroids
- Retinal pigment epithelium
- Retinal nerve fiber layer
- Optic disc
- Optic nerve.

Lesion affecting retina or retinal nerve fiber layer—it produces ipsilateral visual field defect—whose size, shape, extent, position varies according to site of lesion.

Macular disease may produce:

- Metamorphopsia
- Micropsia, photopsia (flushing of light).

To assess the optic nerve related visual field defect —The nerve fiber arrangement should be remembered:

- Fibers from peripheral ganglion cells arrange around peripheral portion of optic disc—fibers from central ganglion cells arrange in the central portion of optic disc.
- Peripheral fibers run peripherally throughout the extent of optic nerve.
- Papillomacular bundle occupies large sector-shaped regions on the temporal side of retina. This bundle runs centrally throughout the optic nerve.
- Nerve fiber arrangement—is same in optic nerve except in lateral geniculate nucleus and optic tract—here there is a rotation of 90°.

Central visual field defect: Unilateral or bilateral due to damage in papillomacular bundle or optic nerve.

Unilateral central scotoma
- Vascular optic neuropathy
- Compressive
- Infiltrative
- Glaucoma
- Early macular disease.

Bilateral central or centrocecal scotoma
- *Hereditary disease*: Leber's hereditary optic neuropathy
- Toxic-nutritional neuropathies
- Bilateral macular lesion
- Compression on optic nerve bilaterally
- Bilateral lesion affecting occipital pole.

Ipsilateral Temporal Hemianopia

- *Early case of chiasmatic lesion:* Filed defect is restricted to temporal field of ipsilateral eye.

  This is due to involvement of ipsilateral optic nerve medially producing damage of ipsilateral nasal fibers but too anterior to affect the crossed nasal fibers from contralateral side.
- Lesion from anterior extent of calcarine cortex produces crescent-shaped field defect of the contralateral temporal visual field (monocular temporal crescent).
- Lesions affecting occipital lobe spare the calcarine cortex in its foremost part and result is contralateral homonymous hemianopia.

Mono-ocular altitudinal defect
Partial lesion of optic nerve produces altitudinal hemianopia with macular sparing.

Causes are:
- Obstruction of distribution of central retinal artery, but macular sparing is due to sparing cilioretinal artery supplying macula.
- Infarction of anterior portion of optic nerve due to ischemia involving posterior ciliary arteries—produce inferior altitudinal defect.
- Choroiditis
- Choroidal coloboma
- Retina detachment
- Glaucoma
- Optic nerve hypoplasia
- Drusen bodies
- Optic nerve trauma
- Masses compressing optic nerve.

Bilateral altitudinal defect: Causes:
- Bilateral lesions in optic nerve and retina.
- Large prechiasmal lesion compresses both nerves inferiorly producing superior altitudinal defect.
- Lesion from below the optic chiasma elevates them against the dural shelves causes bilateral inferior altitudinal defect.
- Bilateral lesion on the medial aspect of lateral geniculate body produces bilateral inferior altitudinal defect.
- Occipital infarct produces altitudinal defect sparing macular vision due to anastomosis of blood vessels—with absence of retinal or optic nerve abnormality.

Bilateral ring defect
Bilateral occipital lesions posteriorly—a vertical step can be identified between two halves of ring.

Bitemporal defect: Causes:
- *Mass lesion affecting optic chiasma:* Pituitary tumor.
- Rapidly progressing hydrocephalus in children.
- Trauma.

True pure bitemporal hemianopia is rare, no lesion except trauma affects the nasal crossing fiber only.

Bitemporal hemianopia: It may be peripheral, paracentral or central.

Certain anatomical relationship is important in evaluating chiasma field defect:
- *Ratio of crossed:* Uncrossed fibers = 53:47
- Uncrossed both ventral and dorsal fibers maintain their relative position in chiasma and optic tract.
- *Dorsal extramacular crossing fibers:* Decussate posteriorly in the chiasma and direct enter dorsomedial aspect of contralateral optic tract.
- *Macular fibers, that cross:* Do so in central and posterior portion of chiasma.
- *Some inferonasal retinal fibers:* Primary peripheral fibers loop in Wilbrand's loop.

In early compressive lesion produced by pituitary tumor—there is defect limited to central parts of upper temporal quadrant. As the lesion increases—the compression area will be increased, as a result uncrossed temporal fibers are involved—

So at first—bitemporal hemianopia.

But later on—bitemporal hemianopia is associated with binasal depression.

Few patients with chiasmal compression—show:
- Bitemporal superior visual depression
- Bitemporal scotoma
- Bitemporal arcuate defect

Chiasmal syndrome: Three syndromes:
1. *Anterior chiasmal syndrome*:
   a. Unilateral optic defect
   b. Superior temporal defect.
2. *Body of chiasmal syndrome*:
   a. *Bitemporal field defect:* Central, peripheral or both
   b. *Macular splitting:* Hemianopic or quadrantic
   c. *Visual acuity:* Normal
   d. *Optic disc:* Normal or pale.
3. *Posterior chiasma syndrome*:
   a. Bitemporal scotoma
   b. Visual acuity—normal
   c. Optic disc—normal.

Tilted Disc

It produces bitemporal hemianopia. This type of defect can be differentiated from chiasmatic lesion—that the field defect in case of tilted disc crosses meridian to nasal field.

Pseudochiasmal Visual Field Defect

Bitemporal field defect cross the vertical meridian—causes:
- Astigmatism
- Coloboma
- Ametropia
- Binasal retinal disease
- Bilateral optic neuropathies.

Central scotoma or central defect with superior temporal defect or other due to involvement of:
- *Optic nerve:* Ipsilateral
- Inferomedial nasal fibers of other eye.

Binasal hemianopia
- *Lesions of retina:*
  - ❖ Retinitis pigmentosa
  - ❖ Retinoschisis.
- *Lesions in optic nerve:*
  - ❖ Chronic papilledema
  - ❖ Glaucoma
  - ❖ Ischemic optic neuropathy
  - ❖ Drusen.
- *Bilateral compression of lateral chiasma:* Hydrocephalus with enlargement of third ventricle producing lateral displacement of optic nerve against supra clinoid portion of internal carotid arteries.

- Empty sella syndrome.
- Suprasellar lesion.

Homonymous hemianopia: It occurs from lesion of:
- Optic tract
- Lateral geniculate body
- Optic radiation
- Occipital cortex.

Optic Tract

Fiber arrangements:
- Macular fibers dorsolaterally
- Upper retinal fibers dorsomedially
- Lower retinal fibers ventrolaterally.

Complete unilateral optic tract lesion
- Macular splitting homonymous hemianopia.
- Visual acuity is normal.

Partial optic tract lesion: Incongruous field defect

Optic tract lesion + Relative afferent papillary defect:
- Homonymous hemianopia
- Afferent pupillary defect in the contralateral eye.

Optic tract lesion + ipsilateral third nerve damage:
- Homonymous hemianopia
- Pupil in ipsilateral to side of lesion is dilated, poorly reactive.

Chronic optic tract lesion
- Homonymous hemianopia
- Bilateral optic atrophy
- Wedge or bow tie pallor in contralateral eye
- More generalized pallor in ipsilateral optic nerve with associated loss of nerve fiber layer in superior and inferior arcuate region.

Hemianopic optic atrophy indicates the damage of postchiasma and preoptic radiations (Optic tract and lateral geniculate body).

Causes of optic tract lesions
- SOL—Meningioma, glioma, pituitary tumor, pinealoma
- AV malformation
- Aneurysm
- Trauma
- Neurosurgical procedure.

Lateral Geniculate Body

Fiber arrangement (Fig. 11.32)
Incoming fibers:
- *Axons of ganglion cells superior to fovea:* These are located medially.

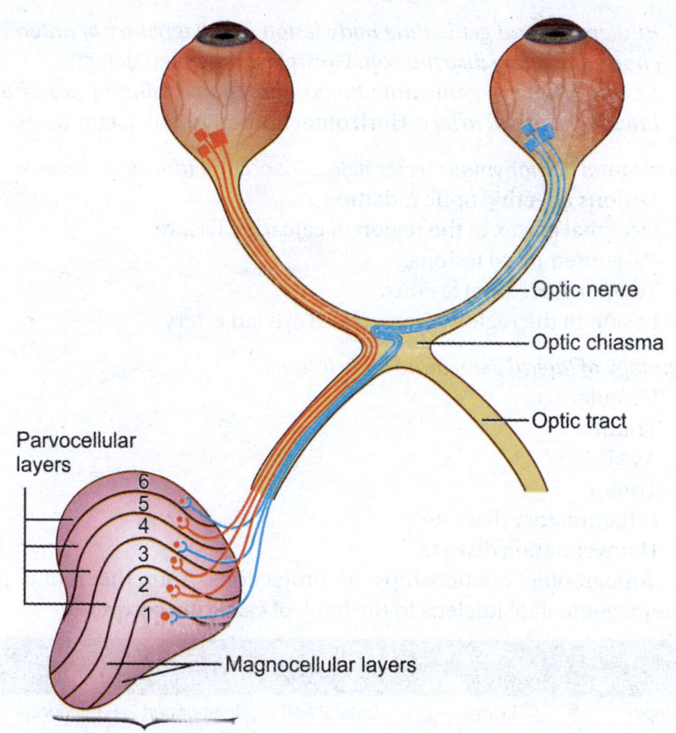

FIG. 11.32   Retinal ganglion cell projection to lateral geniculate body of thalamus. 1, 4, 6 layers receive information from contralateral retina. 2, 3, 5 layers receive informations from ipsilateral retina

- *Axons of ganglion cells inferior to fovea:* These are located laterally.
- Macular fibers are arranged centrally.

Arrangements of outgoing fibers:
- Fibers synapsed with axons of superior retina are located in superior radiation.
- Fibers synapsed with axons of inferior retina are located in inferior radiation.

Lesions of lateral geniculate body: Produces macular splitting homonymous hemianopia.

Focal lesions in lateral geniculate body
- *Lesions in lateral geniculate body in the territory of anterior choroidal artery distribution:* Homonymous hemianopia in upper and lower quadrants with a sparing of horizontal sector (quadruple sectoranopia).

- *Bilateral lateral geniculate body lesion in the territory of anterior choroidal artery distribution:* Hourglass type filed defect.
- *Lesion in lateral geniculate body—due to occlusion of posterior lateral choroidal artery:* Horizontal homonymous sector defect.

Horizontal homonymous sector defect—it occur with—other lesions:
- Lesions affecting optic radiation
- Occipital cortex in the region of calcarine fissure
- Parietotemporal lesions.
- Temporo-occipital lesions.
- Lesion in the region of superficial sylvian artery.

Etiology of lateral geniculate body lesions
- Vascular
- Trauma
- AVM
- Tumor
- Inflammatory disease
- Demyelinating disease.

Topographic relationships of projections from the retina to lateral geniculate nucleus to the bank of calcarine cortex.

Visual field quadrants	Retinal field quadrants	LGN	Optic radiation	Calcarine banks
Upper	Lower	Lateral half	Inferior part	Inferior
Lower	Upper	Medial half	superior	superior

Lesions in Optic Radiations

- *Superior homonymous quadrantic defect:* (pie-on-the sky defect)
  - ❖ Lesion in temporal lobe radiations
  - ❖ Inferior bank of calcarine fissure.
  - *The above lesion:*
  - ❖ If small → produces scotoma
  - ❖ If extensive → produces quadrantic defect.
  - *In temporal lobe lesion:*
  - ❖ *It in usually incongruous:* The inferior margin of sloping border may cross beyond the horizontal meridian.
  - ❖ *In ipsilateral eye:* Nasal field defect is denser and comes closer to fixation than contralateral eye.
- *Inferior quadrantic defect:* (pie-on-the floor defect):
  - *It occurs in parietal lobe lesions:*
  - ❖ It is more congruous.
  - ❖ It produces inferior homonymous quadrantic defect.
  - If the parietal lobe lesion is extensive:
  - It involves whole radiation to produce complete homonymous hemianopia with macular splitting.

- *Parietal lobe lesion may produce:*
  - Somatosensory impairment
  - Impaired position sense
  - Impaired tactile sense, touch and pain sensation.
- *Dominant parietal lobe lesion may produce:*
  - Apraxia
  - Aphasia
  - Acalculia
  - finger agnosia
  - Alexia
  - Right to left disorientation.
- *Nondominant parietal lobe lesion may produce:*
  - Dressing apraxia
  - Constructional apraxia
  - Anosognosia
  - Atopognosia
  - Hemispatial neglect
  - Spatial disorientation.

Occipital Lesions (Fig. 11.33)

In case of unilateral occipital lesion

1. Extra striate cortex: Tumor having irregular margins, it crosses horizontal meridian of extra striate cortex and produces a quadrantic field defect with horizontal border, because areas V_2 and V_3 (extra striate cortex) are divided along the horizontal meridian into separate halves flanking striate (V_1) cortex.

   This type of congruous inferior quadrantanopia with sharp vertical and horizontal border seen in the lesion of superior fibers of optic radiation near contralateral trigone.

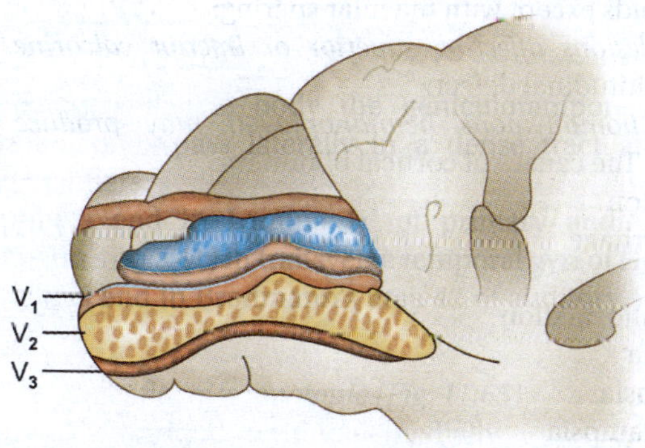

FIG. 11.33 Occipital Lesions

So, this type of lesion is not pathognomonic of extrastriate lesion, it may occur with lesion of striate cortex.

In medial occipital lesion:

When both upper and lower calcarine cortexes are affected—

Complete homonymous hemianopia with macular sparing (sparing of the central 5 degrees of vision).

Macular sparing is due to:

❖ Large macular representation

❖ Dual blood supply.

Lesion:

❖ Due to occipital infarcts in the distribution of posterior cerebral artery—by emboli to basilar apex

❖ Venous infarction

❖ Arteriovenous malformation

❖ Fistulas

❖ Tumor

❖ Abscess

❖ Trauma.

- *Striate cortex:* It can be classified into three locations:
  1. *Anterior location:* It lies adjacent to parieto-occipital fissure—lesion here—produces monocular temporal crescent of the contralateral visual field (Half moon syndrome).
  2. *Posterior lesion:* It affects 50%–60% of visual cortex—including occipital cortex, occipital pole.
     Lesion here affects macular vision (central 10° in contralateral visual field).
  3. *Intermediate lesion:* It affects 10°–60° of macular vision in contralateral visual field.

Bilateral occipital lobe lesion: It produces:

- Bilateral homonymous scotoma with some macular sparing that respect vertical midline.
- Bilateral complete homonymous hemianopia with central key-hole fields except with macular sparing.

Bilateral lesions affecting superior or inferior calcarine cortices: Bilateral altitudinal defect:

Bilateral homonymous hemianopia—It may produce cortical blindness: The causes of cortical blindness:

- Infarction
- Hemorrhage
- Tumor
- A-V malformation
- Hypoxia
- Eclampsia
- Pre-eclampsia
- Hypertensive encephalopathy.

Changes in visual perception

- *Lesions affecting anterior pathways:* It produces difficulty in reading and dimness of vision
- *Altitudinal field defect:* As curtain coming down or sensation of looking over horizon
- *Vertical hemianopic defect:* Patient can see half of the page or half of the keyboard.
- *Micropsia:* Objects appearing as reduced in size. It occurs due to excessive separation of photoreceptors by edematous fluid. It rarely occurs with lesions of optic chiasma.
- *Macropsia:* Objects appearing as larger in size. It occurs due to progressive closer of photoreceptors than normal.
- *Metamorphopsia:* Objects appearing as irregular in shape and size—when photoreceptors are not evenly spaced.
  It occurs:
  a. Scarring of retina
  b. Occipital or temporal lobe disease.
- *Hemimicropsia:* Reduction in size of object in one-half of visual field. It results from—contralateral focal lesion affecting unimodal visual association cortex.
- *Phosphenes:* Sensation of flashes of light when eyes are moving in the dark. This occurs:
  Lesion of optic nerve: In demyelinating disease—due to increased mechanosensitivity of the demyelinating areas of optic nerve—Lhermitte's sign.
- *Dazzle:* Painless intolerance of eye to bright light. It occurs in:
  - Albinism
  - Cone degeneration
  - Achromatopsia
  - Lenticular opacities
  - Corneal opacities
  - Vitreous opacities.
- *Central dazzle:* It may occur with lesion of:
  - Optic nerve
  - Chiasma
  - Thalamus
  - Occipitotemporal region
  - Brainstem
  - Trigeminal nucleus producing trigeminal neuropathy.

Fifth Cranial Nerve

Trigeminal nerve has two components *(Figs 11.34A and B)*
1. Motor innervations
2. Sensory innervations.

Motor Innervations (Fig. 11.34C)

- *Nucleus:* Present at midpontine level—medial to main sensory nucleus of trigeminal nerve.
- Supranuclear control through corticobulbar fibers traveling through corona radiata, internal capsule, cerebral peduncle.
- *Course:* It emerges through anteromedial aspect of pons anterior and medial to large sensory root → passes through posterior fossa → pierces the dura mater → enters the cavity of dura mater overlying the apex of petrous bone. (Meckel's cave) →

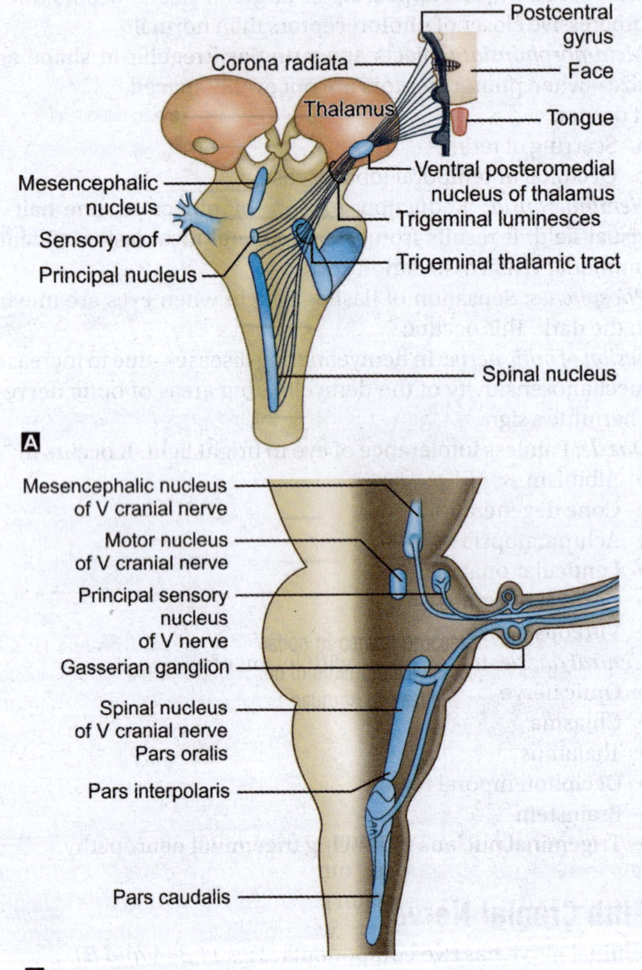

FIGS 11.34A AND B (A) Primary, secondary and tertiary trigeminal afferents; (B) Schematic diagram of trigeminal system

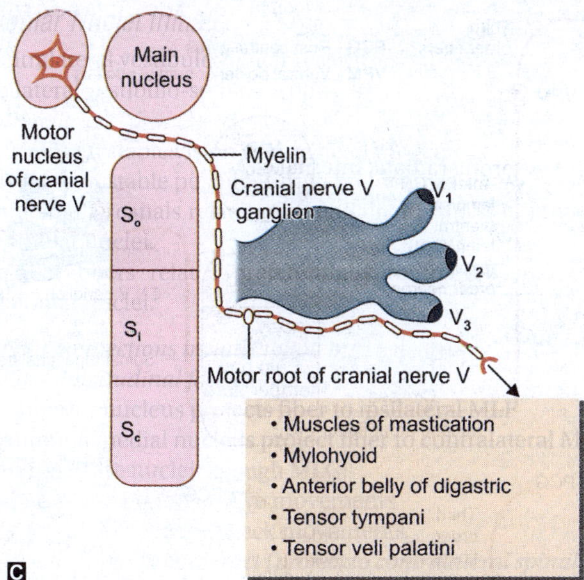

FIG. 11.34C   Motor innervation of trigeminal nerve

travels beneath trigeminal (gasserian) ganglia → leaves through foramen ovale → its motor root joins the mandibular division of trigeminal nerve to form mandibular nerve and supply the masticatory muscles:

- Masseter muscles
- Temporalis muscles
- Medial and lateral pterygoid muscles
- Tensor tympani muscles
- Tensor veli palatini
- Mylohyoid muscles
- Anterior belly of digastric muscle.

Sensory Innervations (Figs 11.35A to C)

Preganglionic sensory fibers terminate in gasserian ganglion near apex of petrous bone.

From this ganglion—postganglionic fibers terminate into three main nuclei:

1. Nucleus of spinal tract of trigeminal nerve
2. Main sensory nucleus
3. Mesencephalic nucleus.

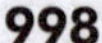

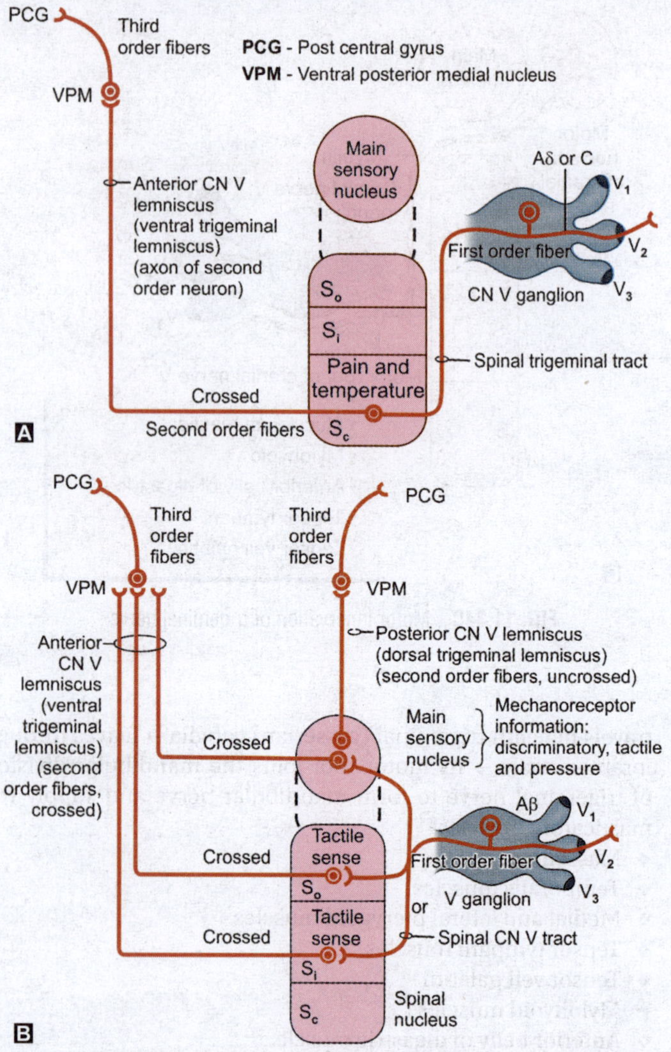

FIGS 11.35A AND B   (A) Trigeminal pathway of pain and temperature; (B) Trigeminal pathway for touch and pressure VPM—Ventral posteriror medial nucleus; PCG–Post-central gyrus; CN = Cranical nerve.

Nucleus of spinal tract of trigeminal nerve is divided into three parts:

1. *Pars oralis:* It extends from mid pons to inferior olive.
2. *Pars interpolaris:* It extends from inferior olive to the apex of fourth ventricle.
3. *Pars caudalis:* This is continuous with Lissauer's tract in spinal cord.

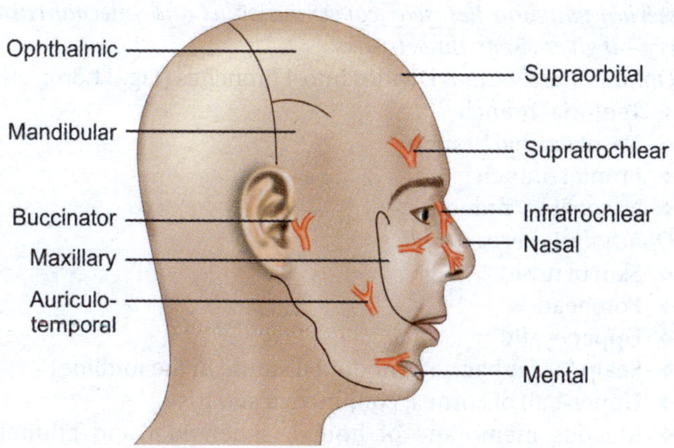

FIG. 11.35C Areas of skin supplying trigeminal nerve

Fibers of ophthalmic division of trigeminal nerve: Terminate in trigeminal nucleus in series with 2nd cervical sensory level—Travelling the most ventral part of spinal tract.

Fibers of mandibular division of trigeminal nerve: Travel through the most dorsal part of spinal tract and terminate in most rostral part of spinal nucleus of trigeminal nerve—Rostral trigeminal nuclei are important for intraoral and dental sensation, nose and mouth sensation.

Caudal nuclei are responsible for lateral facial sensation.

Pattern of termination is responsible for onion-skin pattern of facial sensory loss.

From spinal nucleus of trigeminal nerve, sensation of pain, touch, temperature of face and mucous membrane terminate ipsilaterally in trigeminothalamic tract to terminate into:

- Ventral posteromedial nuclei of thalamus.
- Intralaminar nuclei of thalamus.

Fibers terminating into main sensory nucleus of trigeminal nerve located in lateral pons—It responsible for tactile and proprioceptive sensation.

Postganglionic fibers from main nucleus—pass in two ways:
1. Ventral crossed trigeminothalamic tract.
2. Dorsal uncrossed trigeminothalamic tract.

They terminate into: Ventral Posteromedial nucleus of thalamus.

Third nucleus—mesencephalic nucleus—it receives proprioceptive impulses from (i) masticatory muscles (ii) muscles supplied by other cranial nerves.

Gasserian ganglion lies near cavernous sinus and internal carotid artery—it gives rise to three trunks:

1. *Ophthalmic division*: Divides into 4 branches (Fig. 11.36):
   - ❖ Tentorial branch
   - ❖ Nasolacrimal branch
   - ❖ Frontal branch
   - ❖ Nasociliary branch.

   Ophthalmic nerve supplies:
   - ❖ Skin of nose
   - ❖ Forehead
   - ❖ Upper eyelid
   - ❖ Scalp (as far back a lambdoidal suture in the midline)
   - ❖ Upper-half of cornea, conjunctiva and iris
   - ❖ Mucous membrane of frontal, sphenoidal and ethmoidal sinuses
   - ❖ Upper nasal cavity and septum
   - ❖ Lacrimal canals
   - ❖ Dura mater of anterior cranial fossa
   - ❖ Falx cerebri
   - ❖ Tentorium cerebelli.

2. *Maxillary division*: It leaves through foramen rotundum. Maxillary nerve branches—
   - ❖ *In sphenopalatine fossa:*
     - • Palatine nerves
     - • Middle, posterior and anterior-superior alveolar nerves.

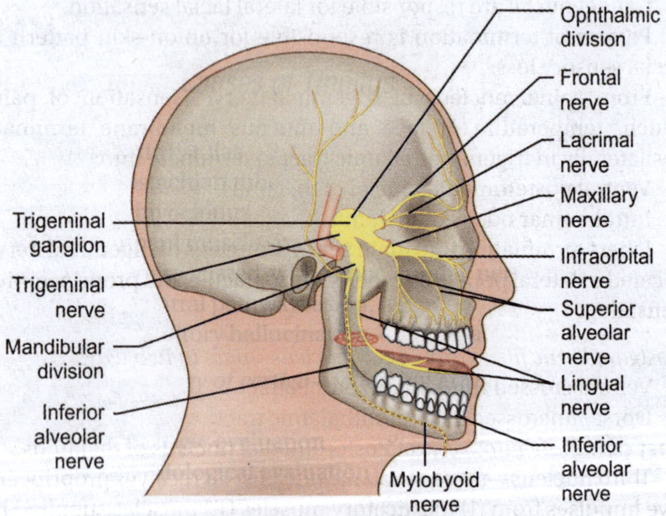

FIG. 11.36 Distribution of trigeminal nerve

❖ *After leaving intra orbital foramen:*
- Inferior palpebral branch
- Nasal branch
- Superior labial branch
- Zygomaticofacial branch.

The areas supplied are:
- Skin of lower eyelid
- Lateral nose
- Upper lip and cheek
- Lower-half of cornea, conjunctive and iris
- Mucous membrane of maxillary sinus
- Lower nasal cavity
- Hard and soft palate
- Upper gum
- Teeth and upper jaw
- Dura mater of middle cranial fossa.

3. *Mandibular division*: It leaves the skill through foramen ovale.

Branches

- Motor branch
- Lingual branch
- Inferior dental branch
- Mental branch.

Area Supplied

Sensory
- Skin of lower lip, lower jaw, chin
- Skin of tympanic membrane
- Auditory meatus
- Upper ear
- Mucous membranes of floor of the mouth
- Lower gum
- Anterior two-thirds of tongue (not taste sensation)
- Teeth of lower jaw
- Dura mater of posterior cranial fossa.

Motor
Muscles supplied: Muscles of mastication.
  i. *Pterygoids:* They move the jaws from side to side while chewing.
  ii. *Masseter:* Clench the jaws
  iii. *Temporalis:* Clench the jaws.

Examination of Sensory Function

Testing of sensations are mainly based on:

- Pain
- Touch
- Temperature
- Vibration sense
- Joint sense.

Three common exercises in evaluating facial sensation
1. Whether sensory loss is organic or nonorganic?
2. What modalities of sensations are involved?
3. Which areas of face are involved?

The following methods can differentiate organic from nonorganic lesion (but they are reliable always):
- Nonorganic sensory loss may have a demarcation of abnormal area at hairline than scalp vertex
- In lower face, sensory loss follow jawline and involves notch over the masseter muscle—functional
- On the trunk—sensory loss—ends short of midline—organic, splitting at midline—nonorganic
- In face—sensory loss may extend to midline—because of less midline overlap in face—organic or nonorganic.
- Corneal reflex and sternutatory reflex normal in nonorganic sensory loss.
- Splitting of vibration sense in midline—nonorganic, because frontal bone and mandible are single bone—so there should not be any difference in vibration sense on either side of mid-line.
- Dissociation of pin prick and temperature—nonorganic.

Examination of reflexes
- *Jaw Jerk (Fig. 11.37)*

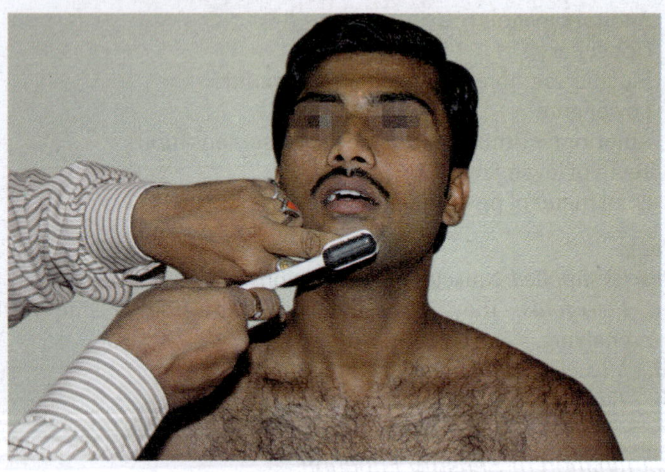

FIG. 11.37 Jaw jerk elicitation

Methods of elicitation:
* ❖ Place the index finger or thumb over the midchin.
* ❖ Mouth will be open in midway with jaw relaxed.
* ❖ Taps the index finger or thumb with hammer.
  Response—upward jerk of the mandible
  This is bilateral repose

If anyone tries to elicit unilateral response (Figs 11.38A and B)
* ❖ Tapping the angle of the jaw by direct tapping.

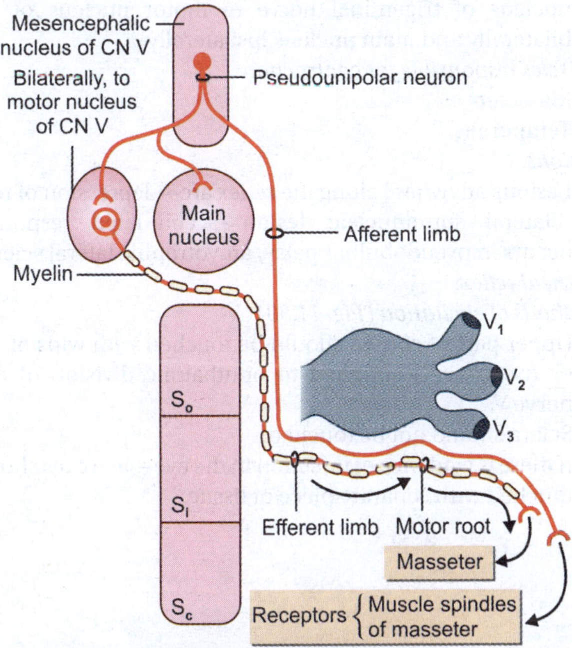

FIG. 11.38A Jaw jerk pathways

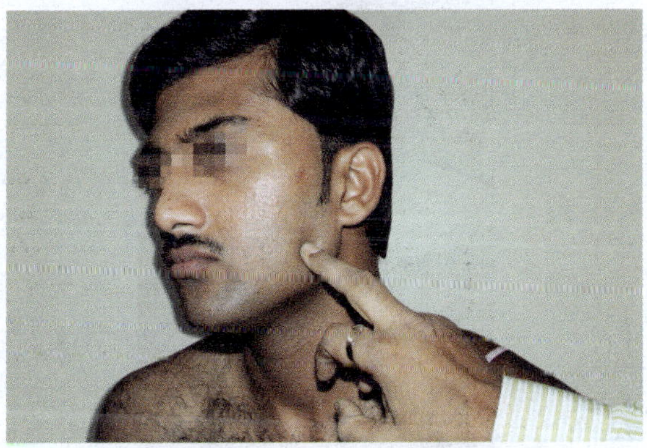

FIG. 11.38B Tapping at the angle of mandible

❖ Placing the tongue depressor over the lower molar teeth along one side and tapping the protruding end.

Response—upward jerk of mandible

Pathways:

❖ Afferent arc is through sensory portion of mandibular division of trigeminal nerve to muscle spindles of masseter muscle.

❖ *Nucleus:* Mesencephalic nucleus of trigeminal nerves.

❖ *Efferent:* Through mandibular fibers originating from motor nucleus of trigeminal nerve to motor nucleus of CN V bilaterally and main nucleus ipsilaterally.

Muscles responsible for contraction:

❖ Masseter

❖ Temporalis.

Lesions:

❖ Lesions anywhere along the reflex arc—depression of reflex.

❖ Bilateral supranuclear lesion—accentuated response. It occurs in pseudobulbar palsy, amyotrophic lateral sclerosis.

2. *Corneal reflex:*

Methods of elicitation (Fig. 11.39)

❖ Upper part of cornea should be touched with wips of cotton or tissue—it is supplied to ophthalmic division of cranial nerve V.

Sclera should not be touched.

❖ If there is evidence of infection in the eye—two eyes should be touched with separate piece of tissue.

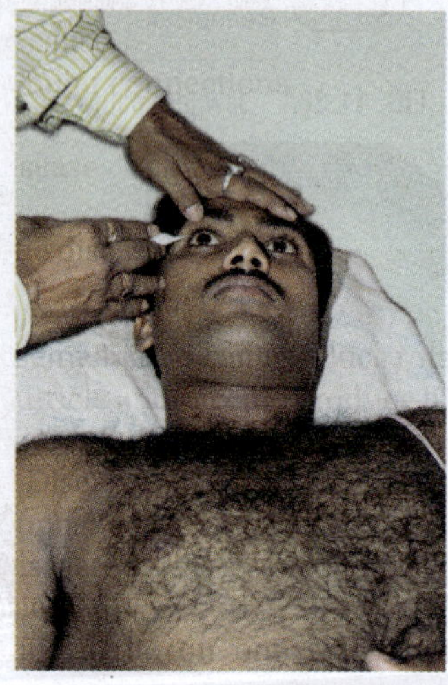

FIG. 11.39   Corneal reflex elicitation

❖ Cornea should not be touched with large blunt object or fingertip.
❖ In response to corneal stimulus, there is ipsilateral and contralateral blinking—direct and consensual reflex.

Pathways (Fig. 11.40):
❖ *Afferent pathway:* It is mediated by ophthalmic and maxillary division of cranial nerve V—mediated via:
    i. Ipsilateral main sensory nucleus of trigeminal nerve
    ii. Ipsilateral and contralateral spinal nuclei of trigeminal nerve.
❖ *Nucleus:* Nucleus of spinal tract of trigeminal nerve and main sensory nucleus of V nerve. From trigeminal nucleus pathway goes to facial nerve nucleus.
❖ *Efferent limb:* Facial nerve—supplying to orbicularis oculi muscles of both eyes.

● *Corneomandibular reflex:*
Methods of elicitation: Corneal stimulation—produces
❖ Bilateral blinking of both eyes.
❖ Brisk anterolateral jaw movement.

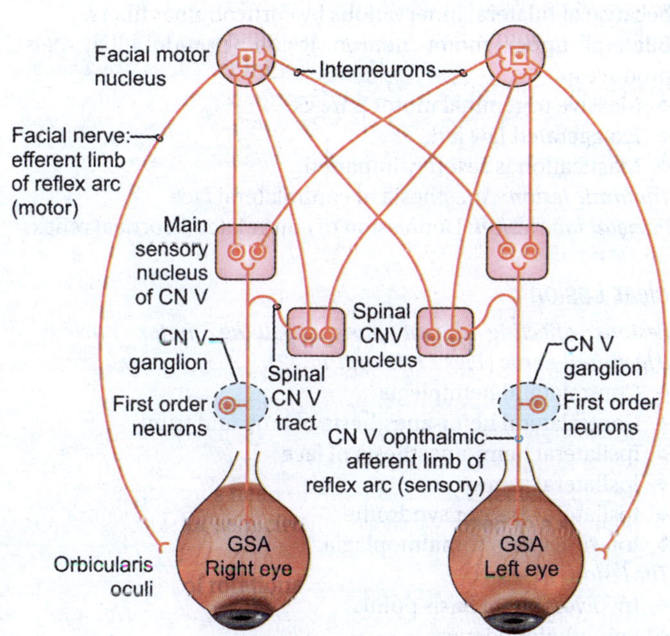

FIG. 11.40 Pathways of corneal reflex GSA—general sensory afferent; CNV—cranial nerve

- *Spontaneous palpebromandibular synkinesia:* Here there is bilateral blinking of both eyes and brisk anterolateral jaw movements, but without any corneal stimulation.
  This occurs in:
  - ❖ Bilateral brainstem lesion above the mid-pons.
  - ❖ Bilateral cerebral lesion.

Spectrum of corneal reflex—according to trigeminal nerve and facial nerve lesion

		Corneal reflex	
Lesion	Stimulation	Direct	Consensual
1. Complete CN-V lesion	involved eye	Absent	Absent
	uninvolved eye	Normal	Normal
2. Complete CN-VII lesion	involved eye	Absent	Normal
	uninvolved eye	Normal	Absent

Localization of Lesion Affecting Cranial Nerve V

Supranuclear Lesion

- Lesion of corticobulbar fibers of one side may result in contralateral trigeminal motor paresis—but paresis may milder because of bilateral innervations by corticobulbar fibers.
- Bilateral upper motor neuron lesion (pseudobulbar palsy) produces:
  - ❖ Massive trigeminal motor paresis
  - ❖ Exaggerated Jaw jerk
  - ❖ Mastication is severely impaired.
- *Thalamic lesion:* Anesthesia of contralateral face.
- *Parietal lobe lesion:* Depression of contralateral corneal reflex.

Nuclear Lesion

- *Lesions affecting dorsal pons involving motor nucleus of trigeminal nerve (Figs 11.41 and 11.42):*
  - ❖ Contralateral hemiplegia
  - ❖ Contralateral hemi-anesthesia of limb and trunk
  - ❖ Ipsilateral hemi-anesthesia of face
  - ❖ Ipsilateral tremor
  - ❖ Ipsilateral Horner syndrome
  - ❖ Internuclear ophthalmoplagia.
  The lesions involve:
  - ❖ Involvement of basis points
  - ❖ Spinothalamic tract
  - ❖ Main sensory nucleus of cranial nerve V
  - ❖ Brachium conjunctive

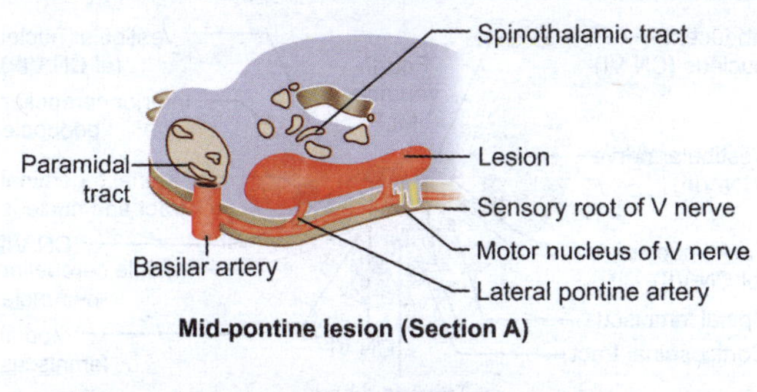

Mid-pontine lesion (Section A)

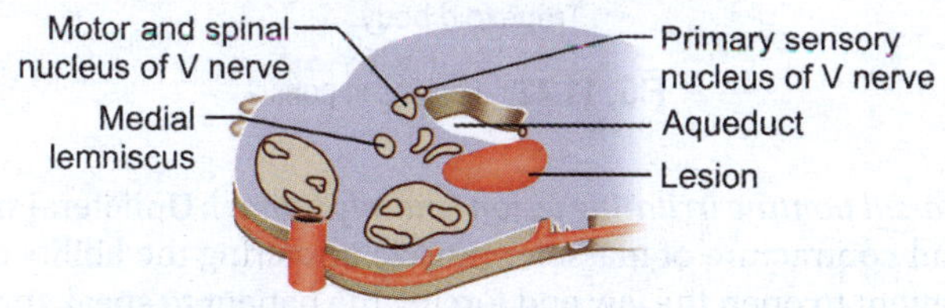

Lesion at upper pontine tegmentum (Section A)

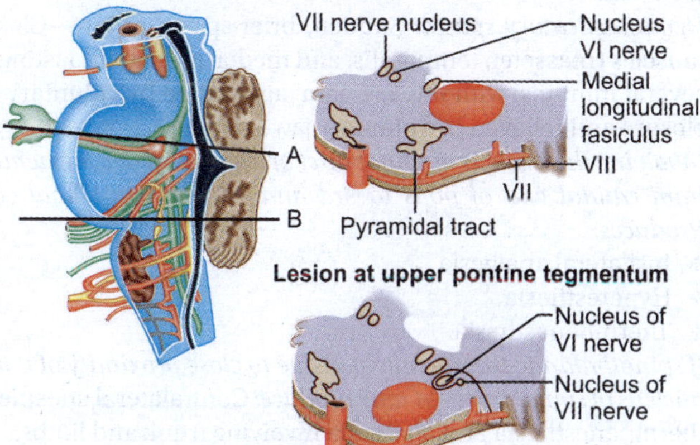

Lesion at upper pontine tegmentum

Paramedian lesion of lower basis pontine (Section B)

FIG. 11.41   Different levels of lesions in brain

- ❖ Descending sympathetic fibers
- ❖ Medial longitudinal fasiculus involvement.
- *Lesions in pontine tegmentum due to involvement of main sensory nucleus of cranial nerve V:* Trigominal sensory neuropathy— producing numbness, paresthesia of half of the face, scalp, ear, tongue.
- *Small left dorsolateral pontine infarct (involving principal sensory nucleus and pars oralis)—produces:* Isolated orofacial sensory defect without any sensory deficit of limb and trunk.

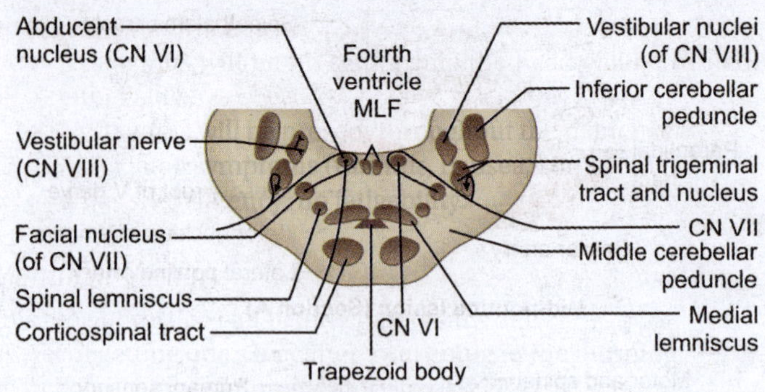

FIG. 11.42 Lesions in pons

- *Dorsal pontine irritating lesion (mainly tumor):* Unilateral spasm and contracture of masseter muscle impairing the ability of the patient to open the jaw and forcing the patient to speak through the teeth.
- *Hemimasticatory spasm:* Sudden, brief spasm of jaw—Closing muscles (masseter, temporalis, and medial pterygoid) lasting for several minutes, with intense pain, aggravated by voluntary jaw closure and relieved by voluntary jaw opening.
- *Involving the nucleus of spinal tract of trigeminal nerve extending from caudal end of pons to 3rd and 4th cervical spinal cord. Produces:*
  - ❖ Ipsilateral analgesia
  - ❖ Hyperesthesia
  - ❖ Thermoanesthesia.

  If spinothalamic tract is involved due to close proximity of it with nucleus of spinal tract—it may produce: Contralateral anesthesia, thermoanesthesia and analgesia involving trunk and limbs.
- *Caudal pontine lesion—involving rostral spinal trigeminal nuclei—produces:* Diminution of intraoral sensation of all modalities, but facial sensation will be unimpaired.
- *Isolated ventral pontine infarction—produces:*
  - ❖ Midfacial ipsilateral sensory loss due to involvement of fibers supplying midfacial areas
  - ❖ Contralateral hemiparesis
  - ❖ Dysarthria.
- *Upper medullary spinal tract lesion—produces:* Entire trigeminal cutaneous distribution will be affected.
- *Lower medullary spinal tract lesion produces:* Sensory loss in forehead, cheek and jaw (onion-skin pattern sensory loss)

  Onion-skin—segmental distribution reflects: Rostral-to-caudal somatotropic arrangement of cutaneous distribution of spinal nucleus—perioral area → rostral and lateral face → caudal area.

- Lateral medullary syndrome—involvement of spinal nucleus of trigeminal nerve.

Preganglionic Trigeminal Nerve Root Lesions

- Preganglionic cranial nerve V involvement may be associated with—other cranial nerves VI, VII and VIIIth nerve.
  Features of cranial nerve V are:
  - ❖ Facial pain
  - ❖ Paresthesia
  - ❖ Numbness
  - ❖ Sensory loss
  - ❖ Depressed corneal reflex
  - ❖ Cranial nerve V motor function loss.
- Idiopathic isolated self-limited trigeminal sensory neuropathy.
- Cerebellopontine angle—Acoustic neuroma, meningioma involve cranial nerve V, VIII. The features of:
  - ❖ Ipsilateral cranial nerve V involvement
  - ❖ Ipsilateral cranial nerve VIII involvement.
  There may be associated following structures involvement:
  - ❖ Facial nerve paralysis
  - ❖ Cerebellar ataxia—ipsilateral
  - ❖ Nystagmus (due to involvement of cerebellar peduncle and cerebellum)
  - ❖ Ipsilateral-lateral rectus paralysis (due to abducens nerve involvement).
  - ❖ Involvement of IX and XII cranial nerve.
- *Trigeminal neuralgia (tic douloureux):* Sudden, lancinating, excruciating, paroxysmal unilateral pain in the distribution of one or more branches of trigeminal nerve.
  Pain lasts for minutes, brief, recurs several times a day.
  It occurs mostly in female, in advanced age, affects right side more than the left.
  It awakens the patient at night.
  Bilateral trigeminal neuralgia: It may occur due to multiple sclerosis.
  Painful paroxysm is triggered by non-nociceptive facial stimulation.
- *Pain of maxillary division:* Referred to upper lip, nose and cheek.
- *Pain of mandibular division:* Referred to lower lip.
- Pain of ophthalmic division is rare.
  The painful facial syndrome may occur due to any pathology affecting brainstem, preganglionic root, gasserian ganglion, peripheral trigeminal nerve.
- The irritating lesion at the entry zone of trigeminal nerve root— multiple sclerosis plaque, brainstem infarction, C-P angle tumor, cavernous malformation

- Meningioma, posterior fossa tumors.
- Brainstem displacement due to type-I Arnold-Chiari malformation or basilar invagination—producing compression of trigeminal nucleus.

Lesions Affecting Gasserian Ganglion

Lesions responsible for damage of gasserian ganglion:
- Tumor
- Sarcoidosis
- Tuberculosis
- Arachnoiditis
- Trauma
- Abscess.

Pain is ipsilateral, severe, hemi-facial or along the distribution of selected branch, starting near midline on the upper lip, chin, progressing laterally to the ear.

Other cranial nerves (VI nerve) may be affected.

Bilateral trigeminal neuropathies along with bilateral abducens paralysis occur in **Tangier disease**.

Bilateral trigeminal neuropathies (sensory) may occur in **connective tissue disease due to vasculitis.**

Trigeminal sensory neuropathy can be distinguished from other conditions associated with facial numbness by following features:
- Sparing the muscles of mastication
- Frequent bilaterality
- Disregard the trigeminal boundaries
- Negative neuroimaging studies.

Trauma to trigeminal nerve may occur—due to—blow in auriculotemporal area—produces complete sensory and motor trigeminal neuropathy.

Raeder's Paratrigeminal Syndrome

Lesions responsible:
- Tumor
- Trauma
- Aneurysm
- Infection.

It has two basic components:
1. *Oculosympathetic paresis:* Produces meiosis, ptosis.
2. *Trigeminal nerve involvement*: Unilateral, head, facial or retro-orbital pain.
- May be associated with IV and VI nerve involvement.

Site of lesion

In the middle cranial fossa in the region between internal carotid artery and trigeminal ganglion near petrous apex.

Gradenigo's Syndrome

Lesions responsible:

- Trauma
- Tumor
- Osteitis
- Leptomeningitis.

Site of lesion

Apex of temporal bone.

Clinical Features

- *Ophthalmic division of trigeminal nerve:* Pain and sensory disturbances in upper part of the face.
- *Abducens nerve paralysis:* Ipsilateral lateral rectus paralysis
- *Oculosympathetic paresis:* Miosis, Ptosis.

Cavernous Sinus Syndrome (Fig. 11.43)

Lesions involve:

- Trauma
- Tumor
- Carotid-cavernous fistula
- Infection.

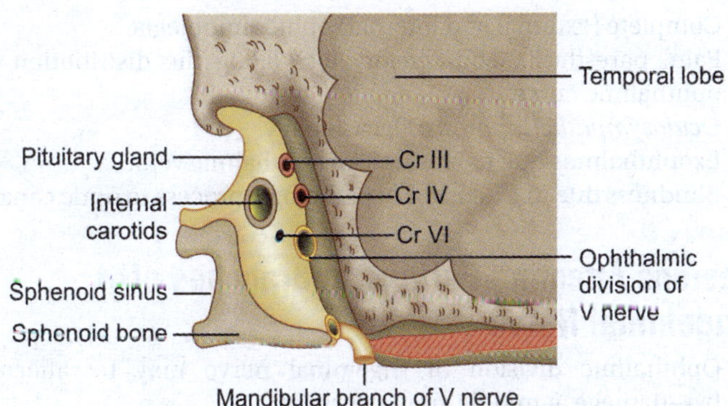

FIG. 11.43   Coronal diagram of cavernous sinus

Nerves involved:
- Ophthalmic and maxillary division of trigeminal nerve
- Abducens nerve
- Oculomotor nerve
- Trochlear nerve.

Clinical Features

- Total unilateral ophthalmoplegia
- *If tumor starts laterally:* Oculomotor palsy
- *If lesions starts from sella:* Pain, paresthesia and sensory loss in the distribution of ophthalmic or maxillary division of trigeminal nerve.

Since mandibular division is no involved no masticatory paresis is evident.

Superior Orbital Fissure Syndrome

The following nerves pass through superior orbital fissure:
- Abducens
- Trochlear nerve
- Oculomotor nerve
- Ophthalmic division of trigeminal nerve.

Lesions responsible:
- Tumor
- Aneurysm
- Infection
- Trauma.

Clinical Features

- Complete (external and internal) ophthalmoplegia.
- Pain, paresthesia and sensory loss along the distribution of ophthalmic nerve.
- *Oculosympathetic paresis:* Occasionally.
- Exophthalmos due to blockade of ophthalmic vein.
- Blindness due to extension of pathologic process to optic canal.

Lesions Affecting Peripheral Branches of Trigeminal Nerve

- Ophthalmic division of trigeminal nerve may be affected by—damage at middle cranial fossa at:
  - Temporal bone apex
  - Lateral wall of cavernous sinus
  - Superior orbital fissure
  - In the face.

- Maxillary division may be affected by:
  - ❖ Lower lateral wall of cavernous sinus
  - ❖ Foramen rotundum
  - ❖ In the pterygopalatine fossa
  - ❖ Floor of the orbit
  - ❖ Infraorbital foramen
  - ❖ On the face.

Numb Cheek Syndrome

Lesion—In infraorbital foramen.

Clinical Feature

Numbness involves: One cheek, upper lip, medial and lateral incisor, canine teeth and adjacent gingival, spares posterior teeth and gum.

Since distal branches of facial nerve are in close proximity to infraorbital branch of cranial nerve V, lesions in face mainly squamous cell carcinoma is associated with:
- Paresis of muscles of upper lip and angle of mouth
- Ipsilateral lower lid droop
  This is called Numb-cheek-limp-lid syndrome.

Trumpet Player's Neuropathy

Trumpet player exerts pressure on the lips with the mouth piece of instrument

↓

Pressure injures anterior superior alveolar nerve

↓

Upper lip numbness and pain.

Mandibular divison: It may be involved by damage of nerve at:
- Foramen ovale
- Zygomatic fossa
- Face.

Numb Chin Syndrome

Causes
- *Systemic cancer:*
  - ❖ Lymphoretricular malignancy
  - ❖ Carcinoma of breast and lung.
  - ❖ Metastasis in jaw producing compression on inferior alveolar nerves.
  - ❖ Base of the skull lesion.
  - ❖ Perineural infiltration of mental nerve.

Mandibular nerve may be affected proximally or distally. This can be differentiated by the following:
- *Involvement of VI and VII cranial nerve in proximal lesion* Involvement of other cranial nerves in distal lesion.
- *Pattern of oral numbness:* Numbness of incisor, canine and bicuspid teeth—due to involvement of incisive nerve—*Distal lesion.*

Dissociative sensory loss with sparing of dental sensation—Proximal involvement.

Tongue numbness—unilateral or bilateral—due to:
- Temporal arteritis
- Ischemia of brainstem or lingual nerve.

Neck Tongue Syndrome

Sudden turning of head produces:
- Pain in upper neck and occiput
- Ipsilateral numbness of the tongue
- Lingual pseudoathetosis.

Cause

Due to irritation of 2nd cervical dorsal root, which also carries proprioceptive fibers through hypoglossal nerve.

Periodic hemilingual numbness

Due to intermittent compression of the lingual nerve by sialolithiasis.

Lingual neuropathy: It involves—hemilingual sensory loss, pain, paresthesia, dysgeusia—due to:
- Wisdom teeth extraction
- Other dental procedure
- Surgery of mandibular ramus
- T-M joint displacement.

Bilateral anterior lingual hypogeusia, hypoesthesia due to:
- Damage of lingual nerve
- Damage of chorda tympani branches of facial nerve—conveying taste sensation.

Motor Evaluation of V Cranial Nerve (Fig. 11.44)

The muscles supplied by the motor branches of V cranial nerve:
- Masseter
- Temporalis
- Medial pterygoid
- Lateral pterygoid.
  - ❖ Clenching of the jaw is done by masseter and temporalis.
  - ❖ Side to side jaw movement is done by lateral and medial pterygoid.

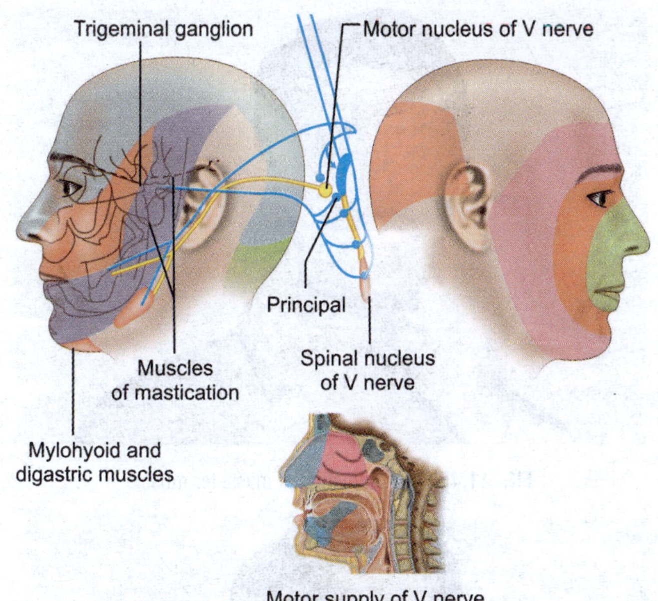

FIG. 11.44 Motor evaluation of V cranial nerve

Motor Function Testing

- *Test of muscle of mastication (Figs 11.45A and B)*
  - Place the fingers over masseter muscles
  - Ask the patient to bite
  - Test the latency, of contraction and force of contraction of masseter muscles bilaterally.

  Similarly, temporalis muscles can be tested.

- *Testing of pterygoids (Fig. 11.46):* While opening the mouth during mastication and jaws are opened, they are pushed forward. Opposing pterygoids are balanced.

  They can be tested in following manner:
  - Symmetry of temporal fossa and angle of jaw should be examined.
  - Ask the patient to open his mouth against pressure below the chin given by you—Watch—Any weakness is present or not. If present—On which side?
  - You place your hands against the sides of the jaw and instruct the patient to push against it.

In case supranuclear lesion: Deviation of jaw occurs towards the opposite side of lesion due to contralateral nucleus involvement.

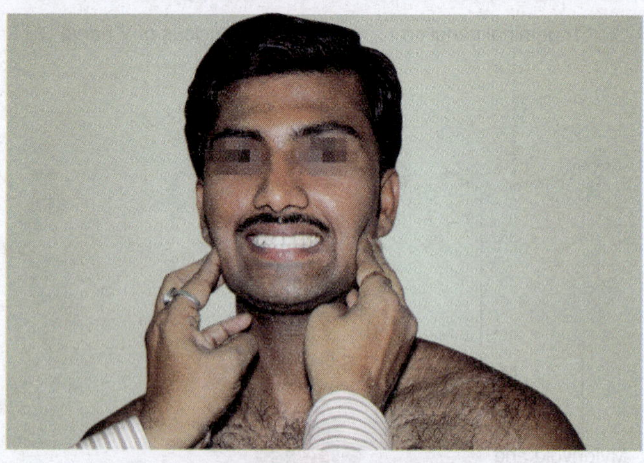

FIG. 11.45A   Examination of masseter muscle

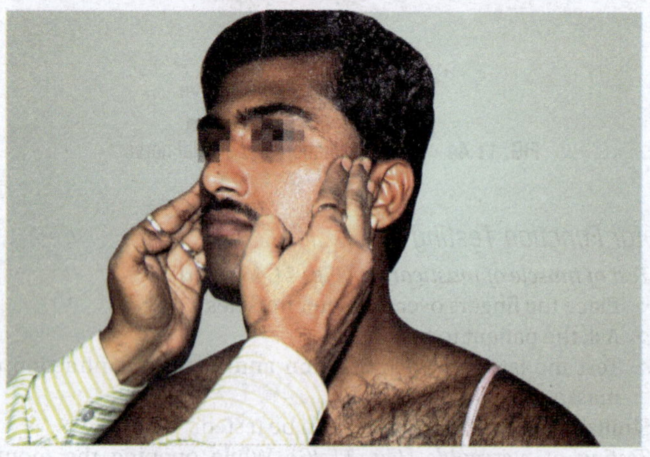

FIG. 11.45B   Examination of temporalis muscles

In case of nuclear lesion: Jaw deviation occurs towards the side of lesion, because masseter, temporalis and pterygoid of the side of lesion are involved.

In lower motor neuron lesions: Fasciculation and atrophy of the affected muscles seen.

Trismus: Inability to open the jaw may be seen in:

- Tetanus
- Acute dystonic reaction
- Polymyositis
- Trauma
- Nemaline myopathy
- Tryptophan associated eosinophilic connective tissue disease.

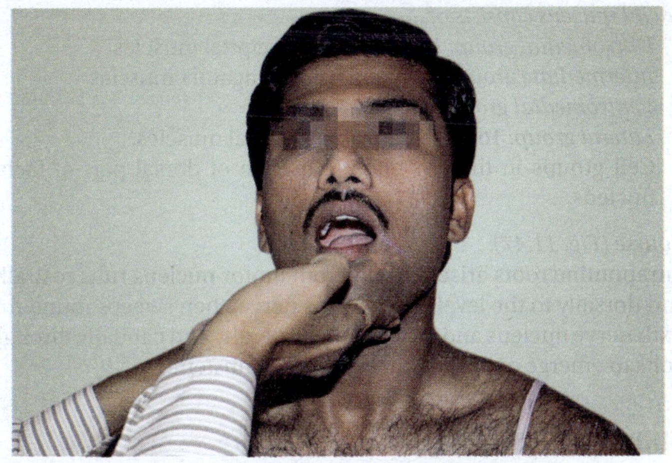

FIG. 11.46 Examination of pterygoid muscles

Intermittent weakness of the muscles of mastication occurs in:

- Myasthenia gravis
- Temporal arteritis
- Takayasu's disease
- Brachial myopathy
- Eaton-Lambert syndrome rarely.

Oromandibular Dystonia

It involves—Jaw opening, jaw closing, lateral movement, bruxism or combinations of above.

Jaw dystonia occurs in:

- Extrapyramidal syndrome due to psychoactive drugs
- Tardive dyskinesia
- Meige's syndrome (combination oromandibular dystonia and blepharospasm)
- Psychosis
- Complex partial seizures.

Painless trismus: Due to fibrosis of masseter in polymyositis.

▇ Facial Nerve

Anatomy: This nerve consists of two portions:

1. Facial nerve proper
2. Nervus intermedius.

   Motor facial nucleus—It present in reticular formation of pontine tegmentum, medial to nucleus of spinal tract of trigeminal nerve, anterolateral to VI cranial nerve nucleus.

Facial nucleus consists of:
- *Dorsomedial group:* Auricular and occipital muscles
- *Intermediate group:* Frontalis and corrugators muscles
- *Ventromedial group:* To platysma
- *Lateral group:* To buccinator, buccolabial muscles.
- Cell groups in the dorsolateral margin of dorsal part of facial nucleus.

Course (Fig. 11.47):
Intrapontine roots arise dorsally from motor nucleus runs rostrally and dorsally to the level of abducens nerve, then sweeps round the sixth nerve nucleus and passes ventrolaterally and caudally through pons to emerge on the lateral aspect of brainstem.

Supranuclear Control

Corticobulbar fibers originating from lower part of precentral gyrus → passes through corona radiata, genu of internal capsule, medial part of cerebral peduncle to reach the pons. Here, the fibers cross to other side and supply contralateral facial nucleus.

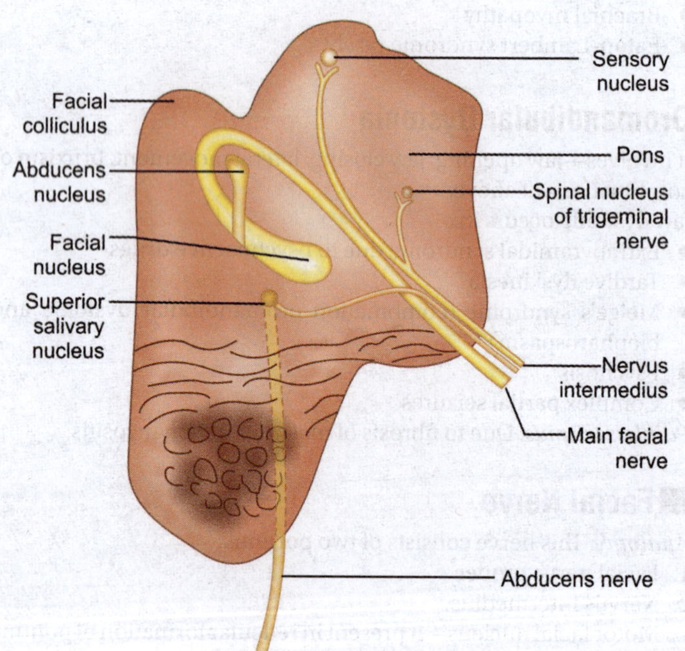

FIG. 11.47   Intracranial path of facial nerve

Distribution of Corticobulbar Fibers (Fig. 11.48)

- Ventral part of facial nucleus—it is supplying lower part of the face, richly supplied by supranuclear fibers—unilateral.
- Dorsal part of facial nucleus, responsible for supply to upper part of face is under bilateral supranuclear control.

Involuntary facial movements are controlled by separate supranuclear pathways. They do not descend in internal capsule.

Right cerebral hemisphere is responsible for controlling supranuclear emotional control.

Nervous Intermedius (Figs 11.49A and B)

It has two parts:

1. *Sensory part*: It receives sensory fibers from geniculate ganglion—which carries sensations from:
   - Anterior two-thirds of tongue
   - Pharynx
   - Nose
   - Palate
   - Skin of external auditory meatus
   - Lateral pinna
   - Mastoid.

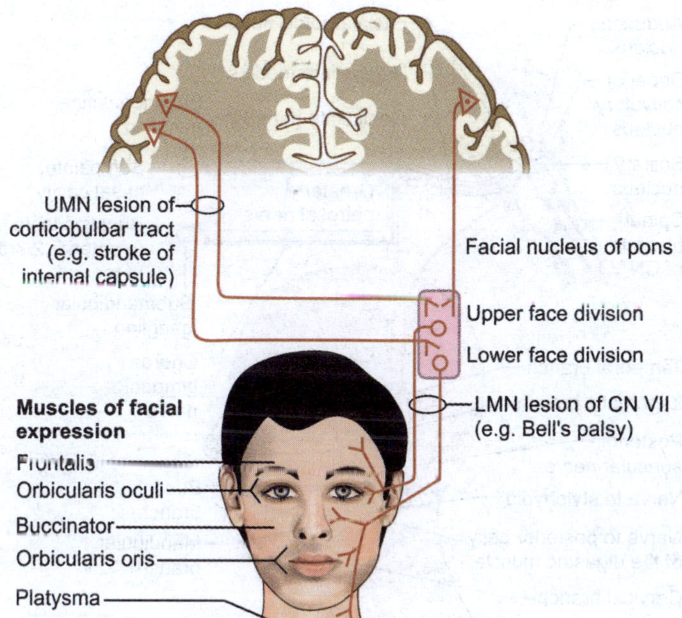

FIG. 11.48 Muscles supplied by facial nerve

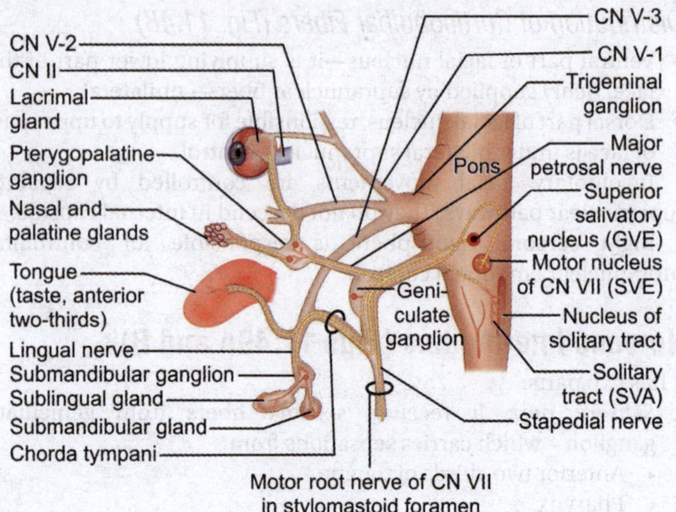

FIG. 11.49A   Course of facial nerve–I

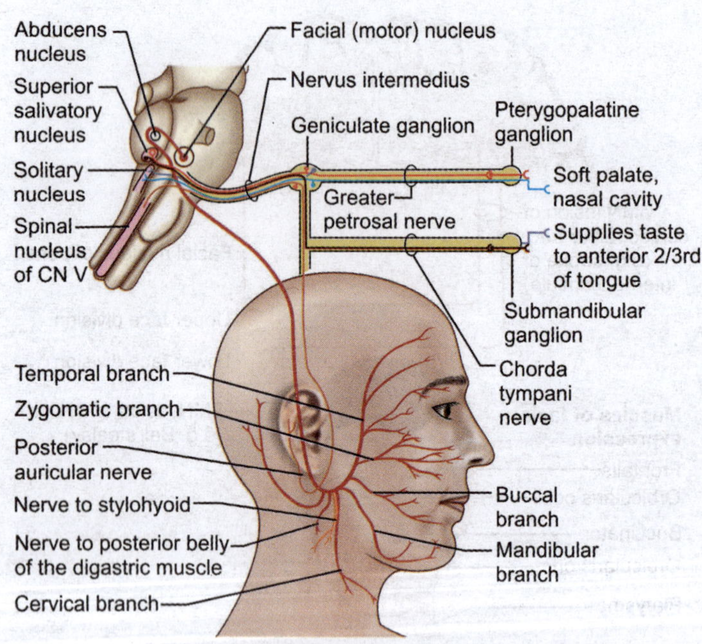

FIG. 11.49B   Course of facial nerve–II

2. *Parasympathetic part:* (Fig. 11.49C)
   - Preganglionic fibers (parasympathetic) to submaxillary ganglion—Postganglionic fibers supply submaxillary gland, submandibular gland and sublingual gland.
   - Preganglionic parasympathetic fibers to pterygopalatine or sphenopalatine ganglion—Postganglionic fibers supply lacrimal gland, nasal and palatal glands.

Nucleus of Nervus Intermedius (Fig. 11.50)

- Parasympathetic fibers arise from superior salivary nucleus.
- Parasympathetic fibers responsible for lacrimation arises from adjacent accessory nucleus—Lacrimal nucleus
- Gustatory afferent nerve ends in nucleus of tractus solitarius.
- Exteroceptive afferent ends in spinal tract of trigeminal nerve.

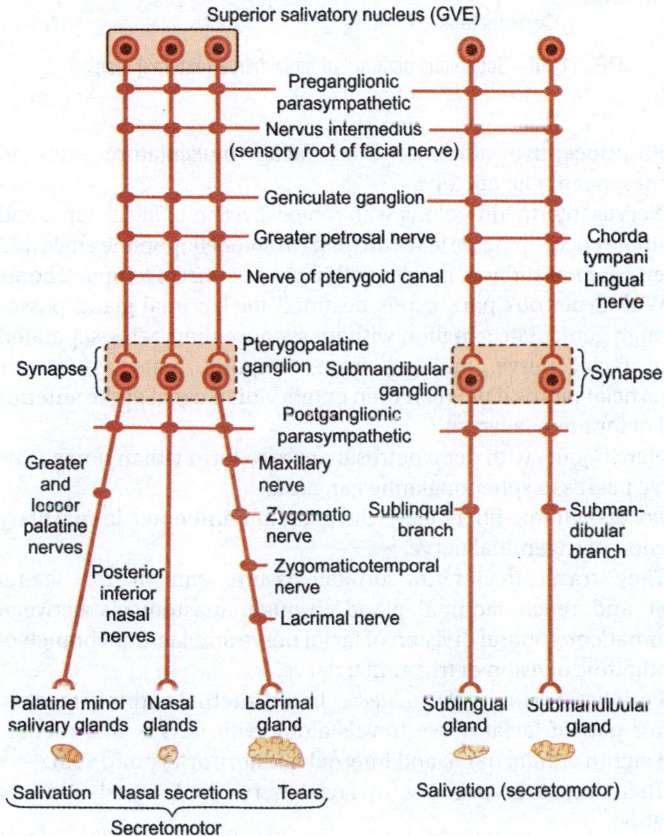

FIG. 11.49C Autonomic part of facial nerve

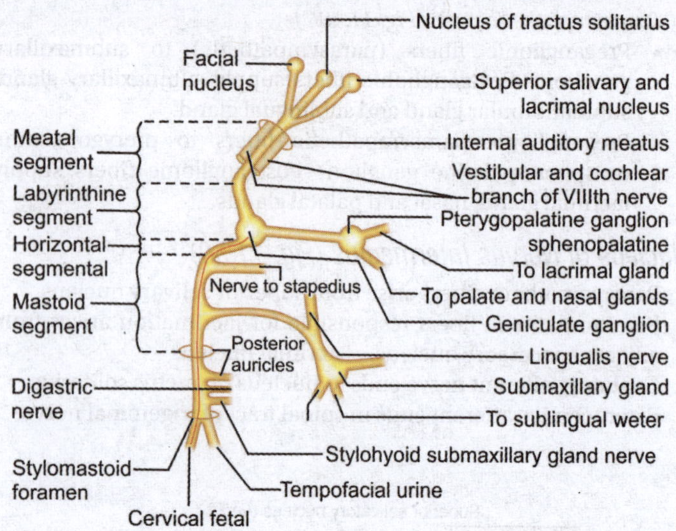

FIG. 11.50   Schematic diagram of facial nerve (external cranial)

- Proprioceptive afferents from facial musculature ends in mesencephalic nucleus.

Nervus intermedius along with motor division of facial nerve and vestibule cochlear nerve leave the pons at cerebellopontine angle and enters internal auditory meatus within petrous part of temporal bone.

Within petrous part, axons destined for lacrimal gland passes through geniculate ganglion without synapse then being separated from facial nerve, emerges from temporal bone as Greater superficial petrosal nerve. It then enters vidian canal at the anterior end of foramen lacerum.

Here it joins with deep petrosal nerve to form vidian nerve. This nerve passes to sphenopalatine ganglion.

Postganglionic fibers leave the ganglion and enter in maxillary division of trigeminal nerve.

They travel to inferior orbital fissure; run in the lateral orbit and reach lacrimal gland through anastomosis between zygomaticotemporal division of facial nerve and lacrimal branch of ophthalmic division of trigeminal nerve.

Peripheral course of facial nerve: In the internal auditory meatus, motor part of facial nerve travels along with nervus intermedius and eighth cranial nerve and internal auditory artery and vein.

There are four portions of facial nerve in internal auditory meatus:

1. *Meatal segment*: Facial nerve runs with nervus intermedius and eighth cranial nerve. There is no branch.

2. *Labyrinthine segment*: In this segment 1st major branch of facial nerve, greater superficial petrosal nerve—Arising from apex of geniculate ganglion—Preganglionic parasympathetic afferent—which innervates lacrimal, nasal and palatal glands.
3. *Horizontal segment*: No major branch originates from this segment.
4. *Mastoid segment*:
   a. From the upper end of this segment—nerve to stapedius arises.
   b. Second major branch—Corda tympani—Joins with lingual nerve. This branch contains preganglionic parasympathetic fibers that innervates submaxillary and sublingual glands through submaxillary ganglion (See Fig. 11.50).
   c. During the exit of facial nerve, it gives rise to following branches:
      i. Posterior auricular nerve (to occipitalis, posterior auricular, transverse and oblique auricular muscles)
      ii. Digastric branches (to posterior belly of digastric)
      iii. Stylohyoid nerve (to stylohyoid muscles).

Facial nerve pierces the parotid gland and is divided into two divisions (Fig. 11.51):
1. Temporofacial branch
2. Cervicofacial branch.

Clinical Evaluation of Facial Nerve Function
Motor Functions
- Symmetry of face
- Symmetry of blinking and lips movements

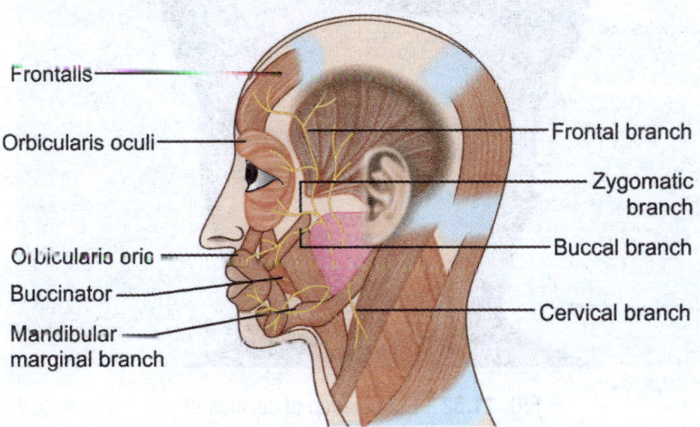

FIG. 11.51 Principal extracranial branches of facial nerve

- Wrinkles of the forehead
- Prominence or absence of nasolabial fold
- Spontaneous movement of the mouth, abnormal movement—like tremor, twitching, myokymia
- Look for atrophy and fasciculation
- Note pattern of spontaneous blinking for frequency and symmetry.

Ask the patient to:
- Frown (Fig. 11.52)
- Close the both eyes forcefully (Fig. 11.53)
- Show his teeth (Fig. 11.54)
- Blow out the cheeks (Fig. 11.55)
- Retract his chin (Fig. 11.56)
- Look upward without elevating his head (Fig. 11.57).

Ask the patient if he has any history of hyperacusis. Weakness of stapedius muscle.

Stylohyoid, posterior belly of digastric, auricular muscles, occipitalis cannot be tested.

But any history of oropharyngeal dysphagia may be due to involvement of:
- Buccinators
- Stylohyoid muscles
- Posterior belly of digastric and perioral muscle weakness.

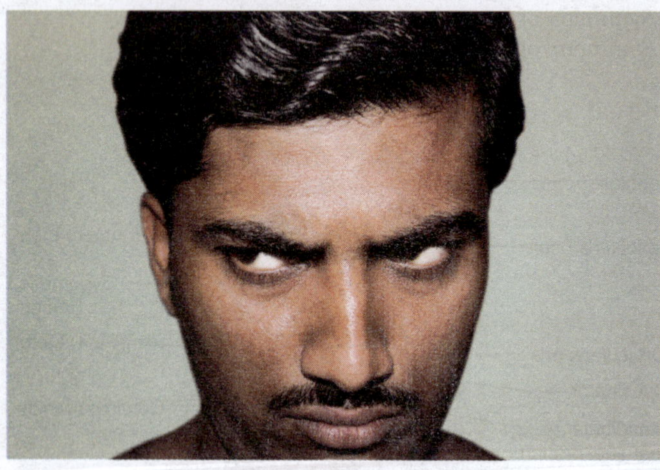

FIG. 11.52   Examination of corrugator

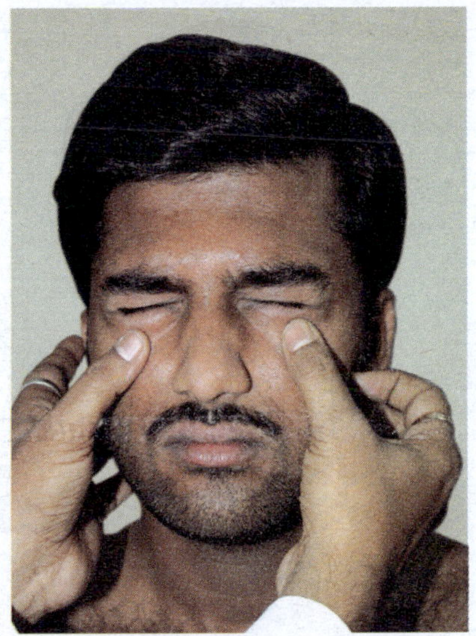

FIG. 11.53   Examination of orbicularis oculi

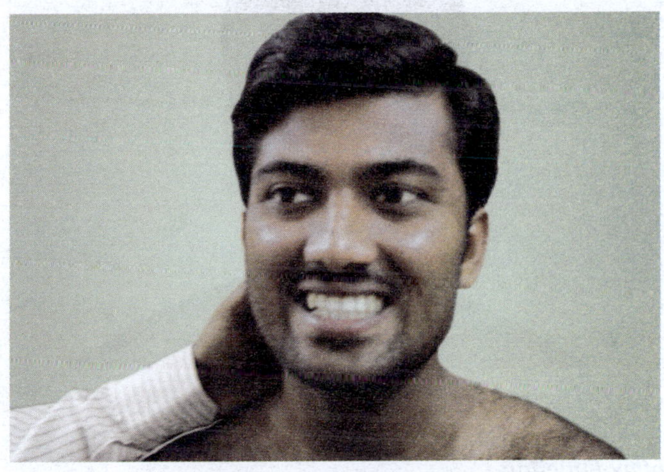

FIG. 11.54   Examination of orbicularis oris

Sensory Function

Taste sensation of anterior two-thirds of the tongue for sweet, sour, salt and bitter taste—each half to be tested separately and find asymmetry.

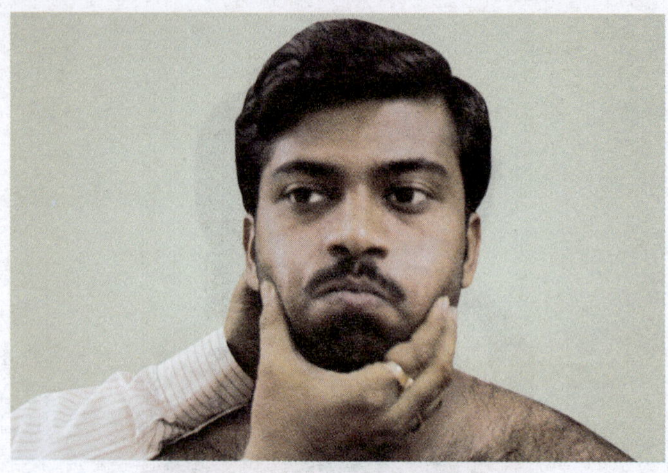

FIG. 11.55   Examination of buccinator

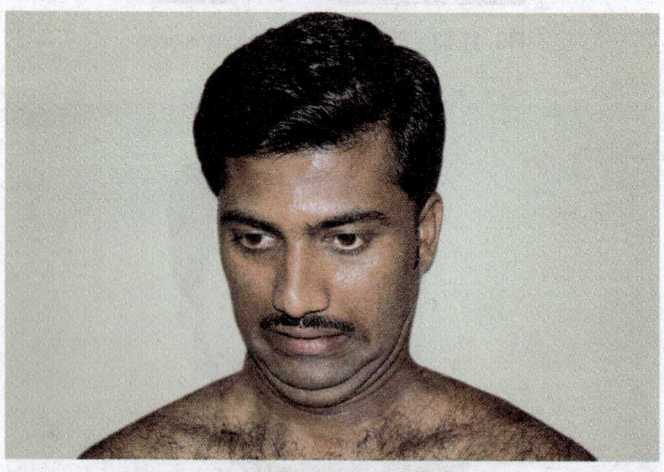

FIG. 11.56   Examination of platysma muscle

Reflex Function

Two important facial reflexes are:
1. Corneal reflex
2. Palpebral reflex.

Parasympathetic Function

Infranuclear lesion is responsible for—increased or impaired lacrimation. This can be tested by—hanging the litmus or filter paper on each lower eyelid (Schirmer's test) (Fig. 11.58).

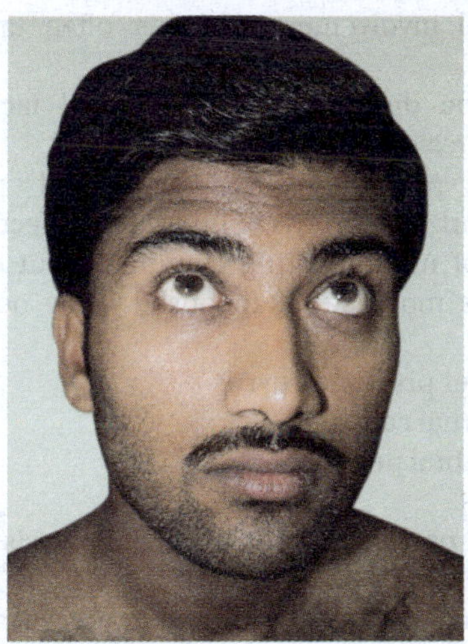

FIG. 11.57   Examination of frontal belly of occipitofrontalis

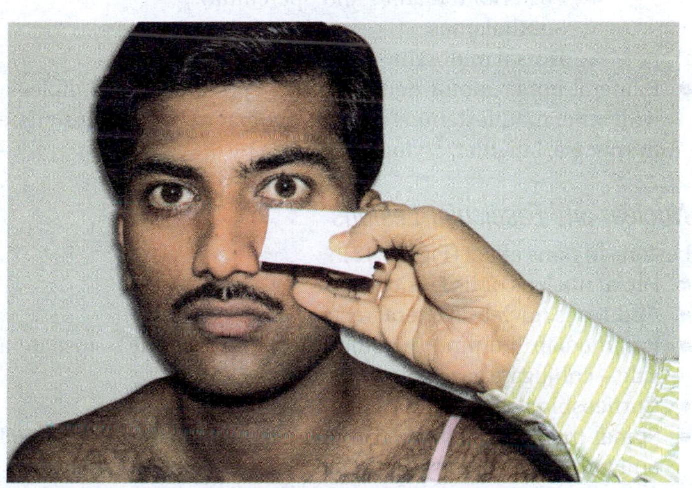

FIG. 11.58   Schirmer test

Localization of Lesion of Facial Nerve

Supranuclear Lesion

- *In supranuclear corticobulbar lesion:* Contralateral paresis of lower portion of face—Because upper portion of face has bilateral innervations with corticobulbar tract, but lower portion of face has only control led by contralateral corticospinal tract.
- ❖ Muscles around mouth are most commonly affected.

- ❖ Occasional involvement of lower often upper orbicularis oculi.
- There may be dissociation of volitional facial paresis and emotional paresis of facial muscles.
  - ❖ Volitional paresis without emotional paresis—(during speaking orbicularis oris of one side is affected, or retraction of angle of mouth during command, but during laughing both sides move simultaneously)—may occur with lesion involving:
    - i. Lower precentral gyrus
    - ii. Internal capsule
    - iii. Cerebral peduncle
    - iv. Pons.
  - ❖ Emotional paresis without volitional paresis will occur—due to lesion:
    - i. Frontal lobe lesion anterior to precentral gyrus
    - ii. Supplementary motor area
    - iii. Thalamus
    - iv. Posterior thalamus and operculum
    - v. Subthalamus
    - vi. Dorsal midbrain.
- Bilateral upper motor neuron lesion—produces facial diplegia, with other manifestations of pseudobulbar palsy (spastic tongue, dysphagia, laughter, crying).

Nuclear and Fascicular Lesions

Lesions in pons affect (Fig. 11.42):
- Facial nucleus or its fascicles.
- Abducens nucleus—lateral rectus palsy.
- Paramedian pontine reticular formation (PPRF)—ipsilateral side—conjugate gaze palsy.
- Corticospinal tract—contralateral hemiparesis.
- Spinal tract of trigeminal nerve—ipsilateral loss of pain, touch and temperature sensation of face.
- Spinothalamic tract—Contralateral loss of sensation of body.
  Unilateral lesion in facial motor nucleus—produces ipsilateral complete facial palsy—characterized by:
- Loss of facial wrinkling.
- Inability to frown.
- Cannot raise the eyebrow, close his eye, blow out his mouth, retract the angle of mouth, show his teeth, and tighten his chin.
- On attempt to close his eye, eyeball will be deviated upward and outward (Bell's phenomenon) it is due to:
  - a. Relaxation of inferior rectus
  - b. Contraction of superior rectus.

- Loss of corneal and palpebral reflexes
- Food will be accumulated between teeth and cheeks due to buccinator paralysis.

There are few syndromes related to facial nerve involvement along with involvement of associated structures (Fig. 11.41):
- *Millard-Gubler syndrome:* Lesion in ventral pons.
  - *Involvement of facial nerve:* Ipsilateral facial paresis
  - *Involvement of abducens nerve:* Ipsilateral lateral rectal paresis
  - *Involvement of corticospinal tract:* Contralateral hemiplegia.
- *Foville syndrome:* Lesion located in pontine tegmentum.
  - *Involvement of facial nerve:* Ipsilateral facial paralysis
  - *Involvement of PPRF:* Paralysis of conjugate gaze to ipsilateral side
  - *Involvement of corticospinal tract:* Contralateral hemiplegia.
- *Eight-and-a-half syndrome:* Lesion involve dorsal tegmentum of caudal pons:
  - *Involvement of PPRF:* Paralysis of conjugate gaze to ipsilateral side.
  - *Involvement of abducens nerve:* Paralysis of ipsilateral lateral rectus.
  - *Involvement of medial longitudinal fasciculus:* Internuclear ophthalmoplegia.
  - *Involvement of facial nerve:* Ipsilateral facial palsy.
- *Isolated peripheral facial and abducens palsy:* Discrete Lesion in caudal tegmental pons:
  - *Involvement of facial fascicle or nucleus:* Ipsilateral facial palsy.
  - *Involvement of abducens nerve:* Ipsilateral lateral rectus palsy.

Posterior Fossa Lesion

Lesions at cerebellopontine angle (Fig. 11.59):
- *Involvement of facial nerve:* Ipsilateral facial palsy
- *Involvement of nervus intermedius:* Loss of taste over anterior two-thirds of the tongue
- *Vestibular nerve involvement:* It produces tinnitus, deafness without hyperacusis.
- *Involvement of pons:* Nystagmus and ipsilateral gaze palsy (PPRF involvement).
- *Involvement of abducens nerve:* Ipsilateral lateral rectus palsy.

Involvement of Facial Nerve in Meatal Canal

- Involvement of facial nerve
- Involvement of nervus intermedius
- Involvement of cight cranial nerves.

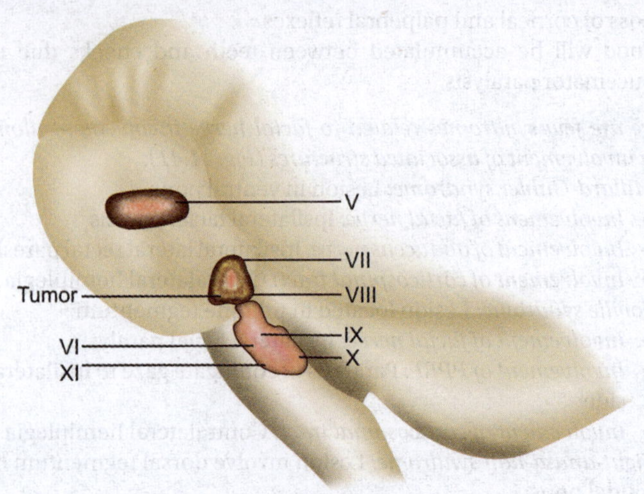

FIG. 11.59   CP angle tumor

Lesion of Facial Nerve within Facial Canal Distal to Meatal Segment but Proximal to Departure of Nerve to Stapedius Muscle

- Facial motor nerve involvement—ipsilateral.
- Nervus intermedius involvement.
- If lesion proximal to greater superficial petrosal nerve—lacrimation is impaired.
- If lesion distal to greater superficial petrosal nerve—lacrimation is normal.
- If geniculate ganglion is involved—due to reactivation of herpes zoster virus, Epstein—Barr virus, mumps, human herpes virus there is hyperacusis, geniculate neuralgia and herpetic vesicles in ear drum, external auditory meatus or palate. (Ramsay Hunt syndrome).

Lesion in Facial Nerve Distal to Departure of Nerve to Stapedius but Proximal to Departure of Chorda Tympani

- Ipsilateral facial nerve paralysis.
- Loss of taste of anterior two-thirds of tongue—ipsilaterally
- Hearing preserved, no hyperacusis.

Lesion Distal to Departure of Chorda Tympani

- Ipsilateral facial motor nerve involvement.
- No loss of taste or hyperacusis.

Lesion Distal to Stylomastoid Foramen

Causes of facial nerve involvement:

- Tumor, infection of parotid gland (sarcoidosis, infectious mononucleosis).
- Lyme's disease.
- Mandibular lymph node.
- Facial trauma—by obstetric forceps.
- AIDS
- Familial syndrome—hyperostosis interna.

Autosomal dominant disorder—recurrent facial nerve palsy with or without cranial nerves I, II, and cranial nerves VIII.

Idiopathic Bell's Palsy

Last trimester of pregnancy is considered to be increased risk (Figs 11.60A and B).

- Women developing Bell's palsy during pregnancy are susceptible to develop hypertension or pre-eclampsia.
- Diabetes.

If one or two facial muscles are involved on name side—it causes may be:

1. Tumor
2. Trauma
3. Perineural spread of skin cancer.

Lesion mainly occurs at the stylomastoid foramen. Patient complains of:

- Retroauricular pain
- Hyperacusis

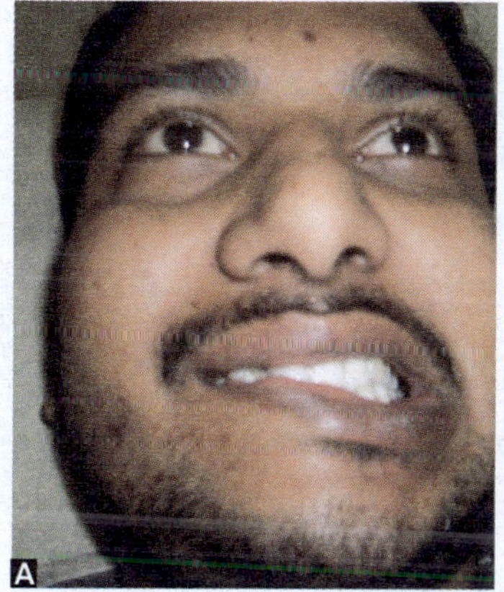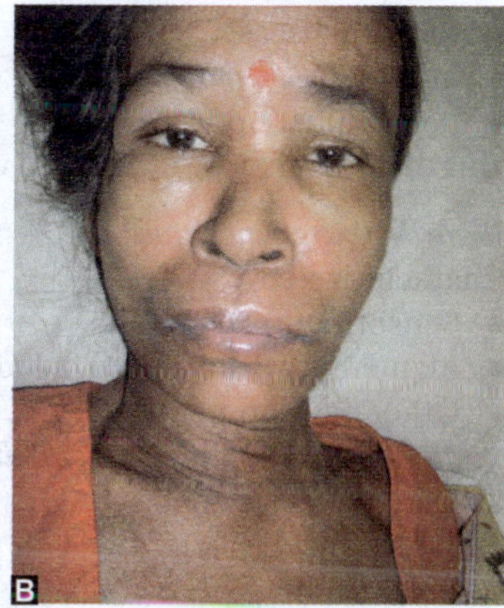

FIGS 11.60A AND B   Bell's palsy

- Dysgeusia
- Decreased tearing.

Retroauricular pain may precede the onset by at least 2 weeks—or maximal at onset—and progresses over 24–48 hours.

Transiently patient may complain of oropharyngeal dysphagia to solid or liquid.

In addition to complete unilateral facial paralysis, patient may develop—corneal ulcerations due to lagophthalmos, may develop epiphora or dry eye.

Progress

- May be favorable prognosis—self-limiting
- If herpes zoster infection, there may be poor prognosis
- Rarely recovery followed by myokymia, blepharospasm like activity.
- Hemifacial muscle mass contraction may be present with normal movement of the face.
- May be aberrant regeneration of nerve fibers, e.g.
  - ❖ Involuntary tearing of involved eye (crocodile tears).
  - ❖ Gustatory sweating due to faulty reinnervation of parasympathetic fibers to sweat glands.
- Recurrence of Bell's palsy.

Melkersson-Rosenthal Syndrome

This is characterized by:
- Recurrent orofacial swelling—affecting lips, face, eyelids
- Unilateral or bilateral facial paralysis
- Scrotal tongue.

This syndrome may be associated with the following disorders:
- Hyperhidrosis
- Acroparesthesia
- Crohn's disease
- Migraine
- Retrobulbar optic neuritis.

This disorder may be associated with:

Waardenburg syndrome
Characterized by:
- Sensorineural deafness
- Pigmentary disturbance in hair and iris
- Other developmental defects.

Bilateral facial paralysis (facial diplegia): Causes are:
- Congenital anomalies
- Infections
- Postinfectious
- Tumor

- Traumatic
- Granulomatous
- Collagen vascular diseases
- Osteopetrosis
- Idiopathic.

Möbius syndrome
It is due to hypoplasia of VI and VII nerve nucleus:
- Bifacial paralysis
- Abnormalities in horizontal eye movements.
Poland's anomaly—Developmental facial diplegia is associated with:
- Unilateral pectoralis muscle hypoplasia
- Ipsilateral breast and upper limb characteristics.

Abnormalities of Tear Secretion

- *Lesion in pons:*
  - ❖ Involvement of superior salivary nucleus—decrease salivary flow.
  - ❖ Involvement of lacrimal nucleus—decrease tears flow.
- *Lesion in brainstem:*
  - ❖ Ipsilateral facial motor paralysis
  - ❖ Sparing of sensory-parasympathetic components—sparing of salivary and tear flow.
- *Lesion in cerebellopontine angle:*
  - ❖ Ipsilateral facial motor paralysis
  - ❖ Loss of taste
  - ❖ Hyperacusis, hearing loss
  - ❖ Loss of lacrimation—dry eye.
- *Acoustic neurinoma in—internal auditory canal:* Asymptomatic tearing on ipsilateral side of the eye.
- *Lesion in floor of middle cranial fossa near gasserian ganglion— due to herpes zoster, tumors, petrositis, internal carotid artery aneurysm:* Impairment of tearing.
- *Extradural in middle cranial fossa—(nasopharyngeal carcinoma):*
  - ❖ Impairment of tearing
  - ❖ Abducens nerve paralysis on the side of lesion.
- *Lesion in sphenopalatine ganglion:*
  - ❖ Impairment of tearing
  - ❖ Dryness of nasal mucosa
  - ❖ Paresthesia or hyperesthesia in the maxillary division of trigeminal nerve.
- Dysautonomia—Riley-Day syndrome, Pandysautonomia, Shy-Drager syndrome reduced secretion of tear.

Abnormal eyelid closure: Two types of blinking are usually occur
- Voluntary eyelid closure—precentral supranuclear control
- Emotional eyelid closure—controlled by extrapyramidal pathways—originating from:
    - Putamen
    - Globus pallidus
    - Thalamus.

Eyelid blinking consists of:
- *Rapid downward phase:* It results from pulse-type firing pattern.
- *Slow upward phase:* It results from pulse—step firing pattern.
    Open eyelid position—in maintained by tonic activity of levator.

Blink results from:
- Inhibition of levator
- Simultaneous contraction of orbicular in oculi
    Down force velocities is two times faster than up phase.
    Blinking is controlled by dopaminergic activity.

So decreased frequency of periodic blinking—occurs in:
- Progressive supranuclear palsy
- Parkinsonism.

Increased frequency of blinking occurs in:
- Drugs induced dyskinesia
- Gilles de la Tourette syndrome
- Schizophrenia.

Insufficient Eye Closure

- *Lesion in precentral gyrus:*
    - Paresis of voluntary eye closure
    - Relative sparing of emotional eye closure.
- *Lesion in nondominant frontal lobe or bilateral frontal lobe lesion:*
    - Compulsive eye closure
    - Unable to initiate voluntary eye closure bilaterally but comprehend the task and presence of intact reflex of eye closure.
- *Apraxia of eyelid closure:*
    - ALS
    - Creutzfeldt-Jakob disease
    - Progressive supranuclear palsy.
- *Bilateral hemispheric or unilateral nondominant hemispheric lesion:* Motor impersistance.
    When the patient is asked to close his eyes and keep them closed—he is unable to maintain closed eyelid, rather he will develop fine tremor followed by reopening.

This usually happens in contralateral eyelid in case of:
- Unilateral hemispheric lesion mainly, right-sided brain damage
- Parkinsonism.

Spasmodic Eye Closure, Blepharospasm

- *Spasmodic eye closure:* Focal seizures (frontal focus).
- *Blepharospasm:* Repeated involuntary, bilateral contracture of orbicularis oculi.
  It may occur with:
  - *Spasmodic dysphonia:* Spasmodic torticolis
  - *Oromandibular dystonia:* Meige's syndrome.

Blepharospasm may occur in:
- Multiple sclerosis
- Bilateral infarction of brainstem, diencephalon, stratum
- Olivo pontocerebellar atrophy.

Unilateral blepharospasm: Frontal cortical infarct of left side
Painful blepharospasm: Eye disease—conjunctivitis
Drug-induced blepharospasm: Tardive dyskinesia
The responsible degenerative diseases for blepharospasm:
- Wilson's disease
- Huntington's disease
- Parkinson's disease
- Progressive supranuclear palsy
- Retinal degeneration
- Apoceruloplasmin deficiency.

Reflex blepharospasm: It occurs:
- After severe hemiplegia
- Nondominant temporoparietal region is usually affected
- It is limited to nonparalyzed side
- It can be evoked when the examiner tries to hold his eye open.

Abnormal Facial Movements

Dyskinctic Movements

Orofacial dyskinesia: It is constellation of movements of face, tongue, jaw, lips—involving following movements:
- Facial grimaces, distortions, expression and twitches
- Pursing, puckering, opening and closing of lips
- Writhing and distorted posturing of tongue
- Wide opening, tight closing of jaw.

Causes
- Idiopathic—elderly
- Side effects of neuroleptics
- Edentulous dyskinesia—lack of dentures
- Extrapyramidal diseases:
  - Huntington's chorea
  - Wilson's disease
  - Neuroacanthocytosis
- Schizophrenia.

Blepharospasm

Bilateral symmetrical involuntary, spasmodic contraction of orbicularis oculi. This may be episodic or sustained.

The causes may be:

- *Extrapyramidal diseases:*
  - ❖ Parkinson's disease
  - ❖ Progressive supranuclear palsy
  - ❖ Tardive dyskinesia
- Thalamic infarct
- Putaminal hemorrhage
- Lower pontine tegmental lesions.

This blepharospasm can be differentiated from other types of facial movements—by the former's symmetrical involvement.

Blepharospasm may be associated by:

- Photophobia
- Foreign body sensation
- If severe, inability to walk or drive.

Meige's syndrome: Blepharospasm associated with oromandibular dystonia which is manifested by grimacing of mouth, jaw clenching, contraction of platysma, and sustained neck contraction, spreading to arm and trunk.

Cause may be—basal ganglia dysfunction.

Brueghel's syndrome: Dystonia of motor components of trigeminal nerve, associated features may be up beating nystagmus, paroxysmal hyperpnea.

Hemifacial spasm: Painless, intermittent, tonic and clonic spasm of orbicularis oculi muscle, progressing downwards to involve orbicularis oris, buccinator, platysma of the affected side.

This spasm may progress from orbicularis oris upwards to involve all facial musculature of same side.

When bilateral, these spasms are asynchronous and asymmetric on both sides. Sometimes it may be alternating from side to side.

Causing of hemifacial spasm

- Lesion cerebellopontine angle
- Intrapontine lesion
- Temporal
- External compression of distal facial nerve within parotid space
- Schwannoma arising from intermediate nerve
- Idiopathic intracranial hypertension.

Postparalytic abnormal movement of facial muscles

Post Bell's palsy following phenomena occurs during recovery:

- Postparalytic hemifacial spasm
- Crocodile tears (eating provocating lacrimation)
- Facial contracture

- Facial synkinesia:
  - ❖ Contraction of the angle of mouth with eye blinking
  - ❖ On full opening of mouth there is eyelid closure or lateral movement of jaw (Marin-Amat syndrome).

The following are the causes:
- Aberrant regeneration of facial nerve on recovery
- One muscle will be innervated by two different cranial nerves during recovery.
  Facial—Trigeminal dyskinesia.
- Abnormal activity of residual motor units.

Facial myokymia: This is characterized by fine, continuous, wave-like, undulating movements (like a bag of worms) associated with muscle contracture.

Causes
- Guillain-Barré syndrome
- Syringobulbia
- Cerebellar and cerebellopontine angle tumor
- Sarcoidosis
- Meningeal carcinomatosis
- Phosgene poisoning
- Timber rattle angle envenomation.

Facial myorhythmia: Ocular, oculofacial or oculomasticatory myorhythmia—due to:
- Whipple's disease
- Use of interferon 2 alfa.

Focal cortical seizure: Clonic movements of the face, spreading to involve other muscles—due to—epileptogenic focus on fontal lobe involving lower precentral gyrus.

Tic and Habit spasm: Sudden, repetitive, stereotyped, involuntary simple or complex movements can be reproduced or inhibited voluntarily—involving muscles outside the distribution of facial nerve of psychogenic origin.

Gilles de la Tourette syndrome: Involuntary tic like movement or vocalization—due to basal ganglia dysfunction.

Fasciculation of facial muscles: Spontaneous twitching of individual muscles fascicles—due to:

Any disease process involving facial nerve nucleus.

Facial fasciculation along with fasciculation of tongue and limbs seen—Kennedy syndrome.

■ Eighth Cranial Nerve

Eighth cranial nerve has two components:
1. Cochlear nerve—it is concerned with hearing
2. Vestibular nerve —it is concerned with equilibrium.

Auditory Pathways (Flow Chart 11.3)

This pathway has four neuronal networks (Figs 11.61 and 11.62).

First Order Neurons

It originates from neuroepithelial hair cells of organ of Corti:

FLOW CHART 11.3 Algorithm of sound pathway

Transmitted via auricle (pinna) and external auditory meatus (canal)

↓

To tympanic membrane (ear drum) producers it to vibrate

↓

Vibration wave passes through malleus, incus and stapes. Causing oscillation of footplate of stapes

↓

Oscillation footplate make attached membrane of oral window to oscillate

↓

This oscillation agitate perilymph of scala vestibuli

↓

Vestibular membrane (Reissner's membrane) begins to oscillate

↓

As a result, generated waves in endolymph of scala media (cochlear duct) oscillate basilar membrane (which supports) organ of corti

↓

Stimulate hair receptor cells

↓

It converts mechanical energy to electrical energy

↓

It stimulates peripheral processes (dendrites) of the bipolar cells (1st order of neuron)—its cell body in with in cochlear ganglion

↓

Impulse in transmitted to central processes (axons) of bipolar 1st order neuron—it forms cochlear nerve

↓

Axons leaves inner ear via internal auditory meatus

↓

It enters posterior cranial fossa

↓

Thin it pierces brain stress at pontomedullary angle of brain stress

↓

It then terminates in cochlear nuclei

↓

Pathway of auditory stimulation from external auditory meatus to cochlear nuclei in brain stress

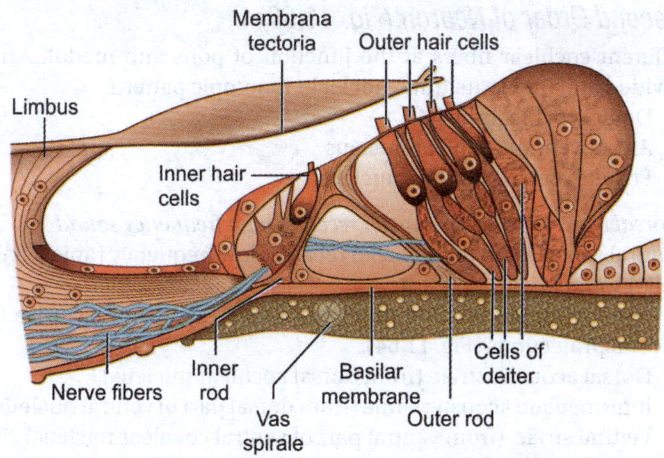

FIG. 11.61 Organ of Corti

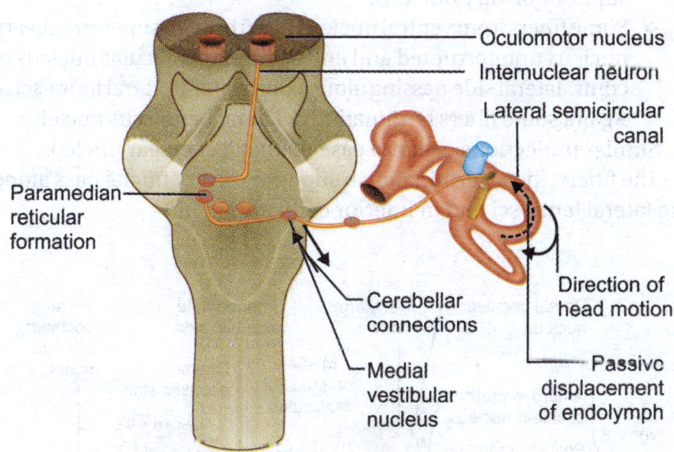

FIG. 11.62 Auditory pathway

- Hair cells at the apex of cochlea are stimulated by low frequency sounds
- Hair cells at the base of cochlea are stimulated by high frequency sounds.

The ganglion of this neuron situated at Rosenthal canal at the base of bony spiral lamina called spiral ganglion of cochlear nerve.

The afferent of this ganglion ends in hair cell of cochlea.

The efferent of this ganglion enters the brainstem at the level of ventral cochlear nuclei as cochlear nerve.

Second Order of Neuron (Fig. 11.63)

Afferent cochlear fibers at the junction of pons and medulla are divided and innervate three nuclei in tonotopic pattern:

- Dorsal cochlear nuclei
- Anteroventral cochlear nucleus
- Posteroventral cochlear nucleus.

Dorsal aspect of all three nuclei receives high frequency sound
Ventral aspect of all three nuclei receives low frequency (apical hair cells) sounds.

From these nuclei, 2nd order of neurons arise and give rise to several projections (Fig. 11.64):

- Dorsal acoustic striae (from dorsal cochlear nucleus)
- Intermediate acoustic striae (from dorsal part of ventral nucleus)
- Ventral striae (from ventral part of ventral cochlear nucleus)
  - ❖ Some fibers from ventral nucleus projects to superior olivary nucleus of same side.
  - ❖ Some fibers from ventral nuclei projects to contralateral superior olivary nucleus.
  - ❖ Some fibers from ventral nucleus pass through superior salivary nucleus uninterrupted and end at inferior collicular nucleus of contralateral side passing along contralateral lateral lemniscus.

Again, some fibers terminating in lateral lemniscus nuclei.
Similar projections occur in case of dorsal cochlear nucleus.

The fibers, those terminated in superior olivary nuclei pass along the lateral lemnisci end in inferior colliculus.

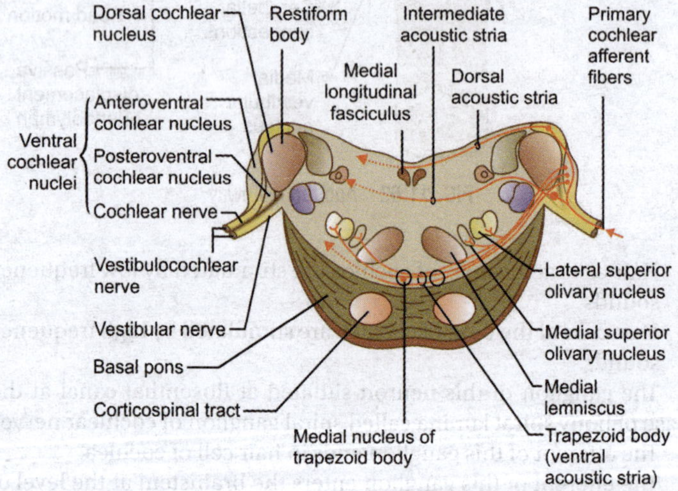

FIG. 11.63 Pathways of VIII nerve

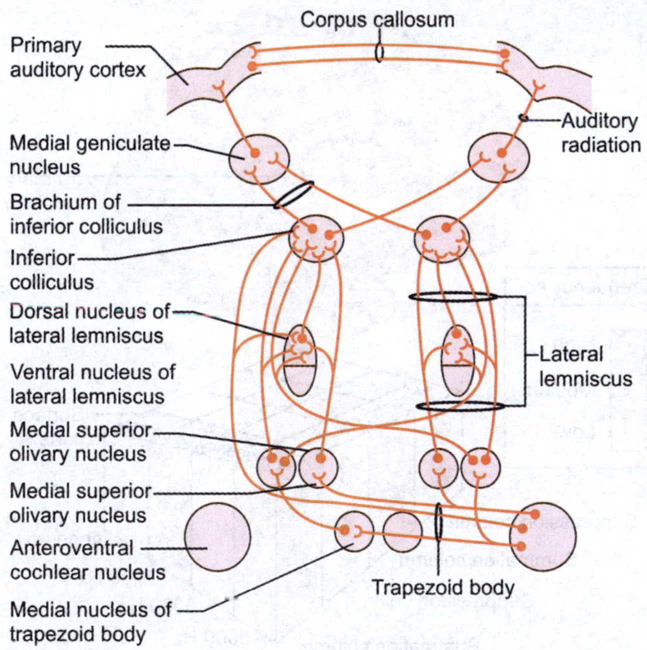

FIG. 11.64   Projection towards auditory cortex

Third Order of Neurons

Inferior colliculus located in midbrain serves as central nucleus of auditory pathways. Fibers from interior colliculus end in medial geniculate body ipsilaterally in a tonotopic manner:

- Fibers containing high frequency sounds terminate in apical and lateral areas of medial geniculate body.
- Fibers containing low frequency sounds terminate in medial part of medial geniculate body.

Fourth Order of Neurons

From medial geniculate body the geniculotemporal fibers or auditory radiations pass laterally in a dense tract and end in following manners:

- Most fibers end in Lamina IV of primary auditory cortex (Brodmann's area 41) in transverse temporal gyri of Heschl.
- Some fibers end in Brodmann's area 42 of auditory association area.

The distribution of fibers is tonotopic (Fig. 11.65)

- High frequency sounds terminate medially
- Low frequency sounds terminate laterally.

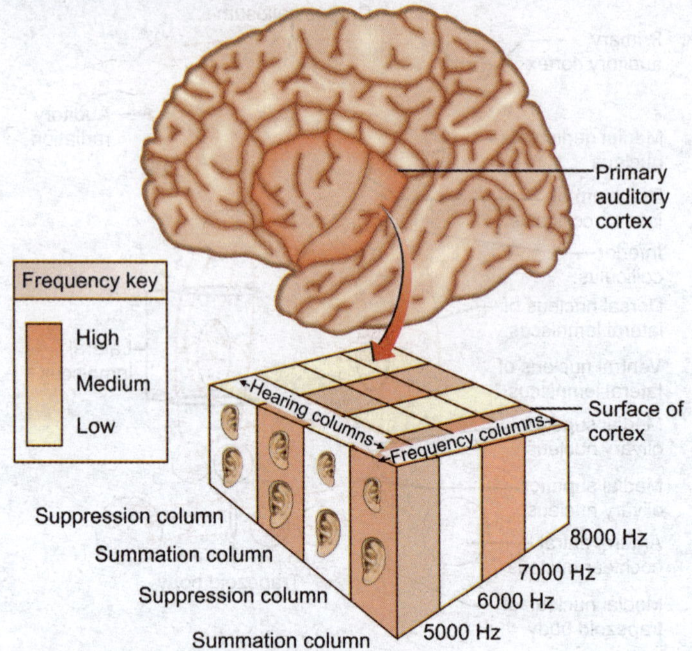

FIG. 11.65   Auditory cortex

The connection between medial geniculate body and Brodmann areas are as follows:

- Area 41 connects with ventral division reciprocally
- Area 42 connects with dorsal division reciprocally.

Following are the connection areas:

In case of unilateral brainstem lesion—bilateral distribution of cochlear nerve are of immense significance.

- The connection between two cochlear nuclei
- The connection between two dorsal nuclei of lateral lemniscus through commissure of probst.
- The connection between colliculus inferior on each side through commissure of inferior colliculus.
- The connections between central nucleus of inferior colliculus and contralateral medial geniculate body through inferior cerebellar peduncle
- From inferior colliculus upwards there are two important projection system:
  - ❖ *Core system:* The connection between portions of inferior colliculus, portions of medial geniculate body and primary auditory cortex → direct auditory pathway.

❖ *Bell projection:* The connection between pericentral inferior colliculus, nonlaminated portion of medial geniculate body and secondary auditory cortex.

The descending auditory pathways are:
- Corticogenicular fibers
- Geniculocollicular fibers
- Corticocollicular fibers
- Collicular efferents
- Efferent cochlear nerves from superior olivary nucleus end in cochlear hair cells of organ of Corti.

Vestibular Pathways (Figs 11.66A and B)

This pathways monitor:
- Position of head in space
- Angular and linear acceleration of head.

The special organ is:

Membranous labyrinth: It consists of:
- Otolith organ—utricle and saccule
- Three semicircular canals.

Linear acceleration is monitored by specialized receptors, macules of utricle and saccule.

Angular acceleration is maintained by specialized receptors, cristae of ampullae of three semicircular canals.

Semicircular canals are three in number—arranged at right angles to one another to detect movement of head. In erect position of head—horizontal canal is almost horizontal.

Utricle and Saccule

- They are arranged at right angle to one another
- Utricle is parallel to base of skull and is stimulated with linear motion
- Saccule is parallel to sagittal plane and stimulated with angular motion.

Mode of Transmission of Stimulation

Transmission from membranous labyrinth is transmitted in two different components of vestibular system:

1. *Superior portion of nerve carries input from:*
   ❖ Horizontal semicircular canal
   ❖ Anterior or superior semicircular canal
   ❖ Utricle.
2. *Interior portion of nerve carries input from:*
   ❖ Posterior semicircular canal
   ❖ Saccule.

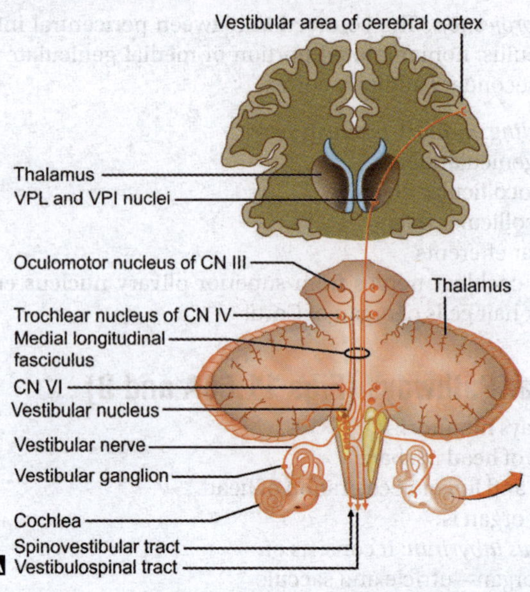

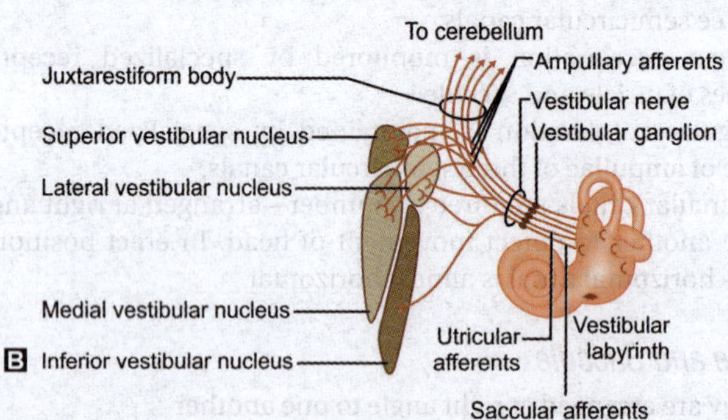

FIGS 11.66A AND B (A) Termination of central processes of VIII cranial nerve in vestibular nuclei and their projection to other cranial nerves; (B) Termination of central processes of 1st order afferent neurons of vestibular ganglion in brain stress vestibular nuclei

The above vestibular nerve enters the brainstem at ponto-medullary level—bifurcates into ascending and descending fascicles and end in the following nucleus:

- Superior nucleus of Bechterew.
- Lateral nucleus of Dieters.
- Medial nucleus of Schwalbe.
- Interior nucleus of Roller.

Vestibular Nuclei Initiate

- Contralateral vestibulo-ocular responses.
- Ipsilateral vestibulo-spinal responses.
  Both reflexes:
  a. Maintain stable vision during head movements.
  b. Maintain stable posture during body movements.
- Semicircular canals relate preferentially to superior and medial vestibular nuclei.
- Macular fibers relates preferentially to inferior and medial vestibular nuclei.

Vestibular connections include following structures:

- *Medial longitudinal fasciculus:*
  ❖ Superior nucleus projects fiber to ipsilateral MLF
  ❖ Interior, medial nucleus project fiber to contralateral MLF.
  Activity: These nuclei through MLC:
  ❖ Control on conjugate eye movements
  ❖ Control on head and neck movements.
- *Medial vestibulospinal tract (project to contralateral spinal cord):*
  This tract receives fibers from:
  ❖ Medial vestibular nuclei
  ❖ Inferior vestibular nuclei—to some extent
  ❖ Lateral vestibular nuclei—to some extent.
    Through this tract, medial vestibular nuclei exert the excitatory or inhibitory effect on cervical cord or upper thoracic level of contralateral spinal cord.
- *Lateral vestibule spinal tract (project to ipsilateral spinal cord):*
  This tract receives fibers from:
  ❖ Lateral vestibular nucleus
  ❖ Inferior vestibular nucleus.
    This tract is responsible for extensor trunk muscle tone and action of antigravity muscles.
- *Cerebellum:*
  ❖ Afferent fibers through vestibulocerebellar tract connect inferior and medial vestibular nuclei with ipsilateral flocculonodular lobe, uvula and fastigial nucleus of cerebellum.
  ❖ Efferent fibers through cerebellovestibular tract connect cerebellar vermis to vestibular nuclei and flocculo-vestibular fibers connect flocculus to vestibular nuclei.
- *Reticular formation:*
  ❖ Through cerebellar projection vestibular nuclei influence reticular formation.
  ❖ Vestibular nuclei also projects fibers back to hair cells in membranous labyrinth—to serve modulating function.

It also receives reciprocal connection with vestibular nuclei including nodular, uvula, flocculus, other areas of cerebellar vermis and fastigovestibular fibers from fastigial nucleus.

Cortical representation of vestibular function is present in:
- Postcentral gyrus near areas 2 and 5 of cerebral cortex
- Frontal lobe (area 6)
- Superior temporal gyrus.

Thalamic Representation of Vestibular Function

Posterior nuclear group of thalamus.

Evaluation of cranial nerve VIII function
Sensory neural deafness is difficulty in perception of tone or speech. This may occur due to lesion in:
- Cochlear nerve
- Central auditory pathways.

This sensory neural deafness may be:
- Bilateral and progressive (otoloxic drugs)
- Unilateral and progressive (acoustic neuroma, Meniere's disease)
- Unilateral and sudden (vascular, viral)

Sensory neural deafness is due to:
- Congenital
- Vascular
- Infection
- Traumatic
- Metabolic
- Structural conditions
- Drugs:
  - Aminoglycosides antibiotics
  - Loop diuretics
  - NSAID
  - Quinine
  - Salicylates
- Cranial radiation
- Drugs used in oncology:
  - Cisplatin
  - Vinca alkaloids

Common causes of conductive deafness
- Blockage of external auditory meatus
- Otosclerosis
- Middle ear disease.

The Interpretation of Tests

In sensory neural deafness
- Weber test—lateralizes to normal ear
- Rinne's test is positive (air conduction > bone conduction)
- Schwabach's test demonstrates—patient's bone conduction is worse than examiner's bone conduction.

In conductive deafness
- Weber test lateralizes to disease ear
- Rinne's test is negative (air conduction < bone conductive)
- Schwabach's test demonstrates is normal or prolonged patient may hear longer than examiner's.

Few Symptoms Related to VIII Cranial Nerve

- *Dizziness:* This can be described as light headedness, presyncope, faintness.
- *Vertigo:* This can be described as sensation of motion, which may be subjective (he/she is spinning) or objective (surrounding environment is moving).

  Vertigo may be associated with—nausea with or without vomiting (related to lesion of peripheral vestibular apparatus) pallor, presence or absence of sweating.
  - *Vertigo associated with hearing loss*—primary ear disease.
  - *Sensation of fullness in the ear*—ear pathology
  - Perception of reverberation of patient's own voice—middle ear disease.
- *Tinnitus:* Sensation of noise in external ear in absence of any stimulus. It may be whistling, ringing, hissing.
  It may be:
  - Paroxysmal
  - Continuous
  - Pulsatile
  - Nonpulsatile
  - Unilateral
  - bilateral.

Paroxysmal or continuous—pulsatile or nonpulsatile tinnitus associated without vertigo—mainly due to peripheral lesions.

Unilateral, pulsatile, fluctuating tinnitus or tinnitus associated with vertigo—It may be due to central or peripheral serious lesions.

Low roaring tinnitus—Meniere's disease

High roaring tinnitus—Acoustic tumor.

Pulsatile tinnitus—It is due to:
- Glomus jugulare tumor
- Aberrant and tortuous artery

- Vascular loops
- Persistent stapedial artery
- Intracranial AV malformation
- Jugular diverticulum
- Carotid artery stenosis
- Meningioma
- Idiopathic intracranial hypertension—
Due to turbulent blood flow from the hypertensive intracranial circulation into low pressure jugular bulb.
Pulsatile tinnitus due to all above causes except idiopathic intracranial hypertension may be decreased by rotating head to ipsilateral side.

Gaze-evoked Tinnitus

This type of tinnitus associated with saccades, vestibulo-ocular eye movements may occur due to aberrant connection between vestibular and cochlear nerve, as a result of sprouting after section of vestibulocochlear nerve following operation of cerebellopontine angle tumor.

Systemic Causes of Tinnitus

- Anemia
- Thyrotoxicosis
- Paget's disease of bone
- Sickle cell anemia
- High cardiac output
- Loud cardiac murmur.

Other Vestibular Causes of Tinnitus

- Labyrinthitis
- Perilymphatic fistulas
- Patulous eustachian tube
- Middle ear myoclonus
- Tensor tympani muscle spasm.
If vertigo is associated with other cranial nerve or brainstem dysfunction—central pathway lesion.
Associated auditory hallucination—temporal lobe disease.

To search for etiology of vertigo—following examinations should be done:
- Complete otologic evaluation
- Complete audiological evaluation
- Blood pressure examination in:
  - ❖ Both arms
  - ❖ Standing and lying down position

- Carotid bruit
- Cardiac murmur and if present, its radiation
- Detailed cranial nerve examination
- Evaluation of vestibular control of balance:
  - ❖ *Romberg test (Fig. 11.67)*
    - Ask the patient to stand both feet together with eye closed
    - Patient tends to fall on the side of vestibular lesion.
  - ❖ *Balance during movement test:* The patient is asked to step forward 3 steps and backward 3 steps with eye closed.
    Result: There is tendency to reeling one side—to the side of lesion.
  - ❖ *To detect any abnormality of distal movement:* The patient is asked to place index finger of his outstretched hand on the examiner's finger-top.

    The patient with hypofunction of vestibular apparatus, moves his arm in an arc from above his head and touches the examiner's finger—on the side of lesion.
- *Provocative test for positional nystagmus:* By:
  - ❖ Postural change
  - ❖ Head turning
  - ❖ Sudden turn while walking
  - ❖ Valsalva maneuver
  - ❖ Caloric testing.

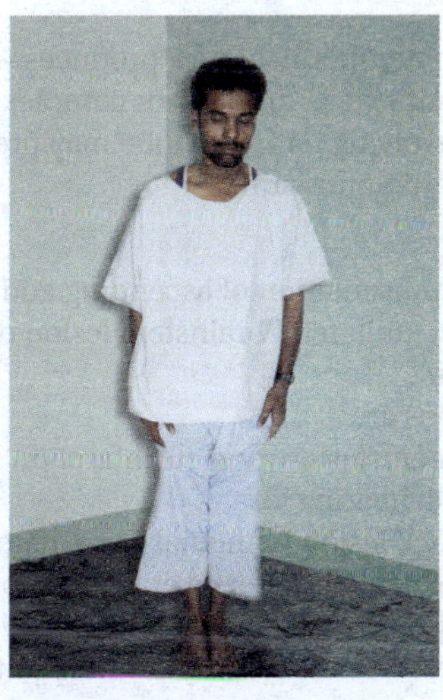

FIG. 11.67   Stands with eyes closed

Localizing Lesions for Producing Vertigo and Deafness

Human auditory cortex comprises of:

Superior temporal gyrus along sylvian fissure: It is subdivided into:

- Audiosensory area—Brodmann area 41
- Audit psychic area—Brodmann area 42, 22.

The following lesions are responsible for different type of hearing loss:

- *Unilateral lesion*—it may produce subtle hearing loss.
- *Unilateral dominant posterior temporal lesion or* bilateral temporal lobe lesion involving Heschl's gyrus—pure word deafness—inability to comprehend spoken language despite normal auditory acuity but naming, writing, reading, non-language word comprehension are intact.
- *Bilateral lesion in auditory cortical region—It produces:*
  - ❖ Auditory agnosia
  - ❖ Selective auditory agnosia
  - ❖ Pure word deafness
  - ❖ Milder disturbance in temporal analysis of sounds
  - ❖ Amusia.
- *Left hemisphere lesion*—impaired speech discrimination. *Right hemisphere lesion*—impair complex speech discrimination.
  - ❖ Severity of lesion depends upon extent or the lesion.
  - ❖ During and after recovery—minor audiometric speech difficulty with varying degree of impairment of interpretating the verbal and nonverbal sounds.

Type of Lesion

Irritative lesion in temporal cortex produces—auditory hallucination—may be simple (e.g. tinnitus) or complex (e.g. music).

Focal seizure involving temporal lobe may present initially with auditory aura or vertiginous aura.

Brainstem lesion

Due to binaural representation of ascending auditory tract—above the cochlear nuclei, unilateral brainstem lesion does not cause any hearing impairment.

The following lesions are:

- Bilateral brainstem lesion due to infarction or hemorrhage—produce bilateral hearing loss.
- Small hemorrhage lesion in medial geniculate body produces—hyperacusis, palinacousis (perseveration of sounds).
- Tumor in midbrain and pineal body—sudden and complete bilateral deafness—because here auditory pathways are closely packed together.

- Lesions in low midbrain and rostral pontine tegmentum—auditory hallucinations associated with hearing loss and clear sensorium.

Peripheral Nerve Lesions

Peripheral cochlear nerve lesion produces:
- Unilateral deafness
- Ipsilateral tinnitus (for high frequency sound).

The causes of lesions:
- Trauma (basal skull fracture)
- Infections (syphilis, bacterial infection)
- Drugs (aminoglycosides)
- Aneurysm (anterior inferior cerebellar artery), tumors (C-P angle tumor, meningioma, vestibular schwannoma, arachnoid's cyst, vascular loops, epidermoid cyst, cholesteatoma)

Other cranial nerves involved are:
V, VI, VII, IX, X, XI, XII cranial nerves.

Cerebellopontine Angle Syndrome

The following are the spectrum of lesion and symptoms according to progressive increase in size of lesion:

First early loss of speech discrimination, tinnitus and sensorineural hearing loss

↓

Sense of imbalance, unsteady gait, vertigo, headache

↓

Widening of internal auditory meatus canal and complete loss of unilateral hearing

↓

Neighboring cranial nerves are involved

↓

Eventually brainstem will be affected

↓

Ipsilateral cerebellar involvement

↓

Tumor enlargement with increase in intracranial pressure and production of hydrocephalus.

- *With anterior extension of tumor following cranial nerves are involved:*
  - ❖ Trigeminal nerve
  - ❖ Abducens nerve.
- *With posteroinferior extension of tumor following cranial nerves are involved:*
  - ❖ Glossopharyngeal nerve
  - ❖ Vagus nerve
  - ❖ Spinal accessory nerve.
- *With eitherward extension—facial nerve is involved.*

Susac's syndrome: Triad of:
- Microangiopathy of brain (encephalopathy)
- Microangiopathy of retina (blindness)
- Hearing loss with tinnitus.
  It occurs exclusively in young women.

Refsum disease
- Autosomal recessive disorder
- Pathology is due to accumulation of phytanic acid in blood.
- *Symptoms and signs:*
  - Sensorineural deafness
  - Cerebellar ataxia
  - Pes cavus
  - Anosmia

Localization of Lesions in Patient with Vertigo

Vertigo syndrome can be categorized by following combination of phenomena:
- Vertigo—perceptual
- Nystagmus—direction specific imbalance in the vestibulo-ocular reflexes.
- Ataxia—postural imbalance due to abnormal activation of vestibulospinal pathways
- Nausea and vomiting—it is due to activation of medullary vomiting center.

Causes
- *Peripheral:*
  - Vestibular
  - Labyrinthine cause.
- *Central:* All vestibular connections
- *Systemic disease:*
  - Endocrine disease
  - Metabolic
  - Hematopoietic diseases.

Peripheral causes of vertigo
- Involvement of semicircular canal induce rotatory sensation
- Involvement of utricle and saccule produce linear sensation.

In acute vertigo due to labyrinthine disease: There are two phases:
1. *Irritative phase:* Disease side is more active, the patient tends to fall to the side opposite the side of lesion.
2. *Paretic phase:* Diseases side is less active. The patient tends to fall to the side of lesion.

The patient tends to lie on one side, with affected side in upper most position in order to decrease the imbalance between semicircular canal.

Peripheral vestibular syndrome has complete and congruent symptoms and signs of peripheral vestibular nerve dysfunction:
- Vertigo
- Nystagmus horizontal, rotatory with slow phase towards the side of lesion inhibited by visual fixation.
- Deviation of patient's outstretched hand
- Romberg sign
- Past pointing.

In case of unilateral total loss of semicircular canal—canal paresis can be detected by following manner:

Ask the patient to fix his eyes on a stational target and rotate his head from side to side.

In normal individual patient's gaze is fixed on target throughout the period.

In patient with canal paresis—there are multiple, small, oppositely directed, compensatory and refixation saccades when the head is rotated towards the side of lesions.

Benign Paroxysmal Positional Vertigo (Figs 11.68 and 11.69)

Acute attack of severe vertigo, nystagmus, autonomic symptom without any cochlear pathology, abate after 3–6 months with at least one exacerbation after initial remission.

This benign paroxysmal positional vertigo (BPPV) occurs due to pathology of any one semicircular canal.

Most commonly involved canal is posterior semicircular canal. The pathology involved are:
- Trauma
- Labyrinthitis
- Meniere's disease
- Inner ear surgery
- Idiopathic—canalithiasis or cupololithiasis.

Otoconial particles—being detached from otoconial layers by the process of degeneration or trauma and are settled on the cupola of posterior canal—it is becoming heavier than surrounding endolymph and sensitive to changes in the direction of gravity.

So, if the patient's head in tilted towards affected ear or head is extended, posterior semicircular canal is moved to a specific plane of stimulation so.
- Development of rotational vertigo
- Concomitant upbeat nystagmus with fast phase towards the down most ear.

If lateral or horizontal semicircular canal is involved, during head movement from side to side along horizontal axis:

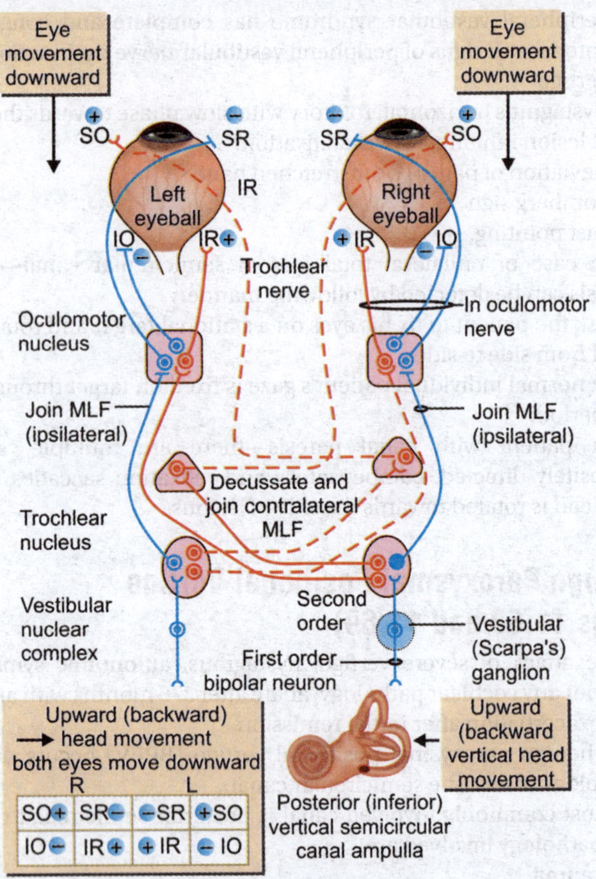

FIG. 11.68   Central connection mediating compensatory vertical (downward) eye movement in response to upward movement of head

- Horizontal linear nystagmus, with fast phase towards the lower most ear induced by rapid turning of head from side to side around longitudinal axis.
- Nystagmus has short latency period, without fatigability.
- Vertigo—it is more prominent on pathologic side.

Most important cause of HC-BPPV is cupololithiasis. Other causes are:

- Trauma
- Infection
- Ischemia, infarction
- Degenerative disease.

Provocative positioning maneuver (Dix-Hallpike or Nylen-Barany maneuvers): The method is as follows:

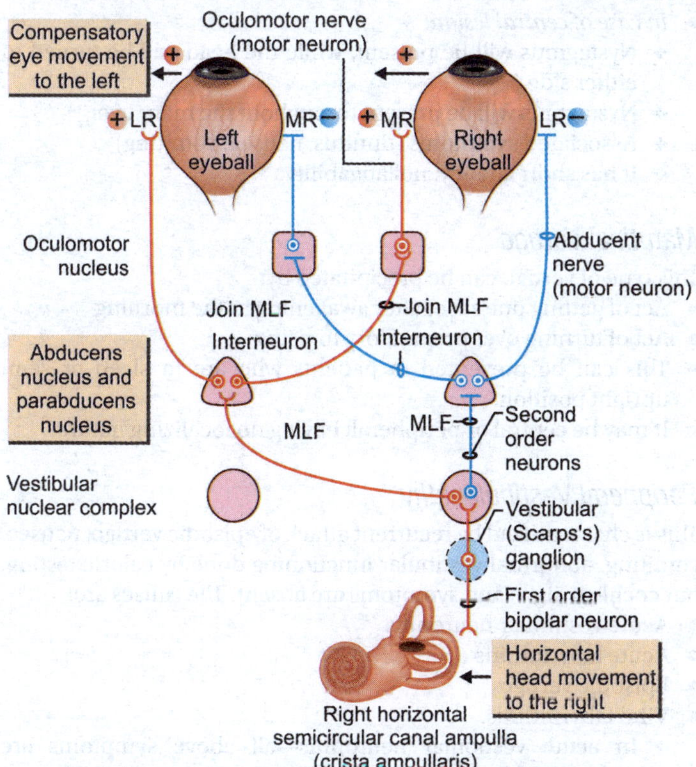

FIG. 11.69 Central connections mediating compensatory horizontal eye movement in response to horizontal head movement

- *The patient is asked to change his position in such a way:*
  - ❖ Head will be hanging 45° below the horizontal plane
  - ❖ Head will be rotated 45° to one side.

Interpretation

- *In a normal person:* There is no nystagmus.
- *In peripheral lesion:*
  - ❖ Vertigo
  - ❖ Nausea
  - ❖ Vomiting
  - ❖ Nystagmus.

Nystagmus has:
  - ❖ 1 to 15 seconds latency after change in position of head
  - ❖ Nystagmus fatigue will occur within 10 seconds of appearance of nystagmus.

As the patient becomes in sitting position the direction of nystagmus will be in opposite side.

- *In case of central lesion:*
  - ❖ Nystagmus will be present, while the head will be turned to either side
  - ❖ Nystagmus will be present throughout the maneuver
  - ❖ Associated symptoms (tinnitus, nausea, vomiting)
  - ❖ It has short latency, no fatigability.

Matutinal Vertigo

This type of vertigo can be precipitated by:
- Act of getting one's feet after awakening in the morning
- Act of turning over preparatory to rising
- This can be prevented in patients who are in sleep or semi upright position.
- It may be central or peripheral; having no localizing nature.

Peripheral Vestibulopathy

This is characterized by recurrent attack of episodic vertigo, nausea, vomiting, abnormal vestibular functioning done by caloric testing, but cochlear signs and symptoms are absent. The causes are:
- Acute vestibular neuronitis
- Acute labyrinthitis
- Episodic vertigo
- Viral labyrinthitis.
  - ❖ In acute vestibular neuronitis—all above symptoms are present—Infection is mainly viral infection.
    - If superior division of vestibular trunk is affected—horizontal semicircular canal paresis
    - If inferior division is affected—posterior semicircular canal paresis.
  - ❖ In acute labyrinthitis—all the above symptoms and signs plus tinnitus and sensorineural deafness will be present.

The causes are:
- Viral (measles, mumps, and rubella),
- Bacterial
- Ototoxic drugs (aminoglycosides, diuretics).

Disabling positional vertigo: This is characterized by disabling positional vertigo, severe nausea, with or without tinnitus—due to intracranial compression of vestibular nerve by aberrant blood vessels.

Episodic Vertigo

It is an autosomal dominant disorder, characterized by episodic vertigo, without any hearing loss, sometime in combination with spinocerebellar ataxia, horizontal vertical or torsional nystagmus, oscillopsia, in association with AV malformation.

Episode—each 15 seconds duration, occurs regularly at 2 minutes interval.

Episodic vertigo: It is due to oculovestibular response, e.g.:
- Walking down the grocery stores
- Driving a car.

In this case, optico-kinetic response is normal. These patients can be treated by acetazolamide.

Meniere's Disease

This is a gradually progressive disorder characterized by:
- Acute and severe attack of vertigo
- Tinnitus
- Fluctuating sensory-hearing loss—at an early stage it affects low frequency sounds, and is intermittent. Later on it affects high frequency sounds and more or less continuous.
- Distortion of sounds.

Pathologically it may be due to: Dilatation of endolymphatic channels. It may be due unilateral or bilateral (20–45%).

Tumarkin's otolithic catastrophe (otolothic crisis): Acute episodes of vertigo, during which muscle tone and power are lost.

Vertigo Related to Central Structures Involvement

- Associated structures of brainstem involvement
- Vestibular syndrome is incongruent and incomplete. Because
  - ❖ Nystagmus is
    - Unidirectional or bidirectional
    - Horizontal, vertical or torsional, rotatory.
    - Not altered by visual fixation
  - ❖ Past pointing, deviation of out stretched hands, Romberg sign may be variable.

Causes
- *Vascular causes of central vestibular syndrome:*
  - ❖ Transient ischemic attack
  - ❖ Labyrinthine stroke
  - ❖ Wallenberg syndrome
  - ❖ Basilar migraine
  - ❖ Subclavian steal syndrome
  - ❖ Cerebellar infarction.
- *Degenerative causes:*
  - ❖ Multiple sclerosis,
  - ❖ Wernicke's encephalopathy.

- *Tumor:* Cerebellopontine angle tumor.
- *Systemic causes:*
  - ❖ Vasculitis
  - ❖ *Hematological disorders*
    - Anemia
    - Polycythemia rubra vera
    - Waldenstrom macroglobulinemia
  - ❖ Hypoglycemia
  - ❖ Hypothyroidism
  - ❖ Hyperventilation syndrome
  - ❖ Drugs
  - ❖ Ocular cause:
    - Glaucoma
    - Extraocular muscle paralysis
    - Use of strong corrective lenses.

■ Ninth Cranial Nerves

Glossopharyngeal Nerve (Figs 11.70 to 11.72)

Course: It emerges from posterolateral sulcus of medulla oblongata close to X and bulbar fibers of XI cranial nerves.

↓

Along with these nerves IX nerve passes through jugular foramen

↓

Distal to the foramen it widens the superior and petrous ganglia

↓

Then it passes along the lateral side of pharynx

↓

It passes in between internal jugular vein and internal carotid artery

↓

It winds round the stylopharyngeus muscle

↓

Penetrates the pharyngeal constrictor muscles and reach the base of the tongue.

It has three components:

1. *Motor component:*
   - ❖ Stylopharyngeus muscle
   - ❖ Pharyngeal constrictor muscles.
2. *Sensory fibers:* These includes:
   - ❖ *Taste afferents:*
     - Posterior third of tongue
     - Pharynx.

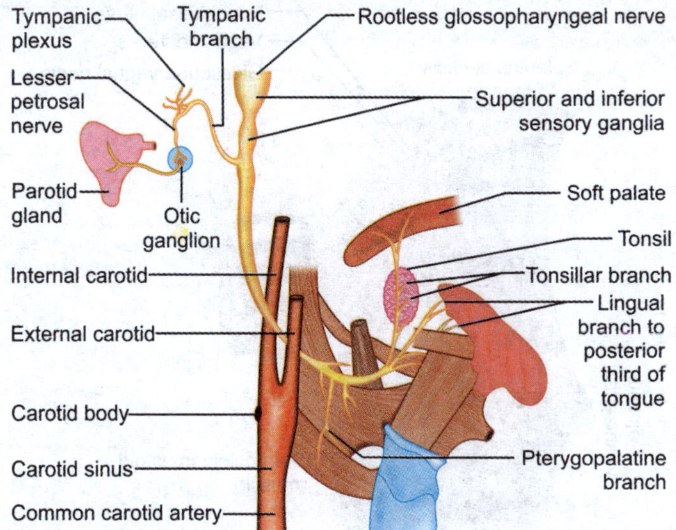

FIG. 11.70   Distribution of glossopharyngeal nerve

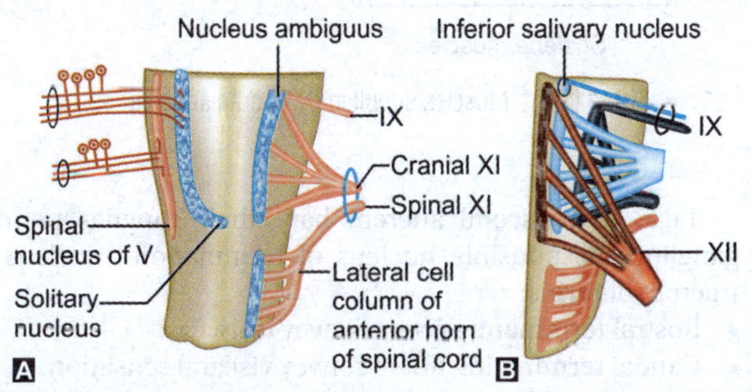

FIGS 11.71A AND B   Sensory nuclei and motor nuclei of cranial nerves IX–XII

- ❖ *Visceral afferents:*
  - Posterior third of tongue
  - Tonsillar region
  - Posterior palatal arch
  - Soft palate
  - Nasopharynx
  - Tragus of the ear
  - By tympanic branch of glossopharyngeal nerve (Jacobson's nerve)—supplies tympanic membrane, eustachian tube and mastoid region.

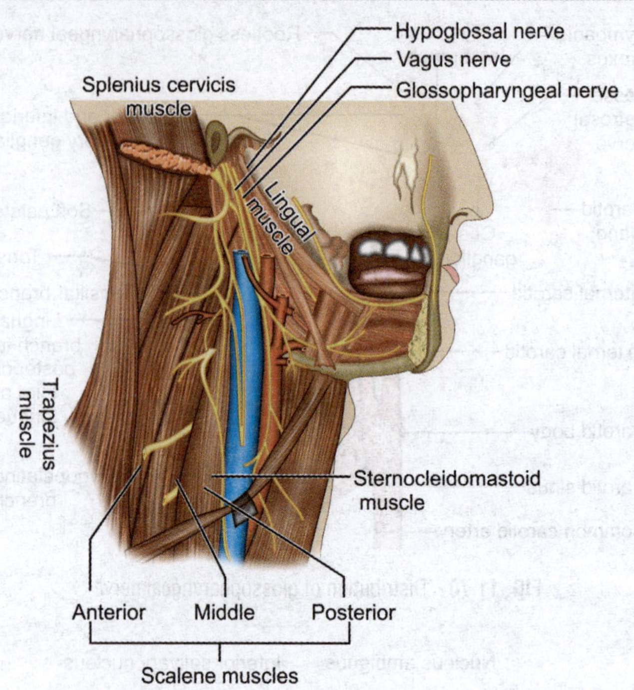

FIG. 11.72   Muscles supplied by XI cranial nerve

Taste and visceral afferent have their ganglia—petrous ganglion. Responsible nucleus of termination—nucleus of tractus solitarius:

- Rostral terminating fibers convey taste
- Caudal terminating fibers convey visceral sensation.

❖ Exteroceptive afferents—through petrous ganglia terminate into spinal tract of trigeminal nerve.

❖ Chemoreceptive afferent from carotid body (chemoreceptor) and baroreceptor afferent from carotid sinus (baroreceptor)— pass sensation by the way of carotid sinus nerve (nerve of Hering).

● *Parasympathetic fibers:*

This fibers originate from inferior salivary nucleus located in periventricular gray matter of rostral medulla

↓

Preganglionic fibers leave the glossopharyngeal nerve at the petrous ganglion

↓

This nerve passes by the way of tympanic branch of Jacobson's nerve and lesser superficial petrosal nerve

↓

Reach the otic ganglion

↓

Postganglionic fibers passes by the way of auriculotemporal branch of trigeminal nerve and carry the secretary and vasodilator fibers to parotid gland.

Clinical Evaluation

- *Motor function:*
  - ❖ Stylopharyngeal muscle is difficult to assess.
  - ❖ Mild dysphagia with weakness of palatal arch.
  - ❖ At rest palatal arch is somewhat lower than the healthy side.
- *Sensory function:*
  - ❖ Taste sensation from posterior third of tongue is lost ipsilaterally
  - ❖ Ipsilateral loss of pain and soft touch on posterior third of tongue, soft palate, tonsillar region, pharyngeal wall.
- *Reflex function:*
  - ❖ *Gag reflex:* Stimulation of posterior pharyngeal wall, tonsillar area and base of the tongue.
    Response: Elevation and constriction of pharyngeal muscle.
  - ❖ *Palatal reflex:* Stimulation of soft palate.
    Response: Elevation of soft palate and ipsilateral deviation of uvula.
    In case of ipsilateral of glossopharyngeal nerve weakness, the above reflexes will be lost.
    Pathways: Afferent is glossopharyngeal nerve. Efferent will be glossopharyngeal and vagus nerve.
- *Autonomic function:* Since parotid gland is innervated by glossopharyngeal nerve, in IX cranial nerve weakness parotid gland secretion will be absent, decrease or paradoxically increased.

Lesions Affecting IX Cranial Nerve

- *Supranuclear lesion:*
  - ❖ *In case of unilateral lesion:* No manifestation of IX cranial nerve weakness, because corticobulbar distribution to nucleus ambiguous is bilateral.
  - ❖ *In case of bilateral lesion or pseudobulbar palsy:*
    - Dysphagia
    - Pathological laughter, spastic tongue

- Explosive dysarthria
- Gag reflex—depressed or severely exacerbated
- Pathological crying.
- *Nuclear in intramedullary lesion:*
  Causes:
  - Motor neuron disease
  - Vascular disease
  - Tumor
  - Syringobulbia
  - Tumor of spinal cord
  - Demyelinating disease.

  Structures involved:
  - Cranial nerve—IX, X, XI cranial nerve
  - Brainstem structures other than cranial nerve.
- *Extramedullary lesions:*
  - *Cerebellopontine angle:* Cause—acoustic neurinoma
    structures involved:
    - IX cranial nerve
    - VIII cranial nerve (vertigo, tinnitus, deafness)
    - V cranial nerve—facial sensory loss
    - Cerebellar involvement
    - Other cranial nerves may be involved.
  - *Jugular foramen syndrome:* Causes:
    - Glomus jugulare
    - Base of skull fracture
    - Meningioma
    - Metastasis to skull base
    - Neuroma
    - Cholesteatoma
    - Gaint cell arteritis.

Structures involved:
- Paresis of ipsilateral and trapezius muscle: It is due to involvement
  of XI cranial nerve.
- Involvement of IX and X cranial nerve producing:
  - Dysphagia
  - Dysphonia
  - Palatal droop on affected side
  - Ipsilateral vocal cord paresis
  - Loss of taste sensation from posterior third of tongue
  - Loss of sensation on posterior third of tongue—ipsilaterally
- Unilateral pain on the affected ear.

Lesions in Retropharyngeal Space or Retroparotid Space

Causes
- Nasopharyngeal carcinoma
- Abscess
- Adenopathy
- Trauma
- Aneurysm.

Structures involved:
- *Collet-Sicard syndrome*: IX, X, XI and XII cranial nerves are involved.
- *Villaret's syndrome*:
  - ❖ Cranial nerve involvement IX, X, XI and XII nerve
  - ❖ Sympathetic chain involvement
  - ❖ Occasionally V cranial nerve involvement.

Glossopharyngeal neuralgia: This is characterized by unilateral, sharp, paroxysmal pain, having abrupt onset.

Site: Throat and ear, larynx, tongue, tonsils, face or jaw may be involved.

Duration: Seconds to minutes.

Triggering factors: Chewing, coughing, talking, swallowing, yawning, eating certain foods.

Associated phenomenon:
- Coughing
- Hoarseness
- Excessive salivation, syncope.

Syncope may be due to reflex bradycardia and asystole due to stimulation of tractus solitarius and dorsal nucleus of vagus by impulses originating from glossopharyngeal nerve.

Causes
- Lesion in posterior fossa
- Tumor, trauma, infection involving IX nerve
- Displaced cerebellar tonsil by Arnold-Chiari malformation.

Tenth Cranial Nerve (Vagus Nerve) (Figs 11.73 and 11.74)

Cranial nerve course: In the cranium:

Six to eight rootlets of vagus nerve emerge from lateral sulcus of lateral medulla oblongata along with glossopharyngeal nerve

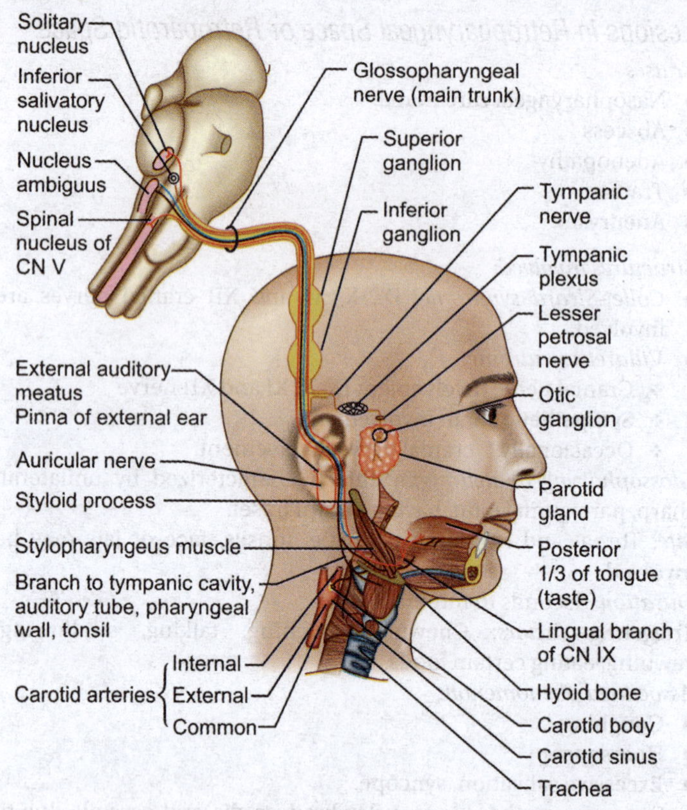

FIG. 11.73   Origin and distribution of vagus nerve

This nerve leaves by the way of jugular foramen in a dural sheath containing spinal accessory nerve

↓

Just inferior to foramen there are two ganglia:

1. Jugular—general somatic afferent
2. Nodose—special and general visceral afferent.
   a. Between two ganglia—auricular ramus—(nerve of Arnold): Innervates skin of concha of the external ear.
   b. At same point—meningeal ramus—to dura mater of posterior fossa.
   c. Pharyngeal ramus:
      i. It forms pharyngeal plexus with glossopharyngeal nerve
      ii. It sends motor fibers to the muscles of pharynx and soft palate except stylopharyngeus (IX nerve) and tensor veli palatini (V cranial nerve)

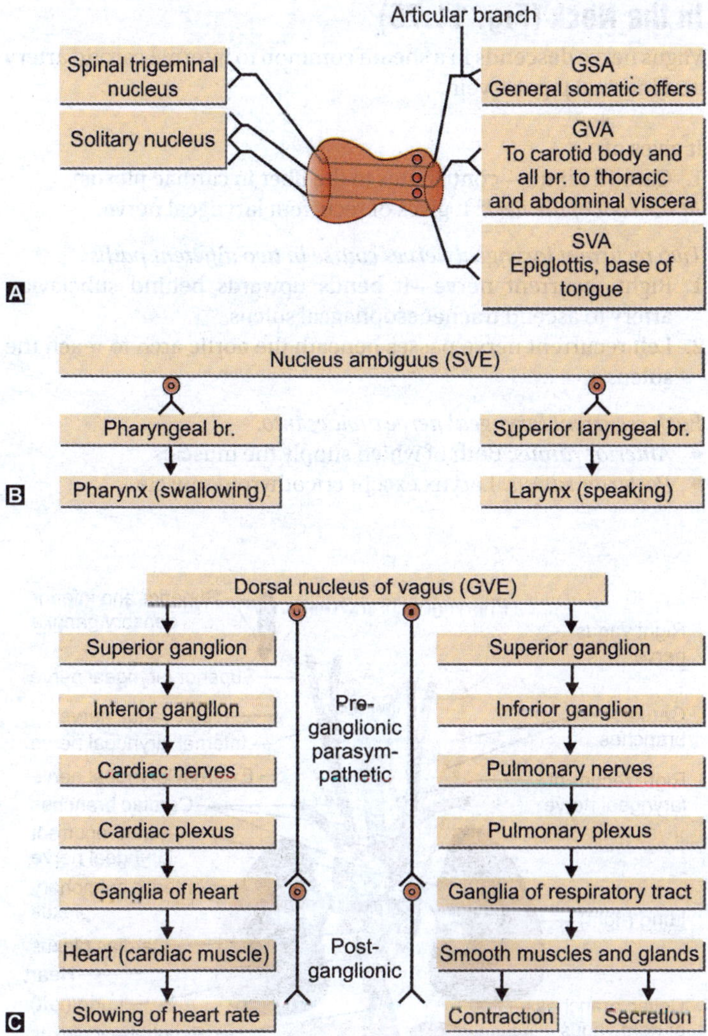

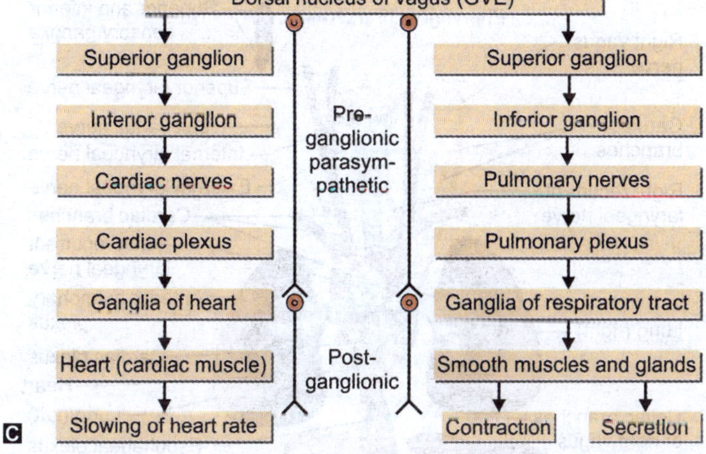

FIGS 11.74A TO C   Innervation of vagus nerve: (A) General somatic efferent; (B) Special visceral efferent; (C) General visceral efferent (GVE)

d   Near nodose ganglion—superior laryngeal nerve arises and is divided into:
  i.   External ramus—to cricothyroid muscle.
  ii. Internal ramus—sends the fiber to larynx.

In the Neck (Fig. 11.75)

Vagus nerve descends in a sheath common to internal carotid artery and internal jugular vein.

↓

It gives of:
1. Carotid ramus—contributes to the fiber in cardiac plexus.

At the root of the neck: It gives of recurrent laryngeal nerve.

Two recurrent laryngeal nerves course in two different paths:
1. Right recurrent nerve—it bends upwards behind subclavian artery to ascend tracheoesophageal sulcus.
2. Left recurrent nerve passes beneath the aortic arch to reach the sulcus.

Each recurrent laryngeal nerve divides into:
- *Anterior ramus:* Both of which supply the muscles
- *Posterior ramus:* Larynx except cricothyroid muscle.

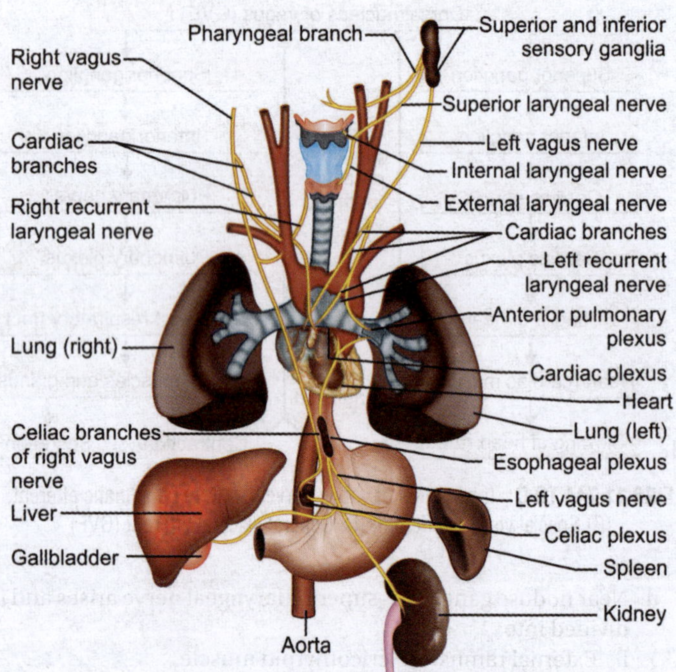

FIG. 11.75 Distribution of vagus nerve

In the Thorax

Vagus nerve enters the thorax after crossing:

- Right subclavian artery in case of right vagus nerve
- Left common carotid and left subclavian artery by left vagus nerve.

In posterior mediastenum: This nerve sends fibers to:

- Pulmonary plexuses
- Esophageal plexuses.

This nerve enters the abdomen through esophageal opening of diaphragm—right nerve behind the esophagus and left nerve in front of esophagus.

After entering abdominal cavity the vagus nerve terminates innervating abdominal viscera.

This nerve has two parts:

1. *Motor fibers*: These fibers arise from two nuclei:
   a. *Dorsal motor nucleus*—situated on the floor of 4th ventricle lateral to hypoglossal nucleus. This nucleus gives rise to preganglionic fibers to the following structures:
      - Pharynx
      - Trachea
      - Bronchi
      - Lung
      - Heart
      - Esophagus
      - Stomach
      - Duodenum
      - Jejunum and ileum
      - Ascending colon
      - Transverse colon
      - Liver
      - Pancreas.
   b. *Nucleus ambiguus*—located in reticular formation in medulla. This nucleus gives rise to fibers supplying all the muscles of pharynx and soft palate except tensor veli palatini and stylopharyngeus.

      Cortical control of the above two motor nucleus are located in lower precentral gyri.

      Supranuclear innervation is predominantly bilateral.

2. *Sensory fibers*:
   - *Nodose ganglion:*
     - Cells are responsible to carrying taste sensation from pharynx, soft palate, hard palate, and epiglottis—

postganglionic fibers end in nucleus of tractus solitarius of the medulla.

- Cells responsible carrying sensation from visceral afferent send efferent fibers to tractus para-solitarius. Jugular ganglion cells responsible for carrying exteroceptive sensations from the concha of the ear sends their postganglionic efferent fibers to descend spinal tract of trigeminal nerve.

Clinical Evaluation of Tenth Cranial Nerve

Motor function

- Ask the patient to open his mouth
- Ask the patient to speak "E"
- Ask the patient to swallow; to cough.

The following things to be notified:

- Watch the position of uvula and soft palate at rest.
- Watch the position of uvula and soft palate during phonation.
- Watch the character of the voice.
- Observe difficulty during deglutition.
- Note the ease of respiration and cough.
- Observe the laryngeal movements during laryngoscopy.

With unilateral vagal lesion:

- Unilateral flattening of palatal arch with phonation.
- Unilateral palate fails to be elevated.
- Uvula will be retracted towards the healthy side.
- There is nasal intonation of voice.
- Ipsilateral vocal cord remains in cadaveric position (midway between abduction and adduction).
- Voluntary coughing will be impaired.

With bilateral vagal nerve lesion:

- Bilateral flattening of palatal arch with phonation.
- No palatal movement.
- Uvula does not move to any side.
- Nasal intonation of voice.
- Pronounced dysphagia—more with liquids.
- Vocal cord in cadaveric position bilaterally.
- Voluntary coughing is impaired.
- Hoarseness of voice.

Sensory function evaluation

Sensory function of vagus nerve cannot be tested because:

- There is overlapping of supply of other cranial nerves.
- Some structures are inaccessible (meninges).

Reflex function
Gag reflex: Afferent nerve is by the way of IX cranial nerve, efferent nerve is by the way of IX and X cranial nerves.

Localization of Lesions Affecting Vagus Nerve

Supranuclear lesion:
- *In case of unilateral cerebral hemispheric lesion (lower part of precentral gyrus):* There is no obvious cause of vagal dysfunction because supranuclear control is bilateral.
- *Involvement of superior segment of corona radiata:* Unilateral palatal paralysis without notable weakness of extremities.
- *Bilateral upper motor neuron lesions:* Pseudobulbar palsy, dysphagia, spastic dysarthria, emotional incontinence, pathologic crying, pathologic laughter, depressed gag reflex.

Nuclear lesions and brainstem lesion:
- *Lesions in nucleus ambiguus:*
  Causes:
  - Vascular
  - Syringobulbia
  - Motor neuron disease
  - Tumor
  - Inflammatory disease.

  Signs:
  - Palatal paralysis
  - Pharyngeal paralysis
  - Laryngeal paralysis
  - Associated involvement of other cranial nerves, roots and long tracts.
- Sites of paralysis according to site of involvement.

Lesions in posterior fossa producing following syndromes

Symptoms		Cranial nerves involved
Jugular foramen syndrome of vernet	–	IX, X and XI
Schmidt's syndrome	–	X and XI
Hughlings-Jackson syndrome	–	X, XI and XII
Collet-Sicard syndrome	–	IX, X, XI and XII

Lesions affecting vagus nerve:
In the neck by:
- Aneurysm of internal carotid artery
- Tumor
- Trauma
- Enlarged lymph node.
  These can produce unilateral vocal cord paralysis.

Lesions affecting superior laryngeal nerve:
Causes:
- Trauma
- Tumor
- Surgery.

Lesion produces:
- Sensory abnormality
- Mild hoarseness of voice due to cricohyoid muscle.

Lesions affecting recurrent laryngeal nerve:
Causes:
- Aneurysm of aortic arch or subclavian artery
- Thoracobronchial abnormal node enlargement
- Mediastinal tumor.

Breast cancer when extends behind carotid sheath at C_6 level produces:
- Recurrent laryngeal nerve palsy
- Paralysis of phrenic nerve
- Paralysis of vagus nerve
- Preganglionic Horner syndrome (Rowland Payne syndrome).

Unilateral recurrent laryngeal nerve palsy: This lesion produces:
- Flaccid dysphonia—voice quality detects hoarseness, short phrases
- Diplophonia—due to vowel prolongation—due to unequal vibratory frequency between two vocal cords
- Unilateral paralysis of all laryngeal muscles
- On laryngoscopy—paralyzed vocal cord lies in paramedian area.

Bilateral paralysis of recurrent laryngeal nerve: It may be seen with:
- Thyroidectomy
- Polyneuropathy
- Carcinoma of thyroid and esophagus. The lesion produces:
  Apposition of both vocal cords produces:
  - ❖ Laryngeal stridor with airway limitation
  - ❖ Dyspnea on exertion
  - ❖ Aphonia

Patient with spinocerebellar ataxia may produce abductor paresis of vocal cord with vertigo, mobbed dysphagia and nocturnal stridor.

■ Eleventh Cranial Nerve (Spinal Accessory Nerve) (Figs 11.76 to 11.78)

Spinal accessory nerve has two roots:
1. *Cranial root*: It arises from caudal part of nucleus ambiguous, in the medulla.

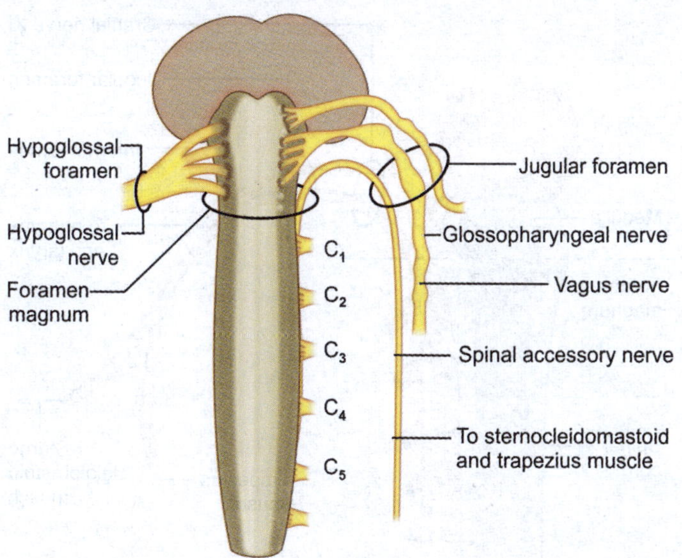

FIG. 11.76 Ventral view of medulla and cranial nerves IX, X, XI, exiting through Jugular foramen

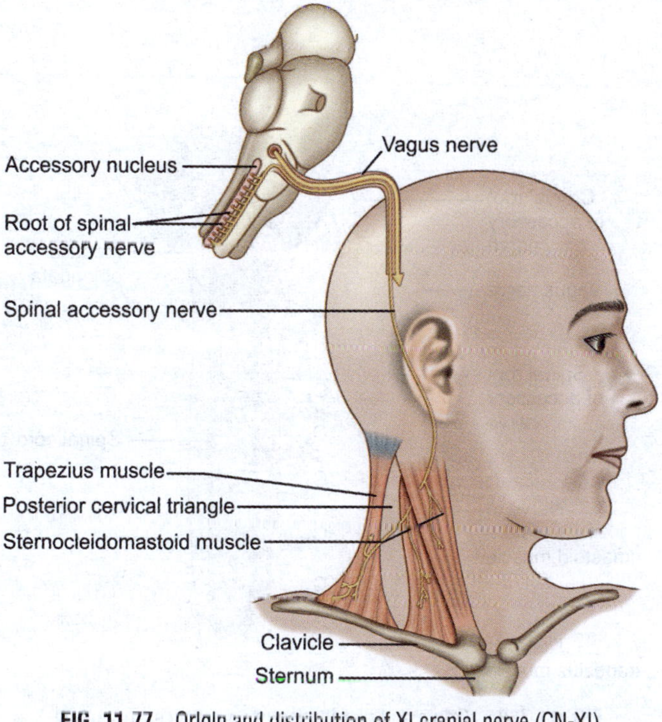

FIG. 11.77 Origin and distribution of XI cranial nerve (CN-XI)

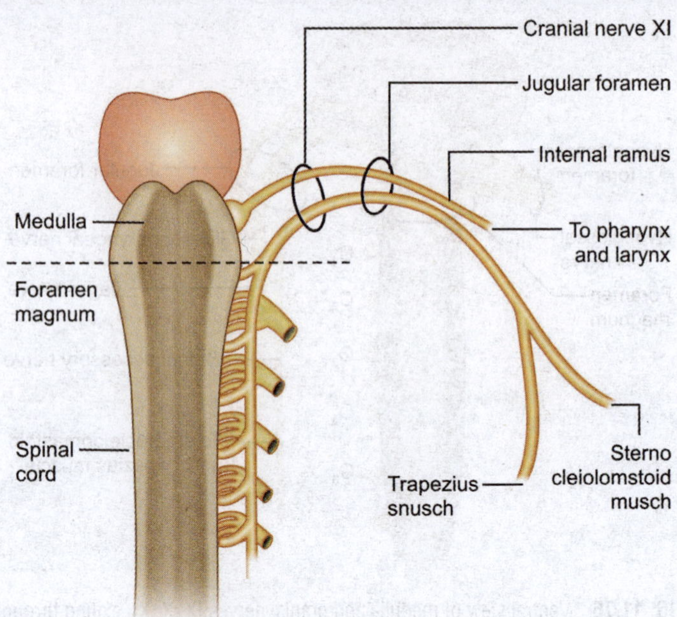

FIG. 11.78A Spinal accessory nerve

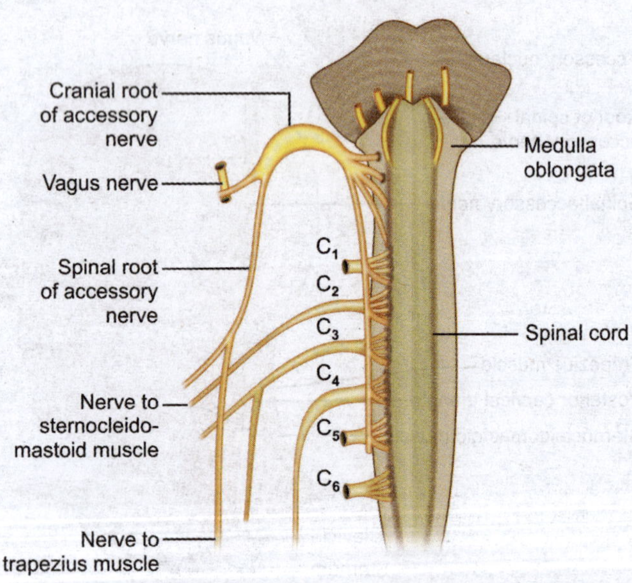

FIG. 11.78B Origin and distribution of spinal accessory nerve

2. *Spinal root*: It arises from column of cells extending from C_1 to C_6 in the dorsolateral part of ventral horn of spinal cord.
   * C_1 to C_2 → innervate ipsilateral sternocleidomastoid muscle.
   * C_3 to C_4 → innervate ipsilateral trapezius muscle.
     Cranial and spinal roots unite and exit from skull through jugular foramen.
     Cranial root branches of as internal ramus and joins the vagus to supply pharynx and larynx.
     Spinal root branches off as external ramus—supply ipsilateral sternocleidomastoid and trapezius muscles.

Supranuclear Innervations Spinal Accessory Nerve

- Corticobulbar fibers supply contralateral nucleus for trapezius
- Croticobulbar fibers for controlling sternocleidomastoid muscle are unknown. But three postulations are:
   * It may be true ipsilateral control.
   * It may be contralateral control— fibers from one hemisphere cross the corpus callosum to the opposite hemisphere and distribute the contralateral sternocleidomastoid muscle.
   * Double decussation may be present—the fibers from one hemisphere cross to opposite pons, then return through C_1 segment to the original side and then distribute to the ipsilateral sternocleidomastoid.

Of two heads of sternocleidomastoid muscle
1. Sternal head has bilateral supranuclear control.
2. Clavicular head has distinct cortical representation.

Following portion should be important
- Eleventh nerve nucleus has rostral and caudal portion.
- Rostral portion receives projections from both hemispheres. Caudal portion is innervated by contralateral hemisphere.
- Caudal eleventh nucleus innervates ipsilateral trapezius and cleidomastoid muscles.
- Rostral eleventh nucleus innervates both sternomastoid muscles.
- Corticobulbar fibers destined for sternocleidomastoid are located in tegmentum of brainstem, and for trapezius are located in ventral brainstem.

Clinical Evaluation of XI Cranial Nerve

Sternocleidomastoid Muscle

- *When muscle of one side contracts (Fig. 11.79)*
   * Chin rotated towards opposite side.
   * Head and occiput is rotated towards the side of contracting muscle.

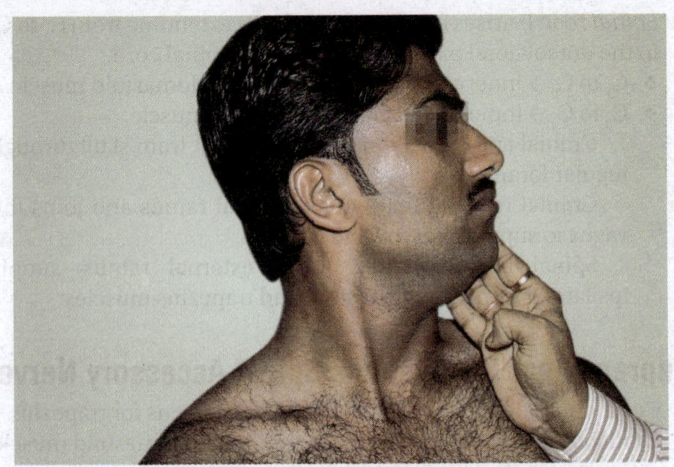

FIG. 11.79   Examination of right sternocleidomastoid muscle

This muscle can be tested by giving resistance from opposite of contracting muscle.

- *If both sternocleidomastoid muscles will contract,* it will flex the head.

This can be tested by exerting pressure on patient's forehead and the patient will forcefully anteflex the neck (Fig. 11.80).

Trapezius Muscle (Fig. 11.81)

- It will retract the head.
- It will elevate, rotates and retracts the scapula.
- It will help in abducting the arm above the horizontal.
- It will elevate the shoulder against resistance.

Unilateral paresis of sternocleidomastoid muscle

- At rest it does not affect the position of the head.
- When the patient's head is flexed, it will be rotated slightly toward unaffected side and chin towards affected side.
- There is weakness in turning the head towards opposite side.

Bilateral paresis of sternocleidomastoid muscles

When the patient try to stand erect, head tends to fall backward.

Unilateral paresis of trapezius muscles

- The shoulder is lower on the affected side at rest
- The scapula is displaced downward and laterally
- There is weakness in shoulder elevation and retraction
- The patient cannot raise the abducted arm above horizontal.

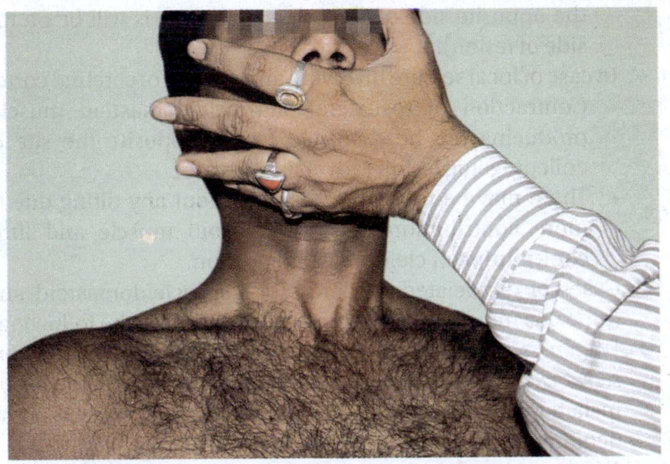

FIG. 11.80 Examination of both sternocleidomastoid muscles

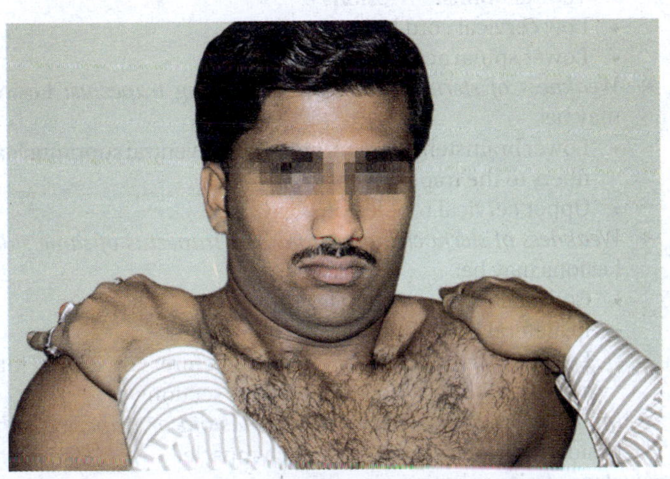

FIG. 11.81 Examination of trapezius muscles

Bilateral paresis of trapezius muscles
- There is weakness in neck extension.
- When the patient tries to stand, his head tends to fall forward.

Since this nerve is completely motor nerve, hence it has no sensory input.

- *In case of supranuclear lesion:*
  - ❖ In hemispheric lesion resulting contralateral hemiplegia
    - Trapezius muscles on the side of hemiplegia will be paretic.
    - Sternocleidomastoid muscles opposite to the side of hemiplegia will be paretic, producing the head turning to

the opposite side of hemiplegia (so paresis will be on the side of lesion).

❖ In case of focal seizure involving area 8 and 9 of cerebral cortex
  - Contraction of ipsilateral sternocleidomastoid muscle, producing the head turned to the opposite the site of epileptogenic lesion (adversive seizure).
  - There may be rotation of head without any tilting due to more contribution of sternomastoid muscle and little contribution of cleidomastoid portion.

Cases of dissociated weakness of sternocleidomastoid and trapezius muscles with neurological lesion are the following:

❖ *Weakness of trapezius muscle on one side and sternocleidomastoid on other side:* Upper motor neuron lesion ipsilateral to involved sternocleidomastoid muscles above oculomotor nucleus.

❖ *Weakness of trapezius muscle, sparing sternocleidomastoid:* Lesions may be:
  - Ventral brainstem lesion
  - Low cervical cord lesion
  - Lower spinal accessory root lesion.

❖ *Weakness of sternocleidomastoid, sparing trapezius:* Lesion may be:
  - Lower brainstem tegmentum, sharing ventral supranuclear fibers to the trapezius.
  - Upper cervical root lesion (C_1–C_2)

❖ *Weakness of sternocleidomastoid and trapezius of same side:* Lesions may be:
  - Contralateral brainstem lesion
  - Ipsilateral high cervical cord lesion
  - Lesions in accessory nerve before division into sternocleidomastoid and trapezius sections.

❖ *Involvement of either sternocleidomastoid or trapezius only:* Lesion is distal to division for each muscle.

- *Nuclear lesion:* Lesion is rare but may occur in motor neuron disease, syringomyelia, spinal tumor. Signs—may be prominent atrophy and fasciculation affecting the trapezius and sternocleidomastoid muscles.

- *Infranuclear lesions:* Spiral accessory nerve enters jugular foramen along with vagus and glossopharyngeal nerve so a lesion in or near jugular foramen produces following syndromes:
  ❖ *Collet-Sicard syndrome*—cranial nerve IX, X, XI, XII
  ❖ *Villaret's syndrome*—cranial nerve IX, X, XI, XII, sympathetic chain.
    VII cranial nerve may be involved.
  ❖ *Schmidt's syndrome*—cranial nerve X and XI

❖ *Jackson's syndrome*—cranial nerve X, XI, XII
❖ *Tapia's syndrome*—cranial nerve X, XI, XII—sympathetic chain may be involved.

The causes may be—tumor infections, vascular, granulomatous disease (sarcoidosis), congenital basilar invagination and, traumatic atlas fracture.

Lesions on Spinal Accessory Nerve in the Neck

Causes are:
● Surgery
● Internal jugular vein cannulation in the posterior triangle of the neck
● Carotid endarterectomy
● Coronary artery bypass surgery
● Trauma
● Radiation.

Signs of ipsilateral sternocleidomastoid and trapezius involvement.

Floppy Head Syndrome

It is characterized by:
● Weakness of neck extension, against gravity.
● Involvement of neck flexion.

Causes may be:
● Myasthenia gravis
● Motor neuron disease
● Demyelinating disease
● Poliomyelitis
● Syringobulbia
● Fasciosacpulohumeral muscular dystrophy.

■ Hypoglossal Nerve (XII Cranial Nerve) (Figs 11.82A and B)

Origin: Hypoglossal nucleus, a longitudinal cell column in medulla near paramedian region.

Fibers from this nucleus travel in ventrolateral direction and emerge from medulla in preolivary sulcus between interior olivary complex and pyramid.

Near its exit it has 10 to 12 rootlets—these unite to form two bundles and pass separately through dura mater and hypoglossal canal.

After its exit from hypoglossal canal, it descends vertically, unite to form single nerve.

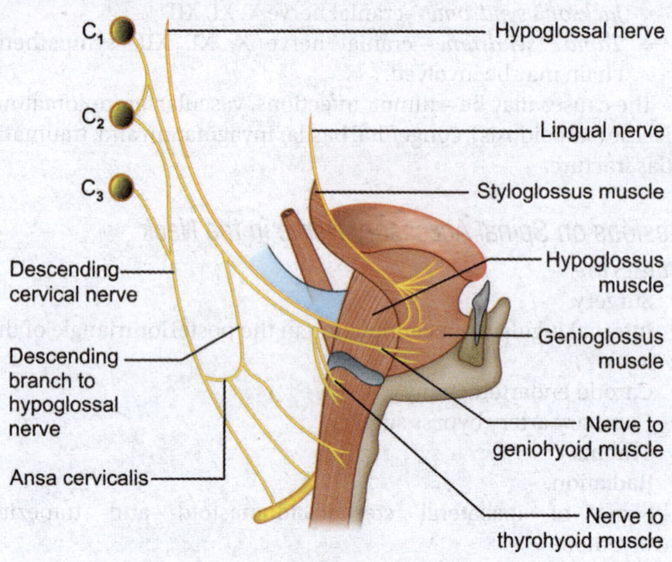

FIG. 11.82A Distribution of hypoglossal nerve

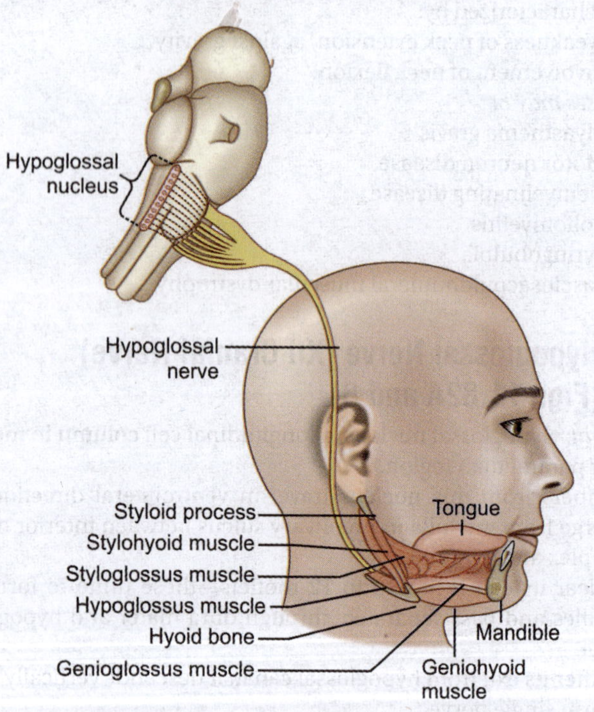

FIG. 11.82B Origin and distribution of hypoglossal nerve

It courses over internal and external carotid arteries to the level of angle of mandible, then passes forward under tongue to supply extrinsic and intrinsic muscles of tongue. The supplied muscles are:

- *Intrinsic muscles:*
  - ❖ Longitudinal muscles
  - ❖ Transverse muscles
  - ❖ Vertical muscles.
- *Extrinsic muscles:*
  - ❖ Hyoglossus
  - ❖ Genioglossus
  - ❖ Styloglossus
  - ❖ Geniohyoid.

Supranuclear Control of Tongue

The higher center responsible is lower part of precentral gyrus around sylvian fissure.

The supranuclear fibers pass along corticobulbar tract through genu, internal capsule and cerebral peduncle.

Corticobulbar fibers supply contralateral genioglossus muscle.

In case of other muscles, cortical representation is always bilateral with contralateral preponderance.

Clinical Evaluation of Hypoglossal Nerve

Look for following features of the tongue:

- Position of tongue at rest, and with protrusion.
- Assessment of strength, bulk and dexterity of tongue.
- Watch for atrophy, fasciculation, and fibrillation
- Watch for deviation of tongue.
- Watch the movement of tongue without protrusion.
- Motor power can be checked by asking the patient to give pressure in inner side of the check by the tip of the tongue and examiner tries to dislodge the tongue. Normally tongue is powerful and cannot be dislodged.
- For more precise testing, sides of protruded tongue are pressed firmly with tongue blade and compare strength of two sides.

In case of unilateral weakness of hypoglossal nerve

- Protruded tongue deviates towards the side of lesion because opposite genioglossus pushes the tongue towards weak side.
- Impairment of ability of the protruded tongue to deviate to nonparetic side.
- Impaired ability of the tongue to push the inner cheek on nonparalytic side.
- Normal power and strength to push the inner cheek on paralytic side.

- Lateral movements of nonprotruded tongue controlled by intrinsic muscles of tongue, may be preserved.
- Inability to remove the food from between the teeth and cheeks on either side.
- Due to extensive interlacing fibers from side to side the unilateral weakness in minimal.
- Tongue fibrillation, fasciculation, and atrophy, present on affected side.

Appearance of tongue during atrophy
- During early stage of atrophy—it is first apparent at the tip and along the borders of tongue.
- In advanced stage–tongue wrinkles, furrowed, smaller, epithelium, and mucous membrane of the affected side are thrown into folds.
- In extreme stage, protruded tongue may curve towards the affected side.
- In amyotrophic lateral sclerosis, progressive bulbar palsy atrophy may be so severe that, tongue will be unable to move, lies inert in the floor of the mouth (glossoplegia).
- In few cases, fine tremor can be present, which can be differentiated from fasciculation by asking the patient to keep the tongue in the floor of the mouth; when tremor will disappear, but fasciculation persists.

Tongue weakness may be due to following types of lesions:
Supranuclear lesion:
In case of unilateral supranuclear lesion
- There is crossed hemiplegia
- Tongue will be moved to the paralytic side
- There is weakness but no atrophy
- There will be dysarthria due to tongue muscle weakness and in coordination.

Lesion may occur in:
- Destructive lesions in cerebral cortex
- Cerebral peduncle
- Pons
- Internal capsule.

In case of bilateral supranuclear lesion
- Bilateral paresis of tongue; but no atrophy and no sign of denervation
- Lateral tongue movements are slow and irregular
- Spastic dysarthric present.

Nuclear Lesions

Usually involves hypoglossal nucleus.

Infranuclear lesion involves
- *Intramedullary site between nucleus and point of exit:* The lesions usually same pathology as that of nuclear lesion.
- *Extramedullary but intracranial course of the nerve may be due to meningeal involvement:*
  - ❖ Infection
  - ❖ Inflammation
  - ❖ Trauma
  - ❖ Neoplasm
  - ❖ Subarachnoid hemorrhage.
  May be due to skull base involvement:
  - ❖ Basilar skull fracture
  - ❖ Basilar neoplasm
  - ❖ Basilar impression
  - ❖ Platybasia.
- *Lesions along the clivus*—produces bilateral hypoglossal palsy.
- *In the extra cranial course:*
  - ❖ Trauma in neck
  - ❖ Surgery in the neck
  - ❖ Carotid aneurysm
  - ❖ Infections in retroparotid end retropharyngeal spaces
  - ❖ Radiation of the neck
  - ❖ Idiopathic
  - ❖ Lesions in tongue base and salivary gland
  - ❖ Guillain-Barre syndrome.
  Symptoms and signs are similar to that of nuclear lesion.

In extrapyramidal disorder
- Tongue movement will be slow
- Thickness of speech
- Difficulty in protrusion of tongue.

In myotonic disorder: To test for this disorder:
- Ask the patient to protrude the tongue
- Place the edge of a tongue blade across the tongue
- Percuss the tongue blade sharply
- Temporally facial contraction along the line of percussion—producing the tongue to become narrow sharply at that point.

Abnormal Movements of the Tongue

- *Course tremor*—Parkinsonism
- *Fine tremor*—Thyrotoxicosis
- *Irregular, jerky movements, inability to keep the tongue in protruded position (snake tongue, trombone tongue)*—Chorea.
- *Esophageal or buccolingual dyskinesia, tardive dyskinesia*—due to psychotropic drugs or antiparkinsonian—levodopa. Meige's syndrome.

- *Abnormal movement*—producing injury to tongue—Seizure—Jacksonian seizure.

Morphologic Changes in the Tongue

- *Macroglossia:*
  - ❖ Acromegaly
  - ❖ Sarcoidosis
  - ❖ Myxedema
  - ❖ Down syndrome
  - ❖ Some myopathies.
- *Atrophic glossitis:* Atrophy of the epithelium and papillae — producing smooth, glossy tongue—vitamin B_{12}, folate and iron deficiency anemia.
- In acute case—scarlet red, swollen, with ulceration, later on smooth and atrophic— Pellagra, niacin deficiency.
- Tongue has purplish or magenta hue with prominent filiform and fungiform papillae—Riboflavin deficiency.
- Fusion and atrophy of papillae and fissuring—geographic and scrotal tongue.
- Burning tongue (glossodynia)—tobacco use, menopausal symptoms, smoke, pellagra.
- Xerostomia and dry tongue—local irradiation.
- Longitudinal lingual fissuring—syphilitic glossitis.
- Ulceration on tongue—syphilis, Behçet disease.
- Parallel fissure in tongue—myasthenia gravis (triple-furrowed tongue).
- Bitten tongue—during seizures.

Galloping Tongue

Episodic, rhythmic, involuntary movements of tongue—at 3 per second waves, having 10 seconds per episode, not accompanied by other body movements or EEG abnormalities—occurred due to head injury.

Continuous Lingual Myoclonus

It occurs after head injury, but EEG is normal. It is a form of branchial myoclonus, without palatal myoclonus.

III, IV, VI Cranial Nerve

Each eye globe is moved by six muscles (Fig. 11.83). These are:

1. *Four recti*: All recti arise from annulus of zinn.
   a. *Medial rectus*: Moves the eyeball medially.
   b. *Lateral rectus*: Moves the eyeball laterally.

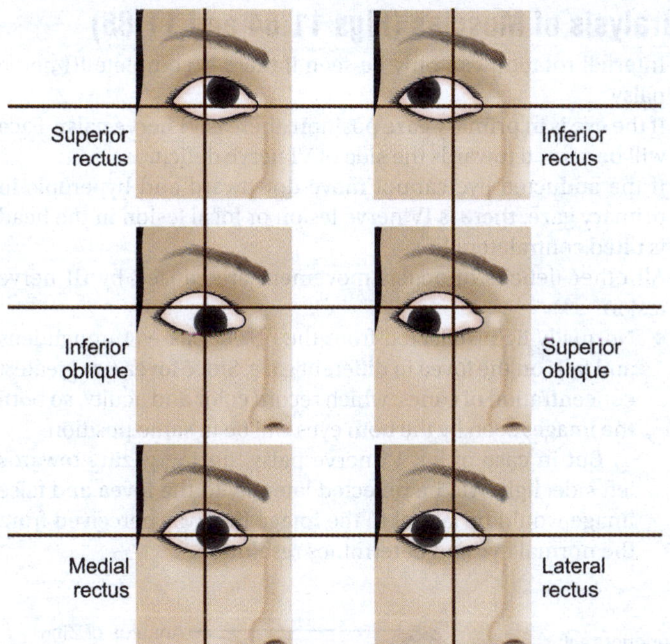

FIG. 11.83   Movement of extraocular muscles

c. *Superior rectus*: Moves the eyeball superiorly, when the eye is abducted.

d. *Inferior rectus*: Moves the eyeball downwards, when the eye is abducted.

2. *Two obliques*: Arise from annulus of zinn.

a. *Superior oblique*: It moves the eyeball downward when eye is adducted, i.e. intorts the eyeball.

b. *Inferior oblique*: It moves the eyeball upward when eye is adducted i.e. extorts the eyeball.

III Nerve Supplies

- Superior rectus
- Inferior rectus
- Medial rectus
- Inferior oblique.

IV nerve supplies—superior oblique muscle.

VI nerve supplies—lateral rectus muscle.

Paralysis of Muscles (Figs 11.84 and 11.85)

- Internal rotation can only be seen if there is complete III nerve palsy.
- If the eye is in primary gaze position, there is VI nerve palsy. Face will be turned towards the side of VI nerve deficit.
- If the adducted eye cannot move downward and hyperopic in primary gaze, there is IV nerve lesion or local lesion in the head is tilted contralaterally.
- All other deficits of ocular movement are caused by III nerve lesion.
  - ❖ Normally light reflected from the object passes through lens and falls on the fovea in different gaze. Since fovea has greatest concentration of cones, which record color and acuity, so both the images seen by the both eyes will be in same position.

    But in case of left VI nerve palsy, during gazing towards left side, light will be reflected laterally to the fovea and false image would be lateral to the image that was perceived from the normal eye and determines resolution.

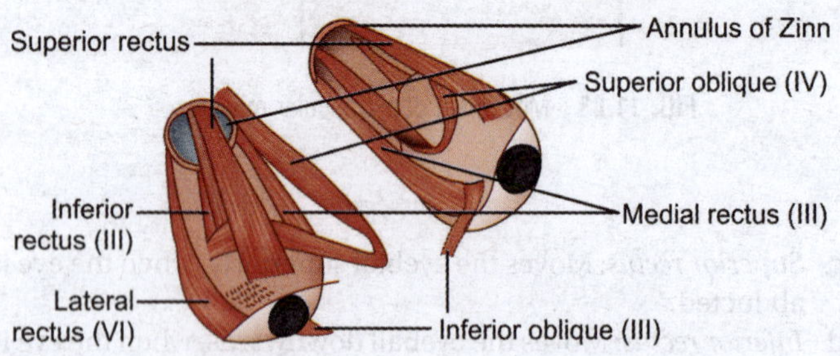

FIG. 11.84 Muscles of eye movements

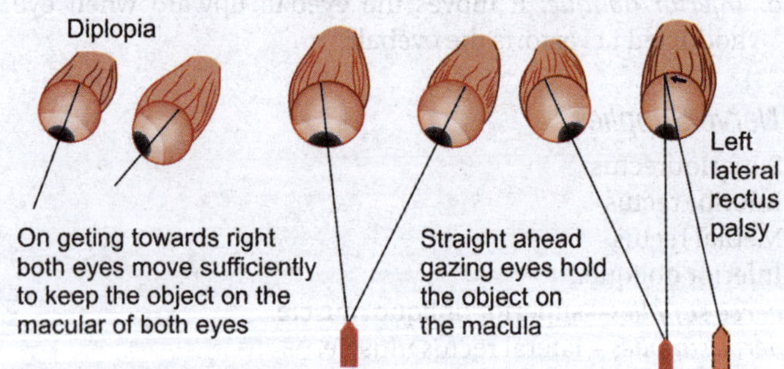

FIG. 11.85 Method of detection of diplopia

Light reflected off from the lens falls on the portion of retina which is rod cells concentrated, so false image is pales and indistinct.

- ❖ Separation of the image is greatest towards the gaze in which the paralyzed muscle has its purest action.
- ❖ False image is displaced in the direction in which weak muscle normally moves the eye, e.g.
  - Horizontally in case of medial and lateral rectus.
  - Vertically for superior rectus, inferior rectus and superior oblique and inferior oblique.

Method of Examination (Figs 11.86 and 11.87)

One eye is covered with red piece of glass or plastic so that the image seen by that eye will be red.

- In each field of gaze, patient is asked whether he or she is seeing one or two.
- *If the patient is seeing two images:*
  - ❖ Whether they are vertically or horizontally displaced?
  - ❖ Which position patient is seeing two images?
  - ❖ Which is red image?
- Cover one eye and asked the patient which image will disappear?

Interpretation of results
- If the images are horizontally displaced, medial or lateral recti are defective.
- If the images are vertically displaced. Superior or inferior recti or oblique muscles are involved.

Muscle pair involved: The position, in which the maximum displacement of image will occur, determines the muscle pair involved.

- *Horizontal displacement on right lateral gaze*, if red plastic on right eye, red image will be in extreme lateral position—if right lateral rectus is involved.

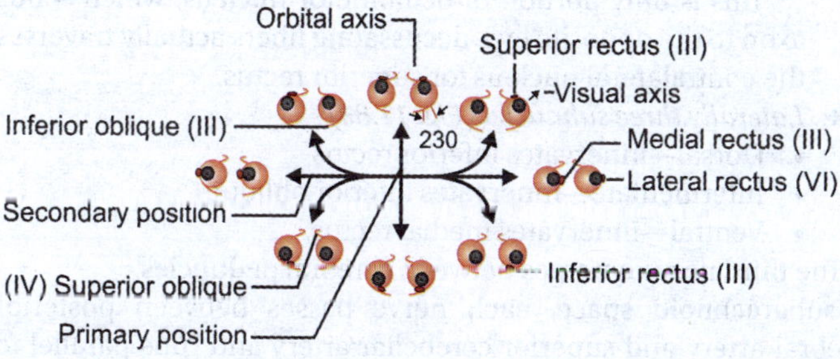

FIG. 11.86 Muscles of eye movements produce position of eyeball in different positions

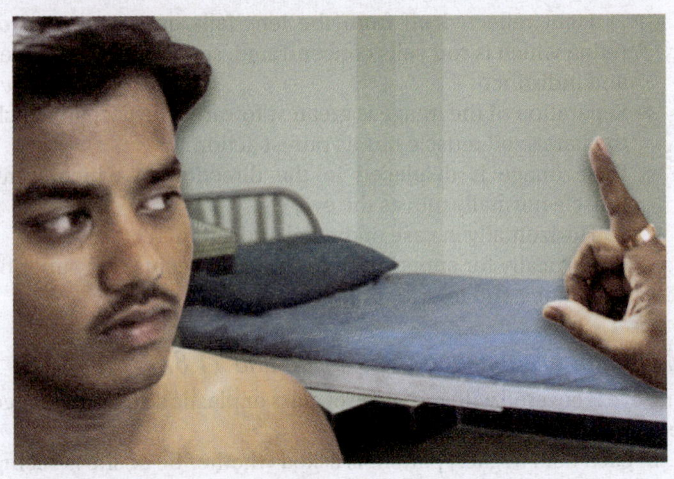

FIG. 11.87 Examination of eye movements

- *If eyes are deviated to the right and upward* and red plastic on right eye (right superior rectus) red image is farthest apart if right superior rectus is paralyzed.

Oculomotor Nerve (III Nerve) (Fig. 11.88)

This third nerve, nuclear complex is present in mid-brain in midline at the level of superior colliculus.

It has one unpaired and four paired nuclei column. They lie ventral to sylvian aqueduct.

- *Unpaired column*—contains visceral nucleus (Edinger-Westphal nucleus) rostrally and subnucleus for levetor palpebrae superior is caudally.
- *Four paired column:*
  - ❖ Most medial column—innervate superior rectus muscle.

    This is only portion of oculomotor nucleus, which sends axon to the opposite eye, decussating fibers actually traverses the contralateral nucleus for superior rectus.
  - ❖ *Laterally three subnuclei (Fig. 11.89):*
    - Dorsal—innervates inferior rectus
    - Intermediate—innervates inferior oblique
    - Ventral—innervates medial rectus.

The third nerve emerges between cerebral peduncles.

In subarachnoid space, each nerve passes between posterior cerebral artery and superior cerebellar artery and runs parallel to posterior communicating artery, courses towards medial edge of uncus of temporal lobe

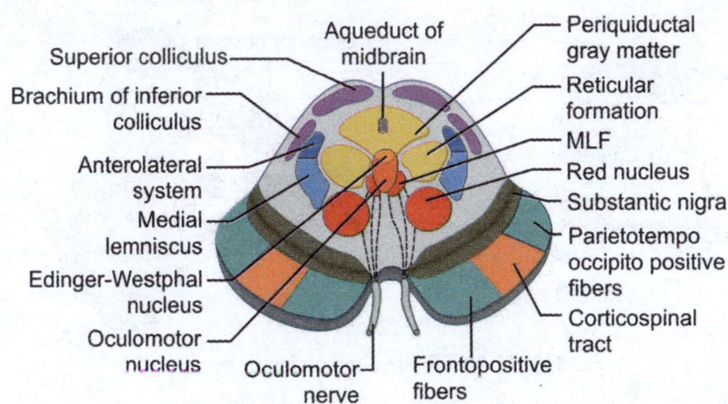

FIG. 11.88 Pathways of oculomotor nerve

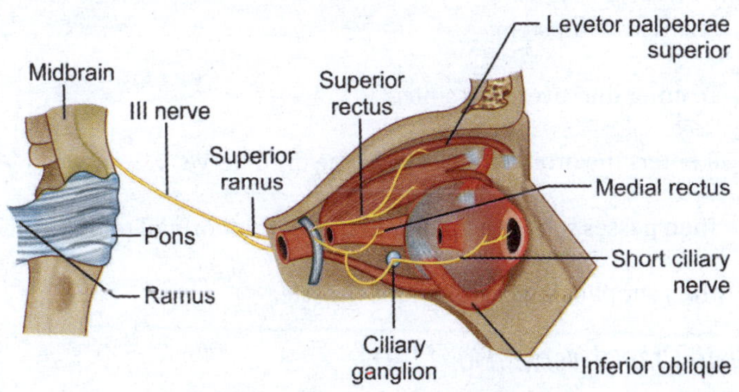

FIG. 11.89   Distribution of oculomotor nerve

Pierces the dura mater and just lateral to posterior clinoid process

↓

Enters the lateral wall of cavernous sinus

↓

The nerve enters through superior orbital fissure

↓

Divides into two branches

1. Upper branch supplies eyelids and superior rectus muscle.
2. Lower branch supplies other muscles and pupil.

Fourth Cranial Nerve (Trochlear Nerve) (Fig. 11.90)

This nerve has few unique features:

- Its nucleus lies on the dorsum of brainstem.
- Fibers cross over in the substance of superior medullary vellum so right nerve originates from left IV nerve nucleus and vice versa.

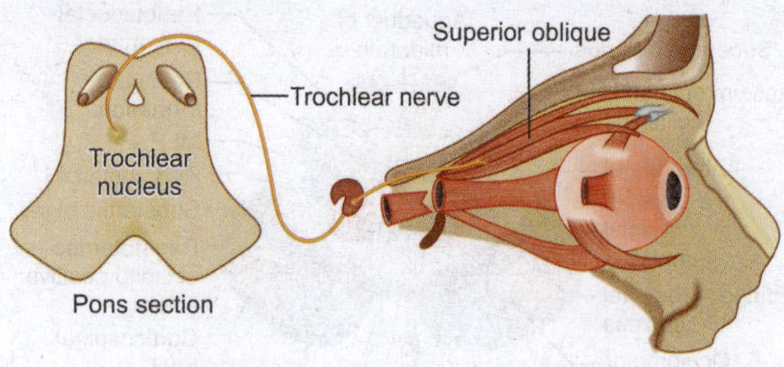

FIG. 11.90 Distribution of fourth nerve

- It runs long course leaving posterior fossa

  ↓

  Encircles brainstem

  ↓

  To enter the cavernous sinus

  ↓

  It enters the orbital roof, crosses the third nerve

  ↓

  Then passes round the pulley in the anterior orbital root

  ↓

  Then supplies superior oblique muscle.

Sixth Cranial Nerve (Fig. 11.91)

Paired nucleus located in dorsal lower portion of pons separated from 4th ventricle by genu of facial colliculus

  ↓

  The nerve emerges from the front of brainstem

  ↓

  If sharply forwards over the tips of petrous bone

  ↓

  Then enters the back of cavernous sinus and lies freely in sinus

  ↓

  Enters the orbit through superior orbital fissure

  ↓

  Supplies lateral rectus muscles.

Before testing diplopia:
- Visual acuity of both eyes
- Lens examination
- Retinal displacement should be examined.

Forced duction test should be performed to differentiate extra-ocular muscle paralysis from mechanical restriction of the globe. This restriction may be due to:

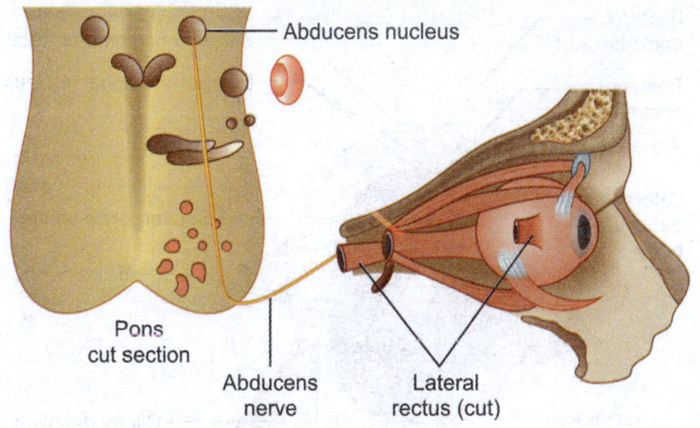

FIG. 11.91 Distribution of sixth nerve

- Thyroid eye disease
- Extraocular muscle paralysis
- Muscle entrapment
- Duane's retraction syndrome
- Carotid—cavernous sinus
- Direct orbital infiltration.

Pupil size is controlled by two types of fibers (Fig. 11.92)

1.	Ring of constrictor fibers—innervated by parasympathetic fibers	Resting pupil size depends upon— 1. Amount of light falls on retina
2.	Radially arranged dilator fibers—controlled by sympathetic nervous system	2. Integrity of parasympathetic fibers
		3. Sympathetic fibers activity—as occurs in anxiety neurosis

Parasympathetic pathways (Fig. 11.93): Intensity of light falling on retina will be conveyed through optic nerve
↓

At the level of optic chiasma impulses split and conveyed through both optic tract to lateral geniculate body of both sides—but without relaying here the impulses go to pretectal nucleus of midbrain both sides around periaqueductal gray matter.

From pretectal nucleus—pretecto-oculomotor tract arises in both sides and ends in parasympathetic nucleus of III nerve (Edinger-Westphal nucleus).

Edinger-Westphal nucleus is also activated by—adjacent III nerve nucleus—controlling activity of medial rectus muscle.

From Edinger-Westphal nucleus parasympathetic fibers are carried in III nerve to the orbit—lie in superficial and dorsal

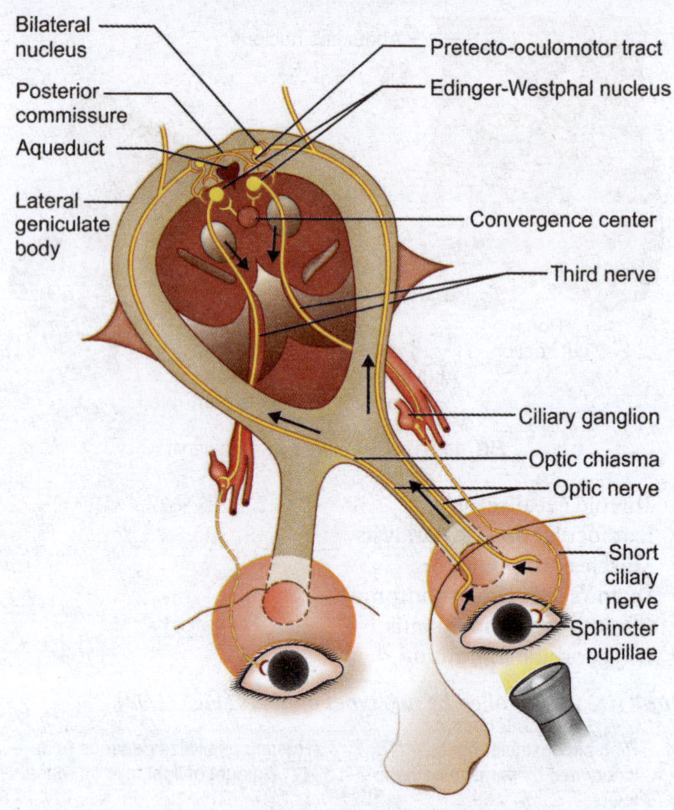

FIG. 11.92   Parasympathetic control of pupil

position—which explain variable amount of abnormalities in the pupil in III nerve palsies.

This preganglionic parasympathetic nerve relay to ciliary *ganglion posterior* to orbit.

↓

From here 8 to 10 short ciliary nerves originate—which subdivide into 16 to 20 branches and supply the constrictor muscle of iris.

- Lesions affecting the parasympathetic control of pupil
  There is no direct light reaction in a completely blind eyes but the pupillary size is same as that of intact eye.
- If both eyes are blind and lesion is anterior to lateral geniculate body, no direct or indirect light reflex in both the eyes and pupils are dilated and fixed to light.
- *If bilateral blindness is due to lesion posterior to lateral geniculate body* or occipital cortex, patient will be completely blind but with preservation of light reflexes in both eyes.

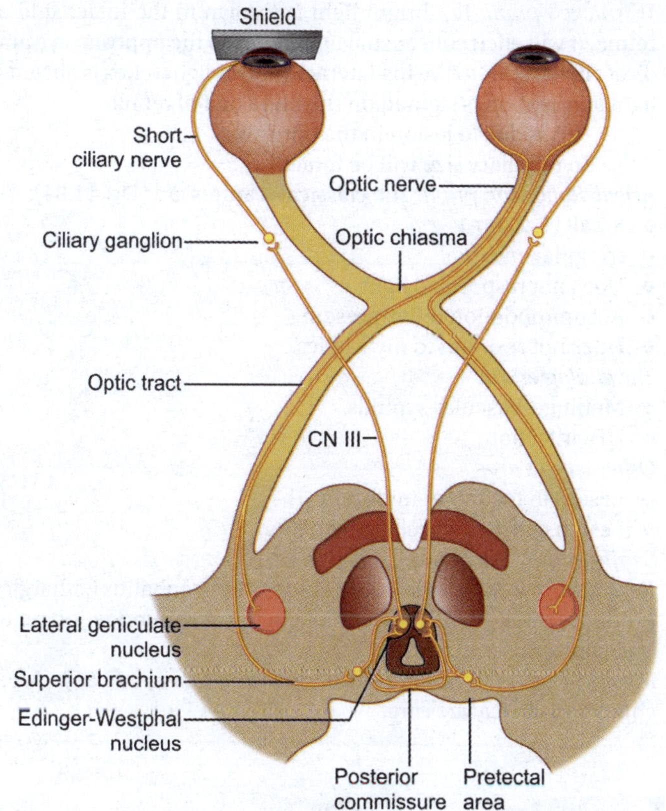

FIG. 11.93 Pupillary light reflex pathway

- *Minimal degree of lesion in retina*, optic nerve, chiasma and optic tract, e.g. due to multiple sclerosis:
  - ❖ When normal eye is stimulated—normal direct and indirect light reflex.
  - ❖ When the affected eye is stimulated with bright light, reaction is slower and incomplete and very brief—this is followed by dilatation of pupil again.

    This type of pupil is called "MURCUS GUNN" pupil.

    This can be tested, if light is rapidly alternated from one eye to another and stimulus will last for 1 second with interval of 2 seconds in between.

    The cause is due to reduction of number of fibers responsible for light reflex on the affected eye. In this case, consensual light reflex will be affected in normal eye.

- *Wernicke's pupil:* If a bright light is thrown to the intact side of retina, it will elicit consensual light reflex to the opposite eye and direct light reflex to the ipsilateral eye. This light reflex is absent if light stimulation is sighted on the blind half of retina.

  This is due to lesion in the optic tract.

  So pupillary size will be intact.

- *Argyll-Robertson pupil:* The classical features are (Fig. 11.94):
  ❖ Small (1–2 mm)
  ❖ Irregular, in equal
  ❖ Does not respond to light
  ❖ Accommodation reflex present
  ❖ Does not respond to mydriatics.

  The etiologies are:
  ❖ Meningo-Vascular syphilis
  ❖ HIV infection.

  Other causes are:
  ❖ Lesion in tectum of midbrain
  ❖ Lesion at the site of ciliary ganglion.

- *Senile miosis:* Small pupil, fixed to light.
- *Reverse Argyll-Robertson pupil:* Epidemic encephalitis Lethargica produces pupil—which reacts to light but accommodation reflex is absent—this is now rare.
- *Myotonic pupil (Holmes-Adie syndrome) (Fig. 11.95):* Most characteristic features are:

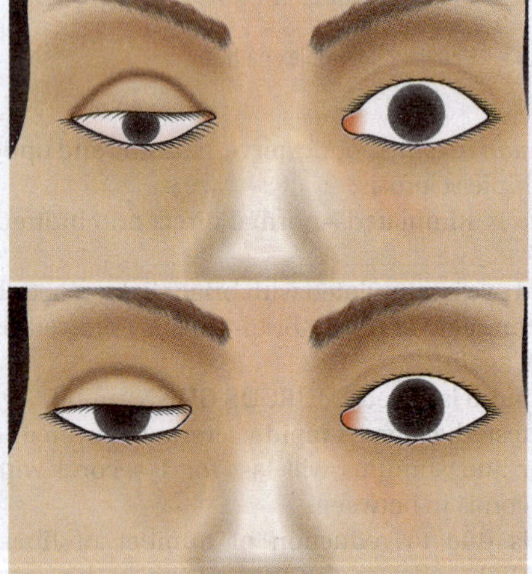

FIG. 11.94   Argyll-Robertson pupil

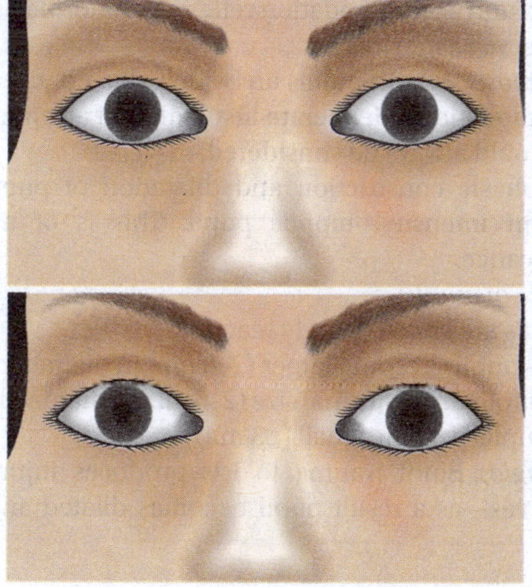

FIG. 11.95   Holmes-Adie syndrome

❖ Widely dilated, circular pupil.
❖ React slowly to very bright light.
❖ Shown more definite response to accommodation. Both above reactions are thought to be produced by slow inhibition of sympathetic activity.
❖ Small dose of 2.5% parasympathomimetics produces brisk constriction response due to denervation super sensitivity.
❖ This is unilateral involvement
❖ *Associated findings:*
  i.   Loss of ankle jerk and knee jerk
  ii. Impairment of sweating.
❖ It is usually discovered in young female, applying cosmetics.
  • *Confirmation of diagnosis*—It can be done by instillation of 2.5% methacholine drops. This chemical is rapidly hydrolyzed by ach esterase to have any effect in normal eye, but in denervated eye, due to denervation hypersensitivity—papillary—constrictor effect is seen.

● *Behr's pupil:* This is slightly dilated unilateral pupil with contralateral hemiparesis.
Causative lesion is optic nerve glioma.

● *Patient with ptosis—two additional features may help in diagnosis:*
  I (a) If the pupil is small—patient has Horner's syndrome.
    (b) If the pupil is dilated—partial III nerve lesion
  II (a) If light reflex and accommodation reflex are normal— Horner's syndrome.

    (b) If light reflex and accommodation reflex are abnormal in partial III nerve lesions.

- *In patient without ptosis:* If both pupils are widely dilated, fixed to light and accommodation—deliberate instillation of atropine drops in that eye should always be considered.
- *Hippus:* There is phasic constriction and dilatation of pupil to light of constant intensity—hippus pupil. This is of no pathological significance.
- *Age variation in size of pupil:*
  - ❖ In infancy—pupils are small—poorly reactive
  - ❖ In adolescence—pupils become larger (7–8 mm in diameter)
  - ❖ In adulthood—pupils are of normal size (2–6 mm in diameter)
  - ❖ In senile age—pupils become small (≤3 mm).
- *Traumatic iridoplagia:* Blunt trauma to iris produces injury to short ciliary nerves—as a result pupil becomes dilated and irregular.

Third Nerve Palsy (Fig. 11.96)

Complete paralysis of III nerve produces:
- Complete paralysis of eyelid-producing ptosis
- Lateral strabismus
- Pupillary dilatation
- Loss of accommodation reflex
- Downward and outward deviation of eye.

    The eye of the affected side moves outward (lateral rectus action) and downwards (secondary depressant action of superior oblique).

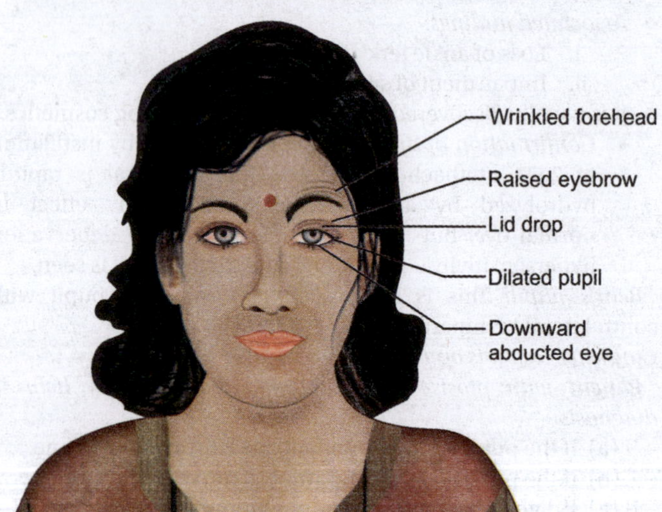

FIG. 11.96 Third nerve palsy

To examine this:
- Lateral gaze of the affected eye should be tested to see the disappearance of diplopia in that direction.
- Normal downward movement of superior oblique cannot be tested because paralyzed medial rectus muscle does not allow the eye to adduct.
- If the patient efforts to look downwards, the eyes rotate further downward (intorsion).

This movement of superior oblique indicates the integrity of IV nerve.

Ocular Sympathetic Pathway (Fig. 11.97)

Ocular sympathetic fibers originate in hypothalamus and remains uncrossed.

- First order of neurons hypothalamus tract pass ipsilaterally to lateral gray column of spinal cord in intermediolateral cell column between spinal segments of C_8 and T_2.
- Second order of neurons exit from the spinal cord through 1st ventral thoracic root, pass through inferior, middle cervical ganglia before terminating into superior cervical ganglion synapsing with post-ganglionic sympathetic neurons.

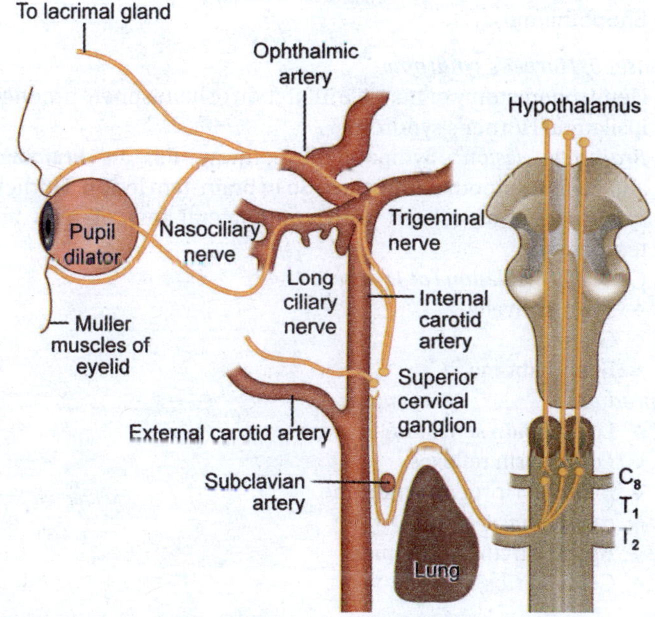

FIG. 11.97   Ocular sympathetic pathway

- Third order of neuron enters the cranial cavity on the surface of carotid artery producing plexus and reaches in following places:
  - ❖ Fibers carried along the III nerve innervate the levator palpebrae superioris of eyelids.
  - ❖ Fibers in nasociliary nerve traverse the ciliary ganglion without synapse to supply blood vessels of eye.
  - ❖ Pseudomotor and vasoconstrictor fibers to the face except those to small area on the forehead running with branches of external carotid artery.
  - ❖ Fibers accompanying internal carotid artery reaches pupil via branches of ophthalmic division of V nerve and reaches eyelids via ophthalmic artery.

    Fibers supplies dilator muscles of iris, and smooth muscles of upper and lower eyelid.

Single physical sign due to damage of sympathetic nerve is Horner's syndrome. The features are:

- Affected pupil becomes smaller than its fellow due to reduced papillary dilator activity.

  This is exacerbated in darkness and minimal in bright light.
- There is variable degree of ptosis. In severe most case—upper eyelid covers the upper edge of pupil.
- Conjunctiva may be slightly bloodshot due to loss of vasoconstrictor activity.
- Sweating of the forehead is impaired.
- Enophthalmos.

Causes of Horner's syndrome

- Hemispherectomy or massive infarction of hemisphere produces ipsilateral Horner's syndrome.
- *Brainstem lesion:* Sympathetic pathway lies in brainstem adjacent to spinothalamic tract. So in brainstem lesion. Horner's syndrome is associated with contralateral loss of pain and temperature.
- *Cervical cord lesion (at D_1 level):*
  - ❖ Syringomyelia
  - ❖ Glioma
  - ❖ Ependymoma.

It produces:
  - ❖ Loss of pain sensation in arms
  - ❖ Loss of arm reflexes
  - ❖ Bilateral Horner's syndrome.
- *D_1 root lesions:*
  - ❖ Apical carcinoma of lung
  - ❖ Cervical ribs

- ❖ Aortic aneurysm
- ❖ Avulsion of lower plexus (Klumpke's paralysis).
- *Lesion in cervical sympathetic chain:*
  - ❖ Thyroid carcinoma
  - ❖ Thyroid surgery
  - ❖ Neoplastic lesion
  - ❖ Local trauma
  - ❖ Surgical extirpation
  - ❖ Malignant lesion in jugular foramen at skull base produces —combination of Horner's syndrome and IX, X, XI and XII nerve lesion:
    - Central lesion produces loss of sweating of head, neck and arm and upper trunk on the same side.
    - Lesion in low neck produces sweating of all over the face.
    - Lesion above superior cervical ganglion may not produce sweating of face, because pseudomotor and vasoconstrictor branches leave below the level of superior cervical ganglion.

Effect of cocaine and adrenaline in pupil with central and peripheral lesions in case of Horner's syndrome (Figs 11.98A to D)

- Decrease in amine-oxidase activity caused by a lesion at or above the superior cervical ganglion sensitizes the pupil to 1:1000 adrenaline instillations.
- Effect of cocaine on pupil depends upon—its blocking effect on amine oxidase. In peripheral denervated pupil—there is depletion of amineoxidase. So there is no effect of cocaine.

Pupillary abnormalities in unconscious patient
- *Normal reacting equal pupils:*
  - ❖ No immediate surgical correction is necessary.
  - ❖ Search for metabolic causes, e.g. diabetic coma, uremic coma, drug overdose.
- *Unequal pupil:* Unilateral dilated pupil indicates herniation of temporal lobe stretches the 3rd nerve on that side and prompt surgical correction is required.
- *Bilateral dilated pupil:* Progressive tentorial herniation produces progressive bilateral dilatation of pupil.

  The chances of recovery of the patient from this stage is remote.
- *Bilateral pinpoint pupil:*
  - ❖ Massive pontine hemorrhage produces pinpoint pupil, spastic tetra paresis and brisk reflexes.
  - ❖ Opiate poisoning produces pinpoint pupil and depressed reflexes.

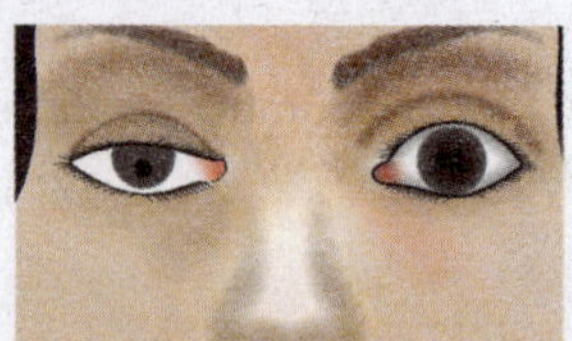

A

No effect due to depletion of amine-oxidase due to postganglionic denervation

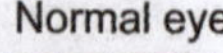

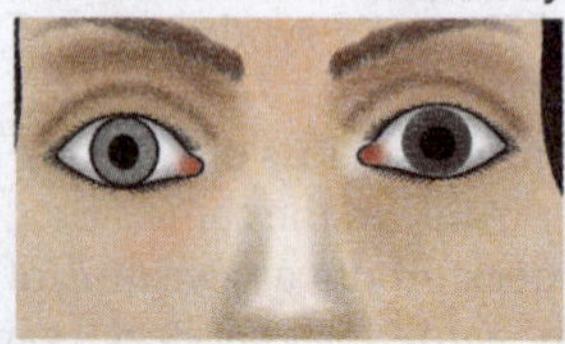

B

Marked effect as adrenaline is not destroyed by amine-oxidase, even the lid will elevate

Rapidly destroyed by amine-oxidase, so no effect

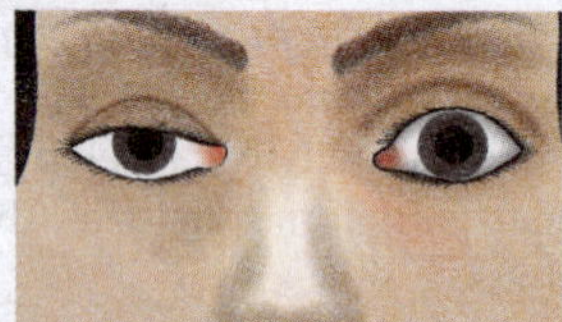

C

Dilates pupil because amine-oxidase is present in pre-ganglionic lesion

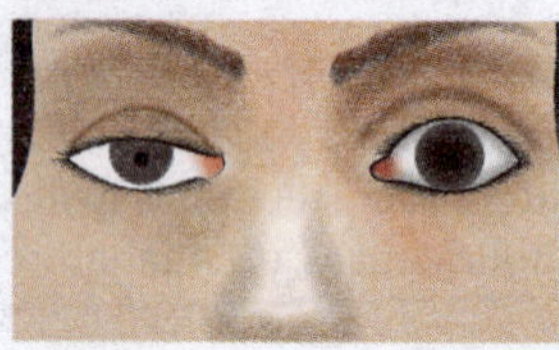

D

No effect as normal amine-oxidase activity presents no effect

No effect on normal pupil

FIGS. 11.98A TO D Effect of cocaine and adrenaline in Horner's syndrome in pupil with (A and B) Peripheral lesion. (above sup. cervical ganglion); (C and D) Central lesion (below sup cerivcal ganglion)

Fourth Nerve Palsy (Fig. 11.99)

It produces superior oblique muscle palsy. In primary position, looking ahead, the eyeball moves outward. Very slight slant of image allow the patient's head to tilt away from the side of affected eye to line it up with the image of normal eye.

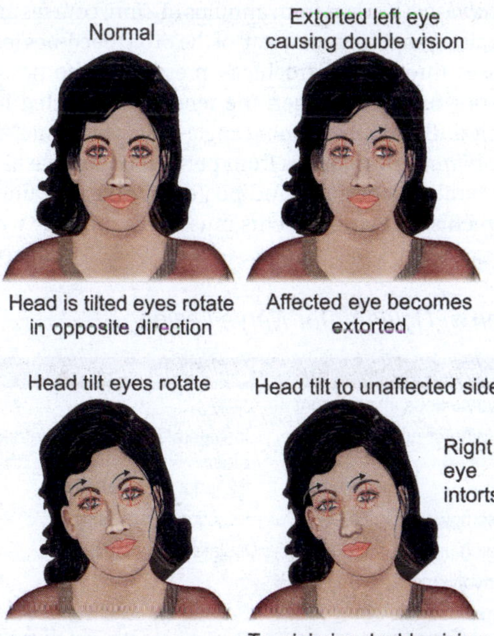

FIG. 11.99   Fourth nerve palsy

Frank diplopia occurs when the patient looks down and away from the side of affected eye.

This can be tested by allowing the patient to read book or newspaper.

Sixth Nerve Palsy

It produces lateral rectus palsy.

There is frank diplopia when looking towards the side of lesion. The patient may compensate by turning the head towards the affected side.

Extraocular Muscle Anatomy

- *Superior rectus:* It originates from annulus of Zinn, courses anteriorly and upward over the eyeball and laterally making 23° with visual axis of eye.
- *Inferior rectus:* It originates from annulus—courses anteriorly, downward and laterally forming angle of 23° with visual axis of eye.

- *Superior oblique:* It arises from annulus of Zinn; courses anteriorly, upwards along superomedial wall of the orbit, becomes tendinous, then passes through the trochlea—present on the nasal side of the superior orbital rim, then the tendon is reflected inferiorly, posteriorly and laterally, forming angle of 51° with visual axis.
- *Inferior oblique:* It originates from periosteum of maxillary bone passes laterally, superiorly and posteriorly passing underneath interior rectus and lateral rectus muscle forming 51° with visual axis.

Localization of Oculomotor Nerve Lesion

Structure involved	Clinical manifestation
• Third nerve nucleus involvement	
❖ Oculomotor nucleus	Ipsilateral II-CN palsy contralateral ptosis Superior rectus paresis
❖ Oculomotor subnucleus	Infection rectus palsy
❖ Isolated, levator subnucleus	Isolated bilateral ptosis
• Fascicle involvement	
❖ Isolated fascicle	Parietal or complete CN-III palsy Pupil may or may not be involved
❖ Paramedian mesencephalon	Ipsilateral ptosis, contralateral eyelid retraction
❖ Fascicles, red nucleus, superior – cerebellar peduncle (Claude's syndrome)	Ipsilateral CN-III palsy, contralateral tremor, contralateral ataxia.
❖ Fascicles, cerebral peduncle	Ipsilateral CN-III palsy, contralateral hemiparesis (Weber's syndrome)
❖ Fascicle, red nucleus/ substantia nigra	Ipsilateral CN-III palsy contralateral choreiform movements (Benedict's syndrome)
• Cavernous sinus involvement	Ipsilateral CN-III, CN-IV, CN-VI, CN-VI palsy, small pupil (Horner's syndrome)
• Lesion in superior orbital fissure	Ipsilateral CN-III palsy, may be or may not be associated with – CN-IV, CN-VI, CN-VI palsy, proptosis

■Convergenic—Accommodation Reflex Pathway (Fig. 11.100 and Flow Chart 11.4)

FLOW CHART 11.4   Algorithm of accommodation reflex pathway

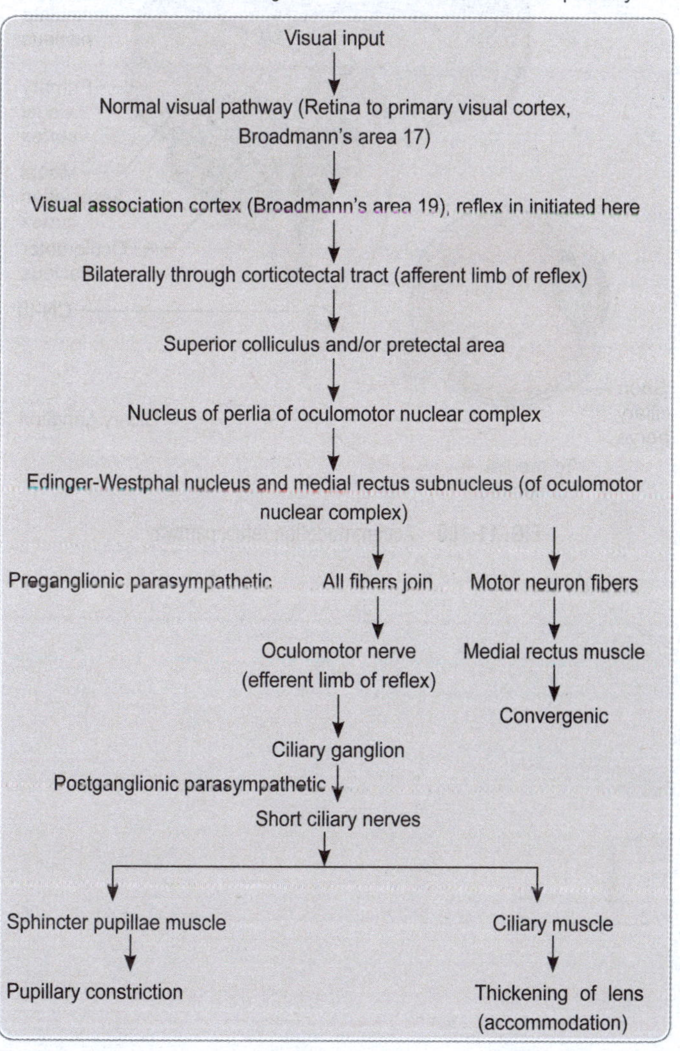

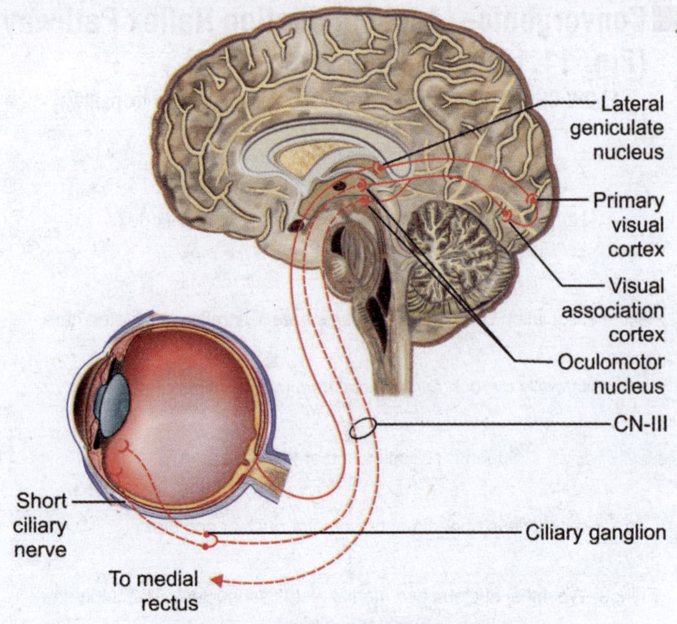

FIG. 11.100 Accommodation reflex pathway

MOTOR SYSTEM

■ Involuntary Movement

During noticing involuntary movement, the examiner must concern the following:

- Which part of the body is affected?
- Whether it is continuous or intermittent?
- Whether it is present at rest of during volition?
- Whether any movement initiates it or abolishes it?
- Whether it is altered by any position of limbs or trunk?
- Whether it is affected by temperature, environment or emotion?
- Whether it is absent during sleep?
- Whether it is suppressed or exacerbated by sleep?

During Questioning, Notice the Following Positions

- Patient utilizes back of the chair to support—indicates cerebellar lesion mainly vermis.
- Patient is rigid and flexed forward—indicates basal ganglia disease.
- Side to side tremor—indicates essential tremor.
- Up and down oscillation of head—indicates ventricular tumor in child and basal ganglia disease in adult.
- Tremor at rest—Parkinson's disease.
- Ties with vocalization with abnormal movements—indicates Tourette's disease.
- Patient is asked to do finger nose test—indicates cerebellar disease.
- Patient is asked to hold the arms steadily flexed—demonstrates postural kinetic tremor from the lesion in cerebellar motor pathways.
- Patient is asked to pick up small objects and performing fine movement—impossible in patient with chorio-athetosis or other dyskinetic disorder.
- The only movement disorder that persists throughout sleep—indicate Huntington's chorea, dystonia.

Epilepsy and Convulsive Movement

The seizure occurs due to paroxysmal electrical discharge from neurons of cortex exception is thalamus in petit mal seizures. *The epileptic seizure depends upon:*

- Afferent and efferent connections in different areas of brain
- Collateral wiring characteristics
- Ease of its depolarization.

Seizurogenic parts in brain are:
- Firstly medial temporal cortex.
- Primary motor and sensory cortex—due to presence of large number of afferent and efferent connection with thalamus and reticular nuclei.
- Parietal, frontal and occipital lobes are less frequently involved.
  - ❖ *Partial seizures involving motor homunculus*—starts—with twitching of thumb, fingers, then angle of mouth, arm—skipping shoulders to feet, then to whole of the body—this is called Jacksonian march.

    If Jacksonian marches will not remit—it will spread to rest of the brain—basal ganglia, substantia nigra, reticular nuclei, thalamus and cerebellum will be involved.

    This will persist for 30 to 40 seconds to 2 minutes.
  - ❖ *Stimulation of large representation of frontal eye field (area 8) produces:*
    - Head and eyes will be deviated to contralateral side
    - Horizontal nystagmus to the contralateral side of lesion.
  - ❖ *Generalized seizure:* It involves following phases:
    - Tonic phase:
      - This persists for 15 to 20 seconds.
      - It involves rigidity of arm and legs. Head and neck deviated to either side.
      - Patient will be unconscious during this phase.
      - It involves thalamic projections bilaterally to motor cortex.
    - Tonic phase is followed by clonic phase: This consists of jerky contraction of face, neck, arm and legs.

      This process is inhibited by intracortical GABA-ergic inhibition from cortical neurones.

      The clonic phase is followed by tonic discharge from reticular neurons of the thalamus.

      Epileptic cry at the onset of seizures is due to expulsion of air through partially opened larynx.

      During seizure, patient becomes cyanotic, dribbling of saliva, biting of lateral side of tongue and urinary incontinence occur.

      Side of tongue biting indicates the lesion will be in contralateral hemisphere.

      Biting of tip of the tongue indicate pseudoseizures.

      The epileptic seizure stops slowly with fewer and fewer jerks, followed by hyperhydrosis and stertorous breathing.

      The total times of seizure are 30 to 90 seconds.

      This is followed by—postictal sleep—it will last for 20 to 30 minutes.

Few major motor seizures are tonic, some seizures are clonic.

If the seizure is bilateral—patient will be conscious and the lesion will be in reticular thalamic nuclei.

❖ *Partial seizures:*
- It affects one extremity, face or one half of the body.
- Patient does not lose consciousness throughout seizures.
- It lasts for hours to days (Menshikoff's syndrome)
- It is caused by:
  - Vascular lesions
  - In children, Rasmussen's encephalitis.

❖ *Seizure from discharge in supplementary motor cortex is characterized by:*
- Speech arrest
- Contralateral dystonia
- Extensor posturing of arm while head is turned to ipsilateral side (seizure focus) with flexed arm (tencer's posture).

❖ *Patient with seizure from temporal lobe may present with:* Automatisms—It has three major components:
1. Arrest of response—in which patient stops of slows motor activity.
2. Autonomic phase—pale and expressionless face.
3. Movement phase—the characteristic movements are:
   - Lip smacking
   - Chewing movements followed by stereotyped hand movements.

   A fugue state lasts for 30 minutes to 1 hour in which patient carries out normal activity, but has impairment of consciousness.

❖ *Petit mal epilepsy:* This is characterized by:
- Frequent episodes of loss of awareness.
- Twitching of eyelids
- Drooping of heads
- Slight jerking of hands
- Repetitive speech
- It occurs several times a day.

The causes are:
Cerebral vasoconstriction accompanied by induced hyperventilation.

Myoclonic Jerk

This is characterized by—sudden jerk-like contraction of flexors of upper limbs and extensors of lower limbs. This movement may be violent suddenly and repetitive.

There are following types of myoclonic jerks according to the site of lesion and causes of lesion:

- *Corticoreticular myoclonus:*
  - ❖ The lesion responsible is diffuse cortical degeneration and absence of cerebral cortical GABAnergic inhibition.
  - ❖ The causes are:
    - i. Stroage disease of childhood and adolescence
    - ii. Creutzfeldt-Jakob disease
    - iii. Lewy body disease
    - iv. Alzheimer's disease
    - v. Anoxic state—e.g. Lance-Adams syndrome—patient may recover from anoxic state, but anoxia produces permanent damage of serotonergic cells of dorsal raphe of thalamus.

    The characteristic presentation: It starts severely from lower limbs then spread all over the body and disrupts sleep.

    This myoclonus is triggered by touch, sounds and loud noise.

    This myoclonus is associated with parasomniac movements and paroxysmal REM sleep disorders.
- *Reticular myoclonus*—localization of lesion—it affects the cells of gigantocellularis of brainstem.

  The causes are—metabolic abnormalities, e.g.—uremia, poisoning, hyperosmotic states.

  The characteristic of lesion: It starts in upper limbs after awakening or shortly thereafter. It occurs in adolescence period.

  It may generalize to motor seizure or remains as epileptic feature.

  Triggering factors: Sound, eye closure, hyperventilation.
- *Segmental myoclonus:* This is of spinal origin. It occurs after:
  - ❖ Use of metrizamide contrast myelography
  - ❖ Segmental arteriography
  - ❖ Hyperosmotic states (nonketotic diabetic coma)
  - ❖ Other metabolic abnormalities.

Opisthotonos

This is characterized by extreme hyperactivity of extensor neurons of spinal cord—in severest form—the back of the head and heel may touch only the floor or bed.

Triggering Factor

In tetanus, it is exacerbated by noise, touch or emotion.

Causes are:
- Tetanus

- In meningeal irritation in children.
- Severe extrapyramidal rigidity.
  In (2) and (3) opisthotonos is maintained.
- In case of transtentorial herniation both the arms are adducted and internally rotated, with extended feet this occurs in:
  - ❖ Basal ganglia lesion
  - ❖ Pontine hemorrhage
  - ❖ Brain tumor
  - ❖ Severe head trauma
  - ❖ Malignant intracerebral edema due to MCA stroke.

■ Chorea (Fig. 11.101)

Chorea is characterized by:

Rapid semipurposeful bizarre movements of the extremities, where two subsequent movements are not equal, associated with irregular respiration, rapid protrusion and retraction of tongue (lizard-like) and peculiar flapping of lip, choreic eye movement which is disorganized also.

Patient may be unable to raise the hand above the head because hand starts pronating.

Patient cannot hold the tongue out of the mouth.

The types of choreic movement:
- *Sydenham's chorea:* It is associated with emotional lability.
- *Huntington's chorea:* It is associated with dementia, choreic eye movements and lurching gait.

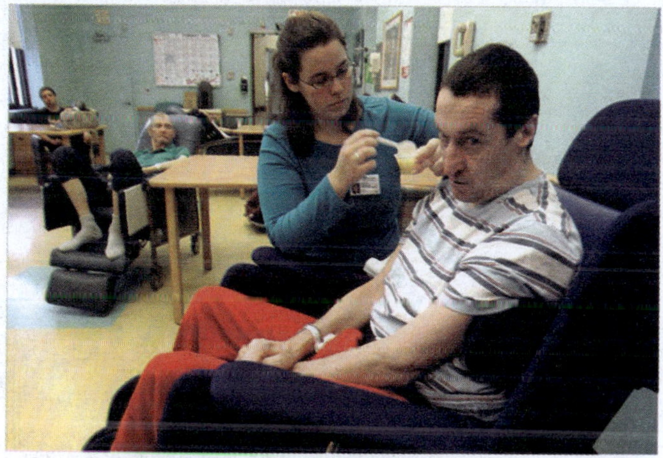

FIG. 11.101   Chorea

- *Chorea with pregnancy:* It is associated with oral contraceptive pills.
- Hereditary chorea.
- Chorea associated with—polycythemia, anoxia.

Athetosis (Fig. 11.102)

This is characterized by slow writhing movements of wrists, fingers, ankles, toes and trunk.

Slowly write with flexed wrist. There is slow adduction and outward abduction.

There is no associated eye movement, respiration is normal, absence of flap in tongue.

But in case of bilateral disease, there is associated facial grimacing.

The causative lesions are—anoxic birth injury, prenatal or perinatal stroke, many heredofamilial syndrome, chorioathetosis.

The combination of chorea and athetosis is more common than either alone. In this case:

Respiratory and tongue movements are affected. This choreoathetosis movement is exacerbated by voluntary movements and reinforcement.

The causes are:
- Anoxic birth injury
- Ataxia telangiectasia
- Multiple heredofamilial syndromes with cognitive impairment
- Neuroacanthocytosis.

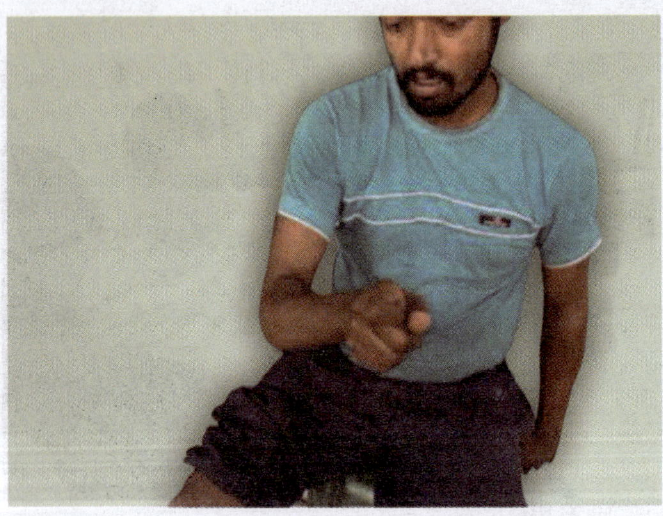

FIG. 11.102 Athetosis

Hemiballismus (Fig. 11.103)

- This is characterized by sudden fling-like movements of the proximal portion of the extremities. It may be constant or intermittent period of repose.
- This is not affected by eye closure, ceases during sleep.
- This is accompanied by hypertonicity and increased reflexes.
- This may be associated with athetotic movements of lower limb.
- The causative lesion is:
  Two-third portion of subthalamic nucleus must be affected to develop hemiballismus. The causes are:
  Embolic or thrombotic infarction produced by blockage of:
  - ❖ Interpeduncular artery from the top of the basilar.
  - ❖ Thalamoperforate artery of P1 segment of posterior cerebral artery.

Idiopathic Generalized Torsion Dystonia

- Dystonia is involuntary and abnormal posture—the lesion responsible is in the putamen and motor thalamus.
- Dystonia may be peripheral or central type.
- *In hereditary forms*—lower limb is flexed and inverted.
- *In peripheral dystonia* due to CRPS- I and II—lower limbs are flexed and inverted, upper limbs are flexed.
- *In severe genetic forms*—trunk and extremities show slow writhing movements, severe proximal joint movement and superimposed quicker movements.
- Affected muscles will be hypertrophied, mainly marked in sternocleidomastoid muscles.

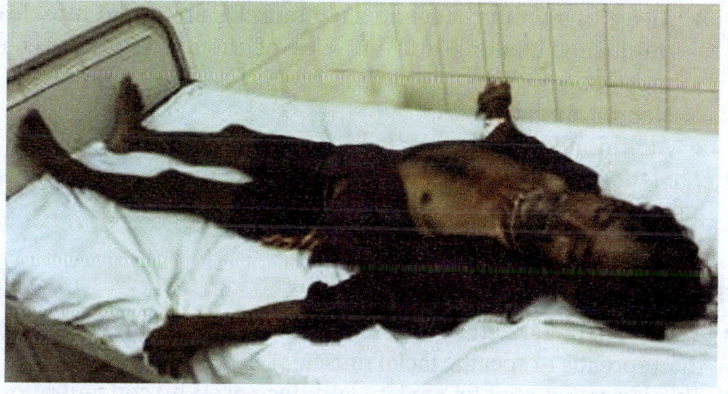

FIG. 11.103   Hemiballismus

■ Truncal Athetoid Movements

- This is characterized by contraction of paraspinal and truncal muscles producing:
  - ❖ Arching of the back
  - ❖ Lateral twisting of torso
  - ❖ Extreme rotations of head and neck.
- It lasts for 5 to 10 seconds
- This is not associated with eye movement, but associated with facial grimacing and protrusion of tongue
- Anxiety increases it and sleep relieves it.

■ Involuntary Movements of Face and Neck

Facial Tics

- This is characterized by stereotype repetitive movements of the face and other muscles of the trunk—unconsciously. These include facial blinking, persing of lips, facial grimacing.
- *There are associated movements:*
  - ❖ Abduction and forward rotation of shoulder
  - ❖ Retraction of the neck
  - ❖ Contraction of platysma
  - ❖ Contraction of pectoral muscles.
- This is exacerbated by anxiety and relieved by concentration.
- This movement occurs in childhood, decreases with adolescence.
- *The causes are:*
  - ❖ *Giller de la taurette syndrome:* This is associated with:
    - Coughing
    - Clearing of throat
    - Barking sound
    - Compulsive sweating.
  - ❖ *Meige's syndrome:* Here affected muscles are eyelid muscles producing blinking and muscles of mouth, e.g. masseter muscles.
  - ❖ Neuroacanthocytosis.
  - ❖ Attentiondeficit disorder.
- *The lesions*—It occurs in putamen, caudate nucleus and globus pallidus.

Hemifacial Spasm

- This is characterized by spasm of orbicularis oculi to start with then spreads to specific facial muscle.
- This is exacerbated by anxiety and decreased by concentration or sleep.
- This spasm starts suddenly and stops suddenly.

- *The causes:*
  - ❖ Aberrant loop of posterior interior cerebellar artery infringes upon the nerve, cured by Jannelta procedure
  - ❖ Tumor at the cerebellopontine angle
  - ❖ Aneurysm of anterior inferior cerebellar artery.
- *Aberrant regeneration of facial nerve produces contractions* of formerly denervated facial muscles, this is most prominent in mentalis muscles, prominent nasolabial fold, fasciculation sometimes maybe observed.
- *Facial seizures:* This is characterized by involvement of muscles of eye and angle of the mouth, movement is slower and coarser and stops slowly.
  This is associated with twitching of thumb and hands.

Facial Myokemia

This is characterized by flickering and undulating movements of facial muscles—unilateral, may be bilateral.

Causative Lesions

- Autoimmune manifestations associated with malignancies.
- Multiple sclerosis
- Vascular lesions of pons
- Genetic conditions.
  Periorbital myokemia is benign, involves orbicularis oculi, does not spread to face.
  This myokemia is associated with fatigue, lack of sleep.

Perioral Tremor

This is characterized by abnormal continuous contraction of orbiculation oris.
The causative lesions are:
- Tertiary syphilis
- Phenothiazine group of drugs.

This tremor is associated with protrusion and retraction (trombone-like movements) of tongue.

Spasmodic Torticollis

- This is characterized by forceful deviation of head to one side, sometimes backwards (retrocolis), chin moves upwards and occiput depressed and rotated.
- Spasm may be sustained or in a rapid series of succession with normal intervals.

- The muscles involved are sternocleidomastoid, scalene group of muscles and strap muscles, which may be hypertrophied.
- There may be associated contraction of platysma and facial muscles.
- Contractions may be so painful that it may be responsible for the development of cervical spondylosis.
- *Lesions responsible:*
  - ❖ Aberrant artery compressing IX nerve
  - ❖ Cervical plexus lesion (C_1 - C_4)—ventral root.

Facial Dystonia

- Bizarre grimacing
- Intermittent protrusion of hypertrophied tongue.
  Associated features of generalized dystonia.

Causative Lesion

- Huntington's dystonia
- Gelles de la taurette syndrome
- Postanoxic state.
  Blepharospasm sometimes to the point of interfering with vision associated with oromandibular dystonia.
  Causative lesion:
  - ❖ Meige's syndrome occurs in adolescence, associated with spasmodic torticollis
  - ❖ Brueghel's syndrome.

Tardive Dyskinesia

- Vertical oscillation of head in upright position, disappears in recumbency:
  Causative lesion: Demyelinative disease that destroys the connection with cerebellum.
  This movement is associated with:
  - ❖ Vermian posture (flexed back)
  - ❖ Sway from side to side.
- Bobble—head tremor—nonstereotyped vertical head tremor
  Causative lesion—third ventricle tumor.
- *Vertical head tremor seen also in:*
  - ❖ Parkinson's disease
  - ❖ Early torticollis.

The patient should be examined in supine, sitting and erect position.
The following points to be examined:
- Congenital abnormalities
- Acquired:

- ❖ Asymmetry
- ❖ Deformities.

Congenital Maldevelopment

- Champagne bottle appearance—atrophy of distal 1/3rd of quadriceps and all muscles below the knee are atrophic.
- A short neck—suggestive of (Arnold-Chiari malformation) may be associated with shallow posterior fossa + cranio-cervical defect.
- Droopy shoulder syndrome—long neck, droopy shoulders and traction on brachial plexus.
- Laurence-Moon-Biedl syndrome—webbed fingers + polydactyly.
- Holt-Oram defect—hand abnormalities from low set thumb + atrial septal defect + brain abscess → trisomy 21.
- Congenital absence of specific muscles—hereditary sensory motor neuropathy, cleido-cranial dysostosis.

Long-standing Neurological Lesions

- *Placenta previa:* Intrauterine stroke due to birth trauma, cocaine—produce contralateral asymmetry of development.
- *Migrational defect:* If neurons fail to migrate from germinal matrix to cerebral cortex this is called migrational defect.
  - ❖ If migration is halted in white matter of the centrum semiovale it is called nodular heteropia (Fig. 11.104). It can be seen in MRI as nodules on left ventricular wall.
  - ❖ Neurons migrate to cortex, but there is failure of apoptosis — it can be seen as double band in the cortex—it is called double cortex syndrome (Lissencephaly) (Fig. 11.105).
  - ❖ Migration is complete but there is disorganization at laminar level—it is called microdysgenesis. It cannot be diagnosed in MRI.

In migrational defect:
  - ❖ Face and arm are smaller and asymmetrical than lower limbs.
  - ❖ Inability to copy the posture (parietal lobe function)

    This asymmetry leads to kyphoscoliosis—as a result: There is traction on nerve root on scoliotic curve as they exit through foramina.

    Severe asymmetry leads to hemiplegia, athetosis, and seizures.

    Acquired defect: In case of surgical lesion – "heavy metal spinal fusions".
  - ❖ Painful at the level of fused interspace.
  - ❖ Painful laterally at the screw level.

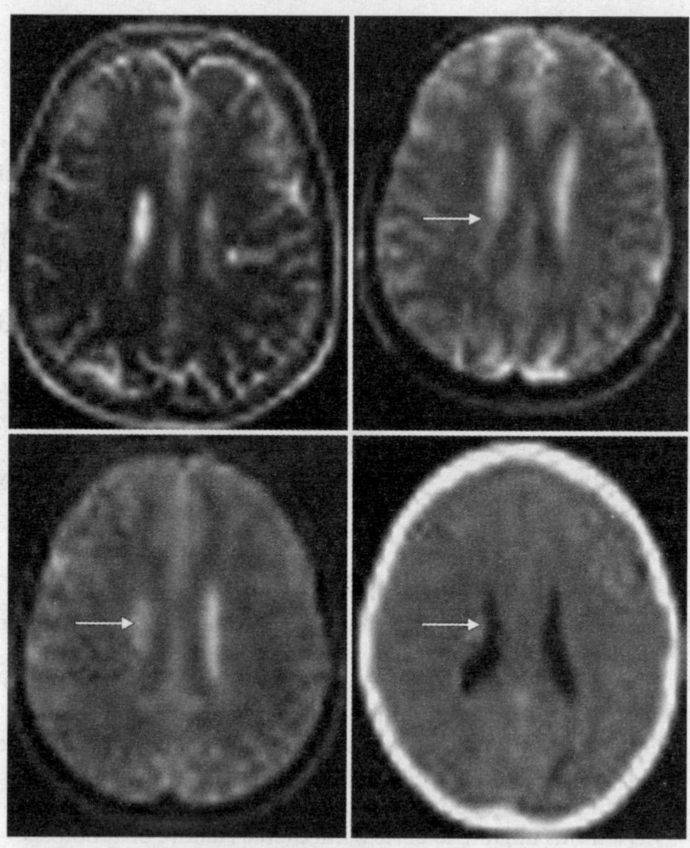

FIG. 11.104 Nodular heteropia

Examination of Joint Movements

- *Charcot's joint (Fig. 11.106):* Denervated and painless joint found in:
  - ❖ Tertiary syphilis
  - ❖ Cervical syringobulbia
  - ❖ Diabetes
  - ❖ Amyloidosis.
- Spinal movement occurs as flexion, extension and lateral rotation.

  In case of lumbar stenosis—flexion is restricted.

  In case of cervical stenosis—extension and lateral movement of the neck are restricted.

In case lumbar spondylolisthiasis
- There is pelvic tilt

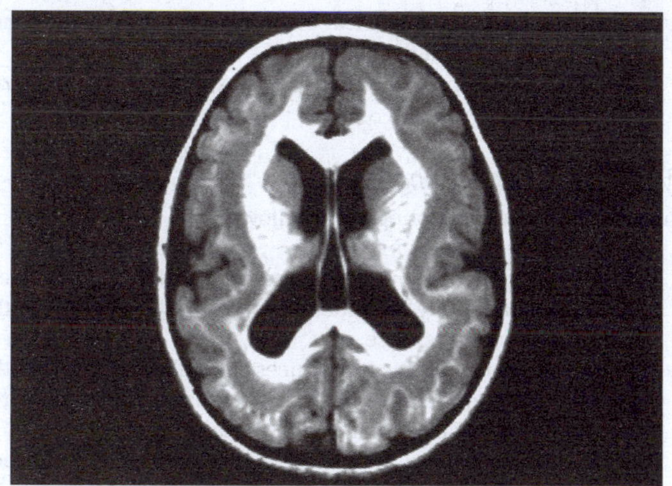

FIG. 11.105   Double cortex syndrome

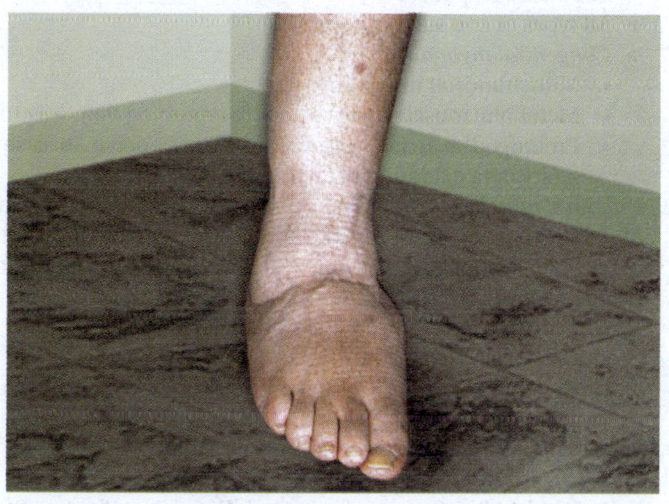

FIG. 11.106   Charcot's joint

- Pain during straight leg rising
- Pain during extension of hip joint.

Evaluation of Wasting of Muscles

Wasting can be measured by:

- Comparison with similar muscle of opposite side

- In case of bilateral symmetrical involvement, comparison done between proximal and distal muscles.
- Comparison in respect of similar age, sex, occupation and size of the patient.

Types of Muscle Wasting

Three types of muscle wasting are as follows:

1. *Generalized muscle wasting:*
   - General systemic illness (congestive cardiac failure, liver failure, renal failure) produces Type II muscle atrophy with proximal preponderance.
   - *Critical care myopathy:* It produces generalized wasting with proximal preponderance. It occurs in those patients who are under mechanical ventilator for long-time.
   - *Critical care axonal neuropathy:* It produces generalized wasting.
   - *Amyotrophic lateral sclerosis:* In later stage, there is severe wasting with fasciculation with hyperactive reflexes and Babinski's response.
   - All types of end stage myopathy.
   - *Congenital myopathy:*
     - Mitochondrial myopathy.
     - Metabolic muscle disease—more cramping than wasting.
     - Prolonged exercise—producing cramps occur in case of faulty beta oxidation of fat, no muscle wasting.

2. *Proximal muscle wasting:* Dystrophin gene present on short arm of X-chromosome, responsible for production of dystrophin, a part of glycoprotein complex called dystrophin-associated protein complex (DAP).

   DAP and dystrophin connect actine with basal laminae to produce muscle contraction.

   If there is deletion of "dystrophin" gene, the muscular dystrophy occurs.

   Causes of proximal muscle wasting are as follows:
   - *Duchenne muscular dystrophy (Fig. 11.107):*
     - Weak at 2 to 3 years of age, waddling gait at 3 to 6 years of age, muscle strength decrease at 11 years and wheelchair bound at 12 years.
     - Difficulty in climbing stairs, jumping, running.
     - Calf muscles are hypertrophied, rubbery in consistency due to acumination of fat and connective tissue.
     - Gowers' maneuver—patients use their hands to push up from the thigh.
     - Neck flexors are weak at all stages.
     - Patient cannot lift his head against gravity.

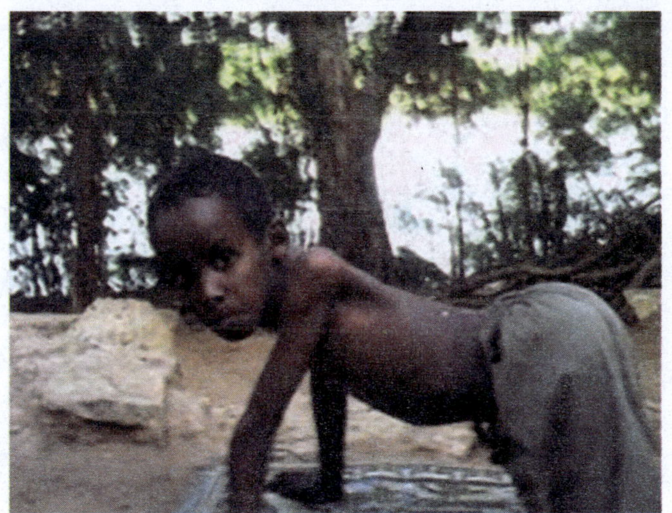

FIG. 11.107 Duchenne muscular dystrophy

- Pseudohypertrophy seen in deltoid, gluteal, masseters and calves.
- Plantar flexors and invertors of feet are strong. Anterior tibialis—weakens—at heels contractures.
- Reflexes are hard to elicit in following pattern—triceps > biceps > knees > brachioradialis and ankle.
- Cardiac—conduction defect.
- Pulmonary disease.
- Cranial muscle and sphincter muscles are spared.
- ❖ *Becker muscular dystrophy*
  - Later age of occurrence.
  - Pelvic and thigh muscles are involved first.
  - Less weakness of tibialis anterior, peroneal muscles, neck muscles.
  - Cardiac conduction defect—less common.
  - Death at 30 to 60 years of age due to cardiomyopathy and respiratory insufficiency.
- ❖ *Emery-Dreifuss muscular dystrophy:*
  - X linked EMD1, autosomal dominant (EMD2).
  - Muscle weakness and wasting—humeroperoneal—distribution—posterior leg wasting, elbow flexion, finger extensions affected.
  - Contracture—quadratus lumborum of low back producing rigid spine; flexion contracture wrist, elbow, ankle, neck.
  - Cardiac involvement—death due to cardiac myopathy.

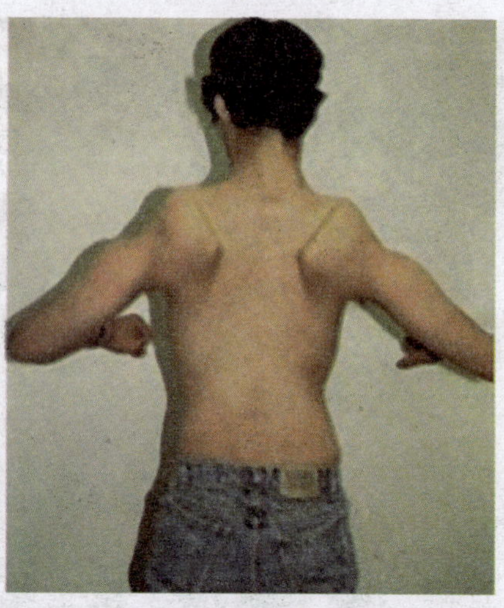

FIG. 11.108   Fascioscapular muscular dystrophy

- ❖ *Fascioscapular muscular dystrophy (Fig. 11.108):*
  - Descending rostral caudal (involving) weakness—facial → shoulder girdle → peroneal → hip single
  - Sparing of deltoids and neck flexors
  - Wasting of biceps and triceps (Popeye appearance)
  - Beevor's sign—lower abdominal muscle weakness
  - High frequency hearing loss and retinal vasculopathy.
- ❖ *Scapuloperoneal syndrome:* Variant of FSMD.
- ❖ *Limb-Girdle muscular dystrophy (Figs 11.109A and B):*
  - Weakness of pelvic girdle, shoulder girdle, or both
  - Calf hypertrophy
  - *Exclusion criteria:* Distal, facial, extraocular muscles
  - Normal lifespan, but may die before middle age.
- ❖ *Motor neuron disease*: It affects shoulder girdle with fasciculation, wasting, weakness.
- ❖ *Cervical spine syrinx*: Dissociated sensory loss, segmental wasting, absent reflexes, weakness in upper extremities, increased reflexes in knee and ankle.
- ❖ *Neuralgia amyotropica:* It is preceded by viral illness, vaccination, involving upper extremity—wasting, may be bilateral, sensory loss in axillary distribution.
- ❖ *Collagen vascular disease:*
  - Polymyositis/dermatomyositis—rash in extensor surface of joint of hand, swallow defect.
  - Scleroderma—periungual telangiectasia.

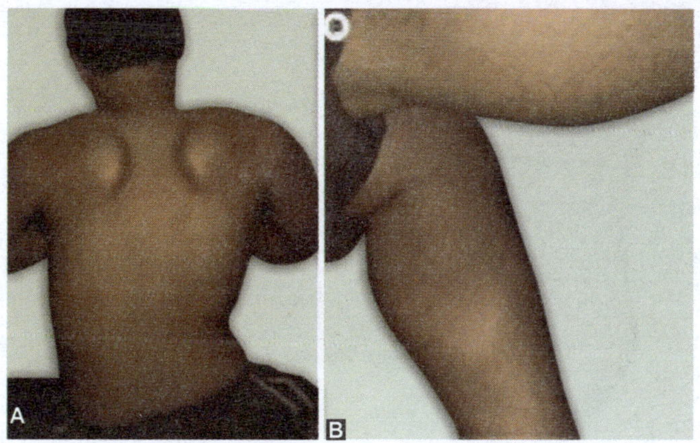

FIGS 11.109A AND B   Limb girdle muscular dystrophy

* *Compressive lesion in C_5 to C_6:* It is deltoid and spinatus atrophy. Loss of bicep reflex, exaggerated triceps jerk and finger flexion reflexes, decreased neck movement.
* *Cauda equina syndrome:*
  * Caused by disc protrusion, cytomegalovirus in patient with HIV
  * Wasting of gluteal muscles
  * Perineal sensory loss
  * Sphincter incontinence.

3. *Distal muscle weakness:*
   To examine distal myopathy—following muscles should be examined:
   * *Anterior tibiulis muscle:* It is rounded adjacent to tibia. So, gentle pressure over the tibia reveals wasting.
   * *Gastronemius muscle:* It should be convex when the leg will be raised from the bed.
   * Extensor digitorum brevis—of lateral side of the foot.
     Here the examiner should note the prominence of the tendons and arch of the foot—It may be increased arch (pes cavus) (Fig. 11.110) in congenital neuropathy or loss of arch (Rocker bottom foot) (Fig. 11.111). Watch the fasciculation of the affected muscles at rest and after induction by percussion.
   * Check the sensory loss.

Causes of distal wasting in case of forearm—lesions usually responsible are from anterior horn cell to the site of innervations. Causes are:

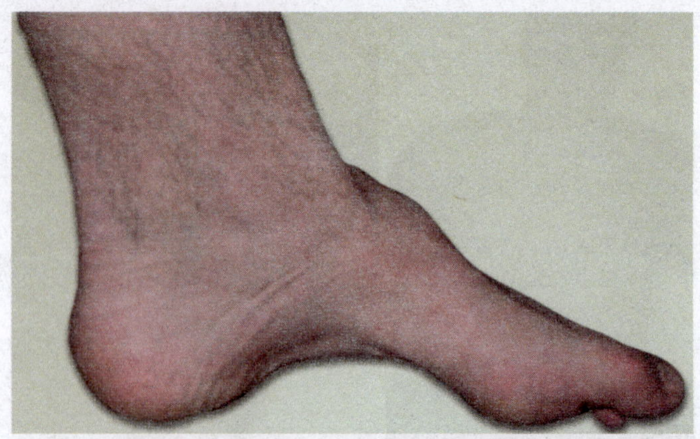

FIG. 11.110 Pes cavus

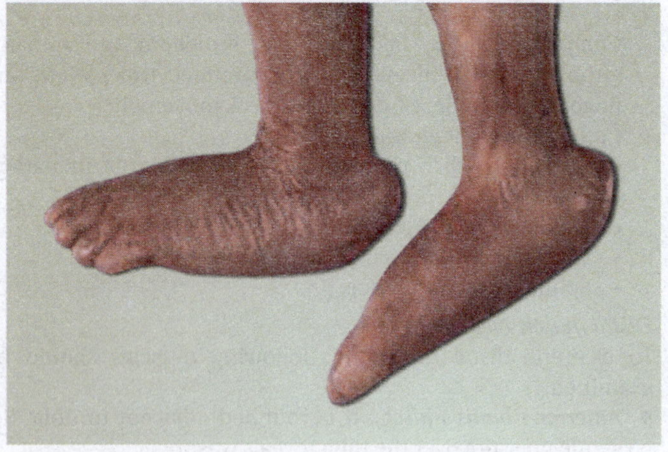

FIG. 11.111 Rocker bottom foot

* *Anterior horn cells of C_8 —for thenar eminence, and T_1—for hypothenar eminence.*
  Causes are:
  * Motor neuron disease
  * Cervical syringomyelia
  * Tumor
  * Rarely poliomyelitis.
* *Ventral roof of C_5 to T_6 involvement by:*
  * Cervical spondylosis
  * Syrinx
  * Tumor.

- Abiotrophies—failure to sustain anterior horn cell survival by lack of trophic factors or genes.
- Inflammation of white matter tracts may affect anterior horn cells directly or may die due to peripheral loss of axons.

❖ *Involvement of brachial plexus—may affect C_8 to T_1:* The causes:
- Trauma
- Autoimmune disease
- Neuralgic amyotrophy.

❖ *Compression of T_1 at thoracic outlet—*in rib-band syndrome of Gilliat (Band).

❖ *Sulcal tumor—*breast carcinoma, bronchogenic carcinoma damage the plexus at the apex of the lung:
The autoimmune neuropathies—are due to:
- Ganglioside M_1 (GM_1) antibodies
- Monoclonal antibody glycoprotein (MAG) antibodies.

❖ *Acute intermittent porphyria—*involves the intrinsic muscles of hand and forearm muscles intermittently, with normalization in between the attack.

❖ *Compression of median nerve at carpal funnel—*wasting of thenar eminence—involved muscles are:
- Abductor pollicis brevis
- Opponens pollicis.

Sensory involvement at the tip of index finger.

❖ *Compression of ulnar nerve at the cubital tunnel (at elbow)—*produces severe wasting of all intrinsic muscle of the hand except abductor pollicis brevis and opponens pollicis.

Compression of ulnar nerve at the Guyon's canal at the wrist—produces no wasting but sensory loss.

Congenital myopathies:
- Autosomal dominant late onset Welander's myopathy — involving weakness of hands, fingers and wrist.
- Autosomal dominant Marksberry/Griggs myopathy—involving anterior leg compartment.
- Autosomal recessive Nonaka myopathy—anterior leg compartment.
- Autosomal recessive Miyoshi distal myopathy— posterior leg compartment.

❖ *Myotonic dystrophy:* Features include:
- Hang jaw
- Facial involvement
- Frontal balding
- Stellate cataract
- Cardiac abnormalities
- Myotonia.

Involving Lower Legs

- Hereditary sensorimotor neuropathies
- Charcot Marie—tooth disease
- L_4 to L_5 radiculopathy—wasting of tibialis anterior
- S_1 - radiculopathy—involving gastrocnemius muscle.

Peripheral Wasting of Upper and Lower Extremities

Metabolic neuropathies due to diabetes, renal, thyroid, liver involvement—symmetrical distal atrophy—sensory loss, loss of reflex, autonomic dysregulation.

■ Muscle Tone

The methods to detect muscle tone:

In Case of Suspicion of Basal Ganglia Diseases

- The examiner flexes and extends the elbow of the patient during conversation with him.
- Examiner rotates the wrist of patient while asking the patient to open and close the opposite hand to reinforce (reinforcement).

  As a result, there is ratchety, jerky tremulous variations in hypertonia, due to superimposed tremor in the examined hand—this is called cog-wheel rigidity.
- In few cases, examiner feels same type of resistance during whole range of flexion or extension if is called lead-pipe rigidity.
- In few cases, during whole range of extension or flexion of arm, there is increased resistance followed by sudden fall in resistance due to inhibitory signal sent to anterior horn cells by tendon of that muscle—clasp knife rigidity.
- By shaking the hand of the patient one can demonstrate hypotonicity.
- In case of bed ridden or unconscious patient, examiner first elevates the limb of the patient and allow it to fall on the bed—watch the speed of fall—it detect hypotonicity.

  Then compare it with the opposite limb.

Testing the Tone of Lower Limb Muscle

- Roll the limb to be examined in between palms of both hands—to detect tone of the musculature.
- Evaluate the side to side movement of the limbs—excess movement indicates—increased tone.
- Place the hands behind the poplitial fossa and elevate the knee of the patient.

  With the elevation of knee, foot will be automatically slided up the bed.

If the foot is off the bed—it is due to increased tone.

Again, in similar manner, foot is allowed to slide back to its original position.

If there is any delay in pushing the foot backwards—it indicates increased tone (Queen Square sign).

Decreased Tone (Hypotonia)

Decreased resistance to passive movement is called hypotonia. There is decreased tendon reflex. It may be due to:
- No input to anterior horn cell
- Decreased firing from anterior horn cell—due to cerebellar disease, spinal or cerebral shock.

Common Causes of Hypotonia
- *Lesions in motor side of reflex are:*
  - Poliomyelitis
  - West Nile fever
  - Primary spinomuscular atrophy
  - Amyotrophic lateral sclerosis
  - Guillain-Barre syndrome
  - Peripheral nerve injury.
- *Lesion in sensory side of reflex are:*
  - Sensory neuropathies
  - Tabes dorsalis
  - Small fiber neuropathies—anti-Hu antibodies in response to tumor antigen
  - Amyloid
  - Pyridoxine.
- *Combined motor and sensory lesion:*
  - Syringomyelia
  - Cord lesion
  - Root lesion
  - *Cerebral shock or spinal shock:*
    - Capsular strokes
    - Hemorrhages.
- *Lesions in muscles:*
  - Acquired myopathies
  - Mitochondrial myopathies
  - *Dystrophic:*
    - Duchenne muscular dystrophy
    - Becker muscular dystrophy
    - Fascioscapular muscular dystrophy
    - Oculopharyngeal muscular dystrophy.
  - Hypokalemic periodic paralysis—due to accumulation of fluid in T tubule system—muscle is tense and swollen, but are flexic and paralyzed.

- *Cerebellar lesion:* Hypotonia is usually associated with of the sings of cerebellar lesions.
- *Chorea:*
  - ❖ Sydenham's chorea
  - ❖ Huntington's chorea.
- *Collagen disorders:*
  - ❖ Marfan's disease
  - ❖ Homocystinuria
  - ❖ Osteogenic imperfecta
  - ❖ Ehlers Danlos Type VI associated with hyperextensibility of distal extremity joint.

Symptoms of Hypotonia
- *Infantile hypotonia (floppy baby syndrome):* Generalized decrease in muscle tone, mainly in neonate.
- *Physiologically* in deep sleep and pathologically in coma.
- *Akinetic epilepsy:* Sudden loss of muscle tone; occurring spontaneously and patient falls into ground.
- *Cataplexy:* Sudden loss of muscle tone precipitated by strong emotions—laughing, crying.
- *Sleep paralysis:* In sleep there is diffuse decrease in muscle tone and unable to move immediately after awakening from sleep.
- Spinal and neural shock.

Increased Tone (Hypertonia)

- *Spasticity*: In this condition, resistance and tone of one group of muscles are greater than the other. This is often called "clasp knife" type hypertonia. Spastic muscles are firm and contracted at rest producing contracture in future. In lower extremities, it frequently occurs associated with ex aggregated jerks and clonus. In upper extremities, there may be supinator catch during supination and pronation of forearm. Increased tone in adductor muscles of lower extremities produces classical scissors gait.
- *Lead-pipe rigidity:* Here the resistances produced by opposing group of muscles are equal throughout the range of motion.

  As a result limbs are flexed, posture is flexed, gait may be apraxia of gait and 'magnetic' foot grasp (Normal pressure hydrocephalus). Gait is cautious and hesitant due to shortened swing phase (Well's dementia gait).
- *Cog wheel rigidity:* This occurs due to alternate contraction of agonist and antagonistic muscles, first appear in proximal muscles, then spread distally.

  There is catch in movement—Negri's sign.

  It is extremely helpful in case of early Parkinson's disease. It is easily observed in wrist which is rotated.

- *Paratonia:* It is an alteration in tone to passive motion— occurs in frontal lobe disease. It can be:
    i. Inhibitory paratonia, and
    ii. Facilitatory paratonia.
- *Gegenhalten:* It is a type of rigidity—where resistance to passive movement given by the patient is directly proportional to force given by the examiner, e.g. harder the examiner pushes, the harder the patient seems to push back.

Method of detection of paratonia
- Examiner elevates the patient's arm and instructs him to relax.
- Then examiner releases the arm and watch whether it remains elevated or not.

If the arm remains in the lifted position in absence of spasticity or Parkinsonism—it dictates paratonia—inhibitory.

In case facilitatory paratonia, patient cooperates much. So in this case, the patient actively assists examiner's passive movements, so, the limb continues to move up even after release of examiner.

Differences between spasticity and rigidity

Spasticity	Rigidity
• Resistance is different throughout the range of movement	• Resistance is uniform throughout the range of movement
• Hypertonia varies greatly from muscle to muscle	• Hypertonia involve all the muscles about same degree
• In case of slow passive movement, there will be little resistance. But if the passive movement is very quick, there will be increased amount of resistance in the form of sudden "catch" in the movement as if the muscle is impacted to be stopped	• Both in slow and increased passive movement resistance will be similar

Muscles involved in spasticity and method of detection
- In upper extremity—Flexors and pronators are involved.
- In lower extremity—Extensors of leg and invertors of ankle adductors of thigh.
  Contracture of adductors of both limbs producing scissor gait.

In upper extremity (Fig. 11.112)
- Patient's elbow will be flexed at 90° and forearm is fully pronated.
- Examiner starts to supinate the forearm:
    ❖ If spasticity is less severe or process of supination is slow there will be no resistance.

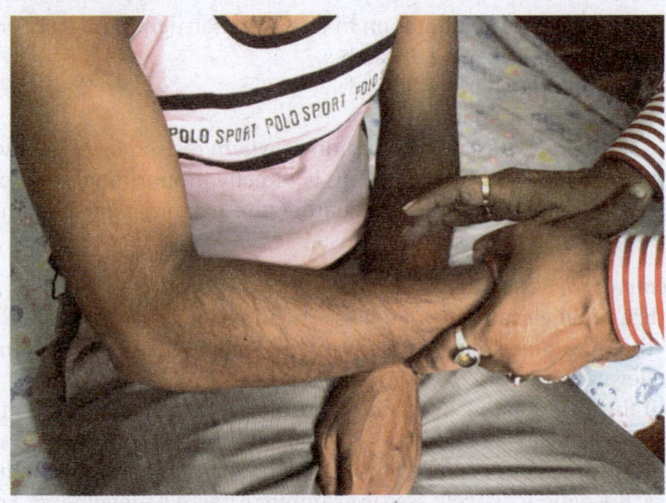

FIG. 11.112 Tone in upper extremity

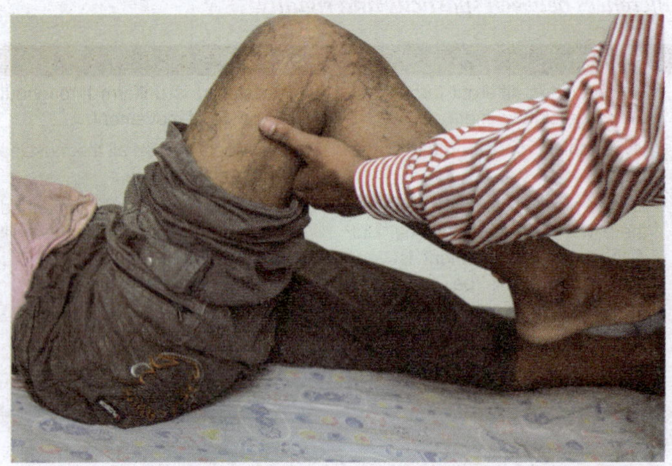

FIG. 11.113 Tone in lower extremity

❖ If spasticity is severe or process of supination is fast there will be sudden catch called "Pronator catch". This catch will relax the muscle and supination process will be completed.
❖ If hypertonia is very severe, there may be pronator clonus.

In case of lower extremity (Fig. 11.113)

● Patient should be in supine and relaxed position.
● Examiner given one hand behind the knee and with other hand slowly flexes and extends the knee of the patient.

If spasticity is less severe or, process is very slow there will be no resistance to passive movement.

If spasticity is fast and process is very fast there will be sudden catch.

- After several slow repetitions, examiners suddenly and abruptly raise the knee upward in fully extended position.

In case moderate to severe spasticity, the foot fires upward in kicking motion (spastic kick).

Heel or Foot Dropping Test (Fig. 11.114)

- Patient's leg is flexed at knee and hip, in this position examiner holds the patient's leg, with one hand behind the knee and other hand supports the foot.
- Now the examiner suddenly release the foot.

In normal patient—foot descent is smooth

In case of spasticity—quadriceps muscles of leg hangs up the foot and drop it in succession of choppy movements.

Ashworth Scale (Grade 1 to 5)

This scale quantifies spasticity.

1 – No increase in muscle tone.

5 – Affected part rigid in flexion or extension.

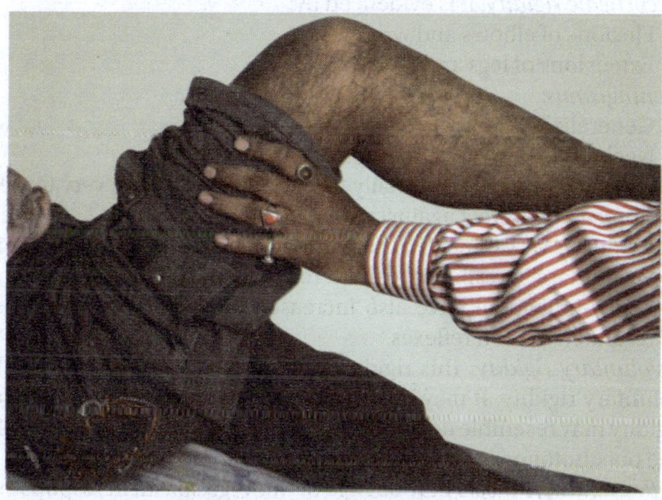

FIG. 11.114   Heel or foot dropping test

In Case of Hemiplegia

Posture
- *Upper extremity:*
  - ❖ Arm is adducted and flexed at elbow
  - ❖ Wrist and fingers are flexed
  - ❖ Forced grasping.
- *Lower extremity:*
  - ❖ Extended and adducted at the hip
  - ❖ Extended at knees and ankle
  - ❖ Inversion and plantar flexion

So there is resistance to extension in case of upper extremity and resistance to flexion in case of lower extremity.

In Case of Bilateral Hemiplegia

Above described tone are present in both sides of upper and lower extremities.

Due to bilateral adductor spasm there is "scissors gait."

Catatonic rigidity: This type of rigidity is comprised of:
- Lead pipe type of rigidity accompanied by posturing
- Bizarre movements and mannerism.
- Psychosis.

Decerebrate rigidity: It is evidenced by:
- Marked rigidity
- Sustained contraction of extensor muscles of all four extremities.

Decorticate rigidity: It is evidenced by:
- Flexions of elbows and wrist
- Extensions of legs and feet.

Meningismus:
- Generalized rigidity
- Neck extension (opisthotonos).

Voluntary rigidity: Occasionally few muscle groups are very tensed and braced to protect against pain.

Again it is very difficult to differentiate whether it is true volitional or involuntary in response to excitement, pain, fatigue.

Tense individual have also increased muscle tension showing exaggerated tendon reflexes.

Involuntary rigidity: This rigidity is nonorganic, reflexic, resemble voluntary rigidity. It may be due to psychogenic origin—hysterical rigidity may resemble decerebrate rigidity or catatonia, occasionally like opisthotonos.

Reflex rigidity: Muscle may be rigid or undergo spasm in response to afferent stimulus—pain.

Muscle spasm is nothing but sustained muscle contraction, sometimes this spasmodic muscle becomes palpable.

Examples:
- Board-like rigidity in peptic perforation.
- Rigidity and extension of neck in meningitis.
- Reflex spasm may be due to cold.
- In some metabolic myopathies (Mac Ardle disease)—painful muscle cramps may occur due to exercise.

Clonus

It is rhythmic contraction of disinhibited muscles caused by supranuclear lesion, mainly pyramidal tract.

It may occur in any muscle, but can be demonstrated in leg in following maneuvers:
- When ankle joint is suddenly dorsiflexed, sudden stretching of tendo Achillis producing clonus.
- In knee, it can be seen in quadriceps muscles when examiner displaces patella sharply downward.
  This clonus may be associated with:
  - ❖ Increased tone of the muscle
  - ❖ Increased reflexes
  - ❖ Babinski's sign
  - ❖ Hoffman's sign.

Lesions Responsible for Increased Tone

- *Corticospinal system (upper motor neuron lesion):* Cortex or spinal cord lesion produces spasticity, increased deep tendon reflexes, loss of abdominal reflexes, Babinski's sign.
  Causes are:
  - ❖ Anoxic birth injury
  - ❖ Vascular disease
  - ❖ Tumor
  - ❖ Degenerative
  - ❖ Demyelinating disease.
- *Akinetic Parkinsonian syndrome produces:*
  Lead pipe rigidity or plastic rigidity: This occurs in:
  - ❖ Nigro-strial degeneration
  - ❖ Progressive supranuclear palsy
  - ❖ Multiple system atrophy
  - ❖ Corticobasal ganglia degeneration.
- *Early stage of Parkinsonian syndrome* may produce cog-wheel rigidity.

Myotonia

It is the state of sudden and sustained contraction of muscles following specific movement, e.g.

- Inability to open his eyes following a cough.
- Inability to open his hand after clenching the fist.
- Percussion over the extensor profundus muscle produces extension of index or long fingers.
- Percussion over thenar eminence produces adduction and dimpling of thumb.

If percussion is hard, it may produce dimpling by the side of dimple.

Myotonia may be with Dystrophic Features

- *Classic myotonic dystrophy:* It is characterized by:
  - ❖ Frontal baldness
  - ❖ Wasting of masseter, temporalis muscles, pterygoid muscles—producing "hanging jaw"
  - ❖ Atrophy of distal sternocleidomastoid muscles
  - ❖ Cataract
  - ❖ IGT (impaired glucose tolerance)
  - ❖ High FSH
  - ❖ Cognitive impairment.
- *Schwartz–Jampel syndrome:*
  - ❖ Dystrophic features
  - ❖ Short stature
  - ❖ Contracture.

Myotonia without Dystrophic Features

- Congenital myotonia—hypertrophied muscles with myotonia without dystrophic feature.
- Several sodium channel myotonias—these are potassium sensitive.
- Paramyotonia congenita—there is myotonia in response to cold.
- Hyperkalemic periodic paralysis.

■ Muscle Power

Muscle power should be tested in individual muscles so the patient is asked to perform a specific movement for a specific muscle by his own without resistance and against resistance given by the examiner.

The following muscle groups are tested for evaluation:
- Flexors and extensors of the neck
- Abductors, adductors and rotators of the shoulder
- Flexors and extensors of elbow, wrist and fingers
- Abdominal muscles
- Extensors of spine
- Flexors and extensors of hip and knee
- Plantar flexors and dorsiflexors of foot
- Flexors, extensors of fingers and toes.

Muscles of Head and Neck

Movement of the neck are:
- Flexion
- Extension
- Rotation
- Lateral bending.

The muscle groups responsible are:
- *Sternocleidomastoid*—flexor and rotator of head and neck
- *Trapezius*—responsible for retraction of neck and lateral bending
- *Paravertebral muscles*— extension and flexion of the neck.

Tests for Neck Extension and Flexion

For Neck-Flexion (Fig. 11.115)

Ask the patient to flex his neck (to touch his chest with chin) actively and passively against resistance, applied by the examiner.

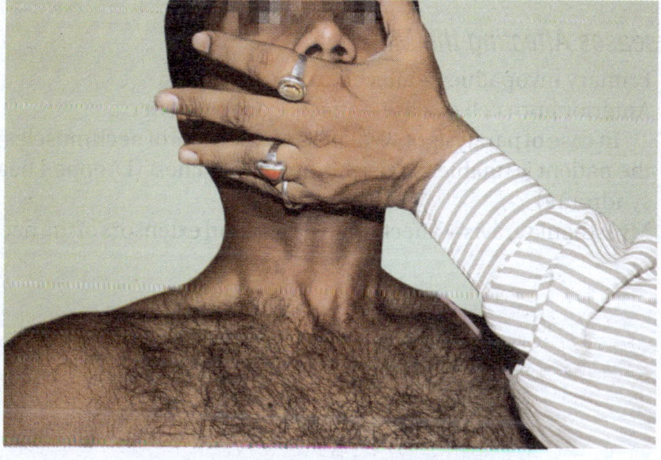

FIG. 11.115   Flexion of neck against resistance

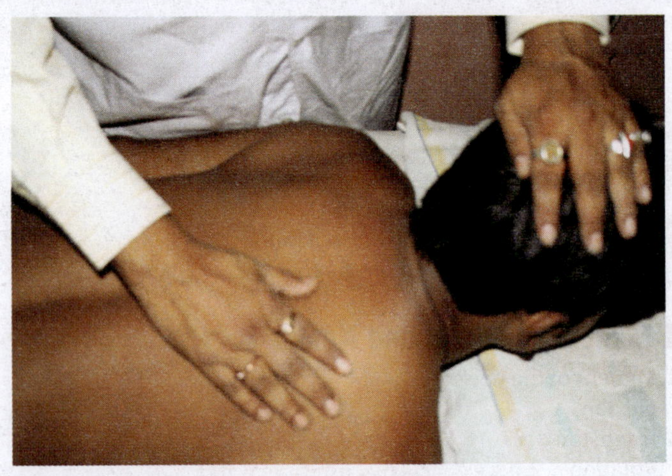

FIG. 11.116 Neck extension against resistance

Sternocleidomastoid, trapezius and other flexor muscles can be palpated.

For Neck Extension (Fig. 11.116)

Ask the patient to extend or elevate his head in prone position actively then passively against resistance applied to occiput by the examiner.

Trapezius and other paravertebral muscles can be palpated.

Neck rotation—contralateral sternocleidomastoid. Splenius capitis and trapezius.

Diseases Affecting the Muscles

- Primary myopathies—affect flexors of the neck.
- Anterior horn cell disease—affects extensor of neck.
    In case of paralysis or weakness of extensors of neck muscles— the patient is unable to raise his head from chest (Dropped head syndrome)
- Myasthenia gravis—affects both flexors and extensors of the neck.

Testing of Muscles of Shoulder Girdle and Scapula
Muscle of Shoulder

Name of muscle	Nerve supply	Test
• Deltoid (Fig. 11.117)	Segment-C5: Peripheral nerve circumflex or axillary nerve	Ask the patient to hold his arm abducted to 60° against examiner's resistance. Palpate the muscle
• Supraspinatus (Fig. 11.118)	Segment-C5: Peripheral nerve: Suprascapular nerve	Ask the patient to initiate abduction of arm against examiner's resistance; first 30° of abduction is done by this muscle. Palpate the muscle
• Infraspinatus (Fig. 11.119)	Segment-C5: Peripheral nerve: Suprascapular nerve	Ask the patient to flex the elbow at 90° position. Hold the elbow to the side of the body and then try to externally rotate forearm against resistance. Palpate the muscle
• Rhomboids (Fig. 11.120)	Segment-C5: Peripheral nerve: Nerve to rhomboids	Ask the patient to keep his hand to the hip. Then ask him to force the elbow backwards against resistance
If this muscle is weak, superior part of scapula is abducted		
• Serratus anterior (Fig. 11.121)	Segment C5–7: Peripheral nerve: Nerve to serratus anterior or long thoracic nerve	Ask the patient to push his arm forwards against resistance (like wall) with arms extended horizontally in front of him
If this muscle is weak, tip of the scapula retracted from the chest wall, medial scapular border remains straight		
• Pectoralis major (Figs 11.122 and 11.123)	Segment-C6–8: Peripheral nerve: Lateral and medial pectoral nerve	Ask the patient to place his hand on the hip and pressing inwards, the sternal part of it can be seen and felt. Ask the patient to raise his arm forwards above 90° and try to adduct it against resistance clavicular part can be seen
• Latissimus dorsi (Fig. 11.124)	Segment-C7: Peripheral nerve: Nerve to latissimus dorsi or thoracodorsai nerve	Ask the patient to elevate his arm to 90° and try to adduct the arm in that position. The muscle can be seen and palpated

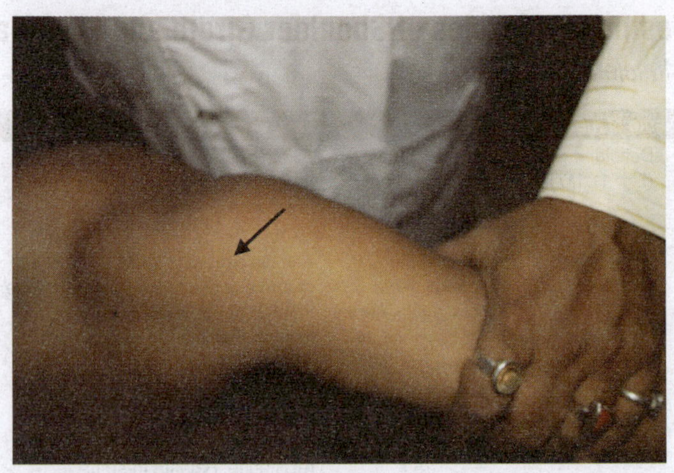

FIG. 11.117 Examination of deltoid muscle

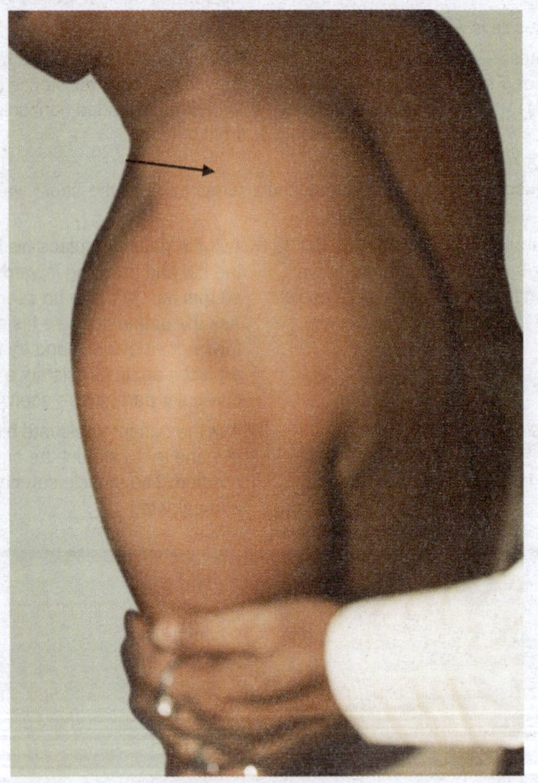

FIG. 11.118 Supraspinatus muscle

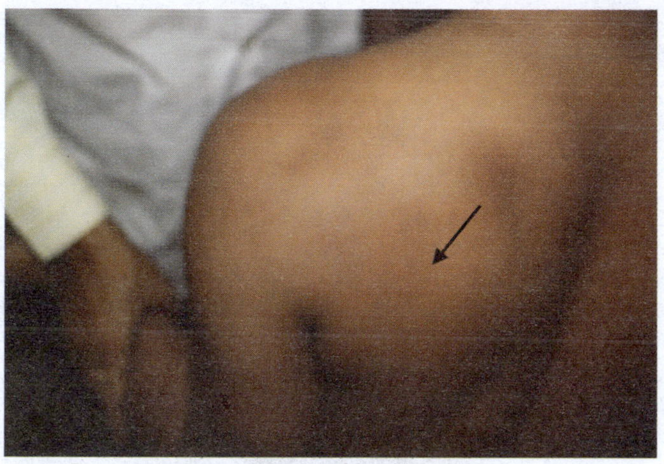

FIG. 11.119   Infraspinatus muscle

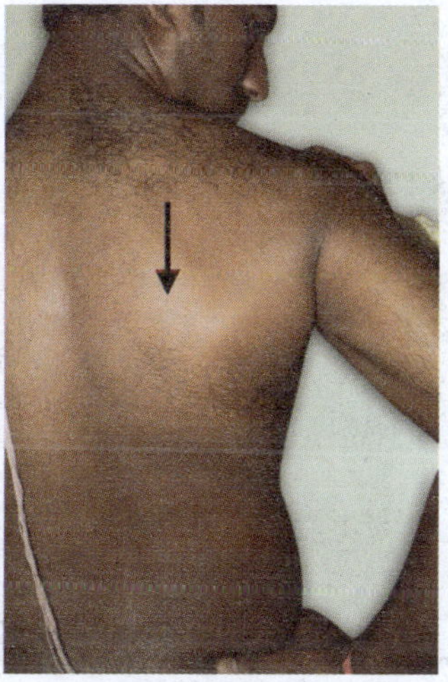

FIG. 11.120   Rhomboid muscle

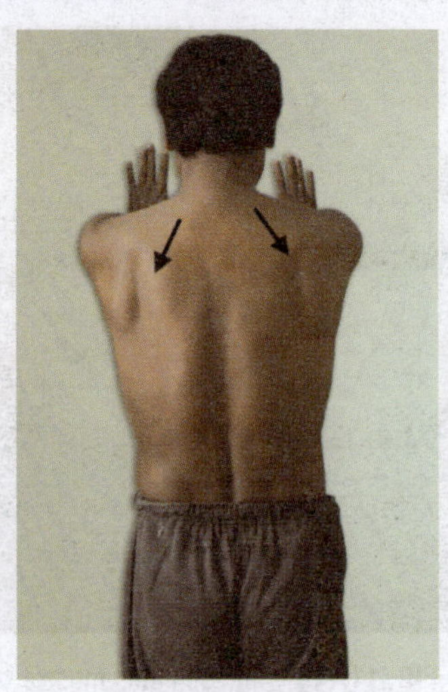

FIG. 11.121   Serratus anterior

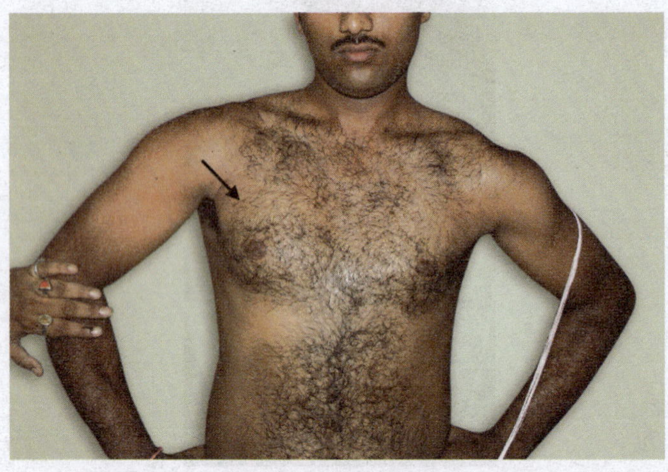

FIG. 11.122   Pectoralis major, sternal part

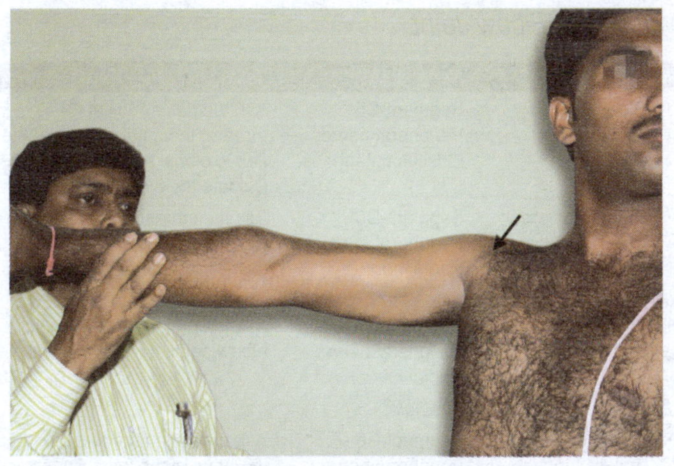

FIG. 11.123 Pectoralis major clavicular part

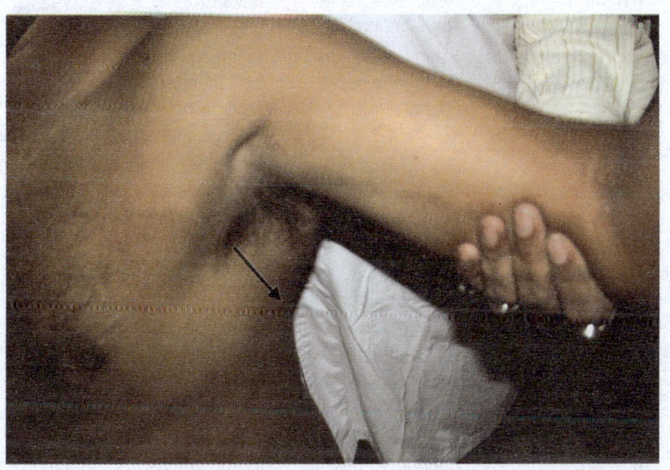

FIG. 11.124 Latissimus dorsi

Muscles of Elbow Joint

Muscles	Nerve supply	Tests
• Biceps (Fig. 11.125)	Segment-C5: Peripheral nerve: Musculocutaneous.	Ask the patient to supine forearm then, ask the patient to flex to elbow against resistance. Palpate the biceps muscle
• Brachioradialis (Fig. 11.126)	Segment-C5: Peripheral nerve: Radial nerve	Ask the patient to pronate the forearm and draw the thumb towards the nose against resistance
• Triceps (Fig. 11.127)	Segment-C7: Peripheral nerve: Radial nerve	Ask the patient to extend his elbow against resistance
Muscles of forearm and wrist joint		
• Extensor carpi radialis longus (Fig. 11.128)	Segment-C6–7. Peripheral nerve: Radial nerve	Ask the patient to dorsiflex the hand at the wrist, fingers partially extended position towards radial side against resistance
• Extensor carpi ulnaris (Fig. 11.129)	Segment-C7. Peripheral nerve: Radial nerve	Same method as above, but towards ulnar side
• Extensor digitorum (Fig. 11.130)	Segment-C7. Peripheral nerve: Radial nerve	Ask the patient to maintain his extended fingers at metacarpophalangeal joint when examiner attempts to flex his fingers as MCP joints
• Flexor carpi radialis (Fig. 11.131)	Segment-C6–C7, peripheral nerve: Median nerve	Ask the patient to flex the wrist towards radial side
• Flexor carpi ulnaris (Fig. 11.132)	Segment-C8 peripheral nerve: Ulnar nerve	
• Abductor pollicis longus (Fig. 11.133)	Segment-C8: Peripheral nerve: Radial nerve	Ask the patient to abduct the thumb against resistance
• Extensor pollicis brevis (Fig. 11.134)	Segment-C8: peripheral nerve: Radial nerve	Ask the patient to extend the thumb against resistance given at metacarpophalangeal joint
• Extensor pollicis longus (Fig. 11.135)	Segment-C8: Peripheral nerve: Radial nerve	Ask the patient to extend the thumb against resistance given at interphalangeal joint

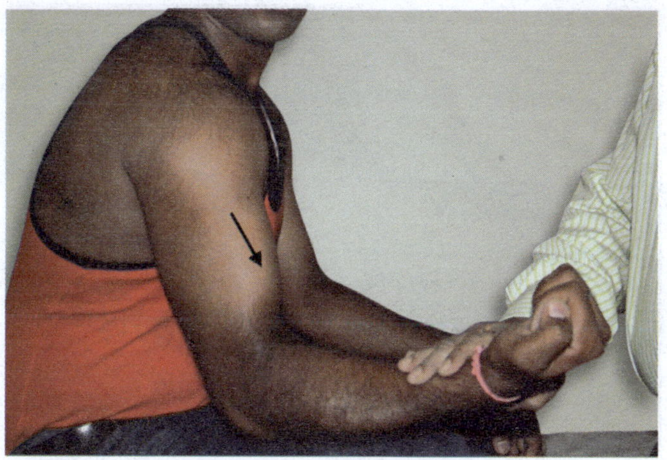

FIG. 11.125   Biceps muscle

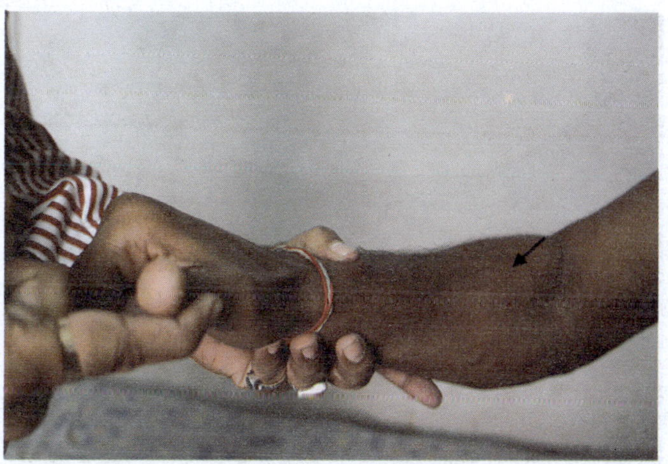

FIG. 11.126   Brachioradialis test

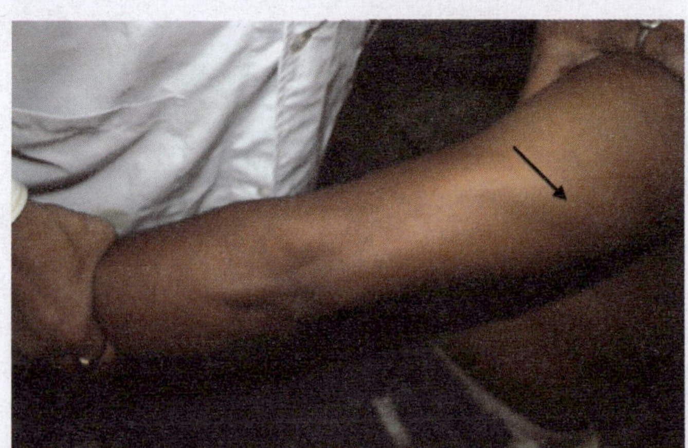

FIG. 11.127   Triceps muscle

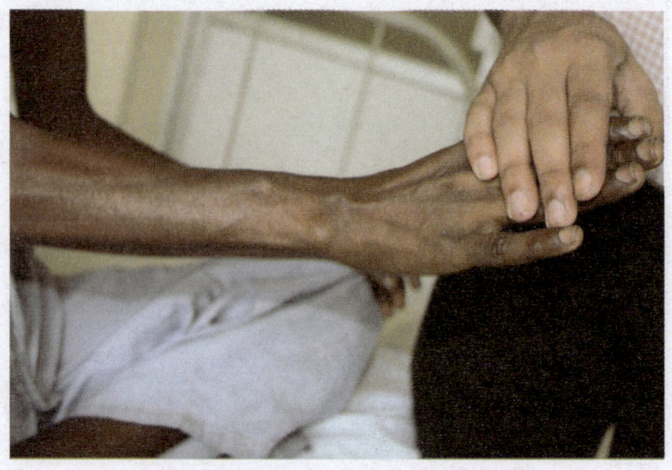

FIG. 11.128   Extensor carpi radialis longus

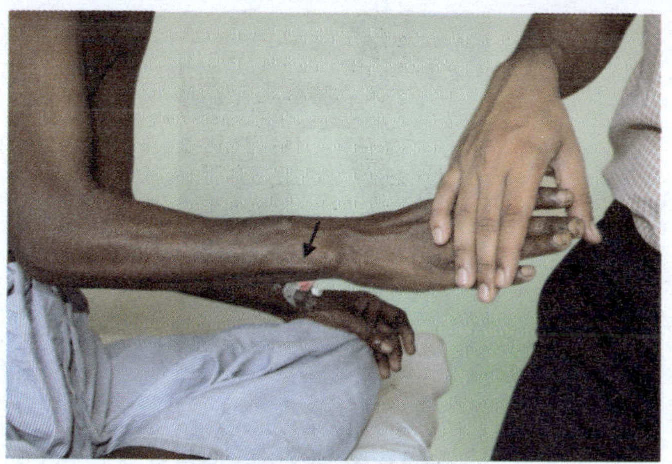

FIG. 11.129 Extensor carpi ulnaris

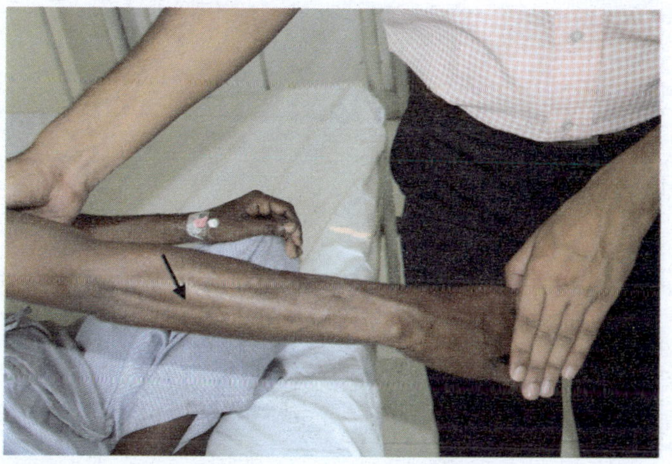

FIG. 11.130 Extensor digitorum

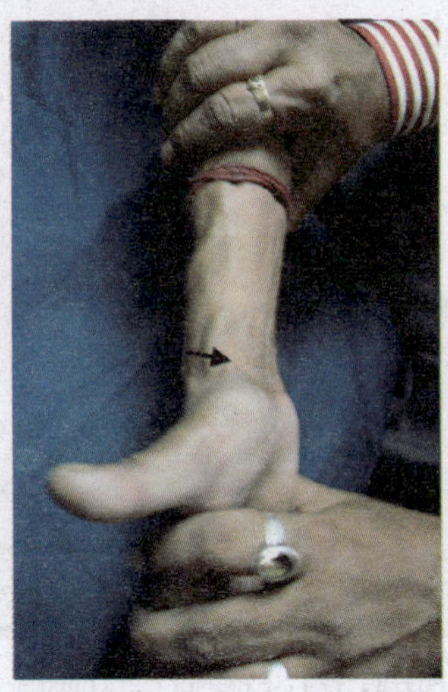

FIG. 11.131 Test for flexor carpi radialis

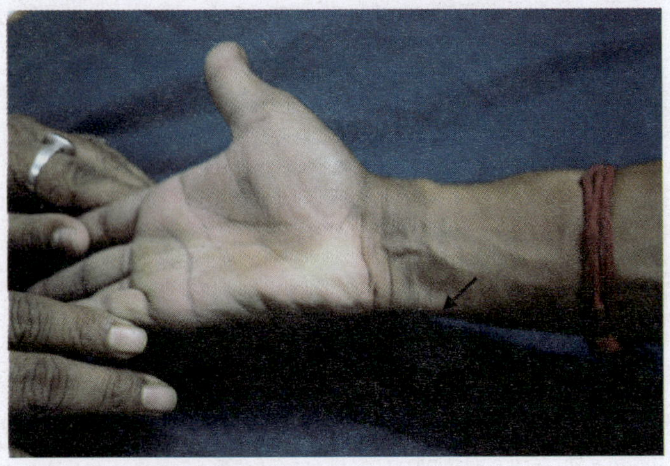

FIG. 11.132 Test for flexor carpi ulnaris

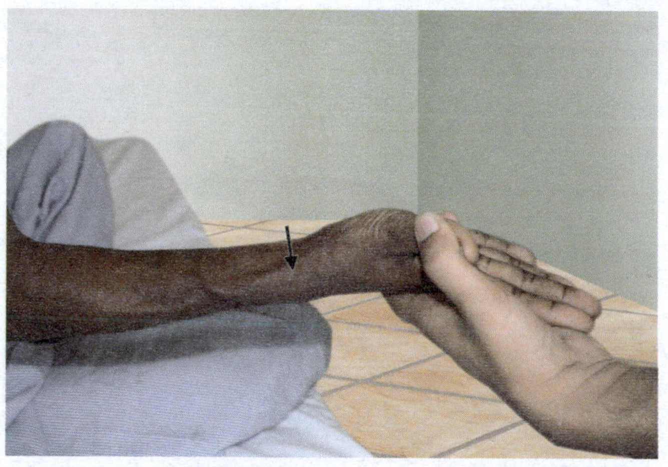

FIG. 11.133 Abductor pollicis longus

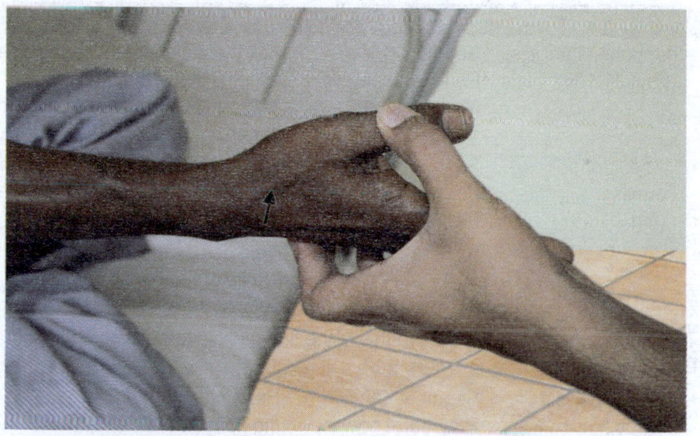

FIG. 11.134 Extensor pollicis brevis

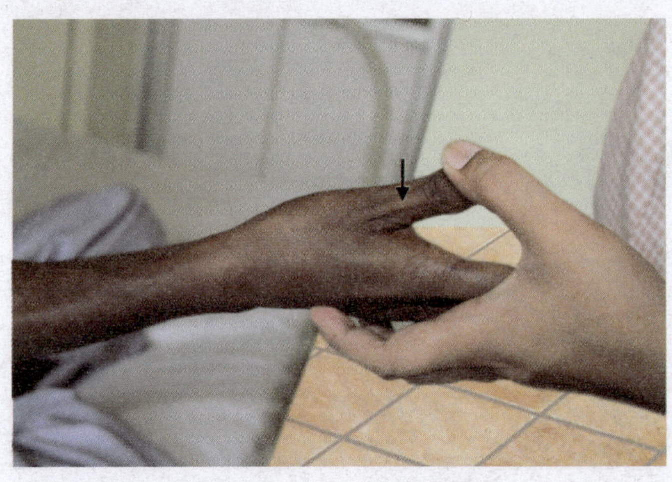

FIG. 11.135 Extensor pollicis longus

Muscles	Nerve supply	Tests
• Opponens pollicis (Fig. 11.136)	Segment-T1: Peripheral nerve: Median nerve	Ask the patient to touch the little finger with the thumb against resistance given at the tip of the thumb
•. Abductor pollicis brevis (Fig. 11.137)	Segment-T1: Peripheral nerve: Median nerve	First place an object in between thumb and the base of forefinger to prevent full adduction
		Next ask the patient to raise the tip of the thumb vertically against resistance
This muscle is important because this is the first muscle to be affected in carpal tunnel syndrome		
•. Flexor pollicis longus (Fig. 11.138)	Segment-C8: Peripheral nerve: Median nerve	Here examiner tries to extend the flexed distal phalanx of the thumb against patient's resistance
• Adductor pollicis (Fig. 11.139)	Segment-T1: Peripheral nerve: Ulnar nerve	Hold the piece of paper in between base of palmar aspect of forefinger and thumb. The examiner tries to pull the paper

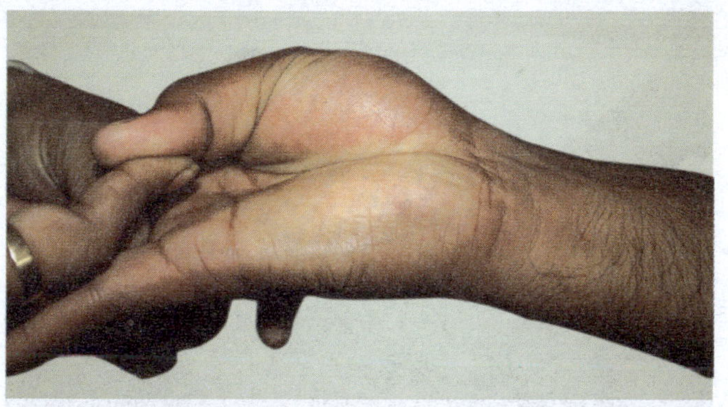

FIG. 11.136   Opponens pollicis

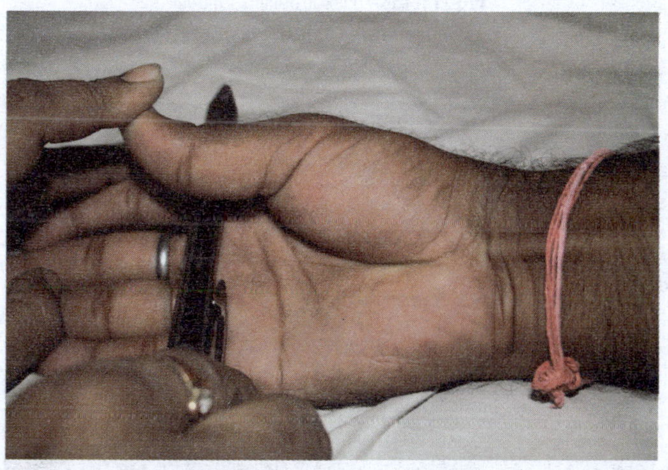

FIG. 11.137   Abductor pollicis brevis

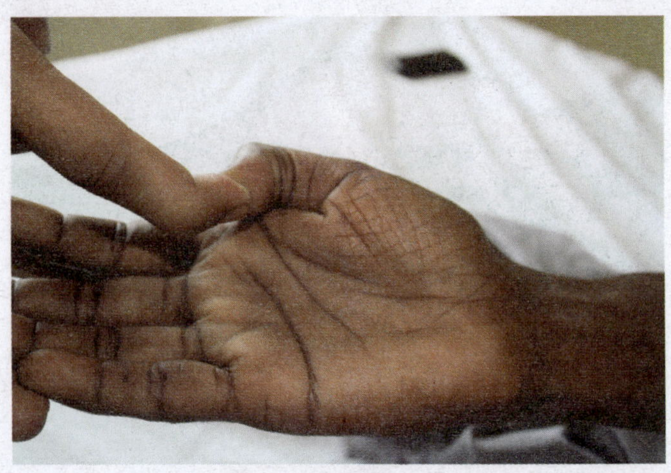

FIG. 11.138 Flexor pollicis longus

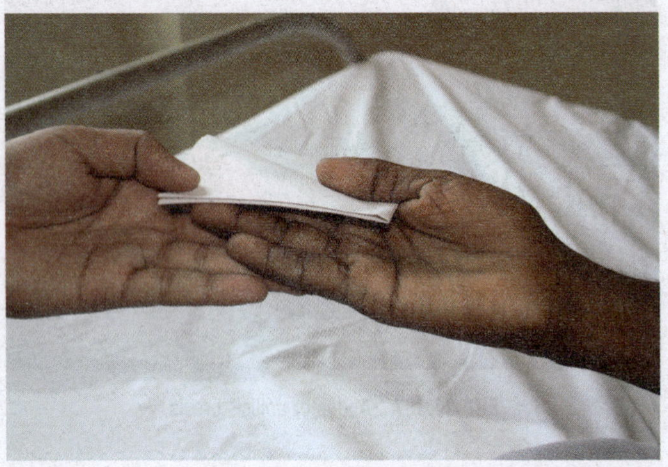

FIG. 11.139 Adductor pollicis

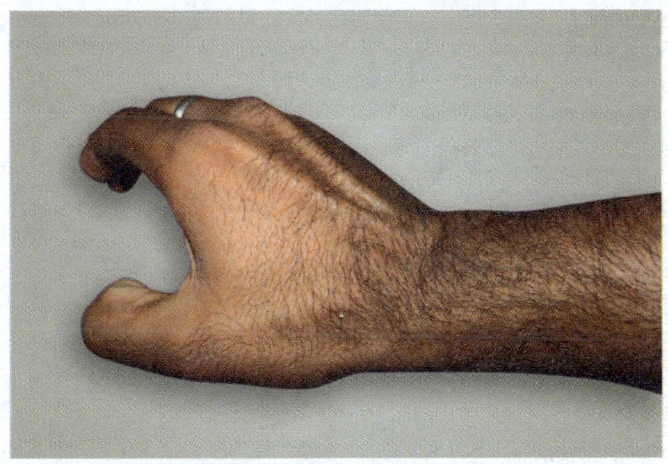

FIG. 11.140 Lumbricals

Muscles	Nerve supply	Tests
Muscles of hand and fingers		
• Lumbricals and Interossei (Fig. 11.140)	Segment-C8 T1 Peripheral nerve: Median (lumbricals I and II) Ulnar (Interossei, Lumbrical III, IV)	• Ask the patient to flex the fingers at metacarpophalangeal joints (Lumbricals) • Ask the patient to keep the fingers in abducted position (interossei)
• First dorsal interosseus and 1st palmar interossei (Fig. 11.141)	Segment-T1: Peripheral nerve: Ulnar nerve	Place the hand on the table. Ask the patient to abduct and adduct the forefinger against resistance
• Flexor digitorum sublimis (Fig. 11.142)	Segment-C8: Peripheral nerve: Median nerve	Ask the patient to flex the fingers except thumb at proximal interphalangeal joints, and examiner put resistance at middle phalanges of all fingers
• Flexor digitorum profundus (Fig. 11.143)	Segment-C8: Peripheral nerve: Median nerve (I and II), Ulnar nerve (III and IV)	Patient is asked to flex the terminal phalanx against resistance given at the tip of the phalanx and middle phalanx is being supported. Each finger is to be tested one by one
• Abductor digit minimi (Fig. 11.144)	Segment-T1: Peripheral nerve: Ulnar nerve	The back of hand to be examined is placed on table. Now little finger is to be abducted against resistance
[In some case, this muscle weakness is the only sign of ulnar nerve lesion.]		

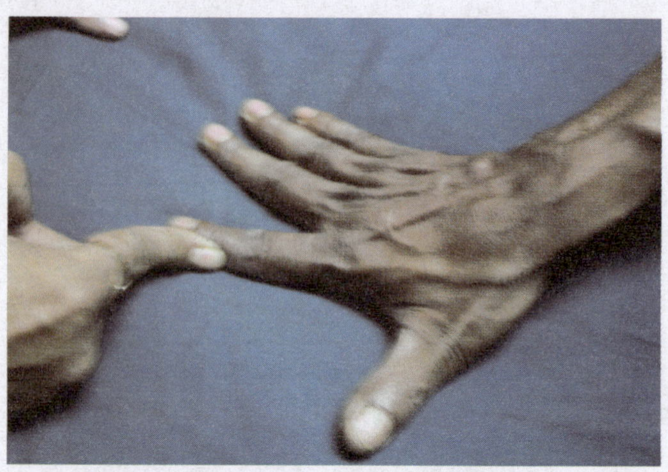

FIG. 11.141 Test for first dorsal interossei

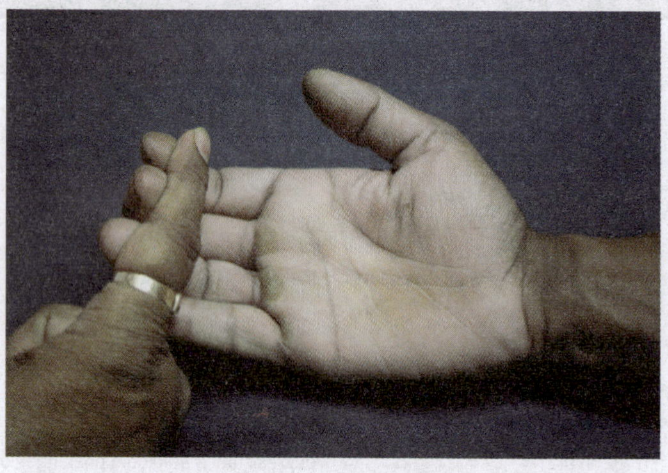

FIG. 11.142 Test for flexor digitorum sublimis

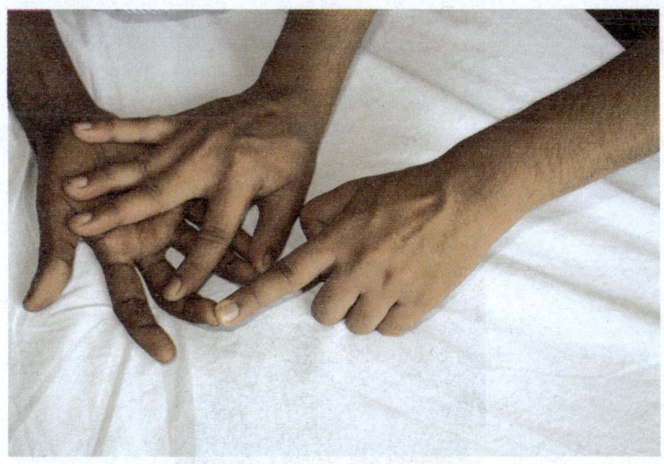

FIG. 11.143   Flexor digitorum profundus

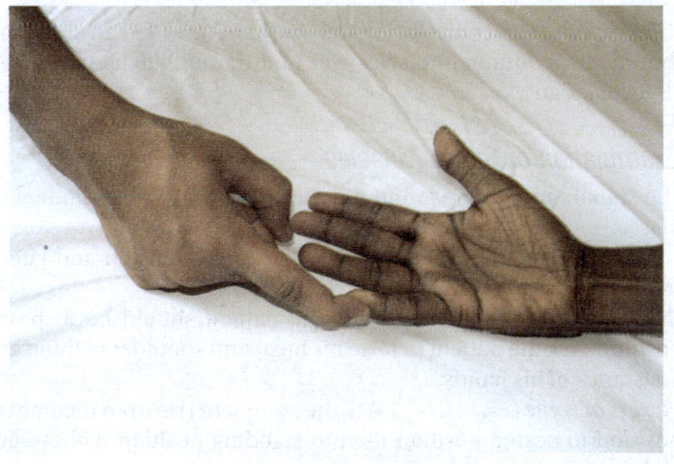

FIG. 11.144   Abductor digiti minimi

Examination of Abdominal Muscles

Weakness of abdominal muscles will not occur in neurological patient.

Abdominal muscles can be tested by asking the patient to raise his head against resistance, or to cough (Fig. 11.145).

Results: If abdominal muscles contract in all quadrants equally, the umbilicus will not move.

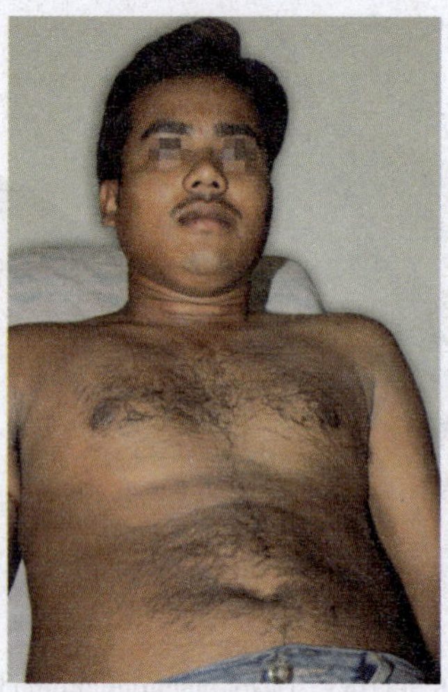

FIG. 11.145 Abdominal muscles

If lower abdominal muscles is paralyzed as in case of T_{10} myelopathy, the upper abdominal muscles will pull the umbilicus upwards—"Beevor's sign".

Examination of Spinal Muscles

The spinal muscles are group muscles—those can be examined en masse.

The movement of the spine are—flexion, extension and lateral rotation.

Extensors of spine (Fig. 11.146): The patient should be in prone position. Ask the patient to raise his head and shoulder without any assistance of his hands.

Flexors of spine (Fig. 11.147): Ask the patient to rise from recumbent position to seated position then to standing position without any assistance of his own hands.

Examination of Muscles of Thorax

The thoracic muscles are:
- *Intercostal muscles:* During inspiration this muscles expanded in anteroposterior and transverse diameter of thorax.
- *Diaphragm:* Vertical diameter of thorax is increased by this muscle.
- *Muscles attached to sternum, clavicles, scapulae:* It acts as accessory muscles of respiration.

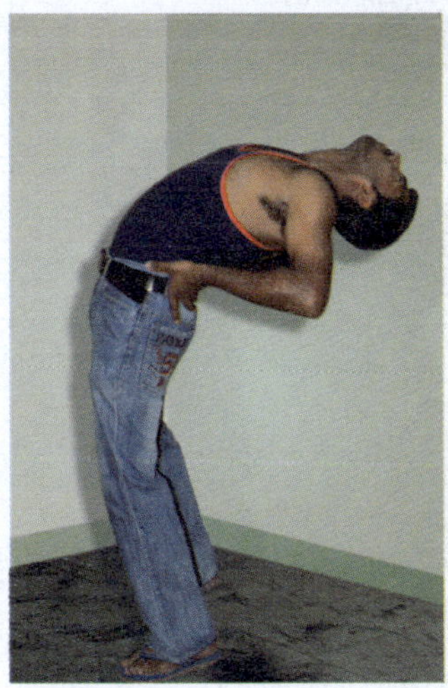

FIG. 11.146   Extension of spine

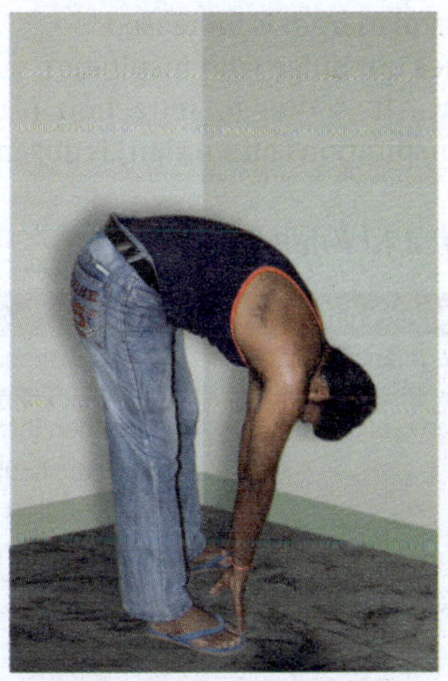

FIG. 11.147   Flexor of spine

In case of weakness of intercostal muscles:
- There is adduction of costal margins
- Diaphragmatic respiration
- Alternate bulging and retraction of epigastria.

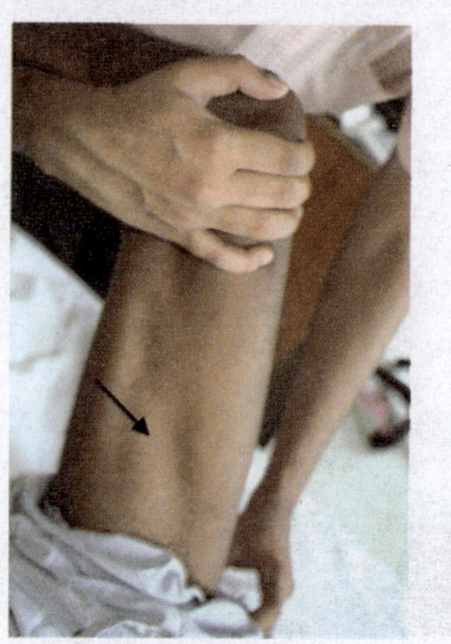

FIG. 11.148   Iliopsoas muscle

With bilateral paralysis of the diaphragm:
- Excursion of costal margin is increased
- Epigastrium does not bulge with inspiration
- Moving shadow—It is due to retraction of lower intercostal spaces during inspiration (Litten sign) is absent.

Muscles of Thigh and Knee

Muscle	Nerve supply	Test
• Iliopsoas (Fig. 11.148)	Segment: L1–L3 peripheral nerve: Femoral nerve	• Patient should lie on his back. Ask the patient to flex his knee and then thigh against resistance
		• Patient should be in sitting position. Hip is now in flexed position. Now ask the patient to further flex his thigh and at the same time examiner should try to push the thigh back to bed
• Adductor femoris (Fig. 11.149)	Segment L5–S1 peripheral never: Obturator	Ask the patient adduct the leg against resistance
• Gluteus medius and minimus (Fig. 11.150)	Segment L2–L3 peripheral nerve: Superior gluteal nerve	Patient is lying down in prone position. First flex the knee, then ask the patient to force the foot outwards against resistance. These muscles also abduct the extended legs

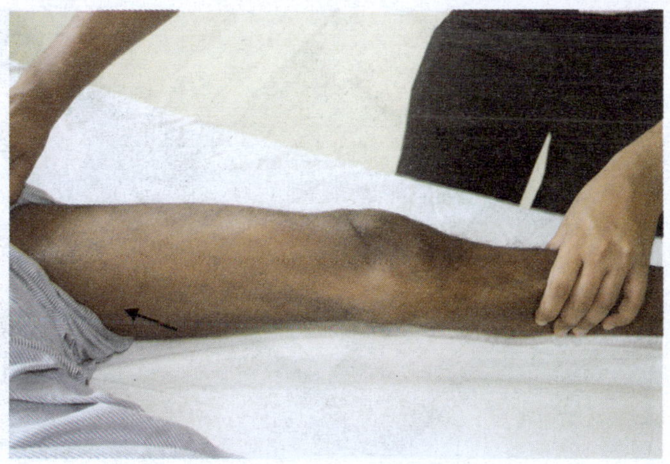

FIG. 11.149 Adductor femoris

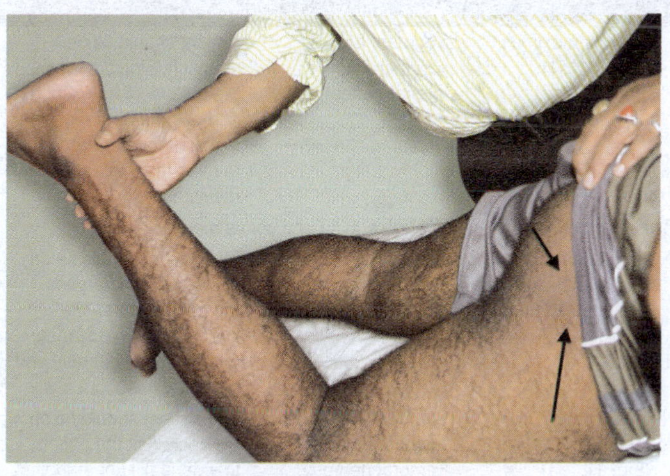

FIG. 11.150 Gluteus medius and minimus

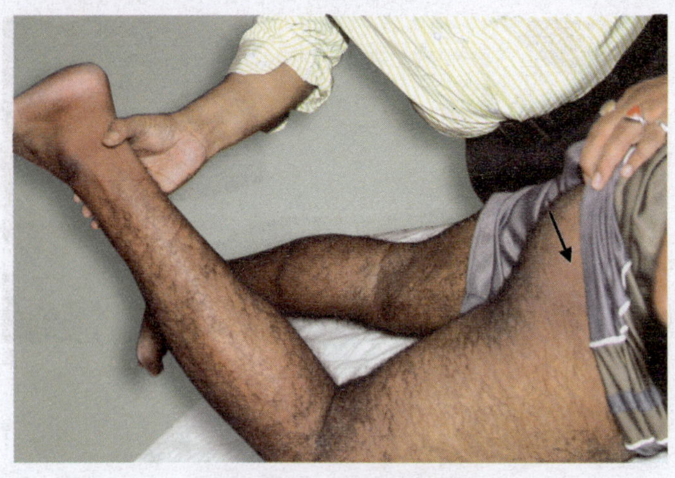

FIG. 11.151 Gluteus maximus

Muscle	Nerve supply	Test
• Gluteus maximus (Fig. 11.151)	Segment L5 – S1 peripheral nerve: Interior gluteal nerve	Patient should lie on stomach. First tightens the buttock of both limbs and palpate both muscles simultaneously. Then try to raise the thigh against resistance
This muscle is important in cauda equina and conus medullaris lesion		
• Hamstrings (Biceps, semimembranosus and semitendinosus) (Fig. 11.152)	Segment L4 L5–S1 peripheral nerve: Sciatic nerve	The patient should lie on his stomach. Then ask the patient to flex the knee against resistance. Bicep is seen laterally and semitendinosus medially
• Quadriceps femoris (Fig. 11.153)	Segment L3–L4. peripheral nerve: Femoral nerve	The patient should lie on his back. Ask the patient to extend his knee against resistance

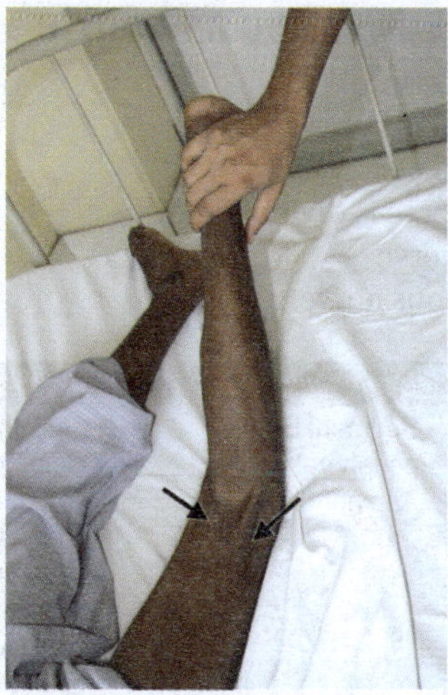

FIG. 11.152 Hamstrings muscles

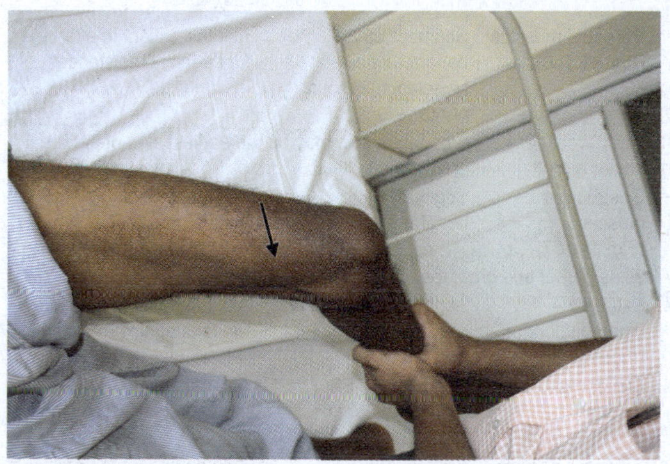

FIG. 11.153 Quadriceps muscle

■ Muscles of Lower Leg and Ankle

Sciatic nerve divides into:

- Medial popliteal nerve
- Lateral popliteal nerve.

Lateral popliteal nerve is divided into:

- Anterior tibial nerve
- Musculocutaneous nerve.

Muscle	Nerve supply	Test
• Tibialis anterior (Fig. 11.154)	Segment L4-L5 peripheral nerve: Anterior tibial nerve	• Ask the patient to dorsiflex the foot against resistance produced by examiner's hand placed on the dorsum of the foot • Examiner press the muscle next to the tibia bone to palpate this muscles
• Tibialis posterior (Fig. 11.155)	Segment L4 peripheral nerve: Medial popliteal nerve	Ask the patient to plantar the foot slightly then invert the foot against resistance given on plantar surface of foot
• Peroneal muscles (Fig. 11.156)	Segment L5-S1 peripheral nerve: Musculocutaneous nerve	Ask the patient to evert the foot against resistance
[Isolated weakness of peroneal muscle may be the earliest sign of peroneal muscular atrophy]		
• Gastrocnemius muscle (Fig. 11.157)	Segment S1 peripheral nerve	Ask the patient to plantar flex against resistance
Muscles of foot and great toe		
• Extensor digitorum longus (Fig. 11.158)	Segment L5 peripheral nerve: Anterior tibial nerve	Ask the patient to dorsiflex the toes against resistance
• Flexor digitorum longus (Fig. 11.159)	Segment S1-S2 peripheral nerve: Medial popliteal nerve	Ask the patient to plantar flex the toes against resistance
• Extensor hallucis (Fig. 11.160)	Segment L5-S1 peripheral nerve: Anterior tibial nerve	Ask the patient to dorsiflex the great toe against resistance
• Extensor digitorum brevis (Fig. 11.161)	Segment S1 peripheral nerve: Anterior tibial nerve	Ask the patient to dorsiflex the great toe against resistance. The triangular muscle is an example of S1 innervated muscle

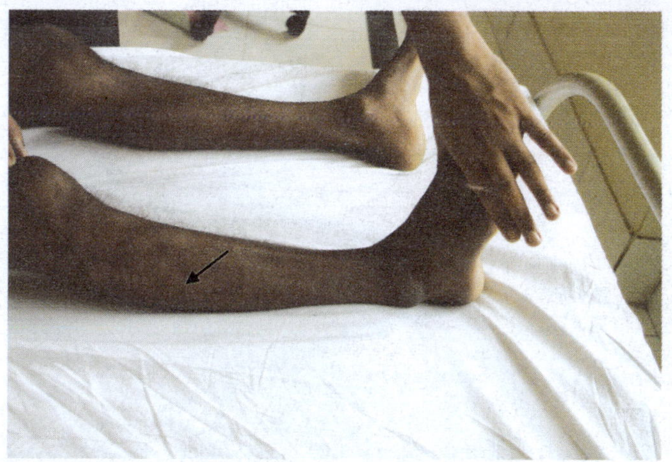

FIG. 11.154   Tibialis anterior muscle

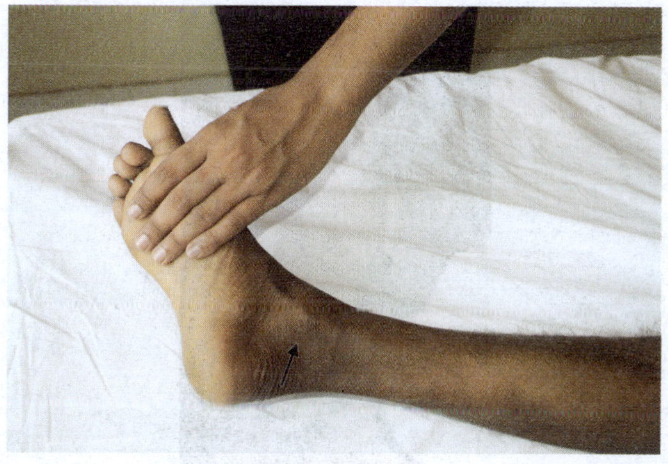

FIG. 11.155   Tibialis posterior muscle

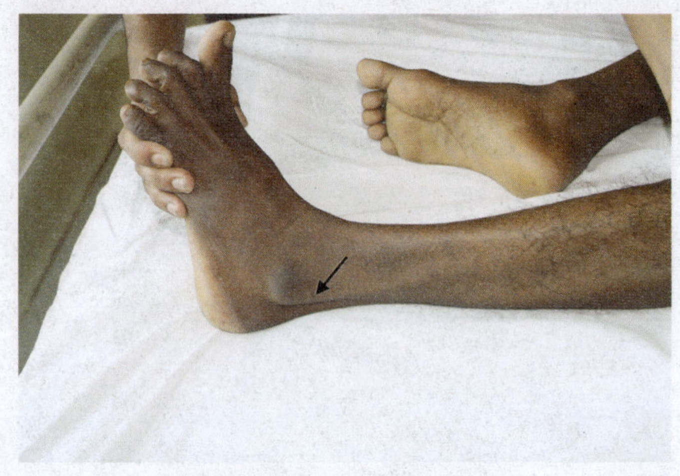

FIG. 11.156 Peroneal muscles

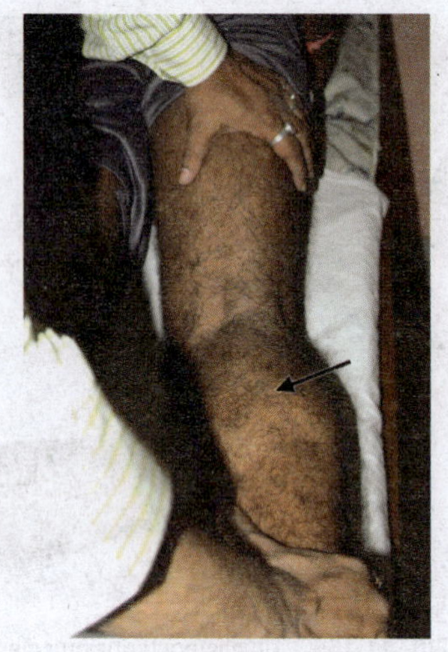

FIG. 11.157 Gastrocnemius muscle

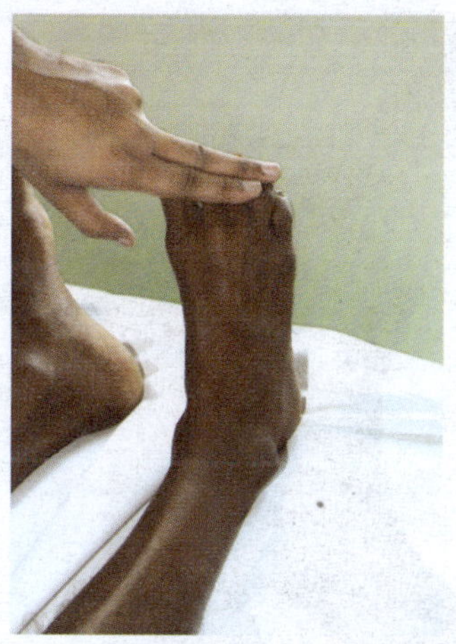

FIG. 11.158   Extensor digitorum longus

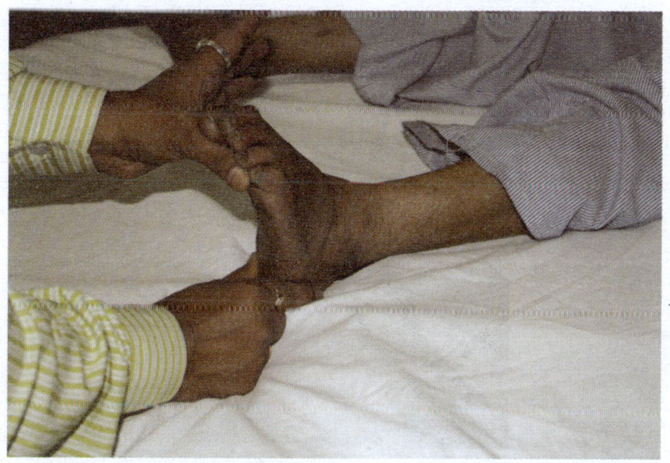

FIG. 11.159   Flexor digitorum longus

Types of Muscles Weakness

- *In case of corticospinal tract lesion:* It involves from motor cortex to anterior horn cell. It affects:
  - ❖ Weakness of abductors and extensors of upper extremity.
  - ❖ If there is weakness of thumb extensors—the lesion will be at cortical level, because hand area is represented in the cortex as motor knuckle (area 4). This area is affected by an embolus

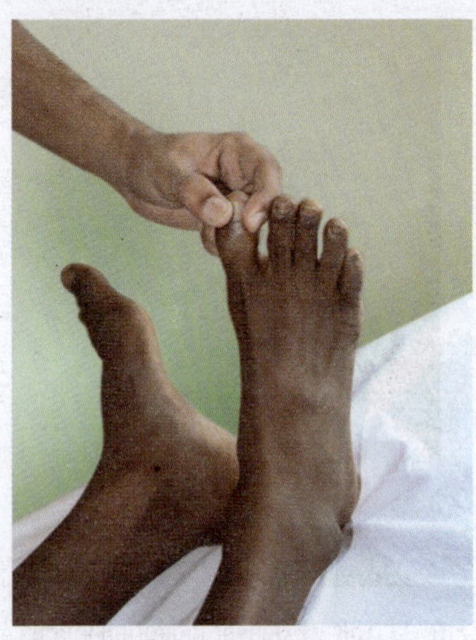

FIG. 11.160 Extensor hallucis

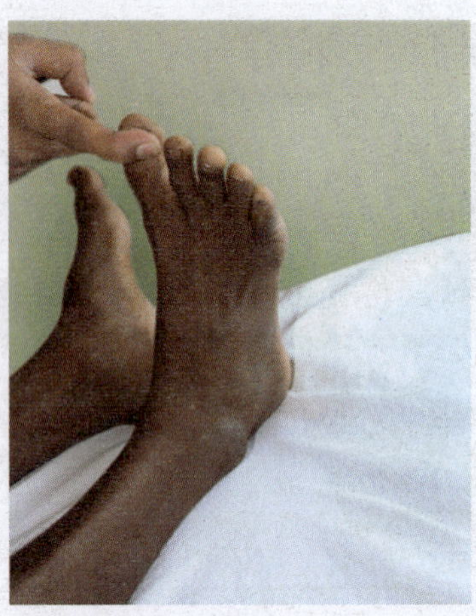

FIG. 11.161 Extensor digitorum brevis

in the central sulcus branch of the superior division of middle cerebral artery.

❖ In case of supranuclear palsy along with wrist drop, there is involvement of finger flexors.

❖ Corticospinal tract lesions. It is associated with more distal weakness than proximal weakness, hemiplegic gait, Babinski's signs.

❖ There is weakness of movement.

- *In case of extrapyramidal lesions:*
  - ❖ No actual loss of strength
  - ❖ Abnormal tone
  - ❖ Inability to sustain initiated movement
  - ❖ Initiation of movement is slow
  - ❖ Rigidity
  - ❖ Decreased reflexes
  - ❖ If the patient is asked to sustain finger movement, it is to be noted that programmed movement becomes smaller and smaller, e.g. if the patient is asked to write his name, each letter becomes gradually smaller and smaller ultimately end of the last letter gradually becomes straight line.
- *In case of lower motor neuron disease:* The key feature of lower motor neuron lesion is atrophy and fasciculation.
  - ❖ The viral illness like poliomyelitis and other neurotrophic virus involves individual anterior horn cell such as intrinsic muscles of the hand.
  - ❖ If the process affects only a group of anterior horn cells wasting is symmetrical and reflexes are absent.
  - ❖ In amyotrophic lateral sclerosis asymmetrical wasting of muscles with hyperreflexia.
  - ❖ If ventral root is involved, all the muscles involved by that root will be wasted, weakened, e.g. in case of cervical spondylosis due to C_5 involvement, deltoid muscle wasting occurs.
  - ❖ In case of peripheral neuropathy (sciatic nerve), all the muscles supplied by that nerve will be involved.
  - ❖ In metabolic, toxic myopathies the muscles involved are distally and symmetrical in arms and legs.
  - ❖ In autoimmune peripheral neuropathy involvement of muscles are asymmetrical and affects upper extremities prior to lower extremities.

Weakness Resulting from Muscular Lesions

- Acquired inflammatory myopathies—proximal
- Inclusion body myositis—distal—forearm flexors.
  Contracture of finger flexors, and distal quadriceps muscles.
- *Distal genetic myopathies:*
  - ❖ Anterior and posterior compartments of lower legs are involved (Welander's myositis, Markesbery)
  - ❖ Sternocleidomastoid
  - ❖ Masseter
  - ❖ Distal extremity (myotonic dystrophy Type 1).

Myasthenia

It involves:

- Ocular muscles
- Muscles of eyelid
- Tongue (triple furrowed tongue)
- Throat
- Larynx
- Muscles of back
- Muscles of shoulders and hand.

Cogan's twitch: It demonstrates subtle weakness superior rectus and inferior oblique muscle.

Patient is asked to gaze up and maintains it for 20–30 seconds, which are produced by superior rectus muscle and inferior oblique muscle. In case of myasthenia, patient is unable to maintain the gaze due to increased fatigability.

Patient is asked to follow the examiner's finger below the horizontal and then back to horizontal.

Normally the lids will be retracted above the iris, and then will be settled to normal position.

But in myasthenia, the lids will the retracted more than necessary.

Eaton-Lambert Syndrome

The weakened muscles get stronger with repetitive stimulation. It occurs in patient with bronchogenic carcinoma.

In this syndrome:

- Ptosis is more common than involvement of extraocular muscles
- Legs are weaker than arms
- Decreased reflexes.

This syndrome occurs in patient with bronchogenic carcinoma (small cell carcinoma).

Motor Power and Strength

Motor strength and power indicates the capacity of muscles to exert force and expend energy.

Decreased strength—It means weakness or paresis.

Absence of muscle contraction—It means paralysis or plegia.

Paresis means

- Loss of speed and rapidity of muscle contraction
- Decrease in range, amplitude of movement of the muscles
- Easy fatigability.

Major criteria of evaluation of muscle strength
Initiation and resisting movement during examination.

In organic weakness
Palpation of either the contraction of muscle belly or movement of its tendon.

In nonorganic weakness
- Contraction of apparently weak muscles may be felt.
- When the patient is asked to contract weak muscle, antagonist muscle may be felt to contract.

Muscle strength may be classified into:
- *Kinetic*: Force exerted in changing position
- *Static*: Force exerted in resisting movement from fixed position.

Strength may be tested by following ways:
- Ask the patient to place a joint in particular position and tell him not to move it in any circumstances.
- Examiner is asked to hold his joint and try to move it.
- Ask the patient to contract a particular muscle against a resistance given by the examiner.

The following factors may complicate the above method of examination:
- Systemic illness
- Inability to understand or cooperate
- Extrapyramidal disease
- Ataxia
- *Impairment of movement due to*:
  - Pain
  - Joint ankylosis
  - Contracture.
- *Psychiatric conditions*:
  - Malingering
  - Hysteria.

Passive movement is very helpful to distinguish decreased motions due to contracture from weakness, muscle spasm.

In contracture, muscles cannot be stretched up to its normal limit without any pain or considerable resistance.

But in weakness and muscle spasm, muscles can be stretched against resistance but with pain.

To assess the strength of the muscle:
- Comparison should be done with the homologous muscles of other side, e.g. comparison of biceps muscles of both arms.
- In cases, e.g. polymyositis, where there is weakness of proximal muscles of both sides, in that case—proximal muscle can be compared with distal muscles of same side.

There is considerable variation in muscle power affecting patient and examiners: For example, age, size, gender, body built and activity level of both patient and the examiners.

- A tall young powerful physician examines short, old, sick patient.
- Little, weak, physician examines large, stout, powerful patient.

Strength of individual muscle is tested and graded—according to Medical Research Council Scale of Muscle strength:

Grade		Muscle strength
0	–	No contraction
1	–	Flickering, or trace of contraction
2	–	Active movement when gravity eliminated
3	–	Active movement against gravity
4 –	–	Active movement against gravity and slight resistance
4	–	Active movement against gravity and moderate resistance
4 +	–	Active movement against gravity and severe resistance
5	–	Normal power

Features of Upper Motor Neuron Versus Lower Motor Neuron Lesion

Features	Upper motor neuron	Lower motor neurons
• Weakness distribution	Corticospinal tract distribution—hemiparesis, quadriparesis, paraparesis, monoparesis	Generalized — predominantly proximal, predominantly distal or focal. No preference for CST innervated muscle
• Sensory loss	Depending upon the site and level of involvement	Nil or glove and stocking distribution. Nerve root or peripheral nerve involvement
• Deep tendon reflexes	In acute stage—absent, in chronic stage—increased. In spinal cord level—at the level of tension—absent	Normal or decreased
• Superficial reflexes	Absent	Normal
• Muscle tone	Increased	Normal or decreased
• Pain	Absent	Sometimes present
• Pathological reflexes	Present	Absent
• Sphincter control	Impaired	Normal
• Other CNS sign	May be present	Absent

Pattern of Weakness According to Lesions in Different Sites of Neuraxis

Middle cerebral artery occlusion

- Spastic contralateral hemiparesis or hemiplegia with more involvement of arm and face than leg.
- Superficial reflexes absent, deep tendon reflex (except in acute condition, when it is absent) are increased.
- Sensory loss may be present.
- Aphasia, apraxia, contralateral visual field deficit.
- Gaze palsy.

Anterior cerebral artery occlusions

- Contralateral spastic hemiparesis or hemiplegia involving leg more than the arm and face.
- Superficial reflexes—Absent.
- Deep tendon reflexes—Increased
- Sensory loss may be present
- Cortical sensory loss. Frontal lobe sign
- Incontinence.

Internal capsule

Pure motor stroke:

- Contralateral face = arm = leg.
- Superficial reflexes absent. Deep tendon reflexes (except in acute conditions) exaggerated.
- No sensory loss.

Brainstem

- Contralateral hemiplegia.
- Ipsilateral cranial nerve involvement.
- Deep tendon reflexes exaggerated.
- Sensory loss—according to the level of lesion and cranial nerve involvement.
- Bladder and bowel may be involved.

Cervical cord involvement

- Upper motor neuron type hyperreflexic quadriparesis below the level of lesion.
- Areflexic paresis at the level of lesion.
- Sensory loss (pain, touch, temperature—due to spinothalamic tract involvement and joint and position sensation due to involvement of posterior column).
- Bladder bowel involvement.
- Sexual dysfunction.
- Hyperesthesia at the level of lesion.

Thoracic cord involvement
- Both legs below the level of lesion show hyper-reflexic spastic paresis.
- Other finding are similar to that of cervical cord hemiparesis.

Cauda equina syndrome
- Asymmetric hyporeflexic paraparesis
- Bladder, bowel dysfunction, sexual dysfunction
- Sensory loss.

Anterior horn cell involvement
- In early stage — focal muscle involvement
  Late stage—generalized muscle involvement
- No sensory loss
- Denervation atrophy, fasciculation
- Bulbar weakness.

Single nerve root
- Areflexic paralysis of the muscles innervated by the involved dermatome
- Sensory loss of the affected dermatome
- Pain in the involved dermatome.

Plexus involvement
- Plexus pattern of involvement of the innervated muscle
- Areflexia of the involved muscles
- Sensory loss
- Pain is common mainly in brachial plexus area.

Mononeuropathy
- Muscles of the affected nerve becomes atrophic
- Areflexia, weakness of affected muscles
- Sensory loss along the distribution of affected nerve.

Polyneuropathy
- Distal limb muscles are more involved than the proximal muscles
- Muscles become weak, areflexic
- Sensory involvement along the involved dermatome
- Atrophy is late feature.

Neuromuscular junction involvement
- Proximal muscles are involved. Bulbar muscles may be involved
- No sensory involvement
- Reflexes are normal
- Ptosis, ophthalmoparesis, fatigue with muscles use.

Muscle involvement
- Proximal muscles are more involved than distal muscles
- Reflexes—deep tendon reflexes—normal
- No sensory loss.
- *Different pattern of muscle involvement:*
  - Limb-girdle
  - Facioscapulohumeral
  - Pseudohypertrophy
  - Myotonia.

Posture and Stance (Figs 11.162 and 11.163)

Patient should be evaluated in:
- Standing position with great toe and heal touching the floor and feet together.
- This maneuver should be exercised in eye opened and in eye closed position.

There may be following results:
- *Inability to stand with feet together:*
  - Cerebellar disease
  - Posterior column lesion
  - Vestibular disease.
- Break in stance in closed eyes—posterior column lesion.
- Stands with wide base in closed eyes—vestibular damage.

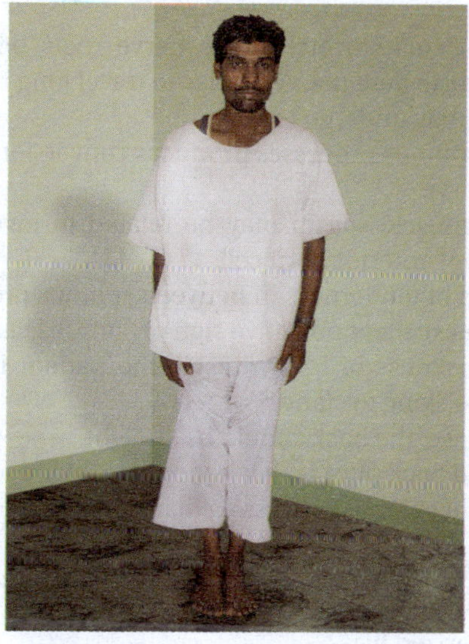

FIG. 11.162   Stands with eyes opened

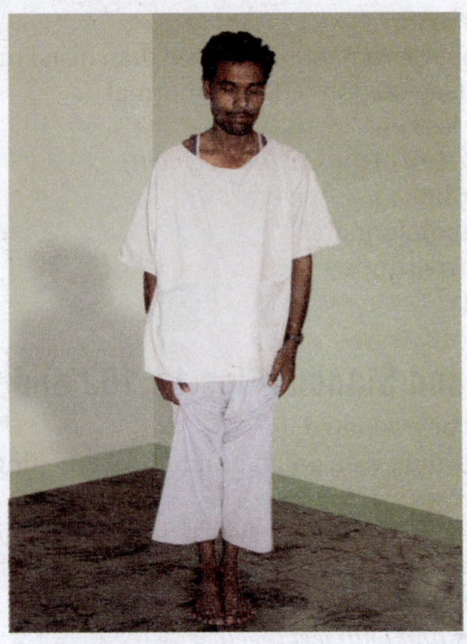

FIG. 11.163 Stands with eyes closed

Back Examination

The back of the patient must be examined for following examinations:

- Lordosis
- Kyphosis
- Scoliosis.

Any type of curve stretches the nerve roots opposite to the convexity, because here the nerve has to travel long route from exit foramina, so it may undergo tension.

- Disease of spinous processes produces conversion of lordosis to a smooth curve.
- Paraspinal muscle spasm may be related to involvement and stimulation of anterior horn cell.
- Localization of tenderness in between spinous processes by the thumb is an excellent objective sign of back disease.
- To elicit weakness of back muscle the patient is asked to sit followed by asking to stand.
  In normal case, the back should be straight.
  In weakened back muscle, back should be blended.
- Percussion of spinous process—elicit spinal tenderness.

Bradykinesia

This is characterized by:

- Slowness of movement
- Slow in initiation

- No or minimal spontaneous movement
- Eye blinking <7/min (normal 14/min)
- Difficulty in turning in the bed
- Difficulty in changing motor program—during walking, the patient freezes suddenly—then utilizes small cautious steps to change direction.

The lesions responsible are:
- Parkinsonism
- Akinetic rigid syndrome.

Position

- *In basal ganglia disease:*
  - ❖ Flexed truncal posture
  - ❖ Flexed arms
  - ❖ Hand flexed at metacarpophalangeal joint
  - ❖ Flexed head.
- *In supranuclear palsy:*
  - ❖ Head extended
  - ❖ Flexed arms
  - ❖ Deep nasolabial furrow.
- *In motor neuron disease, myasthenia gravis, poliomyelitis:* Head falls forward on the chest.
- *In cervical spondylosis:* Desiccation of cervical disc:
  - ❖ Head flexed forward (due to arthritis degeneration of uncovertebral joint)
    If the process is severe:
    - Compression of dorsal and ventral spinocerebellar tract
    - Supinator reflex at C_5- C_6
    - Hyperactive knee jerk.

Kyphoscoliosis

Kyphotic spine—it occurs in:
- Aging
- Emphysema
- Extreme ankylosing spondylosis.

Scoliosis

It can be divided into two types:
1. *C type:* It is due to acquired disease—such as:
   - ❖ Syringomyelia
   - ❖ Tumor—astrocytoma—it may occur on the wall of syrinx
   - ❖ Hemangioma.

2. *S type:* It has compensatory cervical curvature. It is mainly due to hereditary disease. The causes are:
   - Hereditary cerebellar ataxia
   - Neuropathy
   - Late stages of muscle disease—Duchenne muscular dystrophy. Becker muscular dystrophy. Von-Recklinghausen disease.

Severe Kyphoscoliosis Produces

- Spinal cord compression
- Paraplegia
- Lumbar disc irritates ipsilateral ventral roots producing chronic muscular contraction on the side of scoliosis. This is increased with flexion
- Congenital hemivertebra produces scoliosis on forward flexion.

Lordosis

Causes are:
- Asymptomatic,
- *Congenital myopathies:*
  - Duchenne muscular dystrophy
  - Becker's muscular dystrophy
  - Myasthenia gravis
  - Congenital hip disease.

Causes of Rigid Spine

- Type II fiber type disproportion
- Emery-Dreifuss muscular dystrophy
- Limb-girdle muscular dystrophy
- Facioscapulohumeral muscular dystrophy
- Myofibrillar myopathies
- Severe ankylosing spondylosis—entire spine moves en bloc—flexion at hip joint, lumbar spine straight on flexion due to paravertebral muscle spasm.

Spinal Tenderness

It may occur due to following causes:
- *Local bony tumor:*
  - Osteoid bone cyst
  - Hemangioma
  - Articular bone cyst.

- *Diskitis—excruciating pain while the back touching the bed—may occur due to:*
  - ❖ Spinal operation
  - ❖ Intravenous drug user.
- *Epidural abscess:* It involves and spreads over many segments. It can occur due to:
  - ❖ Introduction of epidural catheter for bupivacaine anesthesia
  - ❖ Use of anticoagulant.

Equilibrium

There are following types of abnormalities in equilibrium:
- *Inability to stand upright:*
  - ❖ Lesion in cerebellar tonsils
  - ❖ Lesion in fourth ventricle.

  This posture is out of proportion to limb ataxia.
- *Falling backwards—causes are:*
  - ❖ All types of basal ganglia diseases
  - ❖ Normal pressure hydrocephalus
  - ❖ Progressive supranuclear palsy
  - ❖ Hepatolenticular degeneration.
- *Patient feels as if he is being pushed to one side (lateral propulsion)—causes are:*
  - ❖ Lesion of labyrinth
  - ❖ Destruction of vestibular pathways to brainstem.
- Patient feels as if he is being pushed from back—utricle or saccular disease.
- Patient feels as if he is being pushed away from side of lesion—hemispheric lesion.

Causes and Mechanism of Brainstem Compression

- *Chamberlain's line:* A line drawn from the back of hard palate to the inner table of occipital bone.

  If the odontoid process is 2–3 mm above the Chamberlain's line—it compresses the brainstem.
- Cerebellar tonsils descend and compress the dorsal brainstem.
- Coughing, sneezing and extension of head further compress the medullary pyramids, leading to loss of tone of limbs and collapse.

Romberg Test (Figs 11.162 and 11.163)

This test detects integrity of proprioception from joints of the legs.

Method

Ask the patient to stand with feet together, great toe and heel apposed.

In case of open eye method—patient does not sway and he does not break the stance.

Now ask the patient to close his eyes during stance.

The patient sways from side to side and breaks the stance to wide base stance.

This test is positive in case of following diseases:
- Cervical spondylosis producing compression of spinal cord
- Subacute combined degeneration due to vitamin B_{12} deficiency
- Tabes dorsalis
- HIV myelopathy
- Sjögren's syndrome
- Autoimmune lesion in dorsal root ganglia.

Squatting to Stand Up

The patient when sits or squats, and asked to stand up from squatting position—patient uses Gower's maneuver—pushes himself by placing his hands over the higher part of legs.

The causes are:
- Muscular dystrophy
- Poliomyelitis
- Myasthenia gravis
- Peripheral neuropathy.

Few Special Methods of Testing of Muscles

- *Extensor drift:* On the side opposite to the side of lesion thumb adducted, wrist drops. It may be due to pseudoradial palsy from motor neuron lesion.
- *Alter's sing:* On the side opposite to the side of lesion, ring finger cannot be adducted, and drifts outward.
- *Lengthening test:* The patient is asked to extend his flexed arm. The arm on the opposite to the side of lesion cannot be extended.
- *Leg drift:* On the side opposite to the side of lesion, weakness and downward drift of the leg.
- *Arm roll:* Ask the patient to roll one arm over the other. The arm of the side opposite to the side of lesion cannot roll (in case of corticospinal tract lesion).

The arm of the same side of lesion (basal ganglia disease, akinetic rigid syndrome) cannot roll.

Deep Tendon Reflexes

When muscle fibers are being stretched by percussion on attached tendon or the structures (bone, periostium, joints, and fascia) to which muscles or tendon are attached, there is contraction of muscles to resist stretch—this is called deep tendon reflex.

The requirements for eliciting deep tendon reflexes are:

- High quality rubber percussion hammer.
- Hammer strike should be quick, direct, crisp, forceful holding the hammer handle near its end.
- Patient should be comfortable, relaxed and properly positioned.
- If the patient is over conscious, about the examination method; he should be distracted by light conversation with him.
- In few jerk like—angle jerk, tendon should be stretched slightly before stimulus is being applied.
- Adequate stimulus should be applied at proper spot.
- In few cases, where the jerk cannot be elicitated in usual way, reinforcement is very necessary.
- In order to compare the reflex on both sides of the body, positions of extremities should be symmetric.
- During reflex examination, position of head must be straight, because looking towards one side may after the muscle tone, especially in the arms (tonic neck reflex).
- The examiner can palpate the contraction or see the contraction. So during elicitation of reflex it is sometimes necessary to place one hand on the muscle to palpate contraction where the muscle contraction too insufficient to see, e.g. contraction of quadriceps.

  Contraction and activity of reflexes can be judged by:
  - ❖ Speed of contraction
  - ❖ Duration of contraction
  - ❖ Range of movement
  - ❖ Vigor of responses.

Deep tendon reflexes (DTRs) are usually seen in following muscles with segmental level and peripheral nerves

Reflexes	Segmental level	Peripheral nerve
• Biceps	C5–C6	Musculocutaneous nerve
• Triceps	C7–C8	Radial nerve
• Brachioradialis	C5–C6	Radial nerve
• Quadriceps	L3–L4	Femoral nerve
• Achilles (Gastrocnemius)	S1	Sciatic nerve

Gradation of reflexes can be done and they are graded as absent, sluggish or diminished, normal, exaggerated, markedly hyperactive.

They can be designated as 0–5

0 = absent

1+ = sluggish or diminished

2+ = normal

3+ = increased but not necessary pathological.
4+ = markedly hyperactive.
'+' sign is traditional than informative, so it can be omitted.
'+' sign indicates subtle asymmetry.
In few case,
'5'+ = extreme spasticity associated at clonus.

Few Special Type of Elicitation of Reflexes

- In few cases, contraction of one muscle may be accompanied by contraction of other muscles—this is called irradiation of reflexes. Examples are:
  - ❖ In presence of spasticity, contraction of biceps or brachioradialis reflex is accompanied by flexion of the fingers and adduction of the thumb.
  - ❖ Extension of knee may be accompanied by adduction of hip or bilateral knee extension.
- In few cases, response to percussion tendon may be absent but, muscles supplied by adjacent spinal cord segments contract (inverted brachioradialis reflex).
- In few cases, DTRs are markedly diminished, but obviously no evidence nervous system disease. In these cases— reinforcement is necessary to elicit the reflex response:
  - ❖ *Jendrassik maneuvers (Fig. 11.164):* Ask the patient to pull the hands apart with finger flexed and hooked against others, palm facing—during this maneuver reflex (lower limb) should be elicitated.

    The effect is brief—1 to 6 seconds, occasional 300 milliseconds.

    This maneuver is responsible for elicitation of lower limb jerk.
  - ❖ Ask the patient to clench his teeth, firmly grasps the arm of the chair, or grasp the side of bed during this jerk elicitation.
  - ❖ Coughing, squeezing the knees, deep breath, read loud, and looking towards ceiling.
  - ❖ By loud sudden noise, painful stimulus elsewhere the body —pulling the hair.
  - ❖ *Procedures other than distraction:* Slight steady contraction of the muscle whose tendon is being tested:
    - Slight plantar flexion by pushing ball of the foot against the floor or examiner's hand—reinforce ankle jerk (Fig. 11.165).
    - Patient may extend the knee—produces tensing of quadriceps against resistance—reinforce knee jerk.

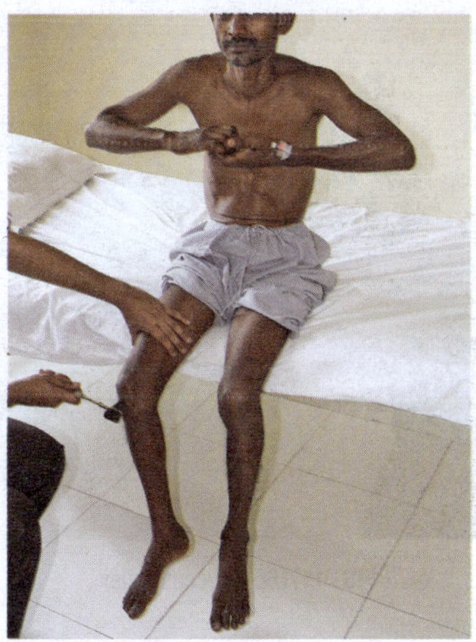

FIG. 11.164   Jendrassik maneuver

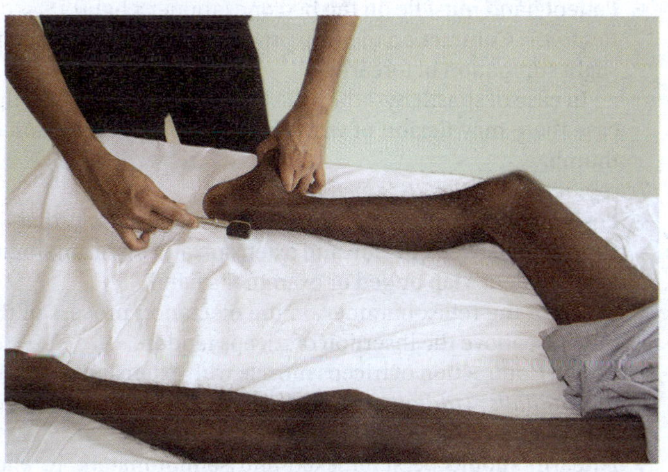

FIG. 11.165   Reinforcement in ankle jerk

Description of following reflexes: Upper limb reflexes
- *Biceps reflex (Fig. 11.166) method:*
  - ❖ Forearm should be slightly pronated and flexed in the midway between flexion and extension.
  - ❖ Examiner places his palmer surface of extended thumb or other fingers on the tendon of biceps.

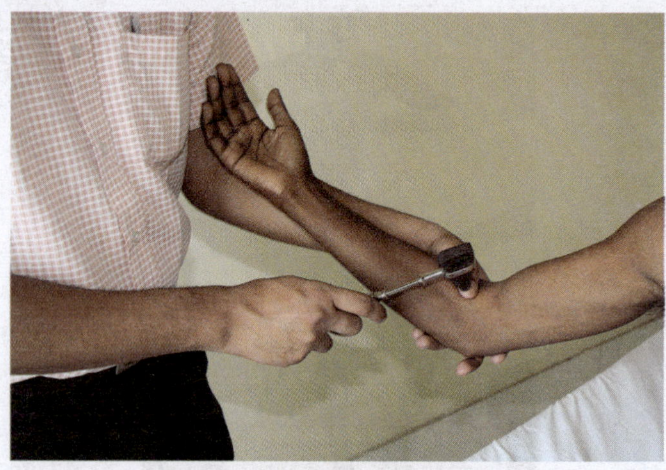

FIG. 11.166 Biceps reflex

- ❖ Strike the extensor surface of the thumb with the reflex hammer. Pressure should by light, because firm pressure against the tendon may fail to elicit the reflex.
- ❖ Patient hand must lie on the bed or examiner's hand.
  Response: Contraction of bicep produces flexion of elbow and slight supination of forearm.
  In case of spasticity—the reflex will be exaggerated. In this case there may flexion of wrist and fingers and adduction of thumb.
- • *Triceps reflex (Fig. 11.167) method:*
  - ❖ Position the hand to be examined in such a way that—it should be between flexion and extension and forearm, should lie on patient's lap or bed or examiner's hand.
  - ❖ Tap with the reflex hammer on the olecranon process of the ulna just above the insertion of triceps tendon.
    Result: Contraction of triceps muscle with extension of elbow.
- • *Brachioradialis (radial periosteal or supinator) reflex (Fig. 11.168):* Method:
  - ❖ Forearm should be semiflexed and semipronated. To elicit better reflex, forearm should be more extended and more pronated.
  - ❖ Muscle is brachioradialis.
  - ❖ Percussion should be done at its insertion on the lateral aspect of base of styloid process of radius or at the junction between mid-third with distal-third of the forearm or at its origin at lateral epicondyle of humerus.

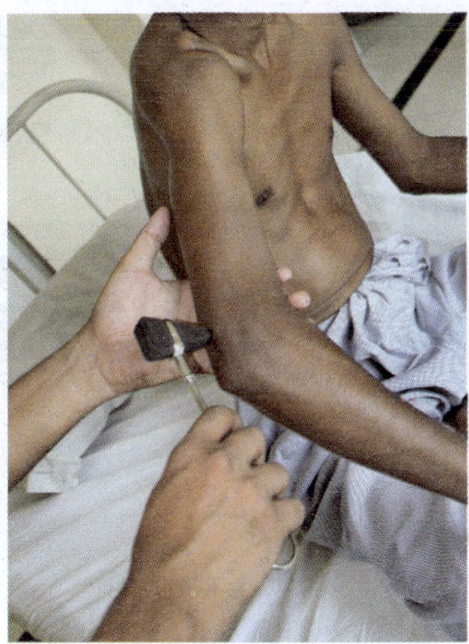

FIG. 11.167   Triceps jerk

Response:
* Flexion of elbow and variable supination.
* In case of hyperreflexia or spasticity—reflex will be exaggerated producing flexion of the wrist and fingers and adduction of forearm.
* In case of impairment due to involvement of afferent limb, there may be twitching of flexors of hand and fingers but no flexion or supination of elbow.
* *Finger flexor reflex (Wartenberg sign) (Fig. 11.169):* Method:
  * Ask the patient to keep his forearm on a table in such a position that hand should be supinated and fingers slightly flexed.
  * Examiner should keep his own fingers against patient's fingers in such a way that palmer surface of examiner's finger should lie against palmer surfaces of patient's fingers.
  * Now tap the extensor aspects of examiner's finger with the reflex hammer.
  Response: Contraction of small muscles of fingers and thumb producing flexion of fingers and distal phalanx of thumb.
  This can be reinforced by slightly less flexing the fingers as the blow is delivered.

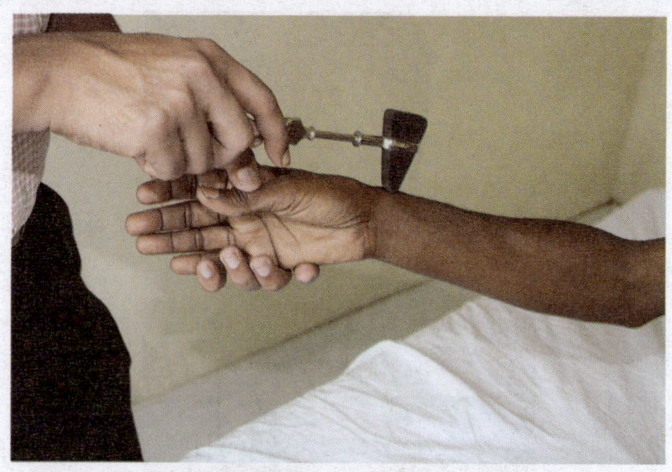

FIG. 11.168 Supinator reflex

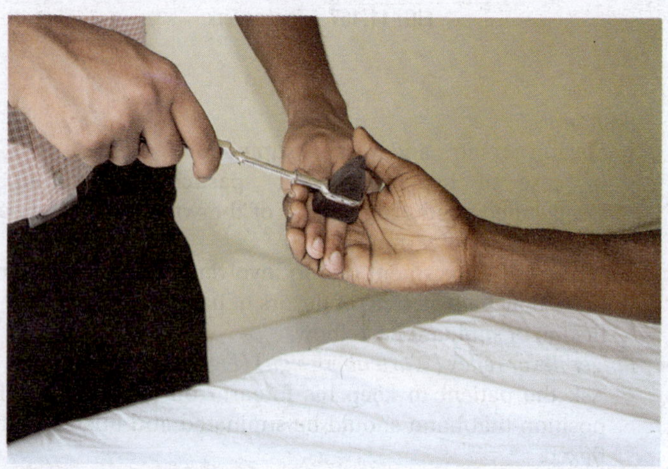

FIG. 11.169 Finger flexion reflex

Lower limb reflexes
- *Patellar reflex (Quadriceps reflex, knee jerk) (Figs 11.170 and 11.171):* Method:
  - ❖ *Position:*
    - Patient sits on a chair with slightly extended knee with heel resting on the floor, or

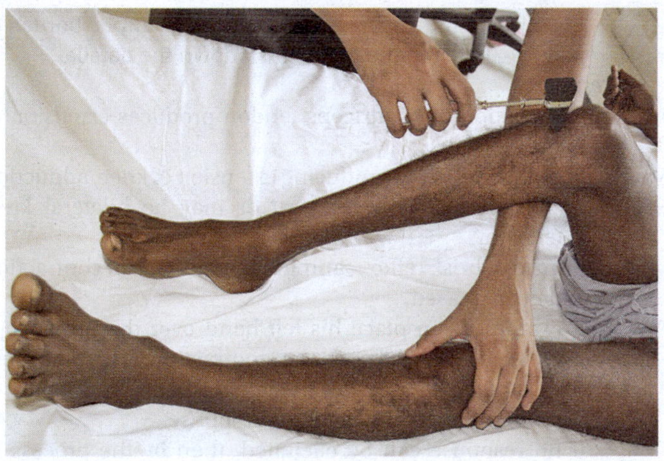

FIG. 11.170 Patellar reflex

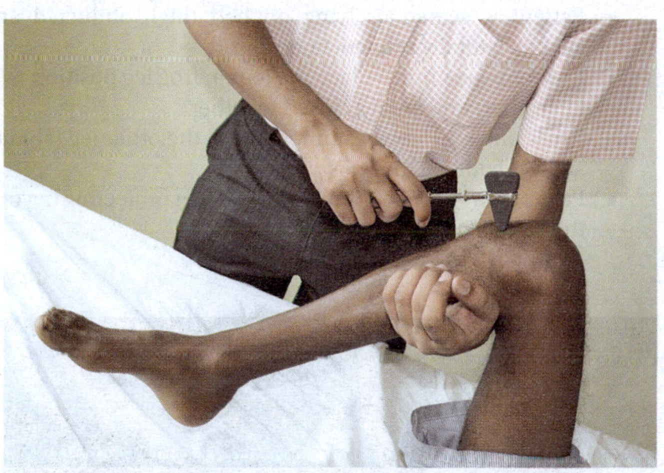

FIG. 11.171 Knee jerk

- Patient may sit on an examination table with leg dangling, or
- Patient is lying on the bed the examiner slightly flexes the knee and placing his hand behind the knee.
- ❖ *Site of tapping:* Tapping with reflex hammer can be done on:
  - Patellar tendon just beneath the patella
  - Just above the patella (suprapatellar or epipatellar reflex)
  - Tendon of the muscle directly

- Examiner's index finger placed on the upper border of patella—here tap the finger push down the patella.
- ❖ *Response:*
  - Contraction of quadriceps tendon produces extension of knee.
  - Spreading of reflex producing extension of knee, adduction of hip, occasionally bilateral or may be bilateral knee extension.
  - In case of brisk reflex—amplitude and force of contraction will be increased.
  - If examiner can place his left hand over the quadriceps muscle, he can palpate the contraction. This can help the examiner to measure the latency between the time of stimulus applied and resulting response.
  - If no response can be elicitated, then by the process of reinforcement described above, the jerk can be revealed.
- **Achilles reflex (Ankle jerk) (Figs 11.172 and 11.173):** Method:
  - ❖ *Position of patient:*
    - Patient is seated or lying on bed thigh abducted and slightly laterally rotated, knee flexed.
    - In supine position—place the legs in frog leg position with knee apart and ankles closed together.
    - Cross one leg to be examined above the other leg (shin or ankle) (figure of four position).
    - Patient may kneel on the chair with feet projecting beyond the chair at right angle.

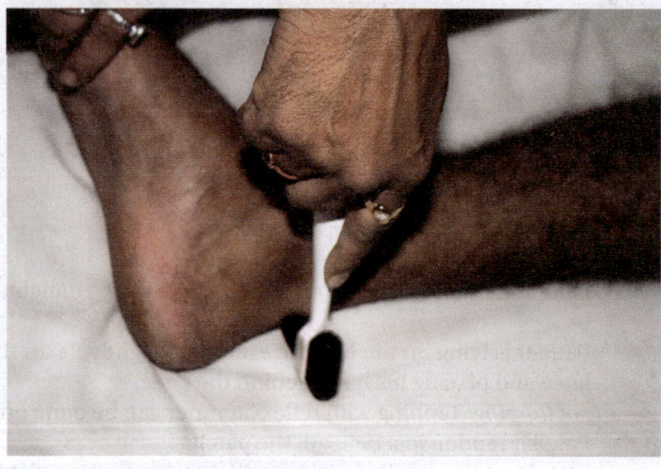

FIG. 11.172 Ankle jerk

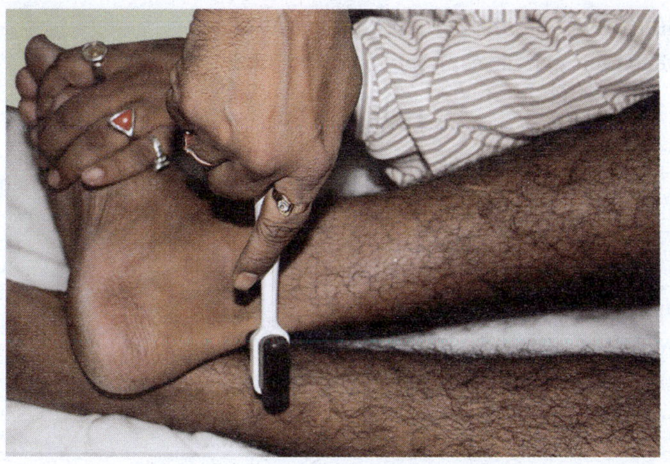

FIG. 11.173 Ankle jerk (2nd method)

Tapping:
- Place your finger under the sole of foot, slightly dorsiflex the ankle and tap with reflex hammer on tendon.
- Direct tapping on the ball of the foot while patient in lying position.
- Tapping over the examiner's hand placed on the sole of the foot.
❖ *Response:*
- Contraction of gastroenemius, soleus and plantaris produces plantar flexion of foot at the ankle.
- If jerk cannot be elicitated— reinforcement can be done to elicit this reflex.
- It may be diminished in elderly but it should be bilateral.

Importance of DTRs

The activity of DTRs can be measured by:
- Latency
- Speed
- Duration of contraction
- Vigor
- Range of movement.

Among all the latent period between time of application of stimulus and onset of contraction is most important.

Abnormalities in Deep Tendon Reflexes

Deep tendon reflexes should be compared:
- Between both sides
- Arms to legs
- Knees to ankles
  - ❖ Slight difference may be permissible, but pronounced difference is not permissible.
  - ❖ Proximal to distal gradient may be significant.

Hypoactive Reflexes

Hypoactive reflexes means:
- Sluggishness in response
- Diminution in the range of movement
- Repeated trigger is necessary to elicit reflex
- Reinforcement may not elicit reflex.

Causes of hypoactive reflexes
- *Involvement of afferent limb—lesion in:*
  - ❖ Sensory nerve
  - ❖ Posterior or dorsal root
  - ❖ Dorsal root ganglia
  - ❖ Intramedullary pathways between dorsal root ganglia and anterior horn cell (Syrinx).
- Abnormalities in motor unit and final common pathways producing efferent limb:
  - ❖ Radiculopathy
  - ❖ Peripheral nerve lesion.

Hyperactive Reflexes

Hyperactive reflexes are characterized by:
- Decrease in reflex threshold
- Decreased latency, time between tendon percussion and reflex contraction
- Increase in range of movement
- Increased area of reflexogenic zone
- Prolongation of reflex contraction.

Decreased reflex threshold: Minimal stimulus may evoke the reflex contraction, may be even light percussion.

Increased area of reflexogenic zone
- Application of stimulus in an area distant to normal area of stimulus
- Tapping the fibula
- Tapping on the dorsum of foot—produces knee jerk— exaggerated.

Biceps jerk may be exaggerated by:
- Tapping the clavicle
- Tapping the scapula.

Lesion in corticospinal tract from cerebral motor cortex to lesion in spinal cord just above the segment responsible for reflex arc—produces
- Exaggerated flexor reflexes in upper limbs
- Exaggerated extensor reflexes in lower limbs.

In psychogenic disorder (anxiety, fright, agitation):
- Reflexes may be diminished, normal or exaggerated.
- During elicitation of knee jerk, the foot may be kicked so far into the air, and held in this position for a time.
- The response may be bilateral.
- Superfluous jerking, of remote parts—whole body jerk.
- Irregular repeated jerky movements (spurious clonus) will be present.

Reflex patterns in different neurological disorders

Site of lesion	Muscle stretch reflex	Superficial reflex	Pathological reflexes	Associated movements
Neuromuscular junction	Normal or decreased	Normal	Absent	Absent
Muscle	Normal or decreased in proportion to weakness	Normal	Absent	Absent
Peripheral nerve	Decreased or absent	Normal or decreased along the region supplied by the nerve	Absent	Present
Corticospinal tract	Hyper-reflexia	Absent	Present	Present
Cerebellar lesion	Pendular	Normal	Absent	Present
Extrapyramidal system	Normal or slightly increased	Normal	Absent	Present
Psychogenic	Normal or increased	Normal	Absent	Bizarre movement

Perverted Reflexes

Inverted reflexes or perverted reflexes are contraction—opposite of those expected, e.g.

- Inverted triceps and patellar reflexes produce elbow and knee flexion instead of extension respectively.
- Inverted brachioradialis reflex—produces perverted response like finger flexion.

Superficial Reflexes

Superficial reflexes can be elicited by stimulus to skin and mucous membrane.

Skin stimulus is light touch and scratch. Painful stimulus produces defensive reaction.

Differences between superficial and deep reflexes:

Superficial reflexes	Deep reflexes
• It is polysynaptic	• It is monosynaptic
• It responds more slowly to the stimulus	• It responds fast to stimulus
• They fatigue more easily	• They fatigue more slowly
• They are not consistently present	• They are consistently present

Superficial Abdominal Reflexes

Anterior abdominal wall can be divided into four quadrants by one vertical and one horizontal line across the umbilicus (Fig. 11.174).

In each quadrant light stroke or scratch produces
- Contraction of abdominal muscles
- Pulling of linea alba and umbilicus in the direction of stimulus.

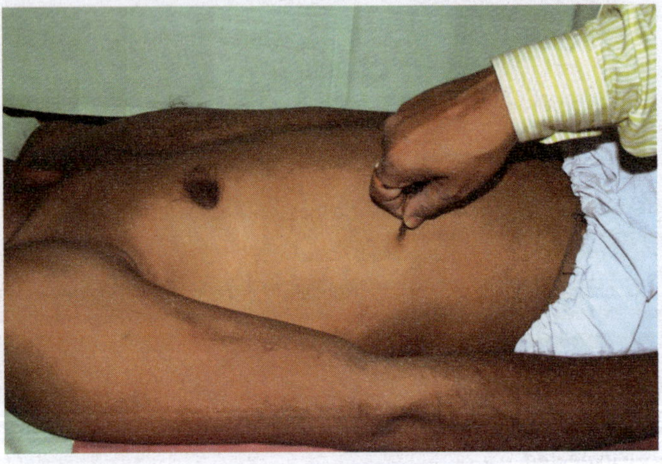

FIG. 11.174 Abdominal reflex

Interpretation
- *Absent in:*
  - ❖ Normal individual with lax abdominal tone
  - ❖ Obese person
  - ❖ Parous women
  - ❖ Corticospinal tract lesion
  - ❖ Motor neuron disease.
- *Increased or brisk in:* Active young individual with good abdominal tone.

Superficial reflexes of lower extremities
- *Cremesteric reflex:* Light scratching on the upper, inner sides of thigh produces:
  - ❖ Contraction of cremesteric muscles
  - ❖ Quick, elevation of homolateral testicle.

  Innervations through:
  - ❖ Ilio-inguinal nerve
  - ❖ Genitofemoral nerve.

  It should not be confused with:

  Scrotal or dartos reflex: Stroking the perineum or thigh, application of cold object to scrotum produces slow writhing, vermicular contraction of scrotal skin and muscles.

  Cremesteric reflex may be absent in:
  - ❖ Patient with hydrocele or varicocele
  - ❖ Elderly males
  - ❖ Patient with orchitis or epididymitis.
- *Plantar reflex (Fig. 11.175):* Light stroke on the plantar surface of foot from sole towards toes—produces:
  - ❖ Plantar flexion of foot
  - ❖ Flexion of toes

    Absent reflex may be present in:
    - Normal person
    - Thick sole

      Pathological reflex is Babinski's sign.

      Deep scratching may produce withdrawal reaction—flexion of hip and knee.
- *Superficial anal reflex:* Stroking or pinching of the skin in perianal region—response—contraction of external anal sphincter.
- *Bulbocavernosus reflex:* In male, grabbing, pinching of glans—produces contraction of external anal sphincter. This can be palpated by introducing the finger into the anal canal—tightening of the sphincter. This reflex is important in showing integrity of:

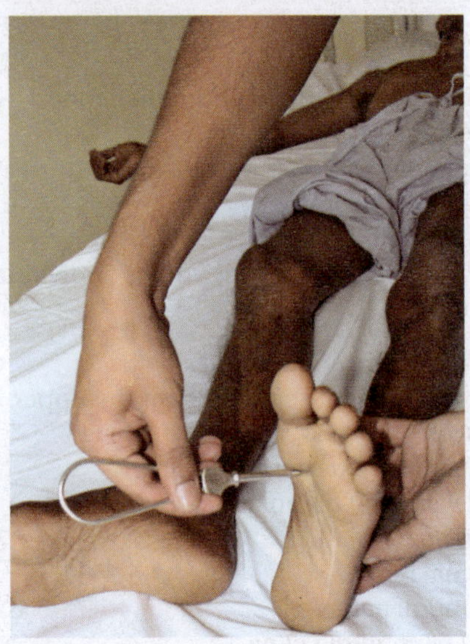

FIG. 11.175   Plantar reflex

- ❖ Cauda equina
- ❖ Lower sacral root and conus medullaris. Lesions anywhere in corticospinal tract—if occurs above decussation—produces contralateral abdominal and cremesteric reflex loss.

If the lesion is below the decussation—the ipsilateral abdominal and cremesteric reflex will be absent.

Pathological Reflexes

- Some are postural reflexes or primitive defense reflexes—these are normally suppressed by cerebral inhibition, but become enhanced when upper motor control over lower motor neuron will be lost.
- Some are normally seen in immature nervous system. With gradual maturity, these will disappear, sometimes persists in normal person or reappear with gross cerebral disease.

Pathological reflexes are related to:

- Corticospinal tract lesions
- CST and associated pathways involvement
- Frontal lobe disease
- Extrapyramidal system lesion.

Pathological reflexes can be divided into two parts:

Pathological reflexes of lower extremities

These are:
- More constant
- Can easily be elicitated
- More reliable
- More clinically important than upper extremities.

Babinski's sign (Fig. 11.175)

Method: Stimulus—applicator stick, handle of hammer, broken tongue blade, blunt end of the key.

It starts from laterally in the distribution of S1 root or sural nerve distribution—beginning from near the heel carried up by the side of the foot, stop at 5th metatarsophalangeal joint, then run medially along the metatarsal pad up to the ball of great toe.

More medial plantar stimulation fails to elicit the positive response.

Most medial stimulation may actually elicit plantar—grasp response.

Response: Extension of great toe and fanning of other toes. With severe and extensive corticospinal tract, lesion the following responses will occur:
- Dorsi flexion of toe, ankle
- Flexion of hip and knee (Triple flexion response)
- Contraction of tensor fascia lata producing internal rotation of hip and adduction of hip.

Position of the patient:
- Patient should be supine, hip and knee extended, heels rests on the bed.
- In case of patient in sitting position, knee should be extended, with foot held either in examiner's hand or knee folded to keep the foot on opposite knee.

In case of serve corticospinal tract disease: Reflexogenic zone will be wider and there will be addition of other components of primitive flexion reflexes. As a result there will be variation of Babinski's sign. These are:
- *Chaddock's sign (Figs 11.176A and B):* Stimulus starting from lateral aspect beginning from little under lateral malleolus runs along the junction of dorsal and plantar skin up to little toe.
  This sign:
  - More sensitive, but less specific
  - Less withdrawal than plantar stimulation
- *Oppenheim's sign (Fig. 11.177):* It can be elicited by dragging the knuckles heavily down the anterolateral surface of tibia starting from infrapatellar region to the ankle.
  This sign:
  - Is slow to elicit
  - Can be seen towards the end of stimulation.

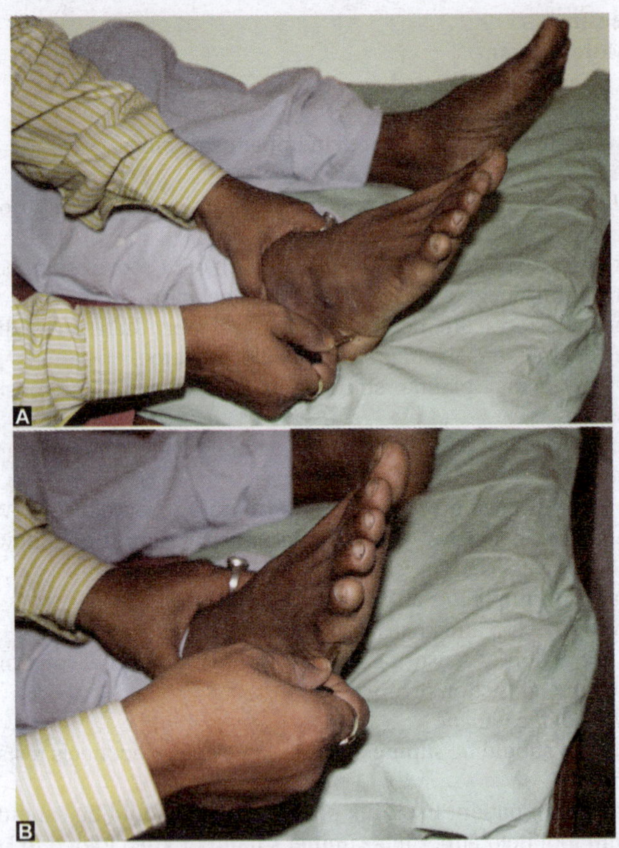

FIGS 11.176A AND B   Chaddock's sign

Sometimes there is spontaneous Babinski's sign, can be seen without any stimulation of the foot.

Sometimes it may be bilateral.

Common error in elicitation of response:

- Insufficient firm stimulation
- If the stimulus is given more medially
- If the stimulus is applied very quickly.

Firm stimulus may produce withdrawal response. Babinski's sign is a part of withdrawal reflex. Withdrawal may be voluntary. The differences between voluntary withdrawal and nonvoluntary withdrawal reflex are:

- Plantar flexion of toes
- Rarely dorsi flexion of ankles seen in voluntary withdrawal reflex.

Nonstructural diseases producing extensor plantar response:

- Physiological dysfunction of corticospinal pathways
- Narcosis

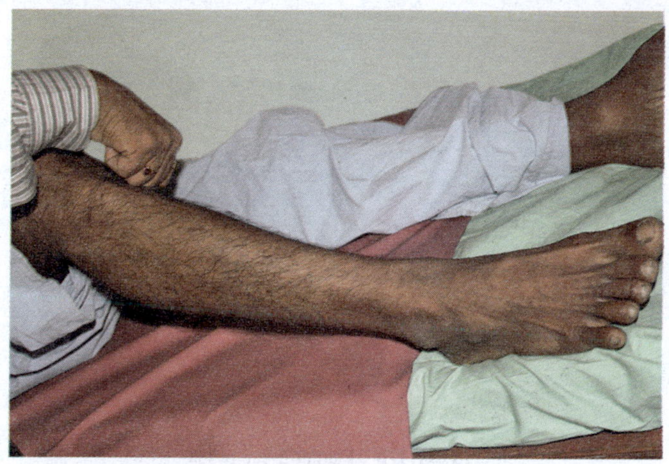

FIG. 11.177 Oppenheim's sign

- Drugs
- Deep anesthesia
- Alcohol intoxication
- Metabolic coma—hypoglycemia
- Deep sleep
- Postictal paralysis.

Plantar Grasp Reflex (Fig. 11.178)

Method: Draw the handle of the hammer from midsole towards toes.

Response: Flexion of toes and adduction of toes and grip the hammer.

It is present at birth, disappear at the end of 1st year, and reappear along with hand grasp reflex in adult in the disease of opposite frontal lobe.

Rossolimo's sign (Figs 11.179A and B)

Method: Tapping the ball of the foot or plantar surfaces of toes stretches the flexor muscles of foot.

Response: Contraction of all the toes.

This response is barely perceptible, but is more obvious in corticospinal tract lesion or disinhibition of spinal cord from higher lesion.

Pathological reflexes of upper extremities: There reflexes are:

- Less constant
- More difficult to elicit
- Less significant.

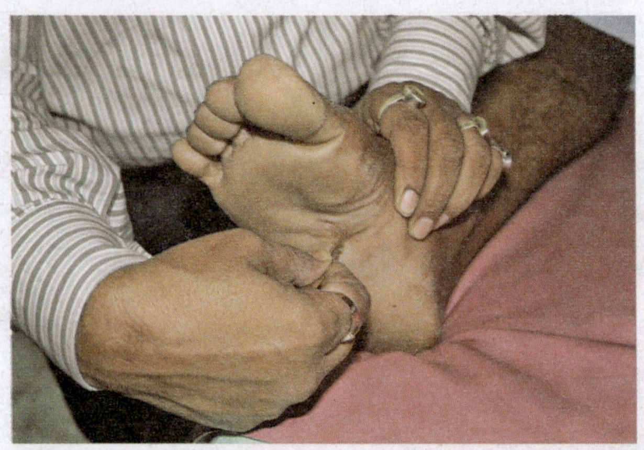

FIG. 11.178 Plantar grasp reflex

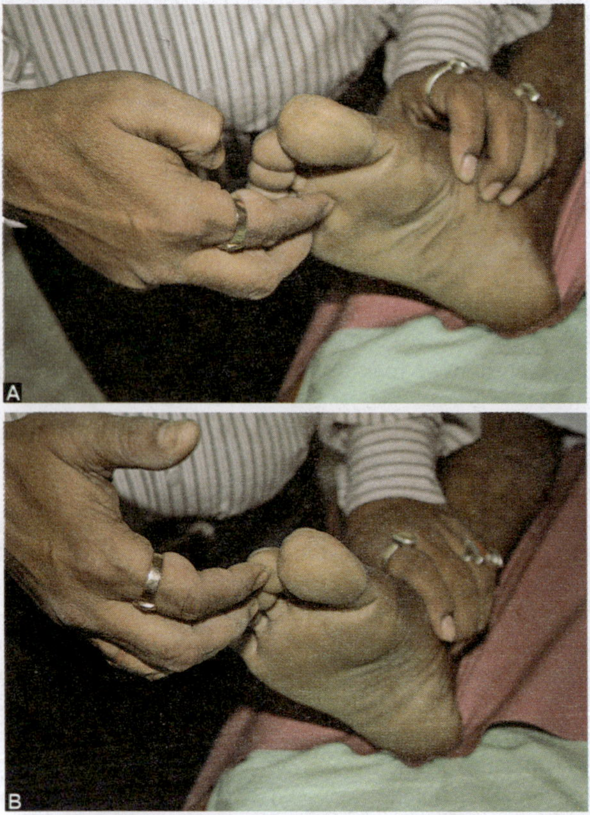

FIGS 11.179A AND B Rossolimo's sign

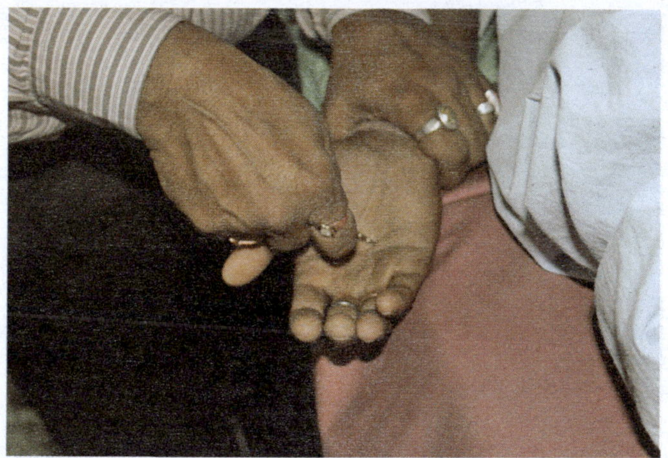

FIG. 11.180   Grasp reflex

These reflexes can be divided into:
- Frontal release signs
- Exaggeration of finger flexion or reflexes.

Frontal release signs
- *Grasp (forced grasping) reflex (Fig. 11.180)*
  Method: Stimulation of skin of the palmer surface of fingers or hand.
  Response: Flexions of fingers and hand.
      This reflex is present at birth, diminished at the age of 2 to 4 months, then again reappears in:
  ❖ Neoplastic lesions of frontal lobe
  ❖ Vascular lesions of frontal lobe
  ❖ Cerebral degenerative disease (contralaterally or ipsilaterally)
  ❖ Corticospinal tract dysfunction.
- *Palmomental reflex (Fig. 11.181)*
  Method: Scratching or stroking over thenar eminence from the wrist towards thumb or vice versa.
  Response:
  ❖ Contraction of mentalis and orbicularis oris causing wrinkle of skin of the chin.
  ❖ Slight retraction and elevation of the angle of mouth. This reflex is present normally in normal persons.
  So only significances of this reflex are:
  ❖ Exaggeration of reflex
  ❖ Asymmetry of reflex on two sides.
      In case of marked exaggeration of this reflex, the reflexogenic area may be increased to hypothenar area.

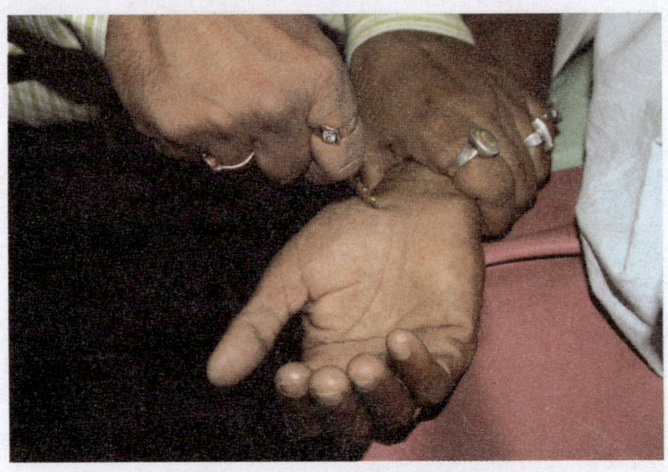

FIG. 11.181 Palmomental reflex

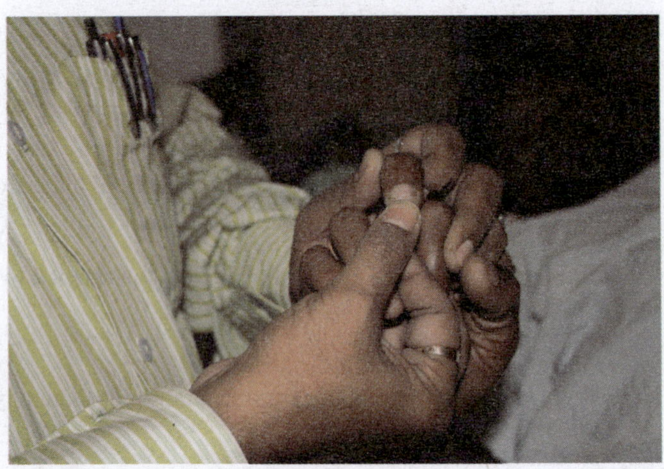

FIG. 11.182 Hoffmann's sign

This reflex may occur with bilateral, ipsilateral or contralateral lesions.

Exaggeration of finger flexion reflexes (Fig. 11.182)
- *Hoffmann's sign:*
  Method: Patient's hand in dorsiflexed at wrist and finger partially flexed to be held by examiner's one hand.
  The partially extended middle finger to be held in between index finger and thumb of examiner's other hand.

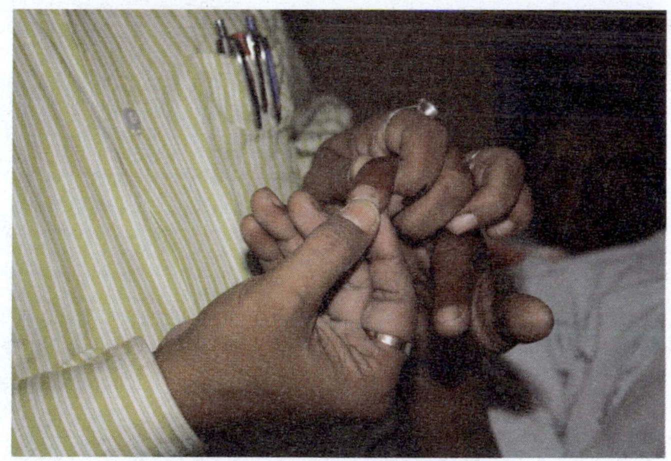

FIG. 11.183   Tromner's sign

By forcible flick by the thumb, the examiner suddenly snaps the nail of the patient's middle finger, forcing distal finger into sharp sudden flexion followed by sudden release.

The rebound of distal phalanx stretches finger flexors.

Response:

* ❖ Flexion and adduction of thumb
* ❖ Flexion of the index finger
* ❖ Flexion of other fingers.

If index finger or thumb responds the sign is incomplete.

* *Tromner's sign (Fig. 11.183)*:

Method: Hold the patient's partially extended middle finger— rest of the fingers and hand are allowed to dangle.

With the other hand, flick or thump the finger pad of middle finger.

Response:

* ❖ Flexion and adduction of thumb
* ❖ Flexion of the index finger
* ❖ Flexion of other fingers.

Snout Reflex (Fig. 11.184)

Method: Stimulation by:

* Backward pressure on the philtrum of upper lip
* Minimal tap on upper lip
* Sweeping the tongue blade across the upper lip.

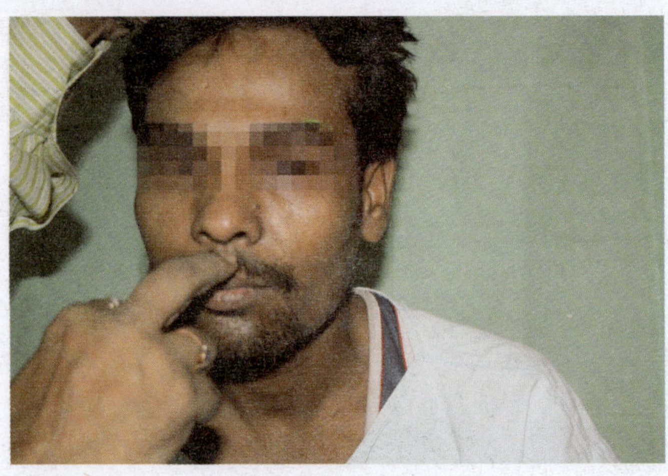

FIG. 11.184   Snout reflex

Response:
- Puckering and protrusion of lower lip
- Depression of the angle of the jaw.

In case of exaggerated response: This extension of response includes:
- Sucking
- Testing
- Chewing and swallowing movement.

Sucking Reflex (Fig. 11.185)

This reflex is normal in infant, but occurs in diffuse cortical degeneration in adult.

Method: Stimulation of perioral region.

Response: Sucking movements of tongue, lips and jaw.

Rooting Reflex (Fig. 11.186)

Method: Stimulus delivered beside the mouth or on the cheek.

Response: Deviation of lips mouth even head retracted towards the side of stimulus.

Glabellar Tap Reflex

In a normal person, when glabella is tapped, patient unusually starts blinking, but after 4 to 5 taps, blinking will disappear. But if it continues, it is pathognomonic. It occurs in Parkinson's disease or other degenerative processes.

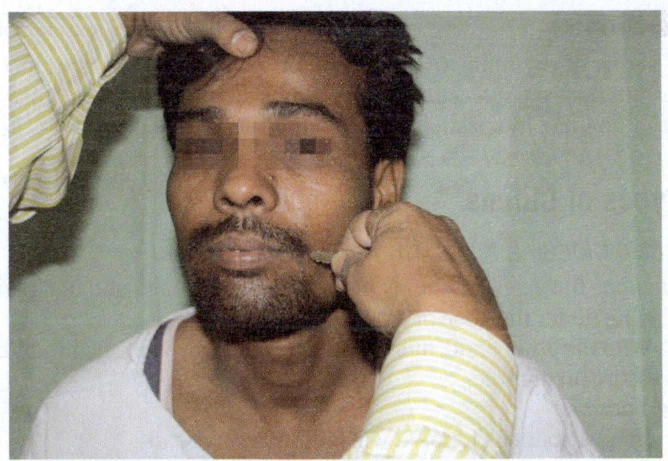

FIG. 11.185   Sucking reflex

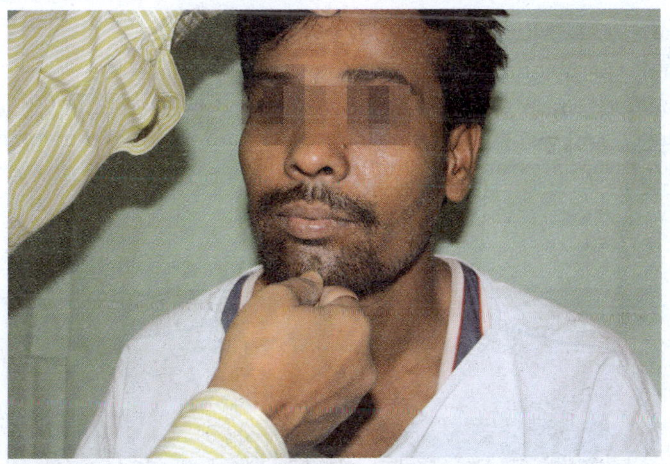

FIG. 11.186   Rooting reflex

Corneal Mandibular Reflex

In an unconscious patient, there is deviation of jaw, if contralateral cornea is stimulated. It occurs due to disinhibition of fifth nerve motor nucleus on a result of structural lesion above the pons.

■ Clonus

A series of rhythmic, involuntary muscular contractions induced by sudden passive stretching of muscles and tendon. This is accompanied by spasticity, hyperactive deep tendon reflexes.

Types of Clonus

Ankle Clonus (Fig. 11.187)

Method: The examiner holds the leg to be examined with one hand placing under the knee or calf.

With the other hand, quickly dorsiflex the foot, while maintaining pressure on the sole.

Response:

- In unsustained clonus, it will fade after few beats.
- In sustained clonus, as long as the examiner continues to hold the foot in dorsiflexed position, clonus will be present—it is never a normal phenomenon. It will be present in UMN lesion. In severe form clonus may occur spontaneous or with slight stimulus.

Patellar Clonus (Fig. 11.188)

Series of rhythmic up and down movement patella.

Method: Grasp the patella to be examined by thumb and index finger, and execute sudden sharp downward thrust and maintain downward pressure. Leg should be extended and relaxed.

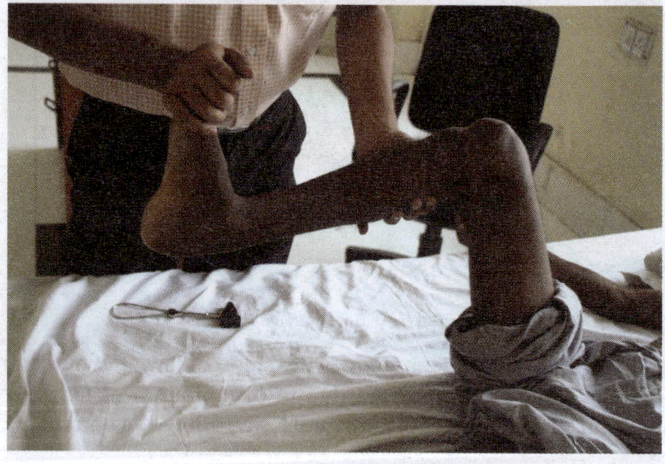

FIG. 11.187   Ankle clonus

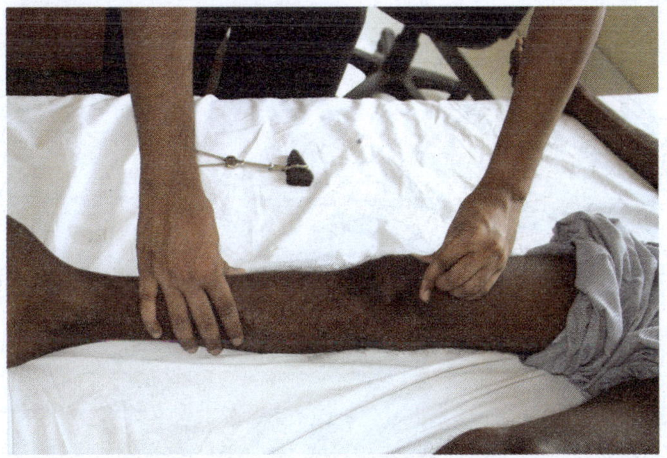

FIG. 11.188   Patellar clonus

Response: Rhythmic up and down movement of patella.

Clonus of wrist: It can be produced by sudden extension of wrist and fingers.

Clonus of jaw: It can be produced by tapping the jaw.

Clonus due to psychogenic origin: This clonus is:
- Poorly sustained
- Irregular in rate
- Irregular rhythm
- Irregular excursion.

Decerebrate rigidity (Fig. 11.189): The posture is like opisthotonos. This is characterized by:
- All four limbs extended
- Head back
- Jaw clenched.

In upper extremity
- Arm internally rotated at shoulder
- Elbow extended and hyperpronated
- Fingers extend at metacarpophalangeal joints and flexed at interphalangeal joints.

In lower extremity
- Legs extended at hip, knee and ankles
- Toes are plantar flexed.

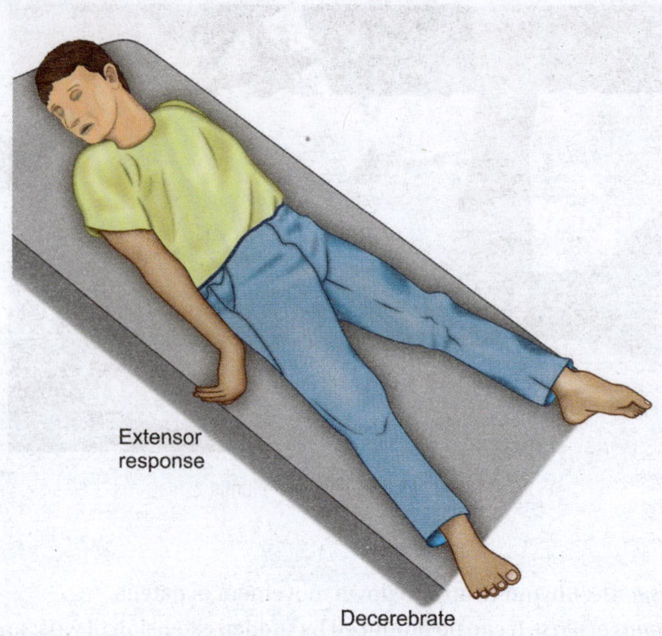

FIG. 11.189 Decerebrate rigidity

Other associated features
Deep tendons reflex—exaggerated, tonic neck reflex and labyrinthine reflexes are present righting reflexes abolished.

Causes of decerebrate rigidity
- Lesion in brainstem at any level between superior colliculi or rubrospinal pathway and rostral portion of vestibular nuclei.
    Integrity of vestibular nuclei is necessary for decerebrate rigidity so these nuclei enhance extensor tone.
- Pontine reticular nuclei and reticulospinal tract lesion.

Decorticate rigidity (Fig. 11.190)
This is characterized by:
- Flexion of wrist and elbows
- Extension of legs and feet.

Causes: Lesion is higher than that causes decerebrate rigidity.
    Preservation of rubrospinal tract increases the flexor tone of upper extremities.

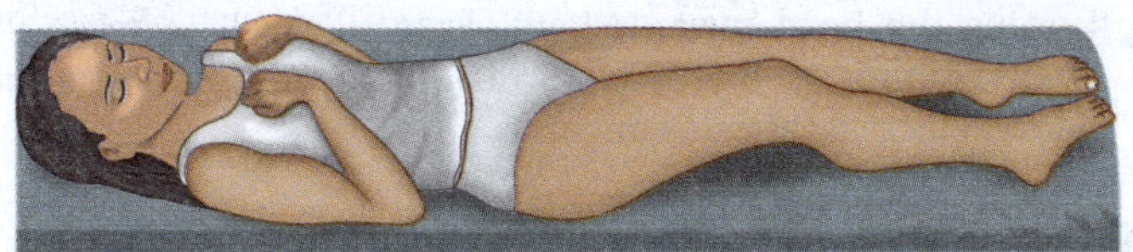

FIG. 11.190 Decorticate rigidity

Associated Movement

This is characterized by unintentional, involuntary, spontaneous, automatic movements, which may be accompanied by voluntary or involuntary movement.

Corticospinal tract controls fine, discrete movement of distal extremities. When there is lesion in corticospinal tract, fine movement of distal extremities will be lost, but does not affect mass movement of proximal muscles.

There are many associated movements which are physiological. These include:

- Pendular swinging of arms when walking
- Facial grimaces with violent exertion
- Movement of the head and neck with movement of the eyes
- Normal extension of the wrist with flexion of the fingers.

Few of the associated movements are lost in extrapyramidal disorders, e.g.

- Masking of face
- Absence of arm swing.

In few conditions, associated movements may be exaggerated and in few conditions new associated movements may appear.

In corticospinal tract lesion, associated movements mainly involve paretic muscle group, which is brought by active movements of other muscle groups as a result, associated movements (AMs) will be slow, forceful, and the limb adopts a new posture.

Generalized Associated Movements

In an attempt of straining, exertion, or to grip with the paretic hand, the involved limb will be spastic, increased flexion of wrist, elbow and shoulder, sometimes accompanied by facial movements on involved side. This posture will be:

- Maintained until grip will be relaxed.
- In autonomic movements like yawn—affected arm extend the elbow, wrist and fingers—new posture will be maintained till yawning will be completed.

- Turning the head towards hemiplegic side will increase the extensor tonus on that side. Turning the head towards normal side will increase the flexion tonus.

Symmetric Associated Movements (Mirror Movement)

In infancy—in case of movement of one limb, there will be involuntary movements of opposite limb. This movement disappears during adolescence—as coordination and muscle power comes in to action. But if this mirror movement is present, it is due to:

- Brain injuries
- Disturbances in cerebral development
- Lesion in upper spinal cord.

In few neurologic disorder, forceful voluntary movement of one limb is associated with similar involuntary movement of opposite limb, mainly paretic limb, e.g. ask the patient to squeeze the hand of examiner with healthy hand; the paretic limb will be flexed.

Similarly, any forceful movement of healthy limb is followed by similar but slow tonic movement of paretic limb.

Coordinated associated movements: This is characterized by involuntary movement of synergistic muscle may be accompanied by voluntary movement of paretic limb.

Types of Associated Movements

Coordinated Associated Movement in Paretic Limb

This is characterized by voluntary movement of involved limb in case of hemiparesis. There are three important signs:

Wartenberg's sign

Active flexion of the terminal phalanges of four fingers against resistance followed by:

- Adduction, flexion and opposition of thumb in paretic limb
- Abduction and extension of thumb in normal limb.

Trunk thigh sign of Babinski

The patient should be lying down in supine position with legs abducted. Ask the patient to sit up keeping his arms crossed on the chest.

- In case of normal person—both the limb will be motionless and heels down.
- In case of hemiparesis—on the affected side, hip and knee flex, trunk flexes, affected limb will be raised with fanning of toes. The unaffected limb will be motionless on the bed.

- In case of paraparesis—both legs rise equally.
- In case of nonorganic weakness, the normal leg rises, paretic one does not.

Ask the patient to sit up with legs hanging by the side of the bed, in case of hemiparesis, hip flexes and knee extended on the involved side.

Tibialis sign of Strumpell

In case of normal person: There is vigorous flexion of hip and knee accompanied by plantar flexion of the foot.

In case of hemiparesis: There is flexion of hip and knee joint accompanied by involuntary dorsiflexion and inversion of the paretic foot.

There may be dorsiflexion of great toe or all the toes. This response is accentuated if movement is carried out against resistance.

Loss of Coordinated Associated Movements

In pyramidal tract lesions—few associated movements are abolished:

- Swinging the arms during walking
- Movements used in rising and sitting down.

The above movements are also lost in disorders of extrapyramidal system.

Cerebellar Function

Cerebrum coordinates the muscular contraction through the activity of cerebellum. In cerebellar lesion, motor activity is uncoordinated, clumsy, tremulous and disorganized.

There are following parts of cerebellum:

	Zone of cerebellum	Clinical manifestation	Possible disorder
1.	Flocculonodular lobe (archicerebellum)	Nystagmus, extraocular movement abnormalities	Medulloblastoma
2.	Vermis (Paleo-cerebellum)	Gait ataxia	Alcoholic degeneration
3.	Hemisphere (Neocerebellum)	Appendicular ataxia	Tumor-stroke
4.	Pancerebellar	All the above	Paraneoplastic

Clinical Manifestations of Cerebellar Disorder

Dyssynergia

Due to proper coordination in the action of agonistic and antagonistic muscles, they contract with proper force, timing, and proper sequence to perform simple or complex activity. Cerebellar activity is instrumental in timing. In case of cerebellar lesion, the muscle movement will be disorganized, disarray, jerky.

Dysmetria

This means error in judging distance, speed, power and direction of movement. So there may be:

- Overshooting (hypermetria)
- Fail to reach the target (hypometria)
- Movement not in straight line in between two points.

Agonist and Antagonist Coordination

It means inability to stop contraction of agonistic muscles and rapid contraction of antagonistic muscles to regulate movements. The disorders of incoordination of muscle movements are:

Dysdiadochokinesia: It means inability to perform rapid repetitive or rapid alternating movements (RAMs). This can be tested by following tests:

- Patting the palm of one hand with palm and dorsum of the other hand alternatively and rapidly (Figs 11.191A and B)
- Tapping the fingers
- Tapping the foot.

Checking movements: It involves contraction of antagonists after release of strong contraction of agonists.

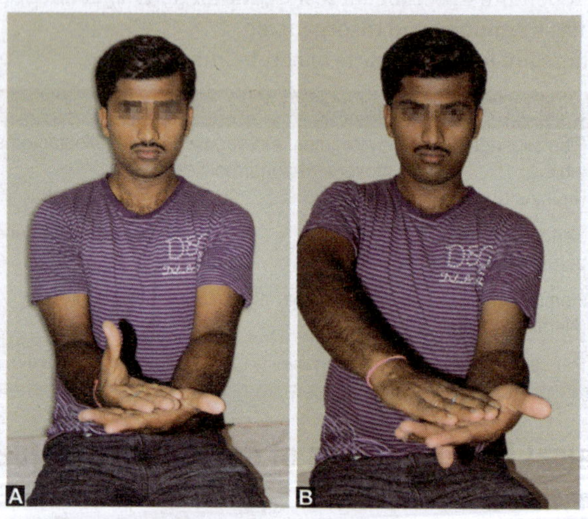

FIGS 11.191A AND B   Dysdiadochokinesia: (A) Patting with dorsum of right hand; (B) Patting with palmer surface of right hand

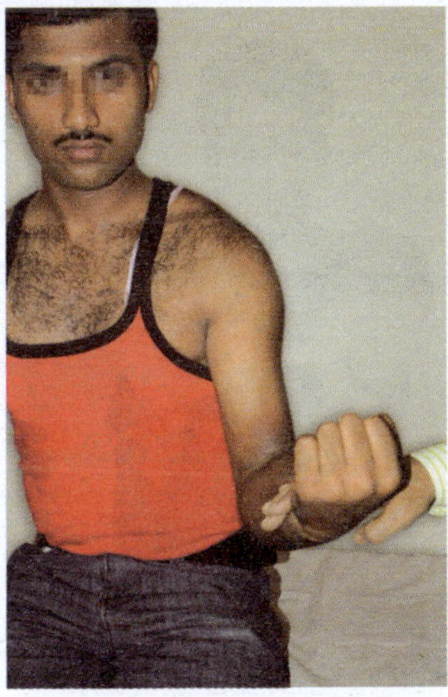

FIG. 11.192   Rebound test

In cerebellar lesion—impairment of reciprocal relationship between antagonist and agonist producing impairment of checking movement.

Holmes (Stewart-Holmes) rebound test (Fig. 11.192)
Ask the patient to abduct the shoulder, flex at elbow, supinate the wrist, firmly clench the fist—in these positions, it will rest on the table.

Now examiner holds his wrist and tries to extend at elbow and asks the patient to resist it.

The examiner suddenly releases the wrist.

In normal people, immediate release of elbow flexor takes place which is followed by contraction of elbow extensors to arrest sudden hitting of hand over the face.

In patient with cerebellar disease, continued contraction of flexor muscles and absence of contraction of extensor muscles takes place—producing the fist to hit the mouth or shoulder. So, examiner should place his free arm in between the patient's hand and face.

Arm-stopping test (Fig. 11.193)
- Patient's arms are outstretched overhead or by his sides
- Examiner holds his outstretched arms horizontally
- Ask the patient to draw his outstretched arm to a level of examiner's outstretched arm, so that the fingertips of examiner and the patient should be as same level.

In case of cerebellar lesion, affected arm often overshoots, then corrects in the opposite direction, or oscillates around examiner's finger before coming to exact point.

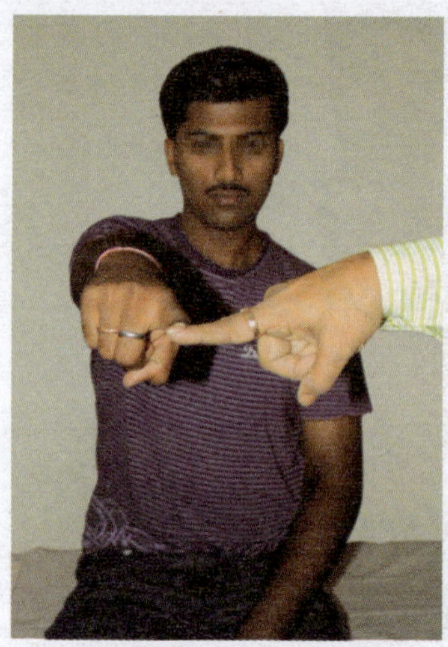

FIG. 11.193 Arm stopping test

Tremor

- *Intention tremor (akinetic, kinetic tremor):* It is absent at rest.
  In upper extremity, when the patient's hand approaches to touch the target, there is irregular, jerky, to and fro movement of the hand.
- *Postural tremor:* This tremor may also occur in patient's outstretched hand, when approaches the target.

Cerebellar Tremor Mainly Involves Proximal Muscles

Severe cerebellar tremor involves entire body and may take myoclonic character.

This tremor may involve cerebellar efferent pathways and connection with red muscles and thalamus (dentatorubral nucleus, dentatothalamic pathways).

Hypotonia

Muscles are flaccid assume unnatural altitude. Stretch reflexes are normal or diminished. Superficial reflexes are unaffected. Jerks are mainly pendular. Tapping the patellar tendon while foot hanging freely by the side of the table, there are to and fro movement of the leg and foot before the limb comes to rest.

There is a characteristic posture in case of cerebellar disease:
- Extended hands because of hypotonia.
- Wrist flexed and arched dorsally, finger hyperextended tendency to over pronation.

Dysarthria

Scanning speech: Slow, ataxic, drawing, jerky and explosive in type.

Staccato speech in Friedreich's ataxia is probably due to cerebellar lesion.

Nystagmus

In case of involvement of connections between cerebellar hemisphere and other centers, there will be gaze paretic nystagmus.

Lesion in one cerebellar hemisphere
- Eyes, at rest, deviates 10 to 30 degrees towards the unaffected side (eyes of involved side).
- When attempting to gaze elsewhere, affected eyes show several saccades towards the point of fixation with slow return to the point of rest.
- This movement is more marked when the patient look towards the side of lesion, amplitude is greater.

When the lesion is in cerebellopontine angle
Nystagmus is coarse, when looking towards the side of lesion fine and rapid when looking towards opposite side (Burns's nystagmus).

Other Ocular Abnormalities in Cerebullar Lesion
- Ocular dysmetria
- Ocular flutter
- Skew deviation of eyes
- Opsoclonus
- Saccadic intrusions.

Rebound nystagmus: In this type of nystagmus, fast component is to the direction of lateral gaze, but direction will be reversed transiently when eyes come back to primary position.

Deviation of head: In unilateral cerebellar lesion, head and neck are deviated to the affected side. Past pointing of extremities towards affected side.

While standing: There is inclination to fall towards the side of lesion.

While walking: There is tendency to deviate towards the side of lesion.

Examination of Coordination and Cerebellar Function

In upper limb:

Preliminary Observation
- Scanning speech (during history taking)
- Ocular dysmetria

- Metacarpophalangeal joints and interphalangeal joints produce over contracture—produced spoon-hand posture
- Cerebellar drift to upwards with eyes closed and arm outstretched
- Broad base gait.

Method of evaluating both pyramidal and cerebellar lesion
Ask the patient to tap the index finger and thumb repetitively.

The examiner evaluates amplitude of each movement and speed with which it is being performed.

This movement can further be evaluated by asking the patient to touch all the fingers with the thumb.

In cerebellar disease: Amplitude and rhythm will be lost.
In pyramidal tract disease:

- Poor facilitation
- Normal rhythm.

Finger-Nose Test

This test can be done in lying down, sitting and standing position.

- Ask the patient to extend his arm completely. Then ask him to touch his tip of the nose with the index finger of the outstretched hand (Fig. 11.194A).
- This execution should be done at first slowly, then rapidly with eyes open and eyes closed.
- Examiner place outstretched hand in different position and in different angles (Fig. 11.194B).
- Again examiner can make this execution much more complex placing his own index finger on the way (Fig. 11.194C).
- Ask the patient to touch the examiner's index finger then to the tip of the nose with the index finger of the patient.

Now watch the smoothness, accuracy, coordination of the movement of patient's finger.

Watch any tremor as the finger approaches the target.

In case of unilateral cerebellar lesion the following can occur:

- If dysmetria, there may be overshoot the mark, bringing the finger to nose with great speed and force, so it may produce trauma. Or there may be undershoot, so the finger may not reach the nose or complete the act slowly.
- If dyssynergia—the act is not smooth, harmonious, there may be acceleration or deceleration of movement.

If the examiner gives some resistance during this act by holding the wrist with his hand or a rubber band there may be ataxia, which may be latent or severe.

In case of unilateral cerebellar lesion ipsilateral limb will be involved.

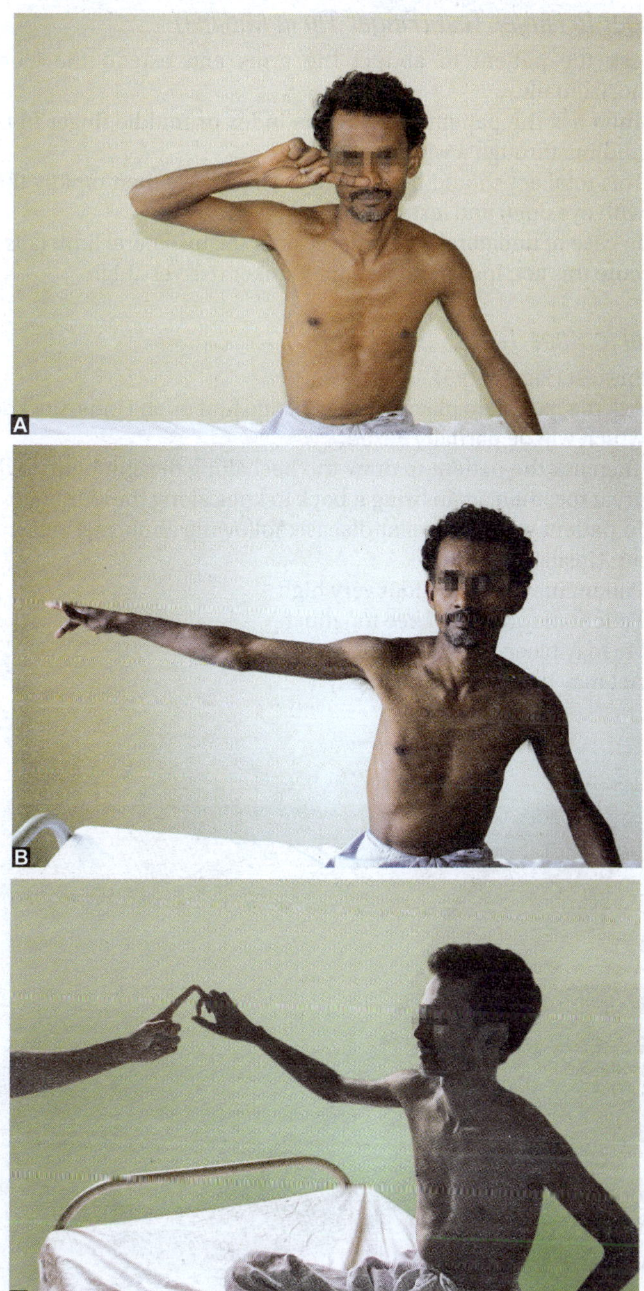

FIGS 11.194A TO C   Finger-nose test

Finger to Finger Test (Finger Tip in Midline)

- Ask the patient to abduct the arms and extend the elbow horizontally.
- Then ask the patient to bring the index or middle finger to the midline through a wide arc.
- This total act should be done first very slowly then rapidly then with eye open and lastly with eye closed.

In case of unilateral cerebellar lesion, the ipsilateral limb fails to execute this act; ipsilateral arm may sinker rise very high.

Heel to Knee Test

In this test (Fig. 11.195)

- Ask the patient to place the heel of one foot on the opposite knee which will be partially flexed.
- Then ask the patient to draw the heel along the shinbone to the great toe, then again bring it back to knee along the shinbone.

In patient with cerebellar disease: following abnormal acts may occur: (ipsilateral side):

- Patient may raise the foot very high
- Patient may flex the knee too much
- He may place the heel above the knee
- Act may be jerky and unsteady.

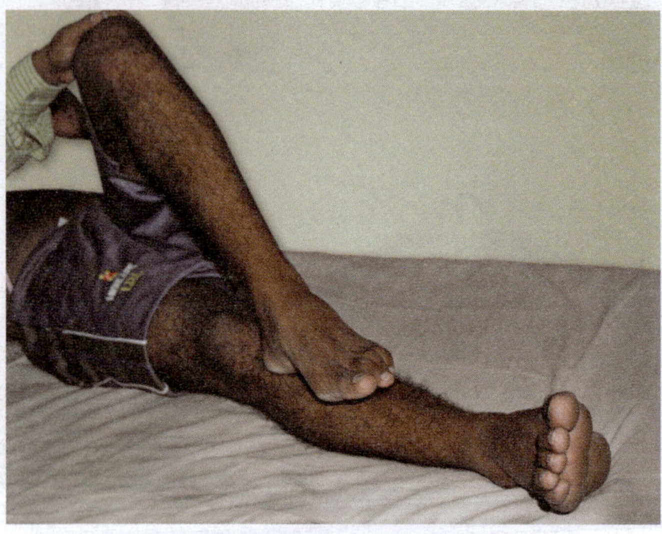

FIG. 11.195   Heel to knee test

With sensory ataxia
- Patient may fail to keep the heel on the shin
- Patient's heel may slip on either side of shin.

Rapid alternating movements: This is called dysdiadochokinesia. In this method—one act cannot be immediately followed by diametrically opposite movements. (Contraction of agonists and relaxation of antagonists and contraction of antagonists and relaxation of the agonist).

Following methods can be done:
- Patting the palm and dorsum of one hand on the thigh or on the palm of other hand.
- Alternate opening or closing the fist.
- Alternate closing and extending the fingers of hand.
- Patting the floor with foot while standing.

In this act, watch the speed, smoothness, accuracy, rate, rhythm, co-ordination, any tremor.

In case ataxia—the whole act is unsteady, dysrhythmic, irregular, clumsy, may be rapidly fatigued.

Two sides have to be compared simultaneously.

Past Pointing and Deviation

- Examiner and the patient should stand or sit facing each other
- Outstretched hand of both people should touch each other horizontally. (Index fingers touch each other).
- Now ask the patient to raise his outstretched hand vertically, upwards or downward, with index finger directed vertically upwards or downwards respectively.
- Then ask the patient to take his hand back to its original position and touch the examiner's index finger. Normally this total act is smooth.
- This total act should be done in eyes opened and eyes closed.

In case of vestibular or cerebellar lesion—past pointing occurs towards the side of lesion first this past pointing occurs —in eye closed position, but in severe cases, it occurs in opened eye position.

Past pointing means the finger pasts the target laterally toward the side of lesion.

When patient try to hold his outstretched hand in space with closed eyes—there may be drift: Three types of drift:
- *Pyramidal drift (Barre sign)*: The arm sinks downward with pronation of forearm (pronator drift).
- *Parietal drift:* The arm usually rises and strays outward (up drift).
- *Cerebellar drift:* The arm drifts outward, either at same level, rising or in sinking.

In case of cerebellar lesion the arm drifts towards the side of lesion.

In case of lower limb
- Patient is lying in supine, raising the leg at a time.

  In case of cerebellar lesion, leg cannot be lifted steadily in a straight line; there may be adduction, abduction, rotation, oscillation or jerky movements.
- When the patient sits on the chair, ask him to elevate the lower limb in space and hold it—in case of cerebellar lesion—the limb will be deviated laterally on ipsilateral side, there may be oscillation of the limb.

Station: It is the patient's attitude, posture and manner of standing. This can be tested in following manner:
- Ask the patient to stand with feet closed together with eyes opened and eyes closed, later on his toes or heels.
- At the same time, he was given a gentle push from back and watch whether he falls to one side, backwards or forwards.

Deviation of station in following lesions:
- *In cerebellar disease*: Patient usually stands on broad base and swaying with eyes opened and closed.
- *In the lesion of vermis (midline lesion):* The swaying occurs forward, backward or side to side.
- *In hemispheric lesion*: Patient may sways towards affected side.
- *In unilateral vestibular lesion*: Patient falls towards affected side.
- *In unilateral cerebellar lesion:* Patient may tilt his head towards affected side and chin towards unaffected side, shoulder of the involved side will be at somewhat higher level.
- *If the patient is being pushed from one side then from the other side*: He may fall when he was pushed towards affected side.
- *If the patient is asked to stand on one foot at a time*: He falls when he tries to stand on the foot of involved side.

Romberg's sign
This sign is positive in case proprioceptive disturbances.

When eyes are opened, the patient can stand, but when eyes are closed, the patient may fail. The essential finding is the difference between standing balance with eyes opened and closed.

The Romberg's sign is very difficult to interpret, e.g. in elderly patient—with eyes closed—minimal amount of sway.

In case of pure cerebellar disease involving spinocerebellar and vestibulocerebellar tract—there is increased instability with eyes closed, but not to that much extent seen in patient proprioceptive disorders. The patient has wide base stance and may be unstable with eyes opened.

In case of vestibulopathy, the patient sways towards the affected side when eyes closed.

Non-neurologic gait disorders
- *Antalgic gait:* It occurs due to pain in lower extremity. Short stance of the involved limb to avoid weight bearing—may occur with hip fracture, dislocation of hip.
- *Lordosis with lordotic gait:* It may occur with ascites, pregnancy and abdominal tumor.
- *Waddling gait:* It may be due to dislocation of hip, advanced pregnancy.
- *Dizziness:* It may occur in severe orthostatic hypotension
- *Marked stooping gait:* It may occur in ankylosis spondylitis simulates fastinant gait of Parkinsonism.
- *A special gait:* It may occur in very weak persons after prolonged bed rest—having generalized weakness.
- *Senile gait:* It occurs in older person—a cautious gait because of uncertainty in balance and postural reflexes. It looks like as if healthy person walks on icy surface—slow velocity, shorten steps.

Hysterical gait
- It is nondescriptable bizarre gait. Patient is afraid of falling but never falls.
- Patient may balance on the stance leg for prolonged period of time.
- Patient may mimic monoparesis, hemiparesis or prepared but in emergency condition, he can use his paralyzed limb.
- Gait may be hoping, dancing and skating characteristics.
- Tremulousness of the extremities may be present.
- Patient is unable to stand upright (astasia) or to walk (abasia)
  Astasia-abasia is characterized by function when recumbent, yet
an inability to walk.

Autonomic Nervous System (Figs 11.196 and 11.197)

From anatomical point of view—Autonomic Nervous System (ANS) can be subdivided into three parts:
1. Sympathetic
2. Parasympathetic
3. Enteric.
Physiologically ANS can be subdivided into two parts:
1. Sympathetic
2. Parasympathetic nervous system.

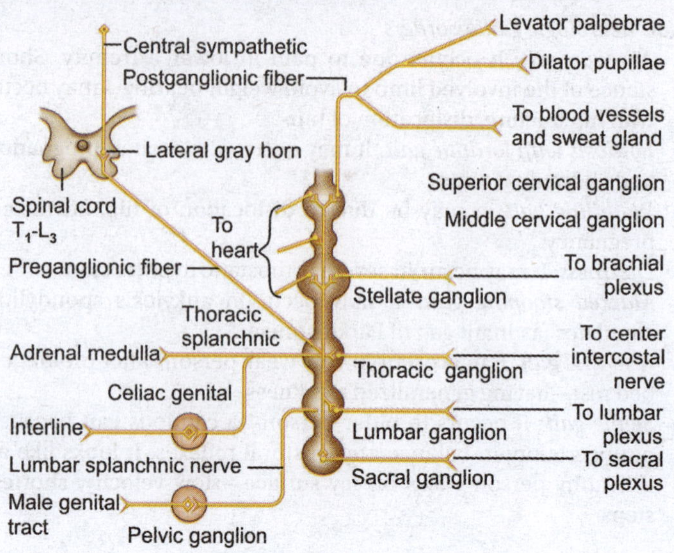

FIG. 11.196 Sympathetic system

Sympathetic Division

This is called thoracolumbar outflow of preganglionic neurons and situated in lateral gray horns of 12 thoracic and first 2 segments of lumbar segments of spinal cord.

Preganglionic fibers arise from these segments run along the anterior root and white rami communicante and end in sympathetic ganglia. From here postganglionic neurons arise and supply— smooth muscle fibers of all visceral organs, like blood vessels, heart, lungs, glands, abdominal viscera.

Sympathetic ganglia have been divided into three groups:

1. Paravertebral sympathetic chain ganglia
2. Paravertebral collateral ganglia
3. Terminal or peripheral ganglia.

Paravertebral sympathetic chain ganglia: It has been subdivided into four groups:

1. *Cervical ganglia*: Eight cervical ganglia arranged in three groups:
   - *Superior cervical ganglia*: Produced by fusion of upper four cervical ganglia—supply fibers to blood vessels, glands and heart through cardiac plexus.

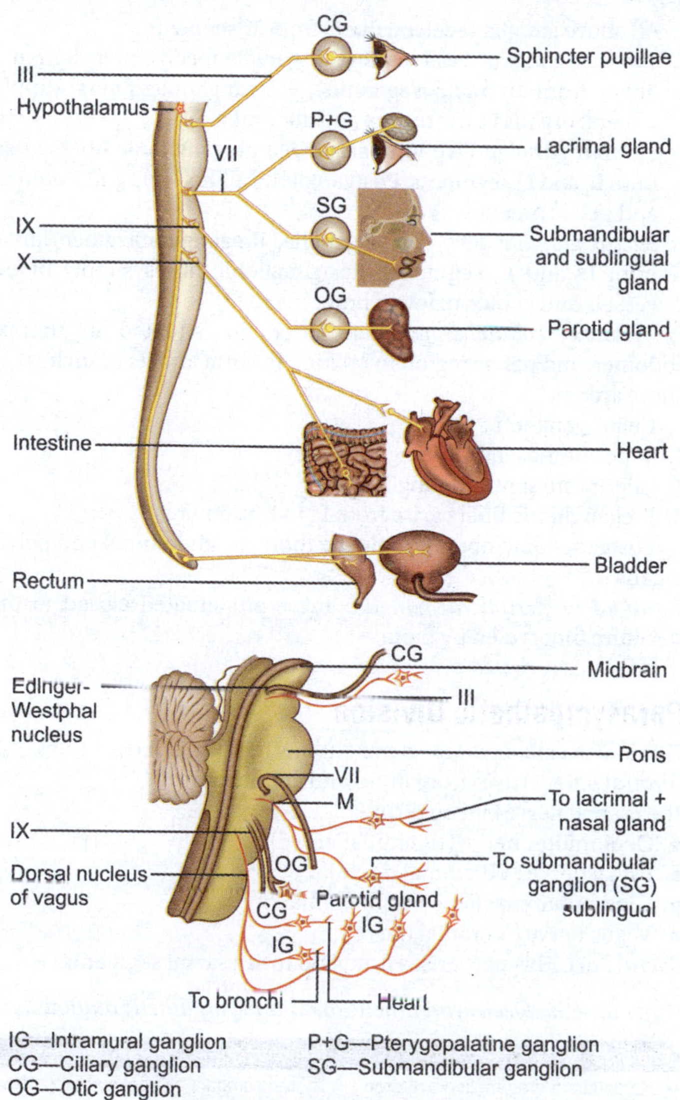

FIG. 11.197 Cranial parasympathetic system

- *Middle cervical ganglia*: It formed by 5th and 6th cervical ganglia—it supplies sweat gland, thyroid gland, parathyroid gland, heart via cardiac plexus.
- *Inferior cervical ganglia*: It formed by fusion of 7th and 8th cervical ganglia. It supplies branches to cardiac plexus.

All above ganglia received fibers from T_1 segment.

2. *Thoracic ganglia*: Twelve thoracic ganglia receive preganglionic fibers from thoracic segments. Postganglionic fibers supply visceral organs in the thorax and abdomen.
3. *Lumbar ganglia*: Five lumbar ganglia preganglionic fibers arise from L_1 and L_2 segments. Postganglionic fibers supply abdominal and pelvic organs.
4. *Sacral ganglia*: Five sacral ganglia. Preganglionic fibers arise from L_1 and L_2 segments. Postganglionic fibers supply blood vessels and glands of lower limb.

Prevertebral collateral ganglia: These are situated in thorax, abdomen and pelvic region in relation to aorta and its branches. These are:

1. Celiac ganglion
2. Superior mesenteric ganglion
3. Inferior mesenteric ganglion.
   Preganglionic fibers arise from L_5 to L_2 segments
   Postganglionic fibers supply the thoracic, abdominal and pelvic organs.

Terminal or peripheral ganglia: These are situated closed to the structure innervated by them.

Parasympathetic Division

This is also called cranio-sacral outflow because it has:

Cranial parts: Arises from brain and cranial nerves.
The cranial nerves involved are:

- Oculomotor nerve (III cranial nerve)
- Facial nerve (VII cranial nerve)
- Glossopharyngeal nerve (IX cranial nerve)
- Vagus nerve (X cranial nerve).

Sacral part: This part arises from 2nd to 4th sacral segments.

Differences between sympathetic and parasympathetic outflow

Features	Sympathetic	Parasympathetic
• Location of preganglionic neuron	Thoracolumbar outflow	Craniosacral outflow
• Location of postganglionic neuron	Away from target organ	Nearer to target organ
• Length of preganglionic fiber	Relatively short	Relatively long
• Length of postganglionic fiber	Relatively long	Relatively short
• Preganglionic neurotransmitter	Ach	Ach
• Postganglionic neurotransmitter	Ach	Noradrenaline

Action of sympathetic and parasympathetic divisions of ANS

Organ	Suborgan	Sympathetic division	Parasympathetic division
• Eye	Ciliary's muscle Pupil	Relaxation Dilatation	Contraction Constriction
• Lacrimal gland		Decrease in secretion	Increase in secretion
• Salivary gland		Decrease in secretion and vasoconstriction	Increase in secretion and vasodilatation
• GI tract	Motility Secretion Sphincters Smooth muscles	Decreased Decreased Constriction Relaxation	Increased Increased Relaxation Contraction
• Gallbladder		Relaxation	Contraction
• Urinary bladder	Detrusor muscle Internal sphincter	Relaxation Constriction	Contraction Relaxation
• Sweat gland		Increased secretion	Decreased secretion
• Heart rate		Increased	Decreased
• Bronchioles		Dilatation	Constriction
• Blood vessels		Constriction except in heart and skeletal muscles	Constriction

Symptoms Related to Autonomic Dysfunction

- *Orthostatic hypotension*: Feeling of light headedness, presyncope, syncope, palpitation, confusion, slurred speech. All appear or worse on standing, postprandially, taking hot bath or ingestion of alcohol.
- *Sweating abnormalities:* Excessive or decreased sweating.
- *GI tract abnormalities:* Dysphagia, early satiety, constipation, diarrhea, weight loss, anorexia, fecal incontinence.
- *Urinary tract related symptoms:* Urinary retention, urgency, urinary tract infection.
- *Sexual abnormalities:* Erectile dysfunction, premature ejaculation, retrograde ejaculation.

Signs Related to Autonomic Dysfunction

- *Assessment of orthostatic hypotension can be done by:*
  - ❖ *Blood pressure measurement:* First in supine position and after standing for variable periods—1, 3 and 5 minutes after standing. Tilt-table testing is more precise.

In normal person, difference in SBP is <20 mm Hg and DBP <10 mm Hg.

If SBP difference >20 mm Hg and DBP difference >10 mm Hg, indicates orthostatic hypotension.

❖ *Heart rate measurement:* In supine position heart rate will be counted and in standing position heart rate will be counted. Normally, heart rate difference is <30 beats/minute above base line on standing.

If it is >30 beats/minute—due to reflex tachycardia—due to fall in blood pressure.

In case of autonomic cardiovascular reflex failure—reflex tachycardia may not occur.

In case of sustained hand grip, cold pressure test—produces increase in DBP 15 mm Hg or increased heart rate >10 beats/min—due to peripheral vasoconstriction.

- *Abnormal dryness:* It may be localized in peripheral neuropathy due to diabetes, or generalized dysautonomia.

  Simple bedside test: Stroking the skin with spoon:
  - ❖ If the stroke is smoothed—skin is dry
  - ❖ If the stroke is irregular and uneven—skin is moist.
- *Other cutaneous signs of dryness:* Skin temperature, color, and mottling, thickening, hypertrichosis, decreased skin wrinkling in water, absence of piloerection, pallor, acrocyanosis, erythema, atrophy.
- *Signs of urinary tract related abnormalities:*
  - ❖ Bladder distension—detected by palpation and percussion.
  - ❖ Bulbocavernosus reflex—somatic motor reflex
  - ❖ Measurement of postvoidal urine.
- *Signs related to GI tract abnormalities:* By insertion of gloved finger into anus—produces constriction of internal anal sphincter.

  If tone is decreased, anus does not close after finger withdrawal.
- *Signs of eye in autonomic dysfunction:*
  - ❖ *By Schirmer's test:* Place a strip of filter paper in lower conjunctival sac—measure the degree of wetting over 5 minutes (Fig. 11.198).
  - ❖ *Eye dryness:* Itching, foreign body sensation.
  - ❖ Ptosis.
- Signs of extrapyramidal, cerebellar signs.
- *Pilomotor response:* Erection of hair occurs due to its follicular base contraction.

  Mechanical stimulus or cold stimulus—heightened the sympathetic activity and piloerection.

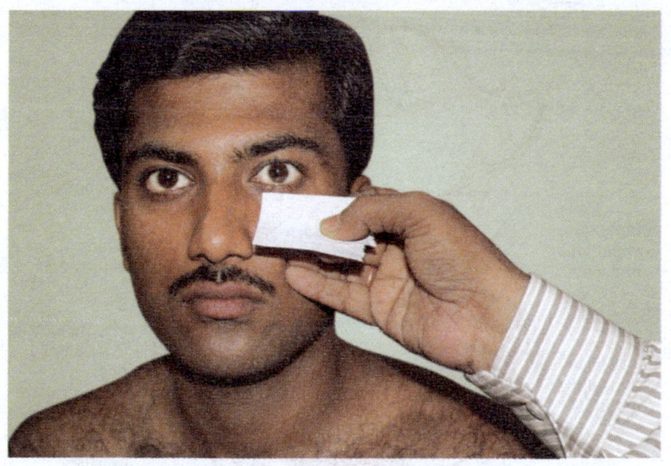

FIG. 11.198   Schirmer's test

- *Scrotal response:* If scrotal skin is touched with cold metal, there is vermicular contraction of dartos muscle, but testes will not be elevated. Only cremesteric reflex will elevate the testicles—scrotal response is absent in sympathetic abnormality.
- *Examination of bladder function (Fig. 11.199).* Voluntary initiation of micturition is generated from 2nd frontal convolution, this is suppressed by paracentral lobule—so a person micturates at proper time and proper place.
  - ❖ *Lesion in frontal lobe and anterior cingulate gyri* produces unawareness of bladder fullness and patient will be incontinent.

    Bladder fibers pass to pontine micturition center, which in turn project into spinal cord micturition center.

    These centers are responsible for coordination between contractions of detrusor muscles of urinary bladder and opening of external sphincter.
  - ❖ *Lesion in frontal lobe:* It may cause spasticity of external sphincter muscle—and produces urinary retention.
  - ❖ *Incomplete upper motor neuron lesion:* It produces neurogenic bladder—a small bladder—its trigone (its sensory component) reflexly contract due to increased pressure given by thick walled small bladder.
  - ❖ *Complete transaction of spinal cord:* It produces paralysis of bladder and overflow incontinence (reflex bladder). Bladder may be emptied by abdominal pressure also.
  - ❖ *Lesion in sacral cord (S_1-S_5) and cauda equina:* It produces flaccid bladder (400–600 mL) with overflow incontinence.

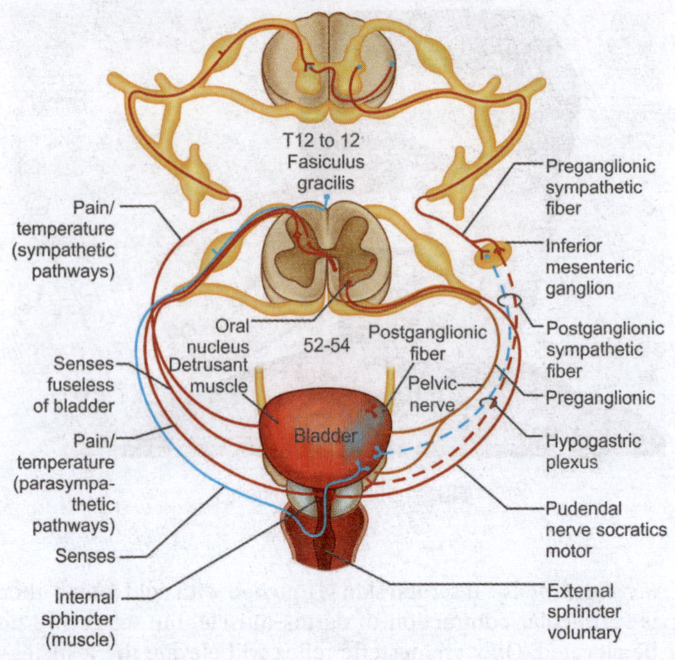

FIG. 11.199 Spinal sensory and spinal motor pathways involved in urination. Black solid line indicates sensation of immitext micturition. Black dotted line indicates inhibition of relaxation of urinary bladder permitting postganglionic fibers to cause contraction of urinary bladders

- *In tabes dorsalis:* There is destruction of sympathetic and parasympathetic innervations to bladder—producing painless flaccid bladder with overflow incontinence.
- *Inability to initiate micturition, division of urinary stream, dribbling of urine:* Prostatic dysfunction.
- *Insensible bladder:* Peripheral neuropathy.
  Onuf's nucleus (S_2-S_4) of conus medullaris innervates external sphincter muscle.
- *Lesion in Onuf's nucleus:* It produces inability to interrupt voiding by external sphincter muscle (Involved in multiple system atrophy but not in ALS).
- *Lesion in thoracic and cervical cord demyelization:* Dyssynergia between detrusor or muscle and external sphincter.

Clinical test of detrusor muscle—patient is asked to take deep breath while voiding.

If detrusor muscle is not functioning, stream of urinary flow will be stopped as abdominal pressure is relived.

Bladder of complete lower motor neuron lesion—It will be largely devoid of feeling, does not contract reflexly, straining only can help voiding, but voiding is not complete.

Bladder of upper motor neuron lesion is small, insensible, hyper-reflexic, hypocomplaint and hyperactive reflex.

Associated neurological lesion will clench the diagnosis, e.g.
- *Absent reflexes—peripheral neuropathy*—Primarily to pin price and cold—small fiber neuropathy.
- *Loss of joint and position sense, areflexia, Argyll Robertson pupil*—tabes dorsalis—or pseudotabes (diabetes mellitus).
- *Decreased or loss of bladder sensation*—Cauda equina or conus medullaris syndrome.
- *Cerebral lesions*—Normal pressure hydrocephalus or degenerative disease produces low bladder capacity, may be urinary retention, but never overflow incontinence.

Lesions producing rectal involvement
- *Acute lesions of conus medullaris or cauda equina:*
  - ❖ Fecal incontinence
  - ❖ Laxity of both internal and external and sphincter
  - ❖ Loss of anal reflex.
- *Acute spinal cord injuries*—It produces spinal shock—incontinence of anal sphincter.
- *High spinal or pontine lesion*—Spastic anal sphincters.
- *Major seizures*—Fecal or urinary incontinence.

Lesions producing sexual dysfunction
- *Pituitary prolactinoma*—producing low testosterone level and high prolactin level.
- *Central autonomic failure:*
  - ❖ Shy-Drager syndrome
  - ❖ Striatonigral degeneration
  - ❖ Multiple system atrophy, demyelinating disease, syrinx.
- *Expanding tumor in conus medullaris producing:* Inability to ejaculate but erection is possible or reverse.
- Root disease.
- *Spinal lesions:*
  - ❖ Lymphoma
  - ❖ Polycythemia vera
  - ❖ 5' esterna inhibitor prolonged painful erection.
- *Spinal lesion at T_2 level produces:*
  - ❖ Impotence
  - ❖ Intact reflex erection
  - ❖ Impaired ejaculation.

- *Psychiatric disorder produces:*
  - ❖ Impotence
  - ❖ Intact reflex erection and ejaculation.
    Bulbocavernosus reflex can be evaluated by pinching glans penis causes contraction of bulbocavernosus muscles behind the scrotum.
- *Cauda equina lesion produces:* Loss of:
  - ❖ Ejaculation
  - ❖ Erection
  - ❖ Sexual sensation
  - ❖ Sensation in the perineum.

▮ Sensory System

Three types of sensations are:

1. *Exteroceptive sensation:* It provides information from surrounding external environment.
2. *Interoceptive sensation:* It provides information regarding internal functions.
3. *Proprioceptive sensation:* It provides information of orientation of joints and body in space.

Sensory system has two components:

1. *Conscious component.*
2. *Unconscious component:* It helps to regulate internal environment.

Monitoring limb has two components:

1. *Conscious component:* Posterior column pathways.
2. *Unconscious component:* Spinocerebellar pathways.

Conscious sensory system has two components:

1. Fine touch, joint sense, position sense.
2. Crude touch, pain temperature.

Each sensory modality is carried by different type of fibers. They differ in:

- Diameter
- Length
- Amount of myelination—all in peripheral nerve.

In central tract:

- Location of the tract through which the sensation is carried out.
- Fine touch, position sense and joint sense of body are carried by posterior column (Fig. 11.200).
- Fine touch, position and joint sense of head and neck are carried by trigeminal principal nucleus.

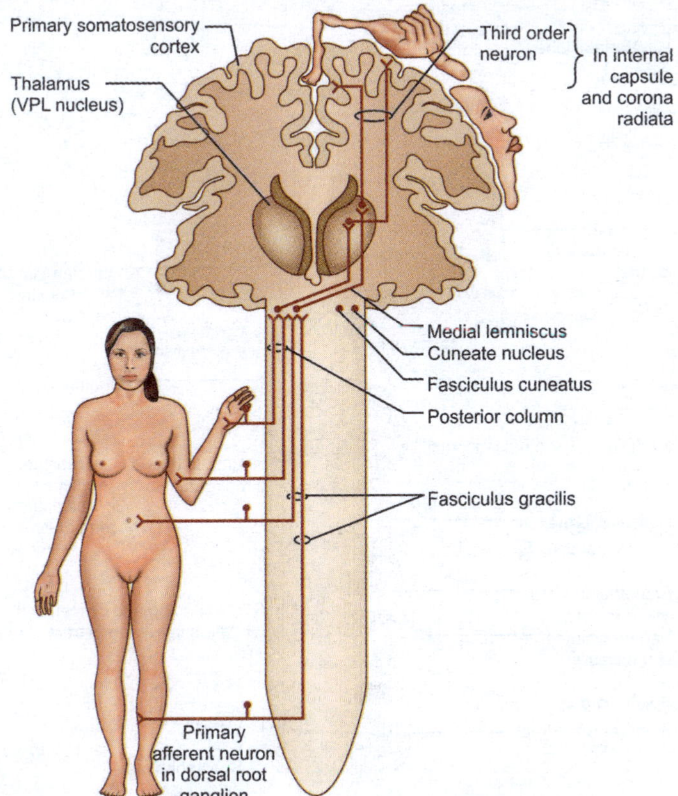

FIG. 11.200 Posterior column carrying sensation of fine touch, vibratory sense, joint sense from the body to sensory motor cortex

- Pain and temperature from body are carried by—spinothalamic tract (Fig. 11.201).
- Pain and temperature from head and neck are carried by—spinal tract and nucleus of trigeminal nerve.

Definitions of a Few Commonly Used Terms

- *Allodynia:* Increased sensitivity to a stimulus producing pain, which normally does not produce pain.
- *Alloesthesia:* Perception of a sensory stimulus at a site other than the site where it is being delivered.
- *Analgesia:* Absence of sensibility to pain.
- *Astereognosis:* Absence of spatial tactile sensibility so inability to identify object by feeling.
- *Anesthesia:* Absence of pain.

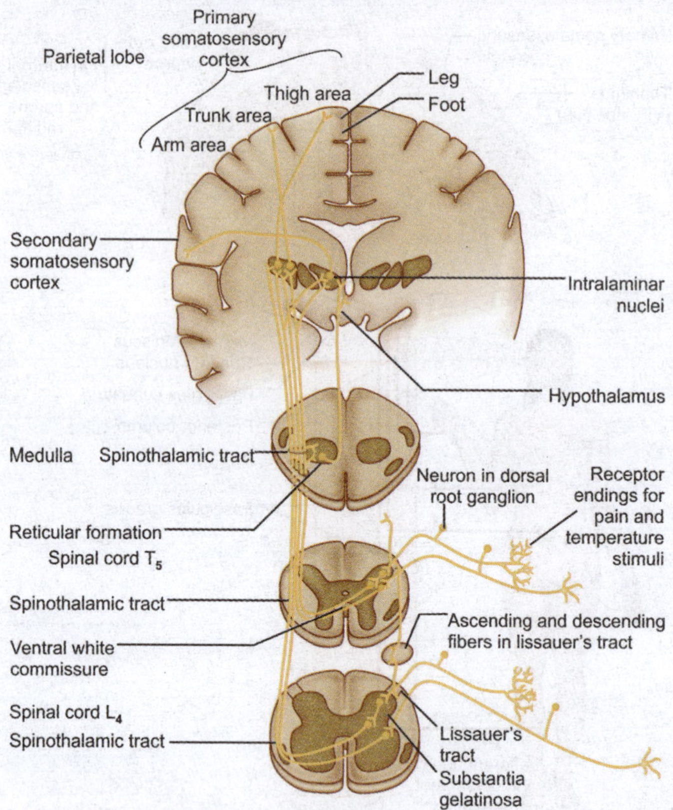

FIG. 11.201 Lateral spinothalamic tract—carrying crude touch, pain, temperature sensation from the body

- *Dysesthesia:* Abnormal unpleasant, perverted sensation either spontaneous or due to nonpainful stimulus.
- *Hypoalgesia:* Decreased sensitivity to pain.
- *Hyperalgesia:* Increased sensitivity to pain.
- *Kinesthesia:* The sense of movement.
- *Pallesthesia:* Vibration sense.
- *Hypopallesthesia:* Decreased vibration sense.
- *Hyperpallesthesia:* Increased vibration sense.
- *Paresthesia:* Abnormal sensation in absence of any stimulus, sensations may be feeling cold, warmth, numbness, tingling, burning, priming, type.

Sensory Examination Performed to Evaluate

- Absent, increase or decrease sensation
- Any radiation

- Type of sensation affected
- Degree of abnormality
- Distribution of abnormality
- Any dissociation of sensations.

Modalities of sensations—those are tested bedside:
- *Pain can be tested by pin:*
  - ❖ Burning pain is carried by 'C' (1 µm) fibers
  - ❖ Sharp pain and cold, lancinating pain is carried by A-delta fibers (1–4 µm) it occurs in roots disease.
- Heat is carried by polymodal C fibers.
- Light touch is carried by A-B fibers (8–10 µm in diameter).
- Deep muscle pressure is carried by A-B fiber.
- Position sense is mediated by large A-Alfa fibers—these fibers innervate muscles, joints, tendon 12 to 22 µm in diameter.
- Stereognosis, two-point discriminations graphesthesia the ability to copy posture, recording of two simultaneous stimuli derive from primary afferent input.

Neurons in Gray Matter of Spinal Cord (Fig. 11.202)

Organization of neurons in gray matter of spinal cord is described as follows:

Nuclei

- *Posterior horn:*
  - ❖ Dorsomarginal nucleus —I
  - ❖ Substantia gelatinosa of Rolando—II

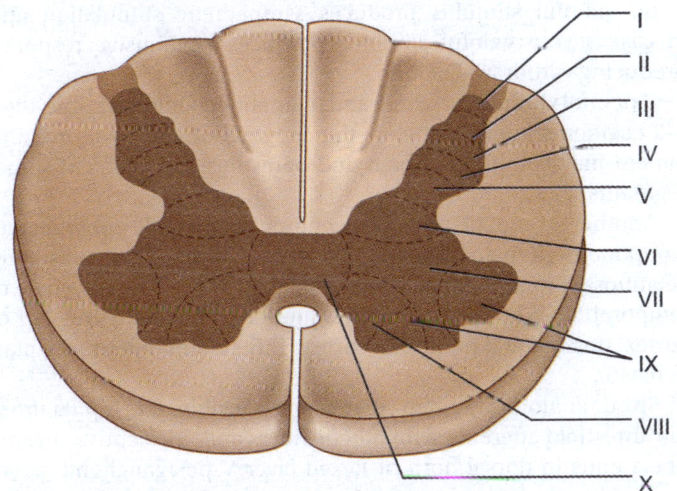

FIG. 11.202 Gray matter in spinal cord

- ❖ Nucleus proprius—III and IV
- ❖ Chief sensory nucleus—VI
- ❖ Dorsal nucleus of Clarke—VII.
- *In lateral column:* Intermediolateral nucleus—VII
- *In anterior gray horn:*
  - ❖ Commissural nucleus—VIII
  - ❖ Alfa motor neuron—IX
  - ❖ Gamma motor neuron—IX
  - ❖ Renshaw cells. These are inhibitory neuron—X.

White matter in spinal cord is divided into three columns:
1. Anterior or ventral column
2. Lateral column
3. Posterior column.

Pain fibers mediate through two major systems:
One system involves the recording of location and frequency of pain firing of activated and delta-A fibers.

Second system involves effect of pain behavior.

First group enters through posterior horn and synapse with neurons in Rexed layer 1 of substantia gelatinosa of the dorsal horn—ascend through brainstem to the ventral posterolateral nuclei of thalamus then to primary sensory nucleus of cerebral cortex.

Few fibers after entering dorsal horn, ascend or descend 1–2 segments above or below and segment they innervate by Lissauer's tract of spinal cord.

They send their collaterals to intermediolateral horn cells and anterior horn cells (Motor neurons) of Rexed layer IX.

So, painful stimulus produces sympathetic stimulation and in case severe painful stimulus produces nocifensive response producing withdrawal of limb.

If painful stimulus is severe and maintained for longer time then 1–2 segments above or below the segment of entry will fire and patient may complain of pain and paresthesia of adjacent spinal segments.

Another group of pain nociceptors responsible for effectual component of pain innervate in Rexed layer II of substantia gelatinosa. From here postganglionic fiber projects to amygdale of temporal lobe, brainstem nuclei, anterior cingulated gyrus, SII of cortex, dorsolateral prefrontal cortex. This system determines pain behavior.

Third anatomic system that is responsible for inputs from low threshold afferents sympathetic fibers and nociceptive specific fibers ends in dorsal horn of Rexed layer V postganglionic fibers cross below the central canal in conjunction with axons from Rexed layer I and II to form anterior spinothalamic tract. This system has rich collaterals from brainstem nuclei, periaqueductal gray matter in midbrain, lateral aspects of reticular formation at all levels, intralaminar thalamic nuclei. These axons project to SI and SII of the cortex bilaterally. Major component is contralateral.

Spinothalamic tract (STT) is lamellated (Figs 11.201 and 11.203A and B) in such a way that sacral fibers most laterally followed by lumbar fibers, arm and hand fibers are most medial. The fibers of this tract cross midline at the level of entry to reach contralateral side and ascends lateral to posterior column (carrying fibers for joint sense, position sense and discrete touch).

Pain fibers from face project to V nerve nucleus, then cross midline in the medulla and pons and joins spinothalamic fibers in pons.

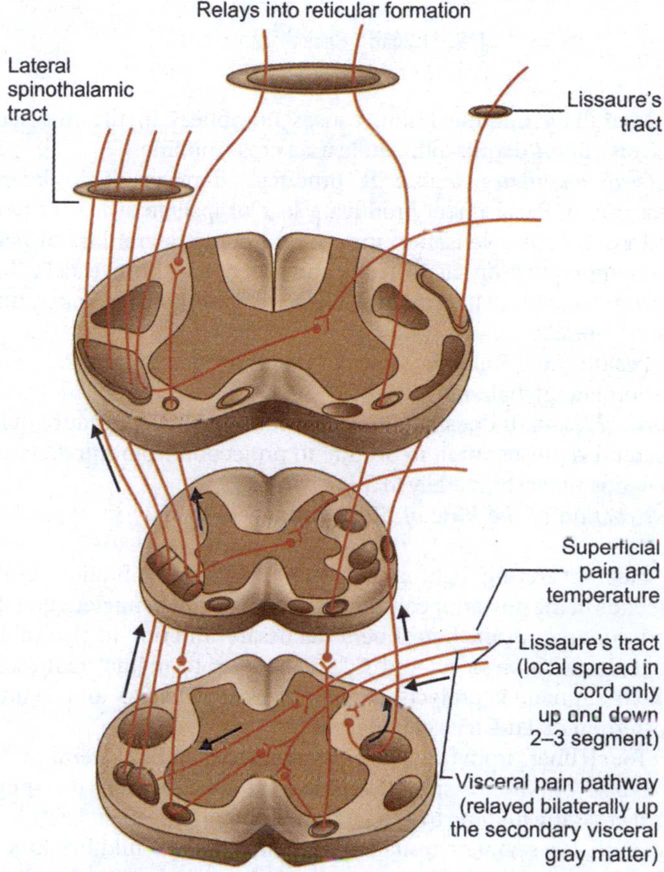

FIG. 11.203A   Temperature (lateral spinothalamic tract)

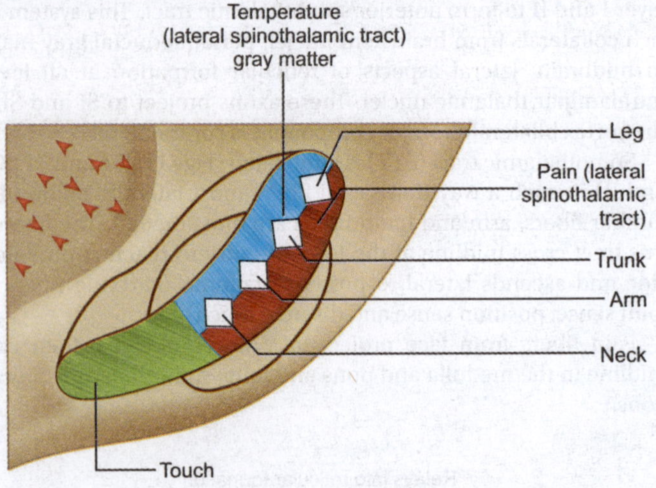

FIG. 11.203B Spinothalamic tract

Medullary midline lesion causes numbness in the mid face because fibers of quintothalamic tract cross midline.

Lateral medullary lesion: It produces damage of ipsilateral descending facial fibers producing loss of ipsilateral loss of pain and temperature sensation in face and contralateral loss of pain and temperature on sacral, trunk and arm below the level of lesion.

Lesion in pons: It produces loss of pain and temperature contralaterally.

Lesion in thalamic nuclei (ventral poster medial and posterolateral thalamic nuclei).

Cortical lesion: It does not affect the pain sensitivity because of its bilateral representation in SII due to projection from intralaminar thalamic nuclei bilaterally to SII of cortex.

Destruction of the base of SII: It produces inability to appreciate pain.

Fibers carrying light touch, joint, position, vibration sense ascends in the posterior column ipsilateral to end in nucleus gracilis and cunatus. From here fibers decussate anterior to pyramidal tract decussation at C_1 and C_2 and project to medial lemniscus which ultimately projects to ventral posterolateral and ventral posteromedial nucleus of thalamus.

Touch fibers from face joins ipsilateral tract in brainstem.

Fibers of anterior spinothalamic tract after entering the spinal cord cross the midline to join lateral spinothalamic tract. Few fibers ascends 2–3 segment ipsilaterally then cross the midline to join contralateral spinothalamic tract. Central cord lesion damage fibers affecting pain and temperature but not the light touch.

Lateral cervical nucleus (C_1–C_4 levels) projects both touch and proprioceptive information to contralateral thalamus—then to S_1 of cortex.

Fasciculus gracilis—it contains input from lower half of the body with fibers arise from lowest segments located most medially.

Fasciculus cuneatus contains input from upper half of the body, with fibers from lower (thoracic) segments are more medial than those from high cervical ones.

So, posterior column contains fibers—(Fig. 11.204) from medial to lateral distribution—sacral, lumbar, thoracic, cervical.

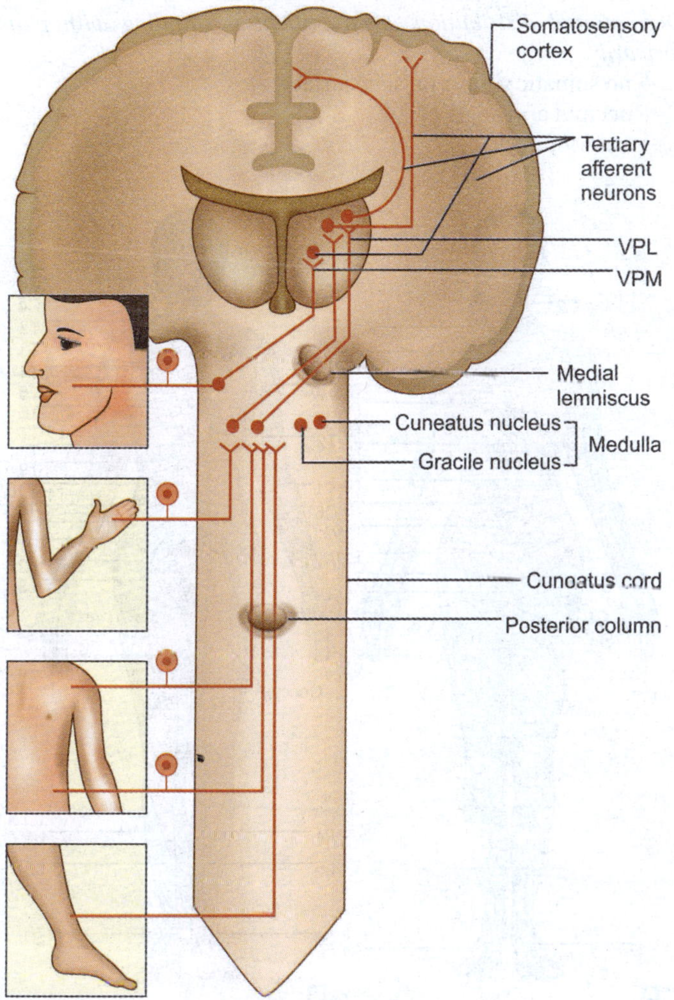

FIG. 11.204 Posterior column

In anterior spinothalamic tract—fibers distribution from medial to lateral—cervical, thoracic, lumbar and sacral.

In lateral spinothalamic tract—fibers distribution from medial to lateral—cervical, thoracic, lumbar.

Because lowest–most fibers are pushed laterally as they cross the midline.

Sensory Dermatome (Figs 11.205A and B)

Sensory root overlaps one segment above and one segment below the level of entry into the spinal cord.

Dermatomal distribution when patient is standing with palms forward:

$C_1 \rightarrow$ no somatic supply on skin surface
$C_2 \rightarrow$ occiput and angle of jaw
$C_3 \rightarrow$ anterior neck

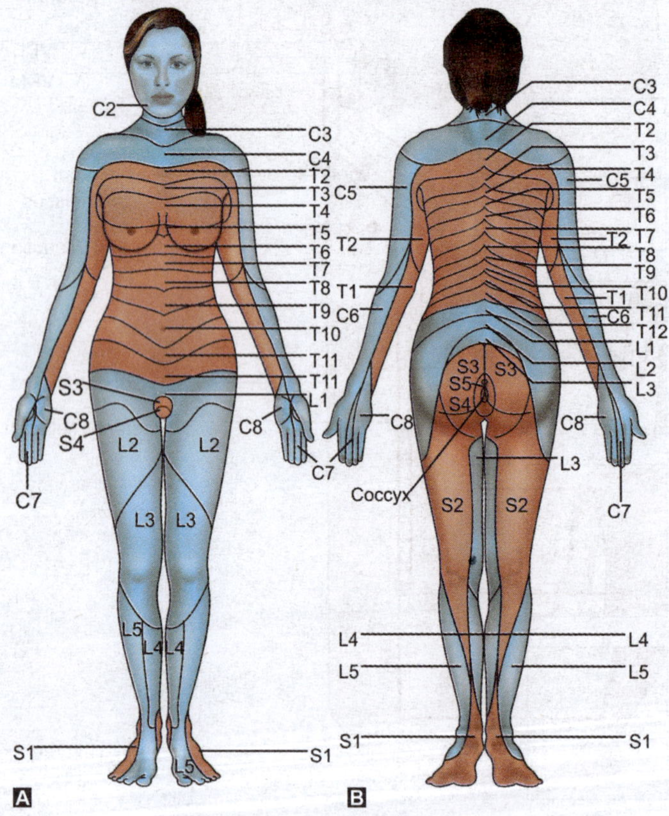

FIGS 11.205A AND B Sensory dermatome

$C_4 \rightarrow$ trapezius ridge
$C_5 \rightarrow$ outer aspect of shoulder tip
$C_6 \rightarrow$ lateral forearm, thumb and index finger (rare)
$C_7 \rightarrow$ triceps, middle finger
$C_8 \rightarrow$ fourth and fifth fingers
$C_8 - T_1 \rightarrow$ sympathetic fibers of eye (superior cervical sympathetic ganglia)
$T_2 \rightarrow$ sympathetic supply to arm (along lower trunk of brachial plexus)
$T_4 \rightarrow$ level of the nipple
$T_6 \rightarrow$ tip of the scapula (notalgia from upper trunk of brachial plexus)
$T_8 \rightarrow$ rib of the margin
$T_{10} \rightarrow$ umbilicus
$T_{12} \rightarrow$ pelvis
$L_1 \rightarrow$ groin
$L_3 \rightarrow$ middle knee
$L_4 \rightarrow$ inner knee, medial leg, band sensation around the ankle.
$L_5 \rightarrow$ lateral thigh, scrotum (projected radiation, anterior thigh—(dural radiation of L_5—recurrent nerve of spurling), lateral knee (part of recurrent nerve of Gonyea, a branch of posterior—tibial nerve).
$S_1 \rightarrow$ lateral side of bottom of the foot, small toe, tip of penis, groin, inside the vagina-unilaterally.
$S_3 - S_5 \rightarrow$ concentric rings around the anus.

Major nerves are:
- Median nerve
- Radial nerve
- Ulnar nerve
- Intercostobrachial (derived from medial cord of brachial plexus)
- Sciatic nerve
- Peroneal nerve
- Saphenous nerve
- Plantar nerve.

Method of Pain Sensation

- Ask the patient to close his eyes.
- Gentle pin prick to be given on both sides in same areas and ask whether the feeling on both areas are same.
- In case of neurologically normal patient, pain sensation on both sides is equal. But in case of real sensory loss, patient may answer—5% or 25%.
- Examiner can deliver alternatively the sharp end and blunt end of a safety pin on skin and ask the patient whether sharp or dull end has been touched. In case of subtle sensory loss—draw the

pin lightly over the skin, ask the patient whether there is change in sensation. Cooperative patient can discriminate the alteration of sensation from normal area to involved area. By this method, examiner can map the area of sensory loss.

If there is hypoalgesia—stimulation should be moved from area of decreased sensation to normal area.

If there is hyperalgesia—Stimulation should be moved from normal area to hyperalgesic area.

Sometimes there is an area of hyperalgesia in between hypoalgesic area and normal area—this indicates the level of lesion, e.g. in spinal cord myelopathy.

If testing is done too rapidly, it produces temporal summation. If testing is done too close, it produces spatial summation.

Stimuli should be given at irregular interval to avoid patient's anticipation.

Tests for Temperature Sensation

- Test tube containing warm and cold water to be taken
  Cold stimuli—5–10°C (41–50°F)
  Warm stimuli—40–45°C (104–113°F)
    Extremes of free flowing water, usually between 10°C and 40°C.
    Temperature below 5°C or above 45°C—usually produces pain rather than warm or cold sensation.
    Normally one can detect difference of 1°C around 30°C.
- Handle of tuning fork may be used instead of water.
  It is sufficient to determine whether the patient can distinguish hot and cold stimuli.

Usually hot and cold sensivity are equally impaired. Occasionally one modality is more involved than the other.

In case of sensory system—pain and temperature are equally involved.

Method of Testing Tactile Sensation

- Light touch sensation can be tested by wisp of cotton, feather, tissue paper, soft brush (Fig. 11.206).
- More detailed evaluation of touch can be done by—Semmes-Weinstein filaments or aesthesiometer. These methods employ filaments of different thickness to deliver varying grade of intensity.

Stimuli should not be heavy enough to produce pressure on subcutaneous tissue.

Ask the patient to tell only "yes" or "no" when the devices are applied on skin.

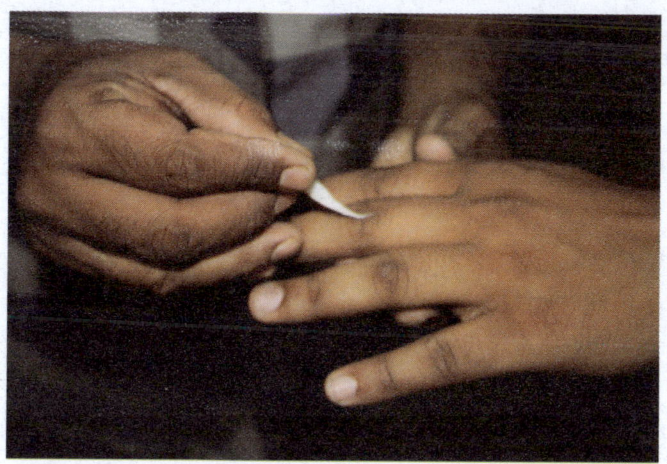

FIG. 11.206 Light touch

If patient says "yes", then ask him to detect the area where stimulus has been employed.

In case of too hairy skin, this stimulation should be avoided, because due to hair motion, examiner may confuse with the stimulus applied.

Methods to Detect Sense of Motion and Position

Sense of motion consists of awareness of position of body or any parts in space; this sensation depends upon impulses from joints and muscles shortening.

Motion and position sense can be tested by passively moving a part of the body and noting the patient's:
- Appreciation of movement
- Direction of movement
- Range of movement
- Minimum angle of movement
- Ability to judge the position of part in space.

Testing should be done:
- In lower extremity—at metatarsophalangeal joint of great toe
- In upper extremity—distal interphalangeal joints.

  No need of testing proximal joints to be tested.

  Test should be done with eyes opened and eyes closed.

  Instruct the patient detail about the examination and ask the patient to answer —"yes", "no", "up" or "down".

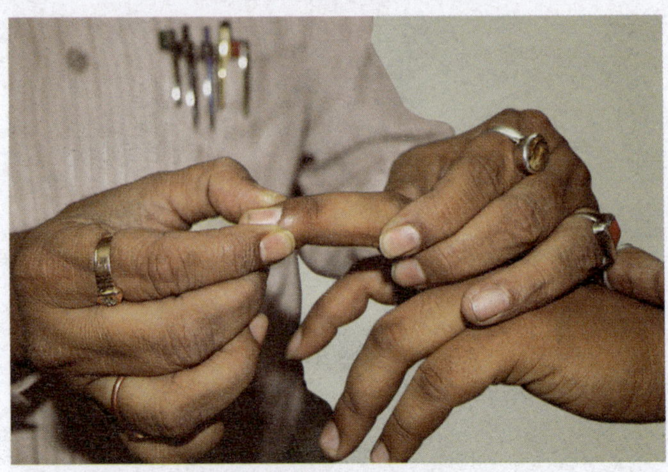

FIG. 11.207   Joint sense

Method (Fig. 11.207)

- Hold the completely relaxed finger on the sides away from neighboring digits parallel to the plane of movement.
- Patient must be relaxed. Ask him to do no active movement of that digit.
- Now the proximal interphalangeal (PIP) joint phalanx should be held with one hands of the examiner.
- Now the distal phalanx should be moved up and down and ask the patient whether the phalanx is up or down or in previous position.
- Quick movement is more easily detected than slow ones.
  - ❖ Healthy young individual can detect the movement of great toe by 1 mm.
  - ❖ Minimal impairment of position sense causes first loss of position of the digits then motion.
  - ❖ In the foot, sensation is lost in smaller toes before disappearance in great toe.
  - ❖ In the hand, involvement of little fingers is first followed by involvement of ring, middle, index and thumb.
  - ❖ If sense of motion and position sense are lost in digits then proximal joints are to be tested, because their involvements are usually associated with ataxia.

Other Methods

- With the hands out stretched, in eye closed position, hand will droop.

- Foot should be moved to new position. Now with eye closed, the patient is asked to point great toe or heel.

  The patient with severe proprioceptive deficit may have ataxia and incoordination—which may be confused with cerebellar lesion—but in former case—it will be worse in eye closed position. So, visual input is responsible for correction of errors and allows the patient to compensate for proprioceptive loss.

  Romberg test is also positive in case of severe proprioceptive loss.

Method of Detection of Vibration Sense

Vibration sense: It consists of perception of presence of vibration when oscillating tuning fork is placed over bony prominences—bone acts as resonator. Impulses are coded in the form of sinusoidal wave, which produces action potential.

These impulses are relayed through:

- With proprioceptive and tactile sensation through medial division of posterior root.
- To fibers in dorsolateral funiculus it may be the most important pathway for sub serving vibration sense.

Loss of position sense and vibration sense do not always parallely involved, e.g.

- *In subacute combined degeneration:* Vibration sense loss is too much than position sense.
- *In tabes dorsalis:* Position sense is much more involved than vibration sense.

Method

- Tuning fork is 128 Hz, weighed ends.
- *Sensations to be tested on bony prominences:*
  - On the great toe
  - Metatarsal head
  - Malleoli
  - Tibia
  - Anterosuperior iliac spine
  - Sacrum
  - Sternum
  - Clavicle
  - Spinous process of the vertebrae
  - Knuckle
  - Styloid process of radius and ulna
  - Finger joints.

- The intensity and duration of vibration sense depends upon:
  - ❖ The force with which the tuning fork is struck
  - ❖ The interval between times it is set in motion and the time of application on bony prominences.
- Tuning fork is struck and placed it on the bony prominence—great toe, interphalangeal joint.
- Hold it in that position till the patient no longer feels the vibration.
- Measure the time during which patient felt the vibration of tuning fork.
- In case of loss of vibration sense: It must be lost mostly in distal extremity and ascends progressively upwards.

Vibration sense is impaired or lost in lesions of:
- Peripheral nerve
- Nerve root
- Dorsal root ganglia
- Posterior column
- Medial lemniscuses.

In posterior column lesion—vibratory sense is lost distally than proximally—lower extremities more involved than upper extremities.

The finding of normal vibratory threshold in distal lower extremities usually obviates the need for testing proximally or in upper extremities.

Difference between lower and upper extremities is usually significant.

Cerebral Sensory System

Cerebral sensory function involves:
- Primary sensory cortex for perception of stimulus.
- Sensory associated areas responsible for interpretation of the stimulus.

Combined sensation describes perception as integration of formation from different modalities for recognition of stimulus.

Functions of parietal lobe are to:
- Analyze, synthesize the varieties of sensations
- Correlation for the perception with memory of past stimuli—whether there is any similarity or not
- Interpretation of the perception
- Refining the perception.

Parietal lobe is not concerned with crude sensation, pain and temperature, which is controlled by thalamus.

Cortical modalities of clinical importance are:

Stereognosis

It can be described as perception, understanding, recognition and identification of the nature of object by touch. Failure of all the above is called astereognosis.

If cutaneous and proprioceptive sensation is intact, only then astereognosis can be diagnosed.

There are following steps of object recognition:

- *Size perception* can be tested by taking objects of some shape but of different sizes.
- *Shape perception* of objects of simple shape (circle, square, and triangle).
- *Form perception* of objects by taking different forms (ball, pyramid and cube).
- *Recognition of objects* by taking the object in hand (key, button, coin, comb, etc.).
- *For more precision*: Ask the patient to know different types of coins, or different alphabet.
- *If there is weakness or incoordination of hand;* examiner can rub the patient's hand over the object.

   Stereognosis should be compared in both hands—whether it is unilateral or bilateral.
- *Recognition of different texture*—and recognize the difference between the textures like—cotton, wool, silk, etc.

Graphesthesia

Recognition of figures—written on the skin with the pencils, dull pin or similar objects (Fig. 11.208).

- Testing to be done over the finger pads, palm and dorsum of the feet.
- Letter should be 1 cm in height written on finger pad.
- Early identifiable dissimilar number (3 and 4 not 3 and 8) should be used.
   Loss of sensory ability is known as a graphesthesia.
- Direction of movement of light scratch stimulus drawn 2 to 3 cm across the skin (directional kinesthesia) may be sensitive indicator of function of posterior column and primary sensory cortex.

Two-Point Discrimination (Fig. 11.209)

This can be described as ability to differentiate cutaneous stimulation by one point to two points while eyes are being closed.

- The instrument used is two-point discriminator—Electrocardiogram calipers, compass.

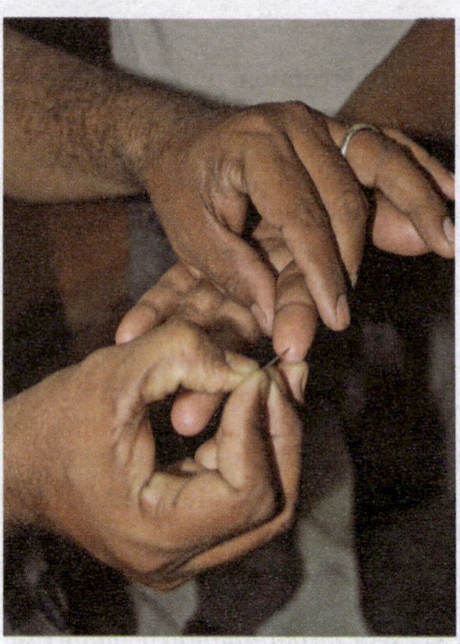

FIG. 11.208 Pin touch

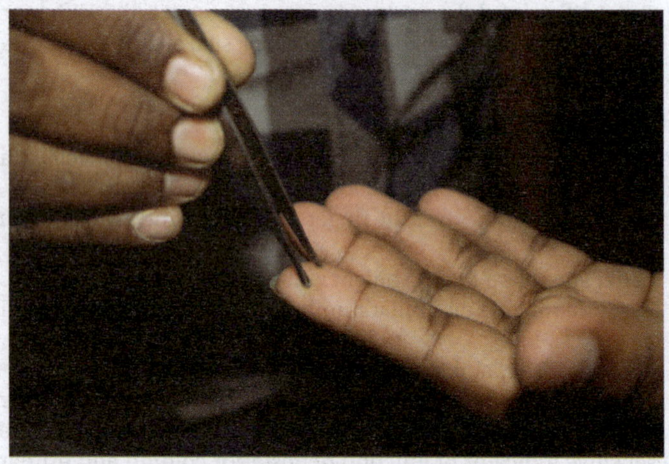

FIG. 11.209 Two-point discrimination

- *Two types of two-point discrimination:*
  a. *Static discrimination*: The instrument is held in place for few seconds on the skin area to be tested.
     i. Start with two-point stimulus—points should be further apart (patient can recognize the two-point discrimination).

ii. Then bring the two points closer and closer until the patient recognize the two points as single point. Measure the distance between two points.

The normal two-point discrimination is:
- 1 mm on the tip of the tongue
- 2 to 3 mm on the lips
- 2 to 4 mm on the fingertips
- 4 to 6 mm on the dorsum of the fingers
- 8 to 12 mm on the palm
- 20 to 30 mm on the back of the hand
- 30 to 40 mm on the dorsum of the foot.

iii. Greater separation is necessary for differentiation on the forearm, upper arm, back, thigh and legs.

b. *Moving two-point discrimination*: This is similar to static discrimination, except, instrument will be drawn across the test area (e.g. in case of finger pad, the discriminator should be drawn from distal interphalangeal crease to tip of the finger).

Two-point discrimination pathways are mainly through posterior column and medial lemniscuses.

Sensory Extinction of Inattention

This can be described as inability to recognize two stimuli applied simultaneously on homologous sites on two sides of the body, the stimulus is touch. When one of the applied stimuli cannot be recognized—this is called extinction.

- Generally more rostral area is the dominant site, e.g. in case of stimulus applied to face and hand simultaneously, dominant site will be face, hand will be site of extinction.
- Severity of extinction can be estimated by increasing the intensity of the applied stimulus.
- Sensory extinction can occur due to lesion in parietal lobe, thalamus and sensory radiation.

Autotopagnosia (Somatotopagnosia)

It can be described as inability to recognize body parts, or orientation of body and relation of individual part.

- Patient may fail to recognize the limbs or one-half of the body.
- Patient may drop his hand from the table to his lap and recognize that an object falls on his lap may not be aware that it is his own body parts.
- *Finger agnosia:* Inability to recognize or name his finger—it may be a part of Gertsmann syndrome (acalculia, agraphia, finger agnosia, fail to right to left discrimination).
- *Anosognosia:* It may be due to lesion in parietal lobe.

■ Sensory Localization

- Primary modalities may be impaired due to lesion in:
  - ❖ Peripheral nerve
  - ❖ Sensory root
  - ❖ Spinal cord
  - ❖ Brainstem
  - ❖ Thalamus.
- Cortical modalities can be impaired in parietal lobe lesion.
- Primary modalities (pain, touch and temperature) pass along the spinothalamic tract. Fine touch, proprioceptive sensations passed through posterior column. But both the tracts converge in thalamus and fibers of cortical representation. So, any lesion in this area produces total loss of sensations in one-half of the body.

  In spinal cord, two tracts run upward as diverging tract, here any lesion may (Syringomyelia) produce dissociative sensory loss.

  In spinal root and in peripheral nerve, the fibers lie close together. So, in spinal root and in peripheral nerve lesion—total loss of sensory modalities.

The following lesions are responsible for dissociative sensory loss:
- *Lateral medullary syndrome:* Loss of pain and temperature of ipsilateral face due to involvement of spinal nucleus of V nerve and contralateral body due to involvement of lateral spinothalamic tract, but light touch may be spared due to spare of posterior column and medial lemniscus.
- *Syringomyelia in spinal cord:* Firstly it involves lateral spinothalamic tract where they decussate in anterior commissure, but spare the posterior column in case of early lesion, which carries light touch.
- *Anterior spinal artery stroke:* It involves anterior two-thirds of the cord, spare the posterior column, which is supplied by posterior spinal artery.
- *Brown-Séquard syndrome:* It is example of extreme dissociation, where pain, touch and temperature of one side of the body is involved and light touch and proprioceptive sensation of other side will be involved.
- *Occasionally in generalized polyneuropathies* involving small and large nerve fibers, can cause differential involvement of pain and temperature as opposed to touch and pressure.

There are several types of distribution of sensory loss
- *In hemidistribution*—due to involvement of cortex or thalamus.
- *In brain system disease*—there is crossed deficit affecting face on one side and body on other side.

- Deficit in sensation below a certain level suggests spinal cord disease.
- *Spinal cord level with sacral sparing*—suggest intraparenchymal spinal cord pathology.
- *Sign suggesting gloves and stocking* distribution of sensory loss—peripheral nerve disease.

  In hemisensory loss—there is certain amount of side to side overlap of innervation in the anterior midline, mainly in the trunk.

- *In lesion—involving conus medullaris or cauda equina*—Saddle-shaped distribution of anesthesia.
- *Burns* produces abnormalities of receptors or nerve filaments.
- *In scar or callosities*—decreased sensation due to involvement of end organ or smaller filaments.

High Level of Bladder Control (Fig. 11.210)

- When the bladder is half-full, visceral afferent from stretch receptors in detrusor muscles and in mucous membrane of trigone pass along the opposite spinoreticulothalamic tract to pons, midbrain and thalamus.
- Activity of sympathetic system is stepped up, so bladder compliance is increased, parasympathetic neurons are silenced by α_2 interconnection.
- Spinoreticular fibers synapse with 'L' nucleus in pons, activate onuf nucleus in sacral cord and raises the tone of external urethral sphincter.
- When the bladder is full, but place is not suitable for voiding—areas in inferior frontal gyrus send inhibitory signals to anterior cingulate gyrus via association fibers. Again projection to hypothalamus and midbrain inhibits preoptic area and periaqueductal gray matter.
- Voluntary contraction of entire pelvic floor can be taken place when command is sent from prefrontal cortex to perineal representation on medial side of cortex in paracentral lobule.
- When time and place permits, anterior cingulate gyrus release the prisoners.

  Then preoptic area, periaqueductal gray matter stimulus dictates 'M' nucleus and inactivates 'L' nucleus.

Urinary incontinence is more common with right-sided lesion in brain.

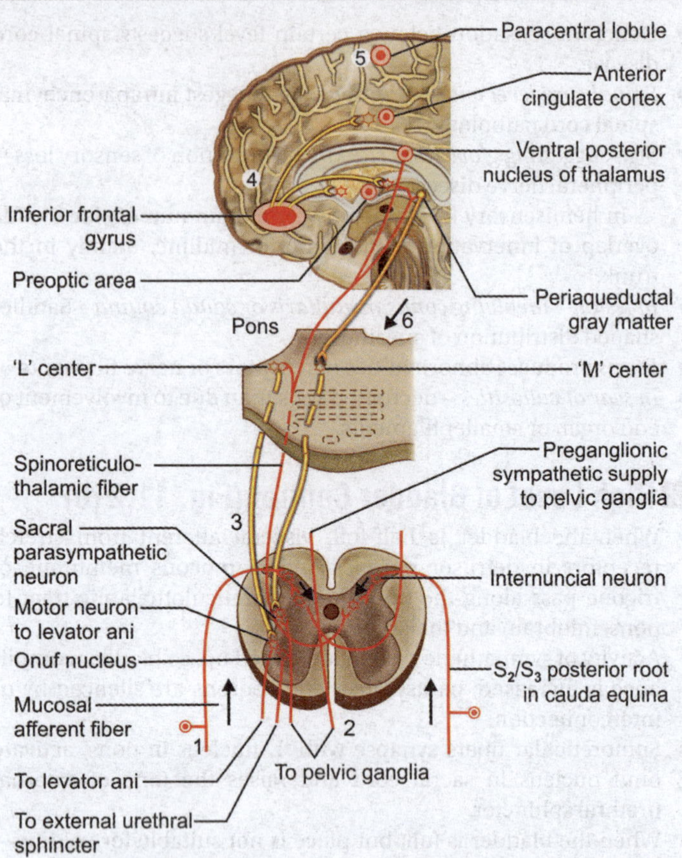

FIG. 11.210   High level of bladder control

NYSTAGMUS (FIGS 11.211A AND B)

Nystagmus can be defined as biphasic ocular oscillations having slow phase, which is responsible for its generic and continuation. Fine nystagmus cannot be detected by simple inspection. This can be diagnosed by fundoscopic examination—the direction in which the retinal venules are seen to oscillate is the opposite of the direction in which the globe oscillates. There are following types of nystagmus.

Oscillopsia

It is illusory movement of environment—may be of following types—(horizontal plane):

- Associated with jerky nystagmus (movement of environment opposite to the movement of slow phase, no movement is received during fast phase due to high visual threshold).
- Associated with pendular nystagmus—(perception of to and fro movement).
- Associated with SOM (Jelly-like quivering).
- Associated with vestibular and labyrinthine dysfunction.

Oscillopsia in vertical plane may be associated with bilateral median longitudinal fasciculus involvement.

Opticokinetic Drum

It is very helpful for detecting pursuits and saccades. When the drum is rotated to right side of the patient, there is slow phase towards right (pursuit) and fast phase towards left (saccade). So, it is helpful in following situations:

- Asymmetry in slow phase in parietal lobe lesion.
- Early saccadic impairment in—Huntington's chorea, progressive supranuclear palsy, olivocerebellar atrophy, congenital ocular motor apraxia, sea-blue histiocytosis.
- Internuclear ophthalmoplegia.
- Vertical rotation in rotatory nystagmus.
- Hysteria or malingering—patient cannot follow the drum.
- Congenital nystagmus—opticokinetic nystagmus.

Normal Nystagmus

- Opticokinetic or vestibular nystagmus.
- Nystagmus on extreme lateral gaze or extreme vertical gaze.

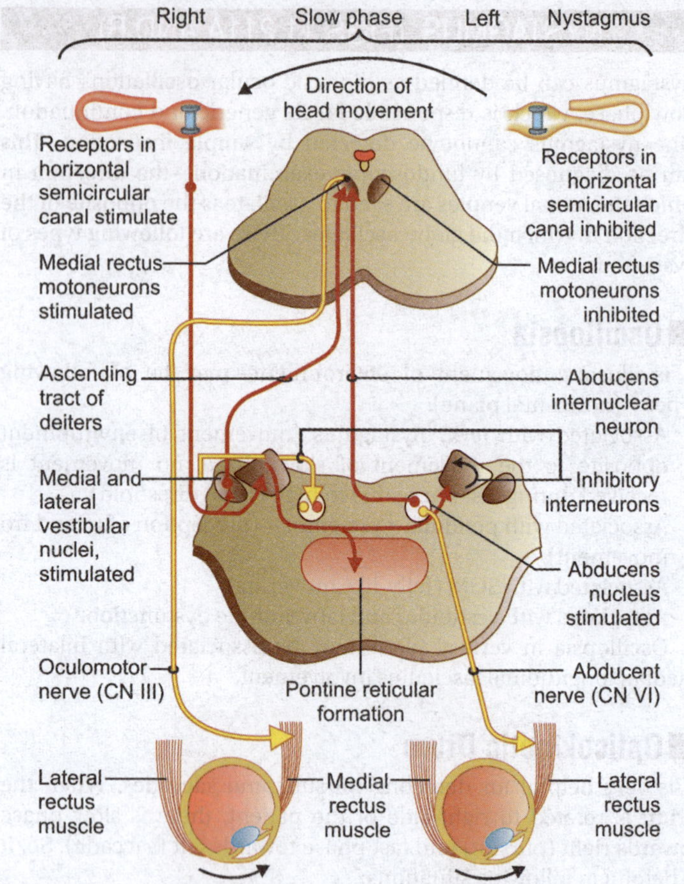

FIG. 11.211A   Nystagmus (slow phase)

Jerky Nystagmus

This type of nystagmus has two components:

1. Slow component and
2. Fast component.

This nystagmus is named according to the fast phase of nystagmus.

This is corrective component.

So, horizontal nystagmus to the right means:

- Corrective phase towards right (saccades)—this brings the eyes back to a position where eyes wish to look.
- Slow phase to the left—analysis of this component is helpful for anatomical diagnosis.

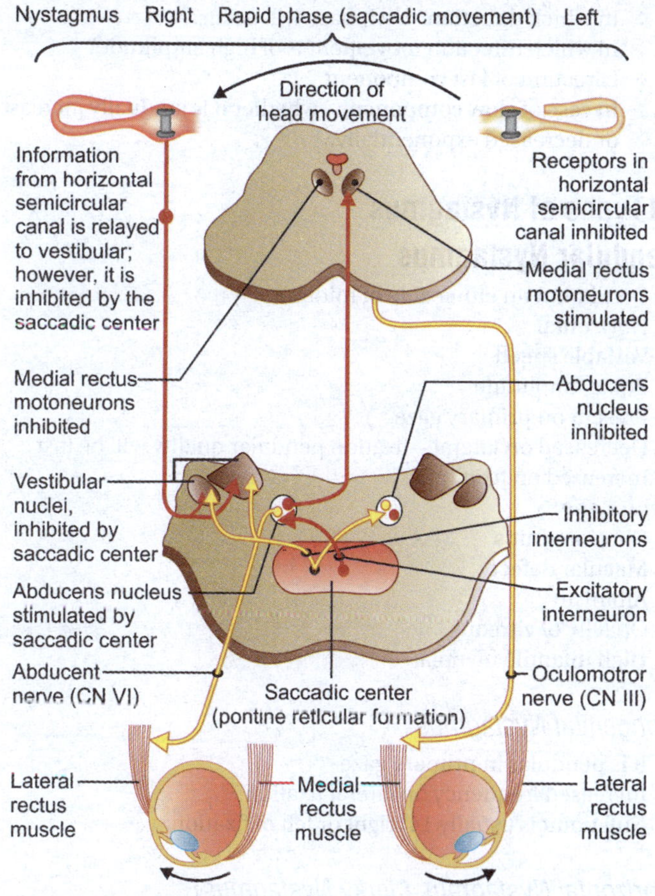

FIG. 11.211B   Nystagmus (rapid phase)

This slow phase may reduce or gain its speed throughout this phase.

Method of Testing for Nystagmus

- Instruct the patient to follow the index finger in all fields of gaze.
- Lateral deviation should be maintained for 3 seconds for nystagmus to develop.
- In any field of gaze extreme deviation should not be done, because it may start spurious nystagmus.
- During examination, followings should be noted by examiner:
  - ❖ In which position, nystagmus will appear?

- ❖ In which direction slow phase will occur?
- ❖ In which direction movement is of high amplitude?
- ❖ Direction of fast component.
- ❖ In case of slow component—whether it is gradually increased or decreased exponentially.

Types of Nystagmus

Pendular Nystagmus

- Oscillation on either side of midline
- Horizontal
- Variable speed
- Equal amplitude
- Present on primary gaze
- Decreased on lateral—fixation pendular quality will be lost
- Increased on fixation.

Causes are:

- Chorioretinitis
- Macular defect
- Albinism
- Opacity of vitreous
- High infantile myopia.

Congenital Nystagmus

- It is pendular in primary gaze
- Increased frequency on lateral fixation
- Null point is usually 14° right or left of fixation.

Horizontal Nystagmus (Jerky Nystagmus)

Vestibular nystagmus

In this type, slow phase is towards the side of lesion and quick phase is away from the side of lesion due to cortical correction.

So, horizontal nystagmus to the left means—slow phase towards right (side of lesion) due to less vestibular input from the right (medial inferior and superior nuclei) to the third and sixth cranial nerve nuclei. So, unopposed left-sided vestibular input drives the eyes to the left (quick phase).

Cortical correction here is from right frontal conjugate eye center, which produces quick component to the left to bring the eye in mid position.

Slow phase of this nystagmus is decreased by fixation and increased in darkness with eye closure or with use of Frenzel lens.

Causes are:

- *Peripheral lesions:*
  - ❖ From labyrinth or cervical joints
  - ❖ Muscle afferents
  - ❖ Eighth cranial nerve to vestibular nuclei or centrally.
- *Central lesions:*
  - ❖ Vestibular nucleus and its connections
  - ❖ Medial longitudinal fasciculus
  - ❖ Lesions in cerebellum.

Cervicogenic nystagmus: This is due to imbalance of proprioceptive input to vestibular nuclei.

Differentiation of nystagmus due to peripheral and central lesion
- *In peripheral lesion:*
  - ❖ Slow component is towards the side of lesion and fast phase is opposite to the side of lesion with greater amplitude.
  - ❖ Associated signs—Tinnitus, vertigo, nausea, vomiting.
  - ❖ In case of cochlear disease or Meniere's disease—Deafness.
- *In case of central (cerebellar) lesion:*
  - ❖ Fast phase is towards the side of lesion with greater amplitude.
  - ❖ In case of cerebellopontine angle tumor, a rotatory component with quick phase having greater amplitude is towards the side of lesion and slow phase with low amplitude is opposite to the side of lesion.

    Pressure from cerebellopontine angle tumor creates pressure on the opposite center for horizontal gaze (PPRF), producing eye to deviate opposite to the side of the lesion (fast phase) followed by cortical correction (slow phase) towards the side of lesion.
  - ❖ Associated signs may be due to involvement of other cranial nerves involvement.

Vertical nystagmus: It consists of (Fig. 11.212):
- Upbeat nystagmus (UBT)
  - ❖ It is usually worse in upward gaze (Alexander's law)
  - ❖ It does not increase on lateral gaze
  - ❖ Convergence may increase or decrease the nystagmus or convert the UBT to DBN
  - ❖ Damage to ventral tegmental pathways linking superior VN to superior rectus and inferior oblique subnuclei making the eye to glide down—resulting UBN
  - ❖ The causes are—lesion in pontomedullary junction and superior vermis.
- Downbeat nystagmus
  - ❖ It is usually worse in downward gaze (Alexander's law).
  - ❖ On upward gaze nystagmus will be decreased or disappear completely.

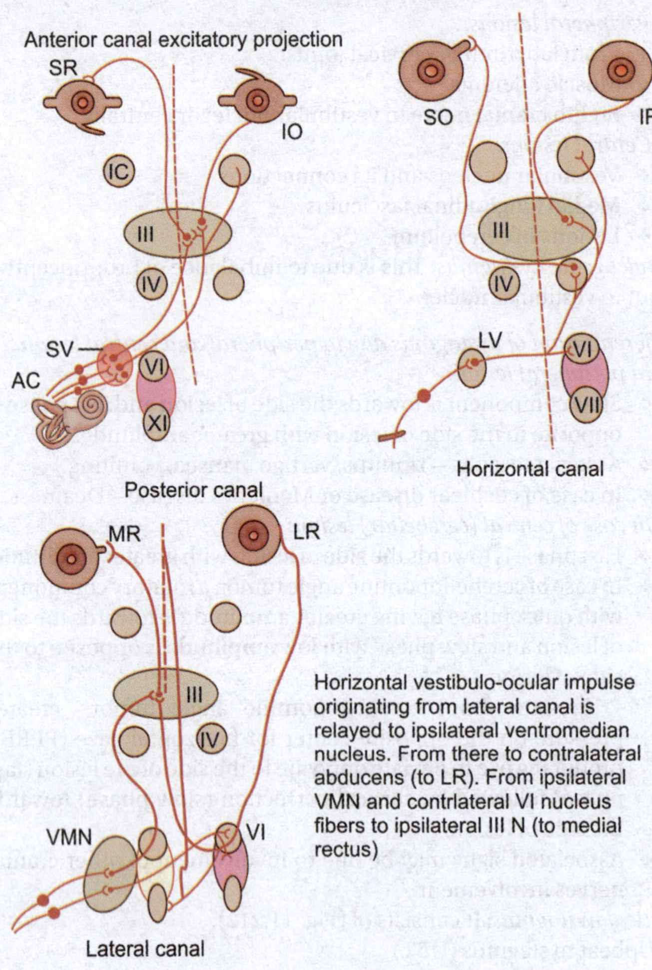

FIG. 11.212　Pathways of myotasis (vestibular)

- ❖ Convergence may increase or decrease the nystagmus or convert DBN to UBN.
- ❖ It may be disjunctive—in one eye, it is more vertical and in other eye it may be torsional.
- ❖ *Causes:*
  - Corticomedullary junction disease
  - Midline medullary lesion
  - Posterior midline cerebellar lesion
  - Diffuse cerebellar disease
  - Olivopontocerebellar atrophy.

- *Vertical:* Combination of up and down beat nystagmus. This may occur in:
  - ❖ Multiple sclerosis
  - ❖ Syringobulbia
  - ❖ Vertebral artery disease
  - ❖ Encephalitis
  - ❖ Basilar invagination with chiari malformation.

Drugs Producing Vertical Nystagmus

- Barbiturates
- Convulsants
- Benzodiazepines.

Rotatory Nystagmus

- In this case, examiner fixes a small blood vessel on the conjunctiva and follow the rotatory component more easily.
- In acute case, it is transient and it occurs in peripheral disorders.
- In chronic case, lesion is in vestibular nuclei (inferior nuclei).
- All cases produce vertical nystagmus.

Seesaw Nystagmus

This consists of:
- In one eye, there is spontaneous upward movement with excyclotropia (rotation in counter clockwise)
- In other eye, there is spontaneous downward movement with encyclotropia (rotation in clockwise).

Lesion responsible is:
- Parasellar lesion
- Anterior third ventricle lesion.

Nystagmus Retractorius

This is characterized by continuous inward and outward movements of the eyes. This can be diagnosed by seeing subtle widening and narrowing of the palpebral fissures.

It can be observed by standing by the side of the patient.

Lesions responsible

- Cyst, glioma or hemorrhage in periaqueductal area.
- Spontaneous contraction of extraocular muscles simultaneously.

Convergent—Retraction Nystagmus

This is characterized by on upward gaze attempt; there are repetitive adducting saccades, which is usually accompanied by retraction of eyes inwards into the orbit.

Lesions
- Mesencephalic lesion involving pretectal region associated with vertical gaze abnormalities
- Midbrain tumor
- Pineal tumor
- Arnold-Chiari malformation
- Whipple disease
- Spasmus nútans.

Divergence Nystagmus

- Repetitive slow divergent movement followed by rapid return to primary position at regular intervals. This is rare class orders.
  Lesion: Coma from hepatic encephalopathy.
- Repetitive fast divergent movement followed by slow return to primary position at regular intervals.
  Lesion:
  - Hindbrain abnormalities
  - Arnold-Chiari malformation.

Oculomasticatory Myorhythmia

This is characterized by pendular vergence oscillation of the eyes associated with concurrent contraction of masticatory muscles.

When this is associated with involvement of nonfacial skeletal muscles—it is called oculofacial—skeletal myorhythmia.

This is characterized by smooth rhythmic convergence of eyes with a frequency of 1 Hz followed by divergence of eyes back to its primary position.

This is associated with rhythmic elevation and depression of mandible synchronizing with ocular movement.

Associated Phenomenon

- Paralysis of verticals gaze
- Progressive somnolence
- Intellectual deterioration.

Congenital Nystagmus

- It may occur in infancy, without any defecation
- It is idiopathic, occasionally familial
- It may be pendular or both pendular and jerky component, or may be vertical
- Jarky nystagmus has slow component, which exponentially increases as the eyes more towards the direction of slow phase
- *Causes*:
  - Lesions affecting visual afferent pathways

- ❖ Joubert's syndrome
- ❖ Chediak Higashi syndrome
- ❖ Paroxysmal disorder.

Latent Nystagmus

It is generally congenital, appears when one eye is covered, both eye developed jerky nystagmus, with slow phase directed towards the nose and quick phase directed towards the sides of fixation.

Head Shaking Nystagmus

This is characterized by development of nystagmus with head oscillation. It may be horizontal or vertical—downbeat or upbeat.

Lesions
- Diffuse cerebellar degeneration
- Focal could cerebellar stroke.

Epileptic Nystagmus

- Nystagmus is usually horizontal
- Epileptiform activity is ipsilateral or contralateral to the slow phase of nystagmus.

Gaze Evoked Nystagmus

Spontaneous binocular conjugate symmetric jerky nystagmus induced by—called gaze evoked nystagmus.

Causes
- Brainstem
- Cercbellar disease
- Drug-induced nystagmus
- Burn's nystagmus.

In gaze evoked nystagmus—velocity of slow component decreases exponentially as the eyes approach mid position.

In cerebellar disease (vestibulo cerebellar lesion) this type of nystagmus is more pronounced when the patient looks towards the lesion.

Brun's Nystagmus

Combination of ipsilateral large amplitude, low frequency nystagmus due to impaired gaze holding and contralateral small amplitude high frequency nystagmus due to vestibular impairment.

Rebound Nystagmus

When eyes are kept eccentric for some time, gaze evoked nystagmus reverse its direction so that slow component is directed centrifugally (centripetal nystagmus), it becomes obvious if the eyes are returned to central position (Rebound nystagmus). This is a reflection of attempting of brainstem or cerebellar mechanism to correct the centripetal drift of gate evoked nystagmus.

Lesions
- Brainstem lesion
- Cerebellar lesion.

Lid Nystagmus

This is evidenced by twitch of eyelids synchronous with fast phase of horizontal nystagmus to the lateral gaze.

Lesion: Lateral medullary disease.

EXAMINATION OF PATIENT IN COMA

Consciousness has two dimensions:
1. *Arousal:* Maintained by deep brainstem and medial thalamic structure.
2. *Cognition:* Maintained by cerebral cortex and important sub-cortical nuclei.

Lowering of Consciousness

- Stupor
- Hypersomnic
- Coma.

Clouding of Consciousness

- Delirium
- Confusion.

Anatomy of Fibers Responsible for Consciousness

- *Reticular activating system (RA)*—arises from:
  - ❖ Paramedian tegmentum of pons and midbrain
  - ❖ Receives fibers from ascending spinothalamic tract
  - ❖ Sends projection fibers—bilaterally to cerebral cortex.

  Fibers of RAS are:
  - ❖ Cholinergic
  - ❖ Adrenergic
  - ❖ Serotonergic
  - ❖ Dopaminergic
  - ❖ Histaminergic.
- *Hypothalamus:* It is important for consciousness—stimulation produces arousal.
- *Thalamic nuclei involves:* Paramedian, parafascicular, dorsomedial, centromedian, intralaminar nuclei (have both cholinergic and GABA minergic cells that regulate activity).

Lesions Responsible for Coma

- Since at cortical level, these are bilateral presentation—damage to one cerebral cortex does not produce unconsciousness. So if, cortical level is involved it must be:
  - ❖ Bilateral—as in case of metabolic cause.
  - ❖ If one cerebral cortex is already involved by previous lesion.
  - ❖ Destructive large lesion is large enough to produce compression of contralateral cerebral hemisphere.

- *In case of brainstem lesion:*
  - ❖ Vascular—involving bilaterally medulla
  - ❖ Trauma
  - ❖ Destruction of dorsal pons by vascular lesion—basilar artery stroke.
    Pressure in periaquiductal gray matter in midbrain.
- *Thalamic nuclei:*
  - ❖ Intralaminar nuclear lesion (acute hemorrhage)
  - ❖ Lesions involving antroventral and dorsomedial nucleus.

Rapidity of Lesion

- Acute lesions (vascular, hemorrhage in tumor, trauma) produce loss of consciousness because brain does not have time to accommodate the new increase. Because there is rapid increase in intracranial pressure.
- Chronic, small lesion may not produce coma at onset only if it is progressively increase in size it may produce unconsciousness.

Mode of Onset of Unconsciousness

It may be acute:
- Due to cardiac arrhythmia, respiratory cause.
- *Neurologic:*
  - ❖ Massive cerebral embolism
  - ❖ Seizures
  - ❖ Intracranial hemorrhage—massive
  - ❖ Subarachnoid hemorrhage—increased blood in third ventricle producing cardiac arrhythmia
  - ❖ Obstruction to third ventricle by intraventricular colloid cyst or tumor producing sudden loss of consciousness by change of position which increases intracranial pressure and internal hydrocephalus.
  - ❖ Carotid artery occlusion.

Vomiting—may occur—in case of unconsciousness
- In case of neurologic cause, vomiting occurs only once because:
  Increased ICP—buffered by over breathing
  ↓
  Produce cerebral vasoconstriction
  ↓
  Decrease in cerebral blood flow
  ↓
  Displacement of spinal fluid into spinal subarachnoid space
  ↓
  Collapse and shift of ventricles
  ↓

Shift of brain cranial vault

↓

Decrease in vomiting

- If there is repeated vomiting—obstruction in upper gastrointestinal tract.
- Vomiting out of proportion to dizziness—brainstem tumor.
- Insidious onset of coma—due to progressively increasing size of tumor.

Premonitory Symptoms in Case of Coma

- *No aura with loss of consciousness*
  - ❖ Cardiac arrhythmia (Mobiz type 1 block, prolonged QT interval).
  - ❖ Rupture of anterior communicating artery aneurysm into third ventricle—producing unconsciousness and death secondary to cardiac arrhythmia.
- Headache, vomiting, lethargy—due to intracranial tumor.
- Associated dizziness ataxia—cerebellar lesion.
- Systemic symptoms—anorexia, weight loss—HIV infection, metastasis.
- Severe depression—drug overdose—in middle-aged person.
- *HIV positive patients*
  - ❖ If there is signs of meningitis—*Cryptococcus*, syphilis, tuberculosis or deep fungal infections.
  - ❖ Signs of basal ganglia involvement in CT scan of brain or basal meningitis or stroke—*Cryptococcus* infection syphilitic infection.
  - ❖ Small stroke with internuclear ophthalmoplegia—mucormycosis.
  - ❖ Lung abscess—aspergillosis.
- *In case of alcoholism:*
  - ❖ Subdual hematoma—progressive increase in unconsciousness from gradual increases in collection of blood in case of subdural hematomas.
  - ❖ Trauma—may occur in patient with or without alcoholism and in case of elderly—due to rupture of dural bridging veins producing unconsciousness.
- Drug-induced (1) coumarin anticoagulant, warfarin, heparin.
- *Nondrug-induced Hematological*
  - ❖ Coagulopathy
  - ❖ Leukemic conditions.
- Raccoon eyes. Battle's sign (discoloration of mastoid)—basilar skill fracture.

- Epidural hematoma—this is 3 hours disease—triphasic course—loss of consciousness then lucid interval followed by increase in unconsciousness, then decortications and decerebration. In CT scan of brain—collection of blood on the convexity of cerebral hemisphere as convex pattern.
- Sagittal sinus thrombosis—dehydration and obstratic cause, hypercoagulable state producing thrombosis.

    Magnetic resonance venous imaging—produces direct evaluation of sinus.

There are the following levels of consciousness:

- *Lethargy:* It is an indicator of future dangerous state of intracranial mass lesion. Patient is slow in process, patient is sleepy. When the patient is being stimulated, he will be completely alert—he can perform simple command, but cannot perform complex command like calculation, fail to perform "face to hand" test.

    If stimulation is withdrawn, patient becomes again unconscious.

    The causes are:
    - ❖ Drug intoxication
    - ❖ Metabolic cause
    - ❖ Early midbrain pressure against tentorium.
- *Obtundation:* External stimulation can arouse the patient to a state of consciousness—during which—the patient can follow command poorly, cannot perform complex actions. Patient will revert to prior stage if stimulation will be ceased

    Eyes will be below the level of horizontal if MLF fibers responsible for upward gaze will be damaged. Pupillary reflexes will be maintained.

    Causes are:
    - ❖ Drug intoxication
    - ❖ Metabolic disease
    - ❖ Compression of upper brainstem.
- *Stupor:* Vigorous stimulation may produce only growing sound of the patient, but response is slow and inadequate.

    Eyes level will be below the horizontal line.

    Patient will lose all defensive maneuvers to avoid painful stimulus, patient is oblivious of the surroundings, and he will fall back into stupors state as soon as the stimulation will be withdrawn.
- *Coma:* Pupillary, corneal and swallowing reflexes will be lost. No voluntary movement, any sleep wake cycles. Glasgow level of coma can identify the level according to verbal, motor response, degree of eye opening.

Specific State of Level of Consciousness

- *Confusion and disorientation*
  - ❖ Patient is fully alert.
  - ❖ He is not aware of his present condition.
  - ❖ Patient has lost the orientation in person, place and time.
- *Delirium*
  - ❖ Patient is usually active, gesticulate, and speak incoherently
  - ❖ Patient may hallucinate
  - ❖ Will be out of touch.

  Causes may be:
  - ❖ Alcohol intoxication
  - ❖ Infection
  - ❖ Toxic states.

  Delirium tremens—due to alcohol withdrawal—produces hallucination—like green insects attack him.

  There may be associated autonomic dysfunction.

  Tachycardia, hyperhydrosis, papillary dilation.
- *Catatonia*
  - ❖ Patient will be immobile, lies mute, unresponsive.
  - ❖ He is unaware of his surroundings.
  - ❖ He has plastic rigidity.

    Lesion:
  - ❖ Frontal lobe lesion.
  - ❖ Hypothalamic lesions.
- *Akinetic mutism*
  - ❖ Patient is motionless and speechless but awake.
  - ❖ Patient's eye can follow the examiner.
  - ❖ Patient is amnesic, normal sleep wake cycle.

  Lesion:
  - ❖ Lesion around the third ventricle.
  - ❖ Involvement in reticular formation in midbrain.
- *Abulia:* Patient initiates nothing, only says "yes" or "no" on interrogation.

  Lesions: Subfrontal lesion due to rupture and repair of anterior communicating artery aneurysm.
- *Locked-in syndrome*
  - ❖ Patient is mute and motionless but remains awake and alert of self, perceives stimulus.
  - ❖ Horizontal eye movement is lost, but vertical eye movement is possible.

    Lesions: Involvement of paramedian pontine reticular formation.

Persistent vegetative state: It can be defined as vegetative state, persists for 1 month after the acute traumatic or nontraumatic brain injury or last for more than 1 month in patient with degenerative or metabolic disorders.

Recovery from nontraumatic persistent vegetative state after 3 months is rare.

Vegetative state: This state can be defined as chronic neurologic conditions characterized by:

- Lack of awareness of self and external stimuli, accompanied by sleep wake cycles.
- Preservation of vital function, e.g. cardiac function, respiratory function, blood pressure.
- Lack of language comprehension.
- Bladder and bowel incontinence.
- Preservation of spinal reflexes and cranial nerves.

General Physical Examination in Coma

Respirations

- *Breath odor*
  - ❖ Acetone—diabetic ketoacidosis
  - ❖ Uriniferous—renal failure
  - ❖ Mousy odor—fetor hepaticus—hepatic failure
  - ❖ Garlic odor—arsenic poisoning
  - ❖ Household gas—carbon monoxide poisoning.
- *Ventilation*
  - ❖ *Hypoventilation*
    - Sedative overdose
    - Myxedema.
  - ❖ *Hyperventilation*
    - Fever
    - DKA
    - Sepsis
    - Hypercapnia
    - Hypoxia
    - Pulmonary embolism
    - Drugs producing metabolic acidosis.
- *Breathing type (Figs 11.213 and 11.214):*
  - ❖ *Cheyne Stokes respiration*
    - Bilateral cerebral disease
    - Transtentorial herniation
    - Metabolic encephalopathy
    - Upper brainstem lesion.
  - ❖ *Cluster breathing*
    - Low pontine lesion
    - High medullary lesion.

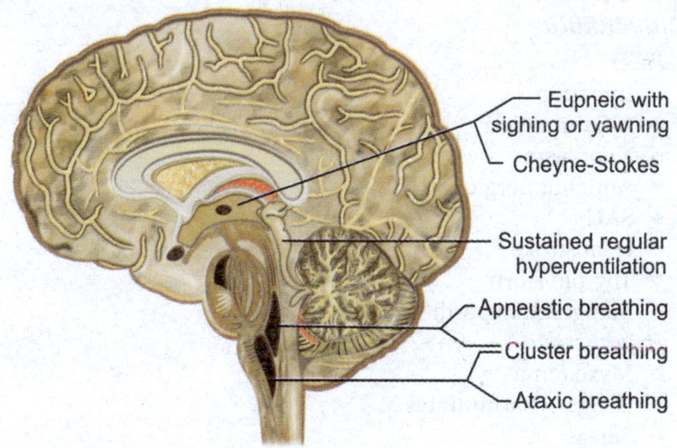

FIG. 11.213   Respiratory patterns in different levels of lesions of brain

1.		Eupneic with sighing or yawning
2.		Cheyne-Stoke
3.		Sustained regular hyperventilation
4.		Apneustic breathing
5.		Cluster breathing
6.		Ataxic breathing

FIG. 11.214   Different types of breathing

- ❖ *Apneustic breathing*
  - Lateral tegmentum of lower pons
  - Transtentorial herniation
  - Metabolic coma.
- ❖ Ataxic breathing—medullary lesion.
- ❖ Ordine's curse—medullary lesion (unilateral or bilateral).

Ondine's curse

- Loss of automatic breathing during sleep
- Respiratory pattern obviously absent in comatose patient.

Temperature

- *Fever*
  - ❖ Infection
  - ❖ Inflammation
  - ❖ Neoplasm
  - ❖ Anticholinergic
  - ❖ SAH
  - ❖ Heat stroke
  - ❖ Thyroid storm
  - ❖ Malignant hyperthermia.
- *Hypothermia*
  - ❖ Myxedema
  - ❖ Drugs → Barbiturates
  - ❖ Sepsis
  - ❖ Shock
  - ❖ Hypoglycemia.

Heart Rate

- *Bradycardia*
  - ❖ Cardiogenic—heat block
  - ❖ Increased intracranial pressure, intoxication.
- *Tachycardia*
  - ❖ Sepsis
  - ❖ Infection
  - ❖ Hypovolemia
  - ❖ Cocaine overdose.

Blood Pressure

- *Hypotension*
  - ❖ Cardiac—ischemia, myocardial infarction
  - ❖ Sepsis.
- *Hypertension*
  - ❖ Stroke
  - ❖ ICH
  - ❖ Hypertensive encephalopathy
  - ❖ Renal disease.

Head and Neck

- Scalp laceration, battle sign and raccoon eyes—trauma
- Stiff neck—SIH, meningitis, cerebellar tonsillar herniation.

Skin

- Needle stick— drug overdose
- Cyanosis—hypoxia, cardiac disease, cyanide

- Cherry red—carbon monoxide poisoning
- Jaundice—hepatic encephalopathy
- Anemia—hemorrhagic shock, syncope
- Petechiae—DIC, TTP, meningococcemia, drugs
- Purplish rash—meningococcemia
- Bruises—trauma, coagulation disorders
- Maculopapular rash—collagen vascular disease. Subacute bacterial endocarditis, toxic shock syndrome
- Sweating—septic shock, fever, hypoglycemia
- Flushing, erythema—polycythemia, alcoholism.

Heart

- Arrhythmia—cerebral embolism
- Murmur—cerebral embolism, SBE.

Lung

Pulmonary edema—acute lung injury. Anoxic encephalopathy, neurogenic pulmonary edema.

GI Tract

- Fecal incontinence—seizures, postictal seizures.
- Stool containing blood—hematochezia, melena.
- Hepatic encephalopathy—bleeding disorder.

Genitourinary

Urinary incontinence—seizures, cerebral cause—cerebral embolism.

Levels of responsiveness: It is wise to describe the patient's state of responsiveness—according a scale, Glasgow coma scale (GES)—according to eye opening, verbal response and motor response.

Glasgow Coma Scale

Eye Opening

- Open spontaneously - 4
- Open only to verbal stimulus - 3
- Only to pain - 2
- Never open. - 1

Best Verbal Response

- Oriented and converses - 5
- Converses, but disorientated, confused - 4

- Use inappropriate words - 3
- Makes incomprehensible sounds - 2
- No verbal response. - 1

Best Motor Response

- Obeys commands - 6
- Localize pain - 5
- Exhibits flexion withdrawal - 4
- Decorticate rigidity - 3
- Decerebrate rigidity - 2
- No motor response. - 1

Alert person with normal eye and motor response—score—15.

Profoundly comatose patient—score—3.

Stimuli applied to diagnose the level of consciousness in patient are painful but not so much, so that it can injure the patient. The following types of stimuli are:

- Supraorbital pressure
- Sternal rub
- Nail bed pressure.

Cranial Nerves

It is not possible to examine the cranial nerves in patient with altered consciousness. So in that case, examinations of pupil and extraocular movements are essential for evaluation of the site of involvement (Fig. 11.215).

- *Bilateral diencephalic dysfunction (metabolic coma):* Small bilateral pupil reactive to light (diencephalic pupil).
- Unilateral hypothalamic damage—myotic pupil and anhydrosis—ipsilateral to the side of lesion.
- Lesion in tectum or pretectal area—affecting posterior commissure:
  - ❖ Loss of light reflex
  - ❖ Midposition and midsize of pupil
  - ❖ Spontaneous oscillation in size of pupil (hippus)
  - ❖ Pupils become larger when neck is pinched (ciliospinal reflex).
- *Lesion in tegmentum of midbrain*—involving third nerve nucleus:
  - ❖ Irregular constriction of sphincter of iris producing unequal irregular pupil or displacement of pupil to one side (Midbrain corectopia).
  - ❖ Reaction to light—absent.
  - ❖ Loss of ciliospinal reflex.
- *Fascicular or peripheral third nerve lesions*
  - ❖ Unilateral or bilateral oval pupil

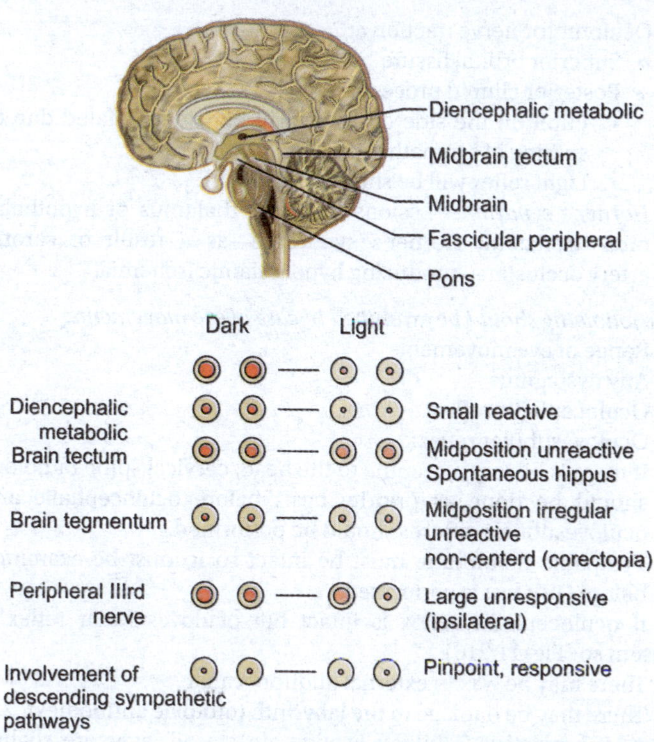

FIG. 11.215 Pupillary responses characteristic of lesions at different levels of brain

- ❖ Reaction to light absent. Oval pupil is due to nonuniform paresis or paralysis of pupillary sphincter with resultant over activity of pupillary dilator.
- *Pontine tegmental lesion (hemorrhage)*—with involvement of descending sympathetic pathways or parasympathetic irritation:
  - ❖ Pinpoint pupil
  - ❖ Reactive to light—this reaction to light is observed by applying magnifying glass.
- Lateral pontine, lateral medullary and ventrolateral cervical cord paralysis—Ipsilateral Horner's syndrome
- Oculomotor nerve compression by
  - ❖ Uncal herniation beneath the tentorial edge
  - ❖ Posterior cerebral artery
  - ❖ Hippocampal gyrus.

Oculomotor nerve traction at
- ❖ Superior orbital fissure
- ❖ Posterior clinoid process:
  - Pupil on the side of lesion will be widely dilated due to sparing of sympathetic fibers.
  - Light reflex will be sluggish or absent.
- *Horner's syndrome:* Lesions involving thalamus or hypothalamus—ipsilateral Horner's syndrome—as a result of carotid artery occlusion—producing hypothalamic ischemia.

The following should be examined in case of eye movements:
- Range of eye movements
- Any nystagmus
- Oculocephalic reflex
- Oculovestibular reflex
- If there is history of trauma to the head, cervical spine radiology should be done as priority basis before oculocephalic and oculovestibular reflexes should be performed.
- Tympanic membrane must be intact so it must be examined before OVR test is performed.

If oculocephalic reflex is intact but oculovestibular reflex is absent so (Fig. 11.216):
- There may be wax in external auditory canal.
- There may be damage to the labyrinth (ototoxic antibodies).
  - ❖ *If brainstem is intact:* Eyelids are closed, eyes are slightly divergent and drift slowly from side to side (roving movement).
  - ❖ Conjugate eye deviation away from paralyzed extremities—destructive frontal lesions.
  - ❖ Conjugate eye deviation towards paralyzed side—brainstem lesion.
  - ❖ Conjugate gaze deviation with jerky nystagmus—it is due to seizure activity due to frontal eye field lesion—side will be the patient looking away from.
  - ❖ *Ping-Pong gaze:* Roving of eyes from one extreme position to other extreme position in horizontal gaze in an oscillating cycle of 2.5 to 8 seconds: (i) Bilateral cerebral lesion, (ii) Hemorrhage in posterior fossa, (iii) Basal ganglia infarction, (iv) Hydrocephalus, and (v) Overdose of MAO inhibitor.
  - ❖ *Repetitive divergence:* In it, primary position of eye is midposition or slight divergent at rest. Then they slowly fully deviated for a brief period then rapidly return to primer position, then repeating this in cycles—hepatic encephalopathy.

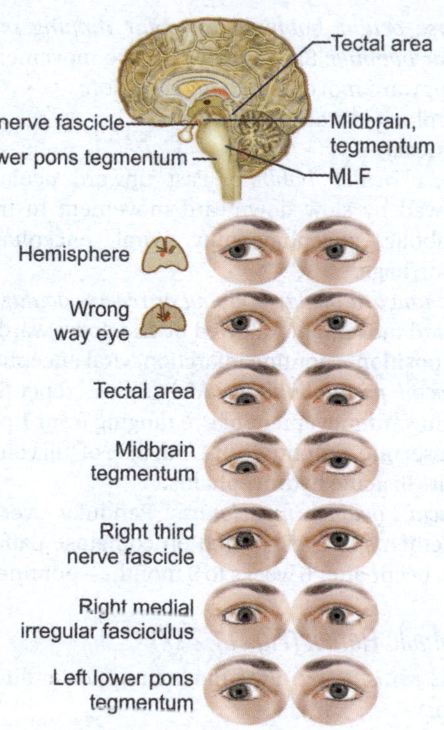

FIG. 11.216   Different eye movements

- ❖ Vertical gaze deviation—Brainstem disease.
  - Sustained downward gaze and deficit in upward gaze — Lesion in upper midbrain and caudal thalamus.
  - Downward gaze deviation—Hepatic encephalopathy.
  - Pontine lesion—Disconjugate rotatory and vertical movement—one eye raises and intorts, other eye falls and extorts.
- ❖ *Electrographic status epilepticus:* Brisk, small amplitude, mainly vertical eye movements—detectable on passive lid elevation—due to anoxia.
- ❖ *Ocular bobbing:* Brisk bilateral downward movement of eyes with slow return to mid position. Cold caloric test increases ocular bobbing:
  - Pontine infarction or hemorrhage
  - Extra-axial fossa masses
  - Diffuse encephalopathy. Unilateral ocular bobbing—it may occur in coexistent unilateral fascicular oculomotor nerve palsy.

- ❖ *Inverse ocular bobbing or ocular dipping or fast upward ocular bobbing:* Slow downward eye movement followed by fast upward movement to mid position:
  - Prolonged status epilepticus
  - Anoxia
- ❖ *Reverse ocular bobbing:* Fast upward ocular movements followed by slow downward movement to mid position—metabolic encephalopathy, viral encephalitis, pontine hemorrhage.
- ❖ *Slow upward ocular bobbing or reverse ocular dipping:* Slow upward movement followed by fast down ward movement to mid position—pontine infarction, viral encephalopathy.
- ❖ *Pretectal pseudobobbing:* Arrhythmic, repetitive downward and inward movement of eye ranging from 1 per 3 second to 2 per second, amplitude of 1/5th to ½ of full voluntary range—occurs in acute hydrocephalus.
- ❖ *Vertical ocular myoclonus:* Pendular vertical isolated movements of eyes—noted on comatose patient, frequency 2 Hz, occur after 6 weeks to 9 months—pontine lesion.

Oculocephalic Reflex (Fig. 11.217)

- *If brainstem is intact:* Eyes move in opposite direction of head rotation.

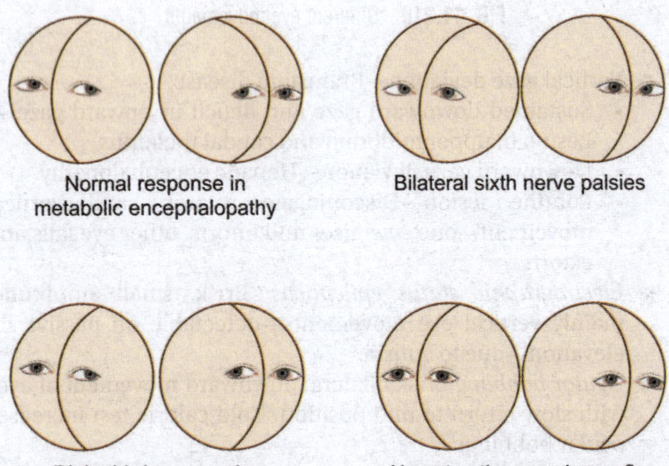

FIG. 11.217   Oculocephalic responses in comatose patient—when brainstem is intact

- *Bilateral sixth nerve palsies:* It is due to paralysis of lateral rectus of both the eyes, in any side of head movement—eyes never go to extreme position in lateral gaze.
- Bilateral third nerve palsies.

Oculovestibular Reflex

Test should be done with cold water and warm water.

- In response to cold water stimulation in coma, tonic deviation of the eyes towards the side of irrigated ear. Warm water response produces opposite effect.
- *Brainstem lesion*—It produces abnormal response to cold.
- *In coma, absent response to cold suggests:*
  - ❖ Sedative intoxication
  - ❖ Structural brainstem lesion.

Position of Eyelid

Watch whether eyes are open or closed, width of palpebral fissure of two sides.

- In comatose patient if eyelids are closed—lower pons is still functioning.
- Asymmetry of palpebral fissure—it indicates upper facial weakness—on the side of width fissure.
- If eyes are completely closed—examiner gently lift the upper eyelids and leave it and watches the rate at which the eyes close again.

    Unilateral orbicularis oculi paresis produces more leisurely closure of the lids.

- In profound weakness, patient may lie with partially closed eyes.
- In deep sleep, patient may lie with partially closed eyes.
- In psychogenic coma, patient may keep the eye tightly closed and resists opening them.

Other Cranial Nerve Examination

- On giving pressure to supraorbital area or sternal area nasolabial furrow will be contracting—since it is very sensitive.
- Pressure to superior orbital fissure—produce facial grimacing of both sides. In case of suspected unilateral weakness, there may be asymmetry of response—no contraction on the side of weakness.
- Blink response to loud noise—crudely asses the auditory function.
- In nonorganic unresponsiveness patient usually resists when examiner tries to open his mouth.
- Presence of gag reflex –palate should rise in midline.

Ophthalmoscopic Examination

- *Papilledema:* Sign of raised intracranial pressure.
- *Normal spontaneous venous pulsation:* It indicates normal intracranial pressure.
- *Subhyaloid hemorrhage:* It occurs in subarachnoid hemorrhage.
- *Roth spot:* Subacute bacterial endocarditis.
- Arteriovenous nipping, cold and hard exudates, flame shaped hemorrhage: Systemic disease.

Examination of Motor Response

- *If paralysis is of sudden onset:*
  - ❖ *Face:*
    - Paralyzed side of the body is flaccid
    - Palpebral fissure will be widened
    - Nasolabial furrow will be shallow
    - Angle of the mouth droop on one side with saliva dribbling
    - Refraction of cheek on inspiration and expiration.
  - ❖ *Upper limb:* If both the arms are lifted and then allowed to fall from a distance on the bed—the paralyzed limb will fall like a flail. Unanalyzed limb will either fall vary slowly to avoid injury or held the arm in same position.
  - ❖ *Lower limb:* If both the lower limbs are lifted to a distance from the bed, and then allowed the limbs to fall on the bed. Paralyzed limb will fall like a log of wood with thigh abducted and externally rotated at hip and extended at knee and at ankle joint.
- *Pinching the skin on unparalyzed side:* The limbs show withdrawal movement.

Pinching the skin on paralyzed side. There is no movement on paralyzed limbs except facial grimacing.

Sensory Examination

If the patient is comatose, he only can respond to painful stimulus by reflex withdrawal of the body or parts of the body away from the stimulus.

So painful stimulus can differential the paralyzed side or unparalyzed side.

Reflexes

- *Plantar response:* It should be tested—it may be extensor (paralyzed UMN lesion) or flexor (normal) or absent (shock or LMN type lesion).
- *Deep tendon reflexes:* It may be exaggerated (UMN) or absent (shock stage or LMN).

- Clonus may be present.
- *Frontal release sign*: (Forced grasping, palmomental reflex, suck reflex, snout response)—it may be present in patient with abnormal mental status.

Meningeal Sign

- *Neck rigidity:* Flex the neck of patient and rotate it from side to side—to detect nuchal rigidity.
- *Kernig sign, Brudzinski sign:* It may be absent in comatose patient in SAH, it requires several hours to develop meningeal signs.

Myoclonus

It is rapid asymmetric movement of extremity or joints. It can be divided into followings:
- Corticoreticular—in which cortical motor spikes precedes the movement
- Brainstem (nucleus gigantocellularis)
- Segmental (origin of spinal cord).

Decerebrate Attack

It may occur spontaneously or with stimulation like tracheostomy. This attack may be reversible or irreversible.

Irreversible causes
- Brainstem compression from transtentorial herniation
- Basilar artery occlusion.

Reversible causes
- Anoxia
- Phenobarbital intoxication
- Hepatic coma.

MISCELLANEOUS NEUROLOGICAL SIGNS

■ Signs of Meningeal Irritation

Meningitis: It means inflammation of meninges. Meningismus: It refers to presence of nuchal rigidity and other clinical signs of meningeal inflammation, which may occur due to:

- Infection
- Foreign body in subarachnoid space (blood).

Meningism can be described as nuchal rigidity without any sign of meningeal inflammation. It occurs in systemic infection particularly in children.

■ Nuchal Rigidity (Fig. 11.218)

Patient is unable to touch his chin to chest, but there is no difficulty in extension of neck. In extreme condition—retraction of neck into a position of opisthotonos. Body assumes a position of Wrestler's bridge or arc de circle position.

Rigidity may be absent in meningitis in severe fulminant or terminal, condition.

These are other condition responsible for neck rigidity:

- Cervical spondylosis
- Osteoarthritis of cervical spine
- Cervical lymphadenopathy
- Retropharyngeal abscess
- Neck trauma

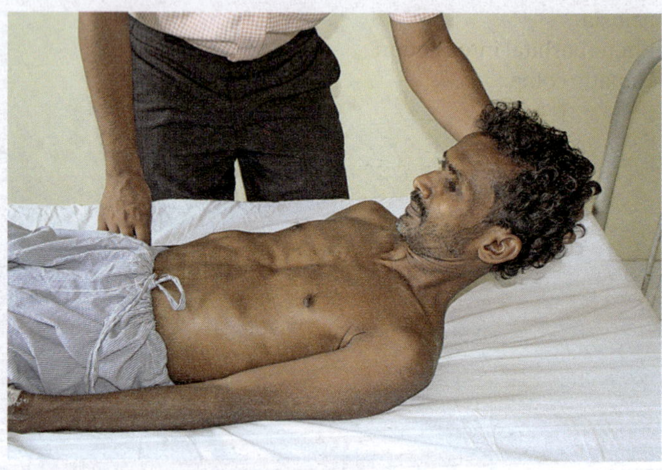

FIG. 11.218 Neck rigidity

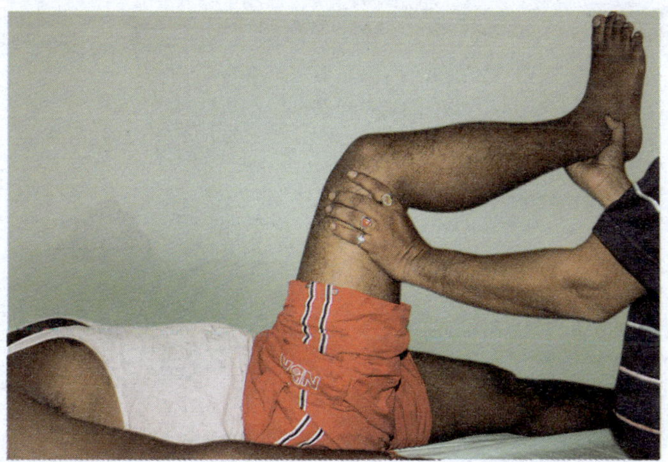

FIG. 11.219   Kernig's sign

- Extrapyramidal disorder
- Progressive supranuclear palsy
- Cerebellar tonsillar herniation.

Kernig's Sign (Fig. 11.219)

Method: Flex the hip and knee at 90°. Then try to extend the knee —
when the knee will be extended to more than 135° (maintain the hip
flexed at 90°)—there will be:

- Pain
- Resistance
- Inability to fully extend the knee.

The positive kernig sign will be present in:

- Meningitis
- Lumbosacral radiculopathy.

The difference between the above two areas:

In meningitis—the positive Kernig's sign will be bilateral. In
radiculopathy the positive Kernig's sign will be unilateral.

Brudzinski's Neck Sign (Fig. 11.220)

Method: Place one hand under the patient's head; flex the mean
while holding down the chest with other hand.
Result: It produces flexion of hips and knees bilaterally.
In severe meningitis: It is not possible to hold the chest down and the
patient may be pulled into sitting position.

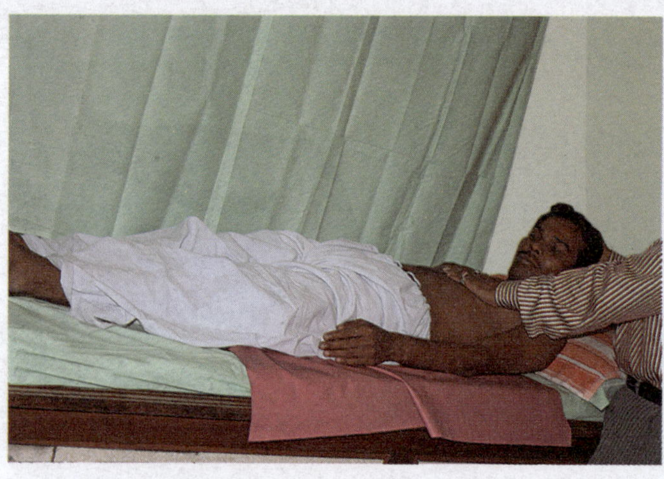

FIG. 11.220   Brudzinski's neck sign

In few cases there may be extension of hallux and fanning of the toes and flexion of arm.

Other meningeal signs: Patient sits on the bed, hand placed far behind, head thrown back, hip and knee flexed and back arched (Tripod sign).

Tetany

The clinical manifestations are:

- Carpopedal spasm with tonic contraction of muscles of wrist, hands, fingers, feet and toes.
- Sensory hyperexcitability of peripheral neurons system.

Produces: Paresthesia of hands and feet and perioral region.

Latent tetany can be revealed by allowing the patient to hyperventilate for few minutes.

Severe tetany can produce—stridor, seizure, laryngospasm and may produce respiratory arrest.

Chvostek's Sign (Fig. 11.221)

Tapping over the facial never at two points:

1. Just below the zygomatic process of temporal bone in front of the ear.
2. Mid position between zygomatic arch and angle of the mouth.

Signal

- *In minimal case:* Slight twitch of upper lip and angle of the mouth.

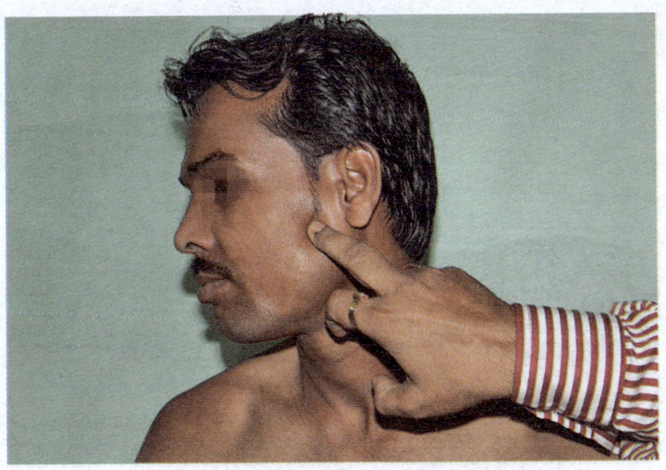

FIG. 11.221 Chvostek's sign

- *In moderate case:* Contraction of alar nasi and entire corner of mouth.
- *In severe case:* Contraction of muscles of forehead, eyelid, cheek. All are the results of hyperexcitabilities of motor nerves.

Trousseau's Signs (Fig. 11.222)

Backgrounds: Ischemia of peripheral nerve produces hyperexcitability and spontaneous discharges.

Compression of the arm can be done by:

- Tourniquet
- Manual pressure
- Sphygmomanometer cuff.

Effect: Distal paresthesias—progressing centripetally followed by:

- Twitching of the fingers, finally
- Contraction of the muscles of fingers—hand, thumb strongly adducted, finger stiffened and flexed at metacarpophalangeal joints forming a cone clustered around the thumb (obstetrician).

Modification of the above method

- Inflate the sphygmomanometer cuff around arm and keep it for 10 minutes and then removes it
- Allow the patient to hyperventilate.

Effect: Titanic spasm occurs on the affected arm.

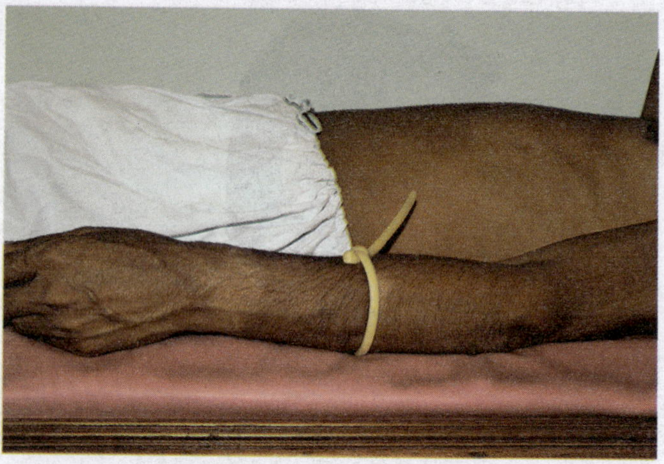

FIG. 11.222 Trousseau's sign

Cervical Radiculopathy

- Radiation of pain on coughing, sneezing and straining—(Dejerine sign).
- Increased pain on shoulder—nonradicular pathology.
- Relieve of pain by resting the hand on the top of head (hand on head sign)—retrieves pain—diagnostic of cervical radiculopathy (CR) (hand on head sign).

Physical Sign

The following assessments are required:
- Range of motion of neck and arms
- Root compression signs
- Detailed examination of muscle strength and reflexes
- Sensory examination
- Areas of muscle spasm or trigger points.

Method of Examinations (Figs 11.223 to 11.226)

Ask the patient to:
- Put his chin on the chest
- Put his chin and ear on both shoulders
- Hyperextend the head in full extension with tilting on both sides.

All the above methods decrease the size of the lumen:
- Putting the ear to the shoulder of affected side—produces pain—suggest radiculopathy.

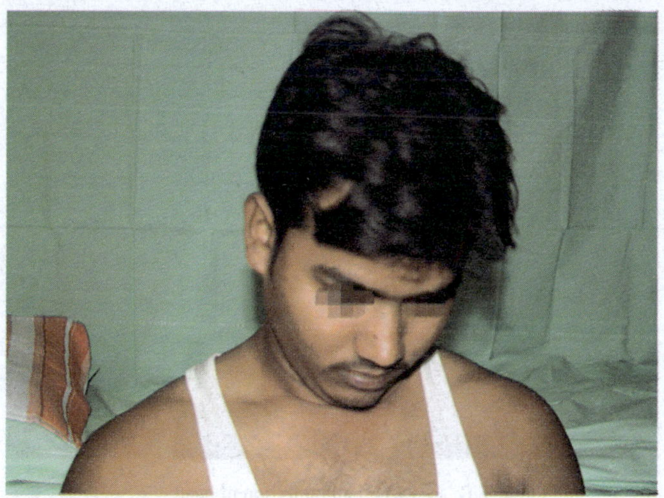

FIG. 11.223   Flexion of head

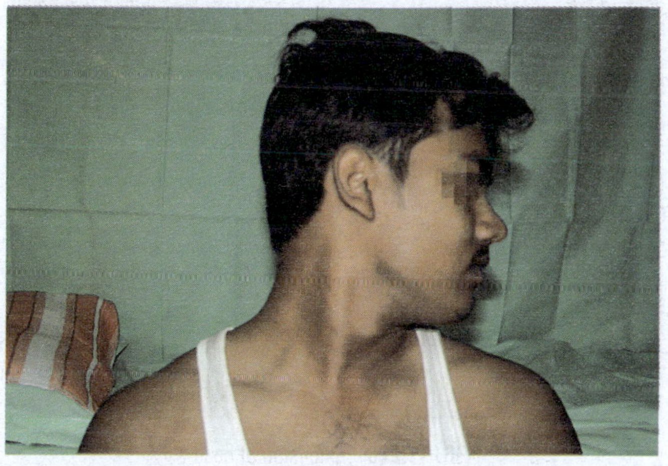

FIG. 11.224   Lateral rotation of head

- Leaning and turning away from the symptomatic side suggest myofacial pain.
- Full extension of head with tilting towards symptomatic side—suggests CR (Spurling sign).

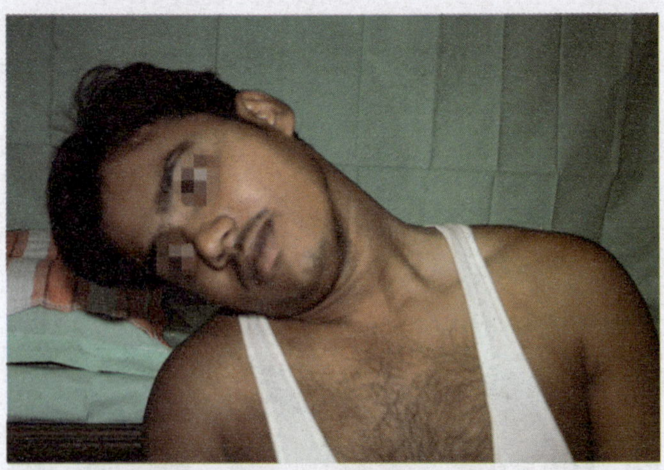

FIG. 11.225 Lateral flexion of head

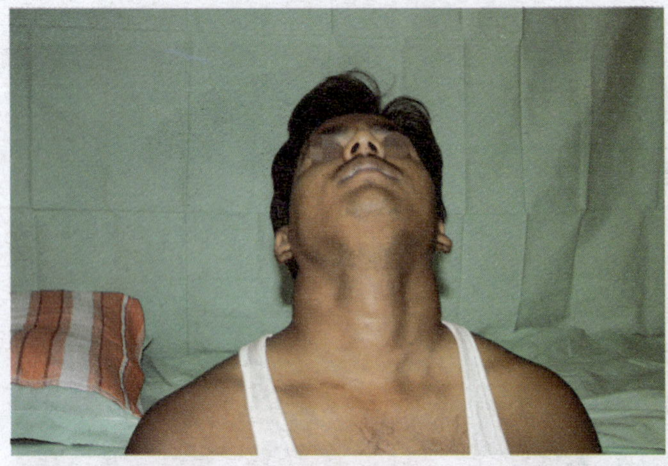

FIG. 11.226 Extension of head

- Valsalva maneuvers—produces cervical radicular pain.
- Light digital compression on jugular vein—until face is flushed and patient is uncomfortable produces:
  - ❖ Radicular pain in shoulders, arm pectoral and scapular region
  - ❖ Radiating paresthesia on arm or hand (Viets signs).

- Blood pressure calf around patient's neck produces
  Jugular venous compression and occlusion (Naffziger sign)
  ↓
  Engorgement of epidural reins
  ↓
  Increased cerebrospinal fluid reservoirs

In case of luminal narrowing | In normal person
(foraminal narrowing) | It is harmless
↓
Nerve root pressure exists
↓
Acute development of symptoms
Viet's sign/Naffziger sign—specific but not very sensitive

- Upward traction of neck with slight flexion of neck—cervical distraction tests
- Decreased pain with shoulder adduction—shoulder abduction relief test.
  - ❖ Flexion of the neck may cause Lhermitte sign—CR.

Lumbosacral Radiculopathy

Straight Leg Rising Sign (Fig. 11.227)

It is mainstay of diagnosis of lumbosacral radiculopathy.
Method: Raise the lower limb (symptomatic) with knee extended slowly during SLR. Tension will be transmitted to nerve roots. So, there may be following results obtained.

- Between 30 and 70°—pain occurs
- Pain less than 30°—nonorganic cause
- Pain in more than 70°—routine and nonsignificant.

There is various level of positivity

- Ipsilateral leg tightness —significant
- Pain in back— more significant
- Radiating pain in leg—most significant
- Rising the asymptomatic leg—it produces pain in symptomatic leg—crossed straight leg rising test. Fajersztajn sign
- In severe condition, SLR causes numbness and paresthesia.

There is various modification of SLR

- SLR in the following position—thigh and leg in adducted position and internally rotated (Bonnet phenomenon)
- SLR can be aggravated by passive dorsiflexion of foot (Bragard sign) (Fig. 11.228)
- SLR can be aggravated by passive dorsiflexion of great toe (Sicardo sign) (Fig. 11.229)

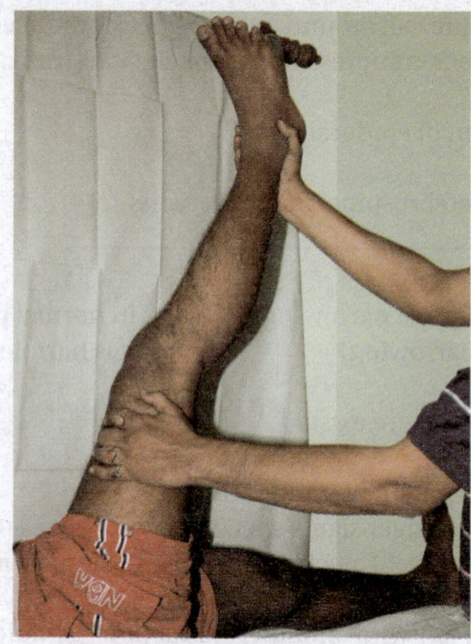

FIG. 11.227 Straight leg rising sign

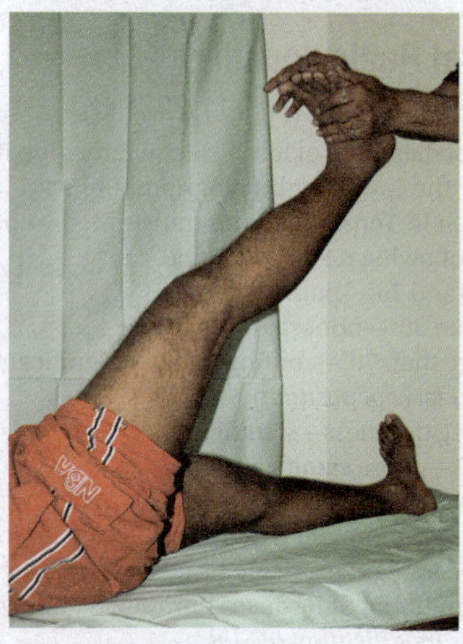

FIG. 11.228 Bragard sign

- A quick snap of sciatic nerve at popliteal fossa as stretch begins to cause pain (Bowstring sign or popliteal compression test) may cause (a) Pain in lumbar region in affected buttock, or radiating along sciatic nerve).

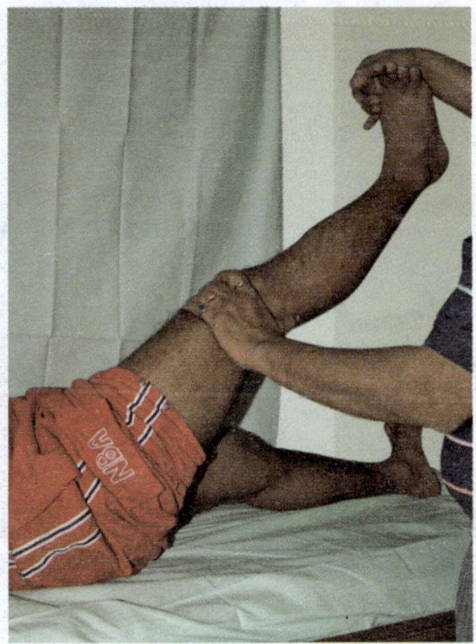

FIG. 11.229   Sicardo's sign

- Mere dorsiflexion of great toe or of the foot in extended leg with patient in supine passion.
- Flexing the thigh just short of that producing pain, then flexes the neck—that may produce acute exacerbation of pain—which would be brought about by further flexion of hip (Brudzinski or Hyndman sign).
- Patient lies in recumbent position with thigh extended passive flexion of neck produces severe pain.
- In sitting position, the patient is able to extend his knee one by one, but extension of both knees at the same time can produce severe pain (Bechterew test).
- *Reverse SLR (femoral stretch test):*
  - ❖ Ask the patient to be in prone position
  - ❖ Then knee is pulled into maximum flexion (Fig. 11.230A)
  - ❖ The examiner pulls the extended knee backward to extend the hip passively (Fig. 11.230B).

Result: Normally persons complain of quadriceps tightness. But in case of patient with CR there will be pain in the back or in the distribution of femoral nerve.

Abnormalities of Posture

- Normal lumbar lordosis will be lost due to spasm of involuntary muscles.

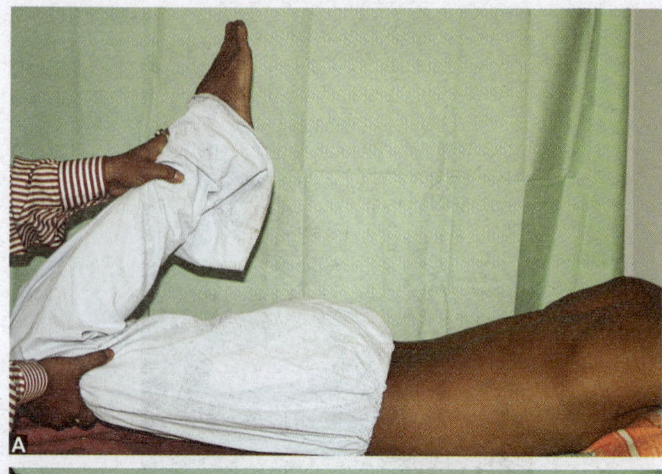

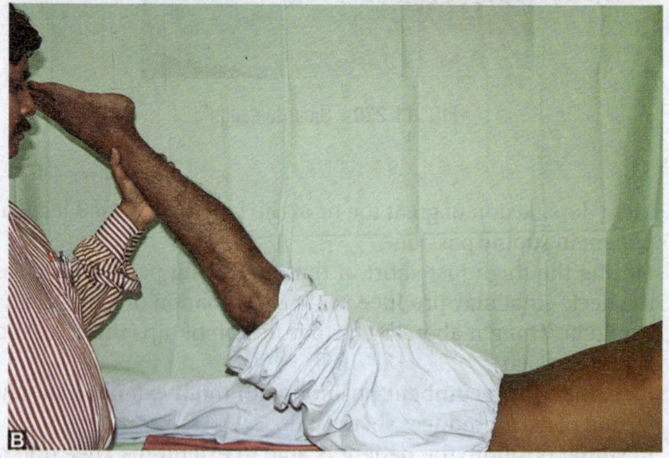

FIGS 11.230A AND B: Reverse straight leg rising (SLR) sign

- Lumbar scoliosis with compensatory thoracic scoliosis to opposite side.
- He attempts to bear weight mostly on the sound leg.
- With severe pain on sciatic nerve, he avoids full extensions of knee and dorsiflexion of foot, so the patients stand on the toes on the floor with knee in semiflexed position.
- Patient's steps will be small.
- In case of bending forward, the patient flexes the knee to avoid stretching of the nerve (Neri sign).
- While sitting, legs will be flexed at knee, rests his weight on opposite buttock.

- During rising from sitting position by supporting himself on unaffected side, bending forward, is placing his hand on the back of the affected side (Minor sign).

Spinsous process: Tenderness can be elicitated:
- Percussion over the spinous process.
- Tenderness just latest to the spinous process.
- With percussion hammer on or lateral to spinous process.
  Spasm of paravertebral muscles hamstring muscles and calf muscles.

Neurological examination including:
- *Power of lower extremity muscle groups*
  - ❖ Dorsiflexors of foot and toes
  - ❖ Everters of foot
  - ❖ Inverters of foot.
- *Trendelenburg position and sign:* Normally pelvis slants upwards towards unsupported leg.
  When Trendelenburg sign is positive—hip moves up and shoulder moves down on the weight bearing side and pelvis sags towards unsupported leg. This sign is positive in:
  - ❖ Weakness of hip abductors (L5 radiculopathy)
  - ❖ Hip dislocation
  - ❖ Fracture of femoral head
  - ❖ Coxa Vera.
- Atrophy and fasciculation to be tested
- Reflexes—knee reflex (L3 – L4), ankle reflex (S1).

Summary of diagnostic criteria for clinical diagnosis of brain death
Prerequisite: Brain death is the absence of clinical brain function when the proximate cause is known and demonstrably irreversible:
- Clinical or neuroimaging evidence of an acute CNS catastrophe.
- *Pupillary response:* Use of bright torch to confirm that pupil fail to respond.
- *Corneal response:*
  - ❖ Gentle application of cotton wool to the cornea—no response
  - ❖ Repeated application produce trauma to cornea.
- *Vestibulo-ocular reflex*
  - ❖ Tympanic membrane must be intact and not obscured by compacted wax.
  - ❖ Insert a soft rubber catheter into external auditory meatus and slowly inject 50 mL of ice cold water. Repeat the test in the other ear.
    There should be no ocular deviation.
- *Motor response in cranial nerve distribution:* Application of painful stimulus to glabella—no response

- *Gag response:* Stimulus to palate or passage of suction catheter into trachea—patient fails to show any response.
- *Respiratory reaction to hypercapnia*
  - ❖ Administer combination of 95% O_2 and 5% CO_2 via respirator – until pCO_2 has risen to 40 mm Hg.
  - ❖ Disconnect the respirator; administer 100% O_2 through a catheter at around 6 liter/minute.
  - ❖ Observe any response occurs when the pCO_2 exceeds 50 mm Hg.

12
CHAPTER
Thyroid Gland

◼ Relation of Thyroid Lobe to the other Neck Structure

Thyroid gland (Fig. 12.1) has two parts:
1. Central isthmus
2. Peripheral two lobes.

Isthmus present in midline just below the cricoid cartilage.

Each lobe extends from isthmus posteriorly around trachea and esophagus, then it ascends backwards and upwards like one hand of 'V'.

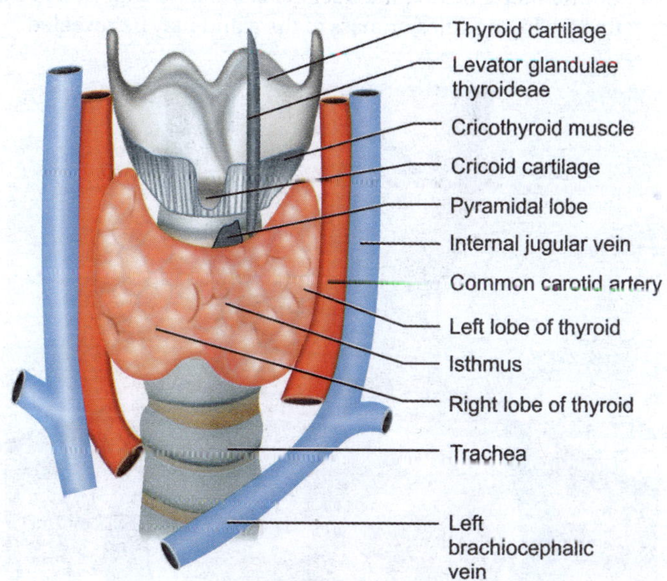

FIG. 12.1 Thyroid gland

Each lobe is 2–3 cm long, lower margin ends 2 cm above the clavicle (5th to 6th tracheal ring).

Upper margin extends upwards in the midline of thyroid cartilage.

Both the lobes are covered with sternocleidomastoid muscles. Isthmus is covered by fascia—it is continuous with pretracheal fascia—hence during deglutition isthmus moves with trachea.

Pyramidal Lobe

It is an upward extension of left lobe of thyroid-normally cannot be palpated, can be detected only in 10–15 percent of nontoxic goiter.

Inspection for Thyroid

In two positions thyroid gland can be inspected:
1. *In front view of the extended neck position (Fig. 12.2):*
   * Ask the patient to sit neck extended to 10° backwards
   * Cervical muscles should be as relaxed as possible.

   The extension of neck is useful for following reasons:
   * It raises the trachea further from suprasternal notch so lower end of low placed thyroid isthmus can be visible
   * It tightens the skin overlying isthmus—helps in visualization
   * Contralateral flexing the neck relax the neck muscles so that underlying nodules or mass of the gland may be revealed.

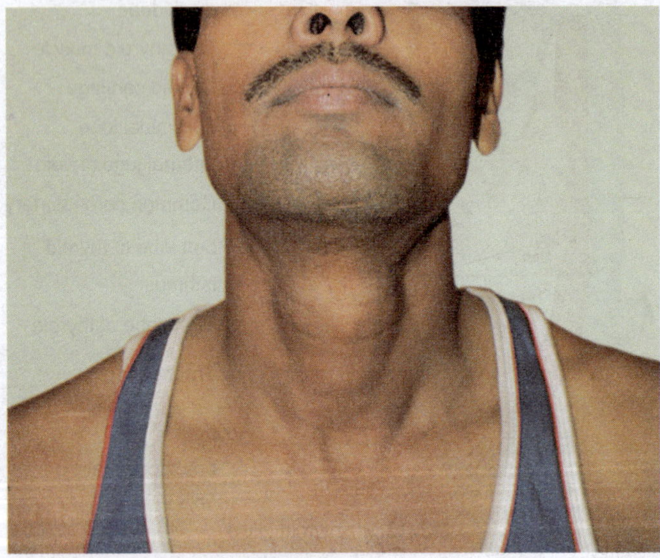

FIG. 12.2   Front view of the extended neck

Following things should be inspected:

- ❖ Midline 2–3 cm above the clavicle should be inspected for isthmus
- ❖ Ask the patient to swallow, to see any swelling that can move upwards and down wards with deglutition
- ❖ Look for superior margin of thyroid lobe
- ❖ Look for enlargement of pyramidal lobe, since normally this lobe cannot be palpated
- ❖ Cross-transillumination test to be done to see the consistency of the nodule in thyroid.

2. *From lateral view of the extended neck (Fig. 12.3):* Observe any swelling present in between cricoid cartilage and suprasternal notch.

Goiter can be ruled out if the thyroid gland is not visible in lateral view and in extended neck position.

Swallowing is important during thyroid gland inspection for following reasons:

- It increases the sensitivity of inspection
- It raises the lower margin of thyroid gland, so that inspection of this gland is more accessible
- During swallowing, the thyroid nodule or mass can be glided under the examiner's hand, improving tactile discrimination

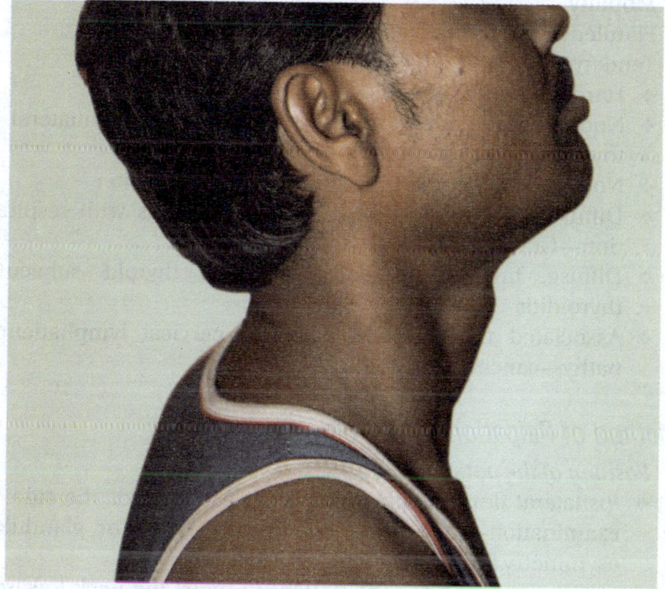

FIG. 12.3   Lateral view of the extended neck

- Swallowing or deglutition can raise the trachea and thyroid by 1.5 to 3.5 cm, this can help to confirm that the nodule is from thyroid gland
- Swallowing a glass of water is more important, because, the upward movement is proportional to amount of fluid to be swallowed.

Maranon's sign: It can be described as red sometimes itchy area of skin overlying thyroid in Graves' disease—described by Gregorio Maranon.

Palpation of Thyroid Gland

Average size of thyroid gland
- Lobes—2 cm wide, 4–5 cm long, 2.5 cm deep
- Isthmus—1.25–2 cm wide, <0.6 cm deep
  15–20 g weight thyroid gland is not palpable
  10–15 g thyroid gland is not detectable
  20–35 g thyroid is palpable.
  Thyroid size is largely determined by dietary iodine supplement.

During palpation the following things should be seen:
- Size
- Shape
- Consistency
- Symmetry
- Mobility
- Flatulence
- Tenderness
  - ❖ Hard nontender thyroid—thyroid cancer
  - ❖ Nodule—nontender, moves with respiration, unilateral—thyroid nodular goiter
  - ❖ Nodules may be multiple—multiple nodular goiter
  - ❖ Diffuse, fine, rubbery in consistency, moves with respiration—Graves' disease
  - ❖ Diffuse, fine tender enlargement of thyroid—subacute thyroiditis
  - ❖ Associated tracheal deviation and cervical lymphadenopathy—cancer.

Method of Palpation of Thyroid

- *Position of the patient:*
  - ❖ Ipsilateral flexion with rotation of neck towards the side of examination—may reveal the mass, nodule or glandular asymmetry (Fig. 12.4).

    For right lobe ask the patient to move the neck towards right side and in flexed position.

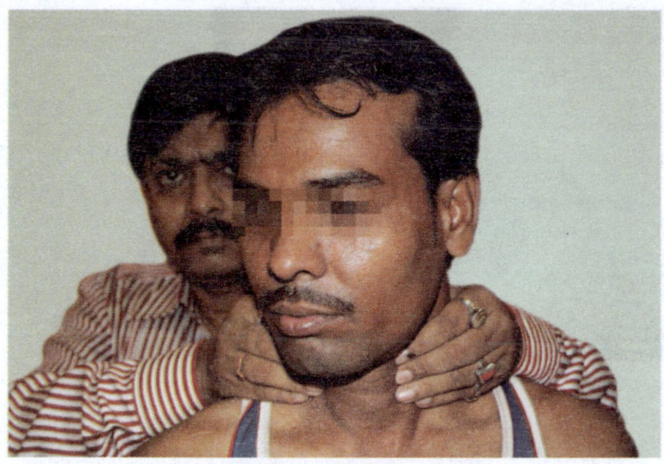

FIG. 12.4   Position of the patient

Both the lobes should be palpated in similar manner.
* In few cases neck should be extended towards 10° to reveal substernal goiter
* During palpation, swallowing should also be done to see mobility of thyroid.
* *Posterior bimanual approach (Fig. 12.5)*
  * Stand behind the patient
  * Place index and middle fingers of both hands midline in the neck, just medial to the medial margin of sternocleidomastoid muscle, this should be 2 cm above the suprasternal notch
  * From that position, locate the thyroid cartilage, then slide down gently to the horizontal groove, which separates from cricoid cartilage
  * This area is covered by cricothyroid membrane, overlying 1st tracheal ring—(area of tracheostomy)
  * Now glide down to 2nd tracheal ring—this is the area of isthmus—it lies between suprasternal notch and cricoid cartilage, it is never palpable
  * Slide your fingers laterally on the isthmus for 2–3 cm along each side—this is the area where the thyroid lobe is present on each side
  * Now you feel the consistency, nodularity, size, mobility
  * Fix the trachea with one hand, and palpate the each lobe separately.
* *Anterior single hand approach (Fig. 12.6)*
  * Sit in front of the patient
  * Use thumb and index finger of one hand to palpate the lobe.

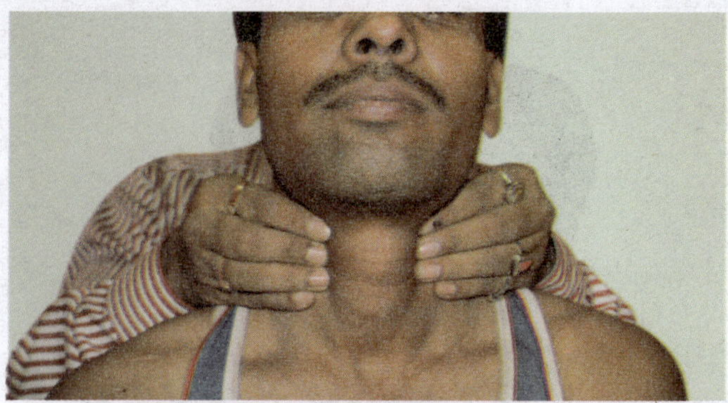

FIG. 12.5 Posterior bimanual approach

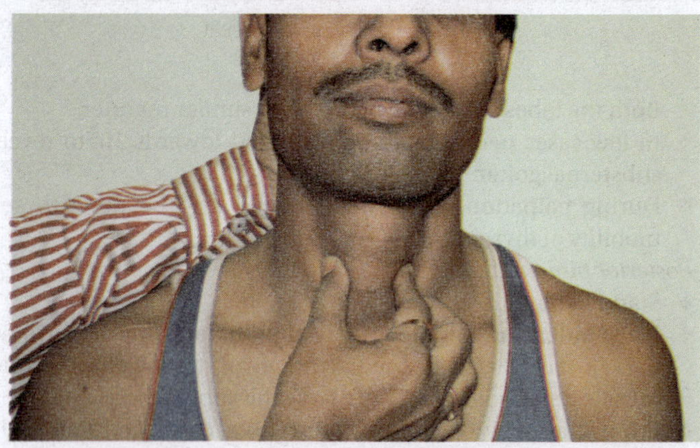

FIG. 12.6 Anterior single hand approach

Variation in size and location of thyroid:
- Female of child bearing age has larger thyroid
- In 1 percent of patient entire left lobe or lower half will be absent
- Right lobe occasionally larger than left lobe
- Sometimes pyramidal lobe appears as triangular projection arising from isthmus toward hyoid
- Posterior, extracapsular and ectopic tissue can occur in 5 percent of gland.

The following the additional findings we are looking for in the neck:
- Scar
- Redness or erythema (Maranon's sign)
- Venous engorgement (Pemberton's maneuver)
- Transillumination test of nodule or cyst

- Auscultation for murmur in case of nodule or hyperactivity of thyroid
- Lymphadenopathy
- Tracheal shift.

Complication of Goiter

All the following complications of goiter due to pressure effect:
- Impaired venous return—facial plethora
- Pressure on esophagus—dysphagia
- Pressure on trachea—stridor, dyspnea
- Pressure by substernal goiter—stridor, tracheal deviation
- Large mediastinal or substernal thyroid—venous engorgement over anterior chest, neck and impaired venous return.

Pemberton's Maneuvers (Figs 12.7A and B)

- Ask the patient to raise his both arms above the head till they touch sides of the head
- In case of positivity, within minutes, face becomes plethoric with cyanosis, respiratory distress—due to venous stasis
- In severe cases, there may be dizziness, stiffness, dyspnea, and hypotension.

Significance of Pemberton's Maneuver

- Diagnostic of increased pressure in thoracic inlet
- *Prognosis:*
  - ❖ More severe disease with airway symptoms
  - ❖ Reduced peak expiratory flow
  - ❖ Thrombosis of right subclavian and axillary veins.

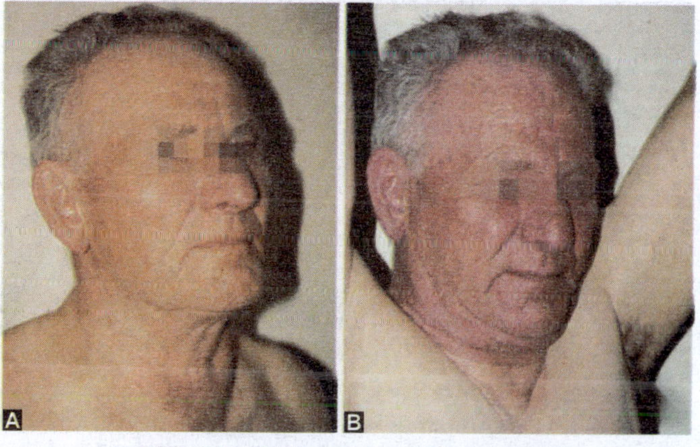

FIGS 12.7A AND B: Pemberton's maneuvers

This maneuver should be used in patient with:
- A large cervical goiter
- Goiter with positional head and neck symptom
- Evidence of substernal extension of the gland.

Pemberton's maneuver can be done in:
- Substernal goiter
- Lymphoma
- Mediastinal tumor
- Thoracic outlet obstruction.
  Bruit (Fig. 12.8) over thyroid can be heard in case of Graves' disease. This can be differentiated from venous hum in following manner:

Venous hum: Heard lower in the neck, suppressed by compression of ipsilateral neck vein.

Carotid bruit: Heard higher, lateral to the thyroid gland.

Transmitted impulses form aortic stenosis and aortic sclerosis
Can be differentiated by associated cardiac examination.

Berry's sign: Absent carotid pulse—due to invasion of vascular bundle by thyroid cancer tissue—sign of malignant thyromegaly.

Most common form of goiter:
- *Euthyroid:*
  - Multinodular goiter
  - Hashimoto thyroiditis.
- *Hypothyroid:* Hashimoto thyroiditis
- *Hyperthyroid:*
  - Graves' disease
  - Multinodular goiter.

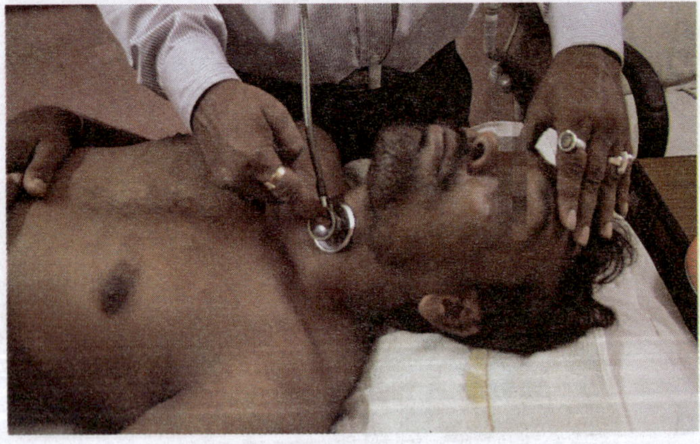

FIG. 12.8 Bruit to be heard over thyroid

Subacute Thyroiditis

Painful modest (1.5–3 times the normal) enlargement of thyroid.

Differentiation of Goiter from Normal Gland

Normally thyroid gland barely visible and slightly palpable due to interference of various surrounding structures, sternocleidomastoid muscles.

Gradual enlargement of thyroid gland is as follows:
- Increase in size of lateral lobes becomes easily palpable
- This is followed by visible enlargement of gland
- Followed by goiter it is large enough to become palpable.

Physical Examinations to Identify Goiter

According to Siminoskin's recommendations:
- Inspection and palpation of thyroid
- *Identify the gland as:*
  - ❖ Normal or impalpable
  - ❖ *Small goitrous:* 1–2 times normal (Fig. 12.9)
  - ❖ *Large goitrous:* >2 times normal (Fig. 12.10).
- In case of small goiter, consider the possibility of over estimation. Look for prominence of neck profile, visibility on frontal view.
- *Place the patient in any of the following categories:*
  - ❖ Goiter—ruled out—normal thyroid size, glands not visible in extended neck position
  - ❖ Goiter ruled it—(large goiter >2 mm)
  - ❖ Inconclusive.

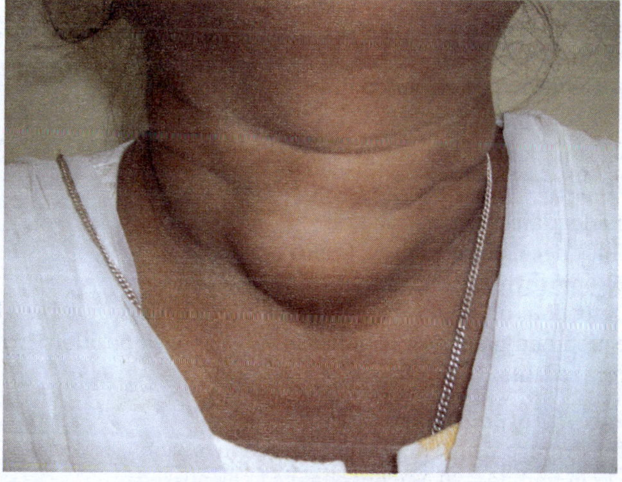

FIG. 12.9 Small goitrous enlargement

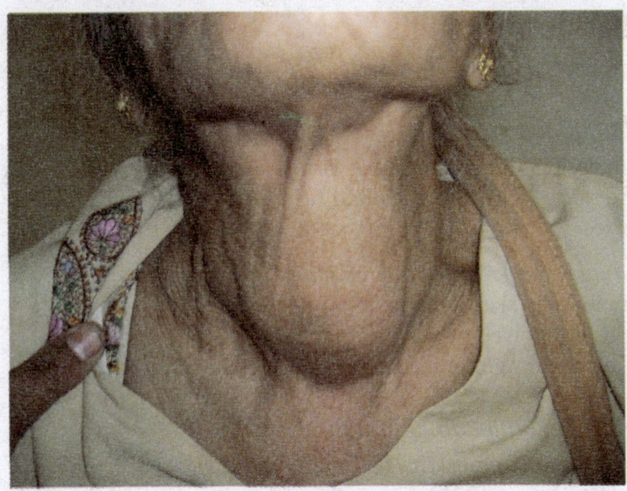

FIG. 12.10 Large goitrous enlargement

False Positive Enlargement of Thyroid

- Accentuated prominence of palpable thyroid gland
- Patient's thyroid gland is misleadingly accessible
- Long curved neck line of the patient makes the thyroid gland more prominent in spite of its normal location and size
- Whose thyroid gland is unusually higher in the neck
- Presence of fat pad anterolateral side of the neck—common in younger women and obese women.
  This fat pad does not rise with swallowing.
- *Anterior neck masses:* This can be differentiated by asking the patient to swallow:
  - ❖ Branchial cyst
  - ❖ Cervical lymphadenopathy
  - ❖ Pharyngeal diverticula.

False Negative Enlargement of Thyroid

- Inadequate examination skill
- Thick neck, obese patient, COPD patient
- Ectopic thyroid—substernal, retroclavicular.

Detection of goiter in extended neck is less reliable than detection and palpation of goiter in normal neck position, which is more reliable.

Average size of palpable nodule:
- The average size of nodule for detection is 3 cm
- <1 cm nodule—90 percent chance to be missed

- <2 cm nodule—50 percent chance to be missed
- 5 percent of thyroid nodule is malignant.

The most common cause of hyperthyroidism is excessive thyroid supplement.

Causes are mainly three:
1. Graves' disease
2. Toxic nodule goiter
3. Thyroiditis.

Manifestation of Hyperthyroidism

- *Hypermetabolism:*
  - ❖ Weight loss
  - ❖ Diarrhea
  - ❖ Sensitive to hot temperature
  - ❖ Amenorrhea.
- *Goiter*—nodular—asymmetric in toxic nodular goiter.
- *Skin:*
  - ❖ Warm and moist skin
  - ❖ Pretibial myxedema
  - ❖ Palmar erythema
  - ❖ Hyperpigmentation at pressure points
  - ❖ Onycholysis
  - ❖ Friable nail.
- *Eyes:*
  - ❖ Lid retraction
  - ❖ Lid lag
  - ❖ Graves' ophthalmopathy.
- *Cardiovascular:*
  - ❖ Tachycardia
  - ❖ Palpitation
  - ❖ Systolic flow murmur.
- *Neurological manifestation:*
  - ❖ Fine tremor (Fig. 12.11)
  - ❖ Anxious, restless
  - ❖ Neuromuscular weakness
  - ❖ Decrease exercise intolerance
  - ❖ Hyperreflexia.

Findings suggestive of hyperthyroidism
- Lid lag
- Lid retraction
- Fine tremor
- Worm and moist skin
- Tachycardia.

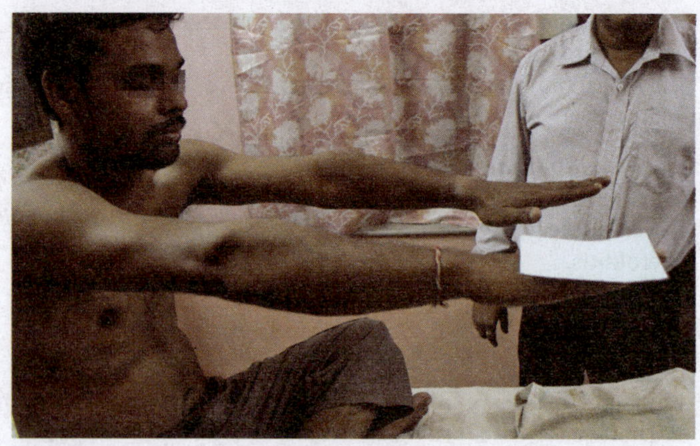

FIG. 12.11 Fine tremor

Presentation in elderly patient with hyperthyroidism:
- *Cardiological manifestations:*
  - ❖ Atrial arrhythmia
  - ❖ Cardiomyopathy
  - ❖ Means-Lerman scratch
  - ❖ Flow murmur.
- *Neurological manifestations:*
  - ❖ Apathy
  - ❖ Proximal muscular weakness
  - ❖ Myopathy.

Three major manifestations of Graves' disease
1. Hyperthyroidism with diffuse goiter
2. Dermopathy
3. Ophthalmopathy.

Pretibial Myxedema

Localized nonpitting edema, well demarcated, raised, bilateral pinkish/brownish nodules on the anterior aspect of shin. This lesion progresses to plaque, may be pruritic or hyperpigmented.

Although it is present in Graves' disease, it is not related to hormone level, so it may be present in euthyroid person.

Pretibial myxedema is localized.

Hypothyroid myxedema in generalized.

Autoimmune findings of Graves' disease
- Premature graying of hair
- Vitiligo
- Hyperpigmentation.

Thyroid acropathy
This is characterized by:
- Clubbing
- Subperiosteal deposition of bones in hands and feet not in long bones—painless and asymptomatic.

This occurs in long acting thyroid stimulating hormone hence it is absent in thyrotoxicosis.

Graves' Ophthalmopathy

Bilateral proptosis (unilateral in 5% cases) in due to edema, lymphocytic penetration of ocular fat, connective tissue, and extra-ocular muscles.

Patient may complain of:
- Gritty sensation in eye
- Tearing from eye
- Diplopia.

Proptosis can be defined as abnormal protrusion of eyeball of more than 18 mm.

Proptosis can be accurately measured by:
Hertel exophthalmometer handheld device to measure that distance between lateral orbital rim and anterior corneal surface.

Characteristics of Graves' Congestive Ophthalmopathy
- Periorbital edema
- Lid edema
- Chemosis (conjunctival edema)
- Ophthalmoplagia.

Eye manifestation of thyrotoxicosis
- *Dalrymple's lid retraction or thyroid stare (Fig. 12.12):* Normally margin of upper lid coves 1 mm of iris, but in lid retraction; upper eyelid is pulled backward, exposing a rim of sclera-hence patient locus staring look
- *von Graafe's sign (Lid lag) (Fig. 12.13):* On looking downward gaze, the eyeball moves downwards briskly. While upper eyelid lags behind, so, sclera between corneal limbus and upper eyelid becomes visible
- *Rosenbach's sign:* Tremor of upper eyelid—when the eyes are closed gently
- *Möbius sign:* Failure of ocular convergence following close accommodations at 5°
- *Stellwag's sign:* Infrequent and incomplete blinking and proptosis

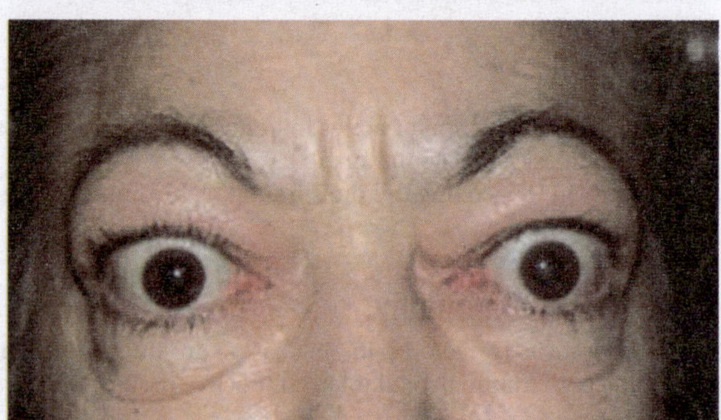

FIG. 12.12   Lid retraction

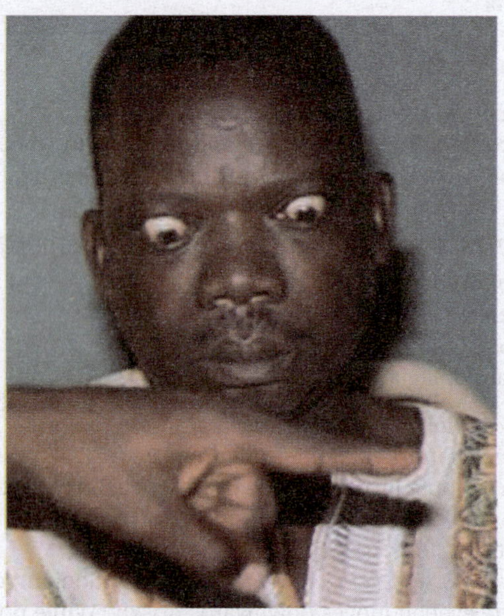

FIG. 12.13   von Graafe's sign

- *Kocher's sign:* In upward gaze upper lids retracts upwards briskly, globe lags behind
- *Joffroy's sign:* Absent wrinkling of forehead during upward gaze
- *Sainton's sign:* On upward gaze, upper eyelid will completely contacts followed by contraction of frontalis muscle
- *Jellinek's sign:* Brownish pigmentation of upper eyelid

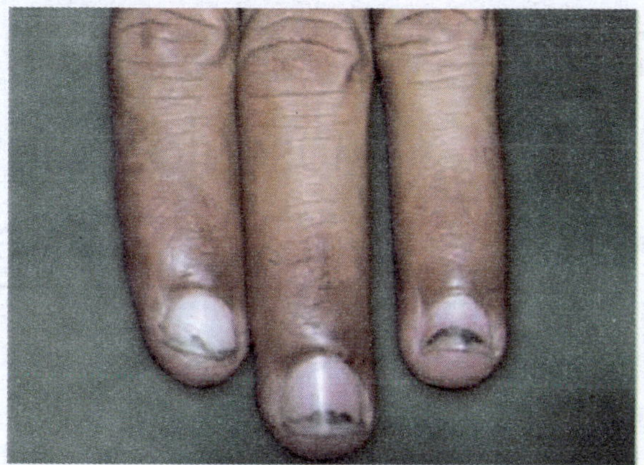

FIG. 12.14 Plummer nail

- *Topolansky sign:* Pericorneal congestion with conjunctival edema in Graves' disease.

Onycholysis

Partial separation of distal and lateral attachments of nail plate form nailbed is called onycholysis. Complete separation of nail plate is called onychomadesis.

It commonly involves ring finger. Beneath the separated nail plate debris are collected.

This type of nail is also called plummer nail (Fig. 12.14).

The causes are:
- Graves' disease
- Psoriasis
- Trauma
- Raynaud's disease
- Phototoxic reaction to tetracycline.

Musculoskeletal System

◼ Bone

It is a living tissue, capable of changing its structure according to the stress it is subjected to. It is hard because of the calcification of extracellular matrix.

Bone exists in two forms:
Compact bone: It appears as solid mass.
Cancellous bone: It consists of branching network of trabeculae.

Classification of Bones

Long Bones (Fig. 13.1A)

They have following parts:
- Tubular shaft—diaphysis.
- Epiphysis—at each end of the bone.
- Diaphysis is separated from epiphysis by epiphyseal cartilage.
- The part of diaphysis adjacent to epiphyseal cartilage is called metaphysis.
- Central part of the shaft is called marrow cavity—containing marrow—bone marrow.
- Outer part of shaft composed of compact bone—covered by a connective tissue sheath—periosteum.
- Long bones found in limbs—humerus, tibia, fibula, radius, ulna, femur, metacarpals and metatarsals.

Short Bones (Fig. 13.1B)

- It is composed of cancellous bone surrounded by compact bone thin layer.
- Short bones are covered by periosteum.
- These are found in hands and feet (scaphoid, lunate, talus and calcaneous).

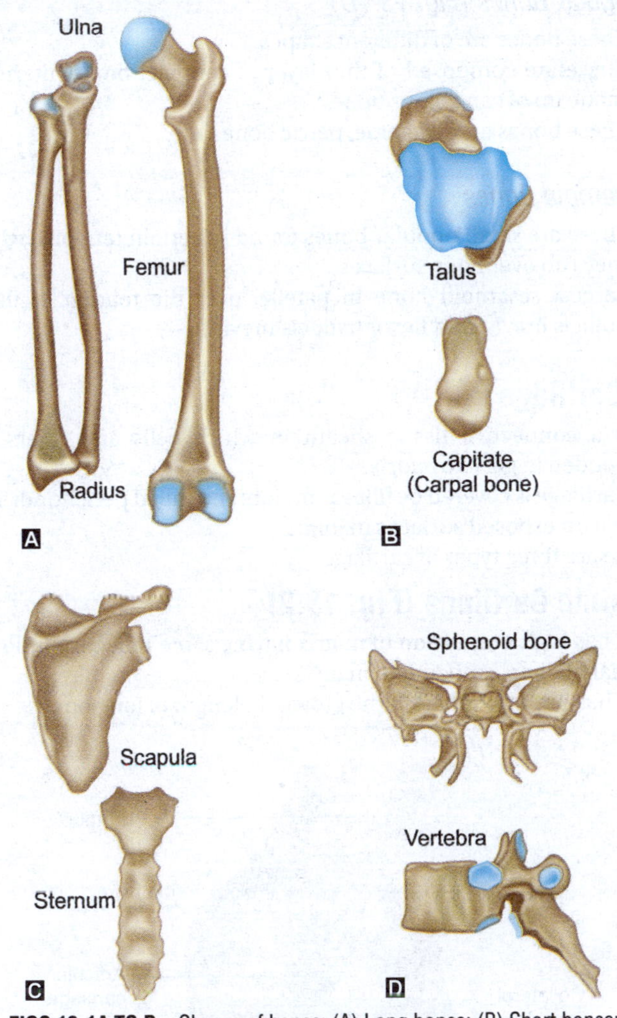

FIGS 13.1A TO D   Shapes of bones: (A) Long bones; (B) Short bones; (C) Flat bones; (D) Irregular bones

Flat Bones (Fig 13.1C)

- Inner layer and outer layer are composed of compact bone—called tables.
- The outer and inner layer is separated by cancellous bone layer—called diploe.
- These bones are found in skull—frontal and parietal bones.

Irregular Bones (Fig. 13.1D)

- These bones are of different shapes.
- These are composed of thin layer of compact bone, interior is made up of cancellous bone.
- These bones are vertebrae, pelvic bones, etc.

Sesamoid Bones

- These are small nodular bones found in certain tendons, where they rub over bony surfaces.
- Largest sesamoid bone in patella, over the tendon of flexor pollicis brevis, and flexor hallucis brevis.

Cartilage

It is a connective tissue sheath in which cells and fibers are embedded in gel like matrix.

Cartilage is covered by fibrous membrane called perichondrium, except on exposed surfaces in joints.

There are three types of cartilage:

Hyaline Cartilage (Fig. 13.2)

- It has high proportion of matrix having same reflective index as that of fibers embedded on it.
- It has important part in the growth in length of long bones.

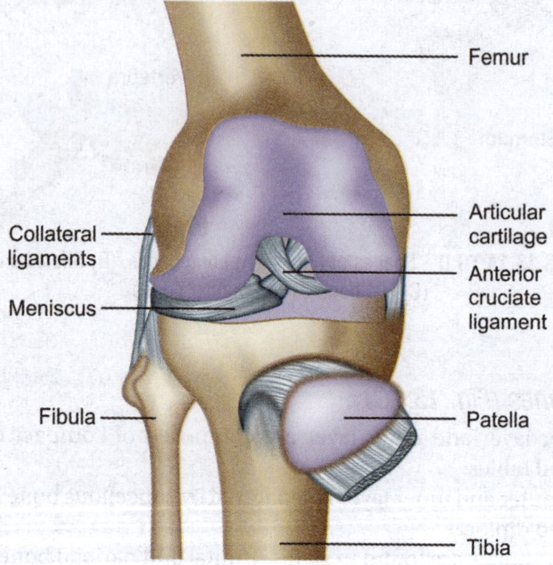

FIG. 13.2 Hyaline cartilage

- It covers the articular surfaces of long bones in all synovial joint.
- It is incapable of repair, when ruptured.

Fibrocartilage (Fig. 13.3)

- A large amount of fibers embedded on small matrix.
- It is found in the disc within the joints (temporomandibular joint, sternoclavicular joint, knee joint) and on articular surfaces of the clavicle and mandible.
- If damaged, repaired by fibrous tissue.

Elastic Cartilage

- Large number of elastic fibers embedded in small amount of matrix.
- It is flexible.
- It is found in auricle, auditory tube, epiglottis.
- If damaged it will be repaired and replaced by fibrous tissue.

Joints

This can be defined by an area where two or more bones come together with or without any movement.

There are following types of joints:

Fibrous Joint (Fig. 13.4)

Where articular surfaces of bones are joined by fibrous tissue.
Examples:
- Sutures of vault of skull
- Interior tibiofibular joint.

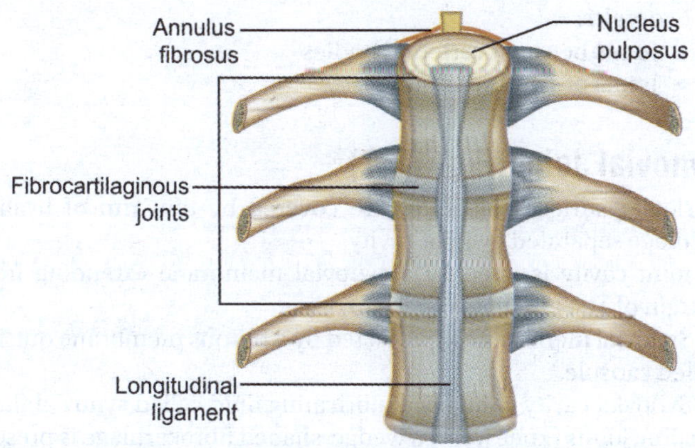

FIG. 13.3 Fibrocartilage

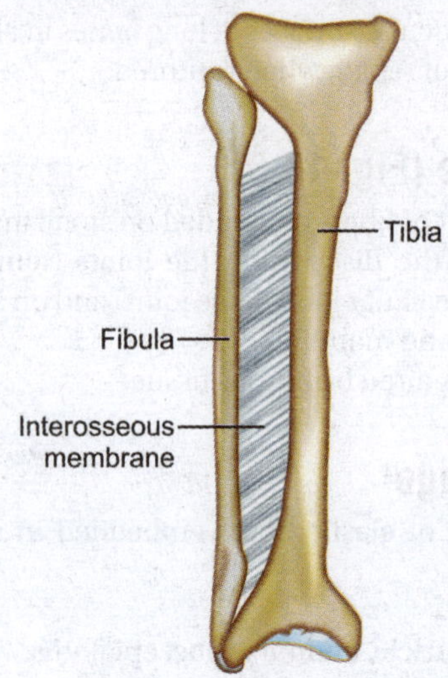

FIG. 13.4 Fibrous joint

Cartilaginous Joint

This can be further subdivided into two types:

1. *Primary cartilaginous joint (Fig. 13.5):* Where two bones are united by a plate or bar of hyaline cartilage.
   Examples:
   * Union between epiphysis and diaphysis of long bones
   * Union between manubrium sterni and 1st rib.
   Characteristics: No movements occur in these joints.
2. *Secondary cartilaginous joint (Fig. 13.6):* Bones are united by fibrous cartilage, but articular surfaces of bones are covered by hyaline cartilage.
   Examples:
   * Joints between vertebral bodies
   * Joints of symphysis pubis.

Synovial Joint (Fig. 13.7)

Auricular surfaces of bones are covered by thin rim of hyaline cartilage separated by joint cavity.

Joint cavity is lined by a synovial membrane extending from margin of one articular surface to other.

Synovial membrane is protected by a fibrous membrane outside called capsule.

Synovial cavity contains a lubricating fluid called synovial fluid. In some joints (knee joint) a wedge-shaped fibrocartilage is present between two articular surface called articular disc.

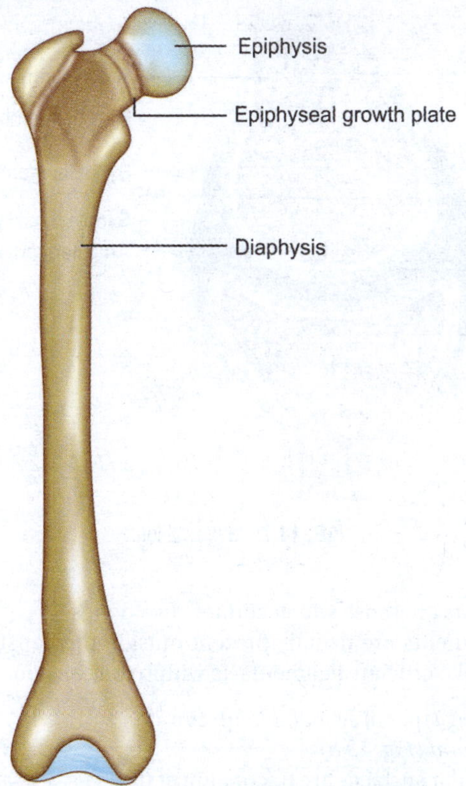

FIG. 13.5 Primary cartilaginous joint

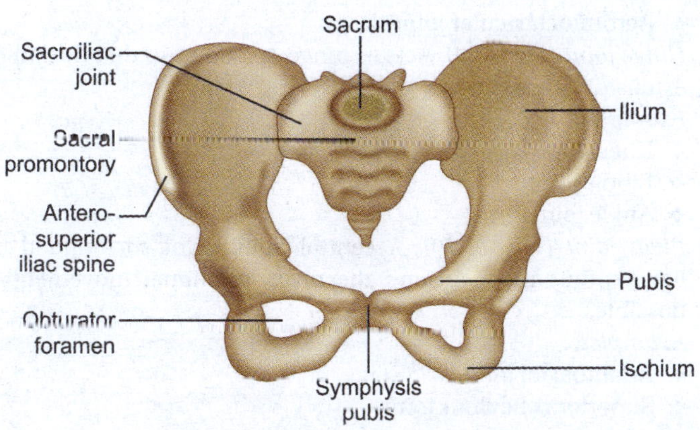

FIG. 13.6 Secondary cartilaginous joint

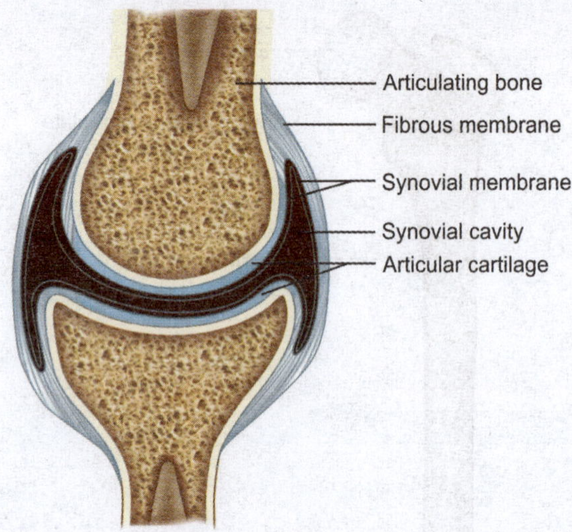

FIG. 13.7 Synovial joint

Ligaments are those which connect two bones.

The ligaments are usually present outside the capsule but few ligaments like cruciate ligaments lie within the capsule.

The following types of synovial joints are:
- *Planar joint (Fig. 13.8)*
  - ❖ Articular surfaces are flat or almost flat
  - ❖ Bones are allowed to slide on one another.
  - *Examples:*
  - ❖ Sternoclavicular joint
  - ❖ Acromioclavicular joint.
- *Hinge joint (Fig. 13.9):* Acts as hinge of a door, so that flexion or extension is possible.
  - *Examples:*
  - ❖ Knee joint
  - ❖ Elbow joint
  - ❖ Ankle joint.
- *Pivot joint (Fig. 13.10):* A central bony pivot surrounded by ligamentous ring—Around the pivot, rotational movement is possible.
  - *Examples:*
  - ❖ Atlantoaxial joint
  - ❖ Superior ridiculous joint
- *Condylar joint (Fig. 13.11):* Here two core surfaces articulate with two concave joints.

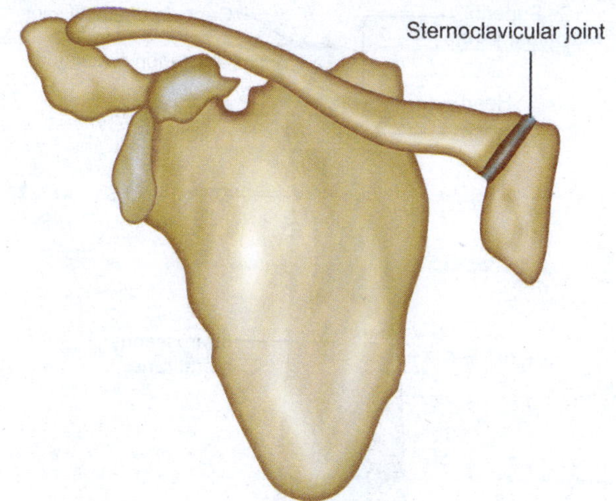

FIG. 13.8 Planar joint

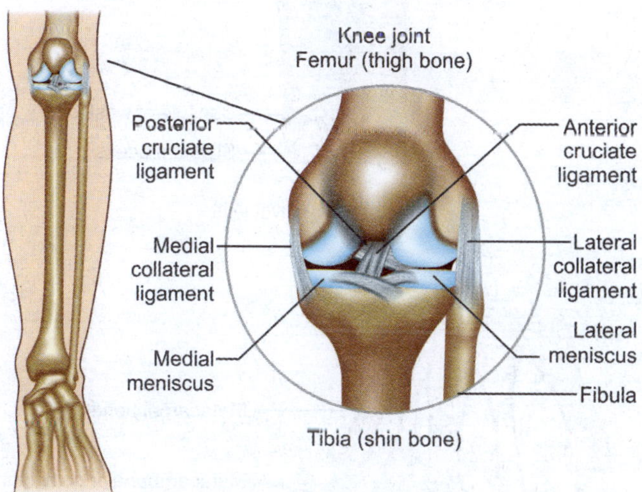

FIG. 13.9 Hinge joint

Movements: Extension, flexion, abduction, adduction and rotation—slight amount.

Example: Metacarpophalangeal joint.

- *Ellipsoid joint (Fig. 13.12):* Here two surfaces are—one ellipsoid convex surface and the other is ellipsoid concave surfaces.

Movements: Extension, flexion, adduction, abduction, no rotational movement.

Example: Wrist joint.

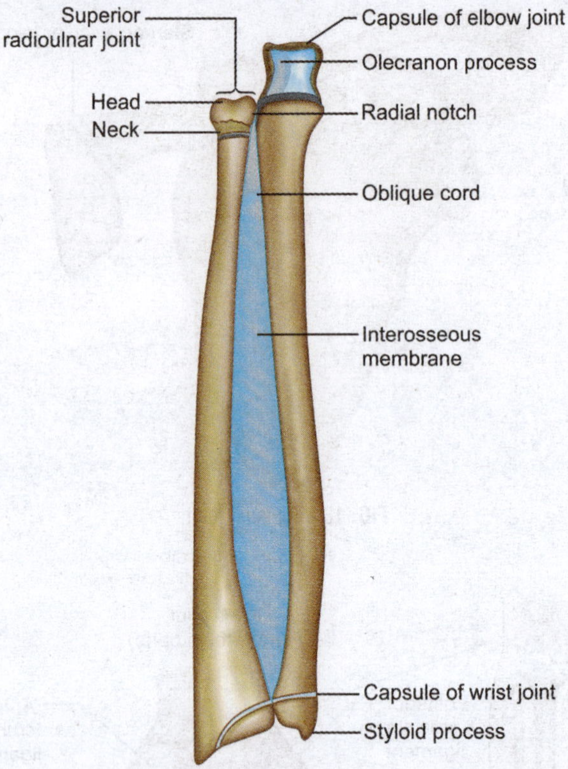

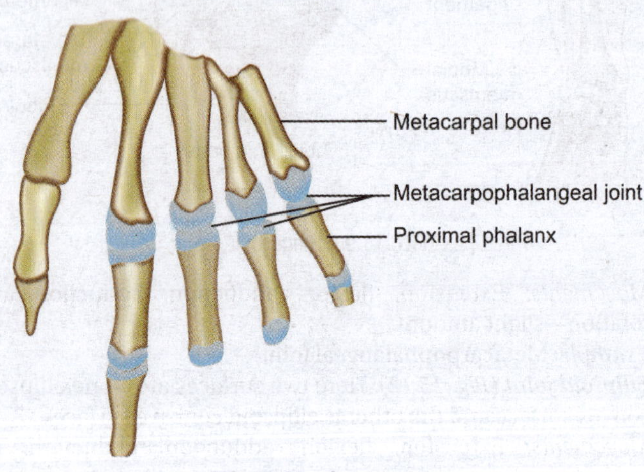

FIG. 13.10   Pivot joint

FIG. 13.11   Condylar joint

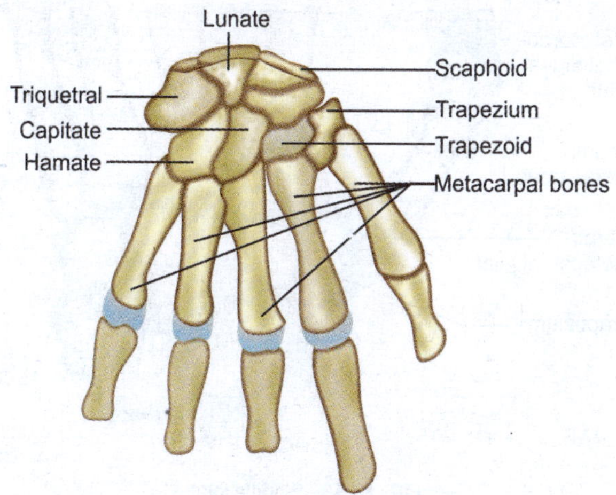

FIG. 13.12   Ellipsoid joint

- *Saddle joint (Fig. 13.13):* Articular surfaces are concavoconvex resembling saddle-shaped on horse back.
  Movements: Extension, flexion, adduction, abduction, and rotation.
  Example: Carpometacarpal joint of thumb.
- *Ball and socket joint (Fig. 13.14):* Here ball shaped head of one bone fits into socket with concavity of another bone.
  Movements: Flexion, extension, abduction, adduction, medial rotation, lateral rotation, and circumduction.
  Examples:
  - ❖ Hip joint
  - ❖ Shoulder joint.

Ligaments

There are two types of ligaments:

1. *Fibrous type of ligament:* It prevents excessive movement in a joint but in severe stress—this ligament can be stretched.
   Example: Plantar arch normally cannot be stretched but in case of stress—this arch will be stretched.
2. *Elastic ligament:* This type of ligament is stretchable and can be reverted back to normal length
   Example: Elastic ligaments of auditory ossicles.

Bursa (Fig. 13.15)

- It is a closed fibrous one lined by delicate smooth membrane containing viscous fluid.

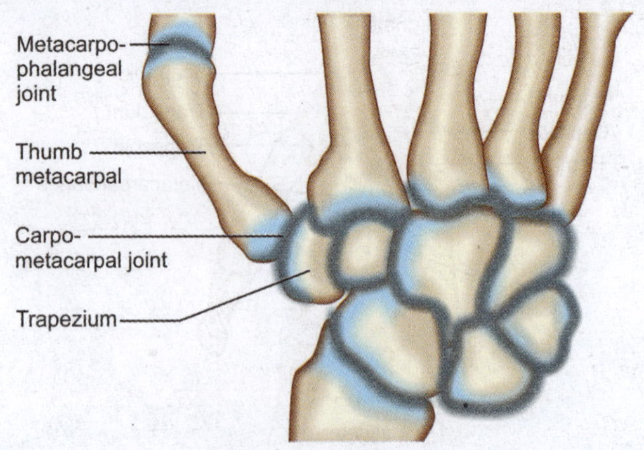

FIG. 13.13   Saddle joint

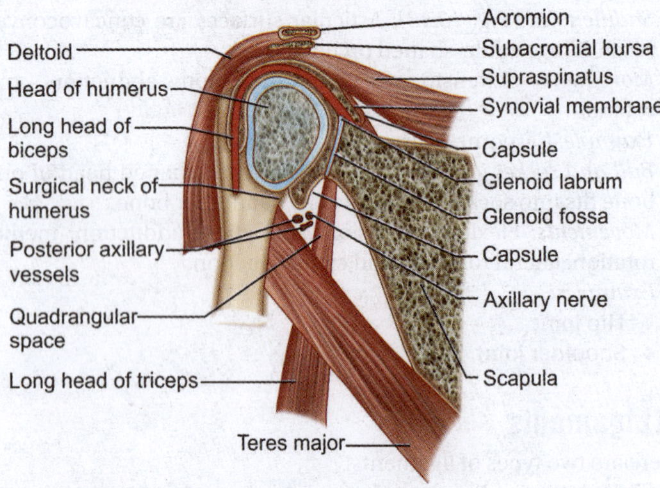

FIG. 13.14   Ball and socket joint

- Bursae are found where the tendon rubs against bones, ligaments or other tendons or skin rubs against bony structure.
  Example: Prepatellar bursa (Fig. 13.16).
- In some cases, bursal cavity communicates with synovial cavity.
  Examples:
  ❖ Subprepatellar bursa communicates with knee joints (Fig. 13.16),
  ❖ Subscapular bursa communicates with shoulder joint.

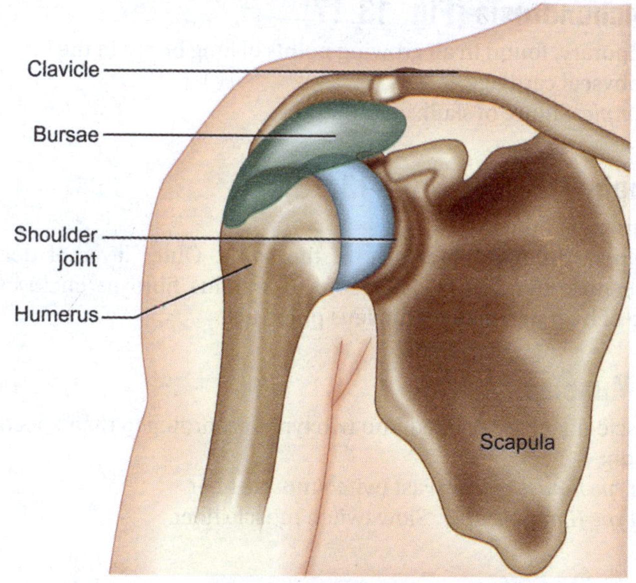

FIG. 13.15 Bursa

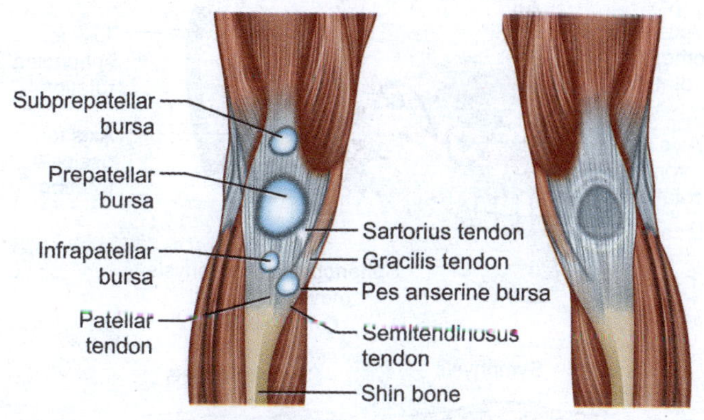

FIG. 13.16 Bursa in the knee

Synovial Fluids

Synovial membrane is one-cell thick.
- One type of cell ingests autologous material entered into joint.
- Another type of cell synthesizes and secrets synovial fluid.

Synovial fluid is plasma dialysate and hyaluronate proteoglycans. It provides nutrition for articular cartilage and help in lubrication of joints.

Synchondrosis (Fig. 13.17)

Temporary, found in all growing points of long bones in the form of epiphyseal cartilage.
Example: Suture of skull.

Amphiarthroses (Fig. 13.18)

Permanent joints.
Example: Intervertebral disc of the spine. Outer layer of dense concentric bundles of collagen, the annulus fibrosus encloses a core of hydrated tissue—nucleus pulposus.

■ Muscles

Muscle fibers are divided into two types according to their speed of action:

1. *Type I muscle fiber:* Fast twitch muscle fiber.
2. *Type II muscle fiber:* Slow twitch muscle fiber.

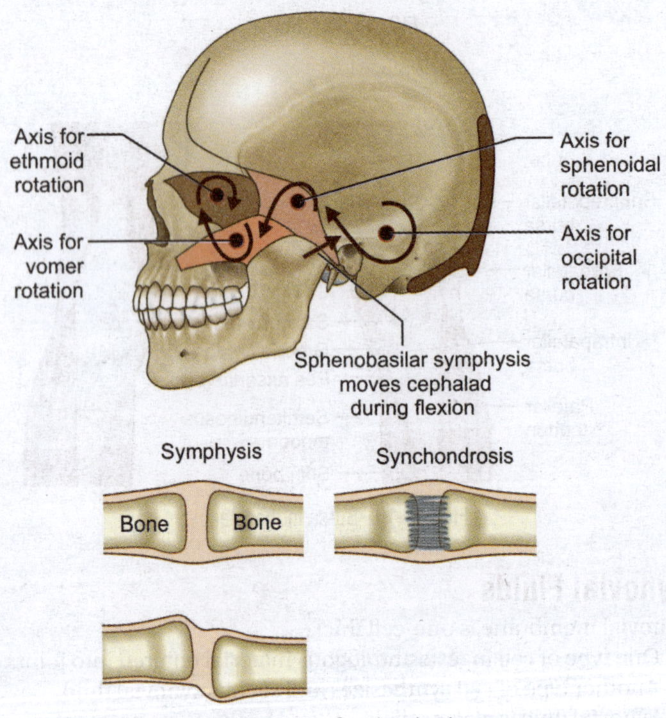

FIG. 13.17 Synchondrosis

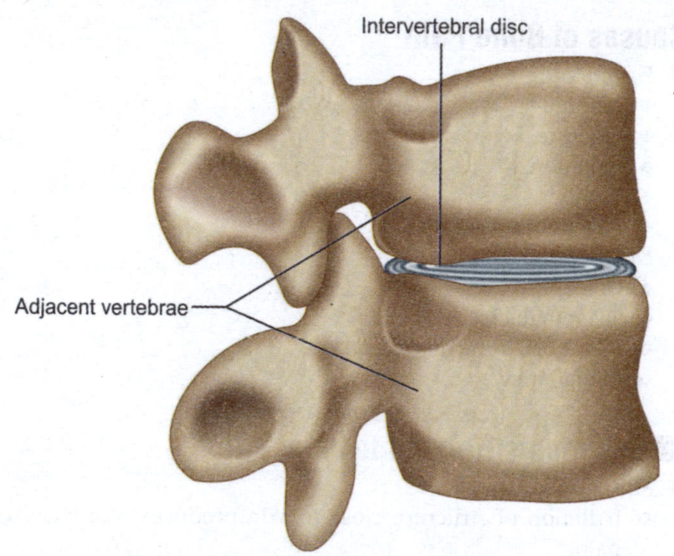

FIG. 13.18 Amphiarthroses

Differences between Two Types of Muscle Fibers

Difference between two types of muscle fibers, i.e. slow twitch and fast twitch muscle fibers.

Slow twitch muscle fiber	Fast twitch muscle fiber
• Innervated by slowly conducting nerve fiber	• Innervated by rapidly conductions nerve fiber
• Have low threshold	• Have high threshold
• Conduct slowly	• Conduct rapidly
• Recruitment begins with slow unit	• Recruitment later progresses to larger units
• Firing frequency ranges from 10–20 Hz	• Firing frequency ranges from 100 Hz
• High myoglobin content	• Low myoglobin content
• Use oxidative mechanism for energy formation	• Use glycolysis for energy formation
• Fatigue resistant	• Fatigable
• It produce sustained muscle contraction	• It produces sudden muscle contraction, short lived

■ Symptoms Related to Bone Pain

Deep boring, localized (in case of trauma, tumor, infection) or generalized (osteoporosis), sharp piercing (fracture).

Aggravated by movement. Relieved by taking rest.

Causes of Bone Pain

- *Focal pain:*
  - ❖ Trauma
  - ❖ Fracture
  - ❖ Infection
  - ❖ Tumor
  - ❖ Paget's disease.
- *Diffuse pain:*
  - ❖ Osteoporosis
  - ❖ Osteomalacia
  - ❖ Metabolic bone disease
  - ❖ Malignancy.

Symptoms Related to Joint Pain

- *Site of pain:*
  - ❖ Irritation of structure close to skin produces well localized pain.
  - ❖ Pain in deeper structures produces poorly localized pain, segmental in distribution called sclerotomal distribution, it differs from specific dermatomal distribution.
- *Radiation of pain:*
  - ❖ Deeper pain may be felt at a point some distance from deeper structure.
  - ❖ Upper cervical pair referred to occipital region.
  - ❖ Disorder of lower lumbar spine may be referred to upper lumbar back pain because posterior longitudinal ligament is innervated by upper lumbar nerves.
- *Severity of pains:*
  - ❖ Acute onset—Gouty arthritis, infective arthritis
  - ❖ Waxing and waning—Rheumatoid arthritis
  - ❖ Progressively increase in pain—infective origin.
- *Aggravating and relieving factors:*
  - ❖ Improving with activity, returning at rest—inflammatory joint disease.
  - ❖ Pain gradually worsen during the course of days— mechanical joint disease (osteoarthritis).
  - ❖ Pain occurs during specific range of movement (at the shoulder).

Swelling and Crepitus

Regarding swelling:
- How long it will be present?
- Whether it is gradually increasing?
- Is there any associated tenderness, redness?

- Is there any fluctuation at that site?
- Is there any restriction of movement or not?

Regarding Crepitations

It is a grating sensation on palpation at the joint site—it may fine or coarse, it may be audible or palpable.

Fine crepitations can be audible then felt.

Presence of crepitus is the diagnostic of degenerative joint disease.

Locking

Locking occurs when foreign material will be accumulated in between two articular surfaces. It mainly occurs in knee cartilages it occurs during particular movement.

Causes of Joint Pain

- *Inflammatory:*
  - ❖ Rheumatoid arthritis
  - ❖ Ankylosing spondylosis.
- *Mechanical:*
  - ❖ Osteoarthritis
  - ❖ Osteoporosis.
- *Infective:*
  - ❖ Pyogenic
  - ❖ Tuberculosis
  - ❖ Brucellosis.
- Traumatic.

Symptoms Related to Muscles Pain

- *Pain and stiffness:*
  - ❖ Deep, constant, poorly localizing pain.
  - ❖ Aggravated by contraction of muscles.
  - ❖ Pain is relieved by rest.
- *Weakness:* Regarding weakness:
  - ❖ *Distribution of weakness:*
    - If it is proximal—polymyositis or myopathies
    - It it is distal weakness—neuropathy myopathy (rare).
  - ❖ *Any pain in the limb*—by polymyositis, trauma, infection.
  - ❖ *Whether weakness is fluctuating*—it weakness worsens during the course of activity—myasthenia gravis.
  - ❖ *If weakness is global*—it is neurotic rather than neuropathy.
  - ❖ *Whether weakness is sudden or gradual and progressive:*

- Sudden entrapment of peripheral nerve (traumatic radial nerve palsy)—it will improve with time
- If the weakness in progressive—Motor neuron disease.

Questions to be asked in case of muscle weakness:
- Whether the weakness is global or focal?
- Whether the weakness is acute at onset or chronic?
- Whether it is progressive?
- Whether it is fluctuating?
- Distribution of weakness.
- Whether the pain and weakness are associated with skin lesion?

- *Wasting and fasciculation:* This can be noticed during history taking as muscle twitching in different muscles or single muscles or calf.

- *Cramp:* It may occur in any muscle mainly in calf muscle—it can be triggered by forceful contraction of muscle.

Following principles to be followed during musculoskeletal examinations are:

Examination of bone:
- Look for limb shortening
- Any local tenderness.

Examination of joints:
- *Inspection:*
  - *Swelling:* Causes may be:
    - Effusions
    - Thickening of synovial tissue
    - Thickening of bony margins.
      - i. Thickening or swelling should be compared with the same joints of other limb.
      - ii. Watch that thickening is mainly due to joint swelling or swelling of adjacent structure.
  - *Deformity of joint:* It may occur from misalignment of the bones forming joint (Fig. 13.19):
    - Deviation of bony part distal to joint away from midline called valgas deformity—in case of knee—genu valgus deformity (Figs 13.20A and B).
    - Deviation of distal bony part of joint towards midline—called varas deformity, e.g. genu varus deformity in case of knee (Fig. 13.21).
    - In case of any other deformity whether it is fixed or mobile—if it is mobile—detect whether it is due to partial loss of contact with articulating surface called subluxation or complete loss of contact with articulating surface called dislocation.

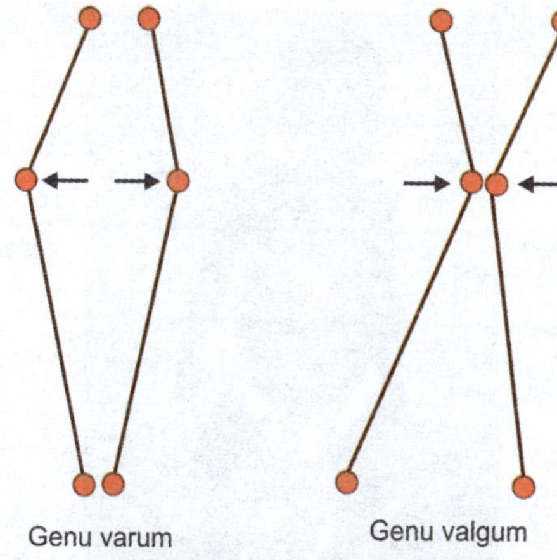

FIG. 13.19 Deformity of joint

FIGS 13.20A AND B Genu valgus

- These are finger deformities (Fig. 13.22)
  - Swan neck deformity (Figs 13.23A and B)
  - Boutonniere deformity (Fig. 13.24)
  - Mallet deformity (Fig. 13.25)

  The above deformities are due to involvement of metacarpophalangeal or interphalangeal joints of hand.
- ❖ *Skin changes*—Watch:
  - Color of skin
  - Temperature
  - Redness
  - Tension around the joint.

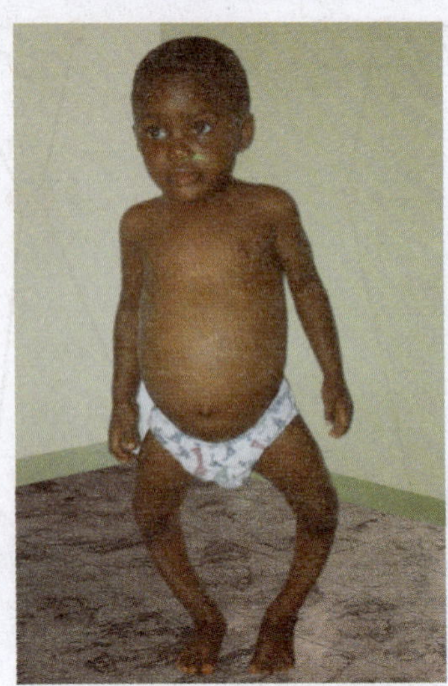

FIG. 13.21 Genu varus

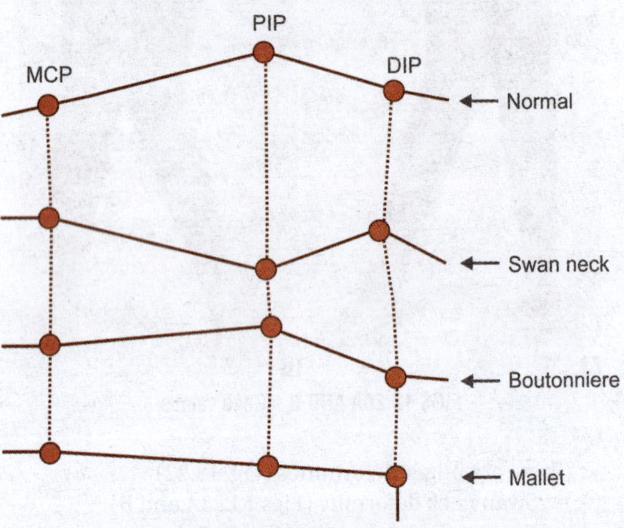

FIG. 13.22 Finger deformities

- ❖ *Changes in adjacent structures:* These include washing of muscles adjacent to diseased joint.
- ❖ Washing of quadriceps around the knee joint.
- • *Palpation:*
  - ❖ *Swelling:* First step to determine consistency of the swelling:
    - • If the swelling is hard bony deformities due to osteo-arthritis involvement of DIP or PIP joints.

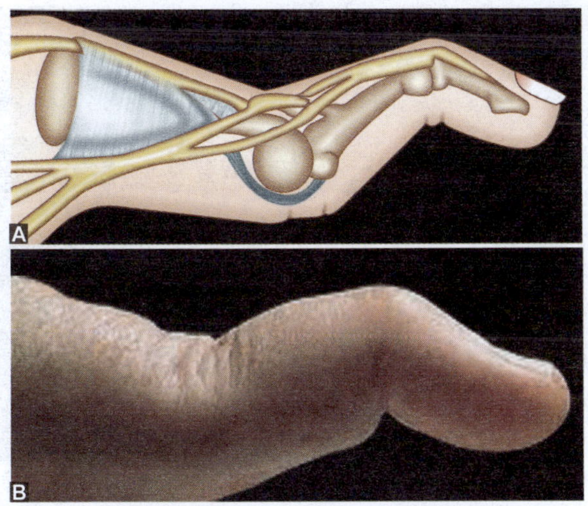

FIGS 13.23A AND B   Swan neck deformity

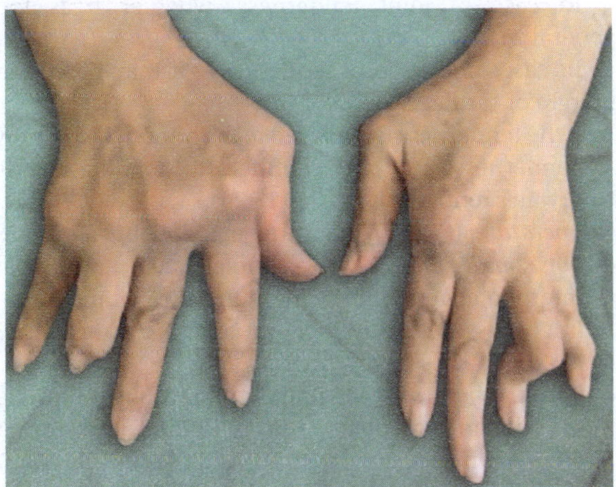

FIG. 13.24   Boutonniere deformity

- Slight spongy boggy swelling suggestive or synovial thickening of rheumatoid arthritis.
- Fluctuation of swelling:
  - Soft fluctuant swelling—suggest bursitis.
  - Harder swelling—rheumatoid arthritis, gout.
- Tenderness of swelling—infective arthritis.
- ❖ *Tenderness:* Tenderness to be elicitated in:
- Joint margin
- Adjacent bony surfaces
- Surrounding ligaments and tendons.

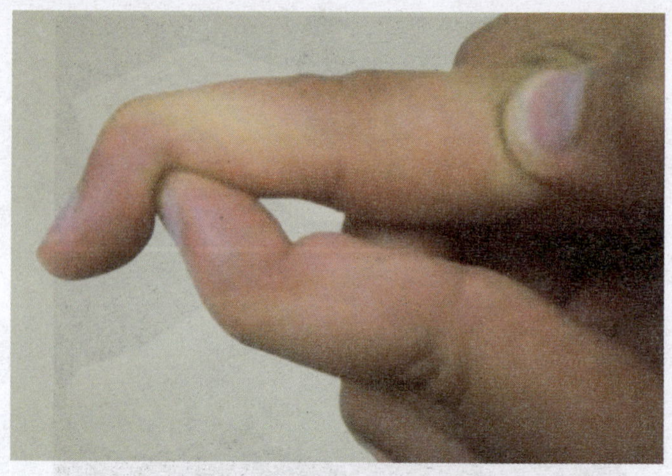

FIG. 13.25 Mallet deformity

In case of joint tenderness—whether it is focal or generalized.

In case of knee joint tenderness—it may be confined to margin of cartilage.

If the tenderness is localized to the bone, it is osteomyelitis. Tenderness may be confined to tendon sheath—De Quervain's tenosynovitis (Fig. 13.26).

❖ *Temperature:* It can be measured in following manners:
  - *For small joint:* For example, metacarpophalangeal, interphalangeal joints measure the temperature with fingertips of the examiner and compare with similar joints of other hands (Fig. 13.27A).
  - *For large joint:* If knee joint or elbow joint—Rub the back of your hand and place it over the joint to be examined and compare it with same joints of other limbs (Fig. 13.27B).
  - If contralateral limb will be affected, measure temperature above or below the joint margin and compare (Fig. 13.28).

● *Movement of joint:* You examine the range of movement and determine whether it is limited by pain or fixed deformity of the joint.
  ❖ *To examine the range of movement, start with joint in the neutral position:*
    - Lower limb extended with feet dorsiflexed to 90° (Fig. 13.29)
    - Upper limb midway between pronation and supination with arms flexed to 90° at the elbows (Fig. 13.30).

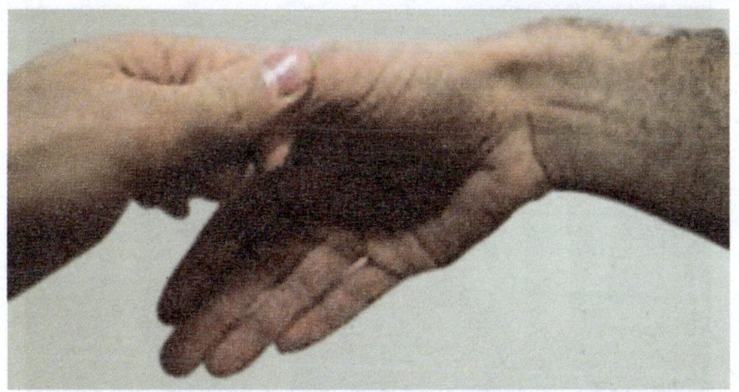

FIG. 13.26   De Quervain's tenosynovitis

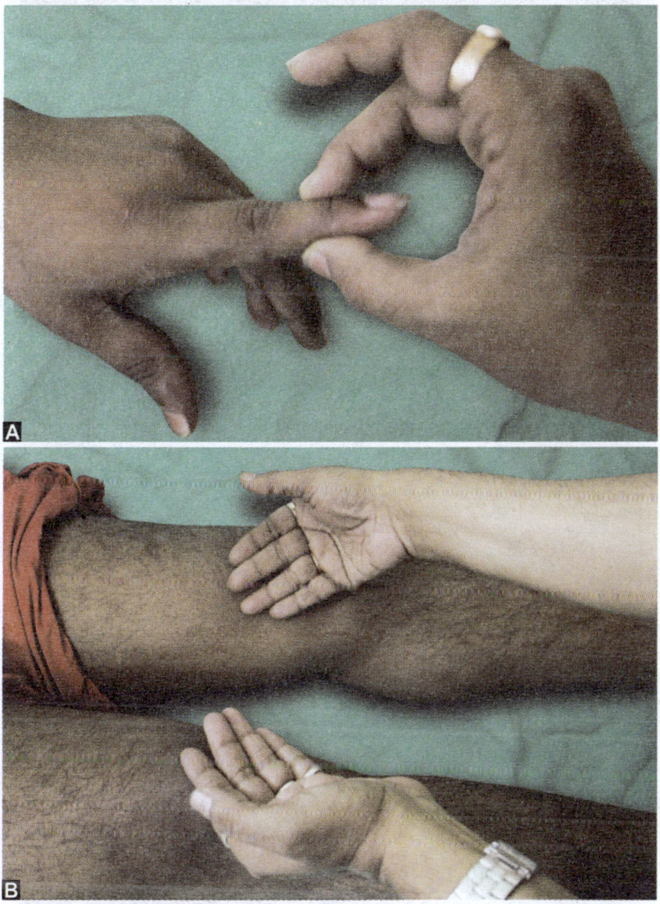

FIGS 13.27A AND B   Temperature measurement in: (A) Small joints;
(B) Large joints

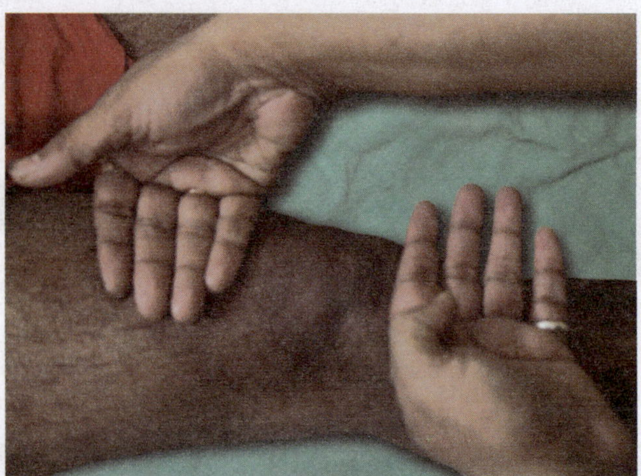

FIG. 13.28 Temperature measurement above or below the joint

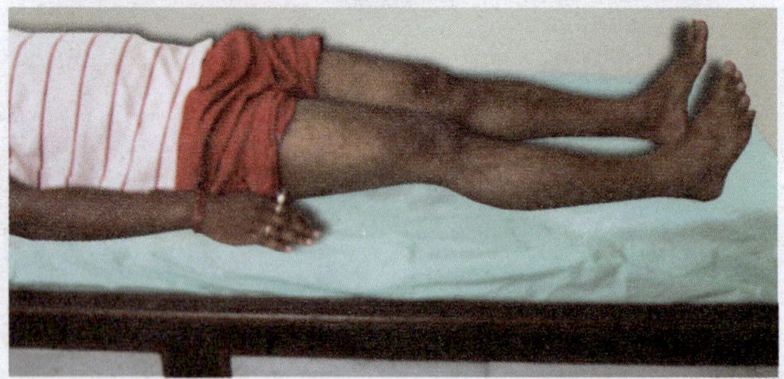

FIG. 13.29 Position of lower limb

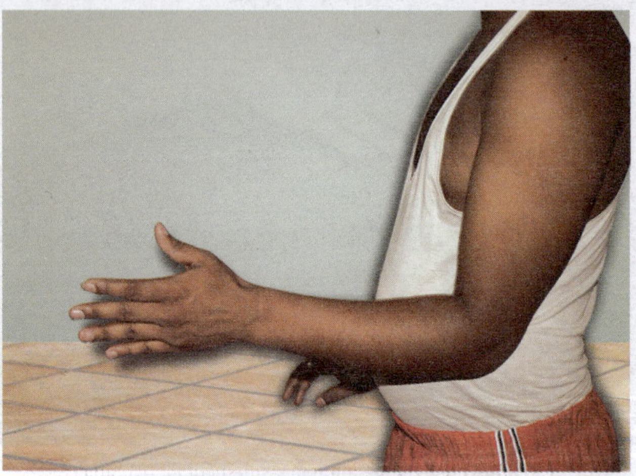

FIG. 13.30 Position of upper limb

- ❖ Examine the active movement of the joint by the patient and passive movement by the examiner.
- ❖ Assess the active movement of the spine and passive movements of the limb joints—its active movement is restricted; it is due to muscle weakness.
- ❖ From neutral position, measure the degree of extension or flexion:
  - In few joints, normally no extension occur. In knee joint, movement of the knee can be described as hyperextension of knee joint.
  - In few cases, there may be restriction of movement.
  - If knee joint falls by 30° to reach extended position— this can be described as 30° flexion deformity or 30° lean of extension.
  - *For ankle and wrist joint:*
    - Extension can be described as dorsiflexion.
    - Flexion can be described as plantar and palmar flexion.
  - *For ball and socket joint:* Flexion, extension, adduction, abduction, internal and external rotation should be examinated. Abnormalities of joint movement:
    - Pain occurs in whole ranges of joint movement.
    - Pain may occur in particular movement of the joint.
    - Damage to particular surfaces or ligaments leads to instability of the joint.

Screening History and Examinations for GALS (Gait, Arms, Legs, Spine)

Screening history
- Is there any stiffness on bone, limbs muscles and joints?
- Can you dress yourself?
- Is he or she able to climb upstairs without difficulty?

Screening examination
- *Gait:*
  - ❖ How patient walks?
  - ❖ How patient turns?
  - ❖ How the patient walks back?
  - ❖ How the patient stands up from sitting position?
- *Arms:*
  - ❖ From in front, ask the patient to place his both hand on the back of the head, and elbows back.
  - ❖ Ask him to place his both hands by the side of the body.
  - ❖ Ask him to place his both hands in front, palms down and finger straight.

- ❖ Ask him to make fist with both hands.
- ❖ Ask the patient to touch the tip of the thumb with each tip of other fingers one by one.
- ❖ Examine squeezes the metacarpal (2nd to 5th) to elicit tenderness.
- *Legs—Inspection from front:*
  - ❖ Observe any abnormality during lying down position.
  - ❖ Ask the patient to flex the hip and knee and observe any crepitus.
  - ❖ At flexed hip position, try to rotate the hip internally to observe any restricted motion or pain during movement.
  - ❖ Push the patella downwards to elicit tenderness.
  - ❖ Push the patella inwards to see any effusion.
  - ❖ Squeeze the small joints (metatarsophalangeal and inter-phalangeal joints) to elicit tenderness, any deformity, any swelling.
  - ❖ Inspect both soles for callosities, tenderness.
- *Spine:* Inspect following motion by viewing the patient from following positions:
  - ❖ From behind
  - ❖ From side
  - ❖ Ask the patient to bend forward
  - ❖ Ask the patient to touch chin on the chest
  - ❖ Ask the patient to touch his chin to the shoulder.

Recording of findings: If gait is normal, records of physical finding obtained from above examinations are usually normal.

Muscles Examination

Wasting: Measure the circumference of limb and compare with the opposite limb.

Washing may be:
- *Associated with joint disease:*
  - ❖ Washing of small muscles of the hand in rheumatoid arthritis
  - ❖ Washing of quadriceps in arthropathy of the knee
- *Without joint disease:*
  - ❖ Primary muscle disease
  - ❖ Myasthenia gravis
  - ❖ Normally in elderly people but not accompanied by weakness.

Increased muscle bulk:
- *The muscles of the body may be truly hypertrophied due to increase in muscle bulk:* It can be seen in a body builder (Fig. 13.31).

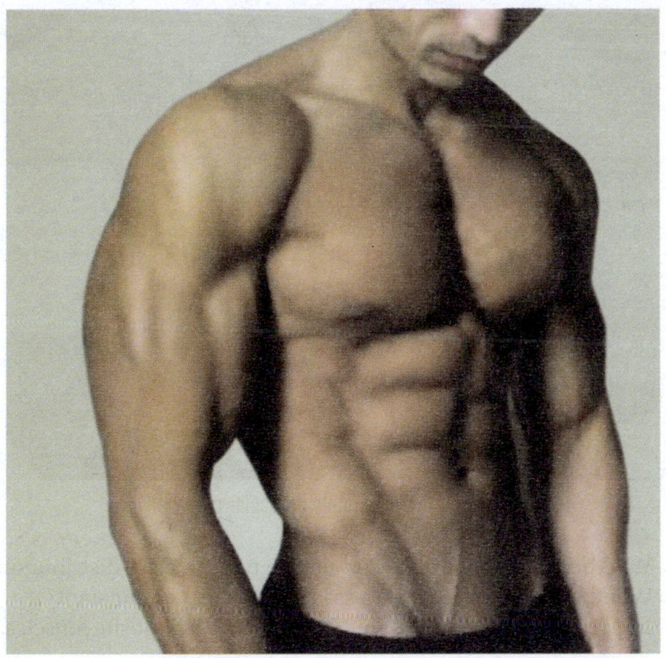

FIG. 13.31 Muscular hypertrophy

- *Muscle bulk may be increased due to fatty infiltration called pseudohypertrophy:* It can be seen in Duchenne's muscular dystrophy (Fig. 13.32).

Spontaneous muscular contraction: Spontaneous movements of the muscles can occur in:

- Upper motor neuron disease—flexor or extensor spasms of legs muscles at hip or at knee.
- Lower motor neuron disease—fasciculation occurs in all the muscles of the body.
- Fasciculation occurs in single muscle may be due to:
  - ❖ Physiologically mainly confined to calves.
  - ❖ Pathologically—cervical radiculopathy.

Palpation of muscles: It is of unlimited value. If the muscle is tender:

- Alcoholic myopathy
- Myositis
- Peripheral neuropathy produced by thiamine deficiency.

Testing of muscle power: Regarding testing of muscle power following questions should be important:

- Whether weakness in focal or global?
- Whether weakness in proximal?

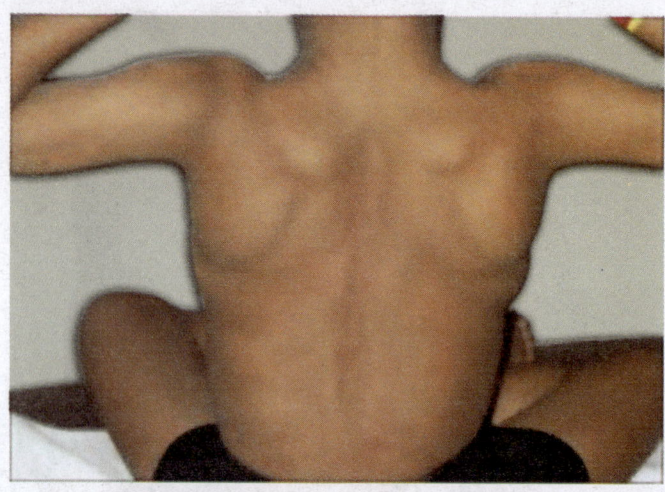

FIG. 13.32 Duchenne's muscular dystrophy

- Whether weakness will occur along a typical nerve distribution?
- Whether the muscle weakness is intermittent or constant?
- In each case comparing should be done with opposite muscles.

Individual Joint Examination

- *Temporomandibular joint (Figs 13.33 and 13.34)*
  Function: It helps to open and close the mouth—there may be side to side movement of the jaw (Figs 13.35 and 13.36)
  Palpation:
  - Place the finger in front and below the tragus.
  - If patient opens his jaw, palpation of the head of the mandible is possible.

  Abnormality:
  - Joint may be tender
  - Dislocation of joint.
- *Spine examination:*
  - *Cervical spine:*
    - Seven cervical vertebrae
    - Five intervertebral disc (C 2/3–C 6/7)
    - C_7/T_1 disc is associated with radicular symptoms
    - Degenerative disease common between C_5 and T_1 disc
    - C_2 and C_3 nerve root covers sensation back of the head, lower jaw line
    - C_4 to T_1 nerve roots produces bacterial plexus.
  - *Thoracic spines:*
    - Thoracic spine moves less than lumbar spine
    - Twelve thoracic vertebrae

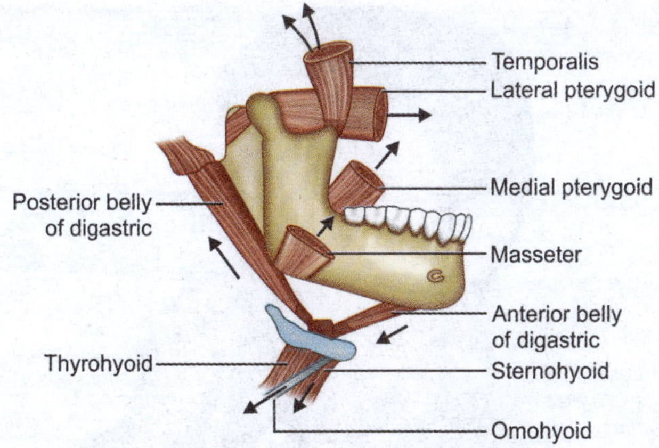

FIG. 13.33   Temporomandibular joint (lateral view)

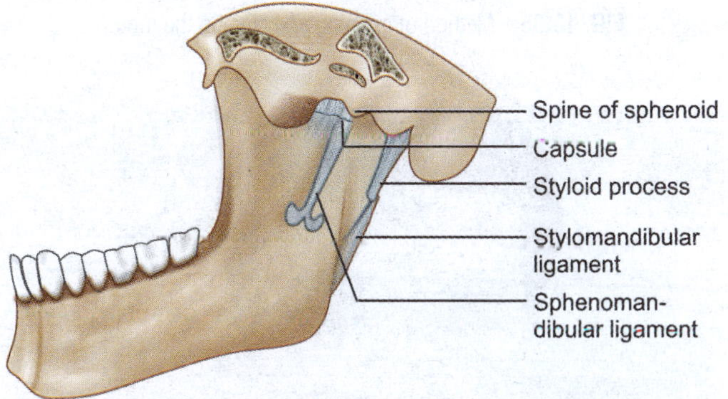

FIG. 13.34   Temporomandibular joint (medial view)

- Segmental movement in any direction is about 6°
- Ribs (1–10) articulate posteriorly with vertebrae at two points—these are both synovial joints
- 11th and 12th ribs do not have costotransverse joints
- Anteriorly ribs join with manubrium sterni.
- ❖ *Lumbar vertebrae:*
  - 5th lumbar vertebrae
  - Transition between mobile lumbar spine and fixed sacrum together with high weight loading combine to make the region highly prone to damage.
  - Sacroiliac joint (sensorial) are held firmly by strong fibrous capsule and tough ligaments. The movement of this joint is inversely proportional to age. Spinal cord ends at L1/L2. Nerves then run individually in the spinal canal—they together are termed as caudal equine.

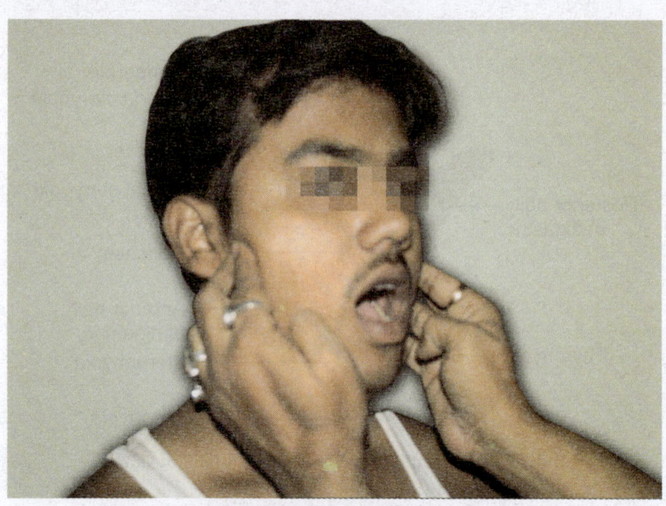

FIG. 13.35 Method of opening and closing the mouth

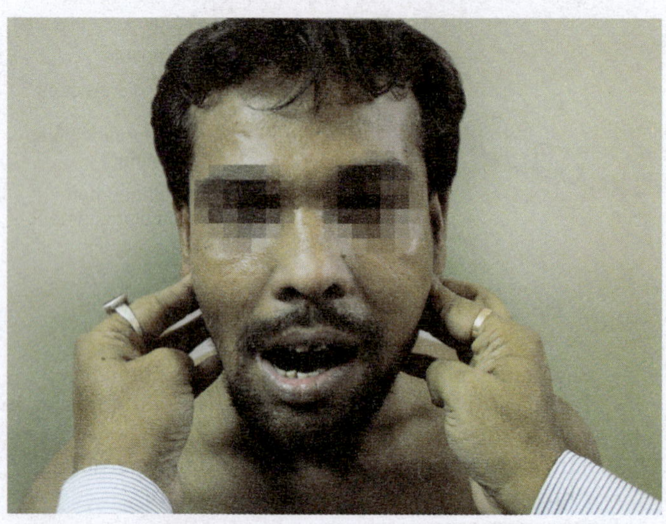

FIG. 13.36 Side-to-side movement of jaw

Primary curvature of spine (Fig. 13.37)
- In cervical and lumbar regions—Lordotic curvature.
  There are secondary curvatures depend upon anterior and posterior aspect of intervertebral disc.
- In thoracic and sacral regions, Kyphotic curvature.
- These are primary curvature—determined by anterior and posterior aspect of intervertebral disc at these levels.

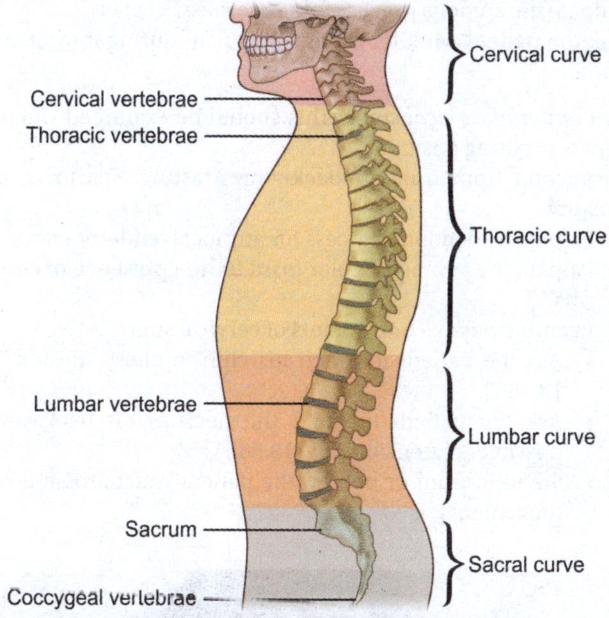

FIG. 13.37   Vertebral column curvature

Nucleus pulpous is responsible for even distribution of force onto annulus fibrosus and hyaline laminae covering vertebral bodies.

Movement of joints
- *Forward flexion and extension*—at all level of spine.
  - ❖ Maximal at the junction of atlas and occipital bone
  - ❖ In lumbar vertebral
  - ❖ Cervical vertebrae.
- *Lateral flexion:*
  - ❖ Greatest at atlantoaxial region
  - ❖ To some extent in lumbar and cervical region
  - ❖ Least movement in thoracic region.
- *Rotatory movement:* Atlantoaxial joints.

Examination of spine at total: Ask the patient to stand erect—watch the posture of the patient:
- Increased flexion   Kyphosis
- Hyperextension—lordosis—Physiological hyperextension occurs in pregnancy.
- Lateral curvature—scoliosis.
- Focal flexion deformity—gibbus.
  As the spinous process rotates towards midline, scoliosis is accentuated when the patient bends forwards.

- Palpate the spinous process for tenderness.
- Ask the patient whether there is any pain during movement of spine.

Examination of cervical spine: This should be examined when the patient is in sitting positions.

- Inspection from front or back—any wasting, spasm or poor posture.
  - ❖ Palpate the spinous process for any local tenderness.
  - ❖ Palpate the supraclavicular fossa for the presence of cervical ribs.
  - ❖ Examine passive movements of cervical spine:
    - Ask the patient to touch his chin to chest—flexion (Fig. 13.38A).
    - Ask the patient to bend the neck as far backward as possible—extension (Fig. 13.38B).
    - Stand in front or behind the patient watch, the following movements:

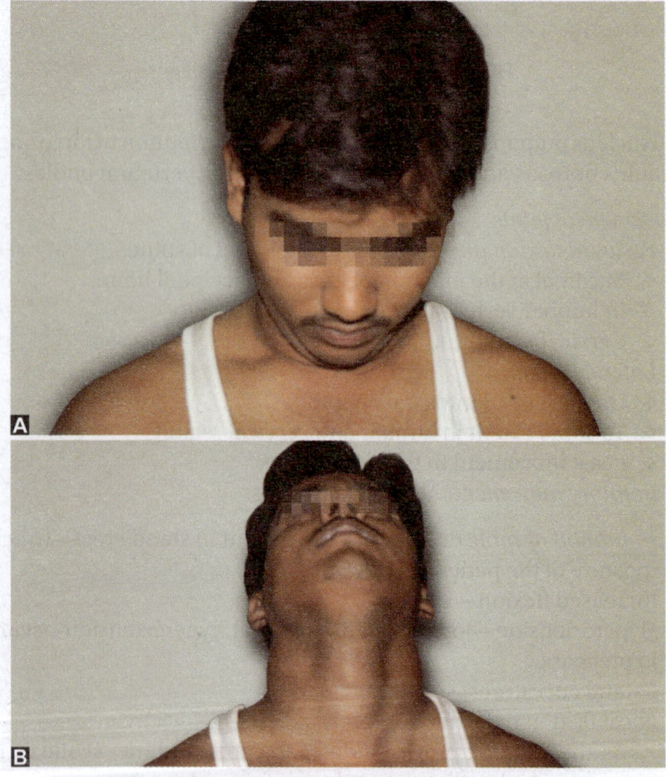

FIGS 13.38A AND B   (A) Flexion of cervical spine; (B) Extension of cervical spine

- Ask the patient to touch his ear towards the shoulder (Fig. 13.39).
First on one side, then on the other side—lateral flexion (Fig. 13.40).
- Ask the patient to look over one shoulder—first on one side, then on the other side—rotatory movements (Figs 13.41 and 13.42).

Remember the movement of neck—the range movements depending on age, sex and ethnicity.

Normal range of lateral flexion is 45° and rotatory movement is 70° in normal middle aged person.

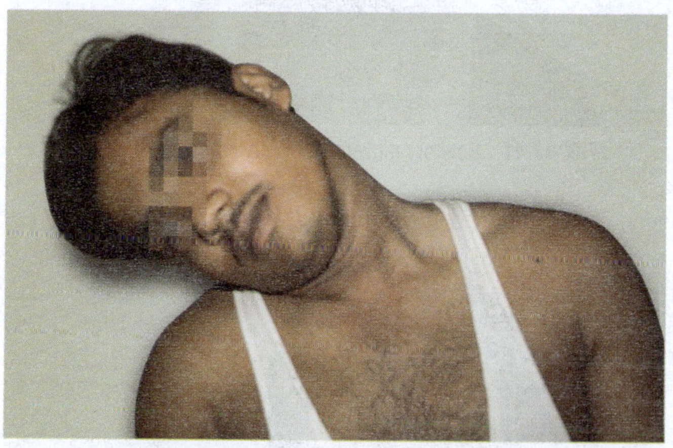

FIG. 13.39   Right lateral flexion of cervical spine

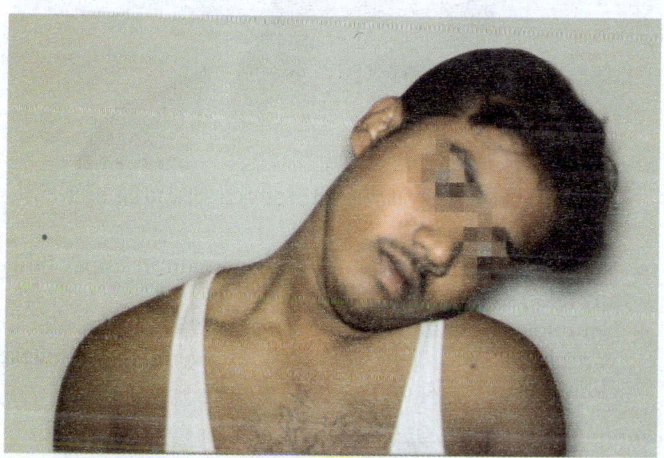

FIG. 13.40   Left lateral flexion of cervical spine

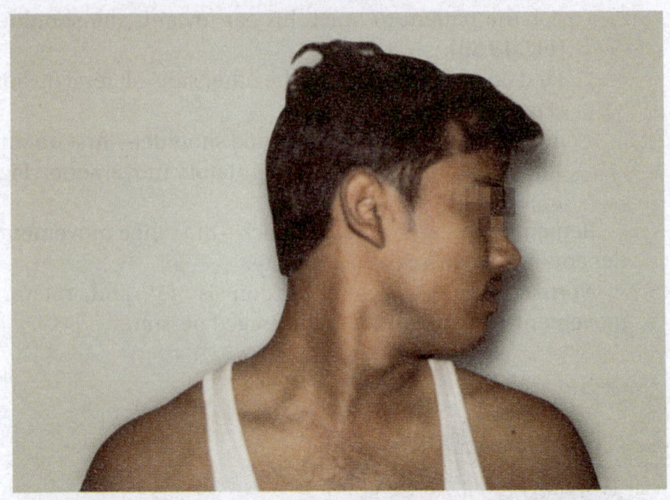

FIG. 13.41   Rotatory movement of cervical spine to the left

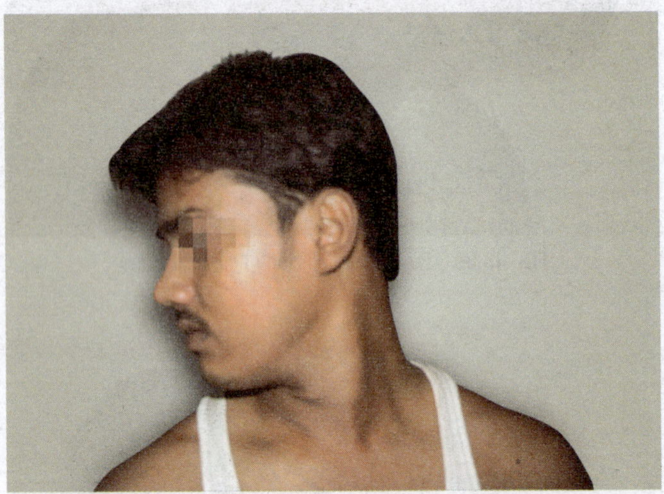

FIG. 13.42   Rotatory movement of cervical spine to the right

- ❖ Note any specific movement triggers pain in upper limb—any referred pain to shoulder.
- ❖ Neurological examination of upper and lower limb for any paresthesia, washing, weakness, exaggeration of reflexes, clonus, plantar response.

Examination of thoracic spine
Inspection: Patient should be inspected from front and back:
- Scoliosis—it may be:

- ❖ Nonstructural due to back pain or abdominal pain, leg length discrepancy
  - ❖ Psychogenic or
  - ❖ Structural—due to bony lesions.
- Kyphosis—normally mild kyphosis is present. Marked kyphosis may be due to:
  - ❖ Osteoporotic vertebral fracture
  - ❖ Degenerative disease.
- Loss of normal kyphosis—flat spine may be due to:
  - ❖ Spondylotic changes
  - ❖ Severe muscle spasm.
- Loose fold on the skin—denote multiple vertebral fractures.
- Costochondral swelling—may be due to:
  - ❖ Costochondritis
  - ❖ Synovits of costosternal joint and sternoclavicular joint.

Palpation: Palpate vertebrae, para vertebral joints, muscles of the back.
- Osteomyelitis of spine—tender, swelling
- Tumor—erythema will be present or not
- Tender costotransverse joints (G5 on from midline)
- Costovertebral joints tenderness can be elicited by manipulation of ribs
- Trigger points in case of myofacial pain
- Tender swelling of sternoclavicular, sternocostal, sternomanu-brial joints suggests spondyloarthropathy or SAPHO (synovitis, acne, pastulosis, hyperostasis and aseptic osteomyelitis).

Movement (Figs 13.43 and 13.44):
- Ask the patient to fold his arm across the chest. Then ask him to twist his body as far as possible from one side to other.
  Range of thoracic movement is:
  - ❖ 30° extension
  - ❖ 20°–40° lateral flexion
  - ❖ 25°–45° flexion
  - ❖ 30°–45° rotation.
  Scoliosis is often associated with rotation of spine.
- Spondylitis may be obvious in case of spinal hypermobility.
- Chest expansion—from forced expiration to forced inspiration can be measured by tape—which is in normal person at least 5 cm.

Other examinations
- Neurological examination of lower limbs to see any sign of spinal cord compression.
- Breast and axillary nodes should be examined.

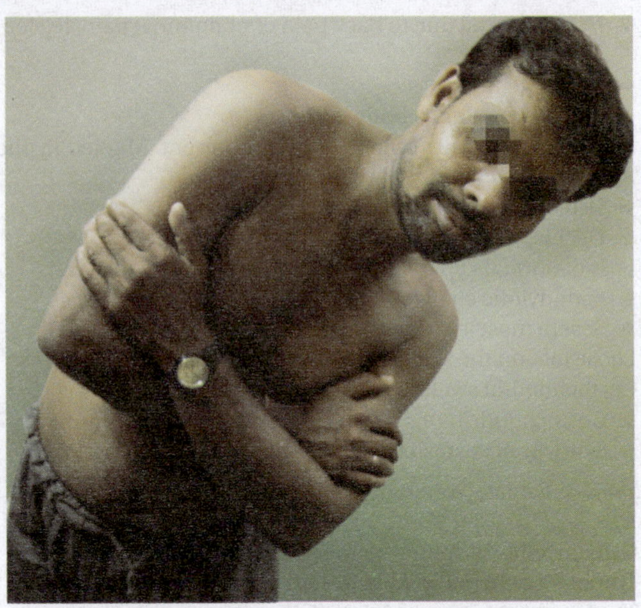

FIG. 13.43   Lateral flexion of thoracic spine

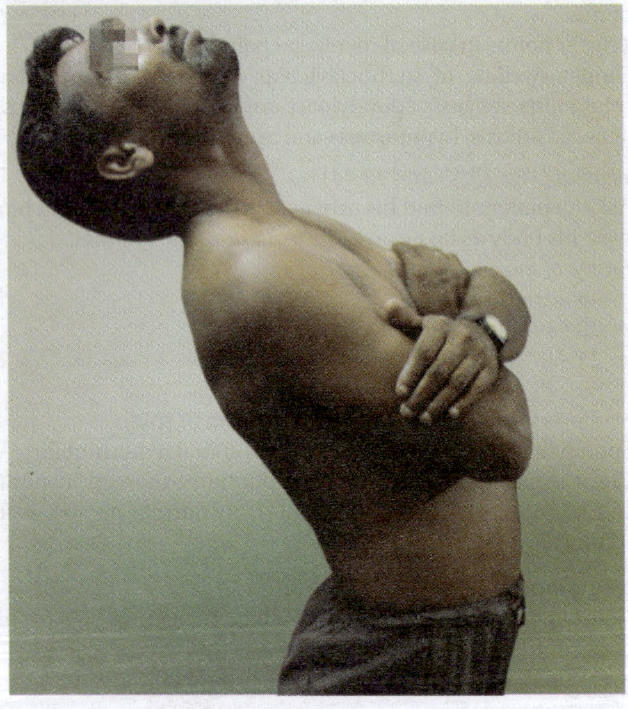

FIG. 13.44   Extension of thoracic spine

Examination of lumbar spine
Inspection:
- Fluidity of movements—when undressed.
- Any swelling, redness, skin markings for osteomyelitis.
- Lipoma, hairy patches, café-au-lait spots, skin tags.
- Multiple skin folds—denotes:
  ❖ Vertebral fractures
  ❖ Spondylolisthesis.
- *Note:*
  ❖ Any hyperlordosis (L5–S1 damage)
  ❖ Prominent thoraco lumbar kyphosis (multiple disc degeneration, vertebral fracture).

Movements of lumbar spine (Figs 13.45 to 13.48)
- *Forward flexion:* Legs straight, slow forward bend to touch his knees or ankles.
- *Extension:* Legs straight, bend backward very slowly as far as possible.
- *Lateral flexion:* Legs and back straight, moves sideways with his hands down the side of the thigh.

Flexion can be mediated by hip joint and extension can be affected by slight pelvic tilt.

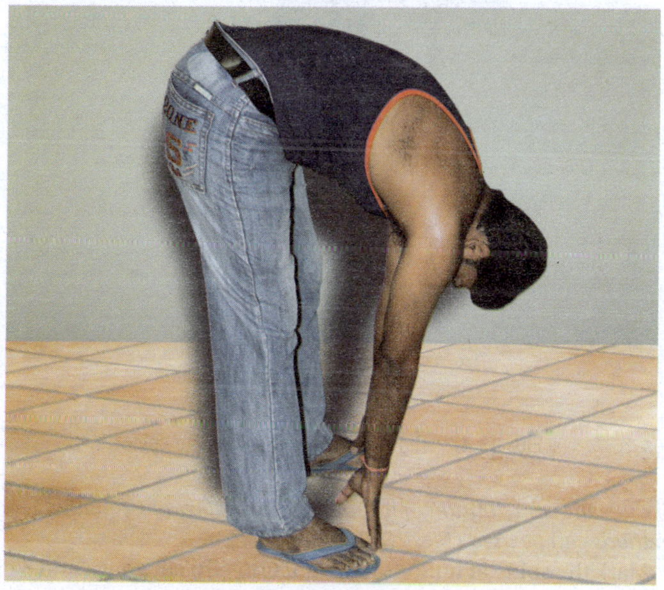

FIG. 13.45   Forward flexion

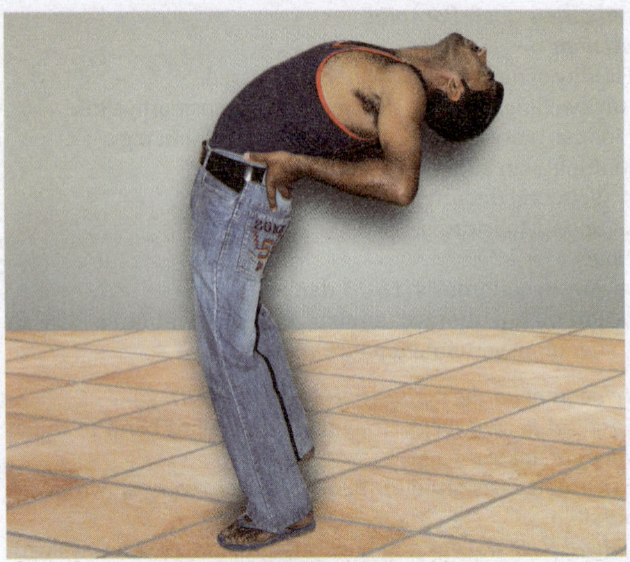

FIG. 13.46 Extension of lumbar spine

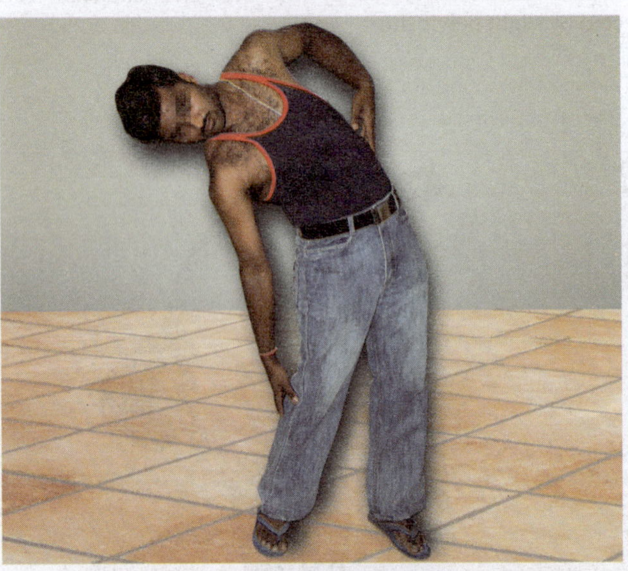

FIG. 13.47 Right lateral flexion of lumbar spine

To asses the contribution of lumbar spine for flexion—following methods can be used (Figs 13.49A and B)

- Mark the spine at lumbosacral junction—10 cm above and 5 cm below the mark—give two additional mark.

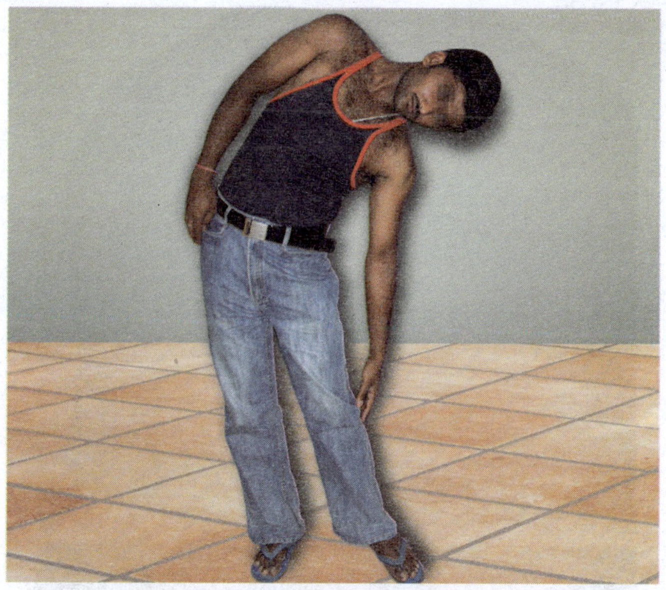

FIG. 13.48   Left lateral flexion of lumbar spine

- On forward flexion distance between the upper two marks is increased by 4 cm approximately.
  But distance between two lower marks remains same.

Disease Interpretation

- *Pain on extension:*
  - ❖ Retrospondylolisthesis
  - ❖ Facet joint arthritis.
- Failure of spinous process to separate during flexion— Parmanent spinal stiffness—ankylosing spondylosis.
- Ask the patient to stand on one foot then to their toes in few occasions—weakness may be due to L5 nerve root entrapment.

Gait pattern
The following are the abnormalities of the gait:
- Antalgic gait
- *Wise base gait:*
  - ❖ Muscular weakness
  - ❖ Cerebellar deficit
- Short shuffling gait—Fastinant gait—Parkinsonism
- Gait of old age—lean forward and small steps
- Flat feet
- Feet valgus
- Genu recurvatum.

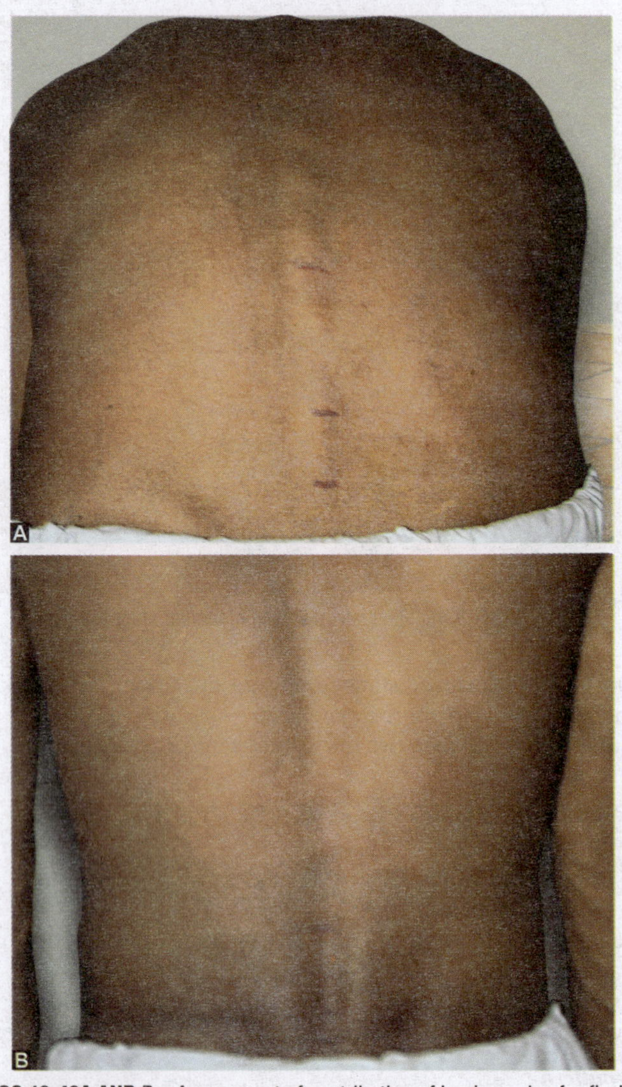

FIGS 13.49A AND B Assessment of contribution of lumbar spine for flexion

If patient is allowed to sit on a chair, pain of lumbar region can be elicited by extension of legs—which stretches the dura—it can elicit root pain or disc prolapse.

Method to elicit sacroiliitis are following:
- *Supine position (Figs 13.50 to 13.52):*
  - ❖ Patient is in supine position. Flex the leg at hip and then extend the legs at knee so that upper leg is vertical.

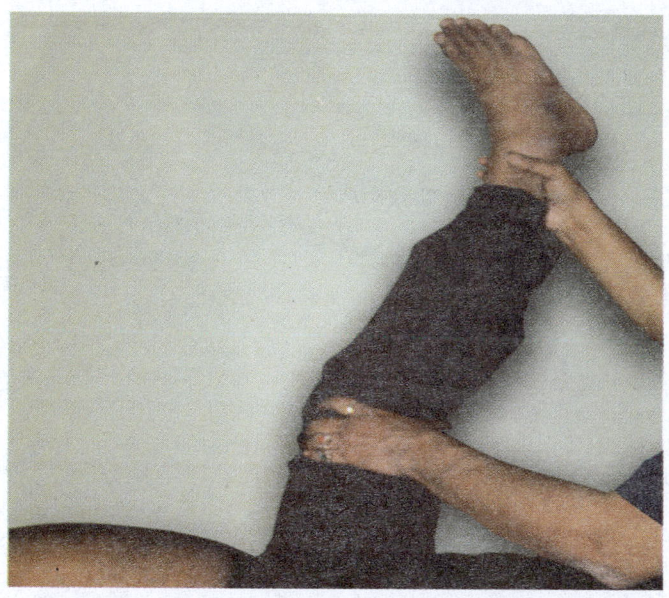

FIG. 13.50   Method to elicit sacroiliitis (supine position) (Step 1)

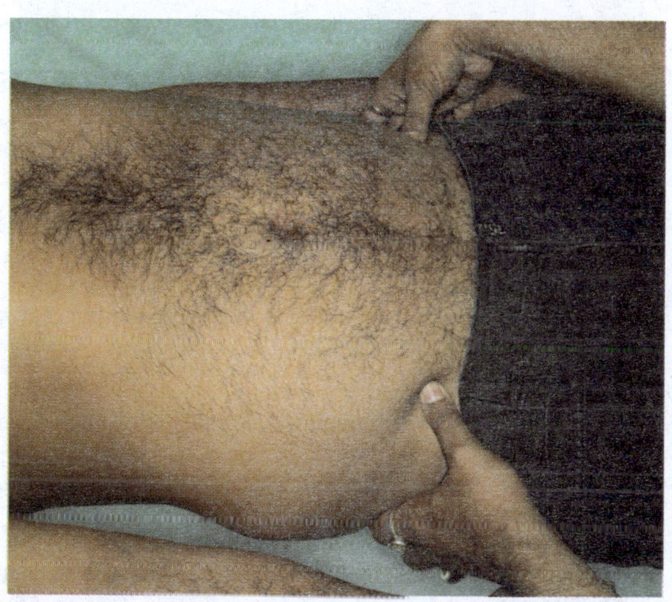

FIG. 13.51   Method to elicit sacroiliitis (supine position) (Step 2)

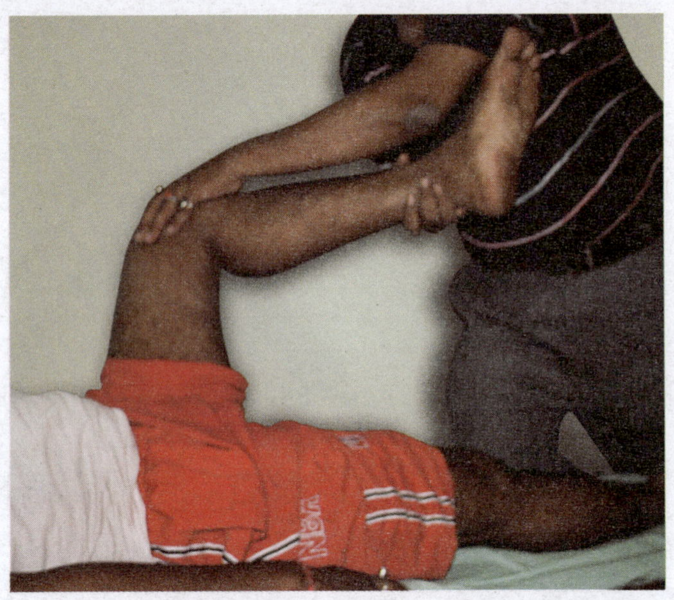

FIG. 13.52 Method to elicit sacroiliitis (supine position) (Step 3)

❖ Press down and out firmly at the anterior superior iliac spine—both at a time.
❖ Lift one leg, flex and abduct at the hip slightly, while other limb kept in extended position.
- *Prone position (Fig. 13.53):* In prone position, press firmly down over the midline of the sacrum.

Nerve stretching test (Lasegue's sign)
- Patient will be in supine position
- Flex the extended at hip
- Normal 80–90° flexion in possible at the hip. Variation may be from 60 to more than 90° in adult.

Deviation from normal
- Normally, there may be tightening due to posterior thigh or calf muscles.
- Raising leg to < 40°—indicates radicular pain in less than 30 years aged persons.
- Cross straight leg rising sign more specific for root lesion.
- To enhance possibility of this sign dorsiflex the foot to stretch the nerve (Bragard's test).

Fallacy
- This test may not be positive even the patient may be suffering from sciatica.

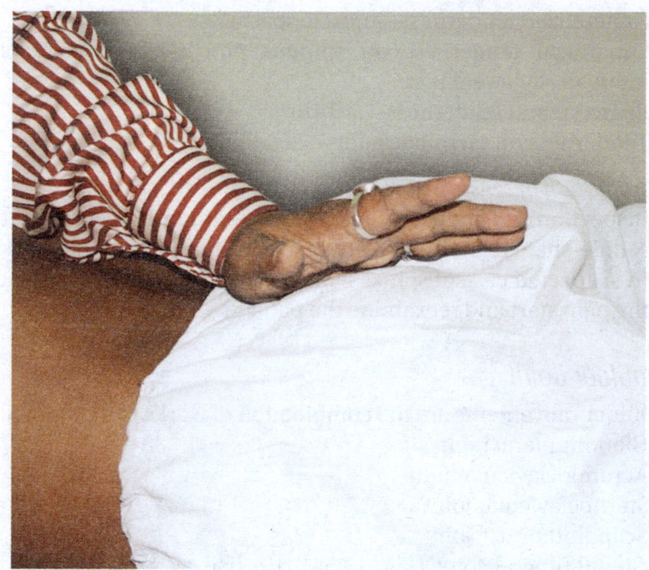

FIG. 13.53   Method to elicit sacroiliitis (prone position)

- This test is negative in patient with foraminal stenosis.
- When central positive dire prolapse occurs—may be negative:

Testing muscles of lower limb:

- ❖ *Hamstrings (L5 S1 S2)—Knee flexion:* Ask the patient to flex the legs at the knee to 45°, and you give resistance from opposite side to flex the knee.
- ❖ *Iliopsoas (Hip flexor and internal rotator)—L1, L2, L3:* Ask the patient to flex the limb at the hip and rotate internally. You resists the limb in opposite direction, e.g. extension and external rotation.
- ❖ Quadriceps fermoris (hip flexor and knee extensor) L2 L3 L4.

  Hold the patient's upper leg from underneath, as a result lower leg falls loosely. Now ask the patient to straighten the lower legs against resistance given by your hands.

  Tibialis anterior (ankle dorsiflexor), L4 L5: Ask the patient to straighten the leg and dorsiflex the foot against resistance given by you.

  Tibialis posterior (ankle inverter and dorsiflexor) L4 L5: Ask the patient to press the toes and great toe against resistance.

  Extensor hallucis longus (dorsiflexor of great toe) L5 S1: Ask the patient to dorsiflex his great toe against resistance.

Examination of patient in prone position: Ask the patient to lie down in prone position and palpation to be done in low back and sacrum:

- Generalized tenderness—muscle spasm.
- Superficial tenderness on spinous process or interspinous interval—ligament tear.
- Paravertebral tenderness—arthritis.
- Tenderness on sacroiliac joint—sacroiliitis.

Examination of sensory system
- Inspection and finding of sensory areas—around lower limbs and saddle-shaped anesthesia—in case of cauda equina syndrome.
- In suspected case of spinal stenosis—ask the patient to walk till the pain start and reexamine the patient.

Shoulder Joint

Shoulder movements are the combination of works of four joints:
1. Glenohumeral joint
2. Acromioclavicular joint
3. Sternoclavicular joint
4. Scapulothoracic joint.

Glenohumeral joint (Fig. 13.54) is a ball as socket joint. The circular fibrocartilaginous labrum increases the articular surfaces of the glenoid cavity.

Coracoacromial arch protects the glenoid cavity from trauma.

Coracoacromial arch and deltoid muscles are separated from capsule by subacromial bursa.

The movement of shoulder and responsible muscles are:
- *Abduction (Fig. 13.55A):*
  - ❖ First 0–30° of movement—contraction of Supraspinatus.
  - ❖ 31–90° of abduction movement—contraction of deltoid.
  - ❖ >90° of abduction movement with rotation of scapula—produced by contraction of trapezius.

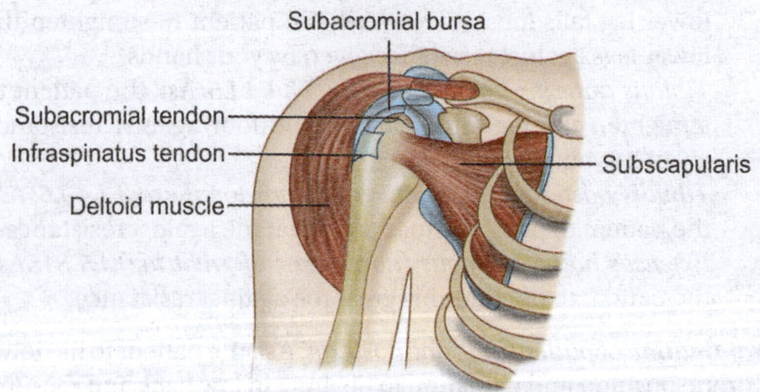

FIG. 13.54 Rotator cuff apparatus of shoulder joint

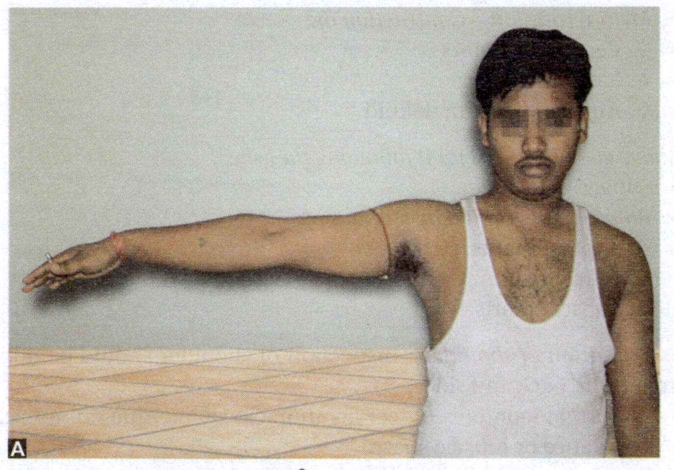

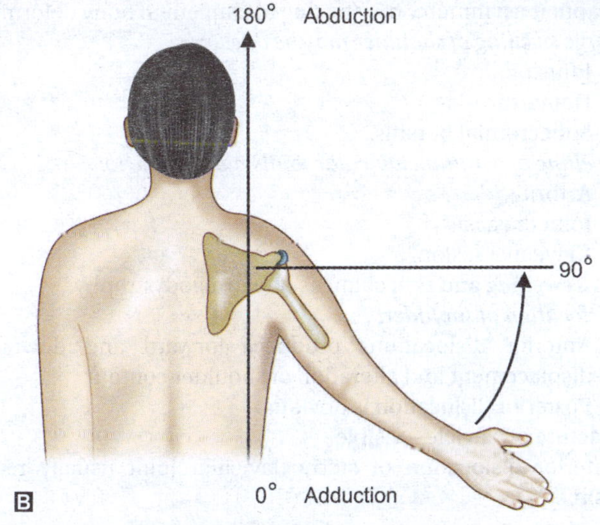

Figs 13.55A and B Shoulder movement

- *Adduction:* Contraction of pectoralis major latissimus dorsi (Fig. 13.55B).
- *Forward flexion—Contraction of:*
  - ❖ Pectoralis major
  - ❖ Anterior fibers of deltoid.
- *Extension—Contraction of:*
  - ❖ Latissimus dorsi
  - ❖ Teres major
  - ❖ Posterior fibers of deltoid.
- *Lateral rotation—Contraction of:* Infraspinatus muscles.

- *Medial rotation—Contraction of:*
  - ❖ Pectoralis majors
  - ❖ Latissimus dorsi
  - ❖ Anterior fibers of deltoid.

Above glenohumeral joint following these lie:
- Subacromial bursa
- *Rotator cuff formed by tendons of:*
  - ❖ Supraspinatus
  - ❖ Infraspinatus
  - ❖ Subscapularis.

Examination of shoulders: Inspection of shoulder should be done from front, back and sides.
- Abnormal contour of cervicothoracic spine due to muscle imbalance or muscle spasm.
- Scapular asymmetry may be due to congenital bony deformity.
- *Large swelling of shoulder may be due to:*
  - ❖ Effusion
  - ❖ Hemarthrosis
  - ❖ Subacromial bursitis.
- *Swelling of acromioclavicular joints may be due to:*
  - ❖ Arthritis
  - ❖ Joint diastasis
  - ❖ Clavicular lesion.
- Arm swelling and skin changes due to algodystrophy.
- *Dislocation of shoulder:*
  - ❖ Anterior dislocations produces forward and downward displacement and alteration of shoulder contour.
  - ❖ Posterior dislocation is obvious.
- Fracture of clavicle—visible.
- Anterior dislocation of sternoclavicular joint usually readily visible.

Method of movement of glenohumeral joint: Shoulder movement examination should be done in all directions by moving upper arm with one of yours hands and place the other hand over the shoulder to palpate:
- Crepitations
- Clunks and resistance to the particular movement.
  - ❖ *Abduction* done from neutral position against resistance arm should be extended at elbow and forearm pronated (Figs 13.55A and B).
  - ❖ *Adduction* is opposite in direction to abduction but in same position of arm and forearm (Figs 13.55B and 13.56).
  - ❖ *Flexion and extension:* Hand should be in semi flexed position at elbow. Then ask the patient to move the arm forward to

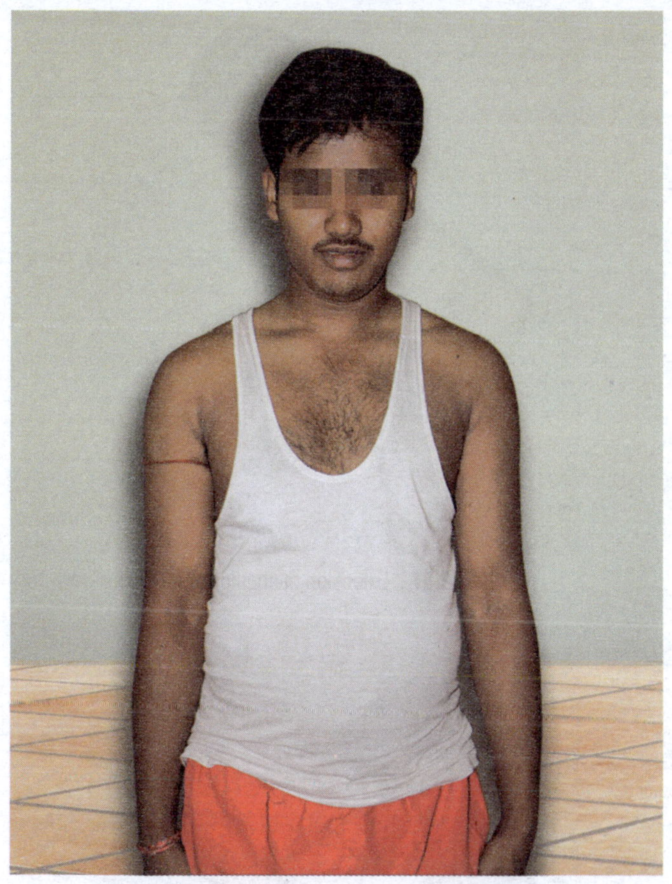

FIG. 13.56   Adduction of shoulder joint

produce flexion and ask the patient to move the arm backward to produce extension (Figs 13.57 and 13.58).

Internal and external rotation: Ask the patient to flex the elbow in such a position as if he is holding a tray, then ask the patient to rotate the arm outward to produce external rotation and to rotate the arm inward to produce internal rotation (Figs 13.59 to 13.61).

Abnormalities of movement of shoulder joint
- If humeral head slides anteriorly without rotation in glenoid cavity—denotes instability.
- Grossly reduced passive shoulder movement—adhesive capsulitis.
- During pulling of arms if both arms moves inferiorly— (sulcus sign)—glenohumeral instability.

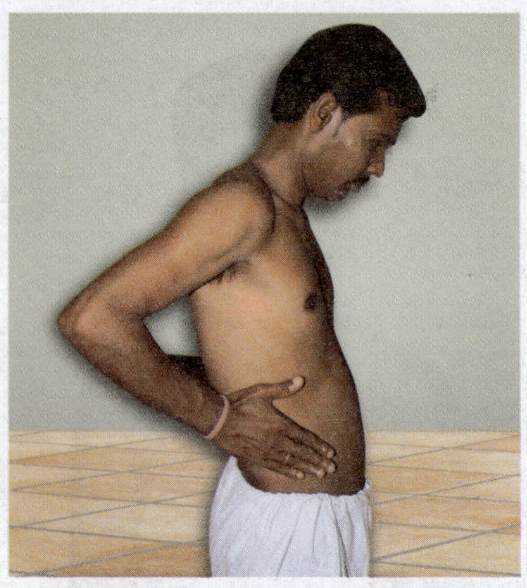

FIG. 13.57   Extension of shoulder joint

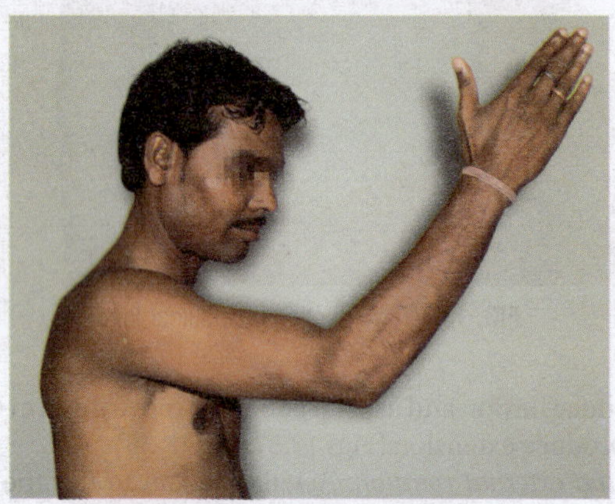

FIG. 13.58   Flexion of shoulder joint

Test for acromioclavicular joint (ACJ) (Fig. 13.62)
Hold the arm in forward flexion (90°). Then ask the patient to draw the hand across the chest. As a result there is compression of ACJ and produces pain in case of arthritis.

Shoulder is examined in supine position for the following detection:
- Anterior cuff deficiency
- Glenohumeral joint laxity
- Labral tear.

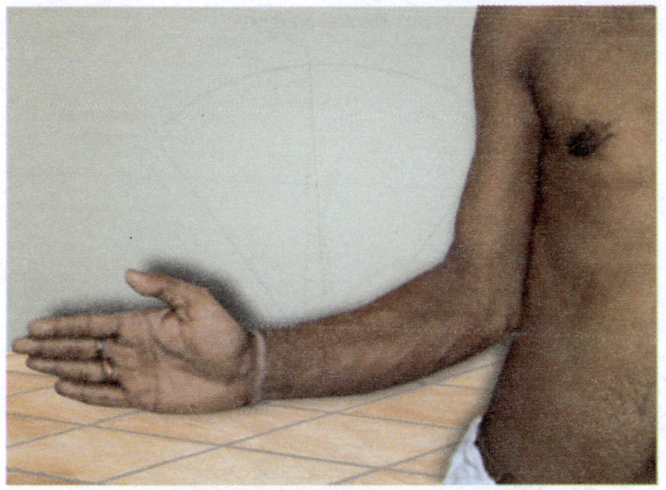

FIG. 13.59   External rotation of shoulder joint

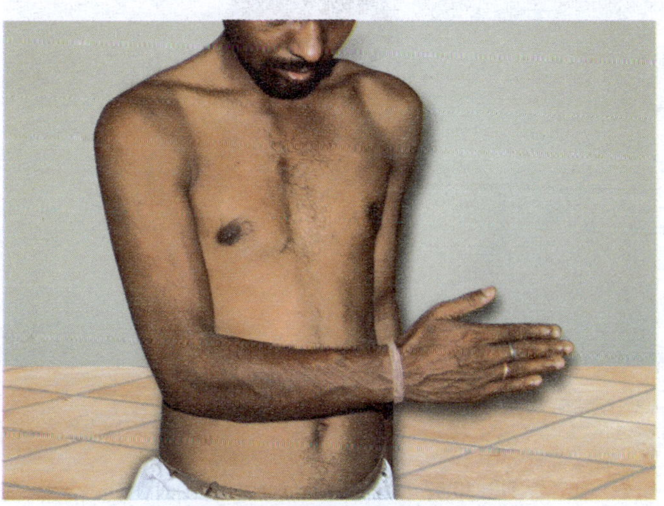

FIG. 13.60   Internal rotation of shoulder joint

Method (Fig. 13.63):
- Hold the arm with elbow flexed at slight abduction and external rotation.
- Then asks the patient to move the arm gently (cranially in coronal plane) and apply gradual external rotation.
  - ❖ In case of anterior cuff deficient there may be chance of anterior dislocation.
  - ❖ In case of labral tear there may be audible clunk.

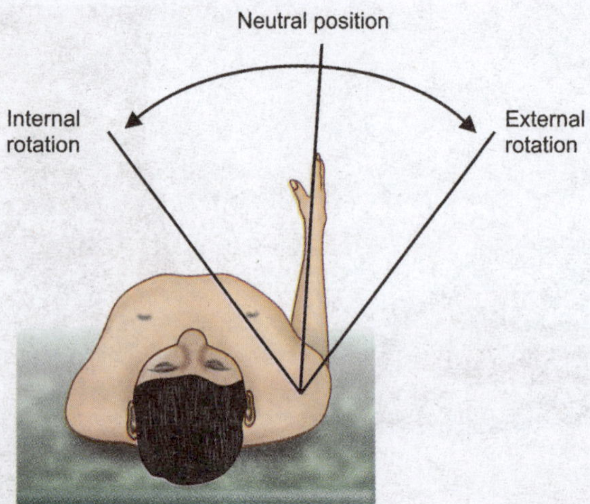

FIG. 13.61   External and internal rotations of a shoulder joint

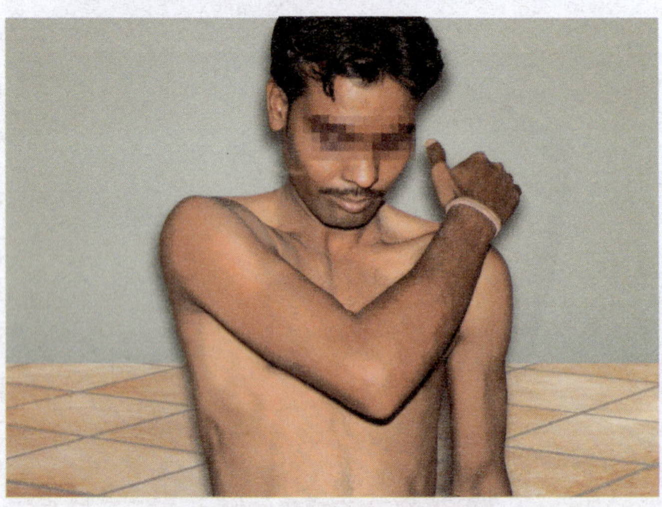

FIG. 13.62   Test of acromioclavicular joint

Painful arc syndrome

Rotator cuff is comprised of—tenders of supraspinatus, infraspinatus and subscapularis which come in contact with underneath of acromian.

Asks the patient to abduct the arm, the following will be happened if there is inflammation of supraspinatus muscle or subacromian bursa:

- Pain is absent initially
- Pain starts when muscles come in contact with underneath of acromian.

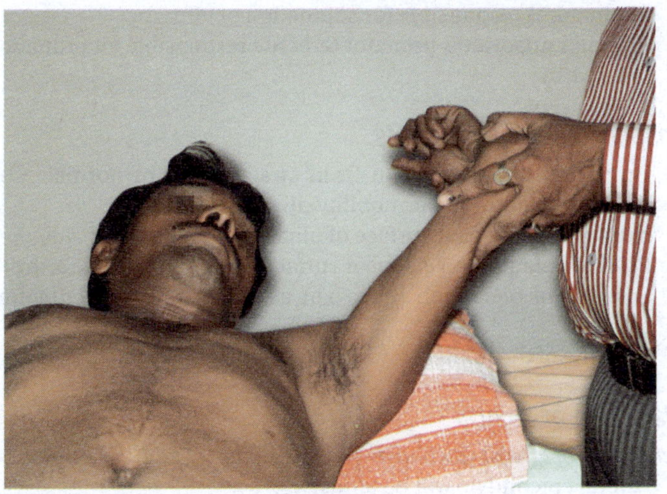

FIG. 13.63   Shoulder examination in supine position

- Disappears in final part of abduction when tendon falls away from acromian.

In case of biceps tendinitis: Pain occurs in anterior aspect shoulder and arm due to tenosynovitis of biceps tendon. Pain occurs when the biceps is allowed to contract.

In case of neuralgic amyotrophy:
- Severe pain occurs around the shoulder.
- Patchy weakness and wasting of the shoulder girdle muscles.

In few cases: There is involvement of long thoracic nerve in thin case—there is winging of scapula as the arm is pushed forwards against resistance.

Elbow joint: This joint comprises two joints:
1. Lower end of humerus with upper end of radius and ulna
2. Upper ends of radius and ulna.

   First joint in responsible for flexion and extension of elbow joint in the range of 150°.

   Second joint is responsible for pronation and supination in the range of 180°.

   In male, forearm is slightly abducted carrying angle will be less. But in female carrying angle will be high due to high abduction of forearm (15°).

The muscles responsible for movement of elbow are:
- Biceps flexes the elbow in supinated arm
- Brachioradialis flexes the supinated or pronated arm
- Triceps is responsible for extension of elbow
- Anconeus is responsible for extension of elbow

- Supinator is responsible for supination of forearm
- Pronator quadratus, pronator teres are responsible for pronation of forearm.

Inspection of Elbow Joints

- Up to 10° hyperextension from straight arm in normal. >10° hyperextension—hypermobility disorder
- Nodules on extensor surface of ulna—rheumatoid arthritis
- Psoriatic plaques on extensor surface of elbow psoriatic arthritis
- Swelling of olecranon bursa—in association with rheumatoid arthritis
- Swelling of the joint—may be due to effusion.

Palpation of Joint

Palpation of lateral epicondyle (Tennis elbow) (Fig. 13.64)

- Lateral epicondyle will be tender
- Pain in the region of elbow
- Tenderness is due to inflammation of radiohumeral bursa—lying under extensor tendon apeunurosis
- First flexing wrist, pronating forearm, then extend elbow—may reproduce pain in lateral epicondyle.

Palpation of medial epicondyle (Golfer elbow) (Fig. 13.65)

- Tenderness suggests—epicondylitis (Golfer's elbow), chronic pain syndrome or enthesitis.
- Stretching the wrist flexors—supinate the forearm then passively extends both wrist and elbow simultaneously—may elicit pain.

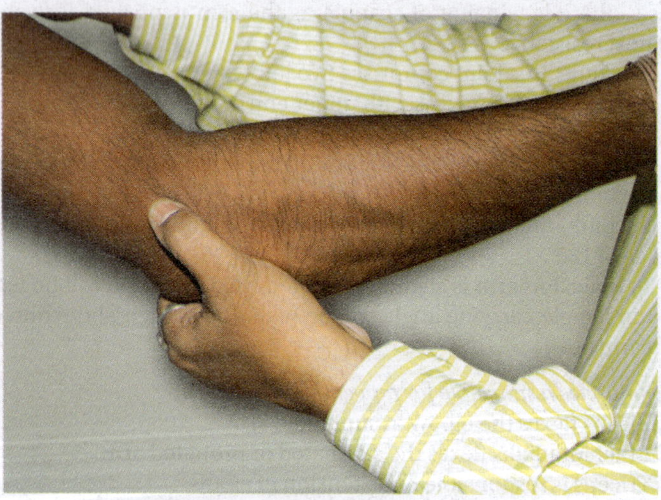

FIG. 13.64 Palpation of lateral epicondyle

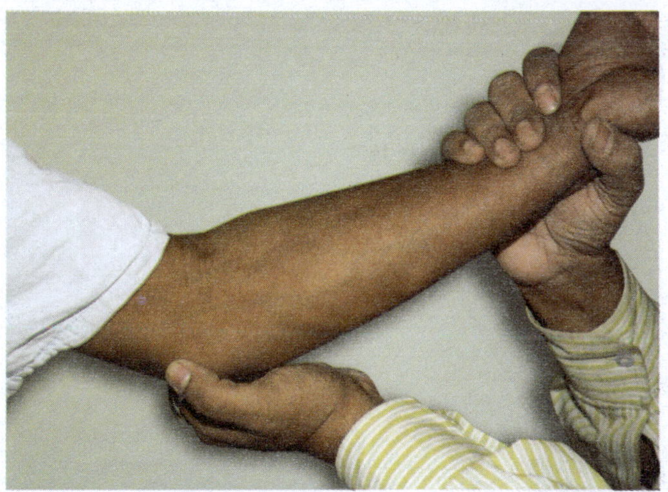

FIG. 13.65   Palpation of medial epicondyle

- Resist palmar flexior at wrist with forearm pronation with elbow extension—produce pain.

Passive flexion and extension of elbow joint (Figs 13.66 and 13.67)
- Any crepitus—due to intra-articular pathology.
- Any locking—loose body in joints.
- Prevention of full flexion or full extension due to bony spur or osteophytes.

Passive supination and pronation of forearm (Figs 13.68 and 13.69): This movement can be done in forearm with flexion of elbow at 90°—pathology may be:
- Crepitations
- Subluxation
- Instability—suggests tear or damage to articular ligament.

Traumatic lesions at elbow joints
- Dislocation.
- Fracture of radial head and distal humerus following fall on outstretched hand.

Dislocation occurs in posterolateral direction producing ulnar and median nerve damage.

Test for peripheral nerve function
- Radial nerve has its course around lateral epicondyle so in case of lateral elbow lesion—radial nerve should be tested.
- Median nerve runs through antecubital fossa may be affected in trauma to elbow.

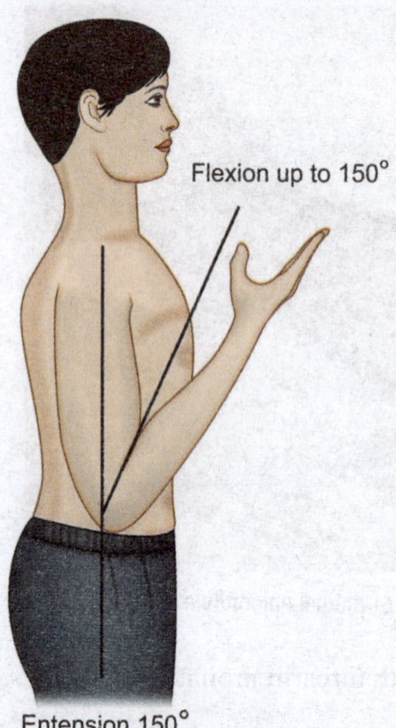

FIG. 13.66 Passive flexion and extension of elbow joint

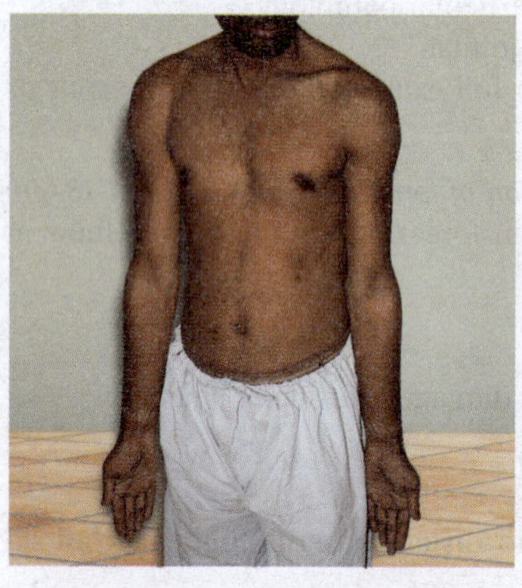

FIG. 13.67 Position of upper limb during examination of elbow joint

- Median nerve passes in between two head of pronator teres (medial epicondyle and coronoid process) and is divided into anterior interosseous and terminal median nerve branches.
- Ulnar nerve lies in the groove behind the medial epicondyle, Bony lesion affect nerve function reduce reaction in little finger and weakness of small muscles of the hand, flexor carpi ulnaris, extensor carpi ulnaris, abductor digiti minimi.

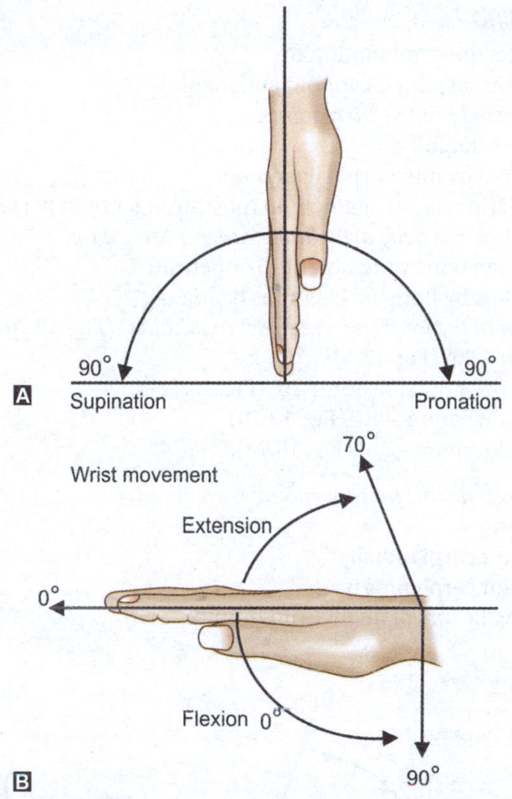

FIGS 13.68A AND B   Passive supination and pronation of forearm

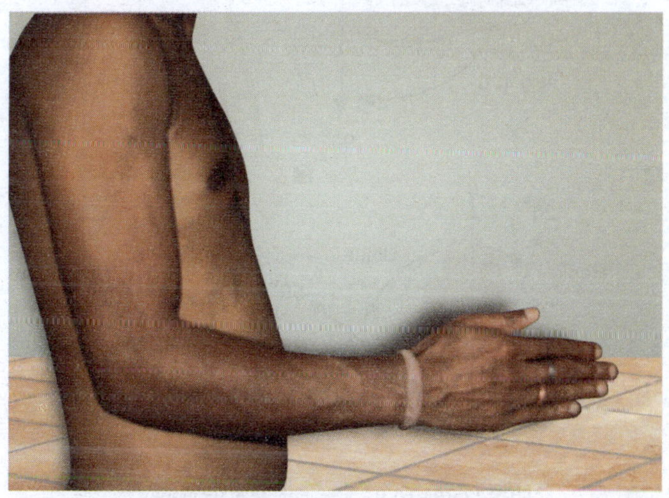

FIG. 13.69   Pronation and supination

Wrist Joints

This joint is the combination of:

- Radiocarpal joint (scaphoid and lunate)
- *Intercarpal joints—these joints:*
  - ❖ Most stable
  - ❖ Joined by intercarpal ligaments
  - ❖ Anterior carpal ligament in most stronger than posterior one.
- *Ulna does not truly articulate, rather attached to:*
  - ❖ Lunate bone by ligament—triquetrum
  - ❖ Radius by fibrocartilaginous ligament.

Movement of the joint (all in respect to midline) (Figs 13.70A to C):

- Flexion—90° (Fig. 13.71)
- Extensor or dorsiflexion—70° (Fig. 13.72)
- Radial deviation—20° (Fig. 13.73)
- Ulnar deviation—55° (Fig. 13.74).

Muscles responsible for movement

- *Flexion:*
  - ❖ Flexor carpi radialis
  - ❖ Flexor carpi ulnaris
  - ❖ Long flexors of fingers and thumb.

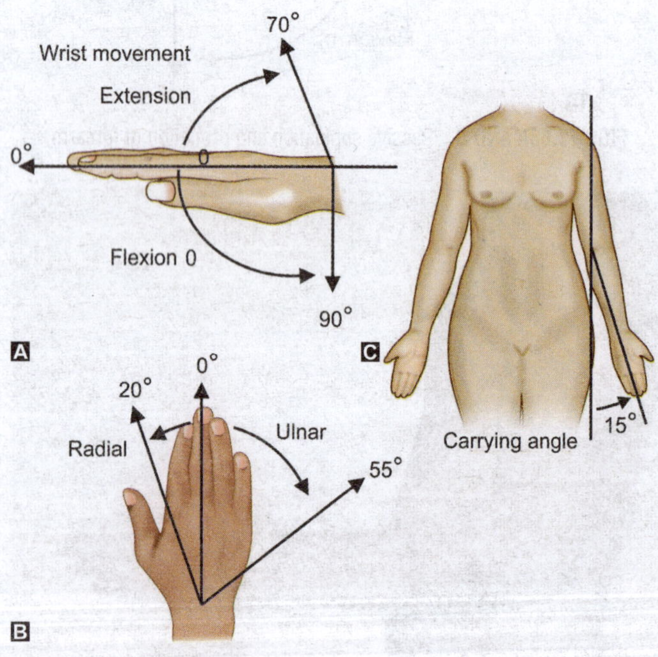

FIGS 13.70A TO C   Movements of wrist joint

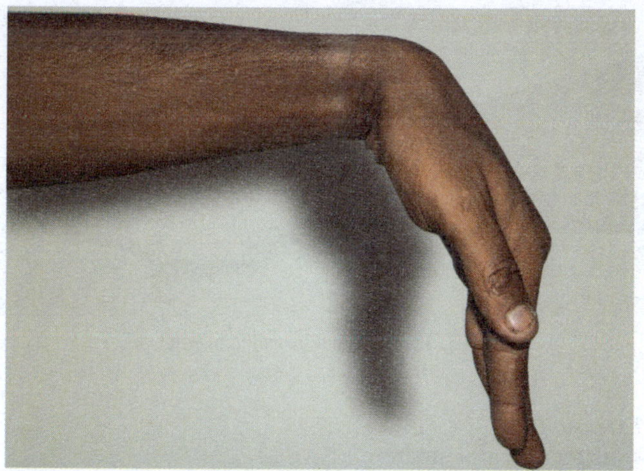

FIG. 13.71   Flexion of wrist

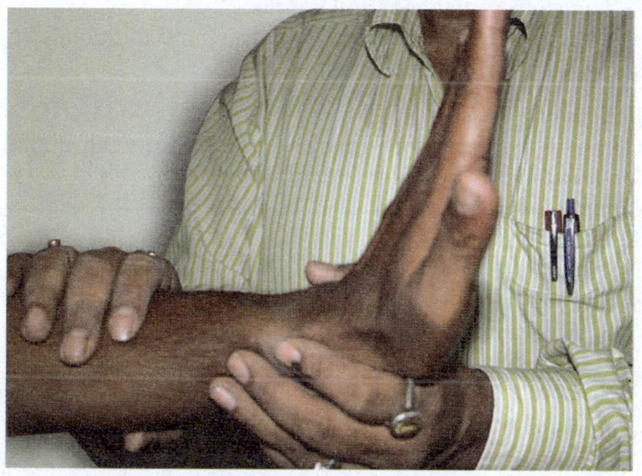

FIG. 13.72   Extension of wrist

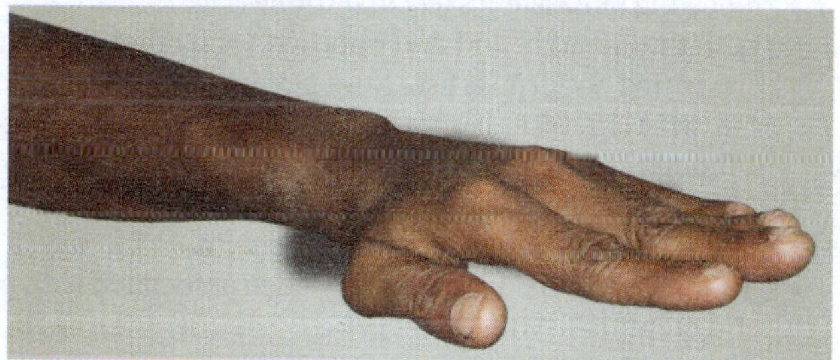

FIG. 13.73   Radial deviation of wrist

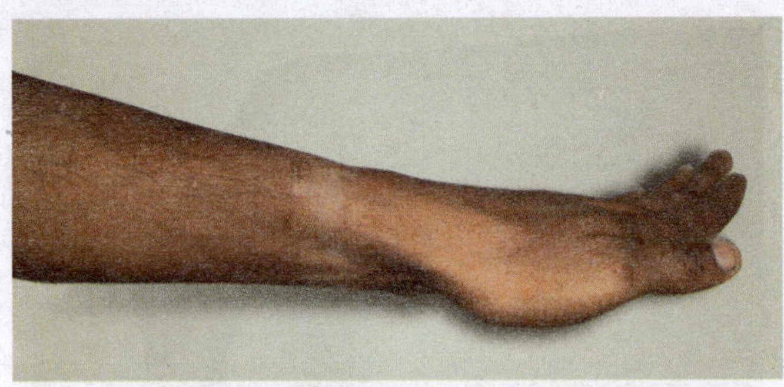

FIG. 13.74 Ulnar deviation of wrist

- *Extension:*
  - ❖ Extensor carpi ulnaris
  - ❖ Extension carpi radialis longus
  - ❖ Extensor carpi radialis brevis
  - ❖ Long flexors of fingers and thumb.

  Long flexors and extensors of fingers and thumb also exert some effect on wrist movement.

Inspection of wrist joint
- Compare the size of forearm of both limbs. Normally dominant forearm tends to be larger and thicker.
- *Compare two wrist for:*
  1. Size
  2. Swelling
  - ❖ Deviation
    - Malunion of distal radial fracture (Colles sign)—extension deformity.
    - Localized tenderness in anatomical snuff box—diagnose saphead fracture.
    - In De Quervain's tenonsinovitis—inflammation of tendon of abductor pollicis longus (APL) and extensor pollicis brevis (EPB)—produce local pain and tenderness—the following Finkelstein's test to be done (Fig. 13.75).
    - With thumb adducted and opposed—the other four finger are curled to form a fist. Now passive ulnar deviation at the wrist stretches abnormal tendons and elicits pain—although semitone but not specific for tendon pain.
    - In case of inflamed tendon of flexors and extensors there is blockage of full range of wrist movement.
    - Abnormal excursion of ulnar styled in associated with pain and crepitus—synovitis.

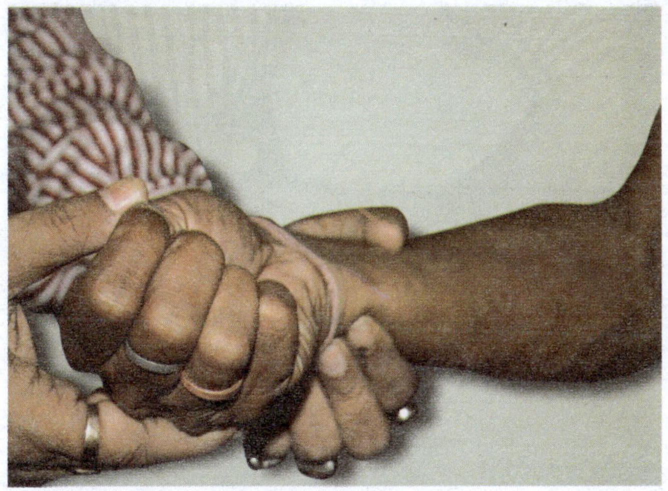

FIG. 13.75   Finkelstein's test

- *Scapholunate dissociation:* This can be demonstrated by (Fig. 13.76):
  - First wrist should be deviated rapidly from starting position to ulnar deviation
  - Forearm pronated
  - Then give firm pressure on the distal pole of scaphoid bone
    ↓
    There is dorsal subluxation of proximal pole of scaphoid.
- Tenderness at the base of the thumb may be due to:
  - Synovitis
  - Carpal, carpo—1st metacarpal osteoarthritis
  - Tenosynovitis
  - Ganglion
  - Tendon lesion.

Joint Movement Testing (Figs 13.77 to 13.81)

- Ask the patient to press the palm together while elevating the elbows to maintain the two forearms in straight line.
  By this mechanism dorsiflexion of wrist can be tested.
- Palmar flexion of the wrist can be tested by—pressing the back of the both hands against each other.
- Radial and ulnar direction of wrist can also be tested.
  In rheumatoid arthritis—these may be flexion deformity of the fourth and fifth digits—due to rapture of their extensor tendons.

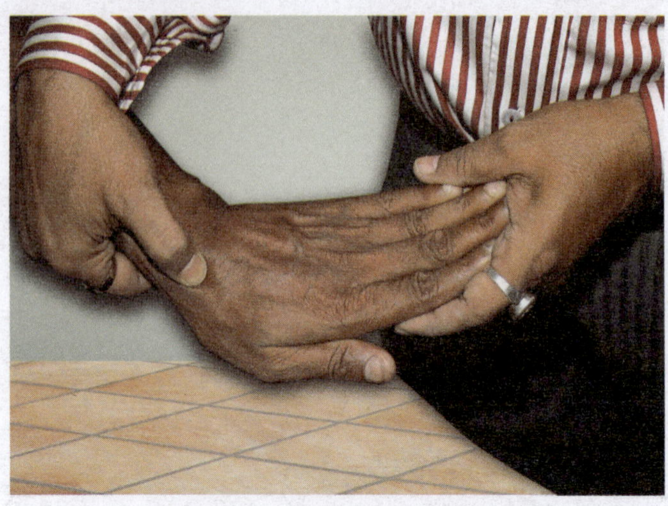

FIG. 13.76   Scapholunate dissociation

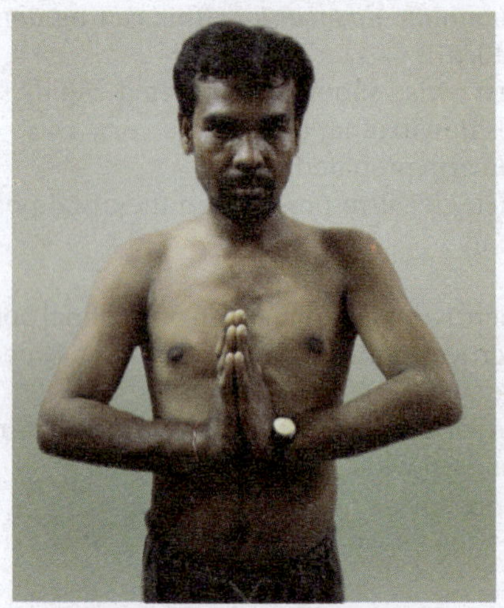

FIG. 13.77   Dorsiflexion of wrist

Traumatic lesion
- Fracture at 1–2 cm above the distal end of radius—Colles' fracture—dorsal displacement occurs.
- Smith's fracture—occurs at same site—displacement occurs on ventral side.
- Carpal-Tunnel syndrome.

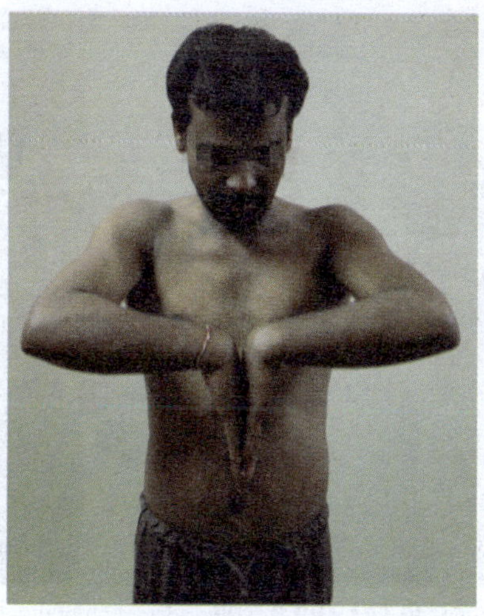

FIG. 13.78   Palmar flexion of wrist

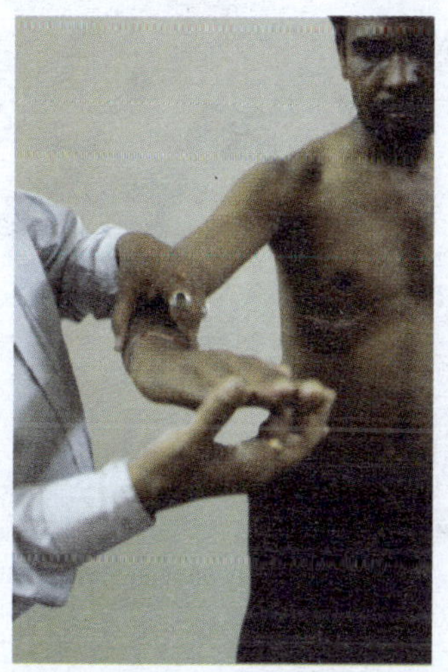

FIG. 13.79   Radial deviation of wrist

Muscle funciton
- *Involvement of C7 roots:*
  - ❖ Triceps and wrist extensors and finger extensors
  - ❖ Sensory loss in middle fingers.
- *Radial nerve involvement in radial groove:* Weakness of Supinator, brachioradialis, wrist extensors, finger extensors.
- Sensory loss in the area of anatomical snuff box.

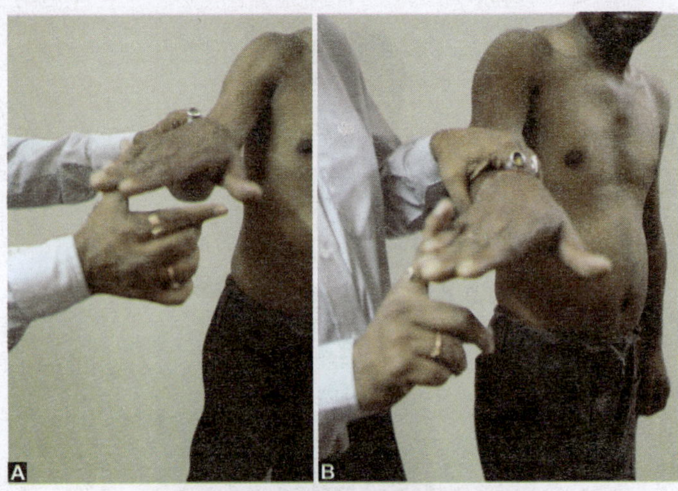

FIGS 13.80A AND B   Ulnar deviation of wrist

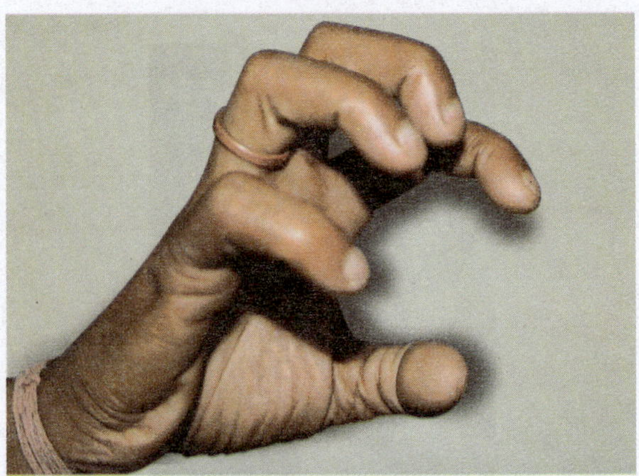

FIG. 13.81   Flexion deformity of wrist in rheumatoid arthritis

Hands

Power of the digits are provided by:

- *Flexors arising from forearm:*
  - ❖ Flexor digitorum superficialis—Flexes proximal inter-phalangeal joints, weakly metacarpophalangeal joints
  - ❖ Flexor digitorum profundus—flexes distal interphalangeal joints, weakly proximal interphalangeal joints and meta-carpophalangeal joints.
  - ❖ Flexor pollicis longus—flexes proximal interphalangeal joints of thumb.

- *Powerful digital extension arising from forearm:*
  - ❖ Extensor digitorum—arising from lateral epicondyle, split at the wrist to insert each dorsal digital expansions (2nd, 3rd, and 4th digits)—these expansions are attached to all phalanges of the digits.
  - ❖ Fifth digit has additional tendon, extensor digits minimum—it also arises from lateral epicondyle.
  - ❖ Extensor pollicis longus—extends the thumb.
  - ❖ Extensor pollicis brevis—extends the thumb.
  - ❖ Abductor pollicis longus—abduct the thumb.
  - ❖ Extensor indicis—arises from posterior border of ulna distal to extensor pollicis longus and inverts extensor digitorum tendon.

Muscles of thenar eminences
- Abductor pollicis brevis
- Flexor pollicis brevis
- Opponens pollicis.

Muscles of hypothenar eminence
- Abductor digits minimi
- Flexor digiti minimi
- Opponens digits minimi.

Intrinsic Muscles of the Hand

- Lumbricals—Four in number—Originates from flexor digitorum profundus—inserted into extensor expansion of medial four fingers.
  Actions: They flex metacarpophalangeal joints and extend interphalangeal joints.
- *Interossei:* Two sets:
  Palmar interossei: Four in number.
  Origin: First one arises from base of 1st metacarpal. Other three arise from anterior surface of shaft of 2nd, 4th and 5th metacarpal bones.
  Insertion: They are inserted into proximal phalanges of thumb, index, ring and little fingers, and dorsal expansion of each finger.
  Action: Adduction of fingers toward centers of 3rd finger.
  Dorsal interossei:
  Origin: Contagious sides of shafts of metacarpal bones.
  Insertion: Proximal phalanges of index, middle and ring finger.
  Function: Abduct finger of insertion from center of third finger.
  Actions of combined interossei: Flex the metacarpophalangeal joints and extend interphalangeal joints.

Mechanism of Grip
- Dorsiflexion at wrist, with slight adduction.
- Contraction of long digital flexors.

For hook grip (Fig. 13.81)
- Extension of thumb.
- Extension of metacarpophalangeal joints.
- Flexion of proximal and distal interphalangeal joints.

For more precise grip: Varying degrees of thumb adduction, abduction and flexion with opposing the thumb an any of the four digits.

Examination
Inspection—Nail and fingers:
- Pits and/or ridges in nails—psoriatic arthritis
- Splinter hemorrhage—traumatic, infective endocarditis rheumatic vasculitis.
- Cuticle damage and punctate cuticular erythema—dilated capillary loops—Raynaud's phenomenon.
- Periungual erythema—connective tissue disorders, autoimmune disorder.
- Multiple telangiectasias—scleroderma.
- Erythematous or violaceous scaly papule of MCP and ICP joints—dermatomyositis.
- Diffuse finger thickening (dactylitis) due to:
  - ❖ Diffuse tendon thickening
  - ❖ Scleroderma.

But bony soft tissue should be discriminated.

Palm and dorsum of the hand inspection
- *Palmar erythema:*
  - ❖ Autoimmune disease
  - ❖ Alcoholic cirrhosis
  - ❖ Connective tissue disorders.
- Thickening of the ulnar side of palmar fascia—Dupuytren's contracture.
- Nodule appears in the DIP joint—Heberden's node in osteoarthritis.
- Nodule at PIP joint—Bouchard's node in osteoarthritis.
- Rheumatoid nodule—appears anywhere on the dorsum of the hand and extensor surface of the elbow.
- Tophi of gout—rubbery and relatively fixed.
- Swelling around the joint—boggy feeling—may be an autoimmune arthropathy.

- Ganglion occurs anywhere in the tendon sheath.
- Nodule formation on a flexor tendon can lead to tendon being caught in a localized narrowing of sheath—Trigger finger.

Diffuse swelling in the hand: It may be seen:
- Rheumatoid arthritis
- Juvenile arthritis
- Algodystrophy.

■ HIP JOINT

Anatomy of Bones and Muscles

Two innominate bones (ileum and ischium)—Joins together:
1. Anteriorly—symphysis pubis.
2. Posteriorly—with sacrum at sacroiliac joint.

Sacroiliac joint is synovial joint to start with, later on it will be turned into a fibrocartilaginous joint.

Symphysis pubis is a fibrocartilaginous joint to start with.

Posterior pelvis is strengthened by several ligaments
- Sacroinnominate ligament
- Lumbosacral ligament
- Lumboiliac ligament.

While the patient is in standing position, the center of gravity passes through the head of the femur, which is already stabilized by fibrous labrum ligament.

Bursae

Ischial bursa separates gluteus maximus from ischial tuberosity.

Anatomy of the Muscles around the Joint (Figs 13.82 and 13.83)

There are usually three groups of muscles around the hip joint:
1. *Gluteus:*

   Gluteus maximus—L5, S1, S2.

   Origin: From ileum and sacrum.

   Insertion: Into posterior femur—20 percent, into tensor fascia lata—80 percent.

   Function: It extends and externally rotates the femur, aided by hamstring.

   Gluteus medius—L4, L5, S1

   Origin: It lies deeper and lateral to gluteus maximus.

   Insertion: Lateral to greater trochanter.

   Function: It abducts and internally rotates the hip.

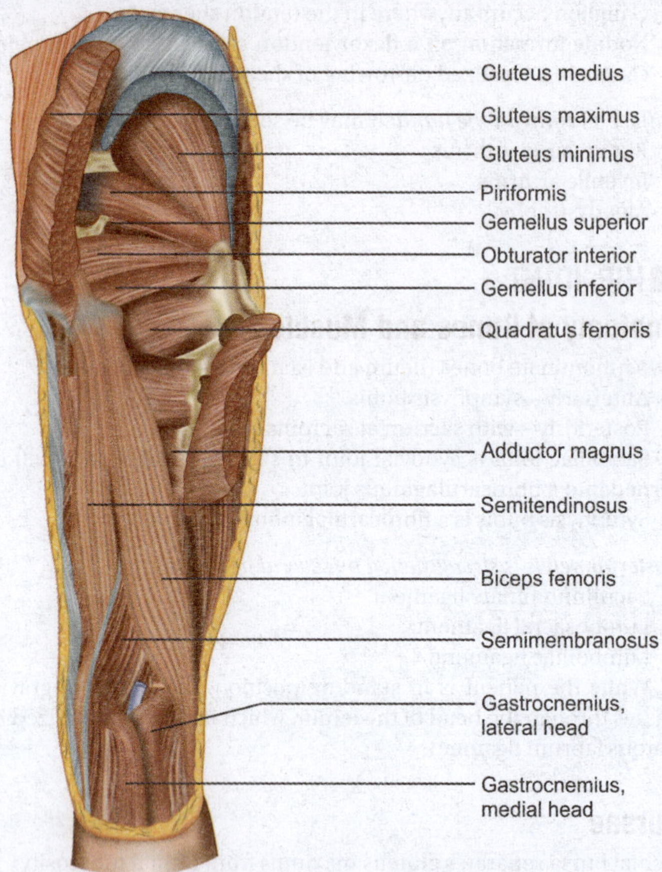

FIG. 13.82   Muscles around the hip

Piriformis, obturator internus, quadratus femoris:
Origin: Deep to the pelvis.
Insertion: Into the greater trochanter.

2. *Flexor group:*
Psoas major: It is a massive muscle. It arises from:
   a. Lateral part of vertebrae
   b. Intervertebral disc
   c. Lateral process of the lumbar vertebrae.
Iliacus:
Origin: In side the iliacus blade.
Insertion both above muscles: Lesser trochanter of femur.
Function: Both muscles flex the thigh.
Psoas muscle internally rotates the thigh and hip.

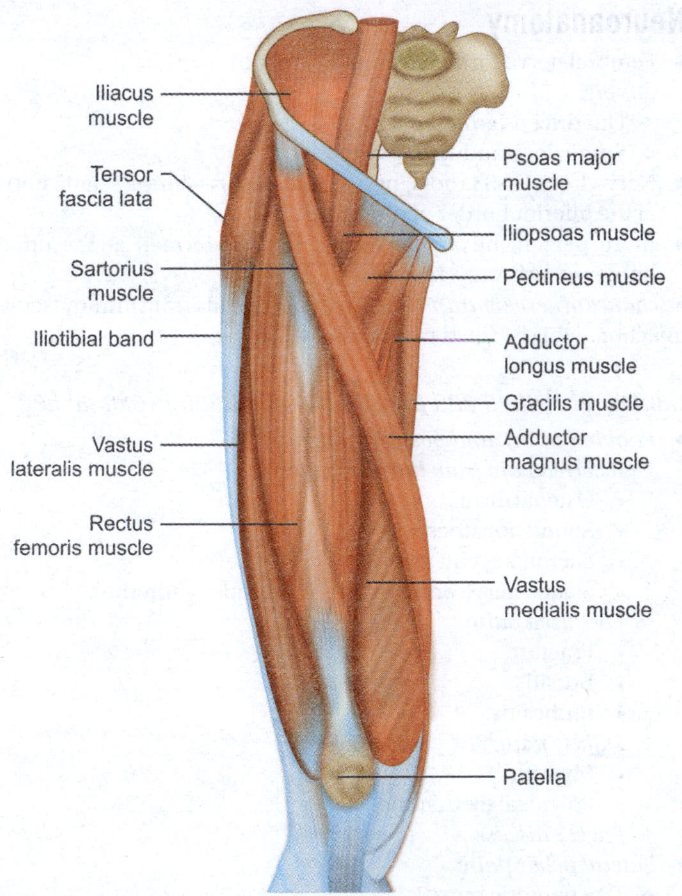

FIG. 13.83   Muscles around the hip (superficial view)

Adductor muscles—Adductor longus and gracilis: These are adductor muscles.

Insertion—Into the:

- ❖ Shaft of the femur
- ❖ Pes anserinus (below the knee).

3. *Adductor magnus:* Largest of deeper adductors.

Inserts into medial femur or shaft of femur.

Function and range of movement around the joint:

- ❖ With knee flexed—Hip flexion at 35°
- ❖ Hip extension—30°
- ❖ Abduction—45°–60°
- ❖ Adduction 20–30°.

Neuroanatomy

- Femoral nerve formed by root L3, root L4
  Supply:
  - ❖ Quadriceps group
  - ❖ Some deep adductor group
- Nerve from L4-S3 roots; nerve from plexus—forms sciatic nerve at the inferior border of piriformis.
- In 10 percent of people sciatic nerve is formed at the upper border of piriformis muscles.

So chance of nerve entrapment in case of: Trauma from intramuscular injection—this is called piriformis syndrome.

Causes of Pain in and around Hip Joint and Proximal Leg

- *Pain in buttock and posterior thigh:*
  - ❖ *Referred pain from lumbar spine:*
    - Osteoarthritis
    - Spondylolisthesis
    - Sacroiliac joint arthritis
    - Sciatic nerve entrapment (Piriformis syndrome).
  - ❖ *Localized pain:*
    - Fracture
    - Bursitis
    - Enthesitis.
  - ❖ *Diffuse pain:*
    - Myositis
    - Polymyalgia rheumatica.
  - ❖ *Paget's disease*
- *Lateral pelvic pain:*
  - ❖ Trochanteric bursitis
  - ❖ Gluteus medius tear
  - ❖ Referred pain from lumbosacral spine
  - ❖ Any local osteophyte.
- *Groin pain:*
  - ❖ Adductor tendonitis
  - ❖ Bursitis-psoas
  - ❖ Pelvic enthesitis
  - ❖ Paget's disease
  - ❖ Adductor tendonitis
  - ❖ Osteitis pubis
  - ❖ Trauma.
- *Anterior and median pain:*
  - ❖ Referred pain from lumbosacral spine
  - ❖ Myositis
  - ❖ Polymyalgia rheumatica

- ❖ Adductor tendonitis, osteitis
- ❖ Claudication
- ❖ Trauma.

Examination of Hip

Inspection and palpation
- Ask the patient to lie down with both legs extended on relaxed
  - ❖ *Leg length is discrepancy:*
    - Hip disease
    - Sacroiliitis
    - Dislocation of hip
  - ❖ Leg externally rotated
    - Hip fracture
    - Hemiplegia
    - Skin changes
      - Psoriasis—indicates seronegative arthritis
      - Violaceous colored and tender lesions—dermato-myositis
    - Swelling in groin
      - Lymphadenopathy
      - Varicose vein
      - Hernia, and if reducible (rubbery/hard) and increase in rise with cough)
    - Tenderness in groin—it may be due to
      - *Specific:*
        - Trauma
        - Fracture
        - Intuition
        - Hyperpathia.
          In above cases groin is very painful and very tender to touch.
      - *Nonspecific:*
        - Psoas bursitis
        - Myositis of deep muscles
        - Numbness on anterolateral side of thigh due to involvement of lateral cutaneous nerve of thigh—Meralgia paresthetica.
        - *Palpation of pubic tubercle:* Draw the hand downwards from umbilicus over the bladder, until bone is reached, this is pubic tubercle.
          Adductor longus can be palpable at its origin at pubic tubercle and at its insertion at upper medial part of the thigh.
        - Pain of osteitis pubis—can be increased by producing abdominal rectus contraction (asks the patient to raise his head and shoulders off the bed and place your one finger on pubic tubercle).

Movements of Hip

- Hip flexion: 20°
- Hip extension: 15°
- Hip abduction: 45°
- Hip adduction: 30°
- Hip internal rotation: 35°
- Hip external rotation: 45°.

Special Palpation of Hip

- *Limb length measurements:* Two lengths to be measured:
  - ❖ True length from anterior superior iliac spine to medial malleolus.
  - ❖ Apparent length from umbilicus to medial malleolus.
    If there is difference in true and apparent length without any difference in true length indicates—Lateral till of pelvis due to adduction deformity of the hip.
- *Thomas test:* When the patient uses to lie flat, flexion deformity can be corrected by compensatory lordosis of lumbar vertebrae. *To check this, following maneuver should be done:*
  - ❖ Flex the opposite hip to maximum to eliminate lordosis
  - ❖ Now in case of concealed flexion deformity—the affected legs will be flexed at the hip—this is Thomas test.
- *When the patient lies in supine position:*
  - ❖ Both iliac crest will be in same plane.
  - ❖ Iliac crest is at right angle to spine.
    If the above criteria are not fulfilled—there must be abduction or abduction deformity.
- *Rotational range of hip can be measured by in extension:* Use patella or tibial tubercle as pointer and hold the heel, ask the patient to rotate the straightened leg.
- *Rotational movement of hip can be also tested by:*
  - ❖ Flex the leg 90° at knee joint.
  - ❖ Swing the foot out produces internal rotation of hip (Fig. 13.84).
  - ❖ Swing the foot inwards produces external rotation of hip (Fig. 13.85).
- *Flexion movement of hip can be tested by (Fig. 13.86):* Bending the knee and hip flexed into abdomen.
- *Extension can tested by (Fig. 13.87):*
  - ❖ Ask the patient to stand and you should be behind the patient.
  - ❖ Draw the leg backwards one by one until the point at which pelvis starts rotating.

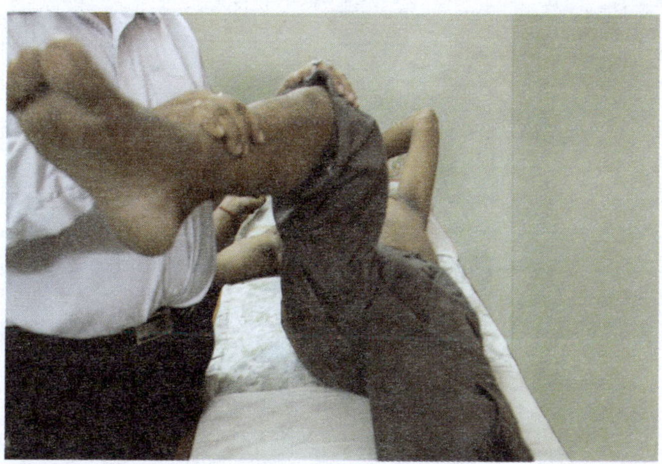

FIG. 13.84 Internal rotation of hip

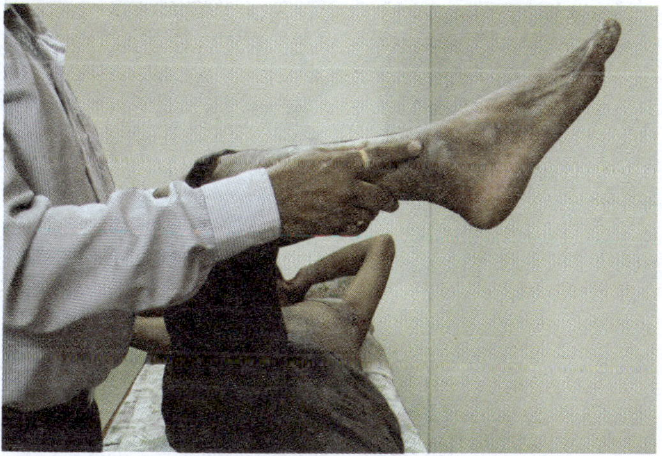

FIG. 13.85 External rotation of hip

- *Adduction and abduction movement of hip can be tested by (Figs 13.88 and 13.89):*
  - ❖ Fix the iliac crest firmly to avoid pelvic tilt.
  - ❖ Asks the patient to abduct the limb to a point or to touch the hand of the examiner.
- *In standing position, following things should be observed:*
  - ❖ Shortening of legs—compensatory scoliotic posture or flexion of lower leg.
  - ❖ Abduction deformity—compensatory flexion of ipsilateral knee.

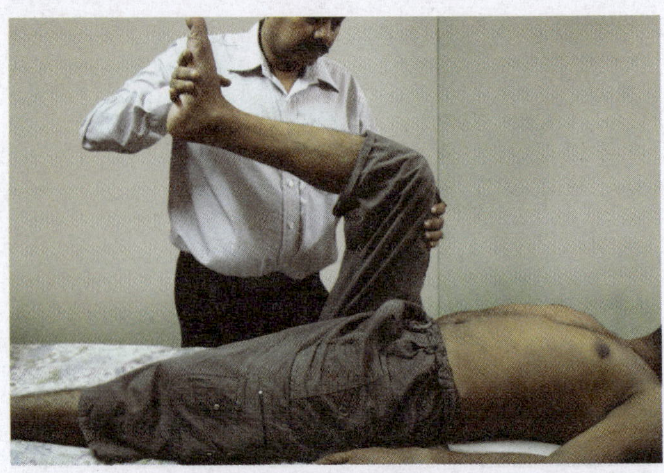

FIG. 13.86 Flexion of hip

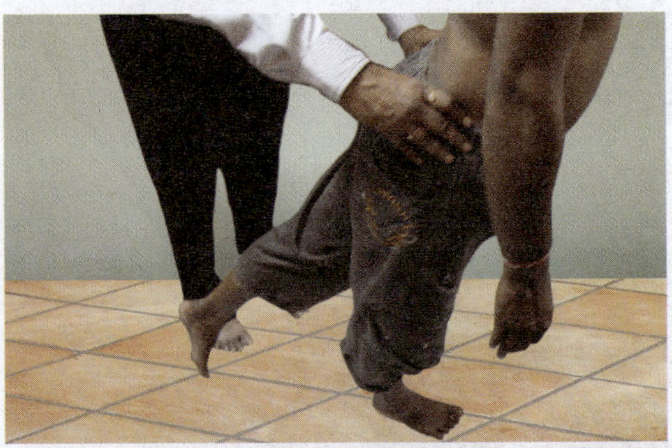

FIG. 13.87 Extension of hip

- ❖ Adduction deformity—compensatory flexion of contralateral knee.
- ❖ Flexion deformity—compensatory exaggeration of lordotic pasture.
- *To detect posterior congenital dislocation of hip—Barlow's maneuver should be done (Fig. 13.90):*
  - ❖ Flex and abduct hip
  - ❖ Exert an axial force into posterior acetabulum demonstrates posterior dislocation of hip.

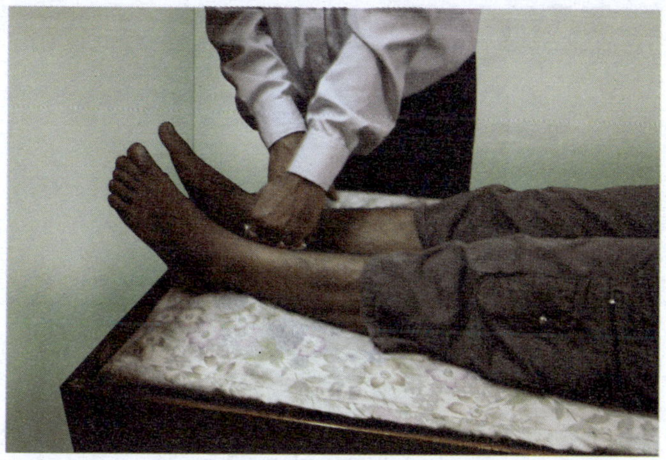

FIG. 13.88   Adduction of hip

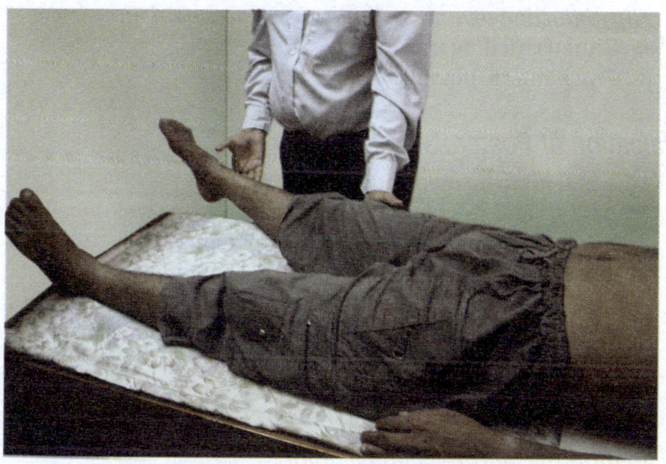

FIG. 13.89   Abduction of hip

Muscles Activation Tests

- *Hip adduction against resistance—produces pain in:*
  - ❖ Osteitis pubis
  - ❖ Hip joint lesion
  - ❖ Soft tissue
  - ❖ Muscle tenderness.
- *Hip flexion and slight internal rotation against resistance produces pain in:*
  - ❖ Psoas bursitis
  - ❖ Infections tracing along psoas muscles.

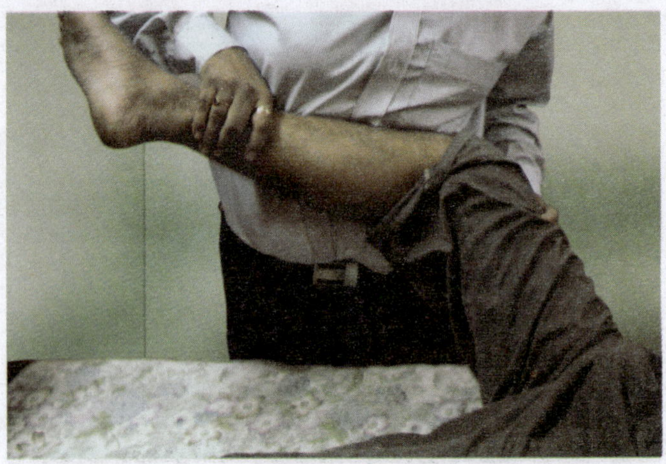

FIG. 13.90 Barlow's test

- *Hip abduction against resistances produces pain in:*
  - ❖ Gluteus medius tear
  - ❖ Trochanteric bursitis.

Palpation of Posterolateral Structures

Ask the patient to lie on position (Fig. 13.91):

- Palpate greater trochanter—tenderness may be well-localized or anterior or posterolateral to greater trochanter
- Ischial tuberosity overlying bursa may be tender
- The area of sciatic nerve exit the pelvis (midway between the ischial spine and greater trochanter) may be tender due to:
  - ❖ Trauma
  - ❖ Piriformis syndrome.

Palpation of Sacrococcygeal Joint

- Ask the patient to lie in left lateral position.
- Enter the index finger in the rectum and place the thumb outside—this two digits hold the coccyx. It may be tender in coccydynia (painful coccyx).

■ Knee Joints

Muscles of the Joint

- *Main extensors are 4 muscles groups:*
  - i. Rectus femoris
  - ii. Vastus medius

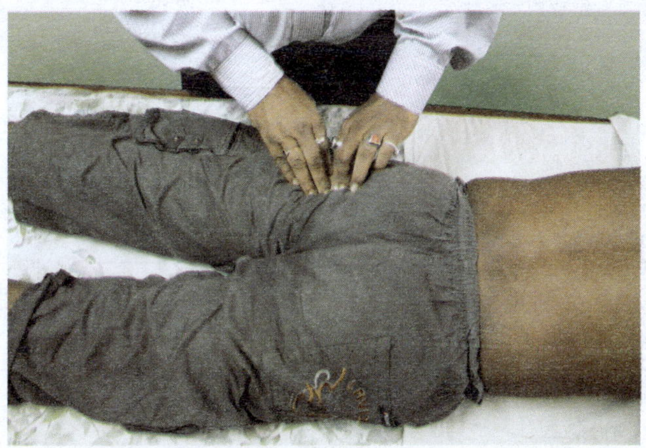

FIG. 13.91   Tenderness in sciatic nerve

  iii. Vastus intermedius
  iv. Vastus lateralis

All above muscles converge to form tendon which encloses patella and inserted into tibial tuberocity.

- *Hamstring muscles 3 muscles group:*
  i. Biceps femoris
  ii. Semimembranosus
  iii. Semitendinosus.

They all arise from ischial tuberosity.

Biceps femoris is inserted around femoral head, other two muscles are inserted into tibia on the medial side.

All muscles flex the knee.

- Femoral condyle articulates with two fibrocartilages on the tibial condyle—called medial and lateral menisci. 10–20 percent of outer part of menisci are vascular, hence can be repaired after trauma.

As the knee will be fully extended, femoral condyle rotates on the tibia, there will be tightening of the ligaments relative to each other.

- As flexion is initiated, small amount of femoral external rotation on the tibia occurs—this unlocking of knee will be done by popliteal muscles—which arrives from posterior surface of tibia to lateral femoral epicondyle.

- *Two cruciate ligaments (Fig. 13.92):*
  i. *Anterior cruciate ligament:* It attaches above to the femoral lateral condyle and is inserted into the tibial spine through a slip attached to the anterior horn or lateral meniscus.
  ii. *Posterior cruciate ligament:* It attaches above to the medial femoral condyle; below it is inserted to the area in between the two tibial condyles.

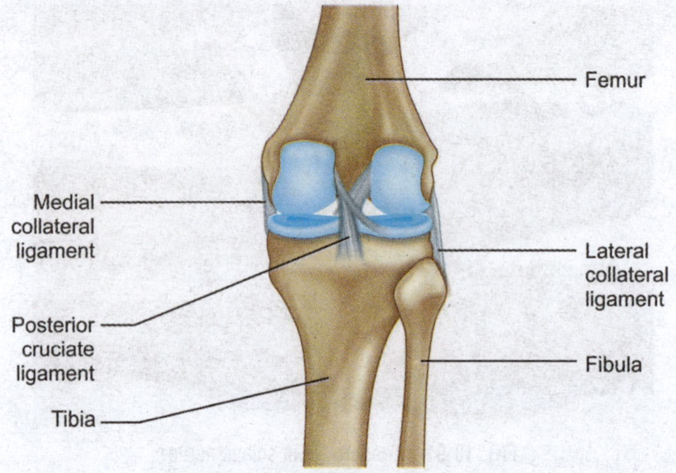

FIG. 13.92 Ligaments around knee joint

Action of anterior cruciate ligament into control the amount of rotation when knee is flexed.

Posterior cruciate ligament actions: It stabilizes the joint by preventing forward displacement of femur relative to tibia.

- *Two collateral ligaments:* There are two collateral ligaments:
    i. *Medial collateral ligament:* It stabilizes the knee from valgus stresses, during flexion.
    ii. *Lateral collateral ligament:* It stabilizes knee on its lateral side.
- *Patella:* It is a sesamoid bone—it is present and articulates with femoral condylar groove, it makes quadriceps action more efficiently.
- *There are four bursae:*
    i.   Between quadriceps tendon and femur—prepateller bursa.
    ii. Between patellar tendon and tibial tubercle—deep to infrapatellar bursae.
    iii. Overlying patella—suprapatellar bursas.
    iv. Patellar tendon inversion—infrapatellar bursa.

Examination of Knee Joints

Inspection and Palpation

In patient with standing position
- *Deformity:*
    ❖ Knock knee—genu valgum where both the knees come in contact with each other (Fig. 13.93).
    ❖ Bow leg—genu varum where both the knees are furthest apart in lower limb in Blount's disease (Fig. 13.94).

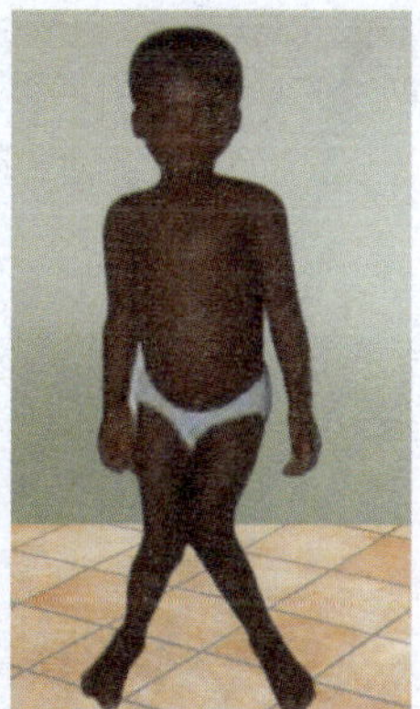

FIG. 13.93 Knock knee

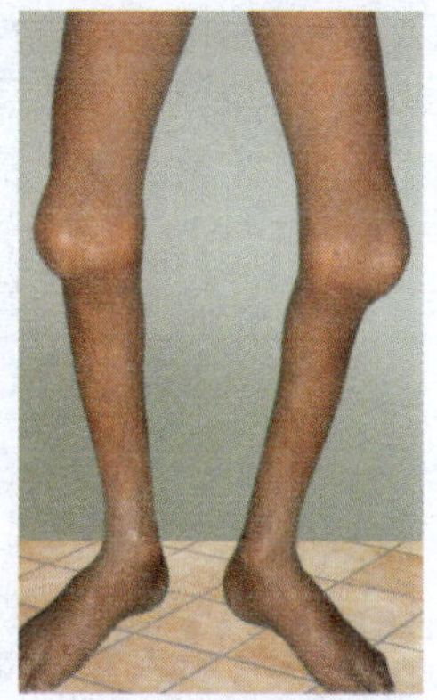

FIG. 13.94 Bow leg

- Patellar asymmetry (Fig. 13.95)
- Prominent tibial tubercles
- Flat feet (Fig. 13.96)
- Hyperextension > 10° (Fig. 13.97)
- Hypermobility (Patellar dislocation) (Figs 13.98A and B)

Examination in sitting patient: Ask the patient to sit on a chair with legs hanging. Now the following should be examined.

- Look for symmetrical patellar alignment.
- Ask the patient to extend the knee actively—the movement should be smooth, pain free.
- Passively rotate the knee externally to its extreme. It will produce pain in the tear of medial meniscus. If rotation is abnormally high, then medial collateral ligament is either deficient or form.
- Wasting of quadriceps by seeing a depression just above the patella (Fig. 13.99).
- *Tenderness to tibiofemoral joint sensitive for:*
  - ❖ Meniscus tear
  - ❖ Appearance of osteophytes
- Patellofemoral joint tenderness can be elicited by giving gentle pressure down the patella.
- Mobilization of patella sick to side—indicates hypermobility.
  Causer of patella femoral joint tenderness:
  - ❖ High patella
  - ❖ Excessive pronation
  - ❖ Weak vastus medialis
  - ❖ Reduced movement at the ankle
  - ❖ Wide Q-angle (Fig. 13.100).

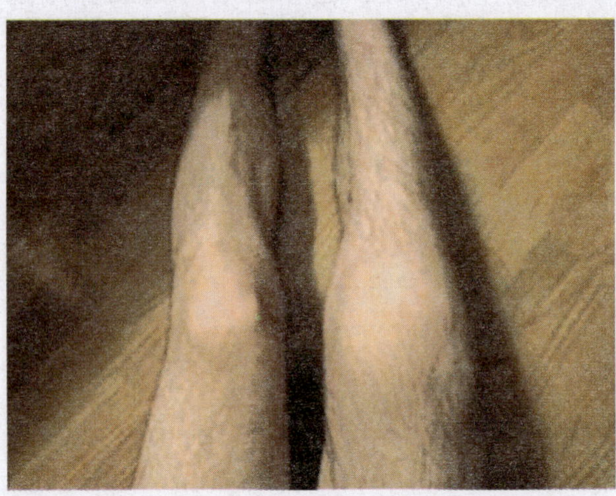

FIG. 13.95   Patellar asymmetry

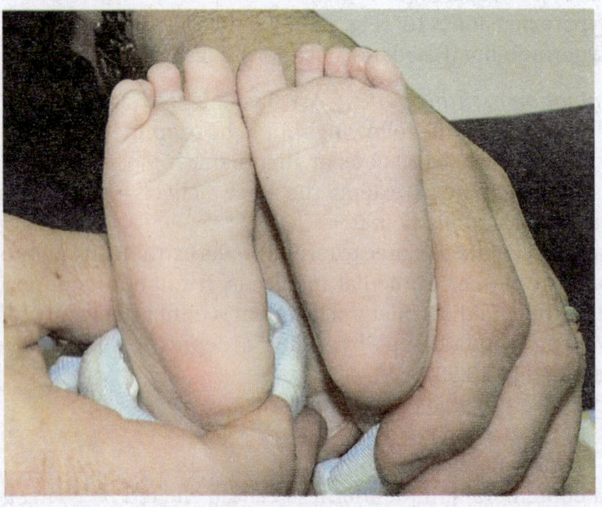

FIG. 13.96   Flat feet

Q-angle: Angle between two lines—one joining anterior superior iliac spine to center of the patella and the other line passing from tibial tubercle through center of the patella.

- Tenderness of femoral condyle—indicates on osteoporosis.

Examine for Joint Effusions (Figs 13.101 and 13.102)

In case of acute synovitis the joint is usually worm, but in chronic synovitis joint is not worm except:

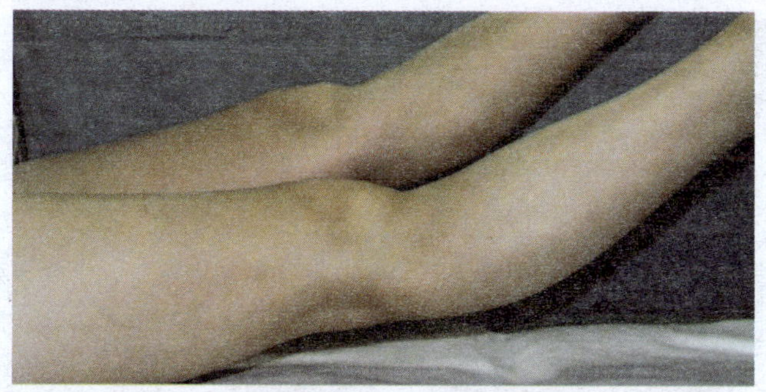

FIG. 13.97 Knee hyperextension

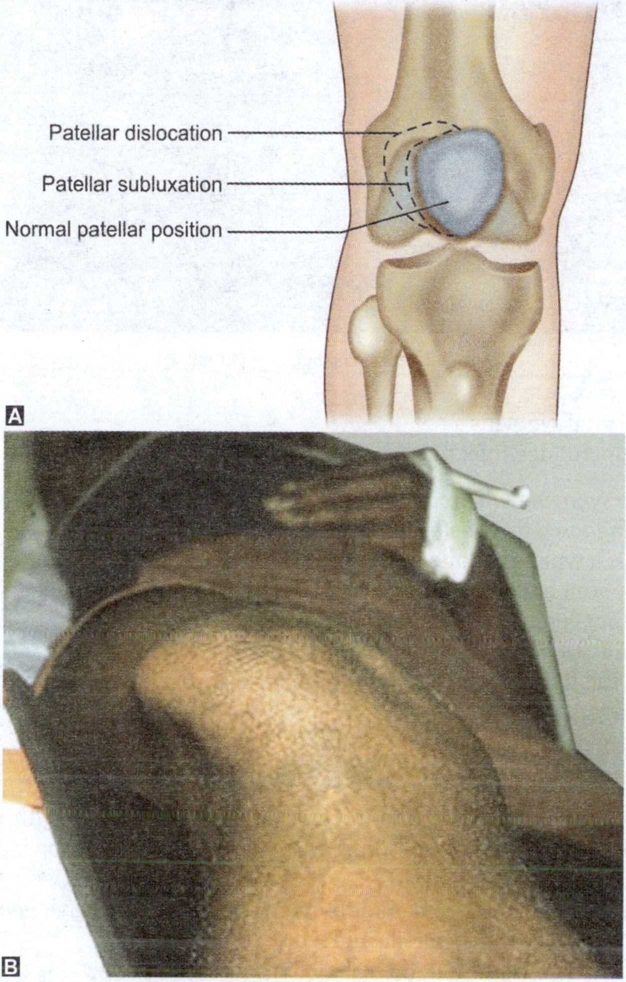

FIGS 13.98A AND B Patellar dislocation

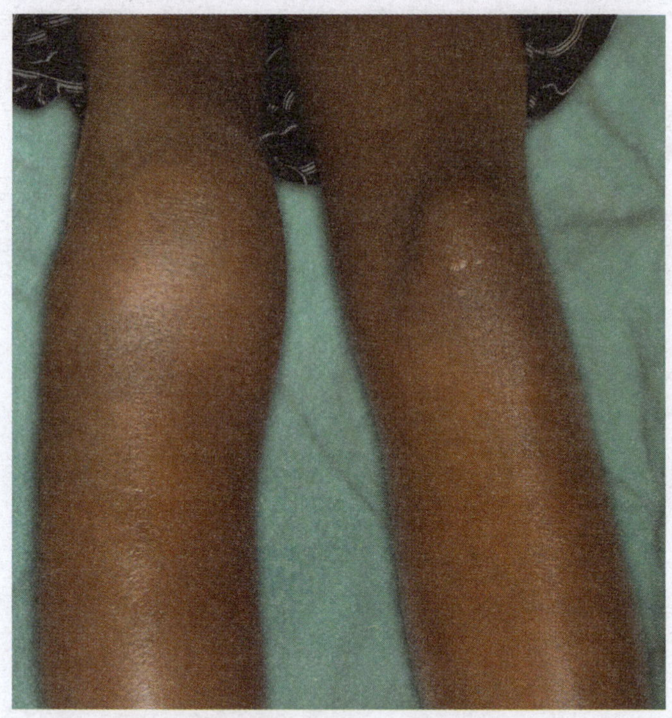

FIG. 13.99   Wasting of quadriceps

- Crystal synovitis
- Superadded infection.

Gross synovitis can produce effusion. It the effusion is large—this can be diagnosed by patellar tap test (Fig. 13.103).
This is a type of ballottement of patella.
- By your left hand force the fluid out of suprapatellar pouch.
- Then gently press the patella into the femur down ward by 2nd and 3rd finger of right hand.
- If the fluid is sufficient, the patella will spring back against your fingers.

If the effusion is small, then this can be diagnosed by 'bulge test' (Fig. 13.104)
- Try to force any fluid out of the suprapatellar pouch with left hand and at the same time anchor the patella with for index finger of same hand.
- Then with index and middle finger of right hand, give gentle stroke in between patella and femoral condyle.
- If effusion is present, then a bulging appears on other side of the knee.

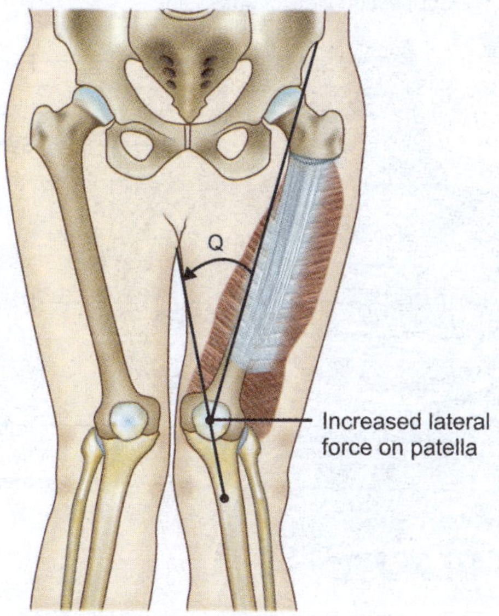

FIG. 13.100 Q-angle

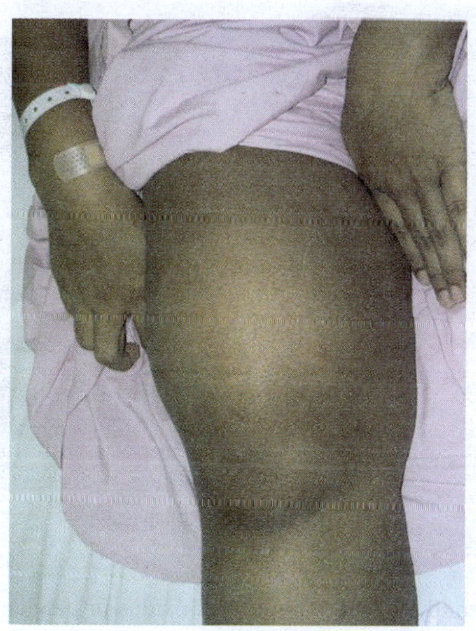

FIG. 13.101 Swollen knee from PVNS

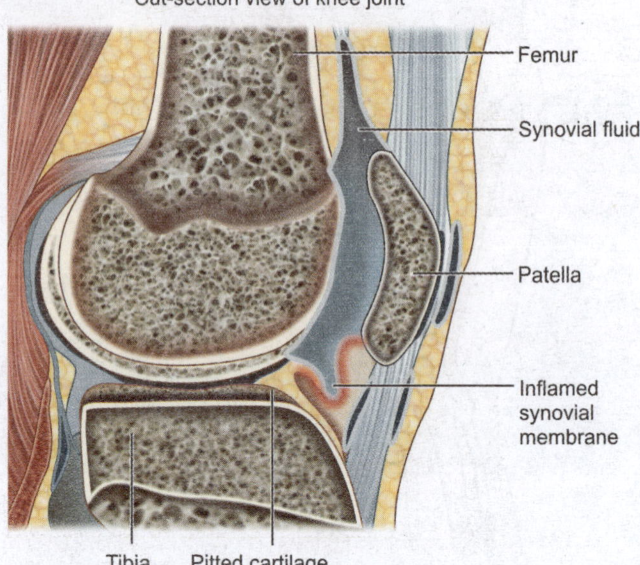

FIG. 13.102   Acute synovitis

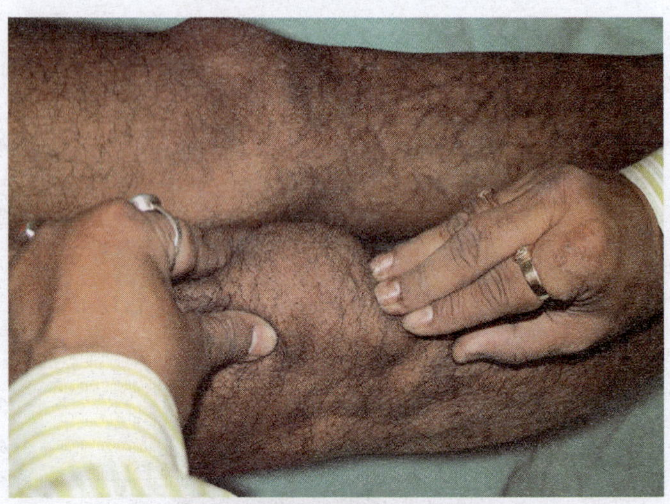

FIG. 13.103   Patellar tap test

- This method will be done for both sides of patella. Thickened synovium can be palpated by wrapping the finger around under the knee in semiflexed position to the knee.

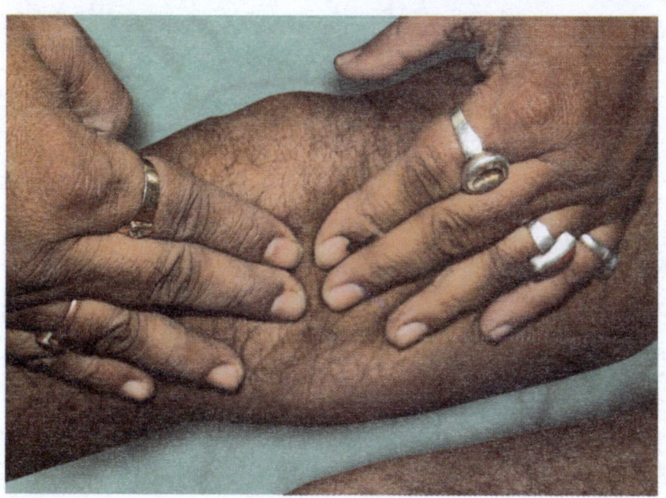

FIG. 13.104 Bulge test

Stability of the Knee Joint

Instability of the knee can be tested by following methods:

- *Lachman test (Fig. 13.105):* This can diagnose anterior cruciate ligament tear.
  - ❖ Ask the patient to flex the knee at 20–30° position.
  - ❖ Grasp the femur and tibia above and below the knee joint.
  - ❖ Now try to move the tibia backwards and forward on the femur.
  - ❖ If there is ligament disruption, there will be clunk and cry for pain.
- *Anterior drawer test (Fig. 13.106):* This can diagnose anterior cruciate ligament tear.
  - ❖ Ask the patient to lie flat with hip flexed and knee flexed at 90°, and foot should be flat on the bed.
  - ❖ Now sit on the foot of the patient and try to draw the upper end of tibia forwards in the line of thigh.
  - ❖ There will be excruciating pain if anterior cruciate ligament is damaged.
- *Posterior drawer test (Fig. 13.106):* This can diagnose posterior cruciate ligament tear or damage.
  - ❖ Ask the patient to lie flat with hip flexed and knee flexed at 90° with foot lie flat on the bed.
  - ❖ Now sit on the foot of the patient and try to push the upper tibia backwards along the line of thigh.
  - ❖ There will be excruciating pain if posterior cruciate ligament is damaged.

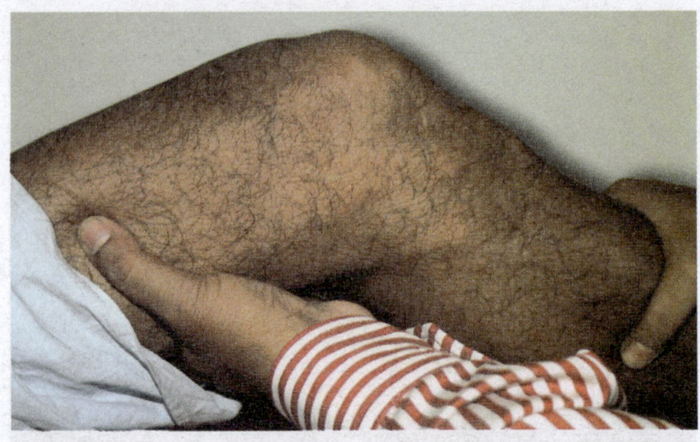

FIG. 13.105   Lachman test

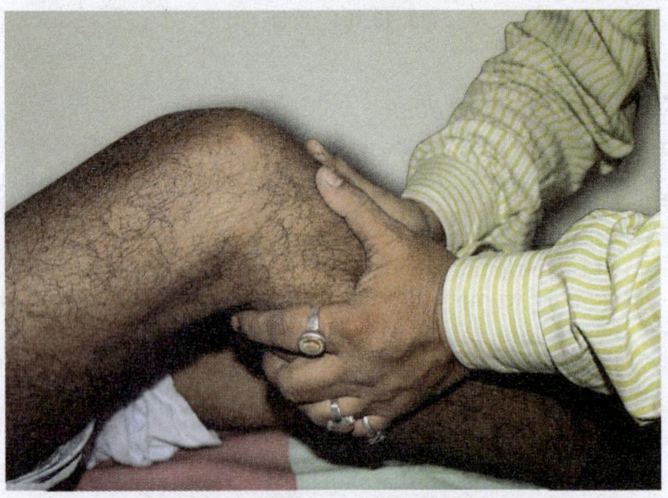

FIG. 13.106   Anterior and posterior drawer test

- To test the collateral ligament attempt to abduct and adduct lower leg—If there is instability of the joint, there may be collateral ligament laxity (Figs 13.107A and B).

Assessment of semilunar cartilage: Cartilage damage is very common in knee joint. Methods of detecting cartilage tear:
- *First method (Fig. 13.108A):*
  ❖ Ask the patient to bend at the hip and knee at 90° position and grasp the heel with your right hand.
  ❖ With other hand (left hand) press the medial end of lateral cartilage. It may produce pain in case of meniscus tear.

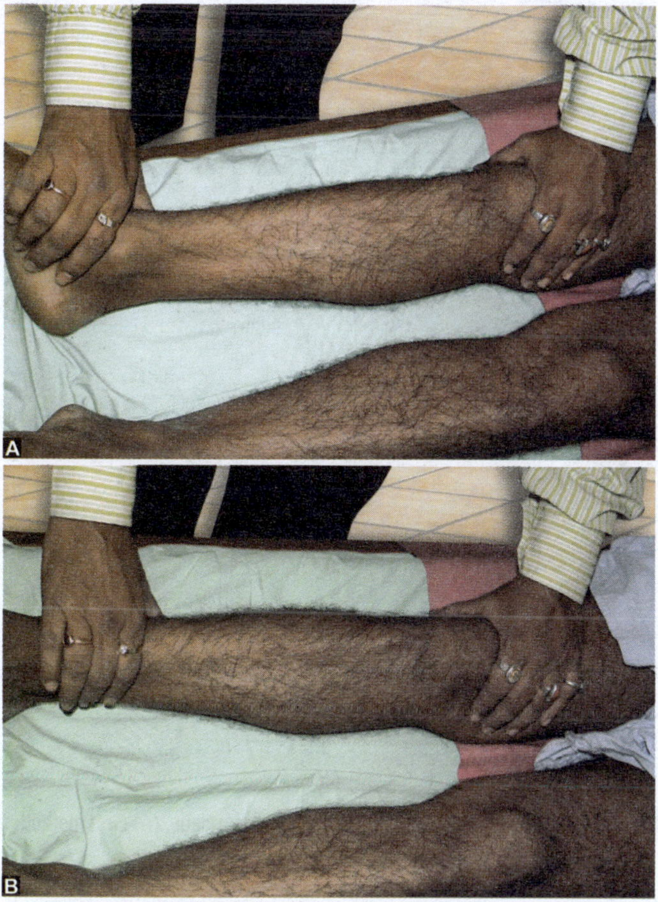

FIGS 13.107A AND B Testing of collateral ligaments of knee

- *Second method (Fig. 13.108B):*
  - ❖ Ask the patient to flex the knee
  - ❖ Rotate the lower leg internally.
  - ❖ If there is cartilage tear—the engagement between femur and tibia during this maneuver produce severe pain and clunking noise, sometimes locking of the joint.
- *Ask the patient to lie on lateral position, and Ober's test can be performed to detect lateral soft tissue injury (Fig. 13.109):*
  - ❖ Ask the patient to lie on lateral side (on the unaffected side) with unaffected limb flexed at the hip.
  - ❖ Upper limb (the affected knee is flexed at 90°, thigh extended and adducted).

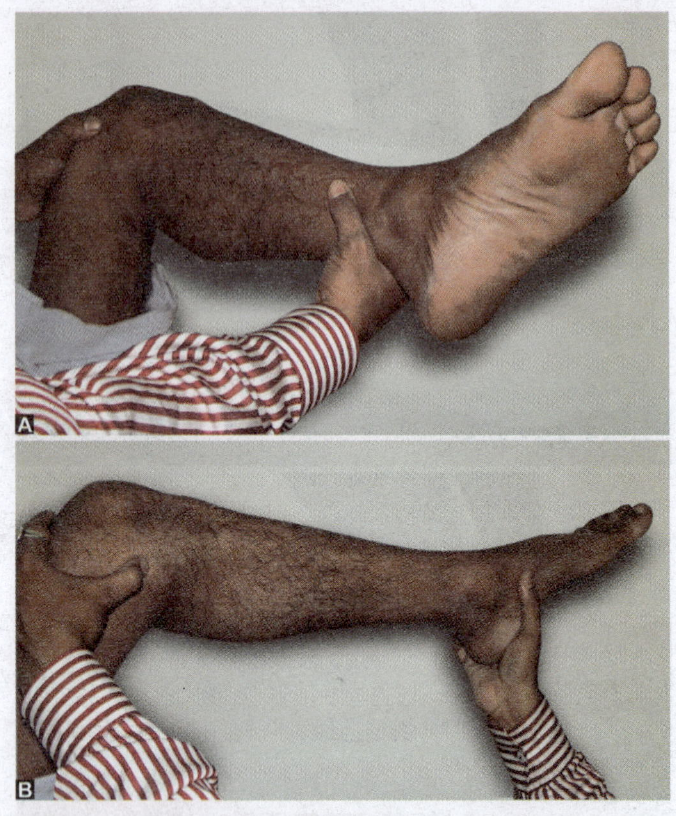

FIGS 13.108A AND B: Assessment of semilunar cartilage: (A) First method; (B) Second method

❖ This test will be positive if—When the examiner's hand will be removed, the hip does not drop down.

In osteoarthritis:

❖ Tenderness at the insertion of capsules and collateral ligament is important.

❖ Later on a bony swelling around the joint is common.

❖ Quadriceps wasting.

Examination of muscles involving the knee joint movement:

● Both quadriceps weakness and wasting—accompanying joint disease.

● If knee joint is normal, quadriceps weakness is due to femoral neuropathy.

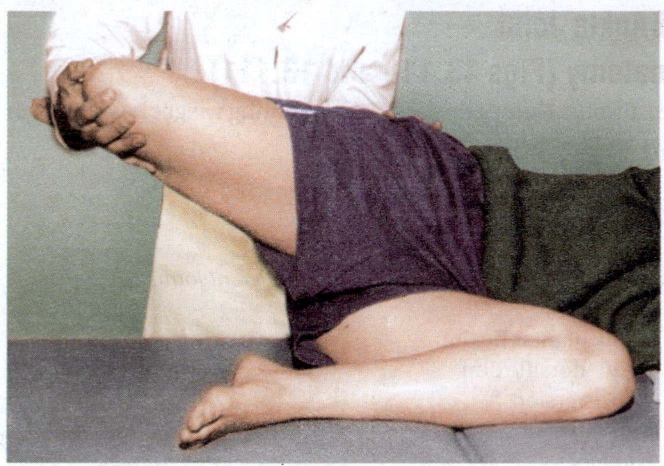

FIG. 13.109 Ober's test

- *If L3 root disease:*
  - ❖ Bilateral quadriceps weakness
  - ❖ Depressed knee jerk
  - ❖ Weakness of the hip adductors.
  - ❖ Sensory changes on the medial aspect of the thigh and knee.

Causes of femoral neuropathy
- Trauma
- Hemorrhage in the psoas sheath
- Diabetes mellitus.

In femoral neuropathy:
- Weakness and wasting of femoral quadriceps
- Loss of knee jerk
- Sensory changes over anterior thigh and medial aspect of lower leg.

In case of obturator nerve palsy:
- Weakness of thigh adductors
- Altered sensation on the inner aspect of the thigh.

Causes are:
- Pelvic fracture
- Surgery
- Secondary to obturator hernia

Meralgia paresthetica: The most common entrapment neuropathy

Causes: Compression of the lateral cutaneous nerve of thigh at the level of groin.

Signs and symptoms: Pain, tingling numbness over anterolateral aspect of the thigh.

■ Ankle Joint

Anatomy (Figs 13.110 and 13.111)

Leg absorbs 6 times the body weight during weight bearing. Strong ligaments—secure:

- Tibiofibular joint at lower end
- Talocalcaneal joint
- Bones of midfoot.

Movement and range of movement in different joints

- *Ankle joint:*
  - ❖ 50° plantar flexion
  - ❖ 20° dorsiflexion
  - ❖ 5° eversion
  - ❖ 5° inversion.
- *Forefoot:*
  - ❖ 30° eversion
  - ❖ 20° inversion.
- *Metatarsophalangeal joint:*
  - ❖ 60° extension (dorsiflexion)
  - ❖ 40° plantar flexion.
- *Interphalangeal joints:* 60° planter flexion.

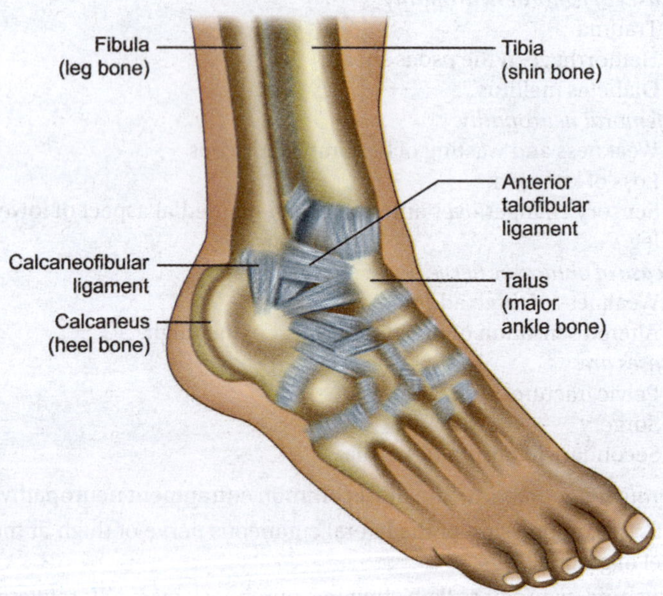

FIG. 13.110 Ankle joint (anterior view)

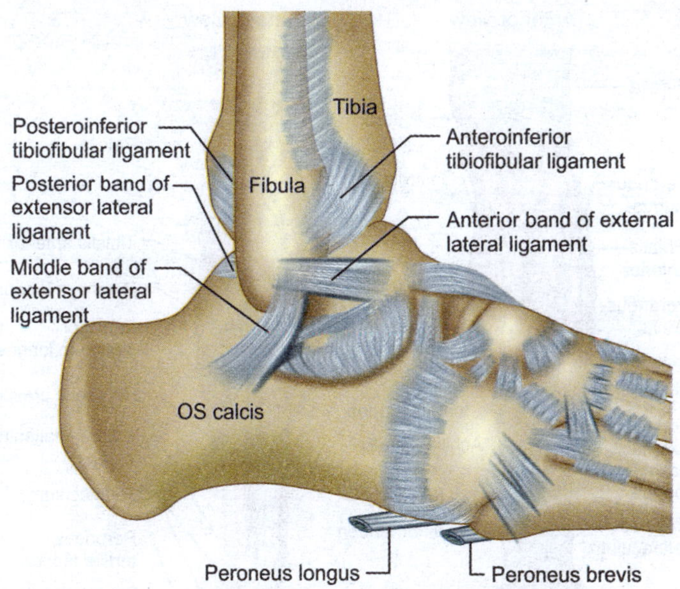

FIG. 13.111   Ankle joint (lateral view)

Muscles, fascia and tendons of lower leg and foot

- Lower end of tibia and fibula are joined by fascia
- Lower leg muscles are compartmentalized by fascia—hence they are prone to pressure effect.

The muscles are grouped as follows:

- *Dorsiflexors (Fig. 13.112)*
  - ❖ Tibialis anterior—bulkiest muscle inserted into medial cuneiform—dorsiflexor and inverter of foot
  - ❖ Extensor digitorum longus—dorsiflex the toes
  - ❖ Extensor hallucis longus—dorsiflex great toes
  - ❖ Peroneus tertius—everter of foot.
- *Plantar flexor (Fig. 13.113)*
  - ❖ Flexor digitorum longus—plantar flexes the toes
  - ❖ Flexor hallucis longus—plantar flex the great toe
  - ❖ Soleus—pure flexor of ankle
  - ❖ Gastrocnemius—plantar flexes both ankle and knee.
- *Evertors of foot*
  - ❖ Peroneus longus—inserts into medial cuneiform—acts as everters of foot
  - ❖ Peroneus brevis—inserts into 5th metatarsal bone—acts as everter of foot.
- *Inverters of foot*
  - ❖ Tibialis anterior
  - ❖ Tibialis posterior.

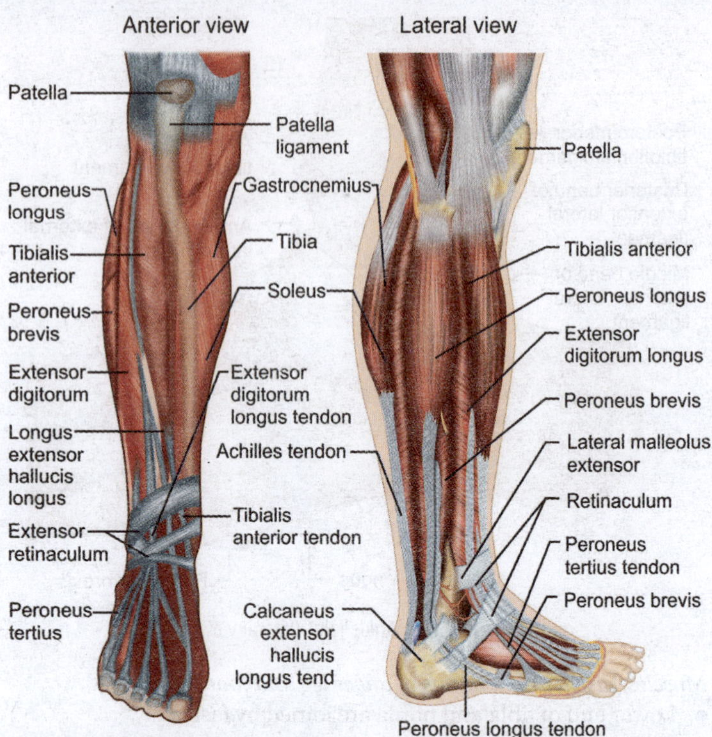

FIG. 13.112   Dorsiflexors of foot

Intrinsic muscles of the foot (Fig. 13.114)
The muscles are arranged in following layers:

1. *Deeper layers*—include:
   ❖ Interossei of forefeet
   ❖ Tibialis posterior
   ❖ Peroneus longus
   ❖ Adductor hallucis
   ❖ Flexor hallucis brevis—it has two insertions into proximal great toe phalanx.

2. *Superficial layers:*
   ❖ Flexor digitorum longus
   ❖ Lumbricals
   ❖ Flexor digitorum brevis
   ❖ Abductor hallucis.

Arches:
- Longitudinal arch—apex at the talus
- Transverse arch—apex at medial cuneiform—It maintain, stabilize the foots.

Neuroanatomy

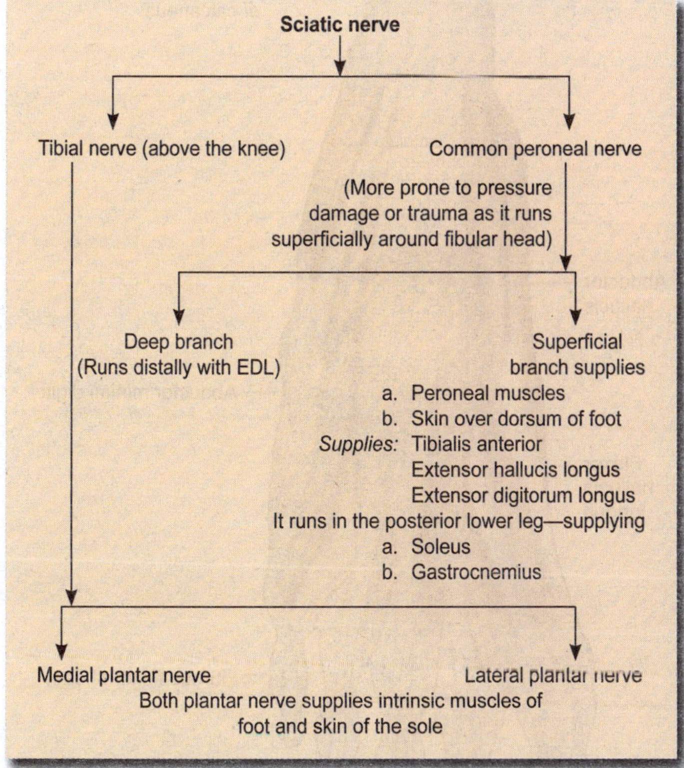

Examinations of Ankles and Forefoot

Examination of the patient when the patient is in standing position:

- *Calf swelling:*
  - ❖ DVT (Fig. 13.115)
  - ❖ Rupture of popliteal cyst
- *Deformity of legs:* Tibia varum (bow legs)
- *Muscles wasting:*
  - ❖ Disuse atrophy
  - ❖ Lower motor neuron disorder—poliomyelitis
  - ❖ Lumbosacral spinal stenosis.
- *Swelling anywhere:*
  - ❖ Trauma
  - ❖ Gout
- *Edema:* Associated with joint swelling.
  Bilateral edema:
  - ❖ Cardiac cause
  - ❖ Vinous congestion

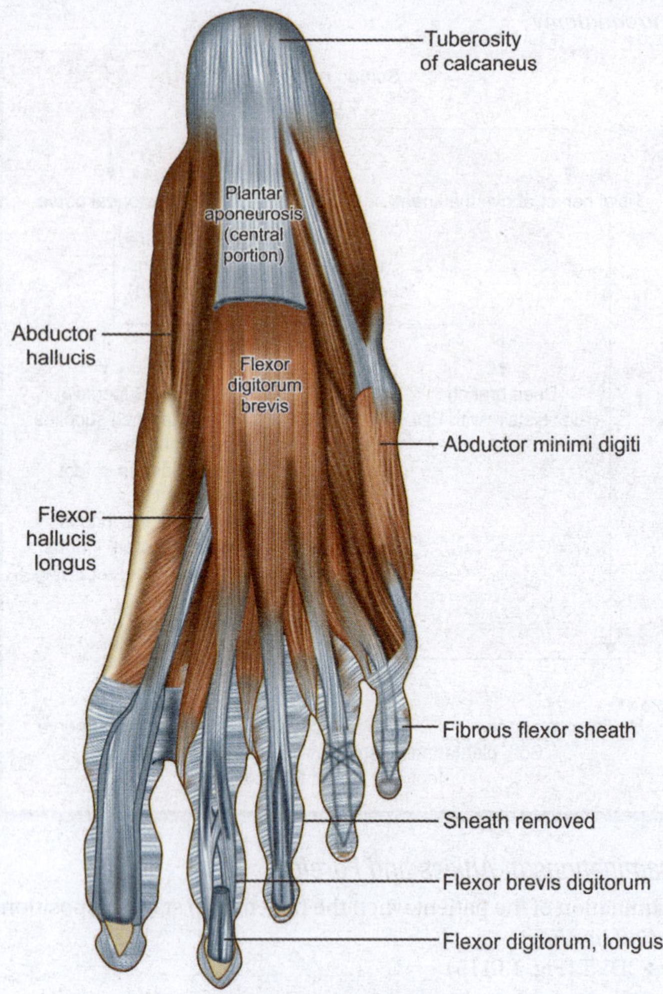

FIG. 13.113 Plantar flexors

* ❖ Hypoproteinemia
* ❖ Lymph edema

Painful edema: Thrombophlebitis.

Unilateral edema:

* ❖ Filariasis (Fig. 13.116)
* ❖ Hypernephroma

Foot deformity:

* ❖ Flat foot (pes planus)—due to loss of plantar arch (Fig. 13.117)
* ❖ High arched foot (pes cavus)—due to high medial arch with hyperextension of toes (Fig. 13.118)

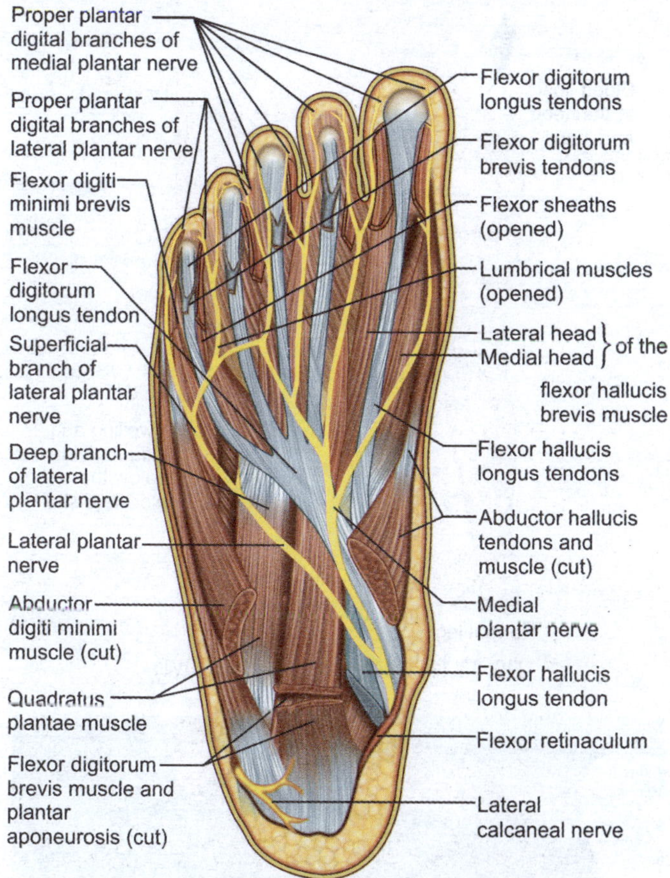

FIG. 13.114 Intrinsic muscles of foot

- ❖ *Hallux valgus (Fig. 13.119):* Abnormal abduction of big toe at metatarsophalangeal joint, with a bursa at pressure point over the head of the 1st metatarsal, more common in women.
- ❖ *Hammer toe (Fig. 13.120):* Hyperextension at metatarsophalangeal joint with flexion of interphalangeal joint. Painful corns may develop over pressure points at proximal interphalangeal joint (Fig. 13.121)
- ❖ Hallux rigidus
- ❖ Claw toes.
- • *Skin:* The following skin lesions can be demonstrable:
  - ❖ Purpura
  - ❖ Panniculitis
  - ❖ Erythema
  - ❖ Pyoderma gangrenosum (mainly seen over shins).

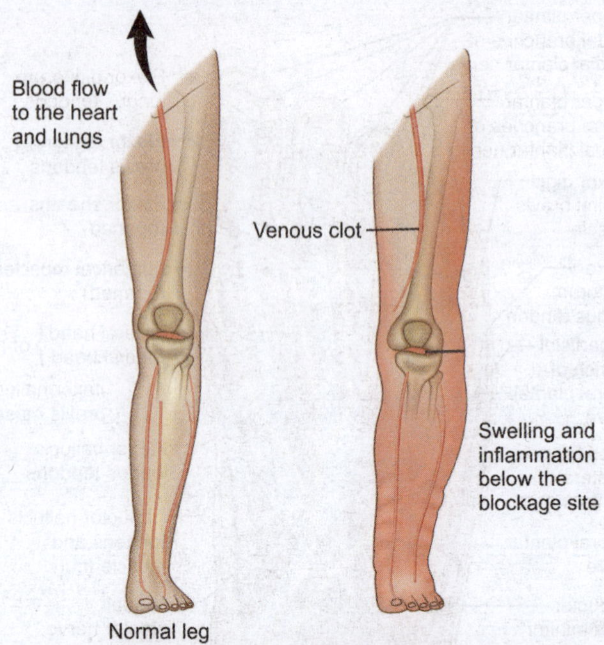

FIG. 13.115   Deep vein thrombosis (DVT)

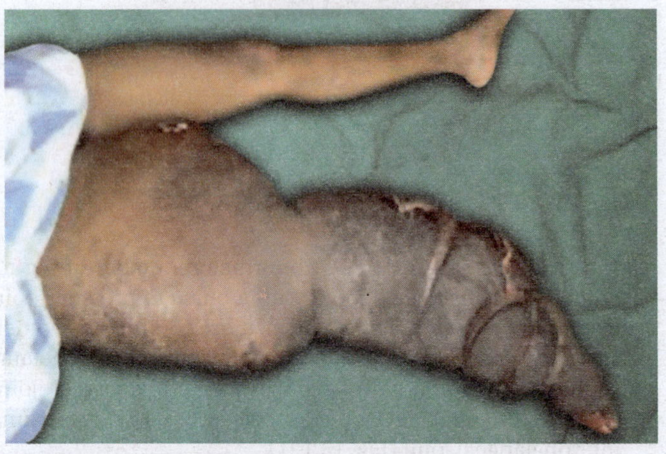

FIG. 13.116   Filariasis

The gait can be demonstrated during walking:
- Antalgic (Limp and wince)—this is nonspecific
- *Wide based gait (>10 cm wider than normal):*
  - ❖ Muscle weakness
  - ❖ Joint instability
  - ❖ Neurological lesion.

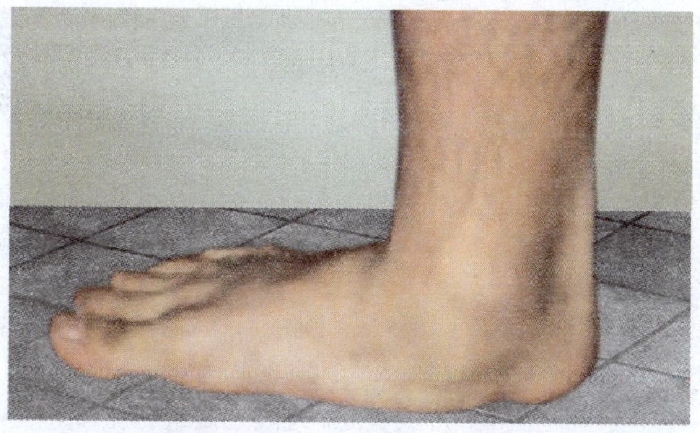

FIG. 13.117 Flat foot (pes planus)

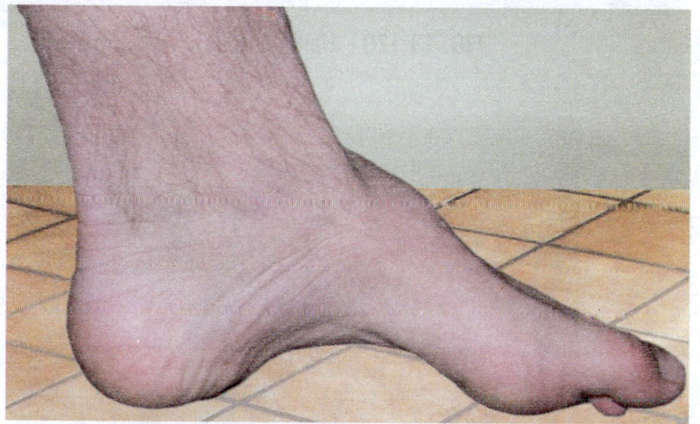

FIG. 13.118 High arched foot (pes cavus)

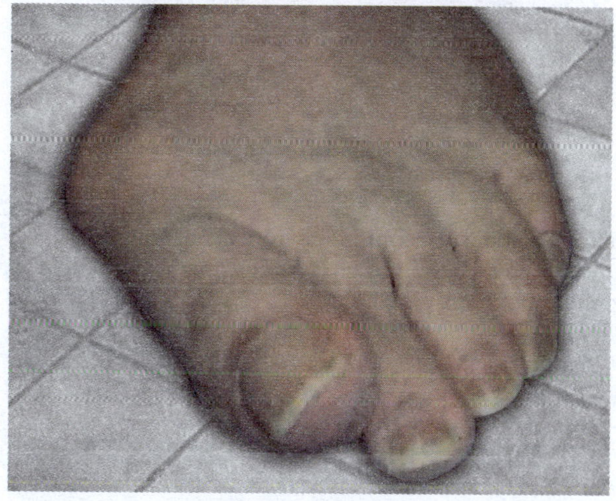

FIG. 13.119 Hallux valgus

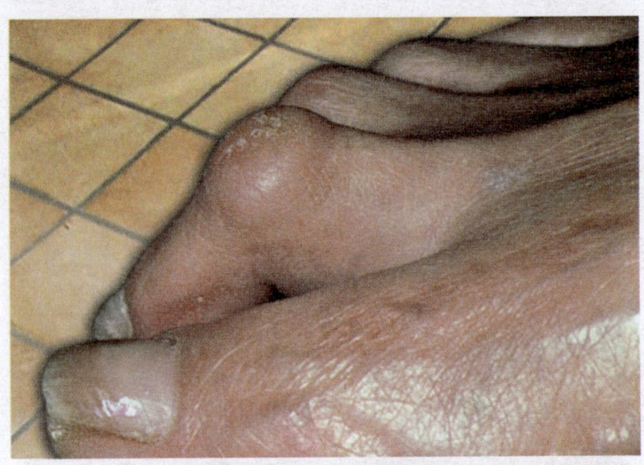

FIG. 13.120   Hammer toes

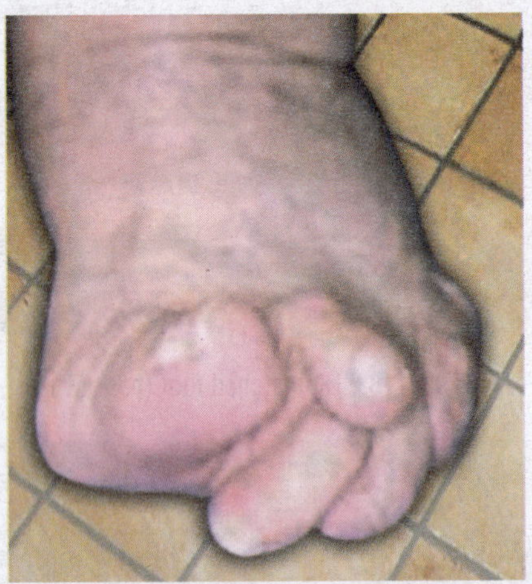

FIG. 13.121   Corn over pressure point

- High stepping gait—common peroneal nerve lesion
- *Lurching gait*—Lesion in L5 (Gluteus medius weakness) and S1 (gluteus maximus weakness)
- Flat foot gait—due to loss of plantar arch in:
  - ❖ Plantar fasciitis
  - ❖ S1 root lesion
  - ❖ Loss of medial arch.

Palpation of lower leg
- *Calf circumference at 10 cm below the tibial tubercle: Tender and swollen and erythematous:*
  - ❖ Rupture of popliteal cyst
  - ❖ Thrombophlebitis

  Nontender swelling—DVT.
- Swelling around the fibular head in patient with foot drop—common peroneal nerve palsy.
- *Tibial tenderness:*
  - ❖ Fracture
  - ❖ Paget's disease (Fig. 13.122)
  - ❖ Pseudofracture in osteomalacia
- Tibial deformity with tenderness—Paget's disease.

Examination of Ankle and Hindfoot

- Thickened tissue around ankle joint and around mutely—ankle joint arthritis (Fig. 13.123).
- If posterior tibial or perineal tendon are inflamed—there is soft tissue swelling of medial and lateral hindfoot, there may be associated involvement of talocalcaneal joint.
- *If there is pain in posterior heel region:*
  - ❖ Tendoachilles tendinitis
  - ❖ Enthesitis
  - ❖ Mechanical damage to the tendon
  - ❖ Retrocalcaneal bursitis.
- *If there is deep tenderness*—trigonum lesion

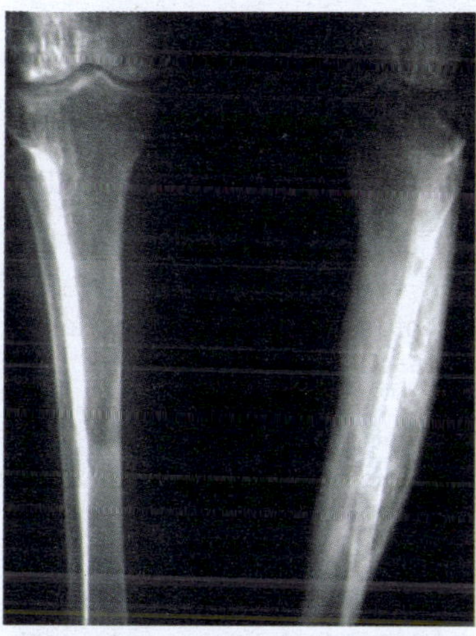

FIG. 13.122   Paget's disease of tibia

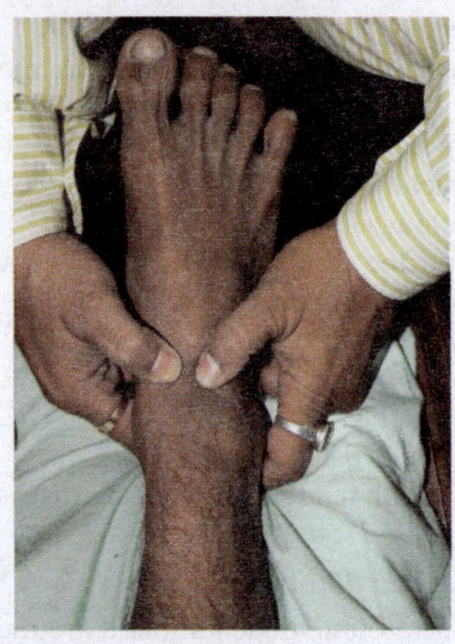

FIG. 13.123   To elicit ankle joint tenderness

- *Loss of passive movement of hindfoot:*
  - ❖ Subtalar arthritis
  - ❖ Any cause involving subtalar joint
- On medial vide—entrapment of tibial nerve is associated with—sensory loss or sole, positive Tinnel's sign.

Examination of Midfoot

- *Twisting of midfoot:*
  - ❖ Rheumatoid arthritis
  - ❖ Spondyloarthropathy, gout
  - ❖ Nonspecific
- Tenderness on bone without soft tissue involvement—does not exclude synovitis
- Midfoot arthropathy—typical of neuroarthropathy of diabetes
- *Exostosis occurs at the site of pressure:*
  - ❖ Head of fifth metatarsal
  - ❖ Distal talus
  - ❖ Dorsal aspect of 1st metatarsophalangeal joint.
- *Swelling, erythema, tenderness:*
  - ❖ Gout
  - ❖ Infection.

In 70 percent of patient Gouty arthritis starts at 1st MTP joint.

Examination of Fore Foot

- *Swelling of soft tissue of whole toe (Dactylitis):*
  - ❖ Spondyloarthropathy
  - ❖ Sarcoid
  - ❖ HIV infection
- *Bony swelling tender suggest bunion (Fig. 13.124):*
  Site:
  - ❖ On dorsal aspect of the toes
  - ❖ 1st metatarsophalangeal joint
  - ❖ 5th metatarsophalangeal joint
- Inter digital separation with splaying of forefoot—suggest interdigital bursitis
- Tenderness in between metatarsal heads—Morton's meta-tarsalgia (Fig. 13.125) associated with interdigital sensory loss
- Uneven callus distribution in abnormal site—abnormal to cussed area of weight bearing.
  Mechanical abnormality.
- *Rashes in role:*
  - ❖ Psoriasis
  - ❖ Keratoderma blennorrhagica (reactive arthritis) (Fig. 13.126)
  - ❖ Arsenic poisoning (Fig. 13.127).

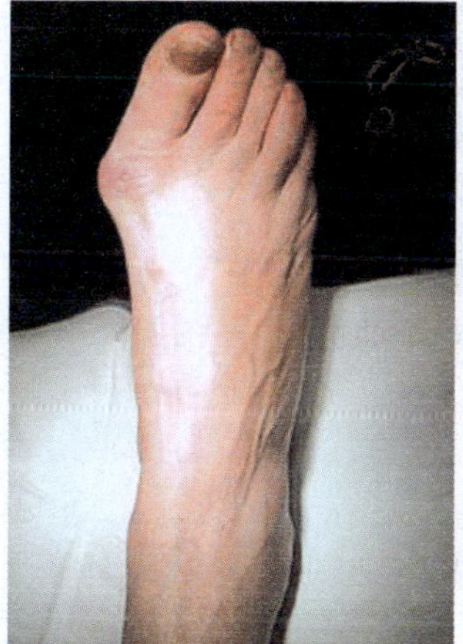

FIG. 13.124   Bunion

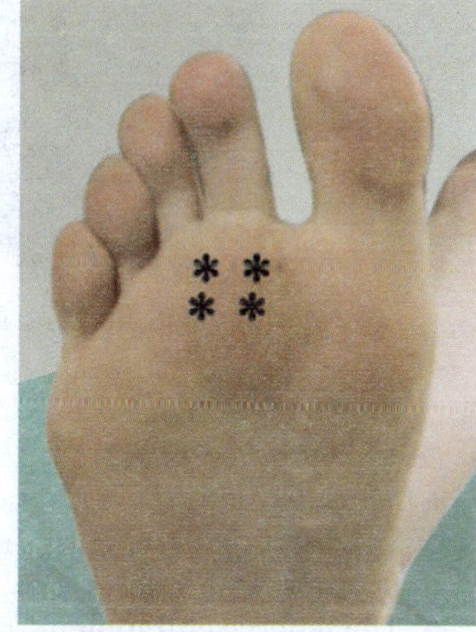

FIG. 13.125   Morton's motatarcalgia

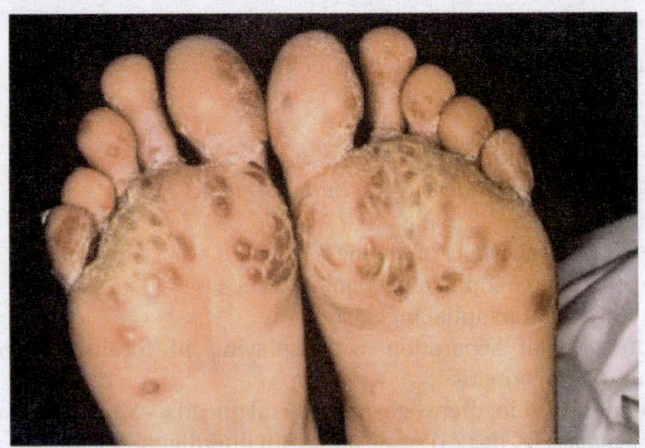

FIG. 13.126 Keratoderma blennorrhagica

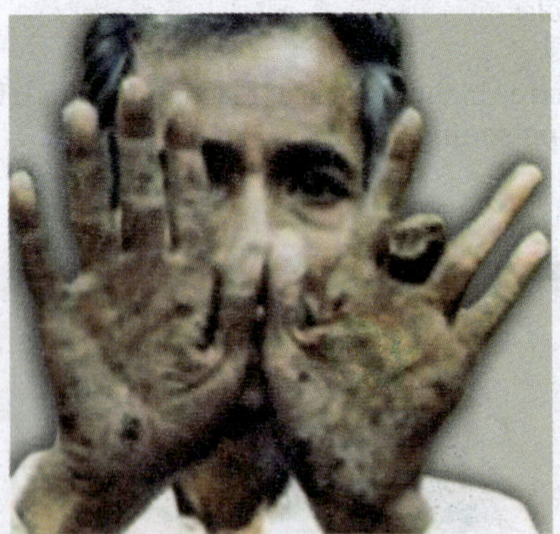

FIG. 13.127 Arsenic poisoning

- *Loss of sensation in the role:*
  - ❖ S1 root lesion
  - ❖ Vasculitis—mononeuritis multiplex
  - ❖ Sjögren syndrome
  - ❖ Tibial nerve entrapment.

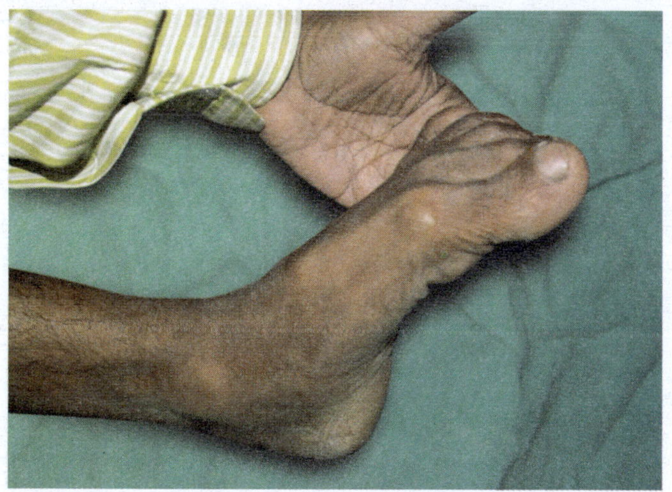

FIG. 13.129   Plantar flexion of foot

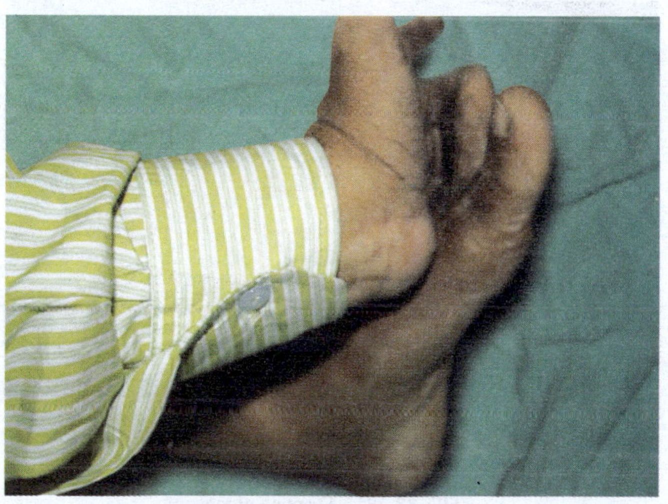

FIG. 13.128   Dorsiflexion of foot

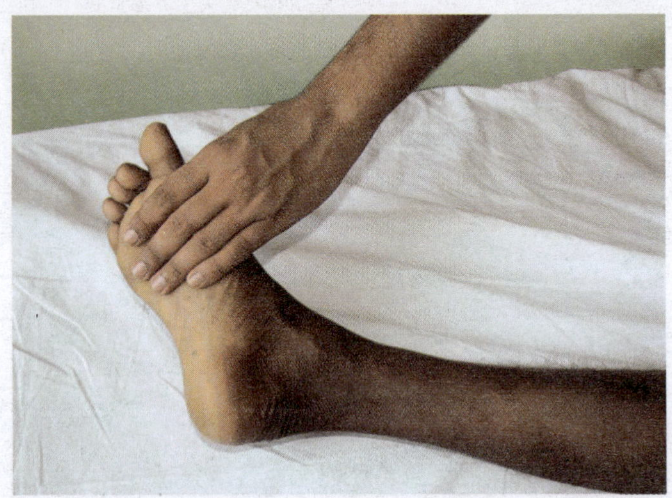

FIG. 13.130 Inversion of foot

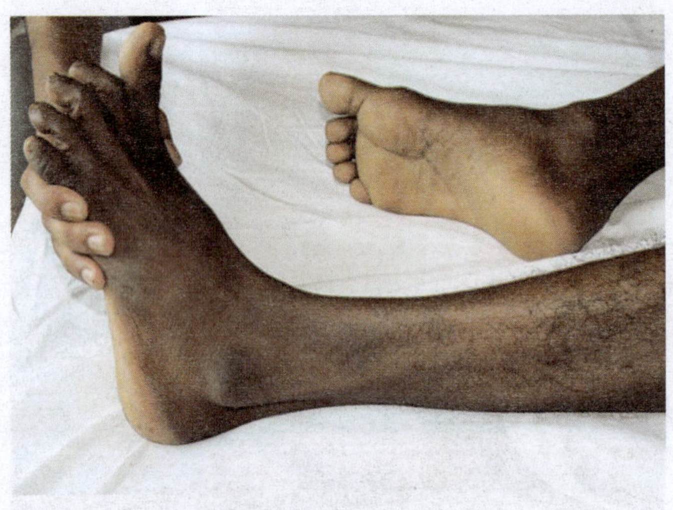

FIG. 13.131 Eversion of foot

Methods of Examinations of Foot

- Dorsiflexion of foot (Fig. 13.128)
- Plantar flexion of foot (Fig. 13.129)
- Inversion of foot (Fig. 13.130)
- Eversion of foot (Fig. 13.131).

Genitalia

■ Male Genitalia

Penis (Figs 14.1 and 14.2) consists of:

- *Shaft:* This contains two juxtaposed spongy vascular erectile tissue called corpora cavernosa. In between there is another tissue, which is a continuation of bulb of penis—called corpora spongiosum

  When if fills with blood temporarily due to stimulus—penis becomes erect.

- *Glans penis:* This is cone-shaped structure called glans It is the distal extremity of penis

  It contains a vertical slit like structure (opening)—called urethral meatus.

- Glans is separated from shaft by a circular sulcus—called corona.

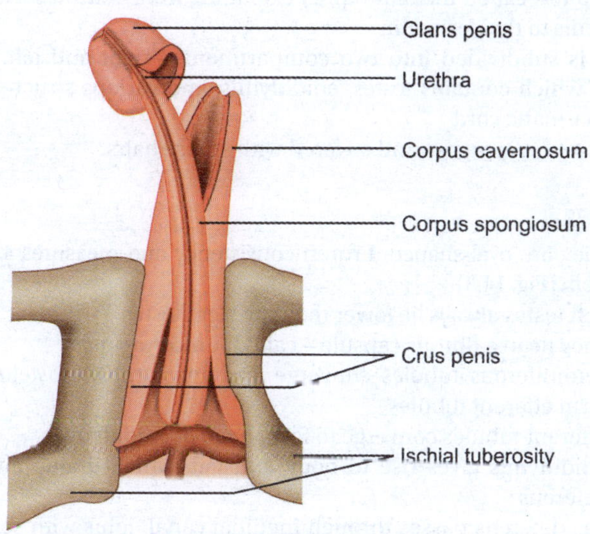

FIG. 14.1 Shaft and glans penis

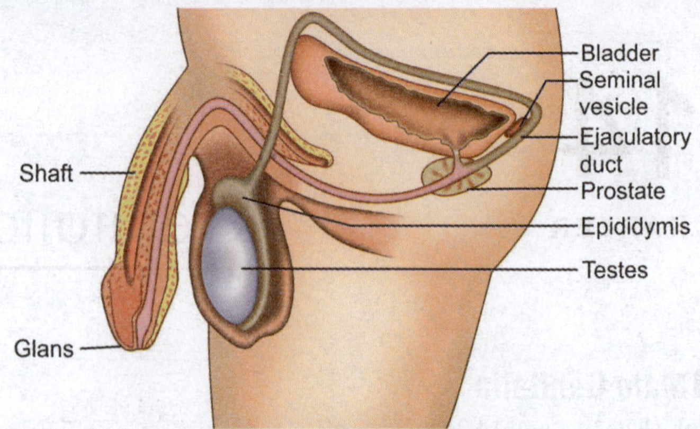

FIG. 14.2 Sagittal section of male genitalia

This is covered by a hood like skin—called foreskin or prepuce. A fold of skin extends from external urethral meatus to the prepuce—it is called frenulum. Prepuce or foreskin covers the glans for a variable distance and it is possible to retract the prepuce over the glans.

Scrotum

- It is a sac, made of skin and fascia—divided in midline by a raphe—called median raphe, extending from ventral surface of penis to the perineum
- It is subdivided into two compartments—right and left, each of which contains testes, epididymis, and various structures of spermatic cord
- Scrotum is rugose and covered with sparse hairs.

Testes

- They are oval-shaped, firm in consistency and measures 4 × 3 × 2 cm (Fig. 14.3)
- Left testes always lie lower than the right testes
- They lie in a fibrous capsule—called tunica vaginalis
- Seminiferous tubules converge and anastomose posteiorly to form efferent tubules
- Efferent tubules converge to form head of epididymis
- Epididymis gives rise to body and tail, which drains into vas deferens
- Vas deferens passes through inguinal canal, joins with seminal vesicles, which converge to form ejaculatory duct

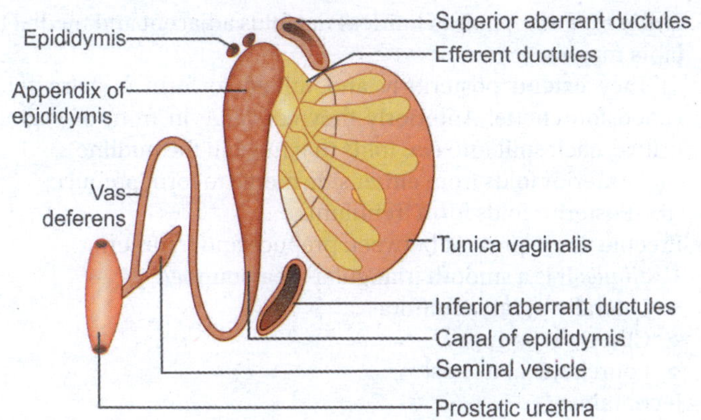

FIG. 14.3 Testes and duct of testes

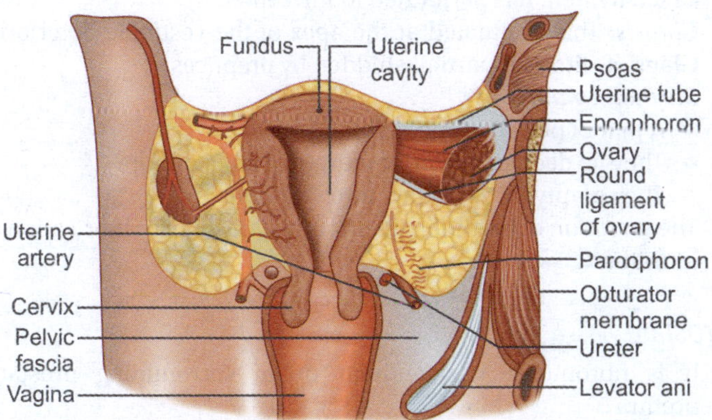

FIG. 14.4 Section of female genital organ

- Both testes and epididymis have vestigial remnants—called appendix testes and hydatid of Morgagni, respectively.

◼ Female Genitalia (Fig. 14.4)

Vulva

It is the external genitalia of female. It consists of:

- *Mons pubis:* It is hairy elevation containing pad of fat overlying symphysis pubis
- *Labia majora:* They are a pair of prominent hairy skin folds extending on either side from mons pubis ends meet posteriorly in the midline in front of anal verge

- *Labia minora:* A pair of hairless flat folds adjacent and medial to labia majora

  They extend posteriorly and united to form a sharp fold, called fourchette. Anteriorly they converge in front of vaginal orifice, each split into two folds that meet in the midline.
  - i. Anterior folds from either side merge to form prepuce
  - ii. Posterior folds form frenulum.

  Erectile tissue present between prepuce and frenulum.
- *Vestibule:* It is a smooth triangular area bounded:
  - ❖ Laterally by labia minora
  - ❖ Clitoris at its apex
  - ❖ Fourchette at its base.

  It contains:
  - ❖ Urethral meatus
  - ❖ Vaginal orifice.
- *Vaginal orifice:* It is protected in virgins by a thin mucosal fold—called hymen. It is perforated in the center.
- *Clitoris:* This is situated at the apex of the vestibule anteriorly. Glans of clitoris is partially hidden by prepuces
- *Bartholin glands:*
  - ❖ A pair of pea size mucous glands
  - ❖ They lie deep to posterior margin of labia minora
  - ❖ They empty through duct into vestibule.

  The secretion of bartholin glands is responsible for lubrication of introitus.

Prostate

- It is fibromuscular, glandular organ surrounding prostatic urethra
- Shape-conical, having base—lies against bladder neck above, apex lying against urogenital diaphragm below
- *Divided into five lobes:*
  - ❖ Anterior lobe—in front of urethra
  - ❖ Median lobe—between the urethra
  - ❖ Posterior lobe—posterior to urethra.
  - ❖ Right and left lobes—on either sides of urethra.
- It secretes acidic fluid—containing citric acid and acid phosphatase—which is added to seminal vesicles fluid at the time of ejaculation.
- *Blood supply:*
  - ❖ Artery—interior vesicle and middle rectal arteries
  - ❖ Vein—prostatic venous plexus.

Ovary

- It lies against the lateral wall of pelvis in a depression—ovarian fossa.
- It is attached to the back of broad ligament by meso-ovarium.
- *Two ligaments:*
  1. Suspensory ligament of ovary—attached with lateral wall of pelvis.
  2. Round ligament of ovary—attached with lateral margin of uterus.
- Ovary is covered with a fibrous capsule—tunica albuginea.
- *Blood supply:* Ovarian artery and ovarian vein.

Uterine Tube

- Four inches long, lies in upper border of broad ligament.
- *It has four parts:*
  1. *Infundibulum:* Funnel-shaped lateral end, fimbriated, fimbriae draped over the ovary.
  2. *Ampula:* Widest part of tube.
  3. *Isthmus:* Narrowest part of tube, lying lateral to uterus.
  4. *Intramural part:* It lies within uterine wall.

Uterus

- Hollow pear-shaped organ, thick muscular walls.
- It measures—3 inch × 2 inch × 1 inch thick
- *It has three parts:*
  1. *Fundus:* It is upper most part, above the origin of uterine tubes.
  2. *Body:* It is the part lies below the entrance of uterine tubes.
  3. *Cervix:* Narrowest part of uterus—divided into:
     - Supravaginal part
     - Vaginal part.
- *Uterine cavity:* Triangular in coronal section.
  Cavity in cervix is called cervical canal—it communicates:
  - With the body through internal os
  - With vagina through external os.
- Blood supply—uterine artery and vein.
- *Uterus covered with peritoneum reflects:*
  - Anteriorly on to the bladder
  - Posteriorly on to the rectum—producing a pouch—pouch of Douglas.
  - Laterally to form broad ligaments.

Vagina

- It is a muscular tube extending upwards and backwards from vulva to uterine cervix
- It is three inches long
- Its anterior and posterior walls are always in apposition
- Its upper end, anterior wall is pierced by cervix
- Its upper half lies above the pelvic floor
- Its lower half lies within the perineum
- Area of vaginal lumen, which surrounds the cervix, is divided into four regions:
    1. Anterior
    2. Posterior
    3. Right lateral
    4. Left lateral.
- Blood supply—vaginal artery, branch of internal iliac artery.

■ Genital Symptoms

Male

- *Penile discharge:* Continuous or intermittent discharge of fluid from urethra. Questions to be asked:
    - ❖ Any history of previous discharge.
    - ❖ If present, color of discharge, clear purulent or mucopurulent of bloody.
    - ❖ Any history of previous sexual contact
    - ❖ If present, is it oral, vaginal or anal contact
    - ❖ Number of sexual partners.

  Blood of discharge:
    - ❖ Ulcerations
    - ❖ Urethritis
    - ❖ Neoplasm.

  Purulent discharge: Thick, yellowish green:
    - ❖ Gonococcal urethritis
    - ❖ Prostatitis.

      Gonorrhea in men starts with dysuria and urethral discharge—2–10 days after exposure.

      In woman—dysuria and vaginal discharge occur days to weeks after exposure—50 percent women become asymptomatic.
- *Dysuria:* If may occur in men with or without discharge.
- *Penile lesion:* History of penile lesions may be suggestive of:
    - ❖ Gonorrhea
    - ❖ Syphilis
    - ❖ Herpes
    - ❖ Trichomoniasis

- ❖ Venereal wart
- ❖ Other sexually transmitted disease.
- ● *Genital rashes:* Male genital rashes are more common.
  - ❖ Some genital lesion may be present only in genitalia.
  - ❖ Some may be extension of rashes present all over the body.

The rashes of genitalia are:
- ❖ *Psoriasis:* Most common, bright red, well-defined, scaling plaques.

  Occasionally scrotum and inguinal folds may be involved.
- ❖ *Contact dermatitis:*
  - • From soap
  - • Disinfectant—itching is major symptom.
- ❖ *Fixed drug eruptions:* It is characterized by multiple, macular, eczematous, bullous patches. Very painful, site is mainly distal penis and glans.

  Drugs are mainly antibiotics, laxatives containing phenolphthalein.
- ❖ *Lichen planus:* Violaceous flat topped papules at the glans penis—Oral mucosa reveals white streaks on buccal mucosa.

Cause of genital ulcerations:
- ❖ *Most common:*
  - • Candidiasis
  - • Trichomoniasis.
- ❖ *Less common:*
  - • Syphilis
  - • Erythema multiforme
  - • Chancroid.
- ❖ *Occasional:*
  - • Lichen sclerosus
  - • Behçet's disease.
- ❖ *Rare:* Vulval carcinoma.

Causes of genital skin lumps:
- ❖ *Most common:*
  - • Molluscum contagiosum
  - • Coronal papillae in men
  - • Vulval papillae in women
  - • Skin tags.
- ❖ *Less common:* Scabies.
- ❖ *Occasional:*
  - • Condyloma lata
  - • Bowenoid papulosis   prostatic intraepithelial neoplasia.
- ❖ *Rare:* Squamous cell cancer.
- ● *Scrotal enlargement:* Questions to be asked:
  - ❖ Is there any enlargement—for how many days?
  - ❖ Is it painful?

❖ Is it recurrent—if so, how many times?
❖ Is there any history of injury?
❖ Is there any problem with fertility?

The enlargement may be:

❖ *Testicular enlargement:*
  • Inflammation
  • Tumor.
❖ *Epididymis:* Inflammation.
❖ *Spermatic cord:*
  • Torsion
  • Spermatocele
  • Hydrocele
  • Strangulation.

● *Groin mass or swelling:*
  ❖ First time of notice.
  ❖ Is it painful?
  ❖ Is it increasing in size progressively or sudden change in size?
  ❖ Any history of venereal disease.

Causes:

  ❖ Hernia
  ❖ Enlarged lymph node
  ❖ Carcinoma penis.

● *Erectile dysfunction:* Persistent inability to achieve and maintain penile erection for sufficient time for satisfactory sexual function:

Causes:

  ❖ *Physiological:*
    • More than 50 years, married
    • Long-term monogamous relationship.
  ❖ *Vascular causes:*
    • Atherosclerotic stenosis of cavernous arteries
    • Vascular problem related to smoking.
  ❖ *Drugs:*
    • Antihypertensive
    • β-blockers
    • Antidepressants
    • Histamine type II blocker.
  ❖ *Systemic disease:*
    • Diabetes
    • Hypertension
    • Hyperlipidemia.
  ❖ *Abuse:*
    • Alcohol
    • Tobacco.

- ❖ Psychological problems.
- ❖ *Neurological cause:*
  - Multiple sclerosis
  - Spinal cord tumor
  - Degenerative disease of spinal cord
  - Local nerve injury.

Questions to be asked:
- ❖ Whether the patient wants to maintain his life in the same way as he is living
- ❖ Whether he is satisfied with his sexual function
- ❖ Whether the relationship with his wife is happy one.
- ❖ Whether his partner is satisfied with his sexual function, if not, why
- ❖ When was the last time he had satisfactory ejaculation?
- ❖ During sexual intercourse, how long he is able to maintain his erection after penetration into vagina?
- ❖ After completion of intercourse, how difficult is to maintain his erection?
- ❖ Constant use of condom—patient often reports that condom split or come off during sex.

For evaluation of erectile dysfunction:
- ❖ Frequency of early morning ejaculation and night-time emissions
- ❖ Whether individual other than his partner arose him
- ❖ Is he able to masturbate for ejaculation?
- *Infertility:* It is inability to conceive or cause pregnancy.

Couples said to be infertile when—after 1 month of normal intercourse, without use of any contraceptive, pregnancy does not occur.

To evaluate the cause of infertility following histories to be taken:
- Mumps
- Injury to testes
- History of exposure
- Diabetes
- Varicocele
- Hypertension
- Exposure to X-ray
- Any surgical procedure
  Diabetic man may be infertile due to—retrograde ejaculation
- Alcohol abuse
- History of intake of drugs
- Sleeping habits
- Type of work he uses to perform.

Physical Examination (Genital System) in Men

Priapism

It is defined as painful protracted erection of penis due to persistent erection of corpora cavernosa of the penis—cause is disturbance in controlling penile detumescence. But corpora spongiosa and glans remain flaccid.

Causes of priapism
- *Local:*
  - ❖ Inflammation
  - ❖ Neoplasm
  - ❖ Hemorrhage.
- *Systemic:*
  - ❖ *Neurologic:*
    - Spinal cord injury
    - Spinal anesthesia.
  - ❖ *Hematological disorders:*
    - Thrombosis
    - Sickle cell anemia
    - Leukemia.
  - ❖ *Infection: Mycoplasma pneumonia.*
- *Drugs:*
  - ❖ *Psychotropic:*
    - Chlorpromazine
    - Trazodone
    - Thioridazine.
  - ❖ Calcium channel blockers
  - ❖ Anticoagulants
  - ❖ *Vasodilators:*
    - Hydralazine
    - Prazosin.
  - ❖ *Others:*
    - Omeprazole
    - Hydorxyzine
    - Testosterone
    - Tamoxifen.

Phimosis

Narrowed opening at the prepuce due to inability to retract the foreskin over the glans penis.

Causes of phimosis:
- *Congenital:*
  85 percent at the age of 1–2 months.
  35 percent at the age of 3 years.

- *Acquired:*
  - ❖ Infection—Balanoposthitis—Chronic
  - ❖ Too forceful retraction of fore skin over the glans
  - ❖ Adhesions due to poor hygiene.

Paraphimosis

Too forcefully retracted skin over the glans becomes edematous and cannot be brought back to its original position—this is called paraphimosis. It is very painful.

Sequelae

If unrelieved, it can cause:
- Urinary tract obstruction
- Venous engorgement
- Edema
- Necrosis of skin.

Causes of paraphimosis

- Too forceful retraction of foreskin over glans
- Poor hygiene
- Catheterization
- Infection chronic balanoposthitis
- Vigorous sexual activity.

Balanoposthitis

This is inflammation of glans and prepuce due to wide variety of organisms.

Pathophysiology

In poor hygienic condition and uncircumcised skin, there is accumulation of smegma (mixture of desquamated epithelial cells, sweat, debris and oils)—which irritate to produce inflammation followed by secondary infection.

Lesion

Moist macular lesion with yellow to black discoloration, having irregular borders and lichenification—due to papilloma virus infection, eventually leading to phimosis.

Causes:

- Bacteria (*Staphylococcus, Gardnerella, Streptococcus pyogenes*)
- *Candida* infection
- Contact dermatitis.

Precipitating factors:

Poor hygiene, poorly retractile skin.

Associated condition:
Ulcerative colitis, Crohn's disease.

Balanitis

In uncircumcised men in poor hygienic condition, accumulation of smegma produces irritation, edema and inflammation of glans—called balanitis.

Balanitis produces adhesion of foreskin producing phimosis.

Predisposing factors
- Diabetes
- Obesity
- Old age
- Edema
- Contact dermatitis
- Seborrheic dermatitis.
  It may be sexually transmitted.

Reiter's syndrome (Fig. 14.5)
It is a reactive arthritis.

Caused by:
- Sexually transmitted organisms (*Chlamydia*, genital mycoplasma, gonococci).
- Enteric organism (*Shigella*, *Salmonella*).

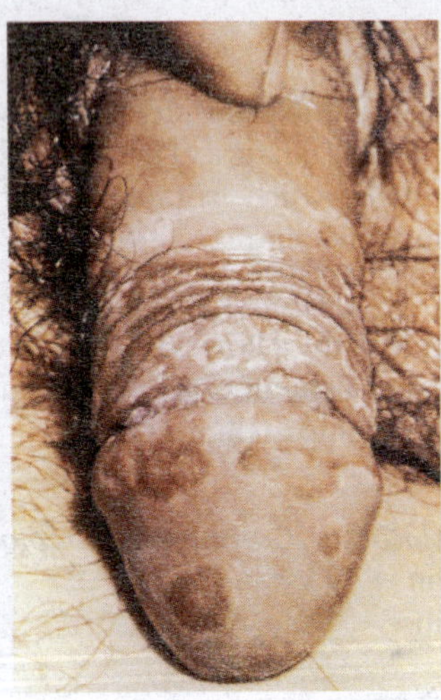

FIG. 14.5   Reiter's syndrome

Clinical manifestation

Arthralgia/Arthritis, conjunctivitis, iridocyclitis, mucocutaneous lesion involves penis—called circinate balanitis—it also involves sulcus and corona.

It will start as painless bleb, ultimately merging into large ring of inflammatory lesion—completely circumscribing glans.

Over hands and feet, lesion may be pustular and scaly resembling psoriasis (keratoderma blennorrhagica).

Skin Lesions in Penis

- *Ulcerating lesions:* These are full thickness loss of epidermis having crater filled up with serum, pus or crust. These are single or multiple.
- *Nonulcerating lesion:* It is divided into:
  - ❖ Papules <1 cm in diameter, raised above surface.
  - ❖ Plaque >1 cm in diameter flat topped surface.

Causes of single ulcerating lesions

- Primary syphilis
- Chancroid (Fig. 14.6)
- Lymphogranuloma venereum
- Granuloma inguinale (Fig. 14.7)
- Penile cancer (Fig. 14.8).

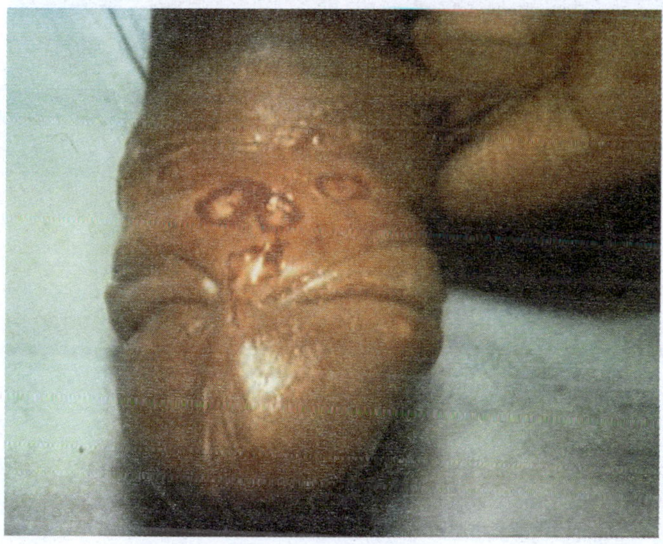

FIG. 14.6 Chancroid

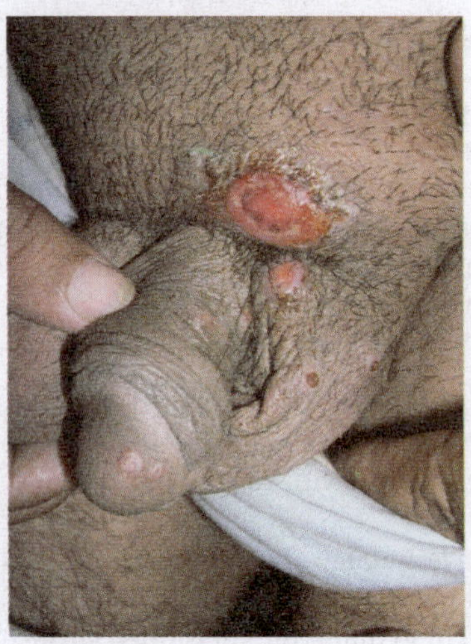

FIG. 14.7   Granuloma inguinale

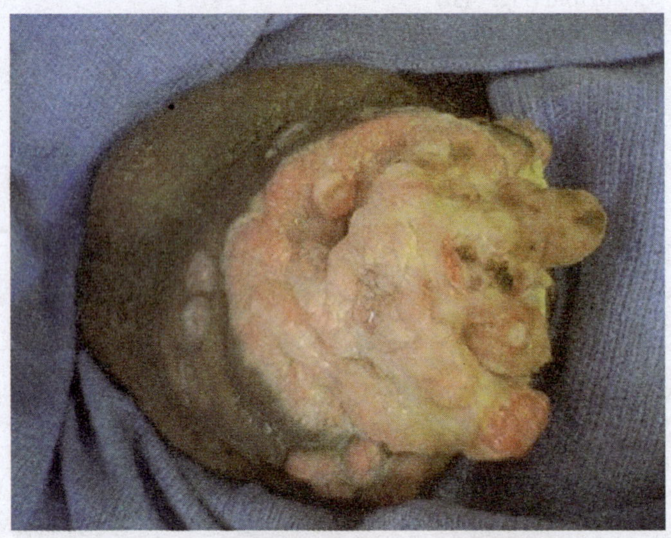

FIG. 14.8   Penile cancer

Causes of multiple ulcerating lesion
- *Acute lesion (<2 weeks):*
  - ❖ Secondary syphilis (Fig. 14.9)
  - ❖ Aphthous ulcers
  - ❖ Herpes simplex.

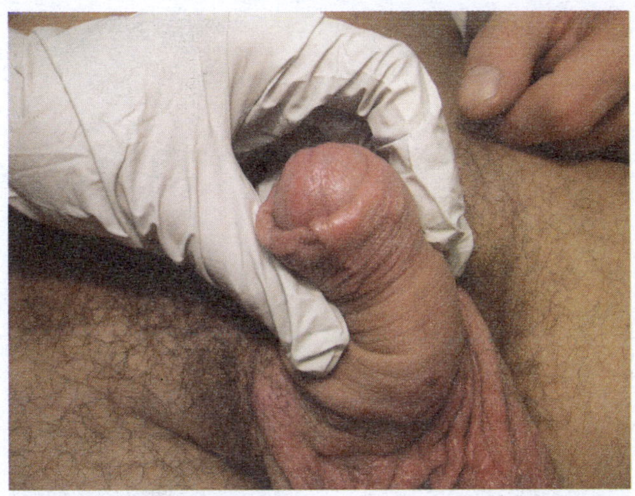

FIG. 14.9   Secondary syphilis in penis

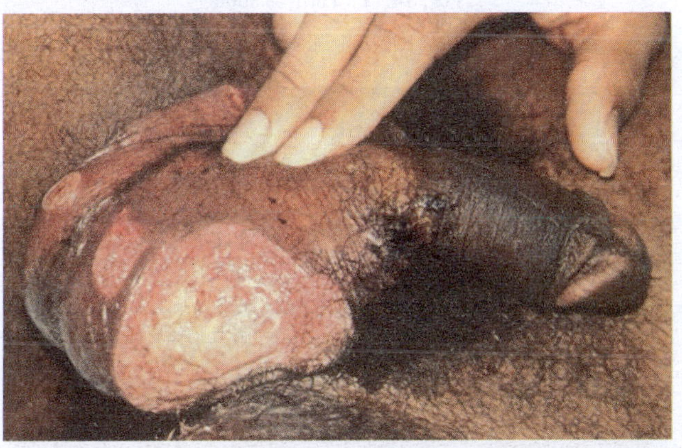

FIG. 14.10   Behçet lesion

- *Chronic lesion (>2 weeks):*
  - ❖ Behçet's lesion (Fig. 14.10)
  - ❖ Reiter's syndrome
  - ❖ Pemphigus.

Causes of nonulcerating lesion
- *Papules:*
  - ❖ Hair follicles
  - ❖ Fordyce spots (Fig. 14.11)

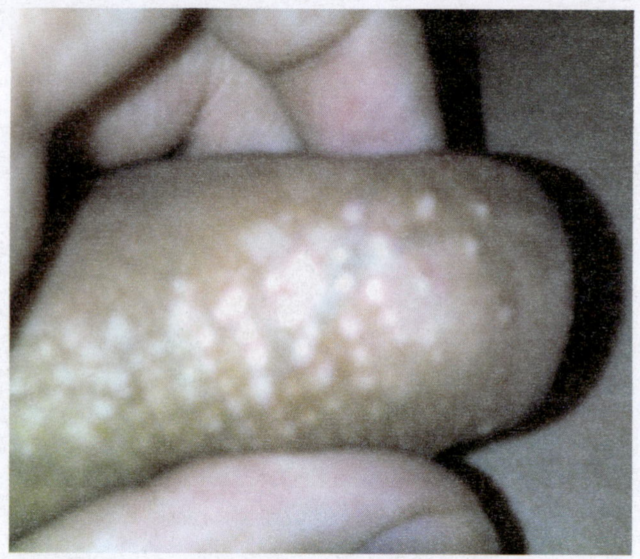

FIG. 14.11 Fordyce spots

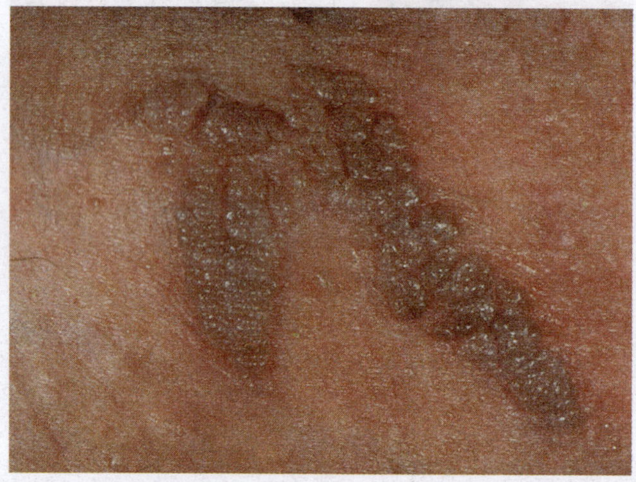

FIG. 14.12 Genital wart (Close view)

- ❖ Molluscum contagiosum
- ❖ Genital wart (Fig. 14.12)
- ❖ Secondary syphilis
- ❖ Pearly penile papule (Fig. 14.13).

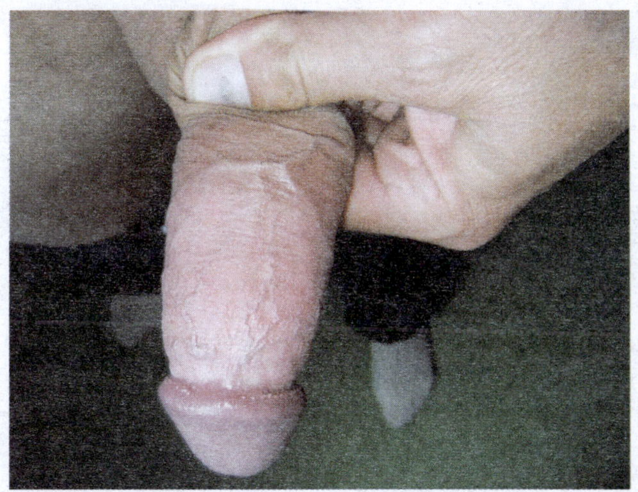

FIG. 14.13 Pearly penile papule

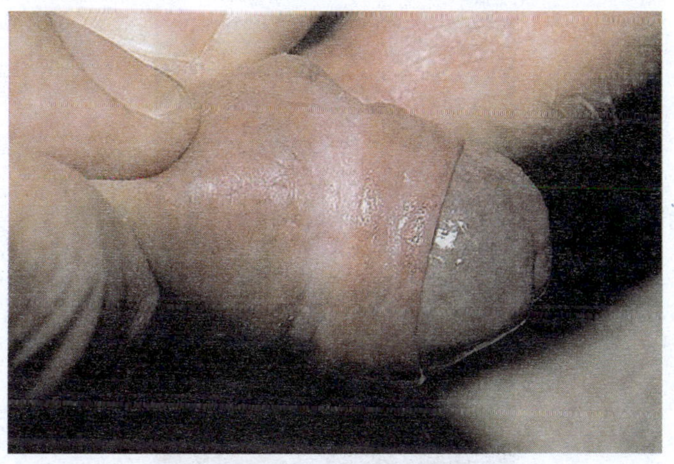

FIG. 14.14 Balanitis

- *Plaques:*
  - ❖ Psoriasis
  - ❖ Balanitis (Fig. 14.14)
  - ❖ Balanoposthitis
  - ❖ Zoon's plasma cell balanitis
  - ❖ Lichen sclerosus
  - ❖ Erythroplasia of Queyrat (Fig. 14.15).

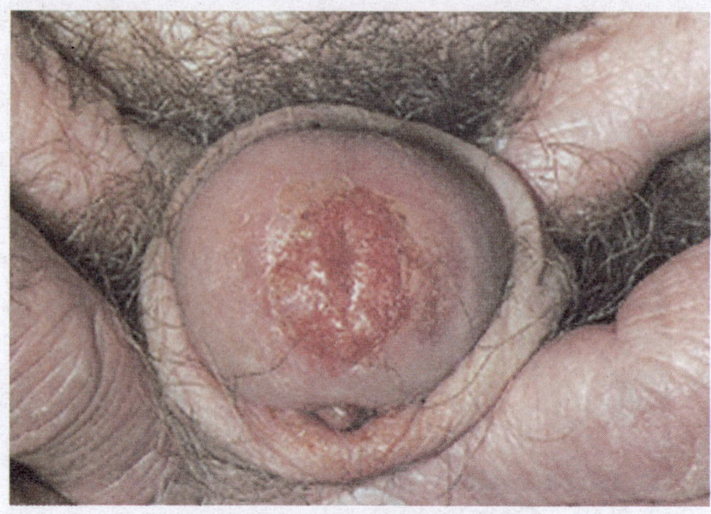

FIG. 14.15 Erythroplasia of Queyrat

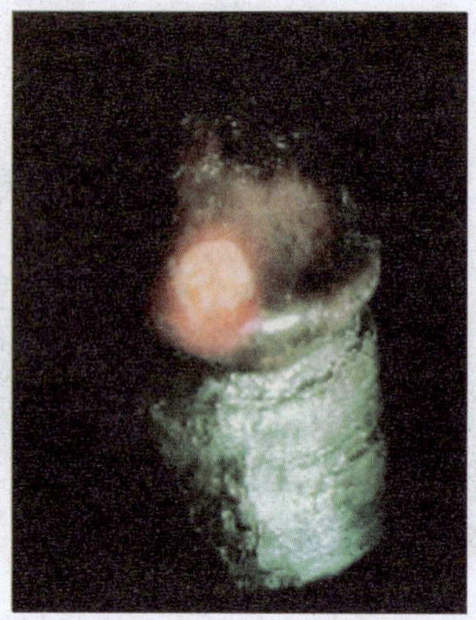

FIG. 14.16 Primary syphilis

Penile Ulcer

Single ulcer is more serious than multiple ulcers.

Penile lesion in primary syphilis (Fig. 14.16)

- Found in genitalia, peri anal region and mouth, well defined, indurated margin and clean base—exudates can be expressed on pressure—chancre.

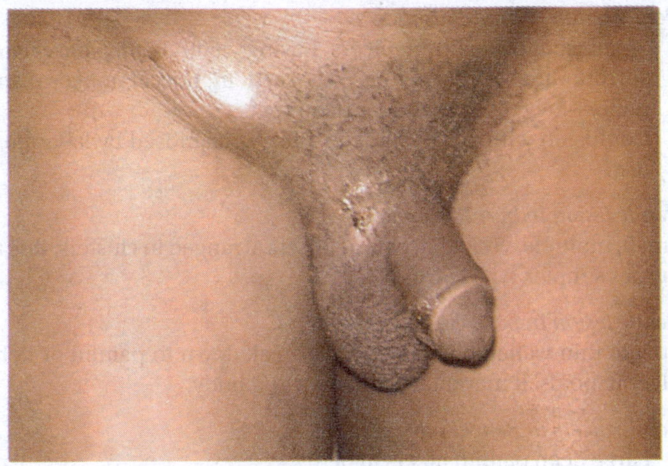

FIG. 14.17 Chancroid

- Ulcer—Round, nontender, painless.
- Bilateral lymphadenopathy.

Painful lesion in chancroid (Fig. 14.17)
- Painful, single, occasionally multiple nonindurated, ragged, undermined edged ulcer, bleeds easily—these are called soft sore.
- Lymphadenopathy in groin, tender, may produce fluctuant buboes. Complication in men—phimosis, partial loss of tissue at glans (phagedenic ulcer).

Penile lesion in granuloma inguinale
- Single, painless ulcer—friable, occurs in anogenital region or hypertrophic lesion—automatically resolved or slowly spread with tissue distraction.
- No lymphadenopathy.

Penile lesion in lymphogranuloma venereum
- Small, nontender, painful ulcer.
- Unilateral tender lymphadenopathy.

Penile ulcers in secondary syphilis
- Multiple, painless, shallow irregular, gray ulcer involving penis—serpiginous ulcers.
- Papulosquamous rose pink, round rash in penis, palms and soles—blotchy. This lesions is followed by coppery popular rash, pustular rash is rare.
- Flu-like illness.

Penile lesion of aphthous ulcer
- Small shallow painful ulcers having central gray base with surrounding erythematous rim seen in buccal mucosa and penis—they resolve without treatment.
- Confusion with herpes simplex ulcer—diagnosed by laboratory test.

Penile lesion in herpes simplex
Small, multiple, vesicular, painful ulcers arranged in clusters, due to herpes simplex type I virus.

Penile lesion in pemphigus
Fragile thin walled blisters—which break down to painful or itchy ulcer in penis. It may attack other parts of body.

Penile ulcers in Behçet's disease
- Large deep painful ulcers in penis.
- This ulcer also may involve scrotum and oral mucosa.
- Skin, joint, eyes, nerves are also involved.

Papular Lesions

- *Hair follicles:* Hair follicles—confused with:
  - ❖ Genital warts—asymmetric, heterogeneous and cauliflower like presentation.
  - ❖ *Molluscum contagiosum:* Flesh, umbilicated, rounded lesions.
- *Sebaceous glands:* Small yellowish nodules, symmetrically distributed in ventral surface of shaft either seen or palpated as lump.
- *Pearly penile papules:* Multiple pearly colored papules present around circumference of glans crown. Occurs in men 20–40 years of age noninfectious, symptomatic, referred to as preputial Tyson's glands.
- *Penile lesion in lichen planus:* Purple or white, ring shaped papular lesion, clustered in circle around penis—They are non-itchy.
- *Penile psoriasis:* The red papules or plaques, well-defined edges, nonirritant, seen on the glans and inner surface of foreskin—this lesion should be differentiated from syphilis.
- *Fordyce lesion:* These are bright red or purple papules present on scrotum, occasionally on glans, noninfectious, but highly vascular, so that they can bleed after minimal trauma or intercourse.

  They may be single or arranged in dusters, may be present in men of more than 50 years of age.
- *Fordyce spots:* Yellowish or white papules—1–3 mm in diameters present on shaft of penis, tongue or vermilion border of lips,

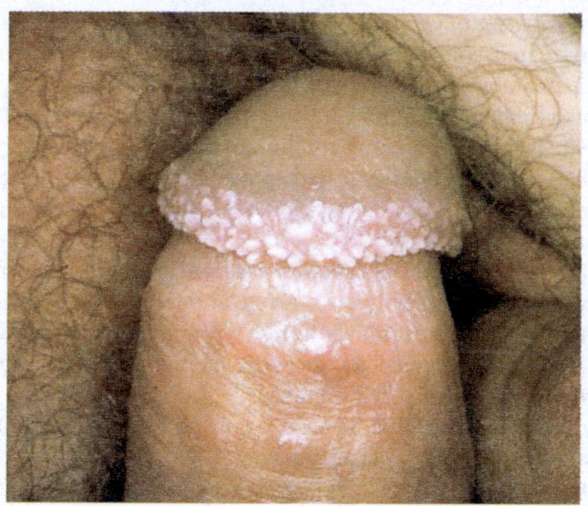

FIG. 14.18 Genital wart

inner surface for cheeks. Usually present at birth, at puberty its size becomes bigger.

They are nothing but the ectopic sebaceous glands.

- *Genital wart (Fig. 14.18):* These are shiny skin colored occasionally enlarges into cauliflower like lesion isolated or arranged in clusters may be latent, subliminal or clinical.

  They are caused by human papilloma virus 6 and 11.

  They are less common with HPV 16 and 18, if they occur—they are usually premalignant.

  These warts are asymmetric present in moist areas (corona or sulcus), penile tip, shaft, and scrotum, inner sides of thigh or lower part of abdomen.

- *Condyloma acuminata:* They are flat topped, soft reddish brown to grayish papules, may be nodules, occasionally cauliflower like, nonindurated, tender.

  Differential diagnosis include—lesions of psoriasis, lichen planus, squamous cell carcinoma, tender Reiter's (nonulcerated penile lesions).

Plaques

- *Zoon's balanitis:* A benign condition characterized by noninfectious, bright red shiny plaques present or either side of glans and inner side of fore skin. It is itchy and recurrent, responding to circumcision.

- *Erythroplasia of Queyrat:* Red, bright painless, nonitchy sharply demarcated, solitary or multiple plaques, scaly, crusty exclusively seen in uncircumcised skin, if not incised, it may progress to invasive cancer. So, it may be described as carcinoma *in situ.*

  Site is mucocutaneous junction of penis or prepuce.
- *Lichen sclerosus:* It is described as atrophic white plaques seen in glans, foreskin or shaft as a result of chronic inflammation—it is asymptomatic.

  Its severe form is balanitis xerotica obliterans—in this condition, affirm, whitish, scarred appearance seen in uncircumcised prepuce. It may interfere with micturition and sex.

  This lesion leads to foreskin depigmentation, atrophy, scarring and eventually phimosis.
- *Peyronie's disease:* This disease is caused by plaques of fibrous tissue around corpora cavernosa.

  In this case, patient is normal at rest, but during erection, the penis becomes bent, deformed and painful.

  So this disease interferes with erection, orgasm, penetration.
- *Hypospadias:* This is a congenital anomaly—where the urethral opening is in undersurface of penis rather than on the glans.

Epispadias

The urethral opening on the upper surface of penis. The above congenital condition is associated with:

- Klinefelter syndrome
- Undescended penis
- Other chromosomal disorder
- Ingestion of estrogen or progesterone
- Congenital adrenal hyperplasia.

Skin Lesions in Scrotum

- *Tinea cruris:* Itchy, scaly lesion ragged margin on the scrotal skin and adjacent to inner surface of thigh.
- *Candida infection:* It can occur in overweight patient, diabetics.
- Lice infestation.
- Scabies infestation occurs in scrotal and pubic areas.

Scrotal swelling: May be:

- *Bilateral:* Diffuse, painless, edema, associated with:
  - ❖ Congestive cardiac failure
  - ❖ Nephrotic syndrome
  - ❖ Cirrhosis.
- *Unilateral:* Local cause:
  - ❖ Varicocele
  - ❖ Testicular involvement—teratoma, seminoma.

Varicocele

This is venous engorgement along the spermatic cord due to incompetence of valves of spermatic vein.

In standing position, this engorged vein appears as nest of worms, but in supine position it will be resolved.

Method of Testicular Palpation

Prerequisite for palpation
- Room must be sufficiently worm so that the scrotal muscles contract to push the testes towards inguinal canal.
- Touch the patient's testes in a gentle way.

Palpation
- By thumb and index finger or by thumb and index and middle finger.
- You can estimate the thickness, tenderness, length of:
  - ❖ Any discrepancy in size, thickness or tenderness
  - ❖ Any irregular swelling on the surface of testes
  - ❖ Any diffuse swelling is present—hydrocele.
- Normally, left testes lies little lower than the right testes. If reverse is true—it indicates situs inversus.
- Patient should be examined in standing and in lying position—in standing position to diagnose:
  - ❖ Varicocele
  - ❖ Hernia.
- Examine upper pole of tests to palpate any swelling near head of epididymides.

Examination of Spermatic Cord

- Follow the head of epididymis to palpate the spermatic cord. It contains:
  - ❖ Vas deferens
  - ❖ Testicular artery and vein
  - ❖ Ilioinguinal nerve
  - ❖ Lymphatic vessels
  - ❖ Fatty tissue.
- Palpate the vas deferens—wire like feeling.
- Note the relationship between testes and inguinal canal.
- Any lumpy feeling in spermatic cord may indicate varicocele because varicocele can be palpated in testes and spermatic cord.

In case of unilateral testicular swelling
It may be solid or cystic and it can be differentiated by following method:

Transillumination Test

- Raise the testes and penis
- Examination room should be dark
- Throw the penlight from the posterior surface the testes
- If there is no transmission of light through the mass—it indicates solid mass
- If the light transmits through the mass—it favors cystic lesion.

Hydrocele

It is collection of serum fluid either in tunica vaginalis or in separate pocket in spermatic cord. It may be unilateral or bilateral, nontender.

Spermatocele

It is sperm filled cyst, nontender, unilateral mobile scrotal mass present above testes.

Cryptorchidism

Failure of tests to descend into scrotum. So, it lies within inguinal canal or abdomen. In these cases:

- They may be atrophied due to high temperature.
- They may undergo neoplastic transformation.

In case of unilateral undescended tests, fertility of the patient remains same.

Small testes

Size is less than 3.5 cm in length—it is called atrophy.
It may be:

- Congenital—Klinefelter's syndrome—it is small and firm.
- Acquired—cirrhosis—in this case testes is small and soft.

Large testes

It is usually testicular tumor or fluid filled testes—can be differentiated by transillumination test.

Epididymitis

Inflammation of epididymis is called epididymitis cause:

- STD
- Prostatitis
- Mump
- Tuberculosis—in this case epididymitis will be nodular, beaded, nontender
- Complication of renal tuberculosis.

Digital Rectal Examination

- *Patient's position:* Patient should be in left lateral decubitus position, knees and hips are flexed towards chest and body as close as possible to the edge of the table.
- Examine the patient's peri anal skin to see any local lesion by spreading the buttock.
- Put on gloves on right hand, lubricate with Xylocaine jelly.
- Inform the patient that you want to examine anal canal and interior by inserting the fingers.
- Ask the patient to bear down as if he was having a bowel movement and at the same time, insert your finger into the anal canal easily because of relaxation of anal sphincter.
- Now ask the patient to constrict the sphincter and estimate the tone.

◼ Genital Symptoms

Female

Questions to be asked:
- Detailing of sexual partner and types of sexual activities should direct the physician to perform proper investigations and swabbing.
- Enquire about type of sex—oral or anal sex, because syphilis and hepatitis B are more common.
- Geographical variations are responsible for types of sexually transmitted infection:
  - ❖ Trichomonal infection is more common in African Caribbean.
  - ❖ Chancroid more common in tropical areas.
- Incubation period, i.e. timing of sexual contact and onset of disease may be important, because:
  - ❖ Short incubation period (4–10 days)—gonococcal infection.
  - ❖ Long incubation period (6–12 weeks)—secondary syphilis.
  - ❖ Asymptomatic for many months genital wart.
- Type of sex—anal, vaginal, oral, receptive or insertive.
- Number of sexual partners.
- Number of intercourses with each sexual partner.
- Whether sexual partner has any sexually contaminated disease or not.
- Whether male partner use condom or not, if yes, whether it splits or comes out during sex.
- *Regarding menstruation:*
  - ❖ Amount of bleeding per menstrual period
  - ❖ Any clot during bleeding
  - ❖ Any foul smelling in bleeding
  - ❖ Duration of bleeding per period

- ❖ How many napkins are used premenstrual period?
- ❖ Whether bleeding occurs in between the period
- ❖ Whether she use contraceptive pills.
- ❖ Any pain is present during or before menstruation
- ❖ If any presence of sweat?
- ❖ Any change in vision
- ❖ Whether the patient is intolerant to heat or cold
- ❖ Is there presence of any headache, nausea.

Amenorrhea: Absence of menstrual bleeding:

Primary:

- Prepuberty
- Menopause
- Pregnancy.

Secondary: Organ related:

- Pituitary
- Thyroid
- Hypothalamus
- Ovary
- Uterus.

Menorrhagia: Excessive bleeding in duration and amount.

Causes:

- Leukemia
- Bleeding abnormalities
- Fibroid.

Metrorrhagia: Uterine bleeding in between menstrual cycles.

Causes:

- Intrauterine devices
- Uterine fibroids
- Ovarian tumor.

Postmenopausal bleeding: Onset of bleeding 6–8 months after onset of menopause.

Causes:

- Uterine fibroid or malignancy
- Cervical cancer
- Ovarian cancer.

Dysmenorrhea: It means painful menstruation. It may be primary or secondary.

Primary dysmenorrhea: It starts after menarche. It is usually colicky uterine contraction preceding menstruation. It is usually subsided after childbirth.

Secondary dysmenorrhea: If may occur due to:

- *Uterus:*
  - ❖ Intrauterine devices
  - ❖ Uterine fibroid or polyp.
- Cervix—Cervical stenosis.
- Pelvic inflammation.

Mass or Lesions

Questions to be asked:
- When the lesion first occurred?
- Whether it is painful or not
- Whether the lesion remits or exacerbates.

The following lesion, may be present:
- Chancre—painless nodule sharply demarcated border.
- Genital herpes—painful nodule.
- Abscess of Bartholin gland—tender mass in vulva.
- Condyloma acuminata.
- Protrusion of vaginal wall through vaginal introitus—due to pelvic relaxation.
- Cystocele—trigger frequency of urination, urinary incontinence.
- Rectocele—produces tenesmus, constipation and incontinence.
- Uterine prolapse may produce sensation of something coming down per vagina.

Vaginal Discharge

Questions to be asked
- Whether any discharge is present or not.
- What is the smell of discharge—foul smelling or fishy?
- What is the color of discharge?
- Is there any associated itching.
- Is there any intake of recent medication?

Causes of vaginal discharge
- *Most common:* Physiological
  - Pregnancy
  - Oral contraceptive pill (OCP)
  - Candidate infection
  - Bacterial vaginosis.
- *Common: Chlamydia*
             Gonorrhea
- *Less common:* Genital wart
                 Genital herpes simplex
- *Rare:*
  - Streptococcal infection
  - Malignancy
  - Foreign body.

Vulval Itching

Questions to be asked
- Whether itch is associated with discharge.
- Time of itching.
- Is there any ulcer?
- Is there any foul smell?

Causes of vaginal itching
- *Most common:*
  - ❖ *Candida* infection
  - ❖ Vulval eczema
  - ❖ Genital herpes.
- *Common:*
  - ❖ Vulval wart
  - ❖ Trichomonas infection
  - ❖ Vulval psoriasis.
- *Less common:* Lichen sclerosus.
- *Rare:* Intraepithelial neoplasia. Vulval leukoplakia, cancer.

Dyspareunia

Pain during penetration of penis into vagina.
If may be due to:
- Vulval soreness, vulval ulcer → during early part of penetration
- Lower abdominal pain in pelvic inflammatory disease, pelvic endometriosis → during deep penetration.
- Dryness of vagina and labia.

Bleeding per Vagina

It may be due to:
- Menstruation
- Penetration into vagina
- Gonococcal cervicitis
- Vaginal ulcer
- *Chlamydia* infection.

Lower Abdominal Pain

Questions to be asked
- Enquire about menstrual period.
- In case of stoppage of menstruation in child bearing age, ask for her last menstrual period.
- Association of pain with menstrual cycle.
- Any history of burning pain during micturition.
- In case of pregnancy, is there any history of sudden bleeding associated with abdominal pain.

Causes of abdominal pain
Acute abdominal pain due to:
Complication of pregnancy:
- Spontaneous abortion
- Missed abortion

- Perforation
- Ruptured ectopic
- Salpingitis
- Oophoritis
- Pain on one side at the time of ovulation—Mittelschmerz
- Acute urinary tract infection.

Chronic abdominal pain may be due to:
- Ectopic endometrial tissue
- Pelvic inflammatory disease of fallopian tube, ovaries
- Pelvic muscle contraction due to protrusion of bladder, rectum, uterus.

Change in Urinary Pattern

Questions to be asked
- Any loss of urine during any type of straining like, cough, sneezing.
- Whether urine is being lost continuously?
- Whether the patient is aware of full bladder?
- If involuntary loss of urine—the amount.
- Aware of weakness of limb.
- Any loss of vision.
- Any history of diabetes.

Stress Incontinence

Incontinence of urine during straining. It is more common in female than men.

In female, urinary bladder and urethra are maintained in good angulation due to pelvic muscles and fascia. Estrogen is responsible for maintaining pelvic support.

In aged female: Stress incontinence occurs because:
- There is loss of estrogen support.
- Repeated vaginal deliveries.
- Strenuous exercise.
- Chronic coughing.

Neurogenic Incontinence

This is due to:
- Cerebral dysfunction
- Spinal cord disease
- Peripheral nerve lesion
- Multiple sclerosis.

Overflow Incontinence

Urinary out flow occurs when urinary bladder pressure exceeds that of urethral pressure. If occurs in:

- Atonic bladder
- Diabetes.

Psychogenic Incontinence

The patient urinates at night in bed to worm themselves.

Infertility

It occurs from:

- Inability to ovulate
- Inadequate function of corpus luteum in patient with cyclic menstrual bleeding.

Questions to be asked

- Whether she has regular menstrual period?
- Any history of STD?
- Intake of any medication to promote infertility?
- Any history of thyroid disease?

■ Signs

Hair Distribution

In case of hormonal disbalance there may be hair less or hair redistribution. The following types of hair distributions are:

- *Hirsutism:* Excessive growth of hair on:
  - ❖ Upper lip
  - ❖ Face
  - ❖ Earlobes
  - ❖ Upper pubic triangle
  - ❖ Trunks
  - ❖ Limbs.
- *Virilization:* It is characterized by:
  - ❖ Excessive hirsutism
  - ❖ Receding temporal hair
  - ❖ Deepening of voice
  - ❖ Clitoral enlargement.

    These are due to excessive androgen production by adrenal gland or ovaries.

- *Polycystic ovarian disease:* This is characterized by:
  - ❖ Hirsutism
  - ❖ Dysfunctional uterine bleeding
  - ❖ Infertility
  - ❖ Obesity.
- *Drugs producing excessive hair growth on the face:*
  - ❖ Minoxidil
  - ❖ Diazoxide
  - ❖ Penicillamine
  - ❖ Cyclosporine
  - ❖ Glucocorticoids.

Hair Loss

Hair loss is called alopecia. Different areas of scalp respond differently to androgen.
- Top and front of the scalp—hair loss due to excess androgen.
- Increased hair growth due to excessive androgen production. High metabolic rate, infectious diseases reduce nutrient available for hair growth resulting decreased hair growth.

Inspection of Female External Genitalia

- Vulval skin for—redness, soreness, nodules, swelling, excoriation, ulceration, leukoplakia
- Mons—lesions, ulceration, swelling
- Hair for lice and nits.
  After spreading labia, the vestibule should be examined as follows:
  - ❖ Urethral meatus for purulent discharge
  - ❖ Skene's glands
  - ❖ Clitoris
  - ❖ Anus
  - ❖ Perineum.

Description of Pubic Hair in Pubis in Male and Female

Pubic hair is triangular in shape.
In female. Apex of the triangle is towards the pubis
In male: Apex of the triangle is towards the umbilicus.

Tanner Stager of Sexual Classification

	Pubic hair	Age range
1.	None	
2.	Straight, countable, increased pigmentation and length on medial border of labia	9–13.5
3.	Darker, begins to curl, increased quantity on mons pubis	9.5–14.25
4.	Increased quantity, course texture, labia and mons well covered	10.5–15
5.	Adult distribution with female triangle and spread to medial thigh	12–16.5

	Breast development	Age range
1.	None	9 – 13
2.	Breast bud present, increased areola size	10 – 14
3.	Further enlargement of breast, no secondary mound	10.5 – 15.6
4.	Secondary mound on areolar area	13 – 18
5.	Mature, alveolar area is a part of breast contour, nipple projects	11 – 14.5

Menarche

Labia Majora and Labia Minora

- Wide variation in shape and size, asymmetrical.
- Asymmetric papules seen in inner side of labia minora—Fordyce's spots.
- White vulval lesion—it may be benign, premalignant or malignant.
- *Benign white lesion:*
  - ❖ Inflammatory dermatitis
  - ❖ Vitiligo.

Premalignant Lesions

Vulval dystrophies (Fig. 14.19)

- *Hyperplastic dystrophy:* Pruritic grayish while plaque not lead to resorption of labia and clitoris. It is nothing but squamous cell hyperplasia.

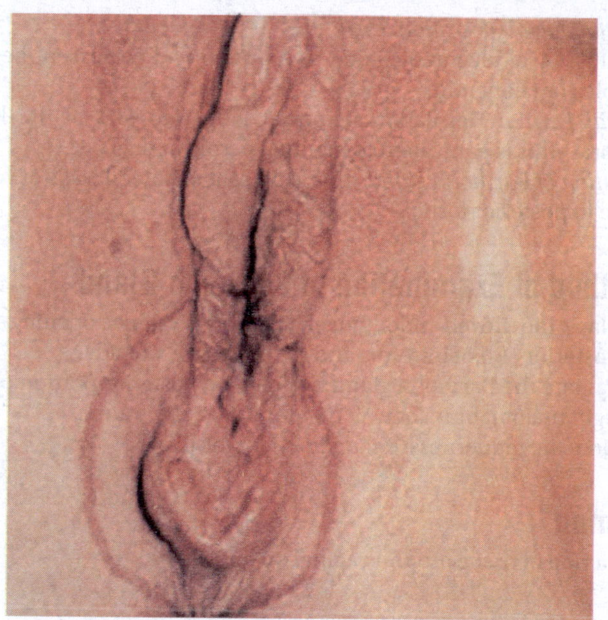

FIG. 14.19 Vulval dystrophies

- *Lichen sclerosus et atrophicus:* Patches of reddened and thin skin evolving into yellowish-bluish papules. They coalesce into areas of atrophic, grayish and wrinkling mucosa.
The lesion is itchy and burning, may be prone to secondary infection. Other symptoms:
- Dyspareunia
- Skin splitting
- Bleeding.
These conditions may lead to resorption of labia and clitoris.

Malignant Lesions

- *Malignant while lesions:*
  - ❖ Intraepithelial neoplasia
  - ❖ Bowen's disease.
- *Other malignant conditions:*
  - ❖ Squamous cell carcinoma
  - ❖ Melanoma
  - ❖ Adenocarcinoma.

Painful vulval ulceration
Painful vulval ulceration—due to ruptured and coalescent herpes simplex or chancroid.
Labial hernia: Herniation of bowel loop into one of the labia majora—this is equivalent to inguinal hernia in male.
Location of Bartholin gland: This is present on lateral walls of vulva, close to posterior fornix.

Method of Examination of Bartholin Gland

- Place the gloved index finger inside the vaginal opening near posterior end of introitus and thumb on the outside.
- Palpate the Bartholin gland by grasping posterior portion of the right major labium between index finger and thumb.
- Note the tenderness, enlargement of the gland.

Hymen

It is a ring of tissue around vaginal opening.

Types of Hymen

- *Annular*—does not completely occlude the introitus.
- *Septate*—one or more bands across the opening.
- *Cribriform*—complete stretching across the opening producing several perforations.
  Bleeding after 1st vaginal penetration is not due to tear of hymen, but due laceration of nearby tissue.

Imperforate hymen: It is a congenital disorder—it is usually asymptomatic until puberty, patient may present with amenorrhea:

If not treated, it may lead to:
- Hematometrium.
- Hematosalpinx.

Clitoris: Normal size—3–4 mm.
Clitoris index: It is calculated by multiplying the sagittal and transverse diameter of the glans:
  Normal range: 9–35 mm.
  Borderline: 36–99 mm.
  Abnormal: >100 mm.
Enlargement of clitoris: Indicate:
  Virilization by testosterone and 17 ketosteroids.

Inspection of urethral meatus
Secretion: Whether it is pus.
  Whether it is foul smelling.
  Whether any mass is present or not.

Condyloma lata: This is wart of secondary syphilis.

Condyloma acuminata: Genital wart due to papilloma virus.

- Flesh-colored papules with cauliflower like papillation.
- It is premalignant condition—The serotype HPV-16, 18, 45 and 56—highest malignant potential.

Process of insertion of speculum

- By left index and middle fingers separate the labia and depress the perineum.
- Ask the patient to take deep breath.
- By your right hand, insert the speculum in closed position, pointing the handle downward at 45°.
- Slide the speculum over left fingers.
- Rotate the speculum downwards to 90°—pointing the handle vertical to the floor.
- Gently open the blades by squeezing the handle.
- This will help to inspect the lateral wall of vagina and cervix, vaginal vault.
- In good position, keep the speculum opened by tightening the screw.

Method of withdrawing speculum

- Open the screw and hold the blades in open position.
- Withdraw the blade for few distance away from the cervix, close the blades.
- During closure, lateral wall of vagina will be inspected for site of any bleeding, ulcer, tumors, any discharge, color and smell of discharge.
- The close the blade and with draw the speculum in closed position.

Colpocele: It is prolapse of vagina post hysterectomy.

Cystocele. A bulging on the anterior wall of vagina—caused by weakening of the wall and protrusion of the bladder.

In severe cases:

- If can be seen at the vestibule.
- If can be palpated.

Rectocele: Bulging on the posterior wall of the vagina due to weakening of the wall and protrusion of rectum.

In severe case: It can be palpated intra vaginally during any type of straining.

Due to the Presence of Rectovaginal Fistula

- Fecal contamination of vagina.
- Fistula can be palpated as indurated area on posterior vaginal wall.

Chadwick's sign: Bluish-violet appearance of vagina or cervix due to mucosal congestion—seen mainly anterior wall of vagina.

Causes:
- Pregnancy
- Pelvic tumor.

Clue to the exposure (prenatal) of diethylstilbestrol on vaginal wall
Adenomyosis—(90% cases): Consists of glandular columnar epithelium of vagina.

   May be associated with clear cell adenocarcinoma.

Gartner's duct cyst: Congenital lesion consists of benign tumor arising in anterior and lateral wall of vagina due to retained epithelial remnants of Wolffian duct.

   Normal vaginal pH is acidic <4.5.

Vaginitis: Inflammation of vagina and vulva—producing pain, itching and discharge.

   Normal vaginal discharge consists of cervical and vaginal mucosal secretion with exfoliation of cells. The secretion is transparent and little odor. If the secretions is foul smelling or purulent—it indicates:
- Infection
- Malignancy.

Few Disease-specific Symptoms and Signs

- *Patient presenting with:*
  - Vaginal discharge
  - Lower abdominal pain
  - Dysuria
  - Postcoital bleeding
  - Dyspareunia.

  Having signs:
  - Foul smelling purulent or mucopurulent discharge
  - Tender during palpation.

  Suggestion: Gonococcal infections of genitalia.

  This disease complicates:
  - Pelvic inflammatory disease—if may precipitates:
    - Ectopic pregnancy
    - Infertility.
  - Abscess of paraurethral glands and Bartholin glands—producing tender swelling.
  - During pregnancy infection may be transferred to baby producing purulent conjunctivitis 3–10 days after delivery — ultimate outcome may be blindness.
- Patient present with offensive vaginal discharge, dysuria, vaginal soreness.

  Sign include:
  - Profuse offensive vaginal discharge
  - Strawberry cervix.

  Suggestion: Trichomonilial infection.

- Patient with immunocompromisation complaining of vaginal discharge—'cottage cheese' like, dyspareunia, itching and soreness in vulva, vaginal fluid pH-4.5.
  Signs—rebleeding of vulva, vagina, excoriated lesion in vulva, and sticky, nonsmelled vaginal discharge.
  Suggestion—consideration of candidiasis.
- Fishy vaginal discharge—increased after unprotected sex, e.g. after ejaculation alkaline fluid makes the amine more volatile.
  Suggestion: Anaerobic bacteria.
  Gardnerella vaginalis. Mycoplasma.
  Urea plasma.

Vulval Signs

- *Genital ulcer:* In women:
  - ❖ It may occur from either trauma or sexually transmitted disease.
  - ❖ It is more painful and chronic than in men, because female genital area is always worm and moist.
  Causes:
  - ❖ *Inflammatory:*
    - • *Infectious:* Herpes simplex type 1 and 2, syphilis, chancroid, lymphogranuloma venereum, lymphogranuloma inguinale, E-B virus, cytomegalovirus.
    - • *Immune:* Behçet syndrome, fixed drug reaction, lichen planus.
  - ❖ *Mechanical:* Inadequate lubrication during intercourse.
  - ❖ *Neoplastic:* Squamous cell carcinoma.
  - ❖ *Idiopathic:* Lichen sclerosus.
- *Vulval rash:* It is acute or chronic, pruritic or painful, dry or moist, whether or not associated with bleeding and may be associated with medication, lotions or creams.
  Causes:
  - ❖ *Immune:* Contact dermatitis
  - ❖ *Endocrine:* Atrophic vulvovaginitis
  - ❖ *Infections:* Candidiasis, fungal infections, abscess of mucosal glands.
  - ❖ *Metabolic:* Diabetes mellitus
  - ❖ *Neoplastic:* Bowen's disease, squamous cell carcinoma
  - ❖ *Psychogenic:* Pruritus vulvae
  - ❖ *Idiopathic:* Lichen sclerosis.
- *Vaginitis.* Skin is red, warm, tender and moist. This may be associated with mucoid or mucopurulent discharge.
  Causes:
  - ❖ Mechanical-tight clothing
  - ❖ Neoplastic-Bowen's disease

- ❖ Metabolic-Diabetes
- ❖ *Immune/Inflammatory:* Contact dermatitis, Lichen planus, Lichen sclerosis.
- ❖ *Infections: Candida*, Fungal infection.
- *Atrophic vulvo vaginitis:* Vulva is thinned, inelastic, easily irritated and inflamed.
  Cause: Estrogen deficiency—Hot flushes—point to diagnosis.
- *Vulval masses:* A mass in vulva.
  Causes:
  - ❖ *Inflammatory:* Granulomatous disease
  - ❖ *Infections:* Condyloma lata, condyloma acuminata, histoplasmosis.
  - ❖ *Mechanical:* Obstruction to Bartholin glands
  - ❖ *Neoplastic:* Bowen's disease, squamous cell cancer.
- *Diffuse swelling of vulva:* Causes
  - ❖ Lymphatic obstruction
  - ❖ Systemic venous pressure is high in case of right ventricular failure or constrictive pericarditis and edema reached above thigh and inguinal ligament.
- *Swelling of labia majora:*
  - ❖ *Hematoma:* Large, painful, bluish swelling—occur, within few hours of trauma.
  - ❖ Cellulitis
  - ❖ *Labial hernia:* Invagination of peritoneal pouch descends from abdomen into labia majus.
  Cause: Failure of obliteration of peritoneal pouch.
- *Absence of greater vestibular gland:* Bartholin gland cyst is very common and asymptomatic. When cyst becomes infected, it produces abscess.

Vaginal Signs

- *Vaginal discharge:* The vaginal fluid is acidic—(pH-4), clear white discharge.
  Contains:
  - ❖ Epithelial cells
  - ❖ Mucus
  - ❖ Commensal bacteria (lactobacilli).
    When vaginal discharge is cloudy containing white blood cells and excessive mucus—it is pathological.
  Causes:
  - ❖ *Inflammatory:* Dermatitis
  - ❖ *Endocrine:* Atrophic vaginitis
  - ❖ *Infections:* Bacterial, Fungal, *Candida*
  - ❖ *Trichomonal: Mycoplasma, Gardnerella*
  - ❖ Vulval and cervical cancer.

- *Vaginitis:*
  Bacterial vaginitis: Most common in women of child bearing age. Fluid is thick, off white, malodorous, fishy smell, pH >4.5, exfoliated vaginal cells.
  Organism: Gardnerella vaginalis.
  Anaerobic bacteria.
  Cytolytic vaginitis: Lactobacillus overgrowth decreases pH of vaginal fluid—leading to breakdown of epithelial cells and inflammation. Vaginal fluid pH will be 3.5–4.5 it contains deformed epithelial cells, polymorphonuclear cells.
  This may be secondarily infected by—*Candida, Trichomonas* and bacteria.

Bluish Vagina

- *Local:* Venous engorgement in
  - ❖ Pregnancy
  - ❖ Tumor
- *Systemic:* Causes of central cyanosis.

Vaginal Mass

It may be:
- Primary
- Secondary to mass in cervix, uterus, rectum, bladder.
- Polyp of vaginal wall or from cervical wall or from stump following hysterectomy.

Rectovaginal Pouch

Mass: It is most dependant pouch in between rectum and vaginal wall. It contains exfoliated cells, mobile mass and fluid from abdomen. Masses are:
- Ovary
- Carcinoma colon
- Bowel loops
- Endometrium
- Ovarian carcinoma
- Accumulation of pus, fluid, blood from abdomen.

Rectovaginal Fistula

It is fistulus opening between rectum and vagina from trauma, carcinoma, Crohn's disease, surgery. Opening can be identified as a patch of induration on the posterior wall of vagina seen through vaginal speculum.

Relaxation of Pelvic Floor

Pelvic floor muscles are pierced by rectum, vagina, and urethra. During vaginal delivery, there is excessive stretching of pelvic floor muscles leads to loss of sphincter functions and prolapse of tissue.

Patient may complain of incontinence, or something coming out of the vagina.

Cervical Signs

- *Cervical cyanosis:* Bluish discoloration of cervix.
  Causes:
  - ❖ Venous congestion due to pregnancy, tumor.
  - ❖ Systemic.
- *Cervical laceration:* It occurs usually during vaginal delivery. Tear may be:
  - ❖ Transverse and bilateral
  - ❖ Unilateral
  - ❖ Stellate shaped. These tears healed by scarring of fissures. Due to scarring of lips of cervix may be everted.
- *Cervical discharge:* Mucopurulent discharge coming out of the cervical os. The lips become inflamed and eroded.

  By palpation—if uterine fundus is not tender—it means pathology lies in cervix.

  Pathophysiology—columnar epithelium of endocervix becomes susceptible to infection with *Candida*, gonorrhea, *Chlamydia*, herpes or *Mycoplasma*.
- *Cervical eversion:* Outward extension of nonulcerated red mucosa through cervical os—due to migration of endocervical tissue onto visible portion of cervix.
- *Cervical ulcer:* The causes are:
  - ❖ Herpes
  - ❖ Chancroid
  - ❖ Tuberculosis
  - ❖ Syphilis
  - ❖ Carcinoma.
- *Cervical hypertrophy:* Lips of cervix of parus woman become elongated and hypertrophic. But funds is in its normal position, cervix retains its normal color in hypertrophy.
- *Cervical polyp:* Pedunculated, red soft benign tumor protrudes through cervical Os.
- *Cervical cyst:* This is a retention cyst of nabothian glands due to occlusion of its duct.
- *Cervical carcinoma:* There is bright red discharge due to a hard palpable mass in cervix.

Index

Page numbers followed by *f* refer to figure